Pediatric Nutrition
Handbook

Fifth Edition

Ronald E. Kleinman, MD
Editor

Library of Congress Control Number: 2002114968
ISBN: 1-58110-109-0
MA0233

The recommendations in this publication do not indicate an exclusive course of treatment or serve as a standard of medical care. Variations, taking into account individual circumstances, may be appropriate.

Committee on Nutrition
2003-2004

Nancy F Krebs, MD, MS, Chairperson

Robert Baker, MD, PhD
Jatinder J. S. Bhatia, MD
Frank R Greer, MD
Melvin B Heyman, MD
Fima Lifshitz, MD
Robert D Baker, Jr, MD, PhD

Former Chairperson
Susan S Baker, MD, PhD

Former Committee Members
William J Cochran, MD
Marc S Jacobson, MD
Tom Jaksic, MD, PhD

Liaison Representatives
Donna Blum-Kemelor, MS, RD, US Department of Food and Agriculture
Margaret P Boland, MD, Canadian Paediatric Society
William Dietz, MD, PhD, Centers for Disease Control and Prevention
Van S Hubbard, MD, PhD, National Institutes of Health
Elizabeth Yetley, PhD, US Food and Drug Administration

Staff
Pamela T Kanda, MPH

Preface

The old maxim that one man's food is another man's poison, if taken literally, would bear particular relevance to pediatric clinical practice these days. The focus of pediatric nutrition support during much of the 20th century was dedicated to identifying and repairing nutrient deficiencies in infants and children. Over the past 25 years, our attention has increasingly shifted toward recognizing the long-term health consequences of an excess of selected nutrients. Thus the scope of this fifth edition of the *Pediatric Nutrition Handbook* has expanded considerably to reflect the new scientific insights into the mechanisms by which nutrients influence and direct growth and development, as well as immediate and long-term health, from birth through the end of adolescence.

As with the previous edition, this handbook is primarily intended to serve as a useful and ready reference for practicing clinicians who care for infants, children, and adolescents. The section on micronutrients and macronutrients provides a discussion of the metabolism and requirements for individual nutrients as well as a general description of methods for assessing nutritional status. This section serves as the basis for other sections that provide evidence-based guidance on feeding healthy infants and children as well as an expanded section on the nutrition support of pediatric patients with acute or chronic health problems. A new chapter on cultural considerations in feeding children addresses this very important aspect of pediatric nutrition support in a multi-cultural society. Within the chapters, every attempt has been made to provide the reader with additional resources, including references to printed materials, agencies, and Web sites that may be useful in practice and for patients to access directly. The appendices are a particularly rich source of practical reference information, including growth charts for very low- and low-birth-weight infants, full-term infants, children, and adolescents.

More than 70 individuals have contributed to the chapters in this handbook. They constitute a broad spectrum of highly respected experts with both scientific and clinical experience in pediatric nutrition. Their work is greatly appreciated by the Committee on Nutrition, which guided the development of this handbook under the expert leadership of Nancy Krebs, MD. I am particularly grateful for this opportunity to work with Dr Krebs and the members and liaisons of the Committee on Nutrition and hope that the readers of this handbook will find it to be a useful and "state-of-the-art" guide.

Ronald E. Kleinman, MD, Editor

Contributors

On behalf of the American Academy of Pediatrics, the Committee on Nutrition gratefully acknowledges the invaluable assistance provided by the following individuals who contributed to the preparation of this edition of the Pediatric Nutrition Handbook.

Steven Abrams, MD, Baylor College of Medicine, Houston, TX

Sue Ann Anderson, PhD, RD, Food and Drug Administration, Washington, DC

Jean Ashland, PhD, Massachusetts General Hospital, Boston, MA

Robert D. Baker, MD, PhD, Children's Hospital of Buffalo, Buffalo, NY

Lori Bechard, RD, Children's Hospital, Boston, MA

Nancy Butte, MD, Children's Nutrition Research Center, Houston, TX

Kattia Corrales, RD, Children's Hospital, Boston, MA

Catherine Cowell, PhD, RD, Columbia University, New York, NY

Scott Denne, MD, Indiana University School of Medicine, Indianapolis, IN

Christopher P. Duggan, MD, MPH, Children's Hospital, Boston, MA

Peter R. Durie, MD, Hospital for Sick Children, Toronto, Ontario, Canada

Johanna Dwyer, DSc, RD, New England Medical Center, Boston, MA

Robert Earl, MPH, RD, National Food Producers Association, Washington, DC

Nancy Ernst, PhD, RD, Nutrition Consultant, Irvington, VA

Drew Feranchak, MD, The Children's Hospital, Denver, CO

Jerry Z. Finkelstein, MD, Long Beach, CA

Marta Fiorotto, PhD, Baylor College of Medicine, Houston, TX

Shahin Firouzbakhsh, RD, Miller Children's Hospital at Long Beach Memorial Medical Center, Long Beach, CA

Jennifer O. Fisher, PhD, Baylor College of Medicine, Houston, TX

Cuthberto Garza, MD, Cornell University, Ithaca, NY

Michael K. Georgieff, MD, Fairview University Medical Center, Minneapolis, MN

Shelley Goldberg, International Food Information Council, Washington, DC

Armond S. Goldman, MD, Children's Hospital, Galveston, TX

William Greenhill, DDS, Children's Hospital Medical Center, Cincinnati, OH

Frank Greer, MD, Meriter Hospital, Madison, WI

Carey Harding, MD, OHSU/CDRC, Portland, OR

Morey Haymond, MD, Baylor College of Medicine, Houston, TX

William C. Heird, MD, Baylor College of Medicine, Houston, TX

Kristy Hendricks, ScD, RD, New England Medical Center, Boston, MA

Marion Hinners, Food Nutrition Service, Alexandria, VA

Van S. Hubbard, MD, PhD, NIH, NIDDK, Bethesda, MD

Kathleen Huntington, RD, OHSU/CDRC, Portland, OR

W. Daniel Jackson, MD, University of Utah School of Medicine,
    Salt Lake City, UT

Thomas Jaksic, MD, PhD, Children's Hospital, Boston, MA

Craig L. Jensen, MD, Baylor College of Medicine, Houston, TX

Susan L. Johnson, PhD, University of Colorado Health Sciences Center,
    Denver, CO

Daina Kalnins, RD, The Hospital for Sick Children, Toronto, Ontario, Canada

John A. Kerner, MD, Stanford University, Palo Alto, CA

William J. Klish, MD, Texas Children's Hospital, Houston, TX

Jill Kramer-Atwood, MS, New England Medical Center, Boston, MA

Richard Kreipe, MD, University of Rochester, Rochester, NY

Ronald M. Lauer, MD, University Hospitals, Iowa City, IA

Bo Lonnerdal, PhD, University of California, Davis, CA

Alan M. Lake, MD, Pediatric Consultants, Lutherville, MD

Rudolph A. Leibel, MD, Columbia University, New York, NY

Carlos H. Lifschitz, MD, Texas Children's Hospital, Houston, TX

Valerie Marchand, MD, Hopital Ste Justine, Montreal, Quebec, Canada

Martin Martin, MD, PhD, UCLA School of Medicine, Los Angeles, CA

Tracie Miller, MD, University of Rochester Medical Center, Rochester, NY

Charles Mize, MD, Food and Drug Administration, Washington, DC

Bruce Z. Morgenstern, MD, Mayo Clinic, Rochester, MN

Pauline Nelson, RD, Mattel Children's Hospital at UCLA, Los Angeles, CA

Aaron Owens, MS, New England Medical Center, Boston, MA

Lois Parker, RPh, Massachusetts General Hospital, Boston, MA

Larry K. Pickering, MD, Centers for Disease Control and Prevention, Atlanta, GA

Michael Rosenbaum, MD, Columbia University, New York, NY

Sylvia Rowe, International Food Information Council, Washington, DC

Hugh A. Sampson, MD, Mount Sinai Medical Center, New York, NY

Richard J. Schanler, MD, Baylor College of Medicine, Houston, TX

Kathleen B. Schwarz, MD, Johns Hopkins University School of Medicine, Baltimore, MD

Robert Shaddy, MD, Primary Children's Medical Center, Salt Lake City, UT

Robert J. Shulman, MD, Baylor College of Medicine, Houston, TX

Katherine M. Shea, MD, MPH, Duke University Medical Center, Durham, NC

Janet Silverstein, MD, University of Florida College of Medicine, Gainesville, FL

Andrea Sitzwohl, RD, St Louis Children's Hospital, St Louis, MO

John Snyder, MD, University of California Medical Center, San Francisco, CA

Ronald J. Sokol, MD, The Children's Hospital, Denver, CO

Virginia A. Stallings, MD, The Children's Hospital of Philadelphia, Philadelphia, PA

Agneta Sunehag, MD, PhD, Children's Nutrition Research Center, Houston, TX

James L. Sutphen, MD, PhD, University of Virginia Medical Center, Charlottesville, VA

Liu Lin Thio, MD, MPH, Washington University School of Medicine, St Louis, MO

Edwin Trevathan, MD, MPH, Washington University School of Medicine, St Louis, MO

John N. Udall, Jr, MD, Children's Hospital, New Orleans, LA

Bradley A. Warady, MD, University of Missouri—Kansas City School of Medicine, Kansas City, MO

William B. Weil, MD, Michigan State University, East Lansing, MI

Elizabeth A. Yetley, PhD, Food and Drug Administration, College Park, MD

J. Paul Zimmer, PhD, Wyeth Nutritionals International, Philadelphia, PA

Table of Contents

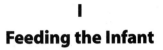

I
Feeding the Infant

1

Infant Nutrition and the Development of Gastrointestinal Function

Swallowing, Sucking, and Gastrointestinal Motility

A fetus starts to swallow amniotic fluid between the third and fifth months of gestation.[1] The volume of swallowed amniotic fluid steadily increases from 18 to 50 mL·kg^{-1}·day^{-1} in the 18-week-old fetus, to 155 mL·kg^{-1}·day^{-1} in the full-term fetus.[2,3] Fetal swallowing regulates the volume of amniotic fluid and controls somatic growth of the gastrointestinal tract.[4] The swallowed amniotic fluid may provide a minimal amount of nutrients to the fetus by absorption of substrates such as amino acids and glucose.

The sucking reflex has been observed after 6 months of gestational age and evolves through 3 developmental stages: mouthing (expression/compression), immature suck-swallow, and a mature type of suck-swallow pattern.[5] The mature pattern is a rhythmic alteration of suction and expression/compression and is acquired in full-term infants within several days of life. However, in premature infants, the first stage may last a month or more; in very small immature infants, the third stage may not appear before the third month.[6,7] There is a wide variation in oral-motor skills at any given gestational age.[6] In infants younger than 3 months, solid food placed in the mouth is forced by the tongue against the palate and is swallowed or forced back out of the mouth. Older infants transfer solid food selectively to the back of the pharynx and then swallow.

The average transit time for a semisolid bolus to travel from the cricopharyngeal area to the stomach increases with age.[8] In full-term infants younger than 12 hours and in premature infants younger than 1 week, esophageal peristalsis is faster than in older and more mature infants.[5] There are an abundance of non-peristaltic pressure waves in the esophagus of very premature infants (26 to 33 weeks of gestational age) that are not associated with swallowing.[9,10] In addition to these non-peristaltic contractions, the normal peristaltic pattern induced by swallowing is generally well developed in very premature infants, resembling the pattern seen in full-term infants. The tone of the lower gastroesophageal sphincter is normal (ranges from

5 to 20 mm Hg) in full-term, premature, and very premature infants. Transient lower gastroesophageal sphincter relaxation is the primary cause of gastroesophageal reflux (GER) in all age groups including very premature infants.

The mean stomach half-emptying time in formula-fed infants (33 weeks of gestational age) was reported as 72 minutes; infants fed expressed breast milk have shorter (32 minutes) mean values.[11] Gastric peristalsis is absent during the first few days of life, and characteristics of the peristaltic waves change during the first 6 months.[5] A delay in antral distention after a bolus feed is seen frequently in very premature infants (23 to 29 weeks' gestation) with feeding intolerance.[12] Immediate antral distention, which is comparable to the pattern seen in term infants and adults, is seen in infants born at 32 weeks of gestation.

Gastrointestinal motor activity is distinct during the fasting and postprandial periods. During the fasting period, the interdigestive migrating motor complex has 3 distinct phases, ranging from no contractions to intense phasic contractions, which recur every 90 minutes. At birth, preterm infants demonstrate only unorganized clusters of motility during fasting, whereas term infants show well-developed migrating motor complexes in addition to nonmigrating cluster activity. The normal migratory motor complexes develop within 10 days of regular feeding in preterm infants.[13,14] The postprandial periods are associated with the presence of continuous contractions in adults and full-term infants that are of higher intensity when compared to phasic contractions seen in the fasting period.[15,16] The majority of premature infants have an immature fed response, characterized by poor motor activity relative to the fasting period. The interstitial cells of Cajal represent the intestinal pacemaker cells and are present along the entire gastrointestinal tract as early as the first trimester, with the network continuing to develop in postnatal life.[17,18]

Digestion and Absorption of Carbohydrates

Digestion of Polysaccharides
The concentration of amylase in saliva is lower in young children than in adults.[19] During the postnatal period, the activity of salivary amylase increases earlier than that of pancreatic amylase. Exocrine pancreatic function, including the synthesis of amylase, is exceedingly low in young infants, and increases considerably during postnatal life.[20,21] Salivary, pancreatic, and breast milk

α-amylase all influence the assimilation of starch and glucose polymers, and produce the di- and oligosaccharides maltose, isomaltose, maltotriose, and maltodextrins.[22,23] Glucoamylase, an intestinal brush border glucan 1,4-α-glucosidase that removes glucose units from the nonreducing ends of molecules of starch and dextran, is present in the developing small intestine at the age of 1 month,[24] with levels of activity that are comparable to those found in young adults.[25] Because of the relative abundance of glucoamylase to lactase in the premature intestine, glucose polymers (polycose) are digested and absorbed better than lactose.[26] Although the digestion of starch in infants is considerable, the tolerance of young infants to large quantities is limited. This limitation may vary in individual infants.[27]

Human breast milk contains an abundance of oligosaccharides that do not differ in either amount or quality in term and pre-term milk.[28] Oligo-saccharides are believed to influence the intestinal microflora (growth factor for *Bifidobacterium bifidum*), and to alter bacterial adhesion to intestinal epithelial cells. Luminal digestion of breast milk oligosaccharides is limited, and their translocation through cellular and paracellular pathways has been recently documented.[29]

Digestion of Disaccharides

Lactase deficiency that results in clinically significant lactose malabsorption is a common finding that results from several underlying causes. Severe lactose intolerance rarely occurs in full-term newborns and generally results from *congenital lactase deficiency*, an extremely rare autosomal recessive disorder.[30] Intestinal lactase activity in the fetus is detectable as early as 12 weeks of gestation, and by 34 weeks is only 30% of the full-term infant.[31,32] Therefore, a relative lactase deficiency can occur in many premature infants, and its contribution to the feeding intolerance that is so common in these young infants remains controversial. Premature infants with low lactase levels experience more bouts of feeding intolerance, compared to those infants with moderate levels.[33] While lactase activity is not inducible by dietary lactose in adults, lactose administered early (<4 days of age) in the life of a premature infant doubles lactase activity by 10 days of age, when compared to those infants who began feeding at 15 days of age.[33] Infants consuming breast milk experience a more significant induction in lactase activity when compared to those fed a premature infant formula. Finally, premature infants who consume a lactose-free formula experience fewer episodes of feeding intolerance compared to those on a standard premature formula.[34]

About 25% of 1-week-old term infants exhibit lactose malabsorption; however, this mild degree of lactase deficiency is generally not associated with clinical symptoms.[35] Lactose not absorbed from the small intestine can be salvaged in the colon after bacterial fermentation in humans at all ages.[36] The intestinal microflora differ between breastfed and formula-fed infants. Species of *Lactobacillus* and *Bifidbacterium* constitute a large proportion of the microflora of breastfed infants, while *Bacteroides* and *Enterobacteria* are the predominant flora in bottle-fed infants.[37] Colonic microflora ferment the unabsorbed carbohydrate to short-chain fatty acids, which promotes water absorption and prevents osmotic diarrhea.[38]

Infectious diarrhea in infancy is frequently associated with a transient (secondary) decline in intestinal lactase activity.[39] Despite lower lactase levels, nearly 80% of children can tolerate full-strength lactose-containing formula during an episode of acute gastroenteritis.[40]

With the exception of humans, all mammals that have been studied experience a decline in lactase levels that correspond to the onset of weaning.[41] Individuals who maintain high levels of lactase throughout life are considered *lactase persistent* and are generally of Western European descent. The persistence of a high level of intestinal lactase activity in adulthood in this population seems to be a product of natural selection in areas where milking and consumption of milk have occurred for centuries. In contrast, a large proportion of the world population goes from a state of lactose tolerance, to a relative lactase deficiency in early to late childhood, a condition frequently referred to as *hypolactasia*.[42] Not all populations show the same rate of decrease of lactose digestion capacity. Finns, white Americans, the Irish, and the British show a small and slow decrease. Children from Thailand and Bangladesh show the earliest decrease, as early as 2 years of age. In African Americans, Asians, and Latin Americans residing in the United States, adult (low) values are found after the first decade of life.[43]

Absorption of Monosaccharides

The absorption of dietary carbohydrates in the intestine is limited to the monosaccharides glucose, galactose, and fructose. The products of lactose hydrolysis, glucose, and galactose are actively transported across the intestinal surface between 10 and 18 weeks of gestation via the sodium/glucose cotransporter, SGLT1.[44–46] Studies in premature infants using ^{13}C glucose show that its absorption and retention increases with postnatal age.[47] The galactose absorption rate reaches adult values between 4 and 8 years of age.[48] The transport of glucose up its concentration gradient occurs in the presence of sodium and results in the absorption of water.[49] The sodium-coupled transport of glucose and water represents the physiologic basis of therapy for infectious diarrhea by oral rehydration solutions.[50] Other sodium-dependent solute cotransporters can also facilitate the absorption of water, and represent the basis of amino acid-based oral rehydration solutions. Over the last half a century, oral rehydration solutions have profoundly influenced the management of infectious diarrhea worldwide, and significantly lowered its mortality rate (see Chapter 26).

Fructose is transported across the brush border membrane by the facilitated transporter GLUT5. An excessive intake of fruit juices containing a high proportion of fructose to glucose, or an excessive amount of the non-absorbable carbohydrate sorbitol, is associated with infant diarrhea and abdominal pain.[51–53] Malabsorption of fruit juices is dose-dependent, with symptoms occurring with the daily consumption of 15 to 20 $mL \cdot kg^{-1}$, and is well tolerated at a dose of 10 $mL \cdot kg^{-1}$.[52]

Digestion and Absorption of Lipids

Lipolytic Activities of the Gastrointestinal Tract

Lipase activity is first found in the stomachs of fetuses after the second month of gestation[54] and increases with subsequent fetal development. Lipase immunoreactivity appears in the pancreas at week 21 of gestation, 5 weeks later than trypsinogen and chymotrypsinogen activity.[55] Postnatally, several lipolytic enzymes are involved in the digestion of fat in the infant. In addition to the classic enzymes originating in the pancreas, other sources (ie, milk, the tongue, and the stomach) provide lipolytic enzymes.

Milk Lipases

Bile salt-stimulated lipase (BSSL) is present in human colostrum[56] and in preterm[57] and term human milk.[58] Properties of BSSL allow it to survive in the stomach with little or no loss of activity and to act in the duodenum when activated by bile acids (eg, cholic acid, chenodeoxycholic acid) in concentrations similar to those found in the infant duodenum.[59,60] The major products are free fatty acids.[59,61] Triglycerides are composed of fatty acids of various lengths that form ester bonds to one of 3 positions (sn) on the glycerol molecule. The outer positions are labeled sn-1 and sn-3, and the inner position, sn-2. The positional nonspecificity (between sn-1, sn-2, and sn-3) of the enzyme enables the BSSL to hydrolyze monoacylglycerol and, thus, makes this enzyme complementary to pancreatic lipase that yields fatty acids and monoa-cylglycerol as its main products. Bile salts not only activate this enzyme, but also protect it against digestion by trypsin and chymotrypsin.[59] Bile salts also reduce the size of the fat globule, enhancing the surface area and improving BSSL-induced hydrolysis. Because efficient absorption of retinol requires hydrolysis, another important role of BSSL is its ability to hydrolyze retinol esters.[62] Bile salt-stimulated lipase also hydrolyzes ceramide, the main sphin-gomyelin (phospholipid) in human milk.[60] The significance of the presence of BSSL for the digestion of milk lipids is supported further by studies of low-birth-weight preterm infants (3 to 6 weeks old) who are fed raw or heat-treated (pasteurized or boiled) human milk. Fat from the former was absorbed more (74%) than was fat from the latter 2, 54% and 46%, respec-tively.[63] Lipoprotein lipase is also present in human milk.[57,64]

Preduodenal Lipases

Lipase activity is present in the gastric fluid of fetuses, preterm and full-term neonates, and adults.[65] Part, but not all, of this lipolytic activity can be attrib-uted to lingual lipase, which is produced by von Ebner serous glands located on the proximal dorsal site of the tongue.[66,67] The activity of gastric lipase is detectable at 10 weeks of gestation, increases to significant levels by the third trimester, and reaches adult levels by early infancy.[54,68] In healthy infants, milk triglycerides are hydrolyzed mainly to diglycerides and fatty acids.[69] Hydrolysis of medium-chain triglycerides occurs 5 times faster than does that of long-chain triglycerides.[70] Preduodenal lipase is stable from both proteolytic diges-tion and the acidity of the gastric mucosa, and is slightly activated by low concentrations of bile salts, but higher concentrations of bile salts lead to almost complete inhibition. These preduodenal lipases exhibit partial stere-ospecificity for sn-3 esters over sn-1 esters.[71,72] Long-chain polyunsaturated fatty acids (LC-PUFAs) are generally hydrolyzed from the sn-3 position of triglycerides by gastric lipase. Dietary LC-PUFAs have been implicated as important substrates for retinal and gastric development.[73,74] Medium-and long-chain triglycerides are hydrolyzed in the stomachs of preterm in-fants, and released medium-chain fatty acids are absorbed directly from the stomach.[75] In premature infants, hydrolysis of fat is more than 2 times higher in breastfed infants compared to formula-fed infants.[76] The difference in fat hydrolysis occurs in the presence of similar gastric lipase synthesis, sug-gesting that breast milk contains several unique properties that facilitate fat digestion.

Pancreatic Lipases

In adults, pancreatic juice contains 2 enzymes that are active against neutral lipids. The so-called pancreatic lipase is more active against insoluble emulsified substrates than against soluble substrates. The second lipase, also called pancreatic carboxylase esterase, is more active against micellar or soluble substrates than against insoluble emulsified substrates. In contrast to the first lipase, it is strongly stimulated by bile salts. Colipase removes the inhibiting effect of bile salts on lipase. The generalized exocrine pancreatic insufficiency present in premature and full-term infants results in limited synthesis of pancreatic lipase.[77] Nevertheless, during the first postnatal month, lipase activity increases linearly in premature infants, reaching 35% of values found in 2- to 6-year-old children.[78] The lipase activity in small-for-gestational-age infants can limit utilization of dietary fat.[79]

Bile Acids

Bile acids are essential to the digestion and absorption of dietary lipids. Several studies show that infants, especially during the first days of life, have a lower concentration of bile acids in the gallbladder and in duodenal fluids than do older children and adults.[80] The bile acid concentrations in duodenal fluid of premature and mature infants increase consistently throughout the first 2 months of life.[81] In these same infants, the relative ratio of cholic acid to chenodeoxycholic acid (CDCA) was highest immediately after birth and gradually declined with increasing age. The concentration of bile acids is similar in preprandially aspirated duodenal juice of small-for-gestational-age infants studied between the third and seventh weeks of life to the concentrations of bile acids in duodenal juice found in appropriate-for-gestational-age infants and are sufficient to activate BSSL in human milk.[79]

As in fetal bile, taurine conjugates predominate in early infancy, whereas in older infants, bile acids are conjugated primarily with glycine.[81,82] Interestingly, a deficiency of dietary taurine during formula feeding does not seem to influence the formation of taurine conjugates during the first month of life.[83] During postnatal development, cholate synthesis and the cholate pool increase. The chenodeoxycholate pool is similar in term infants and children,[84] but is smaller in premature infants. Synthesis of chenodeoxycholate and of total bile acids is several times lower in premature infants than in adults.[85] Bile salt turnover mechanisms are not fully developed postnatally— (1) The ileal mechanism for transport of cholyltaurine in the fetus and newborn is undeveloped; its presence has been demonstrated by 8 months of age.[86] Bile salt reabsorption in the ileum is controlled by the apical sodium-dependent bile acid transporter (ASBT).[87] (2) The primary serum bile acids exhibit transient elevation during infancy,[88] indicating physiologic cholestasis. A steady decline to levels seen in childhood and adult years indicates the continuous maturation of hepatic function.[84] Term infants excrete less bile acid during the first week of life than during the third week of life when adult values are reached.[89] In premature infants of mothers treated prenatally with dexamethasone and phenobarbital, the cholic acid and chenodeoxycholic acid pool and synthesis are increased, as is the duodenal bile salt concentration.[85]

Studies on Fat Absorption

The percent of absorption of fat from breast milk increases slightly during the first month in full-term infants, achieving values of almost 90%.[90,91] In premature infants, absorption values are similar to those found in full-term infants.[92] Fat absorption from cow milk formula in full-term infants also increases postnatally, but values are somewhat lower than those for breast milk in corresponding age groups. The differences disappear around 6 months of age.[93] In premature infants, percent of fat absorption from cow milk formula during the first weeks of life is substantially lower and reaches values of approximately 80% around 10 weeks of age.[92]

Preterm infants (26 to 33 weeks' gestation) retain more fat when fed a 3:2 mixture of infant formula and fresh human milk than do infants fed infant formula only, again supporting a role for breast milk lipase.[94] Furthermore, fat retention is lower in low-birth-weight infants fed a long-chain triglyceride-containing formula nasojejunally than in those fed nasogastrically,[95] reinforcing the importance of lipid processing in the stomach.

Little is known about the cellular processes of lipid absorption during fetal development. The capacity to esterify fatty acids is an important step in the absorption of long-chain fatty acids. The esterification capacity is present in the intestinal mucosa of infants and children; age-dependent differences have not been observed.[96]

Digestion and Absorption of Protein

Proteolysis in the Stomach

Gastric acidity appears in 4-month-old fetuses.[97] Intragastric pH decreases in preterm infants as they mature.[98] The pH of the gastric fluid in infants is substantially influenced by food intake. The entry of milk into the infant's stomach causes a sharp increase in the pH of the gastric contents and a slower return to lower pH values than in older children and adults.[99] These findings not only stress the importance of defining the time after feeding when pH is determined, but also show that the gastric acidity of the newborn is unsuitable for optimal pepsin action. Gastric acid production doubles between 0 to 2 months and 2 to 12 months of age in full-term infants.[100] Hydrochloric acid secretion is much lower in premature infants than in full-term infants.[101] Nevertheless, fasting gastric acid secretion in preterm infants (24 to 29 weeks' gestation) increased with advancing gestational and postnatal age, with gastric pH consistently reaching values of less than 4.[102] In premature and term infants (25 to 42 weeks' gestation), the level of gastric H^+,K^+-adenosine triphosphatase (H^+,K^+-ATPase) increased significantly with advanced gestational age.[103] Moreover, the abundance of the proton pump increased steadily over the first 3 months of life. Nevertheless, the concentration and output of titratable acid after histamine stimulation are normal in the healthy term newborn.[104]

Proteolytic activity is found in fetuses older than 16 weeks of gestation, and gastric pepsin activity does not change significantly between 10 and 20 weeks of gestation.[54,105,106] Results of immunoelectrophoretic analysis of fetal gastric mucosal extracts suggest the appearance of gastrin during the third month and pepsinogen by the fourth month.[107] The output of pepsin is 5 times lower in the 0- to 2-month-old infant than in the 2- to 12-month-old infant.[100] Formula feeding evokes an increase in pepsin activity in the stomach contents of 3- to 4-week-old premature infants fed by the orogastric route.[108]

No substantial digestion of protein is found in specimens of gastric contents taken from 5- to 8-day-old infants,[109] probably because pepsin (which is present in low levels at that time) is almost completely inactivated at the relative high pH levels that are found in the newborn stomach at various intervals after feeding. In older infants (13 to 44 days of age), traces of hydrolyzed protein are found in stomach contents.[110]

Pancreatic Proteolytic Enzymes

Pancreatic enzymes begin to form about the third fetal month,[105] and pancreatic secretion starts at the beginning of the fifth month of gestation.[111] Biochemical studies on the activity of trypsinogen and chymotrypsinogen at various gestational ages have been reported in detail.[112]

Various reports show relatively modest differences in the concentration of trypsin (compared with amylase and lipase) when collected after pancreozymin-secretin stimulation.[20,113] Similarly, no substantial difference is observed in premature infants between 2 days and 7 weeks of age.[114] Levels of trypsin concentration encountered during the first 2 years of life have already been reached by the age of 1 to 3 months.[113,115] The low chymotryptic activity in the newborn gradually increases with age, approaching the levels of older children at about 180 days. From birth, the concentration of chymotrypsin (after pancreozymin-secretin stimulation) increases approximately threefold and reaches adult levels in 3-year-old children.[116]

The *protease inhibitors* in the colostrum and mature milk[117] could influence the processing of protein in the gastrointestinal tract of breastfed infants. Interestingly, they inhibit trypsin and chymotrypsin with no effect on pepsin.

Peptidase Activities in the Small Intestinal Mucosa

The proteolysis of dietary proteins by gastric and pancreatic enzymes results in an intermediate form of oligopeptides that undergo further hydrolysis in the intestine. The epithelial cells of the small and large intestine contain several peptidases, including carboxypeptidase and aminopeptidase N. These brush border enzymes hydrolyze the carboxy and amino termini of small peptides. In contrast, di- and tripeptides are hydrolyzed by intracellular di- and tripeptidases. Aminopeptidase activity is present at high levels in the distal small intestine at 28 to 38 weeks' gestation.[118] Colonic aminopeptidase activity increases to the level seen in the small intestine at term. Detectable enzyme activity of di-, tripeptidase, aminopeptidase, and carboxypeptidase has been established in the small intestine of 17- to 20-week-old fetuses.[119]

Absorption of Proteins and Their Degradation Products

Various studies demonstrate that the small intestine is permeable to minute quantities of intact food proteins during the neonatal period.[120–124] Passage of intact proteins has also been demonstrated in older children and adults. The serum of infants often contains higher titers of antibodies to food antigens than does the serum of adults,[121] which suggests that food proteins are absorbed intact in sufficient quantities for an immunologic response.

The absorption of protein from the duodenum is about the same in 1- to 2-week-old full-term infants and 1- to 4-week-old premature infants, although trypsin values are lower in the 1-week-old premature infant.[125] The protein nitrogen concentration in the ileocecal contents of 1- to 5-month-old infants fed whole cow milk formula is more than 3 times higher than that found in breastfed infants.[126] Analysis of intestinal contents after a feeding with cow milk seems to indicate that the digestion and absorption of cow milk casein increases with age. Adults can digest about 1.6 g of casein $kg^{-1} \cdot hour^{-1}$, whereas the corresponding value in children is 1 g.[127] The colon of infants may also be able to assimilate proteins.[128] About 85% of the food nitrogen in infants is absorbed from the gut—independent of age (birth to 150 days), type of diet, or maturity.

An oligopeptide transporter named Pept-1 has been isolated that transports di and tripeptides across the brush border membrane of the small intestine.[129] Pept-1 is H^+-coupled and is capable of transporting peptide-like drugs (eg, β-lactam antibiotics); however, peptides with more than 3 amino acids cannot be transported. Intracellular di- and tripeptidases are believed to hydrolyze the oligopeptides to single amino acids, which are then transported across the basolateral membrane by specific amino acid transporters. The expression of the oligopeptide transporter has not been characterized in either fetal or newborn intestine.

The brush border membrane of the intestine contains a wide variety of amino acid transporters.[130] Several transport systems such as A, ASC, and L are ubiquitously expressed and exhibit preferences for certain amino acids. For instance, systems A and ASC transport amino acids with small side chains (alanine and serine), whereas amino aids with bulky side chains utilize system L. The expression of several amino acid transporters is limited to certain tissue, like the B system ($B^{o,+}$, b^+, etc), which has broad specificity for neutral amino acids and is produced in the intestine. Other specific amino acids transport systems that are present in the intestine include IMINO (proline and glycine) b^+, (cationic) and rBAT (cystine and dibasic amino acids). Many of these systems have been thoroughly studied in the placenta, yet little is currently known about their expression in fetal and postnatal intestine. Nevertheless, the transport of specific amino acids across the mucosa of the small intestine has been shown in 12- to 18-week-old fetuses.[131,132]

Absorption of Water-Soluble Vitamins

Specific carriers that have recently been identified transport several water-soluble vitamins across the intestinal mucosa. For instance, the Na^+-dependent multivitamin transporter (SMVT) is produced in the small intestine and transports the vitamins biotin and pantothenate.[133] Serum levels of vitamin C (L-ascorbic acid) decline rapidly postpartum in humans. Vitamin C and other antioxidants are believed to be important in diminishing oxidant injury in premature and full-term infants.[134] A recently identified Na+-dependent L-ascorbic acid transporter (SVCT1) has been identified in intestinal epithelial cells.[135] An analysis examining the distribution and presence of either SMVT or SVCT1 transporters in human fetal or neonatal intestine has not been performed.

Mineral Absorption

Most mineral absorption depends on specific carrier-mediated transport and the absorptive capacity of the gastrointestinal tract. Most mineral accretion occurs during the last trimester; the preterm infant, therefore, is at risk for mineral deficiencies because of low stores. The transport of calcium is sensitive to the presence and abundance of other nutrients such as lactose and fatty acids.[136–138] Young animals absorb iron, lead, calcium, and strontium much better than do adults.[136,139] Because human infants readily absorb lead,[140] they are at greater risk than adults for lead toxicity. A divalent cation transporter named DCT1 has been identified as the main iron carrier in the small intestine.[141] While the specificity of the transporter for iron is limited to its reduced ferrous form, the carrier transports other divalent cationic minerals such as zinc, copper, manganese, nickel, lead, cobalt, and cadmium. The expression pattern of this transporter along the small intestine of human infants has not been evaluated.

References

1. McClain CR Jr. Amniography studies of the gastrointestinal motility of the human fetus. *Am J Obstet Gynecol.* 1963;86:1079–1087
2. Pritchard JA. Deglutition by normal and anencephalic fetuses. *Obstet Gynecol.* 1965;25:289–297
3. Abramovich DR. Fetal factors influencing the volume and composition of liquor amnii. *J Obstet Gynaecol Br Commonw.* 1970;77:865–877
4. Ross MG, Nijland MJ. Development of ingestive behavior. *Am J Physiol.* 1998; 274(Pt 2):R879–893
5. Gryboski JD. Suck and swallow in the premature infant. *Pediatrics.* 1969;43: 96–102
6. Lau C, Alagugurusamy R, Schanler RJ, Smith EO, Shulman RJ. Characterization of the developmental stages of sucking in preterm infants during bottle feeding. *Acta Paediatr.* 2000;89:846–852
7. Lau C, Sheena HR, Shulman RJ, Schanler RJ. Oral feeding in low birth weight infants. *J Pediatr.* 1997;130:561–569
8. Shepard R, Fenn S, Sieber WK. Evaluation of esophageal function in postoperative esophageal atresia and tracheoesophageal fistula. *Surgery.* 1966;59:608–617

9. Omari TI, Miki K, Fraser R, et al. Esophageal body and lower esophageal sphincter function in healthy premature infants. *Gastroenterology.* 1995;109:1757–1764

10. Omari TI, Benninga MA, Haslam RR, Barnett CP, Davidson GP, Dent J. Lower esophageal sphincter position in premature infants cannot be correctly estimated with current formulas. *J Pediatr.* 1999;135:522–525

11. Ewer AK, Durbin GM, Morgan ME, Booth IW. Gastric emptying in preterm infants. *Arch Dis Child Fetal Neonatal Ed.* 1994;71:F24–F27

12. Carlos MA, Babyn PS, Marcon MA, Moore AM. Changes in gastric emptying in early postnatal life. *J Pediatr.* 1997;130:931–937

13. Tomomasa T, Itoh Z, Koizumi T, Kuroume T. Nonmigrating rhythmic activity in the stomach and duodenum of neonates. *Biol Neonate.* 1985;48:1–9

14. Berseth CL, Nordyke C. Enteral nutrients promote postnatal maturation of intestinal motor activity in preterm infants. *Am J Physiol.* 1993;264:G1046–G1051

15. Bisset WM, Watt J, Rivers RP, Milla PJ. Postprandial motor response of the small intestine to enteral feeds in preterm infants. *Arch Dis Child.* 1989;64(10 Spec No):1356–1361

16. al Tawil Y, Berseth CL.Gestational and postnatal maturation of duodenal motor responses to intragastric feeding. *J Pediatr.* 1996;129:374–381

17. Vanderwinden JM, Rumessen JJ. Interstitial cells of Cajal in human gut and gastrointestinal disease. *Microsc Res Tech.* 1999;47:344–360

18. Kenny SE, Connell G, Woodward MN, et al. Ontogeny of interstitial cells of Cajal in the human intestine. *J Pediatr Surg.* 1999;34:1241–1247

19. Rossiter MA, Barrowman JA, Dand A, Wharton BA. Amylase content of mixed saliva in children. *Acta Paediatr Scand.* 1974;63:389–392

20. Delachaume-Salem E, Sarles H. Normal human pancreatic secretion in relation to age [in French]. *Biol Gastroenterol* (Paris). 1970;2:135–146

21. Lebenthal E, Lee PC. Development of functional responses in human exocrine pancreas. *Pediatrics.* 1980;66:556–560

22. Heitlinger LA, Lee PC, Dillon WP, Lebenthal E. Mammary amylase: a possible alternate pathway of carbohydrate digestion in infancy. *Pediatr Res.* 1983;17:15–18

23. Lindberg T, Skude G. Amylase in human milk. *Pediatrics.* 1982;70:235–238

24. Eggermont E. The hydrolysis of the naturally occurring alpha-glucosides by the human intestinal mucosa. *Eur J Biochem.* 1969;9:483–487

25. Kerzner B, Sloan HR. Mucosal glucoamylase activity. *J Pediatr.* 1981;99:388–389

26. Shulman RJ, Feste A, Ou C. Absorption of lactose, glucose polymers, or combination in premature infants. *J Pediatr.* 1995;127:626–631

27. De Vizia B, Ciccimarra F, De Cicco N, Auricchio S. Digestibility of starches in infants and children. *J Pediatr.* 1975;85:50–55

28. Kunz C, Rudloff S, Baier W, Klein N, Strobel S. Oligosaccharides in human milk: structural, functional, and metabolic aspects. *Annu Rev Nutr.* 2000;20:699–722

29. Gnoth MJ, Rudloff S, Kunz C, Kinne RK. Investigations on the in vitro transport of human milk oligosaccharides by a Caco-2 monolayer using a novel high performance liquid chromatography-mass spectrometry technique. *J Biol Chem.* 2001;276:34363–34370

30. Savilahti E, Launiala K, Kuitunen P. Congenital lactase deficiency. A clinical study on 16 patients. *Arch Dis Child.* 1983;58:246–252

31. Antonowicz I, Chang SK, Grand RJ. Development and distribution of lysosomal enzymes and disaccharidases in human fetal intestine. *Gastroenterology.* 1974; 67:51–58

32. Raul F, Lacroix B, Aprahamian M. Longitudinal distribution of brush border hydrolases and morphological maturation in the intestine of the preterm infant. *Early Hum Dev.* 1986;13:225–234

33. Shulman RJ, Schanler RJ, Lau C, Heitkemper M, Ou CN, Smith EO. Early feeding, feeding tolerance, and lactase activity in preterm infants. *J Pediatr.* 1998;133: 645–649

34. Griffin MP, Hansen JW. Can the elimination of lactose from formula improve feeding tolerance in premature infants? *J Pediatr.* 1999;135:587–592

35. Douwes AC, Oosterkamp RF, Fernandes J, Los T, Jongbloed AA. Sugar malabsorption in healthy neonates estimated by breath hydrogen. *Arch Dis Child.* 1980;55: 512–515

36. Kien CL, Kepner J, Grotjohn KA, Gilbert MM, McClead RE. Efficient assimilation of lactose carbon in premature infants. *J Pediatr Gastroenterol Nutr.* 1992;15: 253–259

37. Parrett AM, Edwards CA. In vitro fermentation of carbohydrate by breast fed and formula fed infants. *Arch Dis Child.* 1997;76:249–253

38. Topping DL, Clifton PM. Short-chain fatty acids and human colonic function: roles of resistant starch and nonstarch polysaccharides. *Physiol Rev.* 2001;81: 1031–1064

39. Herbst JJ, Sunshine P, Kretchmer N. Intestinal malabsorption in infancy and childhood. *Adv Pediatr.* 1969;16:11–64

40. Practice parameter: the management of acute gastroenteritis in young children. American Academy of Pediatrics, Provisional Committee on Quality Improvement, Subcommittee on Acute Gastroenteritis. *Pediatrics.* 1996;97: 424–435

41. Rings EH, Grand RJ, Buller HA. Lactose intolerance and lactase deficiency in children. *Curr Opin Pediatr.* 1994;6:562–567

42. Northrop-Clewes CA, Lunn PG, Downes RM. Lactose maldigestion in breast-feeding Gambian infants. *J Pediatr Gastroenterol Nutr.* 1997;24:257–263

43. Koldovsky O. Digestive-absorptive functions in fetuses, infants, and children. In: Polin RA, Fox WW, eds. *Fetal and Neonatal Physiology.* Philadelphia, PA: WB Saunders Co; 1992;2:1060–1077

44. Wright EM, Loo DD. Coupling between Na+, sugar, and water transport across the intestine. *Ann N Y Acad Sci.* 2000;915:54–66

45. Koldovsky O, Heringova A, Jirsova V, Jirasek J, Uher J. Transport of glucose against a concentration gradient in everted sacs of jejunum and ileum of human fetuses. *Gastroenterology.* 1965;48:185–187

46. Malo C. Separation of two distinct Na+/D-glucose cotransport systems in the human fetal jejunum by means of their differential specificity for 3-O-methylglucose. *Biochim Biophys Acta.* 1990;1022:8–16

47. Murray RD, Boutton TW, Klein PD, Gilbert M, Paule CL, MacLean WC Jr. Comparative absorption of [^{13}C] glucose and [^{13}C] lactose by premature infants. *Am J Clin Nutr.* 1990;51:59–66

48. Beyreiss K, Rautenbach M, Willgerodt H, Schone S, Al-Rebate I. Besonderheiten der Resorption und des Stoffwechsels von Kohlenhydraten bei Fruh-und Neugeborenen. *Wiss Z Friedrich-Schiller Univ Jena Math-Naturwiss Reihe.* 1972;21:683–693

49. Loo DD, Hirayama BA, Meinild AK, Chandy G, Zeuthen T, Wright EM. Passive water and ion transport by cotransporters. *J Physiol.* 1999;518(Pt 1):195–202

50. Santosham M, Greenough WB 3rd. Oral rehydration therapy: a global perspective. *J Pediatr.* 1991;118(Pt 2):S44–51

51. Nobigrot T, Chasalow FI, Lifshitz F. Carbohydrate absorption from one serving of fruit juice in young children: age and carbohydrate composition effects. *J Am Coll Nutr.* 1997;16:152–158

52. Hoekstra JH. Fructose breath hydrogen tests in infants with chronic non-specific diarrhoea. *Eur J Pediatr.* 1995;154:362–364

53. Smith MM, Davis M, Chasalow FI, Lifshitz F. Carbohydrate absorption from fruit juice in young children. *Pediatrics.* 1995;95:340–344

54. Menard D, Monfils S, Tremblay E. Ontogeny of human gastric lipase and pepsin activities. *Gastroenterology.* 1995;108:1650–1656

55. Carrere J, Figarella-Branger D, Senegas-Balas F, Figarella C, Guy-Crotte O. Immunohistochemical study of secretory proteins in the developing human exocrine pancreas. *Differentiation.* 1992;51:55–60

56. Freudenberg E. *Die Frauenmilch-Lipase: Studien zu ihrer enzymologischen und ernoahrungsphysiologischen Bedeutung.* Basel, Switzerland: S Karger AG; 1953

57. Mehta NR, Jones JB, Hamosh M. Lipases in preterm human milk: ontogeny and physiologic significance. *J Pediatr Gastroenterol Nutr.* 1982;1:317–326

58. Blackberg L, Hernell O. The bile-salt stimulated lipase in human milk: purification and characterization. *Eur J Biochem.* 1981;116:221–225

59. Hernell O. Human milk lipases, III: physiological implications of the bile salt-stimulated lipase. *Eur J Clin Invest.* 1975;5:267–272

60. Nyberg L, Farooqi A, Blackberg L, Duan RD, Nilsson A, Hernell O. Digestion of ceramide by human milk bile salt-stimulated lipase. *J Pediatr Gastroenterol Nutr.* 1998;27:560–567

61. Hernell O, Blackberg L. Digestion of human milk lipids: physiologic significance of sn-2 monoacylglycerol hydrolysis by bile salt-stimulated lipase. *Pediatr Res.* 1982;16:882–885

62. Fredrikzon B, Olivecrona T. Decrease of lipase and esterase activities in intestinal contents of newborn infants during test meals. *Pediatr Res.* 1978; 12:631–634

63. Williamson S, Finucane E, Ellis H, Gamsu HR. Effect of heat treatment of human milk on absorption of nitrogen, fat, sodium, calcium, and phosphorus by preterm infants. *Arch Dis Child.* 1978;53:555–563

64. Wang CS, Kuksis A, Manganaro F. Studies on the substrate specificity of purified human milk lipoprotein lipase. *Lipids.* 1982;17:278–284

65. Gargouri Y, Pieroni G, Riviere C, et al. Importance of human gastric lipase for intestinal lipolysis: an in vitro study. *Biochim Biophys Acta.* 1986;879:419–423

66. von Ebner K. Die acinosen Drusen der Zunge und ihre Beziehungen zu den Geschmacksorganen. In: Hoelliker V, ed. *Handook der Geweblehre des Menschen.* Graz, Austria: Leuschner and Lubensky; 1899:18–38

67. Fink CS, Hamosh P, Hamosh M. Fat digestion in the stomach: stability of lingual lipase in the gastric environment. *Pediatr Res.* 1984;18:248–254

68. Sarles J, Moreau H, Verger R.Human gastric lipase: ontogeny and variations in children. *Acta Paediatr.* 1992;81:511–513

69. Fredrikzon B, Hernell O. Role of feeding on lipase activity in gastric contents. *Acta Paediatr Scand.* 1977;66:479–484

70. Liao TH, Hamosh M, Scanlon JW, Hamosh P. Preduodenal fat digestion in the newborn infant: effect of fatty acid chain length on triglyceride hydrolysis. *Clin Res.* 1980;28:820. Abstract

71. Jensen RG, DeJong FA, Clark RM, Palmgren LG, Liao TH, Hamosh M. Stereospecificity of premature human infant lingual lipase. *Lipids.* 1982;17: 570–572

72. Gargouri Y, Pieroni G, Riviere C, et al. Kinetic assay of human gastric lipase on short- and long-chain triacylglycerol emulsions. *Gastroenterology.* 1986;91: 919–925

73. Agostoni C, Trojan S, Bellu R, Riva E, Giovannini M. Neurodevelopmental quotient of healthy term infants at 4 months and feeding practice: the role of long-chain polyunsaturated fatty acids. *Pediatr Res.* 1995;38:262–266

74. Makrides M, Simmer K, Goggin M, Gibson RA. Erythrocyte docosahexaenoic acid correlates with the visual response of healthy, term infants. *Pediatr Res.* 1993;33(Pt 1):425–427

75. Faber J, Goldstein R, Blondheim O, et al. Absorption of medium chain triglycerides in the stomach of the human infant. *J Pediatr Gastroenterol Nutr.* 1988; 7:189–195

76. Armand M, Hamosh M, Mehta NR, et al. Effect of human milk or formula on gastric function and fat digestion in the premature infant. *Pediatr Res.* 1996; 40:429–437

77. Zoppi G, Andreotti G, Pajno-Ferrara F, Njai DM, Gaburro D. Exocrine pancreas function in premature and full term neonates. *Pediatr Res.* 1972;6:880–886

78. Boehm G, Bierbach U, DelSanto A, Moro G, Minoli I. Activities of trypsin and lipase in duodenal aspirates of healthy preterm infants: effects of gestational and postnatal age. *Biol Neonate.* 1995;67:248–253

79. Boehm G, Bierbach U, Senger H, et al. Activities of lipase and trypsin in duodenal juice of infants small for gestational age. *J Pediatr Gastroenterol Nutr.* 1991;12: 324–327

80. Encrantz J-C, Sjovall J. On the bile acids in duodenal contents of infants and children. *Clin Chim Acta.* 1959;4:793–799

81. Brueton MJ, Berger HM, Brown GA, Ablitt L, Iyngkaran N, Wharton BA. Duodenal bile acid conjugation patterns and dietary sulphur amino acids in the newborn. *Gut.* 1978;19:95–98

82. Boehm G, Braun W, Moro G, Minoli I. Bile acid concentrations in serum and duodenal aspirates of healthy preterm infants: effects of gestational and postnatal age. *Biol Neonate.* 1997;71:207–214

83. Wahlen E, Strandvik B. Effects of different formula feeds on the developmental pattern of urinary bile acid excretion in infants. *J Pediatr Gastroenterol Nutr.* 1994;18:9–19

84. Heubi JE, Balistreri WF, Suchy FJ. Bile salt metabolism in the first year of life. *J Lab Clin Med.* 1982;100:127–136

85. Watkins JB, Szczepanik P, Gould JB, Klein P, Lester R. Bile salt metabolism in the human premature infant: preliminary observations of pool size and synthesis rate following prenatal administration of dexamethasone and phenobarbital. *Gastroenterology.* 1975;69:706–713

86. de Belle RC, Vaupshas V, Vitullo BB, et al. Intestinal absorption of bile salts: immature development in the neonate. *J Pediatr.* 1979;94:472–476

87. Wong MH, Oelkers P, Craddock AL, Dawson PA. Expression cloning and characterization of the hamster ileal sodium-dependent bile acid transporter. *J Biol Chem.* 1994;269:1340–1347

88. Suchy FJ, Balistreri WF, Heubi JE, Searcy JE, Levin RS. Physiologic cholestasis: elevation of the primary serum bile acid concentrations in normal infants. *Gastroenterology.* 1981;80:1037–1041

89. Potter JM, Nestel PJ. Greater bile acid excretion with soy bean than with cow milk in infants. *Am J Clin Nutr.* 1976;29:546–551

90. Roy CC, Ste-Marie M, Chartrand L, Weber A, Bard H, Doray B. Correction of the malabsorption of the preterm infant with a medium-chain triglyceride formula. *J Pediatr.* 1975;86:446–450

91. Tantibhedhyangkul P, Hashim SA. Medium-chain triglyceride feeding in premature infants: effects on fat and nitrogen absorption. *Pediatrics.* 1975;55:359–370

92. Jarvenpaa AL. Feeding the low-birth-weight infant, IV: fat absorption as a function of diet and duodenal bile acids. *Pediatrics.* 1983;72:684–689

93. Weijers HA, Drion EF, Van De Kamer JH. Analysis and interpretation of the fat absorption coefficient. *Acta Paediatr.* 1960;49:615–625

94. Alemi B, Hamosh M, Scanlon JW, Salzman-Mann C, Hamosh P. Fat digestion in very low-birth-weight infants: effect of addition of human milk to low-birth-weight formula. *Pediatrics.* 1981;68:484–489

95. Roy RN, Pollnitz RB, Hamilton JR, Chance GW. Impaired assimilation of nasojejunal feeds in healthy low-birthweight newborn infants. *J Pediatr.* 1977;90:431–434

96. Heubi JE, Partin JC, Schubert WE, McGraw CA. Small intestinal mucosal fatty acid uptake and esterification in infants and children. *Pediatr Res.* 1979;13:781–782

97. Kelly EJ, Brownlee KG. When is the fetus first capable of gastric acid, intrinsic factor and gastrin secretion? *Biol Neonate.* 1993;63:153–156

98. Kelly EJ, Newell SJ, Brownlee KG, Primrose JN, Dear PR. Gastric acid secretion in preterm infants. *Early Hum Dev.* 1993;35:215–220

99. Castberg HB, Hernell O. Role of serum-stimulated lipase in lipolysis in human milk. *Milchwissenchaft.* 1975;30:721–723

100. Mouterde O, Dacher JN, Basuyau JP, Mallet E. Gastric secretion in infants: application to the study of sudden infant death syndrome and apparently life-threatening events. *Biol Neonate.* 1992;62:15–22

101. Mignone F, Castello D. Ricerche sulla secrezione gastrica di acido cloridrico nell'immaturo. *Minerva Pediatr.* 1961;13:1098–1103

102. Kelly EJ, Brownlee KG, Newell SJ. Gastric secretory function in the developing human stomach. *Early Hum Dev.* 1992;31:163–166

103. Grahnquist L, Ruuska T, Finkel Y. Early development of human gastric H,K-adenosine triphosphatase. *J Pediatr Gastroenterol Nutr.* 2000;30:533–537

104. Hyman PE, Clarke DD, Everett SL, et al. Gastric acid secretory function in preterm infants. *J Pediatr* 1985;106:467–471

105. Keene MFL, Hewer EE. Digestive enzymes of the human foetus. *Lancet.* 1924;1:767–769

106. Wagner H. The development to full functional maturity of the gastric mucosa and the kidneys in the fetus and newborn. *Biol Neonate.* 1961;3:257–274

107. Hirsch-Marie H, Loisillier F, Touboul JP, Burtin P. Immunochemical study and cellular localization of human pepsinogens during ontogenesis and in gastric cancers. *Lab Invest.* 1976;34:623–632

108. Yahav J, Carrion V, Lee PC, Lebenthal E. Meal-stimulated pepsinogen secretion in premature infants. *J Pediatr.* 1987;110:949–951

109. Mason S. Some aspects of gastric function in the newborn. *Arch Dis Child.* 1962;37:387–391

110. Berfenstam R, Jagenburg R, Mellander O. Protein hydrolysis in the stomachs of premature and full-term infants. *Acta Paediatr.* 1955;44:348–354

111. Koshtoyants CS. Beitrag zur Physiologie des Embryos (Embryosecretin). *Pfluegers Arch Gesamte Physiol.* 1931;227:359–373

112. Lieberman J. Proteolytic enzyme activity in fetal pancreas and meconium: demonstration of plasminogen and trypsinogen activators in pancreatic tissue. *Gastroenterology.* 1966;50:183–190

113. Boehm G, Bierbach U, DelSanto A, Moro G, Minoli I. Activities of trypsin and lipase in duodenal aspirates of healthy preterm infants: effects of gestational and postnatal age. *Biol Neonate.* 1995;67:248–253

114. Madey S, Dancis J. Proteolytic enzymes of the premature infant: with special reference to his ability to digest unsplit protein food. *Pediatrics.* 1949;4: 177–182

115. Guilbert PW, Barbero GJ. The importance of trypsin in infancy and childhood, II: clinical considerations. *Am J Med Sci.* 1954;227:672–682

116. Bujanover Y, Harel A, Geter R, Blau H, Yahav J, Spirer Z. The development of the chymotryptic activity during postnatal life using the bentiromide test. *Int J Pancreatol.* 1988;3:53–58

117. Lindberg T. Protease inhibitors in human milk. *Pediatrics.* 1979;13:969–972

118. Raul F, Lacroix B, Aprahamian M. Longitudinal distribution of brush border hydrolases and morphological maturation in the intestine of the preterm infant. *Early Hum Dev.* 1986;13:225–234

119. Kushak RI, Winter HS. Regulation of intestinal peptidases by nutrients in human fetuses and children. *Comp Biochem Physiol A Mol Integr Physiol.* 1999;124: 191–198

120. Walker WA. Absorption of protein and protein fragments in the developing intestine: role in immunologic/allergic reactions. *Pediatrics.* 1985;75(suppl): 167–171

121. Roberton DM, Paganelli R, Dinwiddie R, Levinsky RJ. Milk antigen absorption in the preterm and term neonate. *Arch Dis Child.* 1982;57:369–372

122. Tainio VM, Savilahti E, Arjomaa P, Salmenpera L, Perheentupa J, Siimes MA. Plasma antibodies to cow's milk are increased by early weaning and consumption of unmodified milk, but production of plasma IgA and IgM cow's milk antibodies is stimulated even during exclusive breast-feeding. *Acta Paediatr Scand.* 1988;77:807–811

123. Rothberg RM. Immunoglobulin and specific antibody synthesis during the first weeks of life of premature infants. *J Pediatr.* 1969;75:391–399

124. Gruskay FL, Cooke RE. The gastrointestinal absorption of unaltered protein in normal infants and in infants recovering from diarrhea. *Pediatrics.* 1955; 16:763–768

125. Borgstrom B, Lindquist B, Lundh G. Enzyme concentration and absorption of protein and glucose in duodenum of premature infants. *Am J Dis Child.* 1960;99:338–343

126. Hirata Y, Matsuo T, Kokubu H. Digestion and absorption of milk protein in infant's intestine. *Kobe J Med Sci.* 1965;11:103–109

127. Lindberg T. Proteolytic activity in duodenal juice in infants, children, and adults. *Acta Paediatr Scand.* 1974;63:805–808

128. Heine W, Wutzke KD, Richter I, Walther F, Plath C. Evidence for colonic absorption of protein nitrogen in infants. *Acta Paediatr Scand.* 1987;76:741–744

129. Ganapathy ME, Brandsch M, Prasad PD, Ganapathy V, Leibach FH. Differential recognition of beta-lactam antibiotics by intestinal and renal peptide transporters, PEPT 1 and PEPT 2. *J Biol Chem.* 1995;270:25672–25677

130. Palacin M, Estevez R, Bertran J, Zorzano A. Molecular biology of mammalian plasma membrane amino acid transporters. *Physiol Rev.* 1998;78:969–1054

131. Levin RJ, Koldovsky O, Hoskova J, Jirsova V, Uher J. Electrical activity across human foetal small intestine associated with absorption processes. *Gut.* 1968;9:206–213

132. Malo C. Multiple pathways for amino acid transport in brush border membrane vesicles isolated from the human fetal small intestine. *Gastroenterology.* 1991; 100:1644–1652

133. Prasad PD, Wang H, Huang W, Fei YJ, Leibach FH, Devoe LD, Ganapathy V. Molecular and functional characterization of the intestinal Na+-dependent multivitamin transporter. *Arch Biochem Biophys.* 1999;366:95–106

134. Bass WT, Malati N, Castle MC, White LE. Evidence for the safety of ascorbic acid administration to the premature infant. *Am J Perinatol.* 1998;15:133–140

135. Tsukaguchi H, Tokui T, Mackenzie B, et al. A family of mammalian Na+-dependent L-ascorbic acid transporters. *Nature.* 1999;399:70–75

136. Ghishan FK, Parker P, Nichols S, Hoyumpa A. Kinetics of intestinal calcium transport during maturation in rats. *Pediatr Res.* 1984;18:235–239

137. Ghishan FK, Stroop S, Meneely R. The effect of lactose on the intestinal absorption of calcium and zinc in the rat during maturation. *Pediatr Res.* 1982; 16:566–568

138. Barnes LA, Morrow G III, Silverio J, Finnegan LP, Heitman SE. Calcium and fat absorption from infant formulas with different fat blends. *Pediatrics.* 1974;54:217–221

139. Forbes GB, Reina JC. Effect of age on gastrointestinal absorption (Fe, Sr, Pb) in the rat. *J Nutr.* 1972;102:647–652

140. Ziegler EE, Edwards BB, Jensen RL, Mahaffey KR, Fomon SJ. Absorption and retention of lead by infants. *Pediatr Res.* 1978;12:29–34

141. Gunshin H, Mackenzie B, Berger UV, et al. Cloning and characterization of a mammalian proton-coupled metal-ion transporter. *Nature.* 1997;388:482–488

2
Nutritional Needs of the Preterm Infant

Optimal nutrition is critical in the management of small, preterm infants. No standard has been set for the precise nutritional needs of infants born prematurely. Present recommendations are designed to provide nutrients to approximate the rate of growth and composition of weight gain for a normal fetus of the same postmenstrual age, and to maintain normal concentrations of blood and tissue nutrients (Table 2.1).[1–3] Though, in general, the intrauterine growth rate can eventually be achieved, it is not obtained until well after the time of birth and, if catch-up growth occurs, then not until well after the time of discharge.[4] Nearly all extremely low-birth-weight infants (<1000 g birth weight) experience significant growth retardation during their stay in the neonatal intensive care unit (NICU). This is largely a result of the management of acute neonatal illnesses and gradual advancement of feeding to minimize the risk of feeding-related complications, such as necrotizing enterocolitis.

The quality of postnatal growth depends on the type, quantity, and quality of feeding consumed. Preterm infants fed standard infant formulas gain a higher percentage of their weight as fat when compared to a fetus of the same maturity.[5] The use of specially formulated preterm infant formulas and preterm human milk fortifiers results in a composition of weight gain and bone mineralization closer to that of the reference fetus, as compared to infants fed standard formulas for term infants or unfortified human milk.

Randomized prospective trials of specially formulated preterm formulas have shown significant improvements in growth and cognitive development when compared with standard formulas for full-term infants.[6] These findings underscore the need for the clinician to carefully plan and monitor the nutritional care of preterm infants during hospitalization and after discharge. This is even more important in the preterm infant maintained on unfortified human milk after discharge. A consensus recommendation of nutrition experts on specific nutrient requirements in preterm infants summarizes available data and recommendations and should be referred to for more detailed information.[3]

Table 2.1.
Comparison of Enteral Intake Recommendations for Growing Preterm Infants in Stable Clinical Condition

Nutrients per 100 kcal[†]	Consensus Recommendations*		AAPCON[‡]	ESPGAN-CON[‡]
	<1000 g	>1000 g		
Water, mL	125-167	125-167	...	115-154
Energy, kcal	100	100	100	100
Protein, g	3.0-3.16	2.5-3.0	2.9-3.3	2.25-3.1
Carbohydrate, g			9-13	7-14
Lactose, g	3.16-9.5	3.16-9.8	..	...
Oligomers, g	0-7.0	0-7.0	...	...
Fat, g			4.5-6.0	3.6-7
Linoleic acid, g	0.44-1.7	0.44-1.7	0.4+	0.5-1.4
Linolenic acid, g	0.11-0.44	0.11-0.44		>0.055
C18:2/C18:3	>5	>5	..	5-15
Vitamin A, USP units	583-1250	583-1250	75-225	270-450
With lung disease	2250-2333	2250-2333	...	...
Vitamin D, USP units	125-333	125-333	270	800-1600/d
Vitamin E, USP units			>1.1	0.6-10
Supplement, HM[§]	2.9	2.9	...	...
Vitamin K$_1$ μg	6.66-8.33	6.66-8.33	4	4-15
Ascorbate, mg	15-20	15-20	35	7-40
Thiamine, μg	150-200	150-200	>40	20-250
Riboflavin, μg	200-300	200-300	>60	60-600
Pyridoxine, μg	125-175	125-175	>35	35-250
Niacin, mg	3-4	3-4	>0.25	0.8-5.0
Pantothenate, mg	1-15	1-15	>0.30	>0.3
Biotin, μg	3-5	3-5	>1.5	>1.5
Folate, μg	21-42	21-42	33	>60
Vitamin B$_{12}$, μg	0.25	0.25	>0.15	>0.15
Sodium, mg	38-58	38-58	48-67	23-53
Potassium, mg	65-100	65-100	66-98	90-152
Chloride, mg	59-89	59-89	...	57-89
Calcium, mg	100-192	100-192	175	70-140
Phosphorus, mg	50-117	50-117	91.5	50-87

Table 2.1.
Comparison of Enteral Intake Recommendations for Growing Preterm Infants in Stable Clinical Condition *(continued)*

Nutrients per 100 kcal†	Consensus Recommendations*		AAPCON‡	ESPGAN-CON‡
	<1000 g	>1000 g		
Magnesium, mg	6.6-12.5	6.6-12.5	...	6-12
Iron, mg	1.67	1.67	1.7-2.5	1.5
Zinc, μg	833	833	>500	550-1100
Copper, μg	100-125	100-125	90	90-120
Selenium, μg	1.08-2.5	1.08-2.5	...	.
Chromium, μg	0.083-0.42	0.083-0.42	...	..
Manganese, μg	6.3	6.3	>5	1.5-7.5
Molybdenum, μg	0.25	0.25	..	...
Iodine, μg	25-50	25-50	5	10-45
Taurine, mg	3.75-7.5	3.75-7.5	.	..
Carnitine, mg	2.4	2.4	..	>1.2
Inositol, mg	27-67.5	27-67.5	...	...
Choline, mg	12-23.4	12-23.4	...	...

*From Tsang RC, Lucas A, Uauy R, Zlotkin S, eds. *Nutritional Needs of the Preterm Infants: Scientific Basis and Practical Guidelines.* Baltimore, MD: Williams & Wilkins; 1993:296.
†120 kcal/kg/d was used where a conversion was made from per kg recommendations.
‡ AAPCON indicates American Academy of Pediatrics, Committee on Nutrition; ESPGAN-CON, European Society of Pediatric Gastroenterology and Nutrition, Committee on Nutrition of the Preterm Infant.
§HM = human milk.

Energy Requirements

Energy is required for body maintenance and growth. The estimated resting metabolic rate of preterm infants with minimal physical activity is lower during the first week after birth than later. In a thermoneutral environment, it is approximately 40 kcal/kg/d when the infant is parenterally fed and 50 kcal/kg/d by 2 to 3 weeks of age when the infant is fed orally. Each gram of weight gain, including the stored energy and the energy cost of synthesis, requires between 3 and 4.5 kcal.[7] Thus, a daily weight gain of 15 g/kg requires a caloric expenditure of 45 to 67 kcal/kg above the 50 kcal/kg maintenance expenditure.

Estimated average energy requirements of preterm infants during the neonatal period are shown in Table 2.2.[8] It must be noted, however, that these

Table 2.2.
Estimation of the Energy Requirement of the Low-Birth-Weight Infant*

	Average Estimation, kcal/kg/d
Energy expended	40-60
Resting metabolic rate	40-50[†]
Activity	0-5[†]
Thermoregulation	0-5[†]
Synthesis	15[‡]
Energy stored	20-30[‡]
Energy excreted	15
Energy intake	90-120

*Adapted from the Committee on Nutrition of the Preterm Infant, European Society of Paediatric Gastroenterology and Nutrition.[8]
[†]Energy for maintenance.
[‡]Energy cost of growth.

energy requirements have largely been determined in healthy growing preterm infants at 3 to 4 weeks of age. There is very little information about energy requirements of sick and extremely low-birth-weight infants (<1000 g birth weight), especially in early postnatal life.

Activity, basal energy expenditure at thermoneutrality, the efficiency of nutrient absorption, and the utilization of energy for new tissue synthesis vary among infants. These variations may be pronounced in growth-retarded infants. In practice, energy intake by the enteral route of 105 to 130 kcal/kg/d enables most preterm infants to achieve satisfactory rates of growth. More calories may be given if growth is unsatisfactory at these intakes. Lower energy intakes can support growth if the infant is receiving total parenteral nutrition.

Protein Amount and Type
Protein intakes between 2.25 and 4.0 g/kg/d are adequate and not toxic. The estimated requirements based on the fetal accretion rate of protein are 3.5 to 4 g/kg/d. The type and quantity of protein in infant formulas most suitable for preterm infants has been examined in multiple studies.[9–12] In general, infants fed whey-predominant formulas had metabolic indices and plasma amino acid levels closer to those of infants fed pooled, mature human milk. In addition, a protein intake of 2.8 to 3.1 g/kg/d fed at 110 to 120 kcal/kg/d best mimicked fetal growth in the composition and rate of weight gain.

Lactobezoar formation has previously been associated with casein-predominant formulas; however, in a prospective study, Thorkelsson et al found no difference in the rate of gastric emptying between whey-predominant and casein-predominant formulas.[13] Soy-based formulas, as presently constituted, are not recommended for premature infants, because optimal carbohydrate, protein, and mineral absorption and utilization are even less well documented for soy-based formulas than for those based on cow milk.[14]

Fats

Fat provides a major source of energy for growing preterm infants. In human milk, about 50% of the energy is from fat; in commercial formulas, fat provides 40% to 50% of the energy. These feedings provide 5 to 7 g of fat/kg/d. The saturated fat of human milk is well absorbed by the preterm infant, in part because of the distribution pattern of fatty acids on the triglyceride molecule. Palmitic acid is present in the beta position in human milk fat and is more easily absorbed than palmitic acid in the alpha position, which occurs in cow milk, most other animal fats, and vegetable oils. Lingual lipase, acting in conjunction with gastric lipase, facilitates triglyceride digestion in the stomach, and bile salt-activated lipase in human milk-fed preterm infants continues digestion in the duodenum. These lipase activities substitute for the low pancreatic lipase of preterm infants and seem to partly compensate for the low intraluminal bile salt concentration of preterm infants. In formula-fed preterm infants, fat absorption is increased when human milk is mixed with the formula, presumably because of the lipases in human milk.[15]

The recently developed special formulas for preterm infants contain a mixture of medium-chain triglycerides and vegetable oils rich in polyunsaturated, long-chain triglycerides, both of which are well absorbed by premature infants.[1,2] This fat blend meets the estimated essential fatty acid requirement of at least 3% of energy in the form of linoleic acid with additional small amounts of α-linolenic acid. Formulas containing 10%, 30%, and 50% medium-chain triglycerides are well tolerated by preterm infants,[16] with no observed differences in weight gain or fat deposition.

Human milk contains small amounts of the fatty acids, docosahexaenoic acid (DHA), and arachidonic acid (AA), whereas preterm infant formulas available in the United States currently do not provide significant amounts of these fatty acids. Although the capacity for endogenous synthesis of these fatty acids has been thought to be limited in neonates, recent stable isotope studies have demonstrated that both term and preterm infants have the capacity to synthesize DHA and AA.[17,18] It remains unclear whether DHA and AA can be biosynthesized in quantities sufficient to meet the needs of these infants. However, from the results of 5 well-designed, randomized, controlled studies performed to date, no long-term benefit has been demonstrated for preterm infants receiving formula supplemented with DHA or AA.[19–23] There is some evidence that supplementation of formula with DHA increases the early rate of visual maturation in preterm infants, though this advantage does not persist beyond 4 months of age. One can also conclude from available studies that DHA and AA supplements do not impair growth of preterm infants. These fatty acids (derived from a single cell source) have recently been classified as "Generally Regarded as Safe" (GRAS) and may be added to infant formulas in approved ratios after the manufacturer fulfills the requirements of the Infant Formula Act (see Chapter 5).

Carbohydrates

Carbohydrates contribute a readily usable energy source and protect against tissue catabolism. Once the infant's condition is stabilized, the requirement for carbohydrate is estimated at 40% to 50% of calories, or approximately 10 to 14 g/kg/d.

By 34 weeks' gestation, premature infants have intestinal lactase activities that are only 30% of term infants.[24] However, in clinical settings, lactose intolerance is rarely a problem. Human milk is usually well tolerated. This may be because premature infants acquire a relatively efficient capacity to hydrolyze lactose in the small intestine at an earlier developmental stage than do infants in utero.[25] Glycosidase enzymes for glucose polymers are active in small preterm infants, and these polymers are well tolerated by preterm infants. Because glucose polymers add fewer osmotic particles to the formula per unit weight than does lactose, they permit the use of a high-carbohydrate formula with an osmolality below 300 mOsm/kg of water. Special formulas for preterm infants contain approximately 40% to 50% lactose and 50% to 60% glucose polymers, a ratio that does not impair mineral absorption.[26]

Minerals

Sodium and Potassium

Preterm infants, particularly those with a birth weight of less than 1500 g, have high fractional excretion rates of sodium for the first 10 to 14 days after birth, though urinary loss of sodium is also related to total fluid intake.

The low sodium concentrations of human milk, formulas for term infants, or human milk fortifiers designed for the feeding of preterm infants may lead to hyponatremia if these are used initially as the sole source of sodium. Special formulas for preterm infants provide 1.7 to 2.2 mEq/kg/d of sodium at full feeding levels (Appendix H).[27] During the stable and growing period, sodium requirements are usually met with a daily intake of 2 to 3 mEq/kg/d. The potassium requirement of preterm infants seems to be similar to that of term infants—2 to 3 mEq/kg/d.

Calcium, Phosphorus, and Magnesium

During the last trimester of pregnancy, the human fetus accrues about 80% of the calcium, phosphorus, and magnesium present at term. To achieve similar rates of accretion for normal growth and bone mineralization, small preterm infants require higher intakes of these minerals per kilogram of body weight than do term infants.[28] Current recommendations (Table 2.1) reflect the high daily intake requirements for these minerals. However, providing adequate amounts of these nutrients, particularly calcium and phosphorus, to very-low-birth-weight infants during the first few weeks of life is not always possible. As a result, osteopenia is frequent in these infants, and fractures develop in some.[29]

Milk-based formulas used for term infants contain 53 to 76 mg of calcium per 100 kcal and 42 to 57 mg of phosphorus per 100 kcal. The bone mineral content (BMC) in preterm infants consuming these formulas, as determined by photon absorptiometry, is less than normal fetal values.[30] However, the use of formulas specially designed for preterm infants (Appendix H) that contain 165 to 180 mg of calcium per 100 kcal and 82 to 100 mg of phosphorus per 100 kcal may improve the mineral balance and BMC to levels similar to fetal values.[31,32] Preterm human milk contains approximately 40 mg of calcium per 100 kcal and 20 mg of phosphorus per 100 kcal. It has been associated with impaired bone mineralization and rickets. The addition of powdered or liquid human milk fortifiers has improved mineral balance and bone mineralization.[32–34]

Iron

On a weight basis, the iron content of preterm infants at birth is lower than the iron content of full-term infants. Much of the iron is in the circulating hemoglobin; therefore, the frequent blood sampling that occurs with some preterm infants further depletes the amount of iron available for erythropoiesis. The early physiologic anemia of prematurity is not ameliorated by iron therapy, and blood transfusion is common for anemic preterm infants who have apnea of prematurity, a long-term requirement for supplemental oxygen, growth retardation, and patent ductus arteriosus.

During the first months of life, no clear indication exists for iron supplementation. Iron should be provided to human milk-fed preterm infants at 1 month of age at 2 mg/kg/d until 12 months of age. Formula-fed preterm infants may benefit from an iron supplement of 1 mg/kg/d in addition to the iron present in preterm infant and preterm discharge formulas, also continued through the first year of life. There is no role for the use of low-iron formulas; iron-fortified formulas can be used from the first feeding in formula-fed premature infants.

Though the use of recombinant erythropoietin to prevent or treat anemia of prematurity is probably not indicated in most premature infants, its use in the smallest preterm infants (birth weight below 1000 g) remains controversial.[35,36] Oral iron supplementation, up to 6 mg/kg/d, is particularly important when erythropoietin is used because active erythropoiesis requires additional iron as a substrate.[37]

Trace Minerals

During the last trimester of pregnancy, the estimated fetal accretion for zinc is 850 μg/d.[38] Although the zinc concentration of colostrum is high, its concentration in human milk rapidly declines to levels of 2.5 mg/L by 1 month and 1.1 mg/L by 3 months' postpartum. These levels of zinc are inadequate to meet the requirements of the growing preterm infant whose condition is stable, as demonstrated by reports of clinical zinc deficiency among human milk-fed preterm infants.[39] Current enteral recommendations of 600 μg to 1 mg/kg/d (Table 2.1) may result in zinc accretion below that of the fetus. However, higher intakes have not been evaluated for safety and may result in adverse nutrient interactions. Currently marketed preterm and full-term infant formulas as well as human milk fortifiers provide sufficient zinc to meet these recommendations.

Copper retention by the fetus has been estimated to be 56 μg/kg/d. Human milk from mothers of preterm infants contains 58 to 72 μg/dL during the first month after birth. Preterm infants absorb copper at rates of 57% from fortified human milk to 27% from standard cow milk-based formula.[40] Copper absorption is affected by the concentration of dietary zinc. Copper deficiency has been identified among infants primarily fed cow milk or given prolonged copper-free parenteral nutrition. The recommended daily intake (Table 2.1) can be met by using human milk or preterm infant formula.

The iodine content of human milk varies depending on the mother's intake, which is related to the geographic location of her food sources. Transient hypothyroidism has been reported among preterm infants receiving 10 to 30 μg/kg/d of iodine.[41] The recommended iodine intake is 30 to 60 μg/kg/d. All formulas for preterm infants will supply this amount. Powdered human milk fortifiers that are currently available do not contain added iodine. Human milk may not supply enough iodine by itself if the preterm infant is maintained for extended periods on human milk, though the needs for supplementation in this population have not been definitely established.

Deficiency of selenium, chromium, molybdenum, or manganese has not been reported for healthy preterm infants fed human milk. Current minimum recommendations for these microminerals are based on the concentration in human milk (see Appendix A).

Water-Soluble Vitamins
The recommended intake of water-soluble vitamins is based on the estimated amount provided by human milk and current feeding regimens, an understanding of their physiologic functions and excretion, stability during storage, and a limited amount of research data on the vitamin needs of preterm infants (Table 2.1).

The ascorbic acid content of human milk is approximately 8 mg/100 kcal, and that of preterm infant formulas ranges from 20 to 40 mg/100 kcal. Though no reports of deficiency among preterm infants receiving these feedings have been made, no published studies have assessed the ascorbic acid status of enterally fed preterm infants. Because ascorbic acid is essential for the metabolism of several amino acids, its requirement may be increased because of the high level of protein metabolism in the growing preterm infant. Ascorbic acid supplementation of human milk with a human milk fortifier or multivitamins will offset any losses that occur during handling and storage of human milk. Guidelines for ascorbic acid intake vary from 7 to 40 mg/100 kcal.[2,8,42]

Thiamine (vitamin B$_1$) is a cofactor for 3 enzyme complexes required for carbohydrate metabolism, as well as for the decarboxylation of branched-chain amino acids. The thiamine content of human milk is 29 μg/100 kcal, and 200 to 250 μg/100 kcal in preterm infant formulas (Appendix H). Commercially available human milk fortifiers provide an equivalent amount of thiamine when used to fortify human milk to 24/cal/oz. Recommendations for thiamine intake vary from 20 to 250 μg /100 kcal.[2,8,42] Although 200 μg/100 kcal is higher than that provided by human milk, it may be necessary because of the increased metabolic rate of preterm infants.[40]

Riboflavin (vitamin B_2) is a primary component of flavoproteins that serve as hydrogen carriers in numerous oxidation-reduction reactions. Infants with a negative nitrogen balance may have increased urinary losses of riboflavin, and those requiring phototherapy may use their reserves of riboflavin in the photo-catabolism of bilirubin. The riboflavin content is 49 μg/100 kcal in human milk and 150 to 620 μg/100 kcal in preterm formulas (Appendix H).

Commercially available human milk fortifiers provide 250 to 500 μg/100 kcal when used to fortify human milk to 24/cal/oz. Because of the photosensitivity of riboflavin, its content in human milk decreases during storage and handling. Guidelines for riboflavin intake range from 60 to 600 μg/100 kcal.[2,8,42] The higher intake allows for increased losses of riboflavin associated with medical problems commonly found in preterm infants.[42]

Pyridoxine (vitamin B_6) is a cofactor for numerous reactions involved in amino acid synthesis and catabolism. The requirement for pyridoxine is directly related to protein intake. The pyridoxine content of human milk is 28 μg/100 kcal and 150 to 250 μg/100 kcal in preterm formulas (Appendix H). Human milk fortifiers contain the equivalent amount when used as directed. Three preterm infants fed 250 μg/100 kcal for 14 days had blood levels 10 to 20 times higher than cord blood levels.[42] Guidelines range from 35 to 250 μg/100 kcal.[2,3,8]

Niacin (vitamin B_3) is a primary component of cofactors that function in numerous oxidation-reduction reactions, including glycolysis, electron transport, and fatty acid synthesis. Human milk contains 210 μg niacin/100 kcal, and preterm formulas contain 3900 to 5000 μg niacin/100 kcal (Appendix H). Human milk fortifiers contain the equivalent amount when used as directed. No cases of niacin deficiency have been reported in healthy preterm infants using current feeding regimens; however, no studies of niacin status in enterally fed infants are available. Recommended intake ranges from 250 to 5000 μg niacin/100 kcal.[2,8,42]

Biotin is a cofactor for 4 carboxylation reactions and is active in folate metabolism. The only reports of biotin deficiency have occurred in infants supported on biotin-free parenteral nutrition for several weeks.[43] The biotin content of human milk is 0.56 μg/100 kcal, and that of preterm formulas is 3.9 to 37 μg/100 kcal (Appendix H). Powdered human milk fortifiers contain the equivalent amount when used as directed. The recommended daily intake ranges from 1.5 to 5 μg/100 kcal.[2,8,42]

Pantothenic acid is a component of the acyl transfer group coenzyme A that is essential for fat, carbohydrate, and protein metabolism. Human milk provides 250 μg pantothenic acid/100 kcal and preterm formulas contain 1200 to 1900 μg pantothenic acid/100 kcal (Appendix H), which will easily provide the recommended daily intake of 300 to 1500 μg/100 kcal.[2,8,42] Powdered human milk fortifiers contain the equivalent amount when used as directed.

Folic acid is a cofactor that serves as an acceptor and donor of one-carbon units in amino acid and nucleotide metabolism. Deficiency alters cell division, particularly in tissues with rapid cell turnover, such as the intestine and bone marrow. Preterm infants are at increased risk for folate deficiency because of limited hepatic stores and rapid postnatal growth. Studies of preterm infants have shown improved folate status, assessed by red blood cell folate concentrations, among those provided supplemental folic acid.[44-46] On the basis of these studies, recommendations for folic acid intake range from 21 to 60 μg/100 kcal.[2,3,8] When the equivalent of 40 weeks of postmenstrual age is reached, the minimum recommendation for daily folic acid intake is comparable to that for term infants, which equals 4 μg/100 kcal. Human milk provides approximately 7 μg/100 kcal of folic acid. Preterm formulas contain 20 to 37 μg folic acid/100 kcal (Appendix H). Powdered human milk fortifiers will supply up to 30 μg folic acid/100 kcal when used as directed.

Vitamin B_{12} (cobalamine) is a cofactor involved in the synthesis of DNA and the transfer of methyl groups. Clinical symptoms of deficiency have been reported in infants who were exclusively breastfed by vegetarian mothers.[47] Deficiency has not been reported in term or preterm infants born to well-nourished mothers. Vitamin B_{12} is well absorbed from human milk and infant formula. Human milk provides 0.07 μg vitamin B_{12}/100 kcal and preterm infant formulas, 0.25 to 0.55 μg/100 kcal (Appendix H). Powdered human milk fortifiers will provide 0.22 to 0.79 μg/100 kcal when used as directed. Recommended intakes range from 0.15 to 0.25 μg/100 kcal.[2,3,8]

As a group, the body's reserves of water-soluble vitamins are limited, and a continuing supply of these nutrients is essential for normal metabolism. The higher recommended intake for preterm infants compared to that for term infants is based on their higher protein requirements and reduced vitamin reserves associated with shortened gestation. The recommended enteral intake of water-soluble vitamins for preterm infants fed human milk may be achieved by using a vitamin-containing human milk fortifier. Relatively few of these vitamins are provided by standard, oral multivitamin supplements. In formula-fed preterm infants, recommendations may be met by feeding preterm formulas that contain higher levels of water-soluble vitamins than term formulas. Again, standard multivitamin supplements for infants contain only a few of these vitamins.

There are no guidelines for supplementing premature infants with water-soluble vitamins after hospital discharge. However, as they still have potential for increased requirements over the amounts supplied by human milk or formulas, as with iron, supplementation until 1 year of chronological age is not unreasonable. The formulas now available for preterm infants after discharge (Appendix H) generally supply more water-soluble vitamins compared to standard formulas for term infants.

Fat-Soluble Vitamins

Vitamin A is a fat-soluble vitamin that promotes normal growth and differentiation of epithelial tissues. The liver is the primary storage site for vitamin A. At birth, the hepatic vitamin A content of preterm infants is low.[48] Measured values have indicated limited reserves and, in some cases, depletion. In addition, the plasma retinol, retinol binding protein (RBP), and retinol:RBP molar ratios of preterm infants are less than those of infants born at term.[49] The low vitamin A reserves in conjunction with impaired absorption, due to reduced hydrolysis of fats and low levels of intestinal carrier proteins for retinol, place the preterm infant at risk for vitamin A deficiency. The preterm infant's vitamin A status may affect the maintenance and development of pulmonary epithelial tissue. The recommendations for vitamin A intake range from 583 to 1250 IU/100 kcal, or 700 to 1500 IU/kg/d. Supplementation of premature infants with 1500 IU/kg/d results in normalization of serum retinol and RBP.[50] Given their high vitamin A content (10 150 IU/L, 1250 IU/100 kcal [Appendix H]), special formulas for preterm infants will supply this amount. Human milk, with a vitamin A concentration of 2230 IU/L (338 IU/100 kcal), will not supply the recommended intake. The human milk fortifiers, when used as directed, will provide an additional 6200 to 9500 IU/L. Several studies have indicated that normal vitamin A status reduces the incidence and severity of lung disease in the preterm infant,[51,52] although the largest study to date found that the only benefit was a reduction in oxygen requirement among the survivors at 36 weeks' postmenstrual age.[53] Though additional supplementation may be beneficial for preterm infants at risk for lung disease, clinicians must weigh the modest benefits against necessity for repeated intramuscular injections.[54]

Vitamin E is an antioxidant that actively inhibits fatty acid peroxidation in cell membranes. The vitamin E requirement increases with the level of polyunsaturated fatty acids (PUFAs) in the diet. Vitamin E deficiency-induced hemolytic anemia has been reported among preterm infants.[55,56] This syndrome has been associated with the use of formulas that contain high levels of PUFAs with inadequate vitamin E while providing supplemental iron, which functions as an oxidant.[57,58] Current formulas have been designed to provide a vitamin E:PUFA ratio that prevents this problem. The enteral intake of vitamin E should provide a minimum of 0.7 IU/100 kcal with at least 1 IU/g of linoleic acid. Pharmacologic doses of vitamin E for the prevention or treatment of retinopathy of prematurity, bronchopulmonary dysplasia, and intraventricular hemorrhage are not recommended. There is a general consensus in the United States that the preterm infant <1000 g birth weight should receive 6 to 12 IU/kg/d enterally (Table 2.1).[59] The formulas for premature infants will supply 4 to 6 IU/100 kcal/d. As the vitamin E content of mature human milk is quite variable and generally low, powdered human milk fortifiers will supply the equivalent amount per 100/kcal/d.

Overt vitamin D deficiency is rare in the premature infant in the United States given the maternal vitamin D status and the use of supplemental vitamin D in TPN solutions and infant formulas. Vitamin D deficiency has been implicated in the etiology of the osteopenia of prematurity, but it is apparent that the main cause for this condition is a deficiency of calcium and phosphorus.[60] The recommended intake of vitamin D is between 125 and 333 IU/100/kcal/d (Table 2.1). Preterm infants of birthweight <1250 g and gestational age of <32 weeks who receive a high mineral-containing bovine milk-based formula and a daily vitamin D intake of approximately 400 IU maintain normal serum 25-OH vitamin D and appropriately elevated $1,25(OH)_2$ vitamin D for many months.[61] There is no compelling evidence to give the preterm infant any more than 400 IU/kg/d of vitamin D. The human milk powdered fortifiers and special formulas for preterm infants will all supply between 200 and 400 IU/d when fed in typical amounts.

Hemorrhagic disease of the newborn infant, most commonly seen in exclusively breastfed infants, results from vitamin K deficiency.[62] As a preventive measure, an intramuscular injection of vitamin K is routinely provided after birth. In preterm infants who weigh more than 1 kg at birth, the standard dose of 1 mg of phylloquinone is appropriate. Among infants less than 1 kg, a dose of 0.3 mg/kg of phylloquinone is recommended. Formulas for preterm infants provide sufficient vitamin K to meet daily needs thereafter. Human milk has a low vitamin K content. The use of human milk fortifiers that contain supplemental vitamins will provide the additional vitamin K needed to meet the recommended intake of 7 to 9 μg/kg/d (Table 2.1).

There is little information about supplementation of fat-soluble vitamins after hospital discharge. For infants fed human milk, vitamin supplements of A, D, and E are readily available as oral solutions. None of these contain vitamin K. Supplementing formula-fed infants is more problematic, but in general, if premature infants are discharged on standard term infant formulas, they may not receive the recommended amounts of these vitamins, as discussed above, until they reach a weight of 3 kg. Thus, in the "healthy" preterm infant, it is probably not necessary to supplement with fat-soluble vitamins after attaining a weight of 3 kg. On the other hand, the special formulas for preterm infants after discharge should supply adequate amounts of the fat-soluble vitamins (Appendix H).

Energy Density and Water Requirements

The energy density of preterm and term human milk is about 67 kcal/dL at 21 days of lactation. Formulas of this energy density may be used for feeding preterm infants, but more concentrated formulas (ie, 81 kcal/dL [24 kcal/oz]) are often preferred. The increased caloric density allows smaller feeding volumes, an advantage when the gastric capacity is limited or fluid restriction is necessary. Formulas of this concentration provide most preterm infants with sufficient water for the excretion of protein-metabolic products and electrolytes derived from the formula.

Human Milk

Human milk from the preterm infant's mother is usually the enteral feeding of choice. Human milk is generally well tolerated by preterm infants and has been reported to promote the earlier achievement of full enteral feeding compared to infant formula. In addition to its nutritional value, human milk provides immunologic and antimicrobial components, hormones, and enzymes that may contribute positively to the infant's health and development.[63] Nevertheless, once growth is established, the nutritional needs of the preterm infant exceed the content of human milk for protein, calcium, phosphorus, magnesium, sodium, copper, zinc, and vitamins B_2 (riboflavin), B_6 (pyridoxine), C, D, E, and K, and folic acid.[63,64]

Unlike infant formula, the composition of human milk varies within a single feeding (or expression), diurnally, and throughout the course of lactation. Milk from mothers of preterm infants, especially during the first 2 weeks after delivery, contains higher levels of energy and higher concentrations of fat, protein, and sodium, but slightly lower concentrations of lactose, calcium, and phosphorus compared to milk from mothers of term infants.[65] The higher fat content accounts for the higher energy density of preterm milk. The higher protein content of preterm milk expressed during the first 2 to 3 weeks of lactation may be sufficient to match the fetal growth requirement for nitrogen when consumed at very high volumes—180 to 200 mL/kg/d. However, by the end of the first month of lactation, the protein content of preterm milk is inadequate to meet the needs of most preterm infants.[66] Metabolic complications associated with the long-term use of unsupplemented human milk in preterm infants include hyponatremia at 4 to 5 weeks,[67] hypoproteinemia at 8 to 12 weeks,[1,68] osteopenia at 4 to 5 months,[69] and zinc deficiency at 2 to 6 months.[39]

To correct the nutritional inadequacies of human milk for preterm infants, human milk fortifiers are available that provide additional protein, minerals, and vitamins (Appendix H). When these supplements are added to human milk in the first postpartum month, the resultant nutrient, mineral, and vitamin concentrations are similar to those of the formulas developed for feeding preterm infants. Clinical studies of human milk fortified with commercially available powdered mixtures show metabolic and growth effects approaching those of formulas designed for infants with low birth weight.[32,34]

The immunologic and antimicrobial components of human milk have been associated with a reduced incidence of necrotizing enterocolitis.[70] The presence of milk enzymes such as bile salt-stimulated lipase and lipoprotein lipase may facilitate nutrient bioavailability. In addition, the use of a preterm infant's mother's own milk may promote neurologic development. A nonrandomized study found higher developmental scores at 18 months and $7^1/_2$ to 8 years among preterm infants fed their mother's milk than among infants fed term formula.[6] However, there were many confounding variables in this study.

Facilitating Lactation and Human Milk Handling

Mothers of preterm infants should be encouraged to provide their milk for feeding their infants. Even mothers who plan to feed infant formula at discharge are often willing to express their milk for a few days or weeks after delivery. This milk can then be used to establish enteral feeding during the early critical weeks of life when the medical condition is less stable.

Mothers should begin expressing their milk within the first 24 hours after delivery. They should be given verbal and written instructions about appropriate methods for collection, storage, and handling of their milk[71] and assisted in locating a supplier for breast pumping equipment needed to establish and maintain a milk supply. Individual counseling about lactation management issues, such as pumping frequency, methods to facilitate milk letdown, and breast and nipple care, should be readily available.

Fresh milk from an infant's mother may be fed immediately or refrigerated at approximately 4°C. Refrigerated milk should be fed within 48 hours of expression. Any milk that will not be fed within 48 hours should be frozen at –20°C, immediately after it has been expressed. Freezing and heat treatment of human milk alter such labile factors as cellular elements, IgA, IgM, lactoferrin, lysozyme, and C3 complement. However, freezing appears to preserve these factors better than heat treatment. Human milk that has been frozen retains most of its immunologic properties and vitamin content when fed within 3 months of expression. Routine bacteriologic testing and pasteurization of human milk is not necessary when it is fed to the mother's own infant.[71]

Frozen milk should be thawed in cool or lukewarm running tap water or in a basin of warm water. Thawing in a microwave oven is not recommended because it reduces the levels of immunoglobulin (IgA) and lysozyme activity and may produce hot spots in the milk.[72,73] Thawed human milk should be stored in a refrigerator and used within 24 hours.

A limited number of human milk banks in the United States and Canada provide pooled donor human milk to hospitals on prescription.* These donor human milk banks follow specific procedures recommended by the Human Milk Banking Association of North America (HMBANA) for screening potential donors for infectious diseases, medical history, and lifestyle behaviors that

---

*Information about donor human milk banks in the United States and Canada is available from the Human Milk Banking Association of North America, PO Box 370464, West Hartford, CT 06137–0464.

could affect the quality of donated milk. The HMBANA is a nonprofit organization. There are no federal regulations or guidelines for banking human milk. Donor milk is pooled, pasteurized, tested for bacteria, and frozen for storage. Limited supplies of frozen, raw donor milk that meet specific bacteriologic testing criteria are also available for the rare instances in which infants do not tolerate pasteurized milk. Donor milk consists primarily of term human milk and requires fortification when used as a feeding for preterm infants.

As described previously, powdered milk fortifiers are available for supplementing human milk for the preterm infant (Appendix H). These are very similar in content and can be used to supplement human milk for the preterm infant up to 24 cal/oz with a well-balanced fortifier containing protein, minerals, and vitamins. These are designed to be mixed with human milk at the bedside.

Commercial Formulas for Preterm Infants

Commercial preterm infant formulas (Appendix H) have been developed to meet the unique nutritional needs of the growing, preterm infant. In selecting a formula to use for preterm infants, it is important to use a commercially sterile, ready-to-feed liquid formula, as powdered infant formula is not sterile. To minimize the risk of acquiring an infection if a preparation of powdered formula must be used, special precautions must be taken. The Centers for Disease Control and Prevention (CDC) recommends the use of aseptic technique during preparation of powdered formula, which includes refrigeration of prepared formula, discarding any reconstituted formula stored for longer than 24 hours, and limiting the time the formula remains at room temperature to less than 4 hours (http://www.cdc.gov/mmwr). Characteristics of this group of formulas include increased levels of protein and minerals compared with term formulas, carbohydrate blends of lactose and glucose polymers, and fat blends containing a portion of the fat as medium-chain triglycerides. The vitamin levels of these formulas are such that, in general, no additional multivitamin supplementation is necessary.

Preterm formulas are whey-predominant, cow milk-based formulas. Preterm formulas provide from 2.7 to 3.0 g protein per 100 kcal, which promotes a rate of weight gain and body composition similar to that of the reference fetus.[11,74–76]

The higher intake of calcium and phosphorus provided by preterm formulas increases net mineral retention and improves BMC compared with standard term formulas.[31,32] No additional supplements of vitamin D are needed.[60]

The fat blends of preterm formulas have been designed to optimize absorption. Of the fat, 40% to 50% is provided as medium-chain triglycerides. These fats help reduce losses due to low intestinal lipase or bile salt levels. Fat blends providing 40% to 50% of the fat as medium-chain triglycerides may lead to increased plasma ketones and urinary dicarboxylic acid excretion in premature infants, but this has not been shown to be detrimental to date.[77,78]

Traditionally, as formula-fed preterm infants approached discharge, the transition was made to a standard term infant formula for home use. With infants now leaving neonatal units at weights as low as 1500 g, reevaluation of the discharge formula prescription is needed. This is even more important as a recent report documents that even though the rate of intrauterine weight gain is often achieved prior to discharge with our intensive dietary management, catch-up growth itself does not occur until well after the time of discharge.[4] There is a paucity of data on what to feed the preterm infant after hospital discharge. More information is needed, particularly for the preterm infant who is maintained on breast milk whether from the breast or expressed into a bottle. These latter infants need both supplemental vitamins and iron.

The continuation of preterm formulas for a period after discharge provides one solution to this problem[79]; however, the cost and availability of these products may be limiting factors for some families. Intakes of vitamins and minerals become very high as the infants approach a weight of 2500 g. There are 2 preterm discharge formulas (Appendix H) that are now available through retail outlets at a cost only slightly greater than that of term infant formulas. These products provide preterm infants a nutrient intake that is between a preterm and term infant formula. The use of preterm discharge formulas to a postnatal age of 9 months results in greater linear growth, weight gain, and BMC compared with the use of term infant formula.[80–86] As these are iron and vitamin fortified, no other supplements are needed. Preterm infants served by the Special Supplemental Nutrition Program for Women, Infants, and Children (WIC) program can receive preterm discharge formula if they are provided with a prescription that also notes the qualifying diagnosis (eg, prematurity) and duration of treatment.

Enteral Feeding

The method of enteral feeding chosen for each infant should be based on gestational age, birth weight, clinical condition, and experience of the hospital nursing personnel. Specific feeding decisions that must be made by the clinician include age to initiate feeding, type of feeding (formula, breast milk), method of delivery, feeding frequency, concentration of feeding, and rate of advancement.

Enteral feedings have often been delayed when infants require high ventilatory settings or continuous positive airway pressure, have umbilical catheters, or are perceived to be at risk for necrotizing enterocolitis. However, a number of well-designed studies have identified advantages for the early introduction of low-volume, "priming" feedings, even when some of these factors are present.[87-90] Among the benefits reported for early enteral nutrition are a decreased incidence of indirect hyperbilirubinemia, cholestatic jaundice, and metabolic bone disease; increased levels of gastrin and other enteric hormones; fewer days to achieve full enteral feeding; and increased weight gain. These studies have not found an increased incidence of necrotizing enterocolitis among preterm infants receiving early enteral feedings. Based on the available evidence, the institution of early enteral feedings should be considered for all very-low-birth-weight infants.

The route for enteral feeding is determined by the infant's ability to coordinate sucking, swallowing, and breathing, which appear at approximately 32 to 34 weeks of gestation. Preterm infants of this gestational age who are alert and vigorous may be fed by nipple or offered the breast. Infants who are more premature or critically ill require feeding by tube to avoid the risk of aspiration and to conserve energy. Nasogastric and orogastric feedings, the most commonly used tube feedings in the neonatal intensive care unit, may be accomplished with bolus or continuous infusions of formula or human milk. Use of the stomach maximizes the digestive capability of the gastrointestinal tract. Transpyloric feedings provide no improvement in energy intake or growth, and may be associated with significant risks.[91] They should be undertaken only in rare instances, (ie, prolonged gastroparesis or dysmotility) and gastric feedings resumed as soon as possible. Gastrostomy feeding should be considered for infants who will be unable to nipple feed for long periods of time, to decrease negative oral stimulation associated with feeding-tube insertion.

Infants who receive nasogastric, orogastric, or gastrostomy feedings may be fed on an intermittent bolus or continuous schedule. Intermittent feedings every 2 to 3 hours simulate the pattern of feeding the infant will have when advanced to bottle feeding or breastfeeding. A recent large, randomized study demonstrated increased feeding intolerance and decreased growth in premature infants fed continuously compared to those fed by bolus.[90] Although some premature infants may need continuous feedings, bolus feedings over a period of 2 to 25 minutes are generally recommended. Reduced nutrient absorption is also a problem associated with continuous drip feeding.[92] Fat from human milk and medium-chain triglyceride additives tends to adhere to the feeding tube surfaces and reduce energy density.[93,94] Likewise, the loss of nutrients from fortifiers used to supplement human milk is increased when given in a continuous feeding.[95]

When human milk is used to initiate feedings, it is usually given full strength. Infant formulas are started at partial strength or full strength depending on the policies of the nursery. No definitive advantage for partial versus full-strength formula has been identified.

Parenteral Nutrition

Parenteral administration of glucose, fat, and amino acids is an important aspect of the nutritional care of preterm infants, particularly those who weigh less than 1500 g. The high incidence of respiratory problems, limited gastric capacity, and intestinal hypomotility in small preterm infants dictates the need for slow advancement of the volume of enteral feedings. Parenteral nutrition can supplement the slowly increasing enteral feedings so the total daily intake by both routes meets the infant's nutritional needs. When necessary, most nutritional requirements can be met for considerable periods by the parenteral route alone.

Fluid therapy is designed to avoid variations in serum osmolality, dehydration, and overhydration and to provide stable electrolyte and glucose levels and acid-base balance. For preterm infants with birth weights >1500 g, regimens that provide 80 mL/kg on the first day, increasing to 110 to 120 mL/kg by the fourth day, of a solution containing 3 to 4 mEq/kg of sodium as a mixture of chloride and acetate correct acidosis and sodium losses.[96] For infants with a birth weight of 1000 to 1500 g, a similar fluid should be given, with sodium added as serum Na falls below 140 mg/dL. For infants less than 1000 g at birth, much higher fluid intakes are necessary in the first 5 days of life, dependent on urine output and insensible water losses, which may be 5 to 7 mL/kg/h in extreme cases.[97] Once full total parenteral nutrition has been achieved with a weight gain of 15 to 20 g/kg/d, fluid rates will be in the range of 140 to 160 mL/kg/d in most infants. Two 2 to 4 mEq/kg/d of Na and Cl and 1.5 to 2 mEq/kg/d of potassium will be needed for this period of active growth.[98]

Protein is lost at high rates in preterm infants who are receiving glucose alone.[99–102] Multiple studies have clearly documented that these losses can be eliminated by providing intravenous amino acids at 1.1 to 2.2 g/kg/d, even in the face of low caloric intakes (30 to 50 kcal/kg/d).[3] Furthermore, studies have documented no increase in metabolic acidosis, BUN, or ammonia with early amino acid administration.[101,103,104] Intravenous amino acids should be provided to very-low-birth-weight infants at 1.5 to 2 g/kg/d as early as possible (within the first 24 hours of life) to preserve body protein stores.

Positive nitrogen balance, which indicates an anabolic state, can occur with parenteral lipid or glucose energy intakes of 60 kcal/kg/d and amino acid intakes of 2.5 to 3.0 g/kg/d.[105] With nonprotein energy intakes of 80 to 85 kcal/kg/d and amino acid intakes of 2.7 to 3.5 g/kg/d, nitrogen retention may occur at the fetal rate.[106,107] Growth generally requires a minimum parenteral nonprotein energy intake of 70 kcal/kg/d.

Use of glucose as the sole nonprotein energy source presents several problems. Concentrations of glucose higher than 12.5 g/dL cause local irritation of peripheral veins. In addition, very-low-birth-weight preterm infants have poor glucose tolerance during the first days of life, with hyperglycemia (serum glucose >125 mg/dL) occurring frequently when glucose infusion rates exceed 6 mg/kg/min.[108] To avoid the potentially damaging effects of widely varying serum osmolality and the dehydrating effects of an osmotic diuresis from substantial glycosuria, glucose infusion rates should start at a rate less than 6 mg/kg/min (8.6 g/kg/d). Usually a steady increase of the glucose infusion rate stimulates endogenous insulin secretion, and an infusion rate of 11 to 12 mg/kg/min (130 to 140 mL/kg/d of a 13-g/dL solution) is tolerated after 5 to 7 days of parenteral nutrition. Insulin has been administered to achieve an energy intake sufficient for growth.[109-111] However, the use of insulin in this situation is still considered investigational, and it may produce wide swings in levels of blood glucose with resulting periods of hypoglycemia as well as some lactic acidosis.[112]

The availability of intravenous lipid preparations has allowed the provision of energy adequate for growth via peripheral veins. The lipids have a high concentration of calories (2.0 kcal/mL in the 20% preparation) but have the same osmolality as plasma and, thus, do not irritate the veins. Lipid tolerance is clearly superior with 20% compared to 10% solutions because of their lower phospholipid emulsifier content. Therefore, 10% intravenous lipid solutions should not be used.[113] The tolerance for parenteral lipid is less in newborn infants than in older children and is further diminished in the small preterm infant.[114,115] In addition, infants with retarded intrauterine growth have even less parenteral fat tolerance than would be predicted from their gestational ages. Thus, the lipid should be administered continuously over 18 to 24 hours/d at an initial dose of 0.5 to 1.0 g/kg/d and should be slowly increased to a maximum of 2.0 to 3.0 g/kg/d. Fat tolerance can be assessed by determining serum triglyceride levels, which should be kept less than 150 mg/dL. The role of carnitine deficiency in causing the poor tolerance of lipids in the parenterally fed preterm infant is uncertain. Blood and tissue carnitine levels are low in preterm infants.[116] Intravenous carnitine may enhance the preterm infant's ability to use exogenous fat for energy, though clinical studies are contradictory in demonstrating metabolic or physiologic benefit in preterm infants following addition of carnitine to parenteral nutrition solutions.[117,118] Intravenous lipids increase serum-free fatty acid concentrations, which can displace bilirubin from albumin binding sites. However, studies have demonstrated that if parenteral lipids are provided continuously over a 24-hour period, free bilirubin is unaffected, and intravenous lipids do not need to be discontinued in jaundiced infants.[113]

The provision of calcium and phosphorus intravenously can be accomplished more easily with currently used amino acid mixtures with added cysteine because cysteine lowers the pH enough to allow the addition of calcium and phosphorus in increased amounts. Levels of fetal calcium and phosphorus

Table 2.3.
Mineral Supplements for Parenteral Nutrition for Preterm Infants per Kilogram per Day*

Mineral	Recommended Dosage
Calcium	80-100 mg
Phosphorus	43-62 mg
Magnesium	6-10 mg
Zinc	400 μg
Copper	20 μg
Selenium	2 μg
Chromium	0.2 μg
Manganese	1 μg
Molybdenum	0.25 μg
Iodide	1 μg

*From Greene, et al.[119]

accretion cannot be met, but severe metabolic bone disease in preterm infants can be minimized by adding minerals[119] (Table 2.3) to parenteral amino acid solutions containing 2.5 g/dL amino acids and by administering the solution at 120 to 150 mL/kg/d. Each institution should establish Ca and P solubility curves for their parenteral nutrition solutions. Goals for Ca intake are 60 to 90 mg/kg/d, and for P, 47 to 70 mg/kg/d.[120]

When parenteral nutrition supplements enteral feedings or is limited to 1 to 2 weeks, zinc is the only trace mineral that needs to be added. If total parenteral nutrition is required for a longer period, the other trace minerals may be added; however, copper and manganese should be omitted in the presence of obstructive jaundice, and selenium and chromium should be omitted in patients with renal dysfunction.[121]

The recommended dose of parenteral vitamins for preterm infants is 2 mL/kg/d of the currently available single dose vial of the lyophilized multivitamin mixture (MVI Pediatric, Astra Pharmaceuticals) with a maximum daily dose of one vial (ie, 5 μL) (Table 2.4).[119] The mixture given at this dosage will provide the recommended amounts of vitamins E and K, but low levels of vitamin A and D and excess levels of most B vitamins. However, a more appropri-

Table 2.4.
MVI Pediatric Ingredients*

Vitamin	Amount Provided
Ascorbic acid (vitamin C)	80 mg
Vitamin A (retinol)†	2300 USP units
Vitamin D†	400 USP units
Thiamine (vitamin B$_1$) (as the hydrochloride)	1.20 mg
Riboflavin (vitamin B$_2$) (as riboflavin-5-phosphate sodium)	1.4 mg
Pyridoxine (vitamin B$_6$) (as the hydrochloride)	1.0 mg
Niacinamide	17.0 mg
Dexpanthenol (pantothenyl alcohol)	5 mg
Vitamin E (d-α-tocopheryl acetate)	7.0 USP units
Biotin	20 μg
Folic acid	140 μg
Vitamin B$_{12}$ (cyanocobolamine)	1.0 μg
Vitamin K$_1$ (phytonadione)†	200 μg

*MVI Pediatric is a lyophilized, sterile powder intended for reconstitution and dilution in intravenous infusions. Each 5 mL of reconstituted product provides the indicated amounts of the vitamins.
†Fat-soluble vitamins solubilized with polysorbate 80.

ate mixture is not available, and individual vitamins are not available for parenteral use. A practical problem in providing fat-soluble vitamins parenterally is adherence, particularly of vitamin A, to the plastic tubing in intravenous administration sets. This can be overcome in part by administering the multivitamin mixture in the lipid emulsion used for parenteral nutrition.[122]

Conclusion

Nutrition plays a major role in the ultimate well-being of the increasing number of preterm infants who survive, and it is becoming clear that early nutritional intervention can have long-term consequences.[6,123] Because of the potential damage caused by inadequate nutrition during the early neonatal period, the dilemma of feeding the preterm infant is that of attempting to provide sufficient nutrition by enteral and parenteral routes to ensure optimal development without inducing additional morbidity and mortality secondary to the feedings. A recent randomized control trial has demonstrated that early aggressive enteral and parenteral nutrition in sick very-low-birth-weight infants can improve growth outcomes without increasing the risk of all measured clinical and metabolic sequelae.[124] It seems apparent that altering poor nutritional outcomes will require a more sustained effort to provide adequate nutritional support in early postnatal life. Unfortunately, there is still very limited information on the nutritional status of preterm infants after hospital discharge.

References

1. American Academy of Pediatrics, Committee on Nutrition. Nutritional needs of low-birth-weight infants. *Pediatrics.* 1977;60:519–530
2. American Academy of Pediatrics, Committee on Nutrition. Nutritional needs of low-birth-weight infants. *Pediatrics.* 1985;75:976–986
3. Tsang RC, Lucas A, Uauy R, Zlotkin S, eds. *Nutritional Needs of the Preterm Infant: Scientific Basis and Practical Guidelines.* Baltimore, MD: Williams & Wilkins; 1993
4. Lemons JA, Bauer CR, Oh W, et al. Very low birth weight outcomes of the National Institute of Child Health and Human Development Neonatal Research Network, January 1995 through December 1996. *Pediatrics.* 2001;107:e1
5. Reichman B, Chessex P, Putet G, et al. Diet, fat accretion, and growth in premature infants. *N Engl J Med.* 1981;305:1495–1500
6. Morley R, Lucas A. Influence of early diet on outcome in preterm infants. *Acta Paediatr Suppl.* 1994;405:123–126

7. Roberts SB, Young VR. Energy costs of fat and protein deposition in the human infant. *Am J Clin Nutr.* 1988;48:951–955

8. Committee on Nutrition of the Preterm Infant, European Society of Paediatric Gastroenterology and Nutrition (ESPGAN). *Nutrition and Feeding of Preterm Infants.* Oxford, England: Blackwell Scientific Publications; 1987

9. Gaull GE, Rassin DK, Raiha NC, Heinonen K. Milk protein quantity and quality in low-birth-weight infants, III: effects on sulfur amino acids in plasma and urine. *J Pediatr.* 1977;90:348–355

10. Raiha NC, Heinonen K, Rassin DK, Gaull GE. Milk protein quantity and quality in low-birthweight infants, I: metabolic responses and effects on growth. *Pediatrics.* 1976;57:659–684

11. Kashyap S, Schulze KF, Forsyth M, et al. Growth, nutrient retention, and metabolic response in low birth weight infants fed varying intakes of protein and energy. *J Pediatr.* 1988;113:713–721

12. Rigo J, Senterre J. Significance of plasma amino acid pattern in preterm infants. *Biol Neonate.* 1987;52(suppl 1):41–49

13. Thorkelsson T, Mimouni F, Namgung R, Fernandez-Ulloa M, Krug-Wispe S, Tsang RC. Similar gastric emptying rates for casein- and whey-predominant formulas in preterm infants. *Pediatr Res.* 1994;36:329–333

14. Shenai JP, Jhaveri BM, Reynolds JW, Huston RK, Babson SG. Nutritional balance studies in very low-birth-weight infants: role of soy formula. *Pediatrics.* 1981; 67:631–637

15. Alemi B, Hamosh M, Scanlon JW, Salzman-Mann C, Hamosh P. Fat digestion in very low-birth-weight infants: effect of addition of human milk to low-birth-weight formula. *Pediatrics.* 1981;68:484–489

16. Bustamante SA, Fiello A, Pollack PF. Growth of premature infants fed formulas with 10%, 30%, or 50% medium-chain triglycerides. *Am J Dis Child.* 1987; 141:516–519

17. Carnielli VP, Wattimena DJ, Luijendijk IH, Boerlage A, Degenhart HJ, Sauer PJ. The very low birth weight premature infant is capable of synthesizing arachidonic and docosahexaenoic acids from linoleic and linolenic acids. *Pediatr Res.* 1996; 40:169–174

18. Sauerwald TU, Hachey DL, Jensen CL, Chen H, Anderson RE, Heird WC. Intermediates in endogenous synthesis of C22:6 omega 3 and C20:4 omega 6 by term and preterm infants. *Pediatr Res.* 1997;41:183–187

19. Birch DG, Birch EE, Hoffman DR, Uauy RD. Retinal development of very-low-birth-weight infants fed diets differing in omega–3 fatty acids. *Invest Ophthalmol Vis Sci.* 1992;33:2365–2376

20. Carlson SE, Werkman SH, Rhodes PG, Tolley EA. Visual-acuity development in healthy preterm infants: effect of marine-oil supplementation. *Am J Clin Nutr.* 1993;58:35–42

21. Clandinin MT, Van Aerde JE, Parrott A, Field CJ, Euler AR, Lien EL. Assessment of the efficacious dose of arachidonic and docosahexaenoic acids in preterm infant formulas: fatty acid composition of erythrocyte membrane lipids. *Pediatr Res.* 1997;42:819–825

22. Vanderhoof J, Gross S, Hegyi T. A new arachidonic acid (ARA) and docosahexanoic acid (DHA) supplemented preterm formula: growth and safety assessment. *Pediatr Res.* 1997;41:242A

23. Hansen J, Schape D, et al. Docosahexaenoic acid plus arachidonic acid enhance preterm infant growth. In: *Essential Fatty Acids & Eicosanoids: Invited Papers from the Fourth International Congress.* Champaign, IL: American Oil Chemists' Society; 1999:T16

24. Kien CL, Heitlinger LA, Li BU, Murray RD. Digestion, absorption, and fermentation of carbohydrate. *Semin Perinatol.* 1989;13:78–87

25. Kien CL. Carbohydrates. In: Tsang RC, Lucas A, Uauy R, Zlotkin S, eds. *Nutritional Needs of the Preterm Infant: Scientific Basis and Practical Guidelines.* Baltimore, MD: Williams & Wilkins; 1993:47–63

26. Wirth FH Jr, Numerof B, Pleban P, Neylan MJ. Effect of lactose on mineral absorption in preterm infants. *J Pediatr.* 1990;117:283–287

27. Arant BS Jr. Sodium, chloride, and potassium. In: Tsang RC, Lucas A, Uauy R, Zlotkin S, eds. *Nutritional Needs of the Preterm Infant: Scientific Basis and Practical Guidelines.* Baltimore, MD: Williams & Wilkins; 1993:157–175

28. Koo WWK, Tsang RC. Calcium, magnesium, phosphorus, and vitamin D. In: Tsang RC, Lucas A, Uauy R, Zlotkin S, eds. *Nutritional Needs of the Preterm Infant: Scientific Basis and Practical Guidelines.* Baltimore, MD; Williams & Wilkins; 1993:135–155

29. Koo WW, Sherman R, Succop P, et al. Fractures and rickets in very low birth weight infants: conservative management and outcome. *J Pediatr Orthop.* 1989;9:326–330

30. Minton SD, Steichen JJ, Tsang RC. Bone mineral content in term and preterm appropriate-for-gestational-age infants. *J Pediatr.* 1979;95:1037–1042

31. Chan GM, Mileur L, Hansen JW. Effects of increased calcium and phosphorus formulas and human milk on bone mineralization in preterm infants. *J Pediatr Gastroenterol Nutr.* 1986;5:444–449

32. Ehrenkranz RA, Gettner PA, Nelli CM. Nutrient balance studies in premature infants fed premature formula or fortified preterm human milk. *J Pediatr Gastroenterol Nutr.* 1989;8:58–67

33. Schanler RJ, Garza C. Improved mineral balance in very low birth weight infants fed fortified human milk. *J Pediatr.* 1988;112:452–456

34. Greer FR, McCormick A. Improved bone mineralization and growth in premature infants fed fortified own mother's milk. *J Pediatr.* 1988;112:961–969

35. Ohls RK. Erythropoietin treatment in extremely low birth weight infants: blood in versus blood out. *J Pediatr.* 2002;141:3–6

36. Zipursky A. Erythropoietin therapy for premature infants: cost without benefit? *Pediatr Res.* 2000;48:136

37. Franz AR, Mihatsch WA, Sander S, Kron M, Pohlandt F. Prospective randomized trial of early versus late enteral iron supplementation in infants with a birth weight of less than 1301 grams. *Pediatrics.* 2000;106:700–706

38. Widdowson EM, Southgate DAT, Hey E. Fetal growth and body composition. In: Lindblad B, ed. *Perinatal Nutrition.* New York, NY: Academic Press; 1988:3–14

39. Zlotkin SH. Assessment of trace element requirements (zinc) in newborns and young infants, including the infant born prematurely. In: Chandra RK, ed. *Trace Elements in Nutrition of Children II.* New York, NY: Raven Press; 1991:49–64

40. Ehrenkranz RA, Gettner PA, Nelli CM, et al. Zinc and copper nutritional studies in very low birth weight infants: comparison of stable isotopic extrinsic tag and chemical balance methods. *Pediatr Res.* 1989;26:298–307

41. Delange F, Dalhem A, Bourdoux P, et al. Increased risk of primary hypothyroidism in preterm infants. *J Pediatr.* 1984;105:462–469

42. Greene HL, Smidt LJ. Water-soluble vitamins: C, B_1, B_2, B_6, niacin, pantothenic acid, and biotin. In: Tsang RC, Lucas A, Uauy R, Zlotkin S, eds. *Nutritional Needs of the Preterm Infant: Scientific Basis and Practical Guidelines.* Baltimore, MD: Williams & Wilkins; 1993:121–133

43. Mock DM, deLorimer AA, Liebman WM, Sweetman L, Baker H. Biotin deficiency: an unusual complication of parenteral alimentation. *N Engl J Med.* 1981; 304:820–823

44. Burland WL, Simpson K, Lord J. Response of low birthweight infants to treatment with folic acid. *Arch Dis Child.* 1971;46:189–194

45. Kendall AC, Jones EE, Wilson CI, Shinton NK, Elwood PC. Folic acid in low birthweight infants. *Arch Dis Child.* 1974;49:736–738

46. Stevens D, Burman D, Strelling MK, Morris A. Folic acid supplementation in low birth weight infants. *Pediatrics.* 1979;64:333–335

47. Higginbottom MC, Sweetman L, Nyhan WL. A syndrome of methylmalonic aciduria, homocystinuria, megaloblastic anemia and neurologic abnormalities in a vitamin B_{12}-deficient breast-fed infant of a strict vegetarian. *N Engl J Med.* 1978; 299:317–323

48. Shenai JP, Chytil F, Stahlman MT. Liver vitamin A reserves of very low birth weight neonates. *Pediatr Res.* 1985;19:892–893

49. Shenai JP, Chytil F, Jhaveri A, Stahlman MT. Plasma vitamin A and retinol-binding protein in premature and term neonates. *J Pediatr.* 1981;99:302–305

50. Shenai JP, Rush MG, Stahlman MT, Chytil F. Plasma retinol-binding protein response to vitamin A administration in infants susceptible to bronchopulmonary dysplasia. *J Pediatr.* 1990;116:607–614

51. Shenai JP, Kennedy KA, Chytil F, Stahlman MT. Clinical trial of vitamin A supplementation in infants susceptible to bronchopulmonary dysplasia. *J Pediatr.* 1987; 111:269–277

52. Robbins ST, Fletcher AB. Early vs delayed vitamin A supplementation in very-low-birth-weight infants. *JPEN J Parenter Enteral Nutr.* 1993;17:220–225

53. Tyson JE, Wright LL, Oh W, et al. Vitamin A supplementation for extremely-low-birth-weight infants. National Institute of Child Health and Human Development Neonatal Research Network. *N Engl J Med.* 1999;340:1962–1968

54. Darlow BA, Graham PJ. Vitamin A supplementation for preventing morbidity and mortality in very low birthweight infants (Cochrane Review). In: *The Cochrane Library*, Issue 1, 2001. Oxford: Update Software

55. Oski FA, Barness LA. Vitamin E deficiency: a previously unrecognized cause of hemolytic anemia in the premature infant. *J Pediatr.* 1967;70:211–220

56. Ritchie JH, Fish MB, McMasters V, Grossman M. Edema and hemolytic anemia in premature infants: a vitamin E deficiency syndrome. *N Engl J Med.* 1968;279: 1185–1190

57. Williams ML, Shott RJ, O'Neal PL, Oski FA. Role of dietary iron and fat on vitamin E deficiency anemia of infancy. *N Engl J Med.* 1975;292:887–890

58. Gross S, Melhorn DK. Vitamin E-dependent anemia in the premature infant. *J Pediatr.* 1974;85:753–759

59. Gross S. Vitamin E. In: Tsang RC, Lucas A, Uauy R, Zlotkin S, eds. *Nutritional Needs of the Preterm Infant: Scientific Basis and Practical Guidelines.* Baltimore, MD: Williams & Wilkins; 1993

60. Greer FR. Osteopenia of prematurity. *Annu Rev Nutr.* 1994;14:169–185

61. Cooke R, Hollis B, Conner C, Watson D, Werkman S, Chesney R. Vitamin D and mineral metabolism in the very low birth weight infant receiving 400 IU of vitamin D. *J Pediatr.* 1990;116:423–428

62. Greer FR, Zachman RD. Fat soluble vitamins. In: Cowett RM, ed. *Principles of Perinatal-Neonatal Metabolism.* New York, NY: Springer Verlag; 1998:943–976

63. Schanler RJ, Hurst NM, Lau C. The use of human milk and breastfeeding in premature infants. *Clin Perinatol.* 1999;26:379–398

64. Lucas A. Enteral nutrition. In: Tsang RC, Lucas A, Uauy R, Zlotkin S, eds. *Nutritional Needs of the Preterm Infant: Scientific Basis and Practical Guidelines.* Baltimore, MD: Williams & Wilkins; 1993:209–223

65. Atkinson SA. Effects of gestational age at delivery on human milk components. In: Jensen RG, ed. *Handbook of Milk Composition.* San Diego, CA: Academic Press; 1995:222–237

66. Lucas A, Hudson G. Preterm milk as a source of protein for low birthweight infants. *Arch Dis Child.* 1984;59:831–836

67. Engelke SC, Shah BL, Vasan U, Raye JR. Sodium balance in very low-birth-weight infants. *J Pediatr.* 1978;93:837–841

68. Ronnholm KA, Sipila I, Siimes MA. Human milk protein supplementation for the prevention of hypoproteinemia without metabolic imbalance in breast milk-fed, very low-birth-weight infants. *J Pediatr.* 1982;101:243–247

69. Greer FR, Steichen JJ, Tsang RC. Calcium and phosphate supplements in breast milk-related rickets: results in a very-low-birth-weight infant. *Am J Dis Child.* 1982;136:581–583

70. Lucas A, Cole TJ. Breast milk and neonatal necrotizing enterocolitis. *Lancet.* 1990;336:1519–1523

71. Human Milk Banking Association of North America. *Recommendations for Collection, Storage and Handling of a Mother's Milk for Her Own Infant in the Hospital Setting.* West Hartford, CT: Human Milk Banking Association of North America; 1993

72. Quan R, Yang C, Rubenstein S, et al. Effects of microwave radiation on anti-infective factors in human milk. *Pediatrics.* 1992;89:667–669

73. Sigman M, Burke KI, Swarner OW, et al. Effects of microwaving human milk: changes in IgA content and bacterial count. *J Am Diet Assoc.* 1989;89:690–692

74. Putet G, Senterre J, Rigo J, et al. Nutrient balance, energy utilization, and composition of gain in very-low-birth-weight infants fed pooled human milk or a preterm formula. *J Pediatr.* 1984;105:79–85

75. Gross SJ. Growth and biochemical response of preterm infants fed human milk or modified infant formula. *N Engl J Med.* 1983;308:237–241

76. Schulze KF, Stefanski M, Masterson J, et al. Energy expenditure, energy balance and composition of weight gain in low birth weight infants fed diets of different protein and energy content. *J Pediatr.* 1989;110:753–759

77. Sulkers EJ, Lafeber HN, Sauer PJ. Quantitation of oxidation of medium-chain triglycerides in preterm infants. *Pediatr Res.* 1989;26:294–297

78. Ponder DL. Medium chain triglyceride and urinary di-carboxylic acids in newborns. *JPEN J Parenter Enteral Nutr.* 1991;15:93–94

79. Cooke RJ, Griffin IJ, McCormick K, et al. Feeding preterm infants after hospital discharge: effect of dietary manipulation on nutrient intake and growth. *Pediatr Res.* 1998;43:355–360

80. Lucas A, Bishop NJ, King FJ, Cole TJ. Randomized trial of nutrition for preterm infants after discharge. *Arch Dis Child.* 1992;67:324–327

81. Bishop NJ, King FJ, Lucas A. Increased bone mineral content of preterm infants fed with a nutrient enriched formula after discharge from hospital. *Arch Dis Child.* 1993;68:573– 578

82. Hall RT, Wheeler RE, Rippetoe LE. Calcium and phosphorus supplementation after initial hospital discharge in breast-fed infants at less than 1800 grams birth weight. *J Perinatol.* 1993;13:272–278

83. Wheeler RE, Hall RT. Feeding of premature infant formula after hospital discharge of infants weighing less than 1800 grams at birth. *J Perinatol.* 1996;16:111–116

84. Friel JK, Andrews WL, Matthew JD, McKim E, French S, Long DR. Improved growth of very low birthweight infants. *Nutr Res.* 1993;13:611–620

85. Carver JD, Wu PYK, Hall RT, Baggs GE, Blenneman B. Growth of preterm infants fed NeoCare or Similac with iron after hospital discharge. *Pediatr Res.* 1997; 41:229A

86. Chan GM. Growth and bone mineral status of discharged very low birth weight infants fed different formulas or human milk. *J Pediatr.* 1993;123:439–443

87. Berseth CL. Effect of early feeding on maturation of the preterm infant's small intestine. *J Pediatr.* 1992;120:947–953

88. Davey AM, Wagner CL, Cox C, Kendig JW. Feeding premature infants while low umbilical artery catheters are in place: a prospective, randomized trial. *J Pediatr.* 1994;124:795–799

89. McClure J, Newell RJ. Randomized controlled trial of trophic feeding and gut motility. *Arch Dis Child.* 1999;80:F54–F58

90. Schanler RJ, Shulman RJ, Lau C, Smith EO, Heitkemper MM. Feeding strategies for premature infants: randomized trial of gastrointestinal priming and tube-feeding method. *Pediatrics.* 1999;103:434–439

91. MacDonald PD, Skeoch CH, Carse H, et al. Randomized trial of continuous nasogastric, bolus nasogastric, and transpyloric feeding in infants of birth weight under 1400 g. *Arch Dis Child.* 1992;67:429–431

92. Roy RN, Pollnitz RB, Hamilton JR, Chance GW. Impaired assimilation of nasojejunal feeds in healthy low-birth-weight newborn infants. *J Pediatr.* 1977;90:431–434

93. Greer FR, McCormick A, Loker J. Changes in fat concentration of human milk during delivery by intermittent bolus and continuous mechanical pump infusion. *J Pediatr.* 1984;105:745–749

94. Mehta NR, Hamosh M, Bitman J, Wood DL. Adherence of medium-chain fatty acids to feeding tubes during gavage feeding of human milk fortified with medium-chain triglycerides. *J Pediatr.* 1988;112:374–376

95. Bhatia J, Rassin DK. Human milk supplementation: delivery of energy, calcium, phosphorus, magnesium, copper, and zinc. *Am J Dis Child.* 1988;142:445–447

96. Ekblad H, Kero P, Takala J, Korvenranta H, Valimaki I. Water, sodium and acid-base balance in premature infants: therapeutical aspects. *Acta Paediatr Scand.* 1987;76:47–53

97. Costarino AT, Baumgart S. Water as nutrition. In: Tsang RC, Lucas A, Uauy R, Zlotkin S, eds. *Nutritional Needs of the Preterm Infant: Scientific Basis and Practical Guidelines.* Baltimore, MD: Williams & Wilkins; 1993:1–14

98. Arant BS. Sodium, chloride and potassium. In: Tsang RC, Lucas A, Uauy R, Zlotkin S, eds. *Nutritional Needs of the Preterm Infant: Scientific Basis and Practical Guidelines.* Baltimore, MD: Williams & Wilkins; 1993:157–176

99. Denne SC, Karn CA, Ahlrichs JA, Dorotheo AR, Wang J, Liechty EA. Proteolysis and phenylalanine hydroxylation in response to parenteral nutrition in extremely premature and normal newborns. *J Clin Invest.* 1996;97:746–754

100. Mitton SG, Calder AG, Garlick PJ. Protein turnover rates in sick, premature neonates during the first few days of life. *Pediatr Res.* 1991;30:418–422

101. Rivera A Jr, Bell EF, Bier DM. Effect of intravenous amino acids on protein metabolism of preterm infants during the first three days of life. *Pediatr Res.* 1993; 33:106–111

102. Kashyap S, Heird WC. *Protein Requirements of Low Birthweight, Very Low Birthweight, and Small for Gestational Age Infants.* New York, NY: Vevey/Raven Press, Ltd; 1994:133–151

103. Van Lingen RA, Van Goudoever JB, Luijendijk IH, Wattimena JL, Saur PJ. Effects of early amino acid administration during total parenteral nutrition on protein metabolism in preterm infants. *Clin Sci (Lond).* 1992;82:199–203

104. Van Goudoever JB, Colen T, Wattimena JL, Huijmans JG, Carnielli VP, Sauer PJ. Immediate commencement of amino acid supplementation in preterm infants: effect on serum amino acid concentrations and protein kinetics on the first day of life. *J Pediatr.* 1995;127:458–465

105. Anderson TL, Muttart CR, Bieber MA, et al. A controlled trial of glucose versus glucose and amino acids in premature infants. *J Pediatr.* 1979;94:947–951

106. Duffy B, Gunn T, Collinge J, et al. The effect of varying protein quality and energy intake on the nitrogen metabolism of parenterally fed very low birthweight (less than 1600 g) infants. *Pediatr Res.* 1981;15:1040–1044

107. Zlotkin SH, Bryan MH, Anderson GH. Intravenous nitrogen and energy intakes required to duplicate in utero nitrogen accretion in prematurely born human infants. *J Pediatr.* 1981;99:115–120

108. Dweck HS, Cassady G. Glucose intolerance in infants of very low birth weight, I: incidence of hyperglycemia in infants of birth weights 1100 grams or less. *Pediatrics.* 1974;53:189–195

109. Binder ND, Raschko PK, Benda GI, et al. Insulin infusion with parenteral nutrition in extremely low birth weight infants with hyperglycemia. *J Pediatr.* 1989;114: 273–280

110. Collins JW, Hoppe M, Brown K, et al. A controlled trial of Insulin infusion and parenteral nutrition in extremely low birth weight infants with glucose intolerance. *J Pediatr.* 1991;118:921–927

111. Kanarek KS, Santeiro ML, Malone JI. Continuous infusion of insulin in hyperglycemic low-birth weight infants receiving parenteral nutrition with and without lipid emulsion. *JPEN J Parenter Enteral Nutr.* 1991;15:417–420

112. Poindexter BB, Karn CA, Denne SC. Exogenous insulin reduces proteolysis and protein synthesis in extremely low birth weight infants. *J Pediatr.* 1998;132: 948–953

113. Putet G. Lipid metabolism of the micropremie. *Clin Perinatol.* 2000;27:57–69

114. Andrew G, Chan G, Schiff D. Lipid metabolism in the neonate, I: the effects of intralipid infusion on plasma triglyceride and free fatty acid concentrations in the neonate. *J Pediatr.* 1976;88:273–278

115. Shennan AT, Bryan MH, Angel A. The effect of gestational age on intralipid tolerance in newborn infants. *J Pediatr.* 1977;91:134–137

116. Penn D, Schmidt-Sommerfeld E, Pascu F. Decreased tissue carnitine concentrations in newborn infants receiving total parenteral nutrition. *J Pediatr.* 1981; 98:976–978

117. Schmidt-Sommerfield E, Penn D. Carnitine and total parenteral nutrition of the neonate. *Biol Neonate*. 1990;58:81–88

118. Larrson LE, Olegard R, Ljung A, Rubensson A, Cederblad G. Parenteral nutrition in preterm neonates with and without carnitine supplementation. *Acta Anaesthesiol Scand*. 1990;34:501–505

119. Greene HL, Hambidge KM, Schanler R, Tsang RC. Guidelines for the use of vitamins, trace elements, calcium, magnesium and phosphorus in infants and children receiving total parenteral nutrition: report of the Subcommittee on Pediatric Parenteral Nutrient Requirements from the Committee on Clinical Practice Issues of The American Society for Clinical Nutrition. *Am J Clin Nutr*. 1988;48: 1324–1342

120. Koo WWK, Tsang RC. Calcium, magnesium, phosphorus, and vitamin D. In: Tsang RC, Lucas A, Uauy R, Zlotkin S, eds. *Nutritional Needs of the Preterm Infant: Scientific Basis and Practical Guidelines*. Baltimore, MD: Williams & Wilkins; 1993:135–156

121. Reifen RM, Zlotkin S. Microminerals. In: Tsang RC, Lucas A, Uauy R, Zlotkin S, eds. *Nutritional Needs of the Preterm Infant: Scientific Basis and Practical Guidelines*. Baltimore, MD: Williams & Wilkins; 1993:195–208

122. Baekert PA, Greene HL, Fritz I, Oelberg DG, Adcock EW. Vitamin concentration in very low birth weight infants given vitamins intravenously in a lipid emulsion: measurement of vitamins A, D, and E and riboflavin. *J Pediatr*. 1988; 113:1057–1065

123. Lucas A, Morley R, Cole RJ, et al. Early diet in preterm babies and developmental status at 18 months. *Lancet*. 1990;335:1477–1481

124. Wilson DC, Carins P, Halliday HL, Reid M, McClure G. Randomized controlled trial of an aggressive nutritional regimen in sick very low birthweight infants. *Arch Dis Child*. 1997;77:F4–F11

3

Breastfeeding

The American Academy of Pediatrics (AAP) and the Canadian Paediatric Society have strongly recommended that breastfeeding be the preferred feeding for all infants, including premature newborns.[1,2] The success of adequate lactation depends substantially on the knowledge and supportive attitude of professional personnel in pediatrics and obstetrics services, hospital policies and practices that are conducive to the initiation and maintenance of breastfeeding, and the realization by health care providers that although breastfeeding is a natural function, many mothers need instruction and support. A short hospital stay may have a negative influence on breastfeeding, and its effects should be anticipated. Caregivers should observe and document breastfeeding within the hospital and at 3 to 5 days of age. Close follow-up after discharge may mitigate the negative effects of early discharge. There is increased public awareness of the benefits of breastfeeding, which has prompted caregivers to request more formal education in the field.[3] Responses to these requests include the formation of an American Academy of Pediatrics Section on Breastfeeding as well other as programs to support pediatricians' practices and enhance their knowledge.

Rates of Breastfeeding in the United States

Infant feeding practices in the United States have changed substantially over the past several decades. Breastfeeding was the norm in the early part of this century, with the mean duration of 4.2 months in 1931.[4] However, during and after World War II the percentage of babies who were breastfed declined dramatically, probably as a result of 2 factors: (1) the great influx of women into the workforce, and (2) the use of the readily available and widely marketed commercial infant formulas.[5] Recognition of the benefits of breastfeeding by the public and health professionals, however, grew during the 1970s, and breastfeeding initiation rates increased from a low of 24.7% in 1971 to 59.7% in 1984.[6] Rates of initiation of breastfeeding declined again to 52.2% in 1989.[6] Since that time there has been a steady increase in the rates of breastfeeding initiation and duration.[5] In 2001, 69.5% of mothers initiated breastfeeding and 32.5% continued to 6 months.[7]

Unfortunately, the increases in breastfeeding rates have not been distributed equally among all groups. Demographically, formula feeding is more common among less-educated women,[8–10] those who are single[8] or young,[6] and among multiparous women.[8–10] Employment has been associated with lower rates of initiation and duration of breastfeeding in some studies.[5] Furthermore, some research suggests that employment may interfere with breastfeeding only under certain circumstances, particularly when a woman starts early supplementation of breastfeeding with formula and returns to work soon after delivery.[11] Some employers have fostered breastfeeding supportive environments that have resulted in higher rates of sustained breastfeeding among lactating employees. Thus, women who work outside the home need assistance and support in balancing breastfeeding with the demands of the workplace.

Ethnicity is another predictor of feeding choices; as a group, African American and some Hispanic women are significantly less likely to breastfeed.[6,8,9,12] Ethnicity also influences attitudes cited in support of feeding decisions, with some feeding beliefs being culturally specific.[13,14] Hispanic mothers sometimes express concern about transmitting dangerous negative emotions to their babies through their milk.[15,16] In contrast, most Navajo mothers believe that breastfeeding passes on maternal attributes and models proper behavior, thereby ensuring a good life for the infant.[17] One of the Healthy People 2010 goals is to eliminate health disparities among subgroups of the population, including racial and ethnic disparities.[18] Finally, support for breastfeeding from the baby's father,[19] from relatives such as the maternal grandmother,[20] or from friends[21] that influences duration of breastfeeding may also vary by ethnicity.[16]

Attitudes about infant feeding differ according to feeding choice. Women who breastfeed cite health benefits to their infants, greater closeness to their child, the mother's enjoyment, the "naturalness" of breastfeeding, and low cost as reasons for their choice.[15,22–24] In contrast, women who bottle-feed their infants state that they chose this method out of modesty, because breastfeeding is "old-fashioned," for reasons of "convenience," including the ability to share the responsibility of feeding, and the freedom to return to work or school.[15,22–24] In general, however, mothers who choose to bottle-feed acknowledge that human milk is best for the infant but cite other reasons for not breastfeeding.

Current breastfeeding rates are substantially lower than the Healthy People 2000 goals of 75% initiation and 50% duration for 6 months or longer.[25] Efforts to increase breastfeeding to these rates, however, are increasing. The resurgence in breastfeeding in the last decade has been attributed to the support and promotion of breastfeeding by the Special Supplemental Nutrition Program for Women, Infants, and Children (WIC) as the greatest gains in the rates of breastfeeding initiation have been seen in the following groups of women: those with low income, only a grade-school education, African American ethnicity, and WIC participation.[26] The Healthy People 2010 goals continue to advocate for breastfeeding to achieve initiation rates of 75%, and rates of breastfeeding at 6 and 12 months of 50% and 25%, respectively.[18]

The Evidence to Support Breastfeeding

Recommendations for the duration of exclusive breastfeeding remain controversial. The World Health Organization (WHO) recommends human milk as the exclusive nutrient source for feeding full-term infants during the first 6 months after birth.[27] In the past, other organizations have recommended exclusive breastfeeding for approximately 6 months or for 4 to 6 months. For a discussion of the timing of introduction of complementary foods for exclusively breastfed infants, see Chapter 6. Regardless of when complementary foods are introduced, breastfeeding should be continued at least through the first 12 months, and thereafter as long as mutually desired.[1,2,27] The recommendation for feeding full-term and preterm infants with human milk arises because of its acknowledged benefits to infant nutrition, gastrointestinal function, host defense, neurodevelopment, and psychological well-being.

Nutritional Aspects

Human milk has a dynamic nutrient composition. Nutrient contents may change through lactation, over the course of a day, within a feeding, or among women. A tabulation of the range of values for nutrients in human milk, depicted as early and more mature milk, is given in Appendix A.[28] In the first few weeks after birth, the total nitrogen content of milk from mothers who deliver preterm infants (preterm milk) is greater than milk obtained from women who have term infants (term milk).[29] The total nitrogen content in both milks, however, declines similarly to approach what is called mature milk.[30] The protein quality (proportion of whey [70%] and casein [30%]) of human milk differs from that in bovine milk (82% casein, 18% whey). The caseins are proteins with low solubility in acid media. Whey proteins remain in solution after acid precipitation. Generally, the whey fraction of soluble proteins is more easily digested and promotes more rapid gastric emptying. The whey protein fraction provides lower concentrations of phenylalanine, tyrosine, and methionine and higher concentrations of taurine than does the casein fraction of milk. The plasma amino acid pattern in the breastfed infants serves as the model upon which parenteral amino acid solutions may be based.

The type of proteins contained in the whey fraction differs between human and bovine milks. The major human whey protein is α-lactalbumin. Lactoferrin, lysozyme, and secretory immunoglobulin A (sIgA) are specific human whey proteins involved in host defense.[31] Because these host defense proteins resist proteolytic digestion, they serve as a first line of defense by lining the gastrointestinal tract. The 3 proteins are present only in trace quantities in bovine milk. The major whey protein in bovine milk is β-lactoglobulin.

The lipid system in human milk, responsible for providing approximately 50% of the calories in the milk, is structured to facilitate fat digestion and absorption. The lipid system is composed of an organized milk fat globule, a pattern of fatty acids (high in palmitic [C16:0], palmitoleic [C16:1 ω-9], linoleic [C18:2 ω-6], and linolenic [C18:3 ω-3] acids) characteristically distributed on the triglyceride molecule (C16:0 at the 2-position of the molecule), and bile salt-stimulated lipase. Because the lipase is heat labile, the superior fat absorption from human milk occurs only when unprocessed milk is fed. Most manufacturers of infant formulas have modified the fat blends in their formulas to contain a greater quantity of medium and intermediate chain-length fatty acids, in part, to match the superior fat absorption from human milk. However, the mixture of fatty acids in commercial formulas differs from that in human milk. The pattern of fatty acids in human milk also is unique in its composition of very long-chain polyunsaturated fatty acids. Arachidonic acid (AA; C20:4 ω-6) and docosahexaenoic acid (DHA; C22:6 ω-3), derivatives of linoleic and linolenic acids, respectively, are found in human but not bovine milk. Arachidonic and docosahexaenoic acids are constituents of retinal and brain phospholipid membranes and functionally have been associated in the short term with improved visual function and potentially improved neurodevelopmental outcome.

The carbohydrate composition of human milk is important as a nutritional source of lactose and for the presence of oligosaccharides. Although studies in full-term infants demonstrate a small proportion of unabsorbed lactose in the feces, the presence of lactose is assumed to be a physiologic effect of feeding infants with human milk. A softer stool consistency, more nonpathogenic bacterial fecal flora, and improved absorption of minerals have been attributed to the presence of small quantities of unabsorbed lactose from feeding infants with human milk. Oligosaccharides are carbohydrate polymers (also including glycoproteins) that, in addition to their role in nutrition, help protect the infant because their structure mimics specific bacterial antigen ligands (substances that bind to bacteria and permit attachment to intestinal cells) and prevent bacterial and bacterial toxin attachment to the host mucosa.

The concentration of calcium and phosphorus in human milk is significantly lower than in bovine milk and infant formula. The content of these macrominerals is relatively constant through lactation. The macrominerals in human milk are more bioavailable than those in infant formula because of the manner in which they are packaged. In human milk, the minerals are bound to digestible proteins and are also present in complexed and ionized states that are readily bioavailable.[32] Thus, despite significant differences in mineral intake, the bone mineral content of breastfed infants is only slightly lower than that of infants fed formula during the first year of life.[33] It is uncertain if this difference is maintained later in childhood.

The concentrations of iron, zinc, and copper decline as lactation continues,[34,35] but appear adequate to meet the infant's nutritional needs until complementary feedings begin. The concentration of iron will not meet most infants' needs beyond 6 months of breastfeeding.[36] At that time, most authorities agree that iron-containing foods are indicated to prevent subsequent iron deficiency anemia. Vitamin K deficiency may be a concern in the breastfed infant. The content of vitamin K in human milk is low. To meet initial vitamin K needs, in many countries all infants are given a single intramuscular dose of vitamin K at birth.[37] The content of vitamin D in human milk is low; nutrient needs generally are met by "adequate" sunlight exposure.[38] Vitamin D deficiency, however, has been reported in breastfed infants who have dark skin pigmentation and/or inadequate exposure to sunlight,[39] and supplementation of the breastfed infant with 200 IU/d of vitamin D is indicated.

Gastrointestinal Functions

Gastric emptying is faster after infants are fed human milk than when they are fed commercial bovine formula. Many factors in human milk may stimulate gastrointestinal growth and motility and enhance maturity of the gastrointestinal tract. Bioactive factors such as lactoferrin may affect intestinal growth, glutamine affects intestinal cellular metabolism, nucleotides affect fecal flora, and enzymes such as acetylhydrolase block the ischemic injury produced by platelet-activating factor in the pathogenesis of necrotizing enterocolitis.[40] Components such as epidermal growth factor support growth and repair of the intestinal mucosa.

Host Defense

Specific factors such as sIgA, lactoferrin, lysozyme, oligosaccharides, growth factors, and cellular components may affect the host defense of the infant (Table 3.1).[41] The enteromammary immune system is an important part of the protective nature of human milk.[42] In this system, the mother produces sIgA antibody when exposed to foreign antigens and is stimulated to make specific antibodies that are elaborated at mucosal surfaces and enter her milk. By ingesting the milk that contains specific sIgA antibody, the infant receives spe-

Table 3.1.
Selected Bioactive Factors in Human Milk

Secretory IgA	Specific antigen-targeted anti-infective action
Lactoferrin	Immunomodulation, iron chelation, antimicrobial action, anti-adhesive, trophic for intestinal growth
Lysozyme	Bacterial lysis, immunomodulation
6-casein	Anti-adhesive, bacterial flora
Oligosaccharides	Reduces bacterial attachment
Cytokines	Anti-inflammatory, epithelial barrier function
Growth factors	
Epidermal Growth Factor	Luminal surveillance, repair of intestinal epithelium
Transforming Growth Factor	Promotes epithelial cell growth (TGF $\forall$) Suppresses lymphocyte function (TGF $\exists$)
Nerve Growth Factor	Promotes nerve growth
Enzymes	
Platelet Activating Factor (PAF) acetylhydrolase	Blocks action of PAF
Glutathione peroxidase	Prevents lipid oxidation
Nucleotides	Enhances immune response, promotes growth of mucosa
Vitamin A, E, C	Antioxidants
Amino acids: Glutamine	Intestinal cell fuel, promotes immune responses
Lipids	Anti-infective properties

Adapted from Hamosh.[41]

cific passive immunity. The system is active in infants against a variety of antigens. sIgA uniquely resists digestion in the stomach and small bowel.

In both developing and industrialized countries, there is reduction in the incidence of gastrointestinal and respiratory diseases and otitis media that is directly attributed to breastfeeding.[43] In Brazil, for example, infants who were completely weaned had 14.2 and 3.6 times the risk of death from diarrhea and respiratory infections, respectively, compared to exclusively breastfed infants.[44] Optimal breastfeeding would save the lives of an estimated 1 million children around the world who die of these illnesses each year.[44] The data also suggest that human milk protects the preterm infant from infection and necrotizing enterocolitis.[45]

In industrialized countries, many of the early studies of breastfeeding and infectious outcomes have been criticized for methodological flaws including detection bias, poor definition of illness outcomes and of feeding status, and small numbers of patients studied.[44] Another important limitation of some early studies was the lack of adjustment for the substantial differences between mothers who breastfeed and mothers who formula feed, which could account for the differences in the health of their infants. Research conducted over the past decade has been more rigorous in addressing these methodological issues, and several studies in the industrialized world have demonstrated that breastfeeding provides clear health benefits.

Large, prospective studies of otitis media show a protective effect of breastfeeding.[46–49] Infants exclusively breastfed for at least 4 months may experience as few as half the number of episodes of otitis media as formula-fed infants and also half as many recurrent episodes.[46] Recently, the findings have been extended to infants with cleft palate, among whom otitis media is usually unremitting.[50] In many of these studies not only is the incidence of disease diminished with breastfeeding, but the duration of individual episodes is reduced.[51]

Lower respiratory tract illnesses and gastroenteritis also are less common or less severe among breastfed infants. For example, breastfeeding for 1 month or longer has been associated with significantly lower rates of wheezing and lower respiratory tract illness during the first 4 months of life.[52] Interactions existed with breastfeeding and other risk factors for lower respiratory tract illnesses (eg, sharing a room, being Mexican American, and being a boy), so exposure to minimal breastfeeding and another risk factor were associated with significant odds of acquiring a respiratory tract illness.[52]

Infants who were breastfed for at least 13 weeks had significantly less gastrointestinal illness during the first year of life, as well as lower rates of respiratory illness during several periods. Additionally, illnesses in infants who were breastfed for at least 13 weeks seemed to be less severe because the infants were significantly less likely to be hospitalized for gastrointestinal illness.[53] Breastfeeding also confers a strong protective effect against *Haemophilus influenzae* type b infection,[54,55] and this is of particular importance to those infants without access to the vaccine.

Urinary tract infections have been reported to be more frequent among formula-fed infants than among breastfed infants.[56,57] Reduced adhesion to uroepithelial cells by pathogens as mediated by oligosaccharides,[58] sIgA,[59] or lactoferrin[60,61] has been hypothesized as the mechanism for this protective effect.

In a study of infant botulism and its role in sudden infant death, formula-fed infants tended to be younger than breastfed infants at onset of the disease and were more likely to experience severe illness.[62] Formula-fed infants were more likely to have botulism resulting in sudden death, while those hospitalized with the disease were more likely to be breastfed. A number of potential mechanisms for a protective effect of breastfeeding have been hypothesized, including differences in intestinal microflora and earlier detection by mothers who breastfeed due to perceived changes in infant sucking on the breast. The intestinal flora differ between breastfed and formula-fed infants, resulting in a lower pH in the breastfed intestinal tract. Proliferation of *Clostridium botulinum* declines with pH.

Chronic Diseases of Childhood

Perhaps the most provocative although limited observational data are those suggesting that specific chronic disorders have a lower incidence in children who were breastfed as infants. There may be protective effects of breastfeeding against Crohn's disease, lymphoma, specific genotypes of type 1 juvenile diabetes mellitus, and certain allergic conditions.[63–65] There are conflicting data about the protection against allergy afforded by breastfeeding, possibly because in some studies maternal diet did not exclude the potentially offending antigens.[66] Breastfeeding, however, appears to be protective against some food allergies during infancy and early childhood.[67,68] Atopic dermatitis may be lessened in infants whose mothers follow a restricted diet. A lower incidence of atopic conditions is reported in breastfed infants with a family history of atopy.[69]

A relationship has been suggested between artificial feeding and the development of type 1 insulin-dependent diabetes mellitus (IDDM), although this is controversial[65] (see Chapter 30). Insulin-dependent diabetes mellitus was more likely when breastfeeding continued for less than 3 months and bovine milk proteins were introduced before 4 months of age.[65] Elevated concentrations of specific IgG antibody to bovine serum albumin that cross reacts with an islet cell-specific surface protein have been identified in children with insulin-dependent diabetes mellitus,[70] although this may be an epiphenomenon and of no relevance. Further studies are in progress to address this issue.

Neurobehavioral Aspects
Maternal-infant bonding is enhanced during breastfeeding. In addition, improved long-term cognitive and motor abilities in full-term infants have been directly correlated with duration of breastfeeding.[71,72] Improved long-term cognitive development in preterm infants also has been correlated with the receipt of human milk during hospitalization.[73,74] A meta-analysis of studies where a multitude of confounding factors were considered concluded that breastfeeding conferred a benefit to cognitive function well beyond the period of actual breastfeeding.[75] It should be noted, however, that many studies do not take into account actual maternal and paternal IQ or the "nurturing abilities" of the parents as confounding variables. Further study is therefore necessary to understand the true contribution of breastfeeding to short- and long-term cognitive development.

Maternal Benefits
There is a tendency to consider that only the infant benefits from breastfeeding. There are, however, positive effects of breastfeeding for the mother. Postpartum weight loss and uterine involution may be more rapid in women who breastfeed than in non-lactating mothers.[76] Exclusive breastfeeding delays the resumption of normal ovarian cycles and the return of fertility in most mothers.[77] As such, the contraceptive effects of breastfeeding contributes to global child-spacing. The lactational amenorrhea method (LAM) cites 3 criteria that ensure the lowest pregnancy rate: (1) full breastfeeding (round-the-clock), (2) no resumption of menses, and (3) an infant less than 6 months of age.[78] The LAM method is a highly effective global program with efficacy rates of 98.5% to 100%, comparable to the best artificial birth control methods.[78]

Epidemiological studies have identified a decreased incidence of premenopausal breast cancer in women who have lactated, and the greater the duration of lactation, the lower the odds ratio of developing breast cancer.[79] In addition, there are epidemiological studies reporting a decreased incidence of ovarian cancer in women who lactated.[80,81] There also is speculation that lactation might protect against the development of osteoporosis.[81] This observation is of interest because during lactation there is a drain on the maternal skeleton such that maternal bone density declines an average of 5% and cannot be prevented by additional calcium intake. However, maternal bone mineral density in the post-weaning period is normal, suggesting a catch-up mineralization.[82,83] The adaptations necessary to remineralize the skeleton may have an effect on decreasing late-onset osteoporosis.

Societal Impact of Breastfeeding

The economic advantages of breastfeeding can be calculated at the personal and national levels. The obvious personal advantage is in the savings accrued by not buying infant formula, a figure conservatively estimated at $300 per year in 1985, but more likely to be $750 to $1200 today. Although most Americans have health insurance, about one third are uninsured or underinsured. Thus, the increased rates of illness in non-breastfed infants may lead to out-of-pocket expenses for medical care. Ironically, it is those who are self-insured and uninsured that have the lowest rates of breastfeeding in our society.

From the perspective of the national economy, the expected savings for infants in the United States' WIC program who were breastfed exclusively for 6 months were estimated to be over $950 million annually in 1997 compared to infants who were not breastfed for 6 months.[84] These savings would come from a combined reduction in household expenditure on formula, as well as reductions in expenditures for health care. In light of these data, the major gains in breastfeeding prevalence among WIC participants has contributed to the resurgence in breastfeeding in the United States in the last decade.[26] The costs of not breastfeeding also have been computed in a health maintenance organization population. Compared to infants who never breastfed, infants who breastfed for 3 months or more had fewer medical office visits, medications, procedures, and hospitalizations, saving $331 per single infant in short-term acute medical care costs only.[85] In the managed care setting, it has been estimated that full breastfeeding is associated with a 20% reduction in total medical expenses compared to never breastfeeding.[86] Not included in these cost estimates is the fewer absences from work of families who are breastfeeding their infants. Thus, the economic incentives for a society to breastfeed are strong and should be promoted.

Contraindications to Breastfeeding

Few contraindications to breastfeeding exist. Infants with galactosemia should not ingest lactose-containing milk. Therefore, as the principal carbohydrate in human milk is lactose, infants with galactosemia should not breastfeed. Infants with other inborn errors of metabolism, such as phenylketonuria, may ingest some human milk, but the amount is closely monitored and depends on the desired protein intake and other factors. Women in the United States who are infected with human immunodeficiency virus (HIV) and those with human T-cell lymphotropic virus should not breastfeed. Globally, the health risks of not breastfeeding must be balanced with the risk of HIV acquisition. When herpetic lesions are localized to the breast, women should not breastfeed. Women with vaginal herpes, however, should be allowed to breastfeed. Mothers with varicella may continue to breastfeed. Any infant born to a mother who has the onset of a varicella rash 5 days before to 2 days after delivery should receive varicella zoster immune globulin, regardless of the sites of the rash on the mother or the method of feeding. Women with miliary tuberculosis should not breastfeed until they are no longer contagious, approximately 2 weeks after initiation of anti-tuberculosis therapy. Women with breast masses may undergo diagnostic studies including mammograms, ultrasonic studies, MRI studies, and needle or excisional biopsies without interruption of breastfeeding. Women diagnosed with breast cancer should not delay treatment so they can breastfeed. Depending on the therapy, women receiving antimetabolite chemotherapy should not breastfeed. Most other medications are compatible with breastfeeding, or a substitute medication may exist. Women ingesting drugs of abuse need counseling and should not breastfeed until they are free of the abused drugs[87] (see Appendix B, Table B-2). Note that the most recent AAP Committee on Drugs statement does not use the term "contraindicated." Instead, the statement refers to "Drugs of Abuse for Which Adverse Effects on the Infant During Breastfeeding Have Been Reported."

Prenatal Considerations

The successful management of lactation begins early, before and during pregnancy.[88,89] Prenatal visits provide significant opportunities for the obstetrician to support and encourage breastfeeding. The early breast examination serves not only to identify potential problems that could impact lactation, but is an advantageous time to encourage the new mother that she should have no problems with breastfeeding. In some cases, the breast examination may identify conditions that might benefit from some therapy. For example, in some cases, a mother with very inverted nipples may benefit from using a breast shell inside the brassiere in the last months of pregnancy to facilitate eversion. Elaborate exercises and preparations, however, are not necessary for most women and may stimulate early uterine contractions.

Along with the early obstetric visits, the pediatrician should discuss feeding plans and issues of infant care during a prenatal office visit. However, in a recent survey, only 11% of pediatricians said that prenatal visits were a part of their office practice.[3] Therefore, it is important that the details of breastfeeding not wait for a pregnancy, but that education on the functions of the mammary gland begin in secondary school and continue through the reproductive life cycle. Then, at the appropriate time, prenatal classes should provide further information to facilitate an informed choice on infant feeding methods closer to the time of delivery.

The Early Lactation Experience

Physicians should ensure that nursing mothers receive appropriate and professional counseling during the hospital stay. All health care staff should be trained in the understanding of lactation. The early days of lactation are critical to establish a good milk supply and effective letdown reflex. The mother should be offered the opportunity to nurse her infant as soon after delivery as possible, preferably during the first hour of life. She should be offered as much assistance as necessary in positioning herself comfortably and facilitating the infant's proper grasp of the breast. Enough of the areola should be in the infant's mouth to permit the tongue to compress the areola overlying the collecting ducts against the hard palate. This will provide a good seal and proper emptying or milking of the ampullae. Except under special circumstances, the newborn should remain with the mother throughout the recovery period.[1]

After suckling at the first breast, the infant is repositioned on the second breast. The mother should offer both breasts, but alternate the side she offers first at each feeding to enhance the stimulation of milk production. The time for suckling should be unrestricted. The infant will indicate the time to be moved to the opposite breast. The time for complete milk transfer is variable—5 to 20 minutes. Newborns should be nursed whenever they show signs of hunger, at least every 2 to 3 hours or 8 to 12 times every 24 hours, to stimulate milk production and facilitate bilirubin excretion. A healthy newborn is alert and attentive and roots, grasps, and suckles well. It is acknowledged that crying is a late indicator of hunger. Occasionally, however, infants may not demand feeding during the first few days, and parents should be instructed to wake them after 4 hours for feedings. Mother and infant should not be separated unless it is medically indicated. Appropriate breastfeeding is facilitated by continuous rooming-in.

The mother who plans to breastfeed after a cesarean delivery should be encouraged to do so. Most mothers find that nursing in a semirecumbent position in bed is most comfortable. With a standard pillow on the mother's abdomen and the infant lying on the pillow, the full weight of the infant is not on the mother's incision. After vaginal delivery, many mothers prefer positioning on the side or sitting up. Families should have access to sound information on breastfeeding well before the first follow-up visit. They should be encouraged to keep in touch with physicians if questions arise. Formal evaluation of breastfeeding should be recorded in the medical record before discharge from the hospital.

Feeding and Hydration of the Breastfed Infant

In the first few weeks after birth, an infant is likely to be adequately nourished if at least 8 to 12 feedings are received each day. Some infants may feed 12 or more times a day. Infants should not refuse to latch on to the breast or be too sleepy to feed. Long nighttime intervals (>4 hours) without feeding should be avoided. Maternal fatigue and anxiety are important contributors to problems with breastfeeding and should be avoided. Family support should be especially helpful in reducing fatigue and anxiety.

Caregivers, as well as parents, should be taught to assess the adequacy of breastfeeding. In some cases, mothers find it instructive to keep a diary of daily feeding and elimination patterns. The adequacy of milk intake each day can be assessed by counting the number of wet diapers and the number and quantity and color of stools. Caregivers can closely monitor weight changes and provide intervention if losses of >7% are approached. The intervention may consist of reaffirming the feeding frequency and determining whether lactogenesis has occurred. During the first day, no more than 24 hours should pass without the infant having a wet diaper and a stool. On day 3, breastfed infants usually have 3 to 4 wet diapers and 1 to 2 stools that are no longer meconium, but are beginning to appear yellow. Later during the first week after birth, the infant should have about 6 wet diapers per day (pale yellow urine) and a yellow stool with each feeding. Later in the month, the stool frequency may diminish to 3 per day. After this period, several days may pass without a stool for some breastfed infants.

Early hospital discharge programs pose a concern for monitoring the breastfed infant. An early home or office visit at 3 to 5 days of age is important to assess breastfeeding and the clinical condition of the infant. This early visit should assess the adequacy of hydration, milk intake, and weight gain, the presence of jaundice, and anxiety or concerns of the mother. One breastfeeding episode should be observed during this first visit. The next visit should be within 2 weeks of hospital discharge. Telephone contact should be encouraged if questions arise. Families should be made aware of the availability of community, office, or hospital lactation resources.

Recognition of "appetite spurts" in the infant is important.[89] These are characterized by periods of crying and apparent insatiability on the part of the infant, usually occurring at 8 to 12 days, 3 to 4 weeks, 3 months of age, and at variable times thereafter. Frequent nursing will increase milk production to meet these changing needs of the infant.

Growth of the Breastfed Infant
The rate of weight gain in the breastfed infant may be lower than that of the infant fed formula after 3 months of age, but differences generally are not reported between groups for length and head circumference.[90,91] Several factors might explain the differences in weight between breastfed and bottle-fed infants. Most notable is that the growth charts used in the comparison were derived from infants predominantly fed formula, the sample population was relatively homogeneous, the measurements were recorded only every 3 months, and the curve-fitting techniques were outdated.[92] Newer growth charts available in 2000 corrected some of the earlier discrepancies but still, as a national sample, contained few breastfed infants, especially after 6 months. Thus the newer 2000 NCHS growth charts still do not reflect **optimal growth associated with breastfeeding,** but instead reflect heavier growth associated with artificial feeding[92]; that is, breastfed infants demonstrate mean weight-for-age percentiles somewhat lower than those represented by the curves of the NCHS charts. Because breastfed infants do not necessarily "follow the chart," many professionals have assumed that human milk is inadequate, rather than realizing that the curves are inappropriate for human milk-fed infants. Several studies have concluded that breastfed infants' rates of weight gain are normal and appropriate. Indeed, breastfed infants regulate their energy intakes at lower lev-

els than formula-fed infants.[92] Body temperature and minimal observable metabolic rates are lower in breastfed than formula-fed infants.[93,94] Thus, it is argued that the more rapid weight gain in formula-fed infants is excessive and that no deleterious outcomes are associated with a slower rate of weight gain in breastfed infants. Each individual infant's growth must be assessed to document that the infant is in fact healthy and thriving, taking into account many factors other than the growth chart.[91,93] Coupled with the positive health advantages, the growth of the breastfed infant should be considered the norm. It is this consideration that has led WHO to develop a new international growth reference based on the growth of healthy infants breastfed throughout the first year of life, although these are not yet available.[92]

Despite the acknowledged differences in rates of growth between populations of breastfed and formula-fed infants, some criteria are available to determine when to intervene if an individual breastfed infant is not gaining adequately.[95] A newborn infant who is less than 2 weeks of age and whose weight is >7% below birth weight should be evaluated. An older infant that fails to regain birth weight by 2 weeks or is not gaining a minimum of 20 g/d should be evaluated. Older infants should not have a plateau in weight gain or linear growth or decelerate their growth to the extent of crossing several percentiles downward. Interventions in the above scenarios are variable depending on evaluations of the state of health of the infant, the infant's feeding ability, and the milk supply of the mother.[96] The infant should be examined and sucking ability evaluated, and a feeding should be observed. Milk intake can be assessed by test weights (pre- and post-breastfeeding on an appropriate sensitive scale). If there are further concerns about effective milk transfer to the infant, a breast pump can be used to measure any residual milk remaining in the breast after a feeding. Inadequate milk intake should be treated by supplementation with the mother's own expressed milk, formula, or pasteurized donor human milk. This milk can be provided in a bottle or by a feeding device, such as a cup or supplemental lactation device. A supplemental lactation device generally consists of a reservoir or container of milk connected to a small soft catheter that is inserted into the infant's mouth while at the breast. As the infant suckles, milk from the supplemental nursing system flows into the infant's mouth by gravity and suction.

When a breastfed infant is not gaining weight satisfactorily, the maternal milk supply usually requires stimulation by extra milk removal (pumping or hand expression) and possibly the use of galactagogues.

Common Problems of the Breast and Nipple

Breast engorgement, sore nipples, and plugged alveolar ducts are common concerns that can be prevented and treated. Engorgement is the physiologic result of increased blood flow, vascular dilatation, and increased milk storage. Frequent feedings facilitate the establishment of lactation and the relief of excessive engorgement. Persistent sore nipples beyond the first 4 to 7 days of lactation may occur because of improper positioning of the infant at the breast, can be prevented by holding the infant in the correct position (eg, cradle hold, football hold), good latch-on to the areola, and alternating the site of initial latch at different feedings. Localized breast tenderness, commonly due to a plugged duct, can be treated by massaging the affected area, frequent nursing, and moist heat.

The nipple should be kept dry. Ointments and lotions usually are not needed. Soaps and alcohol should not be used. Montgomery's glands in the areola provide the best lubrication for the areola and nipple throughout pregnancy and lactation. If nipple irritation develops, it is best to keep the area as dry as possible. The milk that dries on the breast also may assist healing. Some mothers with cracked or fissured, painful nipples have less discomfort if they breastfeed with a breast shield for a short period.

Discomfort or pain in the mother can impair the letdown reflex. Efforts should be made to reduce discomfort and anxiety. The family should assist the mother and provide support to allow her freedom to care for her newborn infant.

Bottle Feeding and Supplements

No supplements (water, glucose water, or formula) should be given to the breastfeeding infant unless medically indicated.[1] Supplements and pacifiers should be avoided until breastfeeding is well established. Under ideal conditions, an infant should not be bottle-fed for the first 3 to 4 weeks, after which time lactation is usually well established. Infants may be confused by a rubber nipple or pacifier, which require different tongue and jaw motions. Furthermore, if the appetite or the sucking response is partially satiated by water or formula, the infant will take less from the breast, causing diminished milk production, which may lead to lactation failure. Sterile water and glucose water supplements may exacerbate hyperbilirubinemia because they prevent adequate milk (calorie) intake.[97]

All infants, including breastfed infants, must receive a vitamin K supplement at birth. There is little biologically active vitamin D in human milk. With continuing reports of rickets in breastfed infants and because of concerns about the adverse effects of sunlight exposure, it is recommended that all breastfed infants be supplemented with 200 IU/d (5 μg) of vitamin D, beginning within the first 2 months after birth.[98]

The American Academy of Pediatrics recommends:

To prevent rickets and vitamin D deficiency in healthy infants and children and acknowledging that adequate sunlight exposure is difficult to determine, we reaffirm the adequate intake of 200 IU per day of vitamin D by the National Academy of Sciences[4] and recommend a supplement of 200 IU per day for the following:

1. All breastfed infants unless they are weaned to at least 500 mL per day of vitamin D-fortified formula or milk.
2. All nonbreastfed infants who are ingesting less than 500 mL per day of vitamin D-fortified formula or milk.
3. Children and adolescents who do not get regular sunlight exposure, do not ingest at least 500 mL per day of vitamin D-fortified milk, or do not take a daily multivitamin supplement containing at least 200 IU of vitamin D.

Iron absorption from human milk is excellent, but because the concentration of iron is low in human milk and iron stores present at birth are expended, the breastfed infant requires an additional iron source from complementary foods no later than 6 months of age. Fluoride supplementation is not needed during the first 6 months but may be required thereafter, depending on the content of fluoride in the local water supply (see Chapter 48).

Xenobiotics

A number of drugs may be secreted into human milk, but only some are thought to be of concern to breastfeeding (Appendix B).[99] These include chemotherapeutic agents, radioactive isotopes, drugs of abuse, lithium, ergotamine, and drugs that suppress lactation. In addition, anticonvulsants, sulfa drugs, quinolones, and salicylates may have effects on some breastfeeding infants, and antihistamines may reduce milk supply. Secretion of medications into milk is affected by dose schedule and duration of action, feeding pattern of the infant, and the infant's total diet and age. The timing of breastfeeding should avoid peak blood concentrations of selected medications. Herbal preparations are widely available and widely used in the United States, but data are lacking about their use during lactation.[100] The mother should be encouraged to discuss any use of prescription drugs, over-the-counter drugs, or herbal medications with her physician.

Jaundice and Breastfeeding

Jaundice due to unconjugated hyperbilirubinemia is common in most newborns and is usually called *physiologic jaundice of the newborn*. In many breastfed newborns, the duration of physiologic jaundice is increased. This has been termed *breast milk jaundice*, a normal physiologic response to the ingestion of human milk.[101] Of more concern is that inadequate breastfeeding during the first week after birth can increase the intensity of the jaundice.[97,102] This has been termed *breastfeeding jaundice* (or, more accurately, *breast-non-feeding-jaundice*).[101] During the first week after birth, this "jaundice-in-a-breastfed-infant" is related to inadequate milk intake from poor lactation performance. The infant is not feeding adequately and/or there is an inadequate supply of milk. Several factors contribute to the poor lactation performance, including the lack of appropriate lactation education of parents and caregivers, water and glucose water supplements,[103] and failure to recognize inadequate milk intake. The treatment is aimed at decreasing the enterohepatic recirculation of bilirubin by increasing milk intake through more frequent breastfeeding. If serum bilirubin is rising but there are indications that maternal milk production is increasing, then continued frequent breastfeeding can be recommended. If hyperbilirubinemia is advanced and milk production is low, the mother may give the infant formula after each breastfeeding, and a manual or mechanical method for milk expression should be used by the mother to increase her milk supply. When phototherapy is used in advanced stages of hyperbilirubinemia, the feeding of mother's milk does not have to cease.[104] The goal for therapy is to provide appropriate quantities of milk. Conversely, overzealous therapy will increase the chances of early termination of breastfeeding.[105] Other causes of jaundice in a breastfed infant that are not necessarily related to breastfeeding should also be considered, including urosepsis, hemolysis, hemorrhage, hypothyroidism, and inherited defects in bilirubin conjugation.

Breast milk jaundice usually begins insidiously and peaks after the first week and is a normal prolongation of physiologic jaundice of the newborn. Detectable hyperbilirubinemia will be found in approximately two thirds of all breastfed infants during the third week of life and one third of all breastfed infants will be clinically icteric with serum unconjugated bilirubin levels in excess of 5.0 mg/dL. Despite adequate lactation and infant milk intake and growth, the infant remains jaundiced. This entity is thought to be related to one or more factors in human milk or to a combination of milk factors in a susceptible recipient infant. In extreme circumstances, usually when the serum bilirubin concentration exceeds 20 mg/dL, the hyperbilirubinemia can be reduced by using phototherapy, supplementing with formula, or feeding the infant formula for 1 to 2 days instead of breastfeeding. If the latter course is chosen, the mother must be encouraged to maintain her milk supply with a manual or mechanical method. When breastfeeding resumes, the serum bilirubin concentration may rise slightly, but once the cycle is interrupted, the recurrence of severe jaundice is unlikely. Serum bilirubin levels should be monitored during this period and a determination of conjugated bilirubin should be obtained if jaundice persists beyond 2 weeks. As with breastfeeding jaundice, overzealous therapy can lead to termination of breastfeeding.[105]

Nutrition for the Lactating Mother

The nutrient content of human milk by and large remains remarkably constant, regardless of the mother's diet, until her own body stores are severely depleted.[106] In fact, evidence from diverse populations indicates that the capacity to produce milk of sufficient quantity and quality to support the growth of infants is satisfactory even when the mother's dietary supply of nutrients is limited.[107] Thus, the lactating mother's diet must be sufficient to prevent her own body stores of certain nutrients from being depleted.[107,108] During the early weeks of lactation, caloric needs for milk production are obtained largely from maternal fat stores, facilitating the return to prepregnancy weight and body composition. Mothers also should be instructed to drink sufficient quantities of fluid to prevent thirst, but counseled that this will not increase their milk volume. Around the world, vastly diverse diets support adequate milk production. With the exception of extreme dietary deprivation, maternal energy intake seems to have only a weak effect on milk volume.[109] Short-term diet restriction does not compromise milk production.[110] Breastfeeding mothers should maintain the same calcium intake as in the prepregnant state (1400 mg/d) from a variety of foods.

The types of fatty acids in human milk are influenced primarily by the type and proportion of fat in the mother's diet.[111] In general, the milk content of fat-soluble vitamins is unaffected by the vitamin content of the mother's diet, while the content of water-soluble vitamins is somewhat more responsive to maternal diet.[112–114] The vegan mother who eats no animal products is at risk of vitamin B_{12} deficiency. Her breastfeeding infant is also at risk for vitamin B_{12} deficiency and may show signs of deficiency before the mother.[115] The recommended dietary allowances for lactating women are listed in Appendix C, Table C-3. (See also Chapter 11.)

Collection and Storage of Human Milk

There are many instances when mothers will be separated from their infants, and prior knowledge of this separation allows them to select methods to express and store their milk for future use. Return to work or school, illness, and hospitalization are some of the common reasons encountered by mothers who wish to learn about the methods for milk collection and storage. To maintain full milk production, the mother will need to express milk for every missed feeding (approximately every 2 to 3 hours in the newborn period). General techniques for ensuring cleanliness during milk expression begin with good hand washing with soap and water. Hand expression can be very effective once it has been learned and practiced. Many types of breast pumps are available in the United States, with varying costs and effectiveness for individuals.

Bicycle horn-type hand pumps may cause breast trauma and contamination of milk and should not be used. Collection kits should be rinsed, cleaned with hot soapy water, and dried in the air. Dishwasher cleaning also is adequate. Glass or hard plastic containers should be used for milk storage. Milk to be fed within 48 hours of collection can be refrigerated without significant bacterial proliferation.

Freezing is the preferred method of storing milk that will not be fed within 48 hours. Single milk expressions should be packaged separately for freezing and labeled with the date (and name of the infant if the infant is cared for in a child care center or hospital). Unlike heat treatment, freezing preserves many of the nutritional and immunologic benefits of human milk. When frozen appropriately in the rear of the freezer compartment, milk can be stored for as long as 3 to 6 months. Milk should be thawed rapidly, usually by holding the container under running tepid (not hot) water. Milk should never be thawed in a

Table 3.2.
Breast Pump Comparisons*†

TYPE OF PUMP	APPROXIMATE COST	SINGLE OR DOUBLE	MAXIMUM PRESSURE RANGE	CYCLES per MINUTE	AC or Battery	OTHER INFORMATION
HAND PUMPS						
Bulb (Bicycle-horn)		Single	??	Vary	N/A	Not recommended / No suction regulation / Easily contaminated, no means of cleaning bulb
Piston-type	Under $40	Single	0–440	Vary	N/A	
Squeeze-handle	Under $40	Single	0–260	Vary	N/A	
BATTERY	Under $80	Single	0–180	9–28	AC	
MANUAL-CYCLE ELEC	Under $150	Single or double	80–220	9–20	AC	
AUTO-CYCLE ELEC						
For purchase – mini	Under $100	Single (double if you buy 2 pumps)	230	50–60	AC or Battery	Guaranteed 3 months
For purchase – deluxe	Under $300	Double	220	50–60	AC	Guaranteed 1 year / Battery pack available
For rent	Under $50 per month	Double	220	50–60	AC	Battery pack available

*This list represents only a cross section of pumps available. This list does not imply endorsement of any particular products by Wesley Medical Center or the American Academy of Pediatrics.
†Information obtained from: Riordan J, Auerbach KG. *Breastfeeding and Human Lactation.* 2nd ed. Boston, MA: Jones and Barlett Publishers; 1998 and Schrago L. Breastfeeding, Breastpumps, and Returning to Work (handout), 1/7/98.

microwave oven. After milk is thawed, it should not be refrozen. Thawed milk should be used completely within 24 hours.

Experienced personnel should maintain quality control of in-hospital breast pumps and methods of milk fortification for premature infants and ensure appropriate methods of milk delivery to the infant. Because human milk is not homogenized, the fat will separate from the milk upon standing. Efforts should be made to ensure that the separated fat is not left behind when the milk is fed. To ensure the best delivery of fat when continuous tube-feeding methods are used, the feeding syringe should be oriented with the tip upright, the syringe emptied completely after each use, and the shortest amount of tubing used.

Processing of Donor Human Milk

An important advantage of breastfeeding is the relative freedom from bacterial contamination of human milk.[116] However, contamination can be a problem with artificially collected and stored human milk. Standards have been published by the Human Milk Banking Association of North America.[117,118] A variety of bacteria, bacterial toxins, and viruses such as rubella, cytomegalovirus, hepatitis B and C, and HIV may be found in the milk of infected mothers. Human milk also may be a vehicle for transmission of herpes simplex type 1 when lesions are located on the breast.[119] For these reasons, human milk banks processing pooled milk from multiple donors screen all donors and use pasteurization methods to avoid disease transmission. The possibility that maternal T lymphocytes may be absorbed intact through the gastrointestinal tract of newborn infants raises theoretical questions about the possibility of inducing a graft versus host reaction when feeding fresh (unfrozen or unheated) human milk from a mother other than the infant's own mother. Freezing and pasteurization destroy the T-cells.

Hospital Lactation Programs

Because the initial hospital experience may affect the ultimate outcome of breastfeeding, programs have been designed to facilitate maternal decisions to breastfeed. Model programs have been adopted that promote a philosophy of maternal and infant care that supports breastfeeding (Table 3.3).[120] In 1991, the United Nations Children's Fund (UNICEF) and WHO began an international campaign, the Baby Friendly Hospital Initiative, to promote breastfeeding. This initiative incorporated the program described in Table 3.2 into 10 steps for global use. The guidelines are useful for hospitals developing their own programs. Many obstacles to the successful implementation of the Baby Friendly

Table 3.3.
WellStart International Model Hospital Breastfeeding Policies for Full-term Healthy Newborn Infants[120]

1. Hospital administrative, medical, nursing, and nutrition staff should establish a strategy that promotes and supports breastfeeding through the formation of an interdisciplinary team responsible for the implementation of hospital policies and provision of ongoing educational activities.

2. All pregnant women should receive information about the benefits and management of breastfeeding before delivery.

3. Every mother should be allowed to have a close companion stay with her continually throughout labor.

4. Infants are to be put to breast as soon after birth as feasible for both mother and infant, in the delivery room or recovery room; every mother is to be instructed about proper breast-feeding technique and the technique reevaluated before discharge from the hospital.

5. Breastfeeding mother-infant couples are to room-in on a 24-hour basis.

6. The infant is to be encouraged to nurse at least 8 to 12 times or more in 24 hours, for a minimum of 8 feedings per 24 hours.

7. Specific timing at the breast is not necessary. Infants usually fall asleep or release the nipple spontaneously when satiated.

8. Infants should spontaneously finish the first breast and then be encouraged to try the second breast at each feeding.

9. If a feeding at the breast is incomplete or ineffective, the mother should be instructed to begin regular expression of milk in conjunction with continued assistance by an experienced staff member. The colostrum or milk obtained by expression should be given to the baby.

10. No supplementary water or milk is to be given unless specifically ordered by a physician or nurse practitioner.

11. Pacifiers are not to be given to any breastfeeding infant unless specifically ordered by a physician or nurse practitioner. The use of bottle nipples and nipple shields should be discouraged.

12. Breastfeeding mothers are to have breasts examined for evidence of problems at least once during every nursing staff shift.

13. Discharge gift packs offered to breastfeeding mothers should contain only noncommercial materials that provide educational information and promote breastfeeding.

14. All breastfeeding mothers are to be advised to arrange for an appointment for their baby's first examination within 1 week after discharge.

15. At discharge, each mother is to be given a phone number to call for breastfeeding assistance.

16. Policies 1, 2, 4, and 10 through 15 apply when mothers and babies are separated. Mothers who are separated from their babies are to be instructed about how to maintain lactation.

Hospital Initiative in the United States remain. The AAP has been a leader in the promotion of breastfeeding. In its 1997 statement, the AAP reaffirmed its position that the pediatrician should be responsible for infant nutrition. As such, the AAP recommended against direct-to-consumer advertising of infant formula as it would be detrimental to breastfeeding and compromise the physician's counseling to promote breastfeeding. Although the AAP encouraged that a diversity of infant formulas be available for those circumstances where breastfeeding was not practiced, it maintained its policy against the distribution of discharge packages without the advice and council of a health care professional.[121]

Conclusion

Strong evidence continues to demonstrate that human milk is the optimal source of nutrition for the human infant and is associated with lower rates of infectious illness during infancy in developing and industrialized countries. Of particular importance, exclusive breastfeeding for at least 4 months is associated with one third the risk of developing otitis media and half the risk of having a wheezing illness during the first 6 months of life. Indications exist that breastfeeding may have some long-term beneficial effects on maternal and infant outcomes, although the mechanisms behind these effects are unknown. Research continues to identify aspects of breastfeeding to which these findings could be attributed, including hormonal interactions and bioactive factors with immunological and/or growth-promoting properties. Substantial improvements in breastfeeding rates in the United States could result in valuable health gains to many women and their infants in diverse settings.

References

1. American Academy of Pediatrics, Work Group on Breastfeeding. Breastfeeding and the use of human milk. *Pediatrics*. 1997;100:1035–1039
2. Canadian Paediatric Society Nutrition Committee, American Academy of Pediatrics Committee on Nutrition. Breast-feeding: a commentary in celebration of the international year of the child, 1979. *Pediatrics*. 1978;65:591–601
3. Schanler RJ, O'Connor KG, Lawrence RA. Pediatricians' practices and attitudes regarding breastfeeding promotion. *Pediatrics*. 1999;103:e35
4. Hirschman C, Butler M. Trends and differentials in breastfeeding: an update. *Demography*. 1981;18:39–54
5. Wright AL. The rise of breastfeeding in the United States. *Pediatr Clin North Am*. 2001;48:1–12
6. Ryan AS, Rush D, Kreiger FW, Lewandowski GE. Recent declines in breast-feeding in the United States, 1984 through 1989. *Pediatrics*. 1991;88:719–727

7. Ryan AS, Wenjun Z, Acosta A. Breastfeeding continues to increase into the new millennium. *Pediatrics.* 2002;110:1103–1109

8. Rassin DK, Richardson CJ, Baranowski T, et al. Incidence of breast-feeding in a low socioeconomic group of mothers in the US: ethnic patterns. *Pediatrics.* 1984;73:132–137

9. Wright AL, Holberg C, Taussig LM. Infant feeding practices among middle-class Anglos and Hispanics. *Pediatrics.* 1988;82:496–503

10. Hirschman C, Butler M. Trends and differentials in breastfeeding. *Demography.* 1981;18:39–54

11. Wright AL, Clark C, Bauer M. Maternal employment and infant feeding practices among the Navajo. *Med Anthropol Q.* 1993;7:260–281

12. Bee DE, Baranowski T, Rassin DK, Richardson CJ, Mikrut W. Breast-feeding initiation in a triethnic population. *Am J Dis Child.* 1991;145:306–309

13. Scrimshaw SCM. The cultural context of breastfeeding in the United States. In: *Report of the Surgeon General's Workshop on Breastfeeding and Human Lactation.* Rockville, MD: US Department of Health and Human Services; 1984:23–30

14. Baranowski T, Rassin DK, Richardson CJ, Brown JP, Bee DE. Attitudes toward breastfeeding. *J Dev Behav Pediatr.* 1986;7:367–377

15. Shapiro J, Saltzer EB. Attitudes toward breast-feeding among Mexican-American women. *J Trop Pediatr.* 1985;31:13–16

16. Weller SC, Dungy CI. Personal preferences and ethnic variations among Anglo and Hispanic breast and bottle feeders. *Soc Sci Med.* 1986;23:539–548

17. Wright AL, Bauer M, Clark C, Morgan F, Begishe K. Cultural interpretations and intracultural variability in Navajo beliefs about breastfeeding. *Am Ethnologist.* 1993;20:781–796

18. US Department of Health and Human Services. *Healthy People 2010.* 2nd ed. With Understanding and Improving Health and Objectives for Improving Health. 2 vols. Washington, DC: US Government Printing Office; 2000

19. Freed GL, Fraley JK, Schanler RJ. Attitudes of expectant fathers regarding breast-feeding. *Pediatrics.* 1992;90:224–227

20. Mackey S, Fried PA. Infant breast and bottle feeding practices: some related factors and attitudes. *Can J Public Health.* 1981;72:312–318

21. Ekwo EE, Dusdieker LB, Booth BM. Factors influencing initiation of breast-feeding. *Am J Dis Child.* 1983;137:375–377

22. Jones RA, Belsey EM. Brestfeeding in an inner London borough: a study of cultural factors. *Soc Sci Med.* 1977;11:175–179

23. Underwood BA. Weaning practices in deprived environments: the weaning dilemma. *Pediatrics.* 1985;75:194–198

24. Neifert M, Gray J, Gary N, Camp B. Factors influencing breastfeeding among adolescents. *J Adolesc Health.* 1988;9:470–473

25. US Department of Health and Human Services. *Report of the Surgeon General's Workshop on Breastfeeding and Human Lactation.* Rockville, MD: US Department of Health and Human Services; 1984

26. Wright AL, Schanler RJ. The resurgence of breastfeeding at the end of the second millennium. *J Nutr.* 2001;131:421S–425S

27. WHO Expert Consultation. The optimal duration of exclusive breastfeeding. 2001; Available at: http://www.who.int

28. Picciano MF. Representative values for constituents of human milk. *Pediatr Clin North Am.* 2001;48:263–264

29. Schanler RJ. Suitability of human milk for the low-birthweight infant. *Clin Perinatol.* 1995;22:207–222

30. Blanc B. Biochemical aspects of human milk: comparison with bovine milk. *World Rev Nutr Diet.* 1981;36:1–89

31. Goldman AS, Chheda S, Keeney SE, Schmalsteig FC, Schanler RJ. Immunologic protection of the premature newborn by human milk. *Semin Perinatol.* 1994; 18:495–501

32. Neville MC, Watters CD. Secretion of calcium into milk: a review. *J Dairy Sci.* 1983;66:371–380

33. Specker BL, Beck A, Kalkwarf H, Ho M. Randomized trial of varying mineral intake on total body bone mineral accretion during the first year of life. *Pediatrics.* 1997;99:e12

34. Casey CE, Hambidge KM, Neville MC. Studies in human lactation: zinc, copper, manganese, and chromium in human milk in the first month of lactation. *Am J Clin Nutr.* 1985;41:1193–1200

35. Siimes MA, Vuori E, Kuitunen P. Breast milk iron: a declining concentration during the course of lactation. *Acta Paediatr Scand.* 1979;68:29–31

36. Lonnerdal B, Hernell O. Iron, zinc, copper and selenium status of breast-fed infants and infants fed trace element fortified milk-based infant formula. *Acta Paediatr.* 1994;83:367–373

37. Greer FR, Suttie JW. Vitamin K and the newborn. In: Tsang RC, Nichols BL, eds. *Nutrition During Infancy.* Philadelphia, PA: Hanley & Belfus; 1988:289–297

38. Specker BL. Do North American women need supplemental vitamin D during pregnancy or lactation? *Am J Clin Nutr.* 1994;59:4845–4918

39. Kreiter SR, Schwartz RP, Kirkman HN Jr, Charlton PA, Calikoglu AS, Davenport ML. Nutritional rickets in African American breastfed infants. *J Pediatr.* 2000;137:153–157

40. Caplan MS, Lickerman M, Adler L, Dietsch GN, Yu A. The role of recombinant platelet-activating factor acetylhydrolase in a neonatal rat model of necrotizing enterocolitis. *Pediatr Res.* 1997;42:779–783

41. Hamosh M. Bioactive factors in human milk. *Pediatr Clin North Am.* 2001; 48:69–86

42. Kleinman RE, Walker WA. The enteromammary immune system. *Dig Dis Sci.* 1979;24:876–882

43. Heinig MJ. Host defense benefits of breastfeeding for the infant: effect of breast-feeding duration and exclusivity. *Pediatr Clin North Am.* 2001;48:105–123

44. Victora CG, Smith PG, Vaughan JP, et al. Evidence for protection by breastfeeding against infant deaths from infectious diseases in Brazil. *Lancet.* 1987;2:319–322

45. Schanler RJ, Shulman RJ, Lau C. Feeding strategies for premature infants: beneficial outcomes of feeding fortified human milk versus preterm formula. *Pediatrics.* 1999;103:1150–1157

46. Duncan B, Ey J, Holberg CJ, Wright AL, Martinez FD, Taussig LM. Exclusive breast-feeding for at least 4 months protects against otitis media. *Pediatrics.* 1993;91:867–872

47. Aniansson G, Alm B, Andersson B, et al. A prospective cohort study on breast-feeding and otitis media in Swedish infants. *Pediatr Infect Dis J.* 1994;12:183–188

48. Owen MJ, Baldwin CD, Swank PR, Pannu AK, Johnson DL, Howie VM. Relation of infant feeding practices, cigarette smoke exposure, and group child care to the onset and duration of otitis media with effusion in the first two years of life. *J Pediatr.* 1993;123:702–711

49. Teele DW, Klein JO, Rosner B. Epidemiology of otitis media during the first seven years of life in children in greater Boston: a prospective, cohort study. *J Infect Dis.* 1989;160:83–94

50. Paradise JL, Elster BA, Tan L. Evidence in infants with cleft palate that breast milk protects against otitis media. *Pediatrics.* 1994;94:853–860

51. Dewey KG, Heinig MJ, Nommsen-Rivers LA. Differences in morbidity between breast-fed and formula-fed infants. *J Pediatr.* 1995;126:696–702

52. Wright AL, Holberg CJ, Martinez FD, Morgan WJ, Taussig LM. Breast feeding and lower respiratory tract illness in the first year of life. *BMJ.* 1989;299:946–949

53. Howie PW, Forsyth JS, Ogston SA, Clark A, Florey CD. Protective effect of breast-feeding against infection. *BMJ.* 1990;300:11–16

54. Arnold C, Makintube S, Istre GR. Day care attendance and other risk factors for invasive *Haemophilus influenzae* type B disease. *Am J Epidemiol.* 1993;138:333–340

55. Petersen GM, Silimperi DR, Chiu CY, Ward JI. Effects of age, breast feeding, and household structure on *Haemophilus influenzae* type B disease risk and antibody acquisition in Alaskan Eskimos. *Am J Epidemiol.* 1991;134:1212–1221

56. Marild S, Jodal U, Hanson LA. Breastfeeding and urinary tract infection [letter]. *Lancet.* 1990;336:92

57. Pisacane A, Graziano L, Mazzarella G, Scarpellino B, Zona G. Breastfeeding and urinary tract infections. *J Pediatr.* 1992;120:87–89

58. Coppa GV, Gabrielli O, Giorgi P, et al. Preliminary study of breastfeeding and bacterial adhesion to uroepithelial cells. *Lancet.* 1990;335:569–571

59. James-Ellison M, Roberts R, Verrier-Jones K, Williams JD, Topley N. Mucosal immunity in the urinary tract: Changes in sIgA, FSC and total IgA with age and in urinary tract infection. *Clin Nephrol.* 1997;48:69–78

60. Hutchens TW, Henry JF, Yip TT, et al. Origin of intact lactoferrin and its DNA-binding fragments found in the urine of human milk-fed preterm infants. Evaluation by stable isotope enrichment. *Pediatr Res.* 1991;29:243–250

61. Goldblum RM, Schanler RJ, Garza C, Goldman AS. Human milk feeding enhances the urinary excretion of immunologic factors in low birth weight infants. *Pediatr Res.* 1989;25:184–188

62. Arnon SS, Damus K, Thompson B, Midura TF, Chin J. Protective role of human milk against sudden infant death from infant botulism. *J Pediatr.* 1982;100: 568–573

63. Davis MK, Savitz DA, Graubard BI. Infant feeding and childhood cancer. *Lancet.* 1988;2:365–368

64. Koletzko S, Sherman P, Corey M, Griffiths A, Smith C. Role of infant feeding practices in development of Crohn's disease in childhood. *BMJ.* 1989;298:1617–1618

65. Gerstein HC. Cow's milk exposure and type I diabetes mellitus. A critical overview of the clinical literature. *Diabetes Care.* 1994;17:13–19

66. Kramer MS. Does breast feeding help protect against atopic disease? Biology, methodology, and a golden jubilee of controversy. *J Pediatr.* 1988;112:181–190

67. Hanson LA, Adlerberth I, Carlsson B, et al. Host defense of the neonate and the intestinal flora. *Acta Paediatr Scand.* 1989;351(suppl):122–125

68. Hanson LA, Ahlstedt S, Andersson B, et al. Protective factors in milk and the development of the immune system. *Pediatrics.* 1985;75(suppl):172–176

69. Saarinen UM, Kajosaari M, Backman A, Siimes MA. Prolonged breast-feeding as prophylaxis for atopic disease. *Lancet.* 1979;2:163–166

70. Karjalainen J, Martin JM, Knip M, et al. A bovine albumin peptide as a possible trigger of insulin-dependent diabetes mellitus. *N Engl J Med.* 1992;327:302–307

71. Rogan WJ, Gladen BC. Breast-feeding and cognitive development. *Early Hum Dev.* 1993;31:181–193

72. Horwood LJ, Fergusson DM. Breastfeeding and later cognitive and academic outcomes. *Pediatrics.* 1998;101:9

73. Lucas A, Morley R, Cole TJ, Lister G, Leeson-Payne C. Breast milk and subsequent intelligence quotient in children born preterm. *Lancet.* 1992;339:261–264

74. Horwood LJ, Mogridge N, Darlow BA. Cognitive, educational, and behavioural outcomes at 7 to 8 years in a national very low birthweight cohort. *Arch Dis Child Fetal Neonatal Ed.* 1998;79:F12–F20

75. Anderson JW, Johnstone BM, Remley DT. Breast-feeding and cognitive development: a meta-analysis. *Am J Clin Nutr.* 1999;70:525–535

76. Heinig MJ, Dewey KG. Health effects of breastfeeding for mothers: a critical review. *Nutr Res Rev.* 1997;10:35–56

77. McNeilly AS. Lactational amenorrhea. *Endocrinol Metab Clin North Am.* 1993;22:59–73

78. Labbok MH. Effects of breastfeeding on the mother. *Pediatr Clin North Am.* 2001;48:143–158

79. Newcomb PA, Storer BE, Longnecker MP, et al. Lactation and a reduced risk of premenopausal breast cancer. *N Engl J Med.* 1994;330:81–87

80. Rosenblatt KA, Thomas DB. Lactation and the risk of epithelial ovarian cancer. *Int J Epidemiol.* 1993;22:192–197

81. Sowers M. Pregnancy and lactation as risk factors for subsequent bone loss and osteoporosis. *J Bone Miner Res.* 1996;11:1052–1060

82. Kalkwarf HJ, Specker BL, Bianchi DC, Ranz J, Ho M. The effect of calcium supplementation on bone density during lactation and after weaning. *N Engl J Med.* 1997;337:523–528

83. Specker BL, Tsang RC, Ho ML. Changes in calcium homeostasis over the first year postpartum: effect of lactation and weaning. *Obstet Gynecol.* 1991;78:56–62

84. Montgomery DL, Splett PL. Economic benefit of breast-feeding infants enrolled in WIC. *J Am Diet Assoc.* 1997;97:379–385

85. Ball TM, Wright AL. Health care costs of formula-feeding in the first year of life. *Pediatrics.* 1999;103:870–876

86. Hoey C, Ware JL. Economic advantages of breastfeeding in an HMO setting: a pilot study. *Am J Manag Care.* 1997;3:861–865

87. Lawrence RM, Lawrence RA. Given the benefits of breastfeeding, what contraindications exist? *Pediatr Clin North Am.* 2001;48:235–251

88. Lawrence RA. *Breastfeeding: A Guide For The Medical Profession.* 4th ed. St Louis, MO: Mosby-Year Book, Inc; 1994

89. Freed GL, Landers S, Schanler RJ. A practical guide to successful breast-feeding management. *Am J Dis Child.* 1991;145:917–921

90. Butte NF, Garza C, Smith EO, Nichols BL. Human milk intake and growth of exclusively breast-fed infants. *J Pediatr.* 1984;104:187–195

91. Dewey KG, Heinig MJ, Nommsen LA, Peerson JM, Lonnerdal B. Growth of breast-fed and formula-fed infants from 0 to 18 months: the DARLING study. *Pediatrics.* 1992;89:1035–1041

92. Dewey KG. Nutrition, growth, and complementary feeding of the breastfed infant. *Pediatr Clin North Am.* 2001;48:87–104

93. Dewey KG, Heinig MJ, Nommsen LA, Lonnerdal B. Adequacy of energy intake among breast-fed infants in the DARLING study: relationships to growth velocity, morbidity, and activity levels. *J Pediatr.* 1991;119:538–547

94. Butte NF, Smith EO, Garza C. Energy utilization of breast-fed and formula-fed infants. *Am J Clin Nutr.* 1990;51:350–358

95. Powers NG. How to assess slow growth in the breastfed infant: birth to 3 months. *Pediatr Clin North Am.* 2001;48:345–363

96. Neifert MR. Prevention of breastfeeding tragedies. *Pediatr Clin North Am.* 2001;48:273–298

97. Gartner LM. On the question of the relationship between breastfeeding and jaundice in the first 5 days of life. *Semin Perinatol.* 1994;18:502–509

98. Tomashek KM, Nesby S, Scanlon KS, et al. Commentary: nutritional rickets in Georgia. *Pediatrics.* 2001;107:e45

99. American Academy of Pediatrics, Committee on Drugs. The transfer of drugs and other chemicals into human milk. *Pediatrics.* 2001;108:776–789

100. Kopec K. Herbal medications and breastfeeding. *J Hum Lact.* 1999;15:157–161

101. Gartner LM, Herschel M. Jaundice and breastfeeding. In: Schanler RJ, ed. *Pediatric Clinics of North America. Breastfeeding 2001, Part I. The Management of Breastfeeding.* Philadelphia: W.B. Saunders Company; 2001:389–400

102. Lascari AD. "Early" breastfeeding jaundice: clinical significance. *J Pediatr.* 1986;108:156–158

103. Nicoll A, Ginsburg R, Tripp HJ. Supplementary feeding and jaundice in newborns. *Acta Paediatr Scand.* 1982;71:759–761

104. Martinez JC, Maisels MJ, Otheguy L, et al. Hyperbilirubinemia in the breast-fed newborn: a controlled trial of four interventions. *Pediatrics.* 1993;91:470–473

105. Kemper K, Forsyth B, McCarthy P. Jaundice, terminating breast-feeding, and the vulnerable child. *Pediatrics.* 1989;84:773–778

106. Picciano MF. Nutrient composition of human milk. *Pediatr Clin North Am.* 2001;48:53–67

107. National Academy of Sciences Subcommittee on Nutrition During Lactation. *Nutrition During Lactation.* Washington, DC: National Academy Press; 1991: 113–152

108. American Academy of Pediatrics, Committee on Nutrition. Nutrition and lactation. *Pediatrics.* 1981;68:435–443

109. Butte NF, Garza C, Stuff JE, Smith EO, Nichols BL. Effect of maternal diet and body composition on lactational performance. *Am J Clin Nutr.* 1984;39:296–306

110. Strode MA, Dewey KG, Lonnerdal B. Effects of short-term caloric restriction on lactational performance of well-nourished women. *Acta Paediatr Scand.* 1986; 75:222–229

111. Jensen RG. *The Lipids of Human Milk.* Boca Raton, FL: CRC Press; 1989:1–213

112. Butte NF, Calloway DH. Evaluation of lactational performance of Navajo women. *Am J Clin Nutr.* 1981;34:2210–2215

113. Hollis BW, Lambert PW, Horst RL. Factors affecting the antirachitic sterol content of native milk. In: Holick MF, Gray TK, Anast CS, eds. *Perinatal Calcium and Phosphorous Metabolism.* Amsterdam, the Netherlands: Elsevier; 1983:157–182

114. von Kries R, Shearer M, McCarthy PT, Haug M, Harzer G, Gobel U. Vitamin K_1 content of maternal milk: influence of the stage of lactation, lipid composition, and vitamin K_1 supplements given to the mother. *Pediatr Res.* 1987;22:513–517

115. Higginbottom MC, Sweetman L, Nyhan WL. A syndrome of methylmalonic aciduria, homocystinuria, megaloblastic anemia and neurologic abnormalities in a vitamin B_{12}-deficient breast-fed infant of a strict vegetarian. *N Engl J Med.* 1978;299:317–323

116. American Academy of Pediatrics, Committee on Nutrition. Human milk banking. *Pediatrics.* 1980;65:854–857

117. Human Milk Banking Association of North America. *Guidelines for the Establishment and Operation of a Donor Human Milk Bank.* West Hartford, CT: Human Milk Banking Association of North America; 1994

118. Human Milk Banking Association of North America. *Recommendations for Collection, Storage, and Handling of a Mother's Milk for her Own Infant in the Hospital Setting.* West Hartford, CT: Human Milk Banking Association of North America; 1993

119. Ruff AJ. Breastmilk, breastfeeding, and transmission of viruses to the neonate. *Semin Perinatol.* 1994;18:510–516

120. Powers NG, Naylor AJ, Wester RA. Hospital policies: crucial to breastfeeding success. *Semin Perinatol.* 1994;18:517–524

121. American Academy of Pediatrics, Committee on Practice and Ambulatory Medicine. Pediatrician's responsibility for infant nutrition. *Pediatrics.* 1997; 99:749–750

4

Formula Feeding of Term Infants

In the absence of human milk, iron-fortified infant formulas are appropriate substitutes for feeding the full-term infant during the first year of life. Although infant formulas are not identical in composition to human milk, many improvements have been made during the last 70 years. When used as the sole source of nourishment during the first 6 months of life, infant formulas must meet all the energy and nutrient requirements for healthy term infants. After the age of 6 months, formulas still supply a significant part of the infant's nutritional requirements.[1,2]

In a recent survey, approximately 69.5% of all infants born in the United States are breastfeeding in the postpartum period in the hospital.[3] Breastfeeding rates are highest among women who are older (30 years), white, well educated, relatively affluent, and live in the western United States. The lowest rates of breastfeeding are among African American mothers who are younger than 20 years and mothers with low income or who live in the southeastern United States.[3,4] The percentage of infants who still breastfed at 6 months of age is approximately 32.5%.[3] Data from 1991 indicate that almost 80% of infants are fed an infant formula or whole cow milk by 1 year of age.[4] Therefore, commercial infant formulas continue to play a substantial role in meeting the nutritional needs of infants in the United States. Direct advertising of infant formulas to the public is a violation of the World Health Organization code. The American Academy of Pediatrics and other organizations have stated their disapproval of direct advertising because of its implications for shortening or obviating breastfeeding.

The use of infant formulas has 3 indications: (1) as a substitute (or supplement) for human milk in infants whose mothers choose not to breastfeed (or not to do so exclusively), (2) as a substitute for human milk in infants for whom breastfeeding is medically contraindicated,[5] and (3) as a supplement for breastfed infants who do not gain weight adequately.

Formula supplementation for a breastfeeding infant may be necessary if the intake of breast milk is inadequate and the infant fails to gain weight. The mother should be encouraged to continue breastfeeding if formula is used as a supplement, but unless milk production is stimulated, the mother's milk supply will decrease. Introduction of complementary foods into the infant's diet is discussed in Chapter 6. The use of infant formula or breastfeeding for the first year of life instead of feeding whole cow milk reduces the risk of malnutrition during this time.

The composition of infant formulas has evolved over many years, and on-going research continues to improve their acceptability and nutritional quality. Human milk serves as a model for the composition of infant formulas, but at present, formulas still do not duplicate the composition of human milk, which contains hormones, immunologic agents, enzymes, and live cells. Early infant formulas consisted of whole or evaporated cow milk, sugar (corn syrup), and water. The protein content of these formulas was much higher than that found in human milk. The fat was largely saturated, poorly absorbed, and contained few essential fatty acids. The carbohydrate content was a mixture of lactose and sucrose. Each of these components has been modified in currently available preparations to approach more closely the composition of human milk. The protein content has been reduced, butterfat has been replaced by a mixture of animal and vegetable oils, and more lactose or other carbohydrates have been added. Standards for nutrient concentrations in infant formulas are stated in the Infant Formula Act of 1980 (revised in 1986) (see Appendix D and Chapter 5). This act establishes the minimum levels of 29 nutrients and the maximum levels of 9 nutrients and requires that a quantitative label declaration be made for each nutrient. The regulations also require the manufacturer to ensure by analysis the declared level of all essential nutrients in each batch of formula. In general, the concentrations of nutrients in formulas are higher than those in human milk to compensate for the possible lower bioavailability.[6]

Infant formulas are available in 3 forms: ready-to-feed, concentrated liquid, and powder. Potable water to be added to the concentrate or powder should be brought to a rolling boil for 1 minute and then allowed to cool before it is added to the concentrate or powder formula. The different forms are nearly identical in nutrient composition, but small differences may exist for technical reasons. While most infants thrive on formulas derived from cow milk, some infants may exhibit intolerance to formula. Consequently, a number of alternative formulas of special composition have been manufactured for infants with gastrointestinal or metabolic disturbances.[7,8] When a transition from one formula to another is undertaken because of cost, availability, or a specific desire to alter the nutrient composition of the diet, the change can be made abruptly. Generic formulas have recently become available. These must meet the requirements set forth in the Infant Formula Act. Their composition may differ qualitatively and quantitatively from their branded counterparts.

Standard Cow Milk-Based Formulas

Standard cow milk-based formula is the feeding of choice when breastfeeding is not used or is stopped before 1 year of age. All of the presently available formulas have been tested extensively under experimental and field conditions and provide adequate nutrition to the healthy infant when used exclusively for the first 4 to 6 months of life.

Composition

Commercial cow milk-based formulas have many similarities, but also differ substantially from each other in quality and quantity of nutrients. While the different manufacturers offer a rationale for formula composition, often physiologically significant differences have not been clearly demonstrated among the various products. The composition of formulas may change over time and is reflected on the formula label. The composition of currently available standard cow milk-derived formulas for term infants is presented in Appendix E, Table E–1.

Protein

Cow milk-based formulas in the United States contain protein at concentrations varying from 1.45 to 1.6 g/dL, which represents almost 50% more protein than is present in human milk (0.9–1.0 g/dL). The ratio between the predominant types of cow milk proteins (ie, whey and casein) varies considerably among these formulas. While some formulas contain cow milk protein with a whey-casein ratio of 18:82, others have added cow milk whey protein with reduced minerals to achieve a whey-casein ratio of 60:40 (similar to that of human milk). A "standard" infant formula containing 100% partially hydrolyzed whey protein is also available. Nevertheless, there are compositional and functional differences between the predominant whey proteins in cow milk and in human milk.[9] The predominant whey protein in cow milk is α-lactoglobulin, whereas the predominant whey protein in human milk is α-lactalbumin. Whey proteins contain more lactalbumins and more sulfur-containing amino acids than does casein. Compared with breastfed infants, infants fed whey-predominant formula have increased serum levels of threonine, phenylalanine, valine, and methionine.

Fat

Fat provides approximately 40% to 50% of the energy from cow milk-derived formulas. During the preparation process, the butterfat of whole cow milk is replaced with vegetable oils or a mixture of vegetable and animal fats. This replacement improves fat digestibility and absorption, increases the concentration of essential fatty acids, and reduces the level of environmental pollutants. Fat blends are selected to provide a balance of saturated and polyunsaturated fatty acids. Coconut oil provides an excellent source of highly digestible saturated, short- and medium-chain fatty acids. Palm oil is a source of long-chain saturated fatty acids, and soy, corn, and safflower oils provide abundant polyunsaturated fatty acids.[10] Some manufacturers use a genetic variant of safflower oil to increase monounsaturated fatty acids in the fat blend. The concentration and ratio of essential fatty acids (ie, linoleic acid and linolenic acid) meet current guidelines. In contrast to human milk, formulas (prepared with vegetable oils) contain little or no cholesterol. There is no demonstrated value to adding cholesterol to infant formulas.

Determination of the ideal fatty acid composition for cow milk-derived formulas is an area of intense research, particularly with regard to the ω-3 and ω-6 fatty acids and their very long-chain polyunsaturated derivatives (LC-PUFAs), such as arachidonic and docosahexaenoic acids. These fatty acids can be synthesized by premature and term infants and are present in a wide range of concentrations in human milk. Some, but not all, studies have found improved short-term performance in tests of visual and cognitive functions both in preterm and in term infants fed formulas supplemented with LC-PUFAs (see Chapter 17). These fatty acids (derived from a single cell source) have recently been classified by the FDA as "GRAS" (generally regarded as safe) and thus may be added to infant formulas in approved ratios, after the manufacturer satisfies the requirements of the Infant Formula Act.

Carbohydrate

Lactose is the major carbohydrate in human milk and in standard cow milk-based infant formulas. Lactose is hydrolyzed in the small intestine by the action of lactase. This enzyme appears later than other disaccharidases in the developing fetal intestine. Some lactose, even in the mature infant, enters the distal bowel where it ferments, permitting the proliferation of an acidophilic bacterial flora. These microorganisms, which include lactobacilli, produce an acid medium that suppresses the growth of more pathogenic organisms and promotes the absorption of calcium and perhaps phosphorus. In addition to lactose, some formulas also contain starch or other complex carbohydrates.

Iron

The cow milk-based formulas are produced either with low iron concentration ($\leq$6.7 mg/100 kcal; =45 mg/L) or fortified with iron ($\geq$6.7 mg/100 kcal; 100 to 145 mg/L). During the 1950s, in response to a high prevalence of iron deficiency among infants in the United States and in an effort to link iron with a major source of dietary energy, iron was added to infant formulas at a concentration of 12 mg/L. Low-iron formulas continue to exist, in part because iron is perceived by some to cause constipation and other feeding problems. Well-controlled studies have consistently failed to show any increase in prevalence of fussiness, cramping, colic, gastroesophageal reflux, constipation, or flatulence with the use of iron-fortified formulas.

> **The American Academy of Pediatrics** sees no role for the use of low-iron formulas in infant feeding and recommends that all formulas fed to infants be fortified with iron (>6.7 mg/100 kcal; 4 to 12 mg/L).[11]
>
> *Pediatrics.* 1999;104:119–123

Other Nutrients

Some of the major minerals and electrolytes (such as calcium, phosphorus, magnesium, sodium, potassium, and chloride) that are present in these formulas are derived from cow milk; others are added as inorganic salts. Formulas that contain minerals at the lower ranges of the recommended values have a lower renal solute load than those with higher mineral concentrations. Trace minerals, vitamins, and amino acids, such as taurine, are also added. Nucleotides, which have also been added to some formulas, may enhance immune function and gastrointestinal development and promote the development of a less pathogenic intestinal flora. However, further research is needed to confirm these potential beneficial effects.

Prebiotics are nutrients that support the growth of nonpathogenic microbial organisms (probiotics—Bifidobacteria, Lactobacilli) that are normally part of the intestinal microflora of the breastfed infant. Several studies have shown positive health outcomes associated with intestinal colonization of probiotic organisms. More studies are needed before the addition of prebiotics or probiotics to infant formulas can be recommended.

Standard infant formulas (Appendix E, Table E–2) are prescribed with a caloric density of 67 to 70 kcal/dL (20 kcal/oz), similar to human milk, and should be offered ad libitum. The usual intake will be 150 to 200 mL/kg/d for the first 3 months of life. This provides 100 to 135 kcal/kg/d and should result in an initial weight gain of 25 to 30 g/d. Between 3 and 6 months of age, weight gain decreases to 15 to 20 g/d and between 6 and 12 months of age, to 10 to 15 g/d. Formula-fed infants do not need additional water. Vomiting or spitting up is common for the first few months of life and requires no change in the feeding regimen if weight gain is adequate. Constipation with slow weight gain may indicate inadequate intake of formula.

Soy Formulas

During the 1960s, formulas were developed with soy protein and without lactose for infants who could not tolerate milk protein or lactose. For the last 25 years, soy formulas (Appendix F) have constituted approximately 25% of all formulas sold and support growth equivalent to that of breastfed and cow milk-based formula-fed infants.[12] Bone mineralization is similar in infants fed soy and cow milk-based formulas.[13–15] In premature infants, older versions of currently available soy formulas were associated with an increased incidence of osteopenia. Because special formulas have been developed for premature infants, there is no indication for the use of soy formulas in these infants.

Uses

Soy formulas may be used by vegetarians. Many infants who have an immunoglobulin E-associated reaction to cow milk proteins do well when fed soy formulas. These formulas have a similar taste to cow milk and cost less than many protein hydrolysate formulas. Nevertheless, soy milks may be allergenic in infants allergic to cow milk protein.[16] All soy formulas in the United States are free of lactose and are recommended for infants with lactase deficiency or galactosemia.[17] While lactose intolerance is known to occur after acute gastroenteritis, soy formulas are recommended for postdiarrheal refeeding only in patients with signs of clinically significant lactose intolerance.[18] Those who require a formula change should be rechallenged with a lactose-containing formula within 1 month. Intolerances to cow milk-based formulas, such as colic, loose stools, spitting up, or vomiting, sometimes prompt a switch to soy formula. Most of these problems are unrelated to the feeding; occasionally, however, some infants respond positively to soy formulas for reasons not totally understood.

Composition

Methionine is added to compensate for the low concentration of this amino acid in soy protein. The fats in soy formulas are similar to those found in cow milk-based formulas. Lactose, the major carbohydrate of human milk and cow milk-based formulas, is not used in soy formulas to avoid contamination with milk proteins. Soy formulas contain sucrose, cornstarch hydrolysates, or mixtures of these 2 carbohydrates. Minerals and vitamins are added to these formulas, usually in amounts greater than cow milk-based formulas to compensate for lower mineral bioavailability (or absorption) caused in part by substances such as phytate in soy beans. Taurine and, more recently, carnitine have also been added to these formulas. Soy formulas contain phytoestrogens, which have demonstrated physiologic activity in rodent models. No significant effects of phytoestrogens have been found on growth or pubertal development in humans. The formulas are also iron fortified.

Recently, a soy formula has been supplemented with partially fermentable soy fiber and marketed for the dietary management of diarrhea in infancy. A clinical trial of this product demonstrated a shorter duration of diarrheal stools

---

The American Academy of Pediatrics recommends the use of soy formulas for the following:

1. Term infants whose nutritional needs are not met from breast milk. The isolated soy protein-based formulas are a safe and nutritionally equivalent alternative to cow milk-based formula.
2. Term infants with galactosemia or hereditary lactase deficiency.
3. Term infants with documented transient lactase deficiency.
4. Infants with documented IgE-associated mediated allergy to cow milk (most will tolerate soy protein-based formula).
5. Patients seeking a vegetarian-based diet for a term infant.

The use of soy protein-based formula is not recommended for the following:

1. Preterm infants with birth weights less than 1800 g.
2. Prevention of colic or allergy.
3. Infants with cow milk protein-induced enterocolitis or enteropathy.

Pediatrics. 1998;101:148–153

in treated infants compared to the duration in infants in the control group.[19] However, no differences were found in stool weights, wet or dry, between the 2 groups of infants. Further studies with this product are required before its use can be recommended for the routine management of diarrhea.

Protein Hydrolysate Formulas

Uses

These formulas were originally developed for infants who could not digest or were severely intolerant to intact cow milk protein. The protein in some of the hydrolysate formulas is extensively hydrolyzed so the resulting peptides are incapable of eliciting an immunologic response in many infants.[20] Protein hydrolysates are recommended as the preferred formula for infants intolerant of cow milk and soy proteins or for those with significant malabsorption due to gastrointestinal or hepatobiliary disease (eg, cystic fibrosis, short gut syndrome, biliary atresia, cholestasis, and protracted diarrhea). In such cases, protein hydrolysate formulas can be lifesaving and are preferable to the alternative of total parenteral nutrition. Disadvantages of protein hydrolysate formulas include the poor taste of these products (owing to the presence of sulfated amino acids), the greater cost, and the high osmolality. (See also Chapter 34.)

Composition

The unique compositions of the different protein hydrolysates are summarized in Appendix G. The milk protein, either casein or whey, is heat treated and enzymatically hydrolyzed. The resulting hydrolysate, consisting of free amino acids and peptides of varying length, is then fortified with amino acids to compensate for the amino acids lost in the manufacturing process. The various hydrolysate formulas contain differing amounts of peptides of different chain lengths. In general, the more extensive the hydrolysis, the lesser the antigenicity and the greater the price. Unfortunately, no definitive in vitro tests quantify the allergenicity of a product. Studies of antigenicity in animals also do not correlate with studies in infants. The only way to accurately test the allergenicity of these products is by implementing clinical trials. Most protein hydrolysate formulas are free of lactose. Manufacturers use sucrose, tapioca starch, corn syrup solids, and cornstarch in various mixtures. Fat in these formulas contains varying amounts of medium-chain triglycerides (MCTs) to facilitate absorption of fat. The MCT oil is supplemented with a small amount of polyunsaturated vegetable oil to supply essential fatty acids. Products differ significantly from each other; brochures from the manufacturers should be consulted for explanations of the differences.

Other special formulas have been made for low-birth-weight infants (see Chapter 2) and for infants with inborn errors of metabolism (see Chapter 29).

Amino Acid-Based Formulas

Amino acid-based formulas specifically designed for infants are indicated for extreme protein hypersensitivity, when symptoms persist even when extensively hydrolyzed protein formulas are used (Appendix G).[21,22] These formulas are more costly than cow milk and soy protein-based formulas. (See also Chapter 34.)

Follow-up Formulas

Follow-up and "toddler" formulas are now available in the United States. The iron fortification they contain is an advantage for infants and toddlers receiving inadequate amounts in their solid feedings. The composition of these formulas differs from standard formulas (increased protein and minerals, among other differences). They are nutritionally adequate but offer no clear advantage for infants receiving adequate amounts of iron and vitamins in their infant formula and solid food (see Appendix E, Table E–3).

Cow Milk

Full-fat cow milk, skim milk, 1%- to 2%-fat milk, goat milk, evaporated milk, and other "milks" not specifically formulated to meet infant nutritional requirements (see Appendix E, Table E–1) are not recommended for use during the first 12 months of life.[23] Infants fed whole pasteurized cow milk between 6 and 12 months of age are at risk of depleting their iron stores and ultimately developing iron-deficiency anemia[24,25] because of the low concentration and bioavailability of iron in cow milk and possible intestinal blood loss. The higher intake of protein, sodium, potassium, and chloride associated with the use of cow milk inappropriately increases the renal solute load.[26] The limited amount of essential fatty acids, as well as vitamin E, zinc, and perhaps other trace substances, may not be adequate to prevent deficiencies. Skim milks may cause the infant to consume excessive amounts of protein, because large volumes are ingested to satisfy caloric needs.[27]

References

1. Montalto MB, Benson JD, Martinez GA. Nutrient intakes of formula-fed infants and infants fed cow's milk. *Pediatrics*. 1985;75:343–351
2. Martinez GA, Ryan AS, Malec DJ. Nutrient intakes of American infants and children fed cow's milk or infant formula. *Am J Dis Child*. 1985;139:1010–1018
3. 2001 Breastfeeding Data from the Mothers Survey, Ross Products Division, Abbott Laboratories, Columbus, OH

4. Ryan AS, Rush D, Krieger FW, Lewandowski GE. Recent declines in breastfeeding in the United States, 1984 through 1989. *Pediatrics.* 1991;88:719–727

5. Stiehm ER, Vink P. Transmission of human immunodeficiency virus infection by breast-feeding. *J Pediatr.* 1991;118:410–412

6. Sandstrom B, Cederblad A, Lonnerdal B. Zinc absorption from human milk, cow's milk, and infant formulas. *Am J Dis Child.* 1983;137:726–729

7. MacLean WC Jr, Benson JD. Theory into practice: the incorporation of new knowledge into infant formula. *Semin Perinatol.* 1989;13:104–111

8. Klish WJ. Special infant formulas. *Pediatr Rev.* 1990;12:55–62

9. Sarwar G, Peace RW, Botting HG. Differences in protein digestibility and quality of liquid concentrate and powder forms of milk-based infant formulas fed to rats. *Am J Clin Nutr.* 1989;49:806–813

10. Lifschitz CH, Gopalakrishna GS, Nichols BL. Tolerance and fat absorption of a special infant formula. *Nutr Rep Int.* 1986;33:585–593

11. American Academy of Pediatrics, Committee on Nutrition. Iron-fortified infant formulas. *Pediatrics.* 1999;104:119–123

12. Sarett HP. Soy-based infant formulas. In: Hill LD, ed. *World Soybean Research.* Danville, IL: Interstate Printers and Publishers; 1976:840–849

13. Mimouni F, Campaigne B, Neylan M, Tsang RC. Bone mineralization in the first year of life in infants fed human milk, cow-milk formula, or soy-based formula. *J Pediatr.* 1993;122:348–354

14. Hillman LS, Chow W, Salmons SS, Weaver E, Erickson M, Hansen J. Vitamin D metabolism, mineral homeostasis, and bone mineralization in term infants fed human milk, cow milk-based formula, or soy-based formula. *J Pediatr.* 1988; 112:864–874

15. Venkataraman PS, Luhar H, Neylan MJ. Bone mineral metabolism in full-term infants fed human milk, cow milk-based, and soy-based formulas. *Am J Dis Child.* 1992;146:1302–1305

16. Zeiger RS, Sampson HA, Bock SA, et al. Soy allergy in infants and children with IgE-associated cow's milk allergy. *J Pediatr.* 1999;134:614–622

17. American Academy of Pediatrics, Committee on Nutrition. Soy protein formulas: recommendations for use in infant feeding. *Pediatrics.* 1998;101:148–153

18. Brown KH, Peerson JM, Fontaine O. Use of nonhuman milks in the dietary management of young children with acute diarrhea: a meta-analysis of clinical trials. *Pediatrics.* 1994;93:17–27

19. Brown KH, Perez F, Peerson JM, et al. Effect of dietary fiber (soy polysaccharide) on the severity, duration, and nutritional outcome of acute, watery diarrhea in children. *Pediatrics.* 1993;92:241–247

20. American Academy of Pediatrics, Committee on Nutrition. Hypoallergenic infant formulas. *Pediatrics.* 2000;106:346–349

21. Sampson HA, James JM, Bernhisel-Broadbent J. Safety of an amino acid-derived infant formula in children allergic to cow milk. *Pediatrics.* 1992;90:463–465

22. Kelso JM, Sampson HA. Food protein-induced enterocolitis to casein hydrolysate formulas. *J Allergy Clin Immunol.* 1993;92:909–910

23. American Academy of Pediatrics, Committee on Nutrition. The use of whole cow milk in infancy. *Pediatrics.* 1992;89:1105–1109

24. Penrod JC, Anderson K, Acosta PB. Impact on iron status of introducing cow's milk in the second six months of life. *J Pediatr Gastroenterol Nutr.* 1990;10:462–467

25. Tunnessen WW Jr, Oski FA. Consequences of starting whole cow milk at 6 months of age. *J Pediatr.* 1987;111:813–816

26. Ziegler EE, Fomon SJ. Potential renal solute load of infant formulas. *J Nutr.* 1989; 119:1785–1788

27. Ryan AS, Martinez GA, Krieger FW. Feeding low-fat milk during infancy. *Am J Phys Anthropol.* 1987;73:539–548

5

Current Legislation and Regulations
for Infant Formulas

Infant formula is a food that purports to be or is represented for special dietary use solely as a food for infants by reason of its simulation of human milk or its suitability as a complete or partial substitute for human milk. Infant formula that is marketed in the United States is subject to the federal Food, Drug, and Cosmetic Act (the Act)[1] and the implementing regulations of the US Food and Drug Administration (FDA).[2] Generally, the Act provides specific regulatory controls for the production and the nutrient composition of infant formulas (see Appendix D for a listing of nutrient specifications).

The purpose of the infant formula provisions of the Act is to protect the health of infants using infant formula products. In 1978, a major manufacturer of infant formula reformulated 2 of its soy products by discontinuing the addition of salt. This reformulation resulted in infant formula products that contained an inadequate amount of chloride, an essential nutrient for growth and development in infants. By mid–1979, a disorder associated with chloride deficiency, hypochloremic metabolic alkalosis, was diagnosed in a substantial number of infants. Development of this disorder was associated with prolonged exclusive use of chloride-deficient soy formulas. This incident resulted in the passage of the Infant Formula Act of 1980, which amended the Food, Drug, and Cosmetic Act to ensure the adequacy of the nutrient composition of infant formulas. In 1986, as part of the Drug Enforcement, Education, and Control Act of 1985, the statutory requirements for infant formula under the Act were revised to give the FDA broader regulatory authority for infant formulas.[3]

The Act, as amended in 1986, provides specific requirements for the nutrient content and nutrient quantity of infant formula, nutrient quality control procedures, record keeping (including records on product testing), and recall procedures for the removal of unsafe infant formula from the marketplace. In addition, the Act requires manufacturers of infant formula to register and submit information to the FDA before marketing any new infant formula, including any infant formula that has had a major change in its formulation or processing. The FDA has a responsibility under the Act to review the new infant formula submission to ensure that a safe product will be produced. If the information in the submission meets the requirements of the Act, the agency will not object to the marketing of the formula. Although the FDA does not have the authority to approve infant formulas before they are marketed, it has compliance authority if an infant formula is marketed over its objection.

Information in such an infant formula submission must include the quantitative formulation and a listing, with amounts, of all ingredients in the formula. Only food ingredients that have been shown by the manufacturer to be safe and suitable under the applicable food safety provisions of the Act may be used in infant formulas. Some ingredients may qualify for the designation Generally Regarded as Safe (GRAS) after appropriate documentation has been submitted and considered by the FDA. In the submission, a manufacturer must provide assurances that the infant formula meets the nutrient content and quantity specifications and the nutrient quality standards in the Act.

The Act specifies the minimum nutrient levels and, in some cases, the maximum nutrient levels that infant formula products must contain. These specifications for the nutrient composition of commercial infant formulas are based in part on recommendations of the American Academy of Pediatrics that were developed by its Committee on Nutrition. Infant formula manufacturers must demonstrate that a required nutrient is present and available in the formula, and that the formula contains appropriate nutrient levels throughout the shelf life of the product. In addition, manufacturers must demonstrate that no other substance in the formula, such as a contaminant or a required nutrient present in a concentration that exceeds the maximum level allowed by FDA regulations, will make the formula unsafe or adulterated.

In certain cases, exemptions from the nutrient specifications are allowed. These exempt infant formulas are specialty formulas for use by infants with special medical and dietary needs, such as those for children with inborn errors of metabolism or of low birth weight. The exemption allows these infant formulas to be specifically formulated to meet the distinctive nutritional needs of infants with specific medical disorders.

Nutrient quality relates to the bioavailability of a nutrient. Infant formula must not only contain all of the nutrients required to support normal growth and development as the sole source of nutrition, but also provide those nutrients in a bioavailable form. Ordinarily, manufacturers submit documentation from clinical studies showing that the infant formula promotes normal infant growth and development and is suitable as the sole source of nutrients for young infants. The clinical studies are generally conducted in accordance with recommendations specific for infant populations by the American Academy of Pediatrics, together with general recommendations for rigorous clinical trial design, conduct, and analysis.

An infant formula submission also must include assurance that the infant formula complies with the Act and is manufactured in a way that is designed to prevent adulteration. Guidelines and regulations for the manufacturing of infant formula are necessary to ensure that infant formula is produced in a manner designed to prevent adulteration. For example, the FDA has guidelines to prevent microbiological contamination of infant formula during manufacture and market distribution.

The labels of infant formulas must include directions for use, including pictorial instructions; a warning statement informing consumers of the consequences of improper preparation or use of the infant formula; and a statement cautioning consumers to use infant formula as directed by a physician. In addition, the product label of an infant formula must bear a "use by" date that ensures that if the formula is consumed by that date, the infant will receive not less than the quantity of nutrients stated on the product label. Many infant formula labels also contain claims. Although claims must be truthful and not misleading under the Act, no requirement exists that label claims for infant formula be approved by the FDA.

References

1. Federal Food, Drug, and Cosmetic Act, 21 USC §321
2. Code of Federal Regulations. Title 21, Parts 106 and 107. Washington, DC: US Government Printing Office
3. Congressional Record. 99th Congress 2nd Session, Senate S 14042–14047. Washington, DC: US Government Printing Office; 1986;132(130)

6

Complementary Feeding

Introduction

The last century has witnessed remarkable temporal trends in infant feeding in western industrialized societies. Besides the marked decline and more recent renaissance of breastfeeding, vast changes have occurred in the timing and types of foods given to complement human milk and/or infant formula. Some nutritionists have emphasized the distinction between **complementary** versus **supplementary** feeding and have restricted the former term to solid or liquid foods that do not displace (ie, reduce intake of) breast milk. In fact, however, the available evidence indicates that any energy-containing foods will displace breastfeeding and reduce the intake of breast milk to some extent,[1-5] and all such foods are referred to herein as complementary.

This chapter will review the evidence bearing on complementary feeding in the first year of life. Much of it will focus on the optimal timing and types of foods to be introduced into the infant's diet after an initial period of exclusive breastfeeding. A recent systemic review of the evidence bearing on the health consequences of shorter versus longer duration of exclusive breastfeeding was undertaken by the World Health Organization (WHO).[6] The main issues to be considered in discussing recommendations for the introduction of complementary foods include the following: energy requirements and growth; iron, zinc, and vitamin D; infectious morbidity associated with these different regimens; the risks for development of atopic disease; and the long-term impact on neurocognitive development and behavior.

In the 1970s and 1980s, concern was expressed about the so-called "weanling's dilemma" in developing countries.[7,8] The dilemma centered on the risk of infection with the introduction of contaminated complementary foods versus the risk of suboptimal growth with continued exclusive breastfeeding. It is clear that breastfeeding protects against morbidity and even mortality from infectious diseases in developing and developed countries, even into the second year of life.[9-11] Growth faltering is commonly observed in developing countries after about age 3 months,[12-14] and early calculations made by the Food and Agricultural Organization (FAO) and WHO suggested that breast milk alone would be inadequate to meet the energy requirements beyond 3 or 4 months of life.[15] Although more recent studies have shown that the earlier FAO/WHO energy recommendations substantially overestimate true energy requirements in infancy,[16-19] infants who do not consume adequate amounts of breast milk may still require an additional source of energy and other nutrients between ages 4 and 6 months (or even earlier).

The weanling's dilemma does not apply in most developed countries; uncontaminated, nutritionally adequate complementary foods are readily available and growth faltering is relatively uncommon. The resurgence of breastfeeding in developed countries is in part a result of recent epidemiologic evidence showing that breastfeeding protects against gastrointestinal and, to a lesser extent, respiratory infection, and that the protective effect is enhanced with greater duration and exclusivity of breastfeeding.[20-22] Prolonged and exclusive breastfeeding (at least for the first few months of life) in some retrospective and observational studies has been associated with reduced risks of sudden infant death syndrome,[23] atopic disease,[24-26] and chronic conditions such as obesity,[27,28] type 1 diabetes,[29,30] Crohn's disease,[31] and lymphoma,[32,33] as well as acceleration of neurocognitive development[34-37] (see Chapter 3).

One of the concerns about prolonged and exclusive breastfeeding in developed countries has been that data show a deceleration in both weight and length gain relative to the international WHO/Centers for Disease Control and Prevention (CDC) growth reference from approximately 3 to 12 months, with partial catch-up in the second year.[38-42] Unfortunately, however, the WHO/CDC reference is based on the Fels Longitudinal Study, which was conducted several decades ago on infants who were primarily bottle-fed. The World Health Organization has, therefore, embarked on an ambitious international study to establish new growth standards for breastfed infants.[43,44]

Timing of Introduction of Complementary Foods

Recommendations for the optimal duration of exclusive breastfeeding remain controversial. The World Health Organization had recommended exclusive breastfeeding for 4 to 6 months, with the introduction of complementary foods thereafter,[45] whereas the United Nations Children's Fund (UNICEF) preferred the wording "about 6 months."[46] In response to a systematic review of the available evidence for both developed and developing countries,[6] WHO has recently revised its recommendation to promote exclusive breastfeeding for 6 months.[47] The American Academy of Pediatrics (AAP) has supported exclusive breastfeeding for approximately 6 months while recognizing that infants are often developmentally ready to accept complementary foods between 4 and 6 months (American Academy of Pediatrics. *Pediatric Nutrition Handbook.* Kleinman RE, ed. 4th ed. Elk Grove Village, IL: American Academy of Pediatrics; 1998).

The recent systematic review for WHO will be described here in some detail because it is the most current and comprehensive review of the evidence that bears on the timing of the introduction of complementary foods. The review included both controlled clinical trials and observational studies, published in any language, that compared health outcomes in full-term infants and their mothers with exclusive breastfeeding (EBF) for ≥6 months of age versus exclusive breastfeeding for at least 3 months, with continued mixed breastfeeding (MBF) until at least 6 months.[6] Two independent literature searches identified a total of 2668 unique citations. Only those studies with an internal comparison group were included in the review; those based on an external comparison group or reference were excluded. A total of 36 citations (articles or abstracts) were identified that met the selection criteria for the review, comprising 20 separate studies, 9 of which were carried out in developing countries and 11 in developed countries. All 20 studies were evaluated for methodologic quality to assess their control for confounding, losses to follow-up, and unbiased assessment of outcome.

The health outcomes reported in these studies included growth, iron and zinc status, infectious morbidity, atopic disease, neuromotor development, rate of postpartum maternal weight loss, and duration of lactational amenorrhea. The evidence reviewed here focuses on the studies from developed country settings, although occasional references are made to studies from developing countries, and in particular to 2 controlled clinical trials of EBF versus MBF carried out in Honduras.[1,2]

Weight, Length, and Head Circumference

A pooled sample of breastfed infants from 6 developed countries,[38,39] a pooled analysis from 5 countries (2 developed, 3 developing, but in which study women were all literate and of middle- to high-socioeconomic status),[48] and a large cohort study nested within a randomized trial in Belarus,[49] reported on weight gain between 3 and 8 months. One of the WHO studies[48] and the

Belarusan study[49] controlled for size or growth in the first 3 to 4 months and other potential confounders using multilevel (mixed) regression analyses. Except for the Belarusan study, no significant differences were noted in weight gain from 3 to 8 months, which averaged 400 to 500 g per month in both the EBF and MBF groups. In the Belarusan study, however, weight gains were much higher: 641 versus 612 g per month in the MBF versus EBF groups. Given the large weight gains in both groups in the Belarusan study, the higher weight gain in the MBF group is not necessarily beneficial. Parallel findings were observed for length gain from 3 to 8 months, again with the Belarusan study showing slightly but significantly more rapid length gains in the MBF group but with no significant differences observed in the 3 other studies. No significant differences were observed in head circumference in the Belarusan study at 6 or 9 months, although the EBF group had a significantly larger head circumference at 12 months. Thus infants exclusively breastfed for 6 months appear to grow adequately. In one study, infants fed complementary foods before 6 months of age gained more weight and length than their exclusively breastfed counterparts.

Iron and Zinc

There is a paucity of information that met the inclusion criteria for the systematic review regarding the effect of exclusive breastfeeding versus mixed breastfeeding on micronutrient status during infancy. A small Italian study[50] of hematologic outcomes included in the review reported that, at 12 months of age, infants in the EBF group had a statistically significantly higher hemoglobin concentration (117 vs 109 g/L), a nonsignificant reduction in anemia (hemoglobin <110 g/L), a nonsignificantly higher ferritin concentration, and a nonsignificant reduction in the risk of low (<10 μg/L) ferritin concentration. It is difficult to reconcile these results with the first Honduran trial, where the EBF group had a significantly lower hemoglobin concentration at 6 months and a lower plasma ferritin concentration at 6 months with a relative risk of 2.93 for a low (<15 μg/L) ferritin concentration.[1] Thus, the duration for which the iron endowment at birth is adequate varies, and some infants will benefit from additional iron at 4 to 6 months of age. (See also Chapter 19.)

The only data on zinc status were reported from the second Honduran trial; no significant effect of feeding was observed on the proportion of infants with a low (<70 μg/L) zinc concentration at 6 months.[2] It is, however, well known that the concentration of zinc in breast milk declines sharply in the first few months of lactation[51,52] and is independent of maternal zinc intake.[52] The infant's hepatic stores may subsidize the intake from breast milk for several months, but complementary foods (primarily meat) are required beginning between 4 and 6 months to prevent zinc deficiency and its consequences, including slowing of growth.

Infection

The Belarusan study[49] found a significantly reduced risk in the EBF group of one or more episodes of gastrointestinal infection in the first 12 months of life [adjusted Risk Ratio (RR)=0.61 (0.41–0.93)], but not in hospitalization for gastrointestinal infection [RR=0.79 (0.42–1.49)]. Pooled results from the Belarusan study,[49] an Australian study,[26] and a study from Arizona[54] showed no significant reduction in risk of upper respiratory infection, lower respiratory infection, hospitalization for respiratory infection, or otitis media.

Allergy

Both the Belarusan study[49] and a cohort study from Finland[55] recorded on **atopic eczema** at 1 year. The 2 studies showed statistical heterogeneity, with the Finnish study reporting a significantly reduced risk at 1 year of age [RR=0.40 (0.21–0.78)] but no reduction in risk at 5 years. The larger Belarusan study found a much lower absolute risk of atopic eczema in both feeding groups and no risk reduction with EBF. Although the Finnish study also reported a reduced risk of **food allergy** by history at 1 year in the EBF group, double food challenges showed no significant risk reduction,[54] and no reduction in risk was seen at 5 years.[55] Neither the Australian[26] nor Belarusan[49] studies found a significant reduction of recurrent (2 or more episodes) wheezing in the EBF group. In the Finnish study, the reduction of **any atopy** at 5 years in the EBF group was nonsignificant.[55] Both the Finnish[55] and Australian[26] studies reported no reduction in the risk for **asthma** at 5 to 6 years from EBF. Finally, the Australian study found no reduction in risk of a positive skin prick test at 6 years in the EBF group.[26]

Development

No studies from developed country settings have compared neurocognitive development or behavior in EBF versus MBF groups. Two controlled clinical trials from Honduras, however, reported that infants in the EBF group crawled significantly sooner (at an average of 0.8 months [0.3 to 1.3 months]) than those in the MBF group.[56] No difference was seen, however, in the mean age in which infants first sat from a lying position, and the 2 trials differed with respect to walking by 12 months, with a significantly lower proportion of exclusively EBF infants not walking by 12 months in the first trial [RR=0.66

(0.45–0.98)], but a nonsignificantly higher proportion not doing so in the second trial [RR=1.12 (0.90–1.38)]. Given the inconsistency in these results and the potential for biased maternal reporting due to nonblinding, no definitive conclusions can be drawn.

Summary

In summary, the systematic review based on a relatively small number of studies and study subjects that met criteria for inclusion concluded that infants who are exclusively breastfed for 6 months have a lower risk of gastrointestinal infection and show no growth deficits versus those who begin complementary foods (in addition to breastfeeding) at 3 or 4 months. No benefits of prolonged EBF have yet been demonstrated, however, with respect to risk of atopic disease or neurocognitive development. The number of studies that met criteria for inclusion in the review was too few to draw conclusions about nutrient sufficiency (ie, iron, zinc, vitamin D) from EBF in diverse populations.

Thus, the timing of introduction of complementary foods into the diet of the breastfed and formula-fed infant is difficult to define with precision. There is no evidence for harm when **safe, nutritious** complementary foods are introduced after 4 months when the infant is developmentally ready. Similarly, very few studies show significant benefit for delaying complementary foods until 6 months. A significant number of infants in all studies who are "low" breast milk consumers may be at risk for inadequate energy, protein, or micronutrient intake. **It seems reasonable, therefore, to recommend that in developing countries, where the use of potentially contaminated and/or low-nutrient dense foods puts infants at risk for diarrhea and undernutrition, infants should be exclusively breastfed for 6 months. If this is not the case (either in developing or, in particular, developed countries), complementary foods may be introduced between ages 4 and 6 months. This is a population-based recommendation, and the timing of introduction of complementary foods for an individual infant may differ from this recommendation.** *

Vitamin D Supplementation

Although the systematic review identified no studies comparing EBF and MBF with respect to vitamin D status, several case series suggest that breastfed infants living in temperate climates with limited sun exposure are at risk for vita-

---

*There is a difference of opinion among AAP experts on this matter. The Committee on Nutrition acknowledges that the Section on Breastfeeding recommends exclusive breastfeeding for at least 6 months.

min D deficiency and rickets unless they receive vitamin D supplements.[57,58] Because of current concerns about risk of sunlight exposure, even to young infants, all breastfed infants should receive 200 IU of vitamin D per day beginning within the first 2 months of life.

Formula-Fed Infants

No systematic review comparable to that summarized for breastfed infants has been undertaken to provide evidence about the timing and types of nonformula liquid and solid foods added to the diet of formula-fed infants. Infants who are formula-fed from birth should be given iron-fortified formula and need no complementary solid foods before approximately 6 months to meet their nutrient requirements. Given the iron, zinc, and vitamin D content of iron-fortified formulas, continued use of such a formula (in addition to solids) until the first birthday should effectively prevent deficiencies of these micronutrients.

Current Practice

The most recent National Health and Nutrition Examination Survey (NHANES III) data (Figures 6.1 and 6.2) show that almost 30% of breastfed

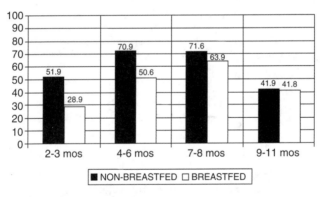

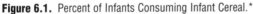

Figure 6.1. Percent of Infants Consuming Infant Cereal.*

*Source of data: National Health and Nutrition Examination Survey (NHANES III) 1988–1994. [Reference: US Department of Health and Human Services (DDHS), National Center for Health Statistics. Third National Health and Nutrition Examination Survey, 1988–1994, NHANES III Examination Data File: CD-ROM series 11 No 1A and No 2A released, July 1997 and April 1998, respectively. Public Use Data File Documentation Number 76200. Hyattsville, MD.]
Breastfed infants consumed >0 g of breast milk with and without infant formula; non-breastfed infants consumed no breast milk in the 24-hour recall.
Study Subjects: Infants aged 2 to 11 months with body weight measurement, and complete, reliable dietary interviews.

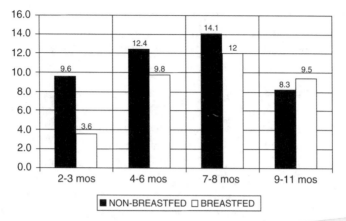

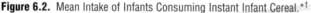

Figure 6.2. Mean Intake of Infants Consuming Instant Infant Cereal.*†

*Grams per day.
†Source of data: National Health and Nutrition Examination Survey (NHANES III) 1988–1994. [Reference: US Department of Health and Human Services (DDHS), National Center for Health Statistics. Third National Health and Nutrition Examination Survey, 1988–1994, NHANES III Examination Data File: CD-ROM series 11 No 1A and No 2A released, July 1997 and April 1998, respectively. Public Use Data File Documentation Number 76200. Hyattsville, MD.]
Breastfed infants consumed >0 g of breast milk with and without infant formula; non-breastfed infants consumed no breast milk in the 24-hour recall.
Mean intake based on infants who consumed only instant infant cereal.
Study Subjects: Infants aged 2 to 11 months with body weight measurement, and complete, reliable dietary interviews.

infants and more than 50% of formula-fed infants consume some infant cereal at 2 to 3 months. By 4 to 6 months, more than 50% of breastfed infants and 70% of formula-fed infants are consuming infant cereal. There is no nutritional indication to add complementary foods to the diet of the healthy term infant before age 4 months.

The general principle should be to introduce one "single-ingredient" new food at a time and not to introduce other new foods for 1 week so as to observe for possible allergic reactions. There is no evidence to support introducing foods in a particular order. The introduction of meat as an early complementary food has the advantage of providing iron and zinc, nutrients that may become limiting from human milk alone, in a highly bioavailable form.

Fruit juices should be limited to 4 to 6 oz/d after age 6 months. Excess juice intake (>250 mL/d) can lead to diarrhea because of the high fructose and sorbitol content of fruit juices.[59] (See also Chapter 7.) Neither breastfed nor formula-fed infants require extra water, even in hot, dry climates and even when febrile. Whole cow milk (and other "milks" not specifically formulated for infants) should be avoided in the first year of life. Among other nutritional issues concerning whole cow milk, the concentration and bioavailability of iron in whole cow milk are extremely low, and this is compounded by the increased occult fecal blood loss, and thus iron loss, that can occur.

Regardless of whether infants are breastfed or formula-fed and of the variety and quantity of complementary foods, each infant must still be managed individually, so that slow growth or other adverse outcomes are detected and appropriate interventions are provided. For breastfed infants, this means ensuring adequate breastfeeding techniques and optimizing breast milk intake and productivity by the mother before introducing complementary foods. Because of evidence that formula displaces breast milk more readily than does solid food,[60] complementary feeding of breastfed infants after 4 to 6 months of age should focus on solid foods, rather than formula. Breastfed and formula-fed infants may have their hemoglobin and mean corpuscular volume tested at 9 to 12 months of age to ensure adequate hematologic status and to initiate treatment if iron deficiency is suggested (see Chapter 19).

In the first year of life, solid foods should be sufficiently mashed or puréed so that they can be swallowed without risk of aspiration. Hot dogs, nuts, grapes, raisins, raw carrots, popcorn, and rounded candies should be avoided in children under age 4 years. Complementary foods should not be prepared with added salt or sugar. Solid foods should be warmed to body temperature but not excessively heated. When a microwave is used, it is important to mix the food thoroughly and for a responsible adult to check the temperature to avoid overheating the food and burning the infant's mouth.

American Academy of Pediatrics Recommendations

In the United States and Canada, processed infant foods have not been implicated in methemoglobinemia associated with food or water intake in infants. Although raw spinach and beets have a higher nitrate content than do other infant foods, one or more protective factors may prevent the extrinsic or intrinsic formation of toxic levels of nitrite from these foods as commercially processed for feeding of infants. Nitrate contamination of drinking water, which may occur from runoff from fields fertilized with nitrates, represents a potential hazard.

References

1. Cohen RJ, Brown KH, Canahuati J, Rivera LL, Dewey KG. Effects of age of introduction of complementary foods on infant breast milk intake, total energy intake, and growth: a randomized intervention study in Honduras. *Lancet.* 1994;344:288–293

2. Dewey KG, Cohen RJ, Brown KH, Rivera LL. Age of introduction of complementary foods and growth of term, low-birth-weight, breast-fed infants: a randomized intervention study in Honduras. *Am J Clin Nutr.* 1999;69:679–686

3. Drewitt R, Paymon B, Whiteby S. Effect of complementary feeds on sucking and milk intake in breastfed babies: an experimental study. *J Reprod Infant Psychol.* 1987;5:133–143

4. Stuff J, Nichols B. Nutrient intake and growth performance of older infants fed human milk. *J Pediatr.* 1989;115:959–968

5. Brown K, Dewey K, Allen L. *Complementary Feeding of Young Children in Developing Countries: A Review of Current Scientific Knowledge.* Geneva, Switzerland: World Health Organization; 1998

6. Kramer M, Kakuma R. *The Optimal Duration of Exclusive Breastfeeding: A Systematic Review.* Geneva, Switzerland: World Health Organization; 2001

7. Rowland MG, Barrell RA, Whitehead RG. Bacterial contamination in traditional Gambian weaning foods. *Lancet.* 1978;1:136–138

8. Rowland MG. The weanling's dilemma: are we making progress? *Acta Paediatr Scand Suppl.* 1986;323:33–42

9. Jason JM, Nieburg P, Marks JS. Mortality and infectious disease associated with infant-feeding practices in developing countries. *Pediatrics.* 1984;74:702–727

10. Feachem R, Koblinsky M. Interventions for the control of diarrhoeal diseases among young children: promotion of breast-feeding. *Bull World Health Organ.* 1984;62:271–291

11. WHO Collaborative Study Team on the Role of Breastfeeding on the Prevention of Infant Mortality. Effect of breastfeeding on infant and child mortality due to infectious diseases in less developed countries: a pooled analysis. *Lancet.* 2001;355: 451–455

12. Waterlow JC, Thomson AM. Observations on the adequacy of breast-feeding. *Lancet.* 1979;2:238–242

13. Whitehead RG, Paul AA. Growth charts and the assessment of infant feeding practices in the western world and in developing countries. *Early Hum Dev.* 1984;9:187–207

14. Shrimpton R, Victora CG, de Onis M, Costa Lima R, Blossner M, Clugston G. Worldwide timing of growth faltering: implications for nutritional interventions. *Pediatrics.* 2001;107:e75

15. FAO/WHO. *Energy and Protein Requirements.* 1973; Rome, Italy: FAO. 52: FAO Nutrition meetings

16. Whitehead RG, Paul AA. Infant growth and human milk requirements. A fresh approach. *Lancet.* 1981;161–163

17. World Health Organization. *Energy and Protein Requirements.* 1985; Report of a Joint FAO/WHO/UNU Expert Consultation ed, Geneva, Switzerland: Technical Report Series. 724

18. Garza C, Butte NF. Energy intakes of human milk-fed infants during the first year. *J Pediatr.* 1990;117:S124–S131

19. Butte NF. Energy requirements of infants. *Eur J Clin Nutr*. 1996;50(suppl):S24–S36

20. Howie PW, Forsyth JF, Ogston SA, Clark A, Florey CD. Protective effect of breast feeding against infection. *BMJ*. 1990;300:11–16

21. Cunningham AS, Jelliffe DB, Jelliffe EF. Breast-feeding and health in the 1980s: a global epidemiologic review. *J Pediatr*. 1991;118:659–666

22. Raisler J, Alexander C, O'Campo P. Breast-feeding and infant illness: a dose-response relationship? *Am J Public Health*. 1999;89:25–30

23. Ford RP, Taylor BJ, Mitchell EA, et al. Breastfeeding and the risk of sudden infant death syndrome. *Int J Epidemiol*. 1993;22:885–890

24. Saarinen UJ, Kajosaari M, Backman A, Simes MA. Prolonged breast-feeding as pro-phylaxis for atopic disease. *Lancet*. 1979;2:163–166

25. Hide DM, Guyer BM. Clinical manifestations of allergy related to breast and cow's milk feeding. *Arch Dis Child*. 1981;56:172–175

26. Oddy WH, Holt PG, Sly PD, et al. Association between breast feeding and asthma in 6 year old children: findings of a prospective birth cohort study. *BMJ*. 1999;319:815–819

27. Kramer MS, Moroz B. Do breast-feeding and delayed introduction of solid foods protect against subsequent atopic eczema? *J Pediatr*. 1981;98:546–550

28. von Kries R, Koletzko B, Sauerwald T, et al. Breast feeding and obesity: cross sec-tional study. *BMJ*. 1999;319:147–150

29. Mayer EJ, Hamman RF, Gay EC, et al. Reduced risk of IDDM among breast-fed children. The Colorado IDDM Registry. *Diabetes*. 1988;37:1625–1632

30. Gerstein H. Cow's milk exposure and type-I diabetes mellitus: a critical overview of the clinical literature. *Diabetes Care*. 1994;17:13–19

31. Koletzko S, Sherman P, Corey M, Griffiths A, Smith C. Role of infant feeding prac-tices in development of Crohn's disease in childhood. *BMJ*. 1989;298:1617–1618

32. Davis MK, Savitz DA, Graubard BI. Infant feeding and childhood cancer. *Lancet*. 1988;2:365–368

33. Davis MK. Review of the evidence for an association between infant feeding and childhood cancer. *Int J Cancer Suppl*. 1998;11:29–33

34. Lucas A, Morley R, Cole TJ, Lister G, Leeson-Payne C. Breast milk and subsequent intelligence quotient in children born preterm. *Lancet*. 1992;339:261–264

35. Lanting CI, Fidler V, Huisman M, Touwen BC, Boersma ER. Neurological differ-ences between 9-year-old children fed breast-milk or formula-milk as babies. *Lancet*. 1994;344:1319–1322

36. Horwood J, Fergusson DM. Breastfeeding and later cognitive and academic out-comes. *Pediatrics*. 1998;101:e9

37. Anderson JW, Johnstone BM, Remley DT. Breast-feeding and cognitive develop-ment: a meta-analysis. *Am J Clin Nutr*. 1999;70:525–535

38. WHO Working Group on Infant Growth. An Evaluation of Infant Growth. Geneva, Switzerland: World Health Organization; 1994

39. Dewey KG, Peerson JM, Brown KH, et al. Growth of breast-fed infants deviates from current reference data: a pooled analysis of US, Canadian, and European data sets. *Pediatrics.* 1995;96:495–503

40. Nielsen GA, Thomsen BL, Michaelsen KF. Influence of breastfeeding and complementary food on growth between 5 and 10 months. *Acta Paediatr.* 1998;87:911–917

41. Hediger ML, Overpeck MD, Ruan WJ, Troendle JF. Early infant feeding and growth status of US-born infants and children aged 4–71 mo: analyses from the third National Health and Nutrition Examination Survey, 1988–1994. *Am J Clin Nutr.* 2000;72:159–167

42. Haschke F, van't Hof MA. Euro-Growth references for breast-fed boys and girls: influence of breast-feeding and solids on growth until 36 months of age. *J Pediatr Gastroenterol Nutr.* 2000;31:S60–S71

43. de Onis M, Garza C, Habicht J. Time for a new growth reference. *Pediatrics.* 1997;100:E8

44. WHO Working Group on the Growth Reference Protocol and WHO Task Force on Methods for the Natural Regulation of Fertility. Growth patterns of breastfed infants in seven countries. *Acta Paediatr.* 2000;89:215–222

45. World Health Organization. Nutrition. Information and attitudes among health personnel about early feeding practices. *Wkly Epidemiol.* 1995;70:117–120

46. United Nations Children's Fund. Facts for Life. New York, NY: UNICEF, WHO, UNESCO, UNFPA; 1993

47. World Health Organization. *Infant and Young Child Nutrition.* Geneva, Switzerland: 2001; Fifty-Fourth World Health Assembly. 54.2

48. Frongillo EJ, de Onis M, Garza C. The World Health Organization Task Force on Methods for the Natural Regulation of Fertility. Effects of timing of complementary foods on post-natal growth. *FASEB J.* 1997;11:A574

49. Kramer MS, Chalmers B, Hodnett ED, et al. Promotion of Breastfeeding Intervention Trial (PROBIT): a randomized trial in the Republic of Belarus. *JAMA.* 2001;285:413–420

50. Pisacane A, de Vizia B, Valiante A, et al. Iron status in breast-fed infants. *J Pediatr.* 1995;127:429–431

51. Jensen R. *Handbook of Milk Composition.* San Diego, CA: Academic Press Inc; 1995

52. Krebs NF, Reidinger CJ, Hartley S, Robertson AD, Hambidge KM. Zinc supplementation during lactation: effects on maternal status and milk zinc concentrations. *Am J Clin Nutr.* 1995;61:1030–1036

53. Duncan B, Ey J, Holberg CJ, Wright AL, Martinez FD, Taussig LM. Exclusive breast-feeding for at least 4 months protects against otitis media. *Pediatrics.* 1993;91:867–872

54. Kajosaari M, Saarinen UM. Prophylaxis of atopic disease by six months' total solid food elimination. Evaluation of 135 exclusively breast-fed infants of atopic families. *Acta Paediatr Scand.* 1983;72:411–414

55. Kajosaari M. Atopy prevention in childhood: the role of diet. A prospective 5-year follow-up of high-risk infants with six months exclusive breastfeeding and solid food elimination. *Pediatr Allergy Immunol.* 1994;5:26–28

56. Dewey KG, Cohen RJ, Brown KH, Rivera LL. Effects of exclusive breastfeeding for four versus six months on maternal nutritional status and infant motor development: results of two randomized trials in Honduras. *J Nutr.* 2001;131:262–267

57. Namgung R, Tsang RC, Lee C, Han DG, Ho ML, Sierra RI. Low total body bone mineral content and high bone resorption in Korean winter-born versus summer-born newborn infants. *J Pediatr.* 1998;132:421–425

58. Kreiter SR, Schwartz RP, Kirkman HN, Charlton PA, Calikoglu AS, Davenport ML. Nutritional rickets in African American breast-fed infants. *J Pediatr.* 2000; 137:153–157

59. American Academy of Pediatrics, Committee on Nutrition. The use and misuse of fruit juice in pediatrics. *Pediatrics.* 2001;107:1210–1213

60. Hörnell A, Hofvander Y, Kylberg E. Solids and formula: association with pattern and duration of breastfeeding. *Pediatrics.* 2001;107:E38

II
Feeding the Child and Adolescent

7

Feeding the Child

After infancy, children experience significant developmental progress that is fundamentally tied to the evolution and establishment of eating behavior. In contrast to infancy, however, the period from 1 year of age to puberty is a slower period of physical growth. Birth weight triples during the first year of life but does not quadruple until 2 years; birth length increases by 50% during the first year but does not double until 4 years. Although growth patterns vary in individual children, children from 2 years to puberty gain an average of 2 to 3 kg ($4^1/_2$ to $6^1/_2$ lb) and grow 5 to 8 cm ($2^1/_2$ to $3^1/_2$ in) in height per year. As growth rates decline during the preschool years, appetites decrease and food intake may appear erratic and unpredictable. Parental confusion and concern are not uncommon. Frequently expressed concerns include the limited variety of foods ingested, dawdling and distractibility, limited consumption of vegetables and meats, and a desire for too many sweets. Parental concern about children's eating behaviors, whether warranted or unfounded, should be addressed with developmentally appropriate nutrition information. Anticipatory guidance for parents and caregivers is key to preventing many feeding problems.

An important goal of early childhood nutrition is to ensure children's present and future health by fostering the development of healthy eating behaviors. Caregivers are called on to offer foods at developmentally appropriate moments—matching the children's age and stage of development with their nutrition needs. (See Cow Milk on page 95.) Appropriate limits for children's eating are set by adhering to a division of responsibility in child feeding.[1] Caregivers are responsible for providing a variety of nutritious foods, defining the structure and timing of meals, and creating a mealtime environment that facilitates eating and social exchange. Children are responsible for participating in choices about food selection and should take primary responsibility for determining how much is consumed at each eating occasion.

Toddlers

Toddlers' eating patterns are characterized by independence both in terms of the physical skills that allow them to become mobile and to self-feed as well as the language skills acquired that enable the toddler to verbally express eating preferences and needs. Physically, the tasks or milestones related to eating include the continued development and coordination of biting, chewing, and swallowing and the mastery of self-feeding with hands or spoons and by drinking from a cup. Bedtime bottles should be strongly discouraged because of their association with dental caries, as should bottles containing juice at any time of the day.[2] At 15 months, the toddler is generally capable of self-feeding prepared table foods and should be weaned to a cup—albeit with less than perfect efficiency and a propensity for spills. Supporting self-feeding is also thought to encourage the maintenance of self-regulation of energy intake and the mastery of feeding skills. Given earlier opportunities for mastery of self-feeding skills, the older toddler (2 years) is ready to consume most of the same foods offered to the rest of the family—with some extra preparation to prevent choking and gagging.

At the beginning of toddlerhood, children typically speak in 1- or 2-word sentences, such as "more" or "no" or "all gone." Between the first and second year, infants move from gross motor skills required for holding a spoon to developing fine motor skills needed to scoop food and bring the spoon to the mouth. Toddlers are continually engaged in understanding the cause-effect relationship. In the eating domain, this translates into using utensils to move foods, using food and eating to elicit responses from the parent. These interactions are part of children's learning about the family's and the culture's standards for behavior; children as young as 2 years of age have demonstrated the ability to evaluate their actions according to the actions' badness or goodness in relation to parental standards for behavior.[3] An example of this type of learning is the toddler's response of "uh-oh" to dropping food or drink on the floor.

Although generally explorative, toddlers tend to go on food "jags," where certain foods are preferentially consumed to the exclusion of others.[4,5] Parents who become concerned when a "good eater" in infancy becomes a "fair to poor" eater as a toddler should be reassured that this change in acceptance is developmentally normative.

Preventing Choking
Gagging and choking are realistic concerns for the toddler. The chewing and swallowing functions are not fully developed until 8 years of age, and a number of precautions should be followed to avoid choking. The toddler should be given foods that gradually build self-feeding skills, starting with soft, mashed,

or ground foods and building to prepared table foods by 15 to 18 months. Foods that may be hard to control in the mouth and may be easily lodged in the esophagus should be avoided, such as nuts, raw carrots, popcorn, and round candy. Other potentially problematic foods, like hot dogs, grapes, and string cheese, may be modified by cutting them into small pieces. The caregiver should always be present during feeding and children should be seated in a high chair during mealtimes. The mealtime environment ideally should be free of distractions like television, loud music, and activities. Eating in the car should be discouraged because (1) aiding the child quickly is difficult if the only adult present is driving, and (2) with obesity prevention in mind, eating should not be encouraged in environments that are not related to family meals (ie, in cars, in front of television/computers). Finally, analgesics used to numb the gums during teething may anesthetize the posterior pharynx. Children who receive such medications should be carefully observed during feeding (Table 7.1).

Preschoolers

The preschooler has more fully developed motor skills, handles utensils and cups efficiently, and can sit at the table for meals. Since growth has slowed, the preschooler's interest in eating may be unpredictable with characteristic periods of disinterest in food or appetite suppression. The attention span of preschoolers may limit the amount of time that they can spend in the

Table 7.1.
Guidelines for Feeding Safety, Preschool Children*

- Insist that children eat sitting down so they can concentrate on chewing and swallowing.
- An adult should supervise children while they eat.
- Foods on which preschoolers often choke, such as hot dogs, peanut butter, hard pieces of fruit, and vegetables, should be avoided for children younger than 3 years.
- Well-cooked foods, modified so the child can chew and swallow without difficulty, should be offered.
- Eating in the car should be avoided because driving the car to the side of the road safely while assisting the child is difficult if the child chokes.
- Rub-on teething medications can cause problems with chewing and swallowing because the muscles in the throat may also become numb. Children who receive such medications should be carefully observed during feeding.

*From Pipes PL, Trahms CM. *Nutrition in Infancy and Childhood.* 5th ed. St Louis, MO: Mosby-Year Book; 1993.

mealtime setting; however, they should be encouraged to attend and partake in family meals for reasonable periods of time (15 to 20 minutes), whether they choose to eat or not.

As children move from toddlerhood to the preschool years, they become increasingly aware of the environment in which eating occurs, particularly the social aspects of eating. By interacting with and observing other children and adults, preschool-aged children become more aware of when and where eating takes place, what types of foods are consumed at specific eating occasions (ie, ice cream is a dessert food), and how much of those foods are consumed at each eating occasion (ie, "finish your vegetables"). As a consequence of this increased attendance, children's food selection and intake patterns are influenced by a variety of environmental cues, including the time of day,[6] portion size,[7] controlling child feeding practices, including restriction and pressure to eat,[8,9] and the preferences and eating behaviors of important others.[10,11]

During the preschool period, most children have moved from eating on demand to a more adult-like eating pattern—consuming 3 meals each day as well as several smaller snacks. While children's food intake from meal to meal may appear to be erratic, total daily energy intake remains fairly constant.[12] Children show the ability to respond to the energy content of foods by adjusting their intake to reflect the energy density of the diet.[8,13] In contrast to their skills in regulation of food intake, young children do not appear to have the innate ability to choose a well-balanced diet.[4,5] Rather, they depend on adults to offer them a variety of nutritious and developmentally appropriate foods and to model the consumption of those foods.

Food Neophobia

Children between the ages of 2 and 5 years become characteristically resistant to consuming new foods, and sometimes dietary variety diminishes to 4 or 5 well-accepted favorites. It should be stressed to families that this is a normal stage of child development that, while potentially frustrating, can be dealt with effectively with knowledge, consistency, and patience. From the standpoint of normal development, the job of the preschool years is individuation through learning. Parents should be advised that food acceptance is facilitated when children are given repeated exposures (between 5 and 10) to new foods and opportunities to learn about food and eating.[14] This requires persistence on the part of the provider and a certain level of trust that, even in the face of temporary rejection, children can learn to like new foods and that children can self-regulate energy intake so that adequate food and energy will be consumed to sustain growth and health.

School-Aged Children

During the school years, increases in memory and logic abilities are accompanied by reading, writing, math skills, and knowledge. This is the period in which basic nutrition education concepts can be successfully introduced. Emphasis should be placed on enjoying the taste of fruits and vegetables rather than to focus exclusively on their healthfulness because young children tend to think of taste and healthfulness as mutually exclusive.[15] Socially, children are learning rules and conventions and also begin to develop friendships. During the period between 8 and 11 years, children begin making more peer comparisons, including those pertaining to weight and body shape. An awareness of the physical self begins to emerge and comparisons with social norms for weight and weight status begin to occur. During this period, children vary greatly in weight, body shape, and growth rate, and teasing of those who fall outside the perceived norms for weight status frequently occurs. Friends and those outside the family can alter food attitudes and choices, which may have either a beneficial or a negative effect on the nutritional status of a given child. Television is another source of influence on young children's eating, given that a majority of US school-aged children watch at least 2 hours of television each day.[16] The more time children spend watching television, the more likely they are to have higher energy intakes, consume greater amounts of pizza, salty snacks, and soda, and to be overweight than children who watch television less.[16–19]

School-aged children have increased freedom over their food choices and, during the school year, eat at least one meal per day away from the home. These choices, such as the decision to consume school lunch or a snack bar meal, may impact dietary quality.[20]

Dieting

Girls as young as 5 years of age possess some understanding of the concept of dieting.[21] Reports of dieting, or attempts to restrict calories, fat, or the intake of specific foods, emerge in children as young as 8 years of age.[22] In general, the restriction of specific foods should be discouraged. Adults can help promote a shift toward healthy eating—increased variety, adequate intake of fruits, vegetables, and calcium-rich foods, and the routine consumption of planned meals and snacks—by making sure those foods are available in the home, continuing to guide children's food choices, and modeling the eating and physical activity behaviors they wish for children to adopt. Children vary extensively in body shape; therefore, references to cultural ideals and popular role models who promote unrealistic goals for thinness should be avoided and countered with examples of successful individuals who exemplify healthy goals for image and weight.

Energy and Nutrient Needs

Current survey data indicate that fruit and vegetable intake among children 2 to 18 years of age is well below current recommendations, while the intake of discretionary fat and added sugar is high.[23,24] Fat intake as a percent of dietary energy decreased from 1988 to 1994 but still remains above current recommendations; only 1 in 4 children currently meet guidelines for fat and saturated fat.[25] Further, low-nutrient-dense foods represent a high contribution to dietary energy and fat intakes; the top 10 foods contributing to energy intakes in 2- to 18-year-old children are milk, yeast bread, cakes/cookies/quick breads/doughnuts, beef, ready-to-eat cereal, soft drinks, cheese, potato chips/corn chips/popcorn, sugars/syrup/jams, and poultry. As a result of this pattern of intake, many children's diets rely on fortified foods to obtain vitamins and minerals.[26] Recent population studies confirm that children in low-income families and homeless children have a higher incidence of inadequate dietary intake.[27,28]

Dietary Reference Intakes (DRIs) are a new set of 4 nutrient-based reference values that can be used for planning and assessing diets of individuals and groups[29] (see Appendix C). They are meant to replace the former Recommended Dietary Allowances (RDAs). The DRIs include data on safety and efficacy, reduction of chronic degenerative disease (rather than the avoidance of nutritional deficiency), and upper levels of intake (where available). The Estimated Average Requirement (EAR) refers to the median usual intake value that is estimated to meet the requirements of one half of apparently healthy individuals of a given age and gender, over time. The RDA refers to the level of intake that is adequate for nearly all healthy individuals of a given gender and age. When the EAR or RDA has not been established, an Adequate Intake (AI) is provided as a standard. The Tolerable Upper Intake Level (UL) is the highest level of continuing daily nutrient intake that is likely to pose no risk of adverse health effects in almost all individuals. The UL, however, is not intended to be a recommended level of intake. Using the age- and gender-specific EAR, it is possible to make a quantitative statistical assessment of the adequacy of an individual's usual intake of a nutrient and to assess the safety of an individual's usual intake by comparison with the UL.

Energy needs are the most variable in children and depend on basal metabolism, rate of growth, physical activity, body size, sex, and onset of puberty. (See also Chapter 15.) Many nutrient requirements depend on energy needs and intake. Micronutrients that are most likely to be low or deficient in the diets of young children are calcium, iron, zinc, vitamin B_6, magnesium, and vitamin A.[30,31]

Supplements

Parents frequently ask health care providers whether their children need vitamin supplements, and many routinely give these supplements to their children. The children who receive the supplements are not necessarily the children who need them most, however, and, in some cases, adequate amounts of the marginal nutrients, such as calcium and zinc, are not included in the supplement. Routine supplementation is not necessary for healthy, growing children who consume a varied diet. For children and adolescents who cannot or will not consume adequate amounts of micronutrients from any dietary sources, the use of mineral supplements should be considered. Children at nutritional risk who may benefit from supplementation include those

- With anorexia or an inadequate appetite or who follow fad diets
- With chronic disease (eg, cystic fibrosis, inflammatory bowel disease, or hepatic disease)
- From deprived families or who suffer parental neglect or abuse
- Who participate in a dietary program for managing obesity
- Who consume a vegetarian diet without adequate dairy products
- With failure to thrive
- Infants that are breastfed unless they are weaned to at least 500 mL per day of vitamin D-fortified formula or milk
- Nonbreastfed infants who are ingesting less than 500 mL per day of vitamin D-fortified formula or milk
- Children and adolescents who do not get regular sunlight exposure, do not ingest at least 500 mL per day of vitamin D-fortified milk, or do not take a daily multivitamin supplement containing at least 200 IU of vitamin D

Evaluation of the dietary intake should be included in any assessment of the need for supplementation. If parents wish to give their children supplements, a standard pediatric vitamin-mineral product containing nutrients in amounts no larger than the DRI (EAR or RDA) poses no risk. Megadose levels should be discouraged and counseling provided about the toxic effects, especially of fat-soluble vitamins. Because the taste, shape, and color of most pediatric preparations are as attractive as candy, parents should be cautioned to keep them out of reach of children. (Refer to Chapters 18 through 21 for more information on vitamins and minerals.)

Dietary Fat

During the past decade, emphasis and educational efforts supporting low-fat, low-cholesterol diets for the general population have increased. A variety of health organizations, including the American Academy of Pediatrics (AAP), recommend against fat or cholesterol restriction for infants <2 years when rapid growth and development require high-energy intakes. For this reason, nonfat and low-fat milks are not recommended for use during the first 2 years of life. Subsequently, fat intake should be gradually decreased during the toddler years so that fat intake, averaged across several days, should provide approximately 30% of total energy.[32,33] Parents should be reassured that this level of intake is sufficient for adequate growth.[34,35] Transitioning children's diets to provide 30% energy from fat can be achieved by substituting grain products, fruits, vegetables, low-fat milk products or other calcium-rich foods, beans, lean meat, poultry, fish, or other protein-rich foods for higher fat foods. Because concerns have been expressed that some parents and their children may over-interpret the need to restrict their fat intakes, a lower limit of 20% of energy from fat has been identified.

Dietary Guidelines

The US Department of Agriculture has developed 2 main nutritional guides that can be used in feeding children. *Dietary Guidelines for Americans*, 5th edition, is intended for children 2 years and older and represents 10 basic principles that fall within 3 main concepts of (1) Aim for fitness, (2) Build a healthy base, and (3) Choose sensibly—for good health.[36]

The second main source of dietary guidance for children is the *Food Guide Pyramid for Young Children*[37] (see Appendix M), which translates the *Dietary Guidelines* into food group-based recommendations for a healthful diet among young children. In addition to helping parents understand the number of servings children need from each food group, this tool can be used to convey basic nutrition concepts for feeding young children such as variety, moderation, the allowance for all types of foods in the diet, and appropriate portion sizes.

Recognition that appropriate child portions are considerably smaller than those for adults is important in light of increasing standard portions[38] and evidence that children increase their intake of foods as the portion size is increased.[7] Table 7.2 gives examples of how appropriate portion sizes differ by age across food groups. One rule for portions that may be followed for preschool children is to initially offer 1 tablespoon of each food for every year of age, with more provided according to appetite.[1]

Because of smaller capacities and fluctuating appetites, most young children fare best when fed 4 to 6 times a day. Snacks should be considered mini-meals and planned so they contribute to the total day's nutrient intake. Healthful snacks accepted by many children include fresh fruit, cheese, whole-grain crackers, bread products (eg, bagels, pita, tortillas, and rice crackers), milk, raw vegetables, 100% fruit juices, sandwiches, peanut butter, and yogurt.

Parenting and the Feeding Relationship

Parenting in the feeding domain can be quite challenging, particularly during the toddler and preschool years. Satter's division of responsibility, in which parents provide structure in mealtime and a healthy variety of foods and opportunities for learning and the child ultimately decides how much and whether to eat on a given eating occasion, represents a sound theoretical basis for implementing appropriate child-feeding practices.[1]

Structure and routine for eating occasions is particularly important for the young child. Children can be moved to a more adult-like eating pattern with opportunities for consumption being centered on meals and snacks (4 to 6 per day) and limited grazing in between. Adults should decide when food is offered or available and the child should be left to decide how much and whether to eat at a given eating occasion. The physical environment should also be structured to promote healthy eating with distractions from television or other activities avoided. Ideally, eating should occur in a designated area of the home with a developmentally appropriate chair for the child. Family meals, where adults are present and eating at least some of the same foods as children, provide occasions to learn and model healthful eating habits as well as opportunities to include the social aspects of eating.

The "job" of early childhood is to learn about the self and the external environment. To facilitate learning in the eating domain, parents should provide

Table 7.2.
Feeding Guide for Children*

Food	Age, y						Comments
	2 to 3		**4 to 6**		**7 to 12**		
	Portion Size	Servings	Portion Size	Servings	Portion Size	Servings	
Milk and dairy	$1/2$ c (4 oz)	4–5 16–20 oz total	$1/2$–$3/4$ c (4–6 oz)	3–4 24–32 oz total	$1/2$–1 c (4–8 oz)	3–4 24–32 oz total	The following may be substituted for $1/2$ c fluid milk: $1/2$–$3/4$ oz cheese, $1/2$ cup yogurt, $2 1/2$ tbsp nonfat dry milk
Meat, fish, poultry, or equivalent	1–2 oz	2 2–4 oz total	1–2 oz	2 2–4 oz total	2 oz	3–4 6–8 oz total	The following may be substituted for 1 oz meat, fish, or poultry: 1 egg, 2 tbsp peanut butter, 4–5 tbsp cooked legumes
Vegetables and fruit		4–5		4–5		3–4	Include one green leafy or yellow vegetable for vitamin A, such as carrots, spinach, broccoli, winter squash, or greens
Vegetables							
Cooked	2–3 tbsp		3–4 tbsp		$1/4$–$1/2$ c		
Raw†	Few pieces		Few Pieces		Several pieces		
Fruit							Include one vitamin C-rich fruit, vegetable, or juice, such as citrus juices, orange, grapefruit, strawberries, melon, tomato, or broccoli
Raw	$1/2$–1 small		$1/2$–1 small		1 medium		
Canned	2–4 tbsp		4–6 tbsp		$1/4$–$1/2$ c		
Juice†	3–4 oz		4 oz		4 oz		
Grain products Whole grain or enriched bread	$1/2$–1 slice	3–4	1 slice	3–4	1 slice	4–5	The following may be substituted for 1 slice of bread: $1/2$ c spaghetti, macaroni, noodles, or rice; 5 saltines; $1/2$ English muffin or bagel; 1 tortilla; corn grits or posole
Cooked cereal	$1/4$–$1/2$ c		$1/2$ c		$1/2$–1 c		
Dry cereal	$1/2$–1 c		1 c		1 c		

*Adapted from Lowenberg ME. Development of food patterns in young children. In: Pipes PL, Trahms CM, eds. *Nutrition Infancy and Childhood*. 5th ed. St Louis, MO: Mosby-Year Book; 1993:168–169. With permission of Times Mirror/Mosby College Publishing.
†Do not give to young children until they can chew well.

repeated opportunities for learning about new foods and about normative eating behavior. Research suggests that it takes many exposures (up to 8 to 10) to help a child accept a novel food and, therefore, patience and consistency are required to facilitate children's acceptance of foods, like vegetables and meat, that are not sweet.[14] However, parental responsibility falls short of "getting" children to eat or like particular foods. Pressuring children to consume foods or rewarding them for consuming specific foods is counterproductive in the long run because it is likely to build resistance and food dislikes rather than acceptance. Instead, considering mealtime from the child's perspective, where everything is new and different, and recognizing that "finicky eating" is a normal stage of development that children outgrow, is a more productive outlook. Parents' concerns can be diminished if the focus becomes the adequacy of children's growth rather than children's behavior at individual eating occasions.

Young children respond well when appropriate maturity demands are made. Children want to learn and want to eat. They also desire to participate in decisions about their own eating. Allowing them the opportunities for mastery of eating, even when it translates into extra work and mess, ultimately promotes self-regulation and autonomy. Experience is the only established predictor of acceptance and liking. Therefore, encouraging learning—using all senses and various modes for learning (eg, food shopping and preparation, reading to children about food, eating and cultures)—can promote more enthusiasm for trying new foods.

Special Topics

Feeding During Illness

A common treatment for acute diarrhea has been a clear liquid diet until symptoms improve. The AAP clinical practice guideline on the management of acute gastroenteritis in young children recommends that only oral electrolyte solutions be used to rehydrate infants and young children and that a normal diet be continued throughout an episode of gastroenteritis.[39] (See also Chapter 28.) Infants and young children can experience a decrease in nutritional status and the illness can be prolonged with a clear liquid diet, especially when it is extended beyond a few days.[40] Continuous or early refeeding has been shown to shorten the duration of the diarrhea. Recommendations for toddlers and preschoolers include reintroduction of solid foods shortly after rehydration. Foods that are usually well tolerated include rice cereals, bananas, potatoes, eggs, rice, plain pasta, and other similar foods. Dairy products in recommended amounts can also be included. During viral illnesses, colds, and other acute childhood illnesses, a variety of foods should be offered according to the child's appetite and tolerance, with extra fluids provided when fever, diarrhea, or vomiting is present.

Breakfast

Breakfast intake among children makes a significant contribution to daily nutrient intake.[41,42] In addition, skipping breakfast or consuming an inadequate breakfast, has been associated with poor school performance.[43,44] Ready-to-eat cereal is among the top contributors to folate, vitamin A, vitamin C, iron, and zinc intakes in young children's diets.[26] United States Department of Agriculture School Breakfast Programs have been shown to improve the nutrient intakes of its participants, who tend to be younger, male, from low-income families, and of African American and Hispanic heritage.[45]

Obesity (see also Chapter 33)

The prevalence of overweight among children has increased dramatically over the past 2 decades and is alarmingly high, where currently 25% of children aged 2 to 18 are overweight.[46] Overweight children are at increased risk of social stigmatization, hyperlipidemia, abnormal glucose tolerance, non–insulin-dependent diabetes mellitus, and hypertension.[47] Environmental influences that promote problematic eating have been given increasing attention in light of the fact that secular increases in overweight have occurred too rapidly to be explained by genetic influences alone.[48,49] Parents have an important role in the etiology of childhood overweight because they provide children with both genes and the environment in which eating and physical activity take place. Evidence of this point is found in the fact that the tracking of childhood overweight into adulthood is particularly strong among children who have one or more overweight parents.[50]

It is recommended that children ≥3 years of age with body mass index (BMI) scores ≥85th percentile with complications of obesity, or with a BMI percentile of ≥95th percentile with or without complications, undergo evaluation and possible treatment.[51] Where possible, guidance to promote healthful eating patterns in the overweight child should be directed to modify the dietary intake patterns and behaviors of the family as a whole rather than targeted specifically at the child. Referring the family for nutrition education and counseling may be useful to help parents discuss behavioral issues involved in child feeding. These discussions should focus on the types of foods that are available in the home, identifying appropriate portion sizes, and incorporating micronutrient rich, low-energy density foods into the child's and family's diet. Parents should also be made aware that highly restrictive approaches to child feeding are not effective, but rather appear to promote the intake of restricted foods[9,52] and contribute to low self-appraisal.[53] Further, parents should be encouraged to exhibit the eating behaviors they would like their children to adopt because children learn to model their parents' eating behavior.[11,20]

Increased physical activity is a critical component of childhood obesity prevention and treatment because low-energy diets may compromise the nutrient status of growing children.[54] Sedentary behavior has been associated with overweight among children[19,55]; practitioners should inquire about the amount of time a child spends in front of television, computers, and video monitors and encourage parents to set daily limits for their children. Caregivers have a central responsibility in this area because they serve as role models for active lifestyles and provide opportunities to children to be physically active. Health care providers should convey the importance of encouraging activity of the family as a whole as well as among individuals within the family. Children should be encouraged to participate in discussions about diet and activity modifications, both to take into account their preferences and allow them a sense of responsibility for decisions about their behavior.

Beverage Consumption

Fruit juices and soft drinks, including fruit-flavored and carbonated drinks, are increasingly common beverages consumed by young children at home and in group settings. These types of beverages provide roughly 10% of energy in 2- to 19-year-old children's diets, with soft drinks providing as much as 8% of total daily energy for adolescents.[25] Soft drinks in particular have been shown to replace milk in the diet, which can have a negative impact on nutrient, particularly calcium, intakes.[56–58] Failure to thrive has been anecdotally associated with excessive intake of fruit juice,[59] and at least one study found carbohydrate malabsorption following consumption of fruit juices in healthy children and in children with chronic nonspecific diarrhea.[60] In addition, excessive weight and adiposity have been linked to excess energy-containing beverage consumption.[25,61] For young children with either chronic diarrhea or excessive weight gain, obtaining a diet history, including the volume of soft drinks consumed, and then providing guidance on limits for these beverages, is useful. Parents should be encouraged to routinely offer plain, unflavored water to children, particularly for fluids consumed outside of meals and snacks.[62]

> **The American Academy of Pediatrics Recommends the following:**
> 1. Juice should not be introduced into the diet of infants before 6 months of age.
> 2. Infants should not be given juice from bottles or easily transportable covered cups that allow them to consume juice easily throughout the day. Infants should not be given juice at bedtime.
> 3. Intake of fruit juice should be limited to 4 to 6 oz/d for children 1 to 6 years old. For children 7 to 18 years old, juice intake should be limited to 8 to 12 oz or 2 servings per day.
> 4. Children should be encouraged to eat whole fruits to meet their recommended daily fruit intake.
> 5. Infants, children, and adolescents should not consume unpasteurized juice.
> 6. In the evaluation of children with malnutrition (overnutrition and undernutrition), the health care provider should determine the amount of juice being consumed.
> 7. In the evaluation of children with chronic diarrhea, excessive flatulence, abdominal pain, and bloating, the health care provider should determine the amount of juice being consumed.
> 8. In the evaluation of dental caries, the amount and means of juice consumption should be determined.
> 9. Pediatricians should routinely discuss the use of fruit juice and fruit drinks and should educate parents about differences between the two.
>
> *Pediatrics.* 2001;107:1210–1213

The Role of Anticipatory Guidance in Promoting Healthy Eating Behaviors

The feeding relationship is vital for its role in promoting healthy growth and development but also for its function in engendering healthy behaviors and habits that can prevent the advent of chronic disease. Beyond physiological outcomes associated with poor eating habits and environments, the feeding relationship is critical for establishing a healthy parent-child relationship. Feeding, at its best, provides opportunities for pleasure, learning, and attaining security, as well as occasions for self-discovery and learning self-control.

A healthy feeding environment requires structure, knowledge, supportive limit setting and parenting, an appreciation of children's developing capabilities and, perhaps most of all, patience. The pediatrician's role includes the timely delivery of information that links children's individual development to their nutrition needs. Each well-child visit can be structured to include nutrition guidance that is relevant to the individual child's development and growth. Information about a child's growth and weight status (by use of BMI curves adjusted for sex and age) and interpretation of the child's growth tracking, over time, is both important and enlightening for parents. Further, anticipating and addressing problematic childhood behaviors (eg, neophobia and preferences for sweet-tasting foods) and framing them in a developmental light often alleviates parental over-concern. Pediatricians can support the families by offering continued encouragement and direction about the benefits of a varied diet, appropriate expectations for children's intake, and the importance of physical activity for children and families.

References

1. Satter E. *How to Get Your Kid to Eat ... But Not Too Much*. Palo Alto, CA: Bull Publishing Company; 1987
2. American Academy of Pediatrics, Committee on Nutrition. The use and misuse of fruit juice in pediatrics. *Pediatrics*. 2000;107:1210–1213
3. Burhans KK, Dweck CS. Helplessness in early childhood: the role of contingent worth. *Child Dev*. 1995;66:1719–1738
4. Davis CM. Self-selection of diet by newly weaned infants. *Am J Dis Child*. 1928; 36:651–679
5. Davis CM. Results of the self-selection of diets by young children. *Can Med Assoc J*. 1939;41:257–261
6. Birch LL, Billman J, Richards SS. Time of day influences food acceptability. *Appetite*. 1984;5:109–116
7. Rolls BJ, Engell D, Birch LL. Serving portion size influences 5-year-old but not 3-year-old children's food intakes. *J Am Diet Assoc*. 2000;100:232–234
8. Johnson SL, Birch LL. Parents' and children's adiposity and eating style. *Pediatrics*. 1994;94:653–661
9. Birch LL, Fisher JO. Mothers' child-feeding practices influence daughters' eating and weight. *Am J Clin Nutr*. 2000;71:1054–1061
10. Birch LL. Effects of peer models' food choices and eating behaviors on preschoolers' food preferences. *Child Dev*. 1980;51:489–496
11. Cutting TM, Fisher JO, Grimm-Thomas K, Birch LL. Like mother, like daughter: familial patterns of overweight are mediated by mothers' dietary disinhibition. *Am J Clin Nutr*. 1999;69:608–613
12. Birch LL, Johnson SL, Andresen G, Peters JC, Schulte MC. The variability of young children's energy intake. *N Engl J Med*. 1991;324:232–235
13. Birch LL, Deysher M. Conditioned and unconditioned caloric compensation: evidence for self-regulation of food intake by young children. *Learn Motiv*. 1985; 16:341–355
14. Sullivan S, Birch L. Pass the sugar; pass the salt: experience dictates preference. *Dev Psychol*. 1990;26:546–551
15. Wardle J, Huon G. An experimental investigation of the influence of health information on children's taste preferences. *Health Educ Res*. 2000;15:39–44
16. Andersen RE, Crespo CJ, Bartlett SJ, Cheskin LJ, Pratt M. Relationship of physical activity and television watching with body weight and level of fatness among children: results from the Third National Health and Nutrition Examination Survey. *JAMA*. 1998;279:938–942

17. American Academy of Pediatrics, Committee on Public Education. Children, adolescents, and television. *Pediatrics.* 2001;107:423–426

18. Coon KA, Goldberg J, Rogers BL, Tucker KL. Relationships between use of television during meals and children's food consumption patterns. *Pediatrics.* 2001;107:E7

19. Crespo CJ, Smit E, Troiano RP, Bartlett SJ, Macera CA, Andersen RE. Television watching, energy intake, and obesity in US children: results from the Third National Health and Nutrition Examination Survey, 1988–1994. *Arch Pediatr Adolesc Med.* 2001;155:360–365

20. Cullen KW, Eagan J, Baranowski T, Owens E, de Moor C. Effect of a la carte and snack bar foods at school on children's lunchtime intake of fruits and vegetables. *J Am Diet Assoc.* 2000;100:1482–1486

21. Abramovitz BA, Birch LL. Five-year-old girls' ideas about dieting are predicted by their mothers' dieting. *J Am Diet Assoc.* 2000;100:1157–1163

22. Hill AJ, Pallin V. Dieting awareness and low self-worth: related issues in 8-year-old girls. *Int J Eat Disord.* 1998:24;405–413

23. Krebs-Smith SM, Cook A, Subar AF, Cleveland L, Friday J, Kahle LL. Fruit and vegetable intakes of children and adolescents in the United States. *Arch Pediatr Adolesc Med.* 1996;150:81–86

24. Munoz KA, Krebs-Smith SM, Ballard-Barbash R, Cleveland LE. Food intakes of US children and adolescents compared with recommendations. *Pediatrics.* 1997;100: 323–329

25. Troiano RP, Briefel RR, Carroll MD, Bialostosky K. Energy and fat intakes of children and adolescents in the United States: data from the national health and nutrition examination surveys. *Am J Clin Nutr.* 2000;72:1343S–1353S

26. Subar AF, Krebs-Smith SM, Cook A, Kahle LL. Dietary sources of nutrients among US children, 1989–1991. *Pediatrics.* 1998;102:913–923

27. US Department of Agriculture. *Nationwide Food Consumption Survey, Continuing Survey of Food Intakes by Individuals: Women 19–50 Years and Children 1–5 Years, 1 Day, 1986.* Hyattsville, MD: Nutrition Information Services, USDA; 1987. Report 86–1

28. Taylor ML, Koblinsky SA. Dietary intake and growth status of young homeless children. *J Am Diet Assoc.* 1993;93:464–466

29. Food and Nutrition Board, National Research Council, NAS. *Dietary Reference Intakes: Applications in Dietary Assessment.* National Academy Press; 2001

30. Alaimo K, McDowell MA, Briefel RR, et al. Dietary intake of vitamins, minerals, and fiber of persons ages 2 months and over in the United States: Third National Health and Nutrition Examination Survey, Phase 1, 1988–91. Advance data. (258):1–28, 1994 Nov 14

31. Federation of American Societies for Experimental Biology, Life Sciences Research Office. Prepared for the Interagency Board for Nutrition Monitoring and Related Research. *Third Report on Nutrition Monitoring in the United States.* Vol 1. Washington, DC: US Government Printing Office; 1995

32. American Academy of Pediatrics, Committee on Nutrition. Statement on cholesterol. *Pediatrics*. 1998;101:141–147

33. Krauss RM, Eckel RH, Howard B, et al. Revision 2000: a statement for healthcare professionals from the nutrition committee of the American Heart Association. *J Nutr*. 2001;131:132–146

34. Obarzanek E, Hunsberger SA, Van Horn L, et al. Safety of a fat-reduced diet: the Dietary Intervention Study in Children (DISC). *Pediatrics*. 1997;100:51–59

35. Butte NF. Fat intake of children in relation to energy requirements. *Am J Clin Nutr*. 2000;72:1246S–1252S

36. US Department of Agriculture. *Nutrition and Your Health: Dietary Guidelines for Americans*. 5th ed. Home and Garden Bulletin No. 232. Washington, DC: United States Department of Agriculture, United States Department of Health and Human Services; 2000:1–44

37. US Department of Agriculture. Center for Nutrition Policy and Promotion. Food Guide Pyramid for Children. 1999

38. Young LR, Nestle MS. Portion sizes in dietary assessment: issues and policy implications. *Nutr Rev*. 1995;53:149–158

39. American Academy of Pediatrics, Provisional Committee on Quality Improvement, Subcommittee on Acute Gastroenteritis. Practice parameter: the management of acute gastroenteritis in young children. *Pediatrics*. 1996;97:424–435

40. Brown KH. Dietary management of acute childhood diarrhea: optimal timing of feeding and appropriate use of milks and mixed diets. *J Pediatr*. 1991;118:S92–S98

41. Morgan KJ, Zabik ME, Leveille GA. The role of breakfast in nutrient intake of 5- to 12-year old children. *Am J Clin Nutr*. 1981;34:1418–1427

42. Preziosi P, Galan P, Deheeger M, Yacoub N, Drewnowski A, Hercberg S. Breakfast type, daily nutrient intakes and vitamin and mineral status of French children, adolescents, and adults. *J Am Coll Nutr*. 1999;18:171–178

43. Murphy JM, Pagano ME, Nachmani J, Sperling P, Kane S, Kleinman RE. The relationship of school breakfast to psychosocial and academic functioning: cross-sectional and longitudinal observations in an inner city school sample. *Arch Pediatr Adolesc Med*. 1998;152:899–907

44. Nicklas TA, O'Neil CE, Berenson GS. Nutrient contribution of breakfast, secular trends, and the role of ready-to-eat cereals: a review of data from the Bogalusa Heart Study. *Am J Clin Nutr*. 1998;67:757S–763S

45. Kennedy E, Davis C. US Department of Agriculture school breakfast program (review). *Am J Clin Nutr*. 1998;67:798S–803S

46. Troiano RP, Flegal KM, Kuczmarski RJ, Campbell SM, Johnson CL. Overweight prevalence and trends for children and adolescents: the National Health and Nutrition Examination Surveys, 1963–1991. *Arch Pediatr Adolesc Med*. 1995;149:1085–1091

47. Dietz WH. Health consequences of obesity in youth: childhood predictors of adult disease. *Pediatrics*. 1998;101:518–525

48. Hill JO, Peters JC. Environmental contributions to the obesity epidemic. *Science.* 1998;280:1371–1374

49. Poston WS, Foreyt JP. Obesity is an environmental issue. *Atherosclerosis.* 1999; 146:201–209

50. Whitaker RC, Wright JA, Pepe MS, Seidel KD, Dietz WH. Predicting obesity in young adulthood from childhood and parental obesity. *N Engl J Med.* 1997; 337:869–873

51. Barlow SE, Dietz WH. Obesity evaluation and treatment: expert committee recommendations. *Pediatrics.* 1998;102:E29

52. Fisher JO, Birch LL. Restricting access to foods and children's eating. *Appetite.* 1999;32:405–419

53. Davison KK, Birch LL. Weight status, parent reaction, and self-concept in five-year-old girls. *Pediatrics.* 2001;107:46–53

54. Goran MI, Reynolds KD, Lindquist CH. Role of physical activity in the prevention of obesity in children. *Int J Obes Relat Metab Disord.* 1999;23:S18–S33

55. American Academy of Pediatrics, Committee on Public Education. Children, adolescents, and television. *Pediatrics.* 2001;107:423–426

56. Harnack L, Stang J, Story M. Soft drink consumption among US children and adolescents: nutritional consequences. *J Am Diet Assoc.* 1999;99:436–441

57. American Academy of Pediatrics, Committee on Nutrition. Calcium requirements of infants, children, and adolescents. *Pediatrics.* 1999;104:1152–1157

58. Fisher, JO, Mitchell DC, Smiciklas-Wright H, Birch LL. Maternal milk consumption predicts the trade-off between milk and soft drinks in young girls' diets. *J Nutr.* 2001;131:246–250

59. Smith MM, Lifshitz F. Excess fruit juice consumption as a contributing factor in nonorganic failure to thrive. *Pediatrics.* 1994;93:438–443

60. Lifshitz F, Ament ME, Kleinman RE, et al. Role of juice carbohydrate malabsorption in chronic non-specific diarrhea in children. *J Pediatr.* 1992;120:825–829

61. Ludwig DS, Peterson KE, Gortmaker SL. Relation between consumption of sugar-sweetened drinks and childhood obesity: a prospective, observational analysis. *Lancet.* 2001;357:505–508

62. American Academy of Pediatrics, Committee on Sports Medicine and Fitness. Climatic heat stress and the exercising child and adolescent. *Pediatrics.* 2000; 106:158–159

8

Cultural Considerations in Feeding Children

Introduction

One of the 2 overriding goals of *Healthy People 2010*, the set of health objectives for the Nation, is to eliminate health disparities by addressing the needs of an expanding culturally diverse population.[1] This goal acknowledges and recognizes the growing number and population of ethnic and racial groups in the United States, including persons from the Caribbean, Central and South America, Asia, Southeast Asia, South Pacific ocean areas, Africa, and Russia and other former Soviet Republic block countries. It is projected that by the year 2050, minorities will represent one half of the population.[2] Newly arriving cultural groups bring and retain their cultural identities and present challenges to health care providers. Their culture encompasses long-held traditions, customs, health beliefs, and behaviors. Food and eating, a part of one's culture, are among the most potent and emotional elements of these traditions, values, and behaviors exhibited by a group.

Culture is a dynamic process that is both learned and shared, and reflects values, practices, and habits passed down from one generation to the next.[3–7] The way one feels about, thinks about, values, and shares food at meal and snack times all are a window of one's culture. Simply defined, culture includes all aspects of daily living—values, religious beliefs, primary language, interactions with others, feelings, health beliefs, food preferences, and when, how, and with whom one eats. Everyone has a culture and, regardless of the culture one identifies with, food and eating are among one of the most deep-seated behaviors in life.

Cultural patterns are significant because the food and beverages consumed, to a degree, determine health and, more specifically, nutritional status. It is recognized that there is a strong link between a healthy child and the child's educational development.[8] This was documented in a unique symposium of health, education, and social service experts who supported a national initiative for an integrated approach toward enhancing the health of young children to better prepare them to be ready to learn. In 1992, it was suggested that health,

education, and social service professionals collaborate to achieve national education goals concurrently, along with achieving some of the pediatric national
health objectives (*Healthy People 2000*).[9] So convincing is this evidence linking
health status and educational readiness that under the umbrella of nutrition,
this initiative was launched based on 8 specific health/nutrition objectives
related to one of the goals of education.[10]

Not only do cultural food patterns impact on the health and educational
readiness of a young child to learn, but on the child's social and emotional
development. Optimum health, which incorporates balanced nutrition, is
a highly significant outcome for an infant to grow as an individual into a
healthy, well-adjusted, and happy adult.[11–13]

Infant Feeding—Foundation of Eating Behavior

Eating is a learned process that begins at birth, starting with the first food and
very first feeding. These practices are reinforced with every subsequent feeding.
For example, for the breastfed infant, there is the physical, emotional, and
social bonding and attachment that begins to evolve between mother and
infant. The numerous and growing evidence of other benefits of breast milk
are detailed and discussed elsewhere in this book. What foods an infant or
young child is fed, the climate or environment in which feeding occurs, and the
feelings and attitudes of the adult who does the feeding all reflect the cultural
practices of both mother and child. Because feeding an infant is defined within
the cultural framework of the mother and family, it is important to understand
the meaning of food and eating within this context, especially its strong role as
a determinant of later food patterns and practices of a child. Cultural food
practices are so strongly embedded for some that it is said that one can tell the
history of a people by their preferred foods. Food practices become internal-
ized and result in being deeply entrenched in one's life.

Challenges for the Pediatrician

The beliefs presented by children and families may be similar to or completely different from those of the pediatrician. To bridge this gap, health care
professionals who are sensitive to the cultural issues of their patients and
willing to learn from them are better able to address their health and nutritional problems. Health care professionals who are knowledgeable in understanding the depth of these practices or who are culturally sensitive will more
likely succeed in counseling patients to improve the health of children and
their families.

Importance of Addressing Cultural Food Practices

Food contains nutrients and calories needed by the body to promote growth and development, especially in children. Protein, carbohydrates, fat, calories, vitamins, and minerals are essential in promoting growth, beginning at birth and continuing through the adolescent years and throughout life. There is evidence that optimal nutrition and physical activity during the critical years can, over time, protect a young child from developing some disease states such as hypertension, heart disease, stroke, obesity, diabetes mellitus, undernutrition, certain types of cancer, hypercholesterolemia, and osteoporosis.[14-16] The recent development and recommendations of the *Food Guide Pyramid for Young Children* (See Appendix M) confirms the need for children ages 2 to 6 to be physically active while consuming a nutritionally sound diet.[17,18]

Therefore, cultural food practices often heavily influence whether children are healthy physically, nutritionally, emotionally, and socially. Clearly, if there is an inadequate intake of calories and essential macro- and micronutrients, an outcome may be poor growth and other related problems such as developmental delay. One example of this occurs in some cultures from the Caribbean. Infants and young children are fed excessive amounts of formula or cow milk from a bottle to which an adult adds sugar.[19-21] This practice probably reflects the setting of a tropical environment of countries where sugar cane is still grown and, therefore, is readily available and accessible. A prolonged period of this practice of large-volume bottle-feedings with added sugar greatly increases the risk of bottle-feeding caries, delay in strengthening jaw muscles needed to chew and swallow coarse textured foods, and rapid weight gain. On inquiry, parents provide a number of reasons for this practice—child sucks more vigorously, so adult feels child really likes milk; it is an accepted practice in their country of origin; sugar cane at one time was a cash crop and was part of the economy, thus it is relatively inexpensive and some feel they are helping the economy. Continuing with sensitive probing, parents reveal that sugar is their way of showing love for their child or confirmation that food is also symbolic. Hence, in a cultural context, sugar denotes a language of food that, in this case, is communicated by equating sugar with love.

Understanding Cultural Food Practices

As families migrate, some begin to change their cultural food patterns, health beliefs, and behaviors. This process of acculturation may occur relatively rapidly, slowly, or not at all. The concept that culture is static is inaccurate. This is documented by historical accounts of cultural groups making changes in the direction of the dominant group to become mainstream.[3,5,11,22] As a result, counseling and advising parents about nutrition and feeding requires listening to what the parent and child are saying and observing responses and reactions to questions asked.

Within every culture there are individuals who do not necessarily embrace the same set of values, beliefs, and behaviors. Thus, some cultural groups are more homogenous than others. Examples of more homogenous groups include some Muslim and Hasidic Jewish sects composed of children and families who adhere to a defined set of religious and dietary laws or customs, like covering their heads at all times, fasting on certain days, or completely avoiding certain foods such as pork and pork products.

The concept of cultural food patterns and practices is complex. A number of factors that are intertwined and overlap are referred to as determinants of these patterns as shown in Table 8.1.

Infant Feeding—Foundation of Food Patterns for Life

Beginning with a total liquid diet of preferably breast milk or iron-fortified formula, the infant makes a transition to a semi-liquid diet sometime between 4 and 6 months of age when developmentally ready for complementary foods. As an infant grows into the toddler years, a wider variety of solid foods of coarser texture, taste, and shapes are fed. During these early years, the toddler embarks on a course of independence by beginning to choose what food and the amount to eat. Upon reaching school age and adolescence, children exert an even greater independence in selecting and eating food.

One caveat for all health care professionals to remember is the dynamic and changing nature of all cultural practices, including feeding, because of the mobility of many and a desire to assimilate the beliefs, behaviors, and practices of the dominant group. This means adopting "popular" food choices (eg, pizza), how one eats a food (eg, hot dog on a roll using one's fingers), and where food is eaten (eg, local street vending cart dispensing local foods). Thus conclusions about feeding practices based on stereotypical behaviors can be very misleading.

To better understand why and what foods are selected by some groups, there are several classifications of food that have evolved.[11,23] For the most part, these classifications are not scientifically based on the nutrient value of the food. Instead, these foods are categorized by social scientists based on the

Table 8.1.
Some Determinants of Cultural Food Practices

Determinant	Description
1. Physiological	Based on gender, age, state of health (pregnant women, infants and young children, the elderly and the sick)
2. Agriculture Production	Kinds of crops, animals grown and locally produced; frequency of harvest; availability of fish
3. Environment/Ecology	Food indigenous to geographical area (climate, rain, soil); use of pesticides, chemicals
4. Food Availability	Access to food markets, distance involved in traveling; packaged food in quantities to meet family needs like rice packaged in 25-lb sacks; clean stores, variety of food
5. Purchasing Power	Ability to buy enough food to feed family (25 lbs rice for some families)
6. Food Storage	Space available to properly store food (pantry, refrigerator, freezer)
7. Fuel for Cooking	Cost of wood, gas, electric to cook
8. Cooking/Eating Equipment/Utensils	Basic pots and pans; eating utensils if used (spoon, fork, knife, cup/glass, plate)
9. Self-image	Individual preference for desired body image
10. Personal	Food likes and dislikes (color, flavor, odor, texture, shape)
11. Historical Significance	Rooted in history (ie, peanuts [ground nuts] from Africa; chocolate from South America; tea from China)
12. Child Rearing	Weaning; introduction of supplemental foods; vitamins and minerals
13. Primary Caretaker	Skill in food preparation; interest or lack of it in cooking; limited time for shopping and preparing food
14. Religious/Faith Beliefs	Ceremonies, traditional rites, and celebrations around food and eating; healing nature of certain foods
15. Health Status	Restricting certain foods during illnesses and disease; use of natural herbs, plants, and other culturally accepted food mixes (gruels) for diseases; use of cultural healers or health providers
16. Community Food and Nutrition Resources	Food distribution systems (including soup kitchens, food pantries, special programs for pregnant women and their babies and young children like WIC [Supplemental Food Program for Women, Infants, and Children], school feeding, and commodity [food] distribution programs)

perceptions, beliefs, customs, and experiences of a cultural group. Among such categories are foods labeled as "staples." These foods tend to be the main source of calories, contain some protein, and are generally widely available to the population. In northern Europe and the United States, wheat is grown and is the dominant grain while corn is the staple food in Central and South America. Rice, especially the polished white kind, is the grain of choice in Asia and Southeast Asia where it is eaten every day at every meal. Other foods are highly desired and prized as so-called "status" foods by some groups. Special milk desserts are considered status foods in India, while chicken is a "status" food in Africa. Some foods are thought to have some "magical" properties or contain special ingredients to improve one's health. One example of this belief is the practice of mixing raw eggs with malta (a beverage containing less than 0.5% alcohol per 12 oz) by Puerto Ricans who believe this drink will enhance a child's appetite and thus promote growth.[24]

Among some groups, a rather complex system of food categories has existed for centuries and is woven into the lives of families based on body image and functions.[22,25,26] Many Asians believe in the YIN/YANG forces. YIN foods are thought to be feminine, cold, and dark, while YANG foods are the opposite—male, hot, and light. The principle of this theory is to bring about balance of body functions by consuming these 2 classes of foods.

A similar concept, the HOT/COLD theory, is a common practice in Central and South America where it is reported to have been introduced by the Spanish and Portuguese during the 16th century. This concept is based on the Hippocratic theory of 4 humors: blood, phlegm, yellow bile, and black bile. When these are in balance, it is thought the result is a positive state of health for an individual. Conversely, disease occurs when there is an imbalance among these humors.[27,28] The label of hot and cold has nothing to do with the temperature of the food but with the properties of food and illness states on body function. Both foods and illnesses are identified as hot, cool, or cold. Hot foods are easier to digest than cool or cold foods, and treatment of an illness consists of using a substance such as a food of one classification that is opposite of the classification of the disease condition. For example, diarrhea is thought to be a hot condition, so cold foods like avocados, coconuts, or bananas are among some of the foods that would be eaten to counteract the diarrhea.

Cultural Practices of Feeding Infants and Young Children

Newborn infants and young children hold a special place in any cultural group where support is given to the mother by a large, extended family located nearby, and neighbors, friends, and informal and formal community networks. There are many infant feeding practices adopted by mothers that may be based on traditions, customs, and information given by grandmothers and older women in a community. These traditions often impact breastfeeding practices and include discarding colostrum and the use of herbal supplements along with breast milk. For example, in the United Arab Emirates, it is reported that some mothers delay breastfeeding until after the first day of life and, instead, provide a bottle containing water, tea, juice, and a local herbal drink (babuny).[29] In another example, foods for first feedings of newborns may function to either purify or clean the "dirty" throat and bowels or prepare the baby for adult life.[30,31]

Sometimes a tea prepared from local plants or bushes (ie, "bush tea") is used in this process of cleansing.[32,33] When extensively practiced, an infant can become seriously ill and need immediate and prompt medical care. In many countries, withholding of colostrum is common practice. Water and sugar are commonly offered in its place.

The resources listed in Table 8.2 provide extensive information for health professionals about the origins and nature of cultural feeding practices.

Intervention Strategies

There are several direct approaches pediatricians can use to obtain information about cultural food practices and health beliefs.[34] It is useful to ask the parents about their child-rearing practices as they relate to feeding and use of "alternative" medicines and dietary supplements. The order in which family members eat is fixed among some groups, so health providers gain important insight into the adequacy or lack of adequate amounts of food, especially for a young child. In some cultures, the father is the first to eat and mothers may eat last. This, of course, may impact the mother's health if she is breastfeeding.

Table 8.3 lists some specific questions and strategies to support optimum nutrition for children of families that have recently arrived in this country or for children who represent a cultural group that the pediatrician has not encountered before.

Because of their growing independence and pressures from their peers, more intense approaches are needed for school-aged children and adolescents. At this time, there usually are changes in the eating patterns of these groups that differ from those of their parents. This causes conflicts in some families, so providers should be aware of family relationships while still supporting a nutritionally sound diet along with daily physical activity.

Table 8.2.
Resources for Cultural Food Practices

Department of Health and Human Services 　Office of Minority Health 　　800/444-6472 　　www.omhrc.gov 　　Check with the 10 Regional Offices of Minority Health and State Departments of Health, 　　　Offices of Minority Health 　Administration for Children and Families 202/401-9215 　　www.acf.dhhs.gov 　Maternal and Child Health Bureau, Division of Child, Adolescent, and Family Health 　　301/443-2250 　　www.mchb.hrsa.gov 　Indian Health Service 301/443-4646 　　www.ihs.gov
The Academy of Breastfeeding Medicine 　www.bfmed.org
Centers for Disease Control and Prevention 　www.cdc.gov
US Department of Agriculture, Food and Nutrition Service 　703/305-2554 　www.fns.usda.gov/fns
National Agricultural Library, Food and Nutrition Information Center 　301/504-5719 　www.nal.usda.gov/fnic
American Dietetic Association 　312/899-0040 　www.eatright.org
Eat 5 A Day 　www.5aday.com
Association of State and Territorial Health Officials 　717/764-7938 　www.astho.org
Federal Citizen Information Center 　202/501-1794 　www.pueblo.gsa.gov
National Maternal and Child Health Clearinghouse 　703/356-1964 　www.ask.hrsa.gov
Society for Nutrition Education 　301/656-4938 　www.sne.org
National Healthy Mothers, Healthy Babies Coalition 　703/836-6110 　www.hmhb.org

Table 8.3.
Strategies for Nutritional Support for Culturally Diverse Pediatric Populations

Age Group	Cultural Considerations	Tips for Counseling
INFANTS		
Breastfeeding	Length of time Initiation of lactation Child rearing practices	Promote benefits of breastfeeding first year of life. Support and compliment mother.
Bottle-feeding	When initiated; how many bottles per day Bottle at bedtime	Encourage exclusive breastfeeding; discourage adding sugar and other foods to bottle. Review schedule of bottles to avoid bedtime bottle; promote oral health to prevent baby bottle disease.
Weaning	Explore patient's under standing of weaning When initiated, and how Customs associated with introduction of new foods Reactions to foods	Encourage introduction of one complementary food at a time and how to feed with a spoon and bowl. Explore for cultural customs of purging/purifying baby's gastrointestinal tract (infusion of teas from plants, other foods/substances). Encourage foods without added sugar, salt, and fat. Cultural remedies (botanicas); make recommendations about benefits or side effects if known.
TODDLERS		
	Feeding practices around milk and beverages (water) Number meals/snacks Location where most meals are eaten	Explore if bottle-feeding occurs; encourage drinking all beverages, including water, from a cup. Promote clean water rather than excessive fruit juices, fruit drinks and ades, punches.
	Toothbrushing patterns Physical activity	How spaced; foods provided; promote healthy snack foods.
		Who does feeding and where; encourage self-feeding with age-appropriate eating utensils and furniture (table and chair).
		Stress toothbrushing and good oral health. Promote health benefits for entire family to engage in physical activity (use *Food Guide Pyramid For Young Children, Ages 2 to 6*).
PRESCHOOLERS		
	Milk drinking pattern	Inquire if any foods still fed by bottle with any added foods; support drinking water, and not other sweetened flavored drinks, from a cup/glass.

Table 8.3.

Strategies for Nutritional Support for Culturally Diverse Pediatric Populations *(continued)*

Age Group	Cultural Considerations	Tips for Counseling
PRESCHOOLERS, continued		
	Meal and snack patterns	Encourage eating a variety of foods including building on some culturally accepted foods Encourage "family" style meals with social interactions between child and other family members.
	Physical activity	Continue to promote age appropriate activities with family.
	Reactions to foods	Explore use of cultural healers and health care providers and cultural remedies (lotions, salves).

Related Policy Statements From the American Academy of Pediatrics

American Academy of Pediatrics Committee on Pediatric Workforce. Culturally effective pediatric care: education and training issues. *Pediatrics*. 1999;103:167–170. Available at: http://aappolicy. aappublications.org/cgi/content/full/pediatrics;103/1/167

American Academy of Pediatrics Committee on Pediatric Research. Race/ethnicity, gender, socioeconomic status—research exploring their effects on child health: a subject review. *Pediatrics*. 2000;105:1349–1351. Available at: http://aappolicy.aappublications.org/cgi/content/full/pediatrics;105/6/1349?full

American Academy of Pediatrics Committee on Pediatric Workforce. Nondiscrimination in pediatric health care. *Pediatrics*. 2001;108:1215. Available at: http://aappolicy.aappublications.org/cgi/content/full/pediatrics;108/5/1215

References

1. US Department of Health and Human Services. *Healthy People 2010*. 2nd ed. With Understanding and Improving Health and Objectives for Improving Health. 2 vols. Washington, DC: US Government Printing Office; 2000
2. United States Census Bureau Projections, April 1996. http//www.census.gov
3. Kittle PM, Sucher K. *Food and Culture in America*. Florenc, KY: Van Nostrand Reinhold; 1990
4. Pelto GH. Cultural issues in maternal and child health and nutrition, *Soc Sci Med*. 1987;25:553–559
5. Williams SR. *Essentials of Nutrition and Diet Therapy*. 7th ed. St Louis, MO: Mosby Inc; 1999:190–191, 203

6. Terry RD. Needed: a new appreciation of culture and food behavior. *J Am Diet Assoc.* 1994;945:501–503

7. Monses ER. Respecting diversity helps America eat right. *J Am Diet Assoc.* 1993; 92:282

8. Novello AC, Degraw C, Kleinman DV. Healthy children ready to learn: an essential collaboration between health and education. *Public Health Rep.* 1992;107:3–15

9. US Department of Health and Human Services. *Healthy People 2000.* Washington, DC: US Government Printing Office; 1990

10. US Department of Education. *Preparing Young Children for Success: Guideposts for Achieving Our First National Goal.* Washington, DC: Department of Education; 1991

11. Story M, Holt K, Sofka D, eds. *Bright Futures in Nutrition Practice.* Arlington, VA: National Center for Education in Maternal and Child Health; 2000

12. Tsang TC, Zlotkin SH, Nichols BL, Hassien JW. *Nutrition During Infancy: Principles and Practice.* 2nd ed. Cincinnati, OH: Digital Educational Publishers; 1997

13. Trahms CM, Pipes PL. *Nutrition in Infancy and Childhood.* 6th ed. New York, NY: WCB/McGraw Hill; 1997

14. US Department of Health and Human Services. *The Surgeon General's Report on Nutrition and Health.* Washington, DC: Department of Health and Human Services, Public Health Service; 1988:2–18, 539–545

15. US Department of Agriculture and US Department of Health and Human Services. *Dietary Guidelines for Americans.* Washington, DC: US Government Printing Office; 2000

16. International Food Information Center. *Summary of Dietary Guidelines 1980–1999.* Washington, DC: International Food Information Council; 1999

17. US Department of Agriculture. *Food Pyramid Guide for Young Children—Ages 2 to 6.* Washington, DC: US Department of Agriculture; 1999

18. Patrick K, Spear B, Holt K, Sofka D, eds. *Bright Futures in Practice: Physical Activity.* Arlington, VA: National Center for Education in Maternal and Child Health; 2001

19. Sanjur D. *Hispanic Foodways, Nutrition and Health.* Needham Heights, MA: Simon and Schuster Co; 1995:43–46, 92–96, 162–164, 285–286

20. Maslansky E, Cowell C, Carol R, Berman S, Grossi M. Survey of infant feeding practices. *Am J Public Health.* 1974;64:780–785

21. Cowell, C, Maslansky E, Grossi M, Dask R, Kayman S, Archer M. Survey of infant feeding practices. *Am J Public Health.* 1973;63:138–141

22. Clark AL. *Culture – Childbearing – Health Professionals.* Philadelphia, PA: FA Davis Company; 1978

23. *Common Health Care Beliefs and Practices of Puerto Ricans, Haitians and Low Income Blacks Living in the NY/NJ Area.* New York, NY: John Snow Public Health Group, Inc (under contract with NHSC/DHHS/Region II); 1985

24. Jelliffe DB. *Child Nutrition in Developing Countries.* Washington, DC: Department of Health, Education, and Welfare, Public Health Service; 1968

25. Risser AL, Mazur LJ. Use of folk remedies in a Hispanic population. *Arch Pediatr Adolesc Med.* 1995;149:978–981

26. Wong C. Yin and yang of nutrition. *Perinatal Nutrition Newsletter.* CA Department of Health Services: April–June; 1985

27. Ikeda J, Wright J. Pediatrics in a culturally diverse society. *Pediatr Basics.* 1996; 76:10–17

28. Harwood A. *Ethnicity and Medical Care.* Cambridge, MA: Harvard University Press; 1981

29. Henderson G, et al. *Transcultural Health Care.* Menlo Park, CA: Addison-Wesley Publishing Company; 1981

30. Al-Mazroui MJ, Oyejide CO, Bener A, Cheema MY. Breastfeeding and supplemental feeding for neonates in Al-Ain, United Arab Emirates. *J Trop Pediatr.* 1997; 43:304–306

31. Lefeber Y, Voorhoeveh H. Indigenous first feeding practices in newborn babies. *Midwifery.* 1999;15:97–100

32. Ghaemi-Almadi S. Attitudes toward breast feeding and infant feeding among Iranian, Afghan, and Southeast Asian immigrant women in the US: implications for health and nutrition education. *J Am Diet Assoc.* 1992;92:354–356

33. Quandt SA. Social cultural influences on food consumption and nutritional status. In: Shils ME, Olson JA, Shike M, Ross AC, eds. *Modern Nutrition in Health and Disease.* Baltimore, MD: Williams and Wilkins; 1999;1783–1800

34. Nutrition Counseling Mothers and Babies Across Cultures. Proceedings of conference Jointly sponsored by The Pediatric Nutrition Practice Group of the American Dietetic Association and Gerber Products Company, New York, NY: Nov 1998

9

Adolescent Nutrition

Approximately 36.5 million people, or 14% of the population in the United States, are 10 to 19 years old. On the basis of dietary histories, some adolescents have insufficient intake of calcium, iron, and vitamins A and C. Special situations, such as pregnancy, chronic disease, and physical conditioning, increase nutritional requirements of the adolescent. Some disorders seen during adolescence, such as anorexia, bulimia, and obesity are associated with insufficient or excessive nutrient intake.

Factors Influencing Nutritional Needs of Adolescents
The onset of puberty, with its associated increased growth rate, changes in body composition, physical activity, and onset of menstruation in girls, affects normal nutritional needs during adolescence. Increased growth rates occur in girls between 10 and 12 years and in boys about 2 years later, although substantial individual variability occurs. Growth in girls is accompanied by a greater increase in the proportion of body fat than in boys and, in boys, growth is accompanied by a greater increase in the proportion of lean body mass (LBM) and blood volume than in girls.

Dietary Reference Intakes
The dietary reference (DRIs) provide guidelines for normal nutrition of adolescent boys and girls in 2 age categories: 11 to 14 years and 15 to 18 years (Appendix C). The recommended dietary allowances (RDAs) for energy (see Table 15.2 in Chapter 15) are based on the median energy intakes of adolescents followed up in longitudinal growth studies. Among adolescents, individual variability occurs in the rates of physical growth, timing of the growth spurt, and physiologic maturation. In addition, individual physical activity patterns vary widely. For these reasons, assessment of energy needs of adolescents should consider appetite, growth, activity, and weight gain in relation to deposition of subcutaneous fat. Restricted food intake in the physically active adolescent results in diminished growth and a drop in the basal metabolic rate and, in girls, amenorrhea. For protein (Table 14.1 in

Chapter 14), vitamins, and minerals, the DRIs are estimates designed to meet the needs of almost all healthy adolescents; therefore, they exceed the requirements for the average person. Because of the rapid growth rate at these ages, the American Academy of Pediatrics Committee on Nutrition recommends that during the first 2 decades of life, fat should constitute approximately 30% of the dietary calories.[1]

During adolescence, increases in the requirement for energy and such nutrients as calcium, nitrogen, and iron are determined by increases in LBM rather than an increase in variable content body weight, with its variable fat content. Based on data from 570 males between 8 and 25 years and 450 females between 10 and 20 years, the male LBM increases from 27 to 62 kg (an average of 35 kg), and the female LBM increases from 24 to 43 kg (an average of 19 kg).[2,3] Assuming that the lean body contents of calcium, iron, nitrogen, zinc, and magnesium of adolescents are the same as those of adults, the daily increments of body nutrients for the growing adolescent can be estimated (Table 9.1).[4] The increments in body contents of these nutrients and the increased nutrient needs are not constant throughout adolescence, but are associated with the growth rate rather than the chronological age.

Table 9.1.
Daily Increments in Body Content of Minerals and Nitrogen During Adolescent Growth*

Mineral	Sex	Average for 10–20 y, mg	Average at Peak of Growth Spurt, mg
Calcium	M	210	400
	F	110	240
Iron	M	0.57	1.1
	F	0.23	0.9
Nitrogen[†]	M	320	610
	F	160	360
Zinc	M	0.27	0.50
	F	0.18	0.31
Magnesium	M	4.4	8.4
	F	2.3	5.0

*Adapted from Forbes.[4]
†Multiply by 0.00625 to obtain grams of protein.

Nutrition Concerns During Adolescence

The National Health and Nutrition Examination Surveys (1971–1974, 1976–1980, and 1988–1991) found that of all age groups, adolescents had the highest prevalence of unsatisfactory nutritional status.[5] On the basis of dietary recall, adolescents' intake of calcium, vitamin A, vitamin C, and iron was below the RDAs. The nutrient intakes of boys were closer to the RDAs simply because they ate relatively more food, whereas girls frequently dieted. Soft drinks, coffee, tea, and alcoholic beverages often replaced milk and juice. Milk intake was diminished in nonwhite adolescents, possibly because of lactose intolerance.

Food habits of adolescents are characterized by (1) an increased tendency to skip meals, especially breakfast and lunch; (2) eating more meals outside the home; (3) snacking, especially candies; (4) consumption of fast foods; and (5) dieting. Some adolescents adhere to vegetarian diets or to extremely restrictive dietary regimens such as Zen macrobiotic diets. Some adolescents follow fad diets and may change their eating habits frequently. These behavioral patterns are explained by the adolescents' newly found independence and busy schedule, difficulty in accepting existing values, dissatisfaction with body image, search for self-identification, desire for peer acceptance, and the need to conform to the adolescent lifestyle. As a result of typical adolescent food behaviors, the following aspects of poor nutrition are related to the adolescent's diet:

1. Energy: The low energy intake by many adolescents creates difficulties in planning diets that contain adequate levels of nutrients, especially iron. The RDAs for energy do not include a safety factor for increased energy needs due to illness, trauma, or stress and should be considered to be only average needs. Actual needs for adolescents vary with physical activity levels and the stage of maturation.
2. Protein: During adolescence, protein needs, like those for energy, correlate more closely with the growth pattern than with chronological age.
3. Calcium: Because of accelerated muscular and skeletal growth, calcium needs are greater during puberty and adolescence than in childhood.
4. Iron: The need for iron for boys and girls is increased during adolescence to sustain the rapidly enlarging LBM and hemoglobin mass; in girls, it is needed to offset menstrual losses as well.
5. Zinc: Zinc is essential for growth and sexual maturation. Growth retardation and hypogonadism have been reported in adolescent boys with zinc deficiency.

6. Vegetarianism: Adolescents who consume no animal products are vulnerable to deficiencies of several nutrients, particularly vitamins D and B_{12}, riboflavin, protein, calcium, iron, zinc, and perhaps other trace elements (see Chapter 20).
7. Dental caries: Although dental caries begin in early childhood, they are a highly prevalent nutrition-related problem of adolescence. Caries are associated with low fluoride intake in childhood and frequent consumption of foods containing carbohydrates (see Chapter 16).
8. Obesity: Results from the 1999 National Health and Nutrition Survey (NHANES) report that 14% of individuals between 12 and 19 years of age were overweight. This was an increase of 3% when compared with the last NHANES report. This major nutrition-related health problem of adolescents is discussed in Chapter 33.
9. Conditioned deficiencies: A number of drug-nutrient interactions have been described[6] (Appendix I). Anticonvulsant drugs, especially phenytoin and phenobarbital, interfere with the metabolism of vitamin D and can lead to rickets and/or osteomalacia; therefore, supplementation with vitamin D may be desirable. Isoniazid interferes with pyridoxine metabolism. Oral contraceptives increase serum lipid values,[7] an effect that may have some clinical significance.
10. Chronic disease: Adolescents may have inflammatory bowel disease, diabetes mellitus, juvenile rheumatoid arthritis, and sickle cell disease, among others. These chronic diseases can profoundly affect nutritional status.

Nutritional Considerations During Pregnancy (see also Chapter 11)
About 500 000 live births per year are reported for girls in their teens; more than one tenth of the girls are 15 years old or younger. Pregnancy is believed to cause additional stress on the nutritional status of the growing and maturing adolescent. Because the adolescent growth spurt is not complete until a few years after menarche, fetal demand for nutrients could place maternal growth in jeopardy. This is especially true in girls who mature early and in girls whose prepregnancy nutritional status is unsatisfactory. However, the nutrient requirements for the adolescent growth spurt, which wanes by the time pregnancy is possible, represent only a small amount above that considered the requirement for a nongrowing pregnant adult. Growing gravidas gain more

weight than do their nongrowing adolescent counterparts. Still, growing adolescents have smaller babies than those who are not growing.[8]

Although the fetus may be protected from the vagaries of maternal diet except in extreme malnutrition, supplementation of inadequate maternal diets with calories and nutrients results in improved maternal weight gain during pregnancy and a reduction in the prevalence of low-birth-weight infants.[9] However, an extensive study of healthy pregnant women showed that protein and energy supplements did not affect birth weight, and the birth weight of infants born to adolescent mothers is similar to those born to older women, when race and maternal stature are considered.[10]

Pregnant adolescents are just as likely as other teenage girls to skip meals, ingest poor-quality snacks, eat away from home, be overly concerned about weight, and have limited food choices.[11] Deficiencies of calcium, vitamins A and C, folate, iron, and zinc most frequently reported in the diets of adolescents may have deleterious effects on the outcome of the pregnancy. Pregnant adolescents should be cautioned against skipping meals, especially breakfast, because skipping meals may increase the risk of ketosis. The pregnant adolescent who is a strict vegetarian may ingest insufficient protein, riboflavin, vitamin B_{12}, vitamin D, and trace minerals. Appropriate vitamin and mineral supplementation is necessary for those who habitually consume inadequate diets. Folate and iron supplementation should be recommended routinely.

A comprehensive health care program for the pregnant adolescent should include proper prenatal care, monitoring of weight gain, nutritional assessment, counseling and support, family planning, and continued schooling. Whenever possible, the parents or other caregiver should be included in the counseling sessions. Many adolescents respond to suggestions that incorporate ethnic foods into their eating patterns. Pregnancy may provide the educator with a unique opportunity to help the adolescent understand and improve her eating habits. Nonnutritional factors can also influence the pregnancy outcome. Pregnant women should be informed of the adverse effects of smoking and of the use of alcohol and nonessential drugs.

References

1. American Academy of Pediatrics, Committee on Nutrition. Statement on cholesterol. *Pediatrics.* 1992;90:469–473
2. Forbes GB. Growth of lean body mass in man. *Growth.* 1972;36:325–338
3. Forbes GB. Relation of lean body mass to height in children and adolescents. *Pediatr Res.* 1972;6:32–37

4. Forbes GB. Nutritional requirements in adolescence. In: Suskind RM, ed. *Textbook of Pediatric Nutrition*. New York, NY: Raven Press; 1981:381–391

5. Caloric and selected nutrient intakes of persons 1–74 years of age. *Vital Health Stat 11*. 1979;209

6. Roe DA. Diet-drug interactions and incompatibilities. In: Hathcock JN, Coon J, eds. *Nutrition and Drug Interrelations*. New York, NY: Academic Press; 1978:319–345

7. Webber LS, Hunter SM, Johnson CC, Srinivasan SR, Berenson GS. Smoking, alcohol, and oral contraceptives: effects on lipids during adolescence and young adulthood—Bogalusa Heart Study. *Ann N Y Acad Sci*. 1991;623:135–154

8. Scholl TO, Hediger ML, Schall JI, Khoo CS, Fischer RL. Maternal growth during pregnancy and the competition for nutrients. *Am J Clin Nutr*. 1994;60:183–188

9. Chez RA. Nutritional factors in pregnancy affecting fetal growth and subsequent infant development. In: Suskind RM, LeWinter-Suskind L, eds. *Textbook of Pediatric Nutrition*. 2nd ed. New York, NY: Raven Press; 1993:1–7

10. Rush D, Stein Z, Susser M. A randomized controlled trial of prenatal nutritional supplementation in New York City. *Pediatrics*. 1980;65:683–697

11. Garn SM, Petzold AS. Characteristics of the mother and child in teenage pregnancy. *Am J Dis Child*. 1983;137:365–368

10

Sports Nutrition

Adolescent athletes see nutrition as a way to enhance their performance. They may seek to improve endurance, alter their percentage of body fat, or lose or gain weight through their diet. Only exercise, in conjunction with good nutrition, can increase muscle mass and strength. Unfortunately, teenagers often obtain nutritional advice from inappropriate and/or inaccurate sources, such as books and magazines (which may promote fad diets) and coaches, trainers, or parents (who may lack specific nutritional knowledge).

The most effective way to provide optimal nutrition for achieving top physical performance is by following a well-balanced diet that provides sufficient nutrients and calories to meet the metabolic demands of the body and promote maximum growth. The well-balanced diet can be achieved by eating adequate amounts of food from the basic food groups of the food pyramid: dairy products, cereals and grains, meat and animal products, and fruits and vegetables. In most persons, intense physical activity probably does not increase the need for specific nutrients, except calories and water, to compensate for the increased energy expenditure and water loss caused by exercise.

Adolescence is characterized by relatively poor eating behaviors. Increased independence leads to erratic eating habits, skipped meals, snacking, and consumption of fast foods. Athletic adolescents, if given sound information, are more likely to eat properly than are nonathletic adolescents. The role of the pediatrician is to provide relevant nutritional information that supports the athlete's goals. To do this, the pediatrician should be familiar with the role of nutrition in exercise physiology. A diet plan for teenagers engaged in strenuous activity must consider the type of activity, whether endurance or sprint (aerobic or anaerobic). It must outline eating strategies for training and for before, during, and after the event.

Physiology

To perform physical work (exercise), muscle derives energy from the oxidative and anaerobic metabolism of carbohydrates, fats, and sometimes protein. With low exercise intensity and adequate oxygen supplies, aerobic combustion occurs, and the main metabolic byproduct is carbon dioxide. However, as exercise intensity increases, muscles begin to use anaerobic metabolism, and the main metabolic byproduct is lactic acid. This point is known as the anaerobic threshold. Anaerobic metabolism allows exercise to continue, but the buildup of lactic acid is ultimately limiting. During low-intensity exercise, a greater proportion of fat is metabolized; as the exercise intensity increases, proportionately more carbohydrate is used. During the initial stages of exercise, muscle glycogen is the main source of this carbohydrate, but as exercise continues, the muscles rely on blood glucose, which is derived from liver glycogen.[1]

Diet for Training

Most athletic activities in which teenagers participate are non-endurance activities in which normal glycogen stores are not completely exhausted. They include physically demanding sports such as football, baseball, swimming, track, gymnastics, and dance. Endurance sports include marathon running, road cycling, triathlons, and long-distance, cross-country skiing. The nutritional demands and requirements for both aerobic and anaerobic athletic activities can usually be met by simply increasing the quantity of a balanced diet.

Calories

The energy requirements during adolescence are extremely variable. This is the result not only of varied activity levels, but also of the extreme variation in size, body composition, stage of sexual maturation, and rate of growth. Two teenagers involved in similar activities can have energy requirements that differ by as much as 1000 kcal. The energy needs of an athletic adolescent can reach astounding levels. For example, the caloric requirement of the 13-year-old athletic boy at the 50th percentile for height and weight is 3500 kcal/d. For a similar teenager at the 95th percentile, the caloric requirement is 4500 kcal/d. The practical implication is the need for calorically dense foods. The most readily available indicator of caloric intake is body weight. Gain in height without gain in weight indicates a negative caloric balance. Because of fluctuation in body composition and because adipose tissue is metabolically less active than muscle, weight is not the most accurate measure to use to estimate caloric needs. Other measures that can be used are weight for height, height, body mass index, and lean body mass (LBM). All of these parameters, with the exception of LBM, are dependent on height. Height is frequently mismeasured, which introduces errors in the calculation of caloric needs. The LBM measurement is difficult to obtain and must be calculated or measured using skinfold calipers or techniques that often are not readily available, such as bioelectrical impedance or dual-beam electron x-ray.

The basal metabolic rate for young adult males averages about 38 kcal/m²/h. Basal requirements are 5% to 10% less for women than men. Children and adolescents have higher metabolic rates per unit of LBM than adults.[2] The energy needs for exercise are added to basal metabolic requirements. A list of the approximate amount of energy expended with various athletic activities is shown in Table 10.1. These values have been derived from measurements in

Table 10.1.
Approximate Energy Costs of Various Activities*

Activity	Calories Expended per Minute of Activity
Cycling, mph	
5.5	4.5
9.4	7.0
13.1	11.1
Dancing	3.3–7.7
Football	8.9
Golf	5.0
Gymnastics	
Balancing	2.5
Abdominal exercises	3.0
Trunk bending	3.5
Arm swinging, hopping	6.5
Running	
Short distance	13.3–16.6
Cross country	10.6
Tennis	7.1
Skating (fast)	11.5
Skiing	
Moderate speed	10.8–15.9
Uphill, maximum speed	18.6
Swimming	
Breaststroke	11.0
Backstroke	11.5
Crawl (55 yd/min)	14.0
Wrestling	14.2

*From the American Association for Health, Physical Education, and Recreation. *Nutrition for the Athlete*. Washington, DC: AAHER; 1971.

adults. Comparable data for adolescents, derived using the same technique for each activity, are not available. Values for energy expended for athletic activities may also vary with body weight. Thus the values provided in this table are intended only to be an approximate comparison of energy expenditures for different activities.

The percentages of calories in a properly proportioned diet for athletes should be 55% to 60% carbohydrate, 25% to 30% fat, and 15% to 20% protein.[3] A slightly higher proportion of fat (up to 35%) may be necessary in the very active adolescent who is unable to maintain body weight with moderate fat intake. Family cardiovascular history and lipid profile should be obtained before advising a diet higher in fat.

Carbohydrates

The source of energy that is used depends on the duration and intensity of exercise and the level of training of the athlete. At rest, most of the energy is supplied by the aerobic metabolism of fat. For intense exercise of very short duration, such as jumping or short sprinting, energy is provided by anaerobic metabolism of glucose to yield adenosine triphosphate and phosphocreatine. As highly intense exercise continues, the muscles operate under anaerobic conditions. The major energy source is glucose in the circulation or stored as muscle glycogen that is metabolized by anaerobic glycolysis. In exercise shorter than a few minutes and of less intensity, the body provides adequate oxygenation to create aerobic conditions in the muscle. Carbohydrates and fats can be metabolized aerobically. With increasing duration, carbohydrates contribute more and fats contribute less of the energy consumed.

Regular training causes an increase in the mitochondrial activity of muscle and in respiratory capacity, resulting in greater fat metabolism during exercise.[4] Fat spares carbohydrates. With greater amounts of glycogen available, endurance may be increased for the final stages of athletic performance. Table 10.2 outlines the energy stores available for exercise.

Glycogen loading is of value for long periods of endurance exercise and activities that take longer than 1 to 2 hours, such as marathons or cross-country skiing races. This method should not be used by children. A low carbohydrate or normal mixed diet is eaten on the first 2 or 3 days while participating in intense exercise. For the next 3 or 4 days before the contest, a high-carbohydrate diet is consumed and exercise is reduced. This method increases glycogen stores in muscle and the liver about twofold, to essentially

Table 10.2.
Average Body Energy Stores of the Nonobese 70-kg Man*

Fuel	Amount Stored, kg	Caloric Value, kcal
Triacylglycerols (adipose tissue)	15.56	140 000
Glycogen		
Muscle	0.35	1400
Liver	0.09	360
Glucose (extracellular fluids)	0.02	80
Protein (muscle)	10.00	40 000
Total	26.02	181 840

*From Felig P, Wahren J. Fuel homeostasis in exercise. *N Engl J Med*. 1975;293:1078–1084.

the same degree but without the undesirable side effects, such as hypoglycemia, nausea, vomiting, fatigue, and diarrhea, that are associated with more prolonged methods.[5] Because 1 to 2 g of water is stored in the hepatocyte or muscle cell with each gram of glycogen, glycogen is a rather inefficient fuel, yielding about 2 kcal/g compared with about 8 kcal/g for fat. The usual glycogen stores last 1 to 2 hours, so glycogen loading makes sense only for longer events and should be discouraged for most teenagers.

Fats
Fat constitutes the largest store of fuel in the human body. The exercising muscle uses endogenous fat and free fatty acids derived from the blood. One of the benefits of training is to allow the muscle to use a proportionately greater amount of fat at any given exercise level. No increase in the requirements for dietary fat is readily apparent in the athletic adolescent, except as a calorically dense source of fuel.

Short- and long-term exercise programs have a beneficial effect on the lipid profile. In later life, physical activity is associated with a decreased risk of coronary vascular disease. Athletic activity during adolescence can help establish lifelong habits of regular exercise and a balanced diet.

Protein
Athletes commonly believe that exercise, especially short periods of intense exercise, breaks down muscle tissue. This "torn-tissue" hypothesis is used as a rationale for a high-protein diet. The effect of non-endurance exercise on protein metabolism has not been determined, and study results conflict. The studies

available indicate that some tissue destruction occurs, thus supporting the torn-tissue hypothesis. However, the studies also suggest that during intense exercise, compensatory increased efficiency in protein utilization occurs. So added dietary protein is not needed to replace destroyed muscle tissue.[6] A small increase in the daily protein intake may be justified to meet the need for building muscle mass and blood volume during training. With a balanced diet, an additional 600 to 1200 kcal will add 22 to 45 g protein/d (1.5 to 2 g/kg/d), a more than adequate intake. The ingestion of a high-protein diet does not seem to improve performance.

Protein metabolism in relation to endurance training has been studied more closely, and results indicate that utilization of protein increases. The studies suggest that endurance exercise is catabolic. This has been interpreted to mean that dietary protein levels should be high for endurance athletes. However, protein metabolism adapts in response to endurance exercise, preventing the net loss of protein over time. These findings are consistent with the observation that endurance athletes, such as marathon runners, do not waste away with time. As with non-endurance training, the slight increase in protein requirement is more than met by the usual amount of protein in the average US diet as well as by an overall increase in food consumption.

Water and Electrolytes

The most essential and often neglected nutrient requirement in an athlete's diet is water. Water regulates body temperature, serves as an essential component of the biochemical reactions involved in energy production, and transports waste products and nutrients. Water is lost from the body by sweating, urination, and evaporation from the respiratory tract during breathing. During intense physical activity, most water is lost through sweating. Perspiration provides a means by which large amounts of heat produced during exercise are dissipated. Water losses increase with greater duration and intensity of exercise and also with higher environmental temperatures. An athlete exercising in hot and humid weather may lose more than 1.0 L/m^2/h through sweating.[7] Thirst is not a reliable indicator of the fluid deficit and often only develops when the athlete is about 3% dehydrated. The average thirst response after exercise will not replace all the water that has been lost. With activity over long periods, water should be taken during the exercise at regularly scheduled intervals to ensure that the athlete is adequately hydrated for the duration of exercise.

Athletes participating in multiple daily exercise sessions in warm environments are at increased risk of dehydration. An effective method to prevent chronic dehydration is to monitor body weight. Weight should be determined before and after workouts, and, for each pound of fluid lost with exercise, 16 oz of water should be consumed. Any decrease in weight that occurs during a period of hours or a few days is almost all water loss. Because of the dangers of heat illness, any athlete who loses more than 3% of body weight during an exercise session should not be permitted to return to strenuous activity until the lost fluid is replaced. A fluid deficit of as little as 2% to 3% of body weight stresses the circulatory system and can substantially impair thermoregulation and endurance capacity. As dehydration increases, the athlete becomes susceptible to problems such as heat exhaustion, heat stroke, and circulatory collapse. Once an athlete has become dehydrated, 24 to 72 hours are needed for rehydration and equilibration of fluids.

Cold water with simple sugars (2.5% to 5%) or glucose polymers is sufficient to restore fluid losses from sweat. It is most rapidly absorbed into the vascular compartment. The rate of fluid absorption depends on gastric emptying and intestinal absorption. Fluids that cause rapid gastric emptying are those that are of low osmolality and of large volume. Cold fluids are advantageous because they contribute to body cooling. An excessive volume of fluid is deleterious. For non-endurance sports, sports drinks have little advantage over cold water. Fluid containing small amounts of sugar will empty from the stomach more rapidly than water. Athletes will spontaneously drink more of a cold, flavored beverage than they will water. On the other hand, sports drinks are expensive. While exercising, the recommended intake of fluid is about 4 to 8 oz every 15 minutes.

During exercise, small amounts of electrolytes, mostly sodium and chloride, are lost in the sweat. Sweat is relatively dilute. Athletes almost always consume enough salt from the diet to replace the losses from exercise. If the athlete loses excessive amounts of fluids (sweat), then some additional salt may need to be consumed in the diet during or after exercise. Salt tablets can induce hypernatremia and increase the need for additional fluids and should never be used.

Calcium and Iron
Because of the increase in the blood volume and skeletal mass, the body's needs for iron and calcium are higher during adolescence than at any other time of life. As much as 45% of the adult skeletal mass is gained during the adolescent

growth spurt. The requirements of exercise and additional losses are added to these growth requirements. Consumption of dairy products decreases during teenage years, possibly because of lactose intolerance or because of natural preferences. Increased calcium losses occur with strenuous exercise. These facts are of particular importance to the female athlete because of the relationship between early calcium accretion and later development of osteoporosis.

Anemia is the most frequently documented nutritional deficiency in adolescent athletes. "Sports anemia" is seen during early training in elite athletes. Hemodilution is the most widely held explanation for sports anemia. Blood volume increases without a commensurate increase in red cell mass. Because this is not truly an anemic state, no implications for performance exist. Iron deficiency is the most common cause of significant anemia in athletes. Iron deficiency occurs because dietary intake is insufficient to compensate for losses. Iron losses can be due to gastrointestinal blood loss, hematuria, and iron loss in sweat. The endurance athlete is most likely to be adversely influenced by these losses. For most athletes, the effect of these losses on total iron stores is not significant. For the adolescent athlete, the most common reasons for anemia are high iron needs and an iron-deficient diet. As for all teenage girls, menstruation is a significant source of iron loss for female athletes. Especially in activities in which weight control is an issue, such as gymnastics, dance, ice skating, long-distance running, and wrestling, caloric intake can be as low as 1800 kcal/d. Under these circumstances, ingesting sufficient iron may be difficult. Anemia adversely effects performance in endurance and non-endurance sports.[8]

The preparticipation physical examination is an appropriate time to screen for anemia and to review the teenager's diet for adequate calcium and iron intake. If the athlete does not ingest sufficient quantities of dairy products (about four 8-oz glasses of milk a day), a supplement should be added. A diet that does not contain sufficient bioavailable iron should be supplemented.

Eating for Training

Perhaps the greatest challenge for the adolescent athlete is to eat well and to stay hydrated during training. The reason this is so important is that the teenager must sustain a high level of awareness for weeks and months at a time. While research suggests that a well-balanced diet taken in regular intervals and in sufficient quantities optimizes an adolescent athlete's training performance, this is not the usual eating behavior of nonathletic teenagers. Thus, to optimize performance, the teenager who is serious about athletics must eat differently from peers. Because of increased energy requirements, an athlete need not, and perhaps should not, eliminate all high-caloric density fast foods that teenagers prefer. Replacing carbohydrates should begin soon after finishing exercise. Glycogen synthesis is augmented during the first hour or 2 after exercise. Thus, food or fluid containing carbohydrates should be ingested within this time. This prescription goes for post-competition replacement of glycogen stores, in which the major concern becomes recovery from the event and a return to training in good condition.

Pre-competition Meal

It is most important for the athlete to eat a full and adequate diet for 2 to 3 days before an event. That said, the goal of the pre-competition meal is to support the athlete physiologically and psychologically. It should provide energy and fluid for the upcoming competition. Eating a meal high in carbohydrates and low in fats about 2 to 4 hours before the event is recommended. The traditional steak and egg breakfast has no place in the pre-competition schema. The prime consideration is that the meal not interfere with the stress of the competition. Therefore, a low-fat, low-protein, high-carbohydrate meal that will empty from the stomach in a short time is advisable. However, meals eaten less than 2 hours before the event have had no detrimental influence. Probably more important than the physiologic aspects of the pre-event meal are the psychological effects of individual and team rituals.

Recommendations for the ingestion of high-calorie supplements immediately before the event have come full circle. At one time, eating chocolate, sugar cubes, or fructose for quick energy was standard practice. This practice was abandoned because it was believed to cause rebound hypoglycemia. Published research suggests that ingesting high-density carbohydrates within 5 minutes of an event can prolong endurance but has no effect on short events.[9] Hydration, with water or a sports drink, should be maintained up to the time of the event.

Nutrition and Hydration During Competition

For non-endurance competition, carbohydrate ingestion does not enhance performance, so the main emphasis should be on maintenance of hydration. As during training, the athlete should know that thirst is not a reliable indicator of hydration status and that fluids should be taken during the competition at regular intervals. Cold fluids will aid in dissipating body heat.

For endurance events, ingesting carbohydrate-containing fluids prolongs time to exhaustion. More important than the ingested carbohydrate, which is probably not available until an hour into the event, is the effect of fluid to maintain hydration.

Eating for a day-long tournament is an important consideration for some adolescent athletes. Tournaments may include 2 or more competitive events. The goals of maintaining hydration and supporting caloric needs while not interfering with the athletic endeavor remain the same. In this situation, a "grazing" approach may be most effective. Eating and drinking small quantities that will rapidly pass through the stomach and be absorbed throughout the day seem to produce the best results.

Weight Control

Many young male athletes want to improve their sports performance by increasing their body weight. An increase in LBM is needed, not excess body fat.[10] This can be achieved only through strength training and an appropriate increase in the intake of calories and nutrients. The use of drugs, hormones, and supplements of protein, vitamins, or other nutrients must be discouraged.[11] Pediatricians should be aware of the widespread use of anabolic steroids among teenage athletes. This practice must be discouraged. Their use threatens not only the health of the individual, but also the integrity of competitive sports at the amateur level. Nutritional ergogenics are substances used to improve performance of the athlete. Popular ergogenic aids are creatine, chromium picolinate, caffeine, ginseng, and amino acid powder. With few exceptions, controlled trials of ergogenic substances have not been conducted,[12] and none have been done in children or adolescents. Uncontrolled reports indicate that the placebo effect may have a large role. Because these substances are considered "nutritional supplements" rather than drugs, they fall under the DISHEA act and do not require FDA approval. Recently the American Academy of Pediatrics Committee on Children With Disabilities published a statement on the use of complementary and alternative medicine (CAM). This statement clearly points out the dilemma of pediatricians dealing with patients who take CAM therapy.[13] Each pound of muscle gained requires a positive energy balance of about 2500 to 3000 kcal. The athlete should attempt to gain no more than 1 to 2 lb per week. A more rapid weight gain is probably from added body fat. The body fat of "Reference Adolescents" for males ranges from 12.7% to 17.2% and, for females, from 21.5% to 25.4%.[14]

Some athletes, particularly females involved in gymnastics, ballet, cross-country running, diving, and figure skating, and males involved in wrestling, may want to reduce body weight for optimal performance or appearance in sports where judging is utilized. In the appropriate situation (the athlete who is overfat), this should be accomplished by reducing body fat and increasing exercise, not merely by ingesting hypocaloric diets. Weight loss should be gradual; more than 1.5% of body weight or 2 to 3 lb per week may result in loss of muscle mass. Further effort to reduce weight results in the loss of muscle tissue, which will reduce physical performance. Too great an emphasis on nutrition and exercise can lead to an eating disorder.[15]

Adolescents involved in sports with weight categories, such as wrestling, boxing, and crew, attempt to lose weight before a competition to compete in a lower weight category. This is called "making weight." It is often accomplished through fluid losses that the athlete then attempts to replace before the event actually begins. While most athletes make weight by exercising and not replacing fluids, drastic methods such as inducing vomiting and ingesting diuretics and cathartics have been used. The effect on the health of cycles of dehydration and rapid rehydration during a season is unknown, but may be detrimental and should be strongly condemned.

References

1. Stanley WC, Connett RJ. Regulation of muscle carbohydrate metabolism during exercise. *FASEB J.* 1991;5:2155–2159

2. Firouzbakhsh S, Mathis RK, Dorchester WL, et al. Measured resting energy expenditure in children. *J Pediatr Gastroenterol Nutr.* 1993;16:136–142

3. Wheeler KB, Lombardo JA. Nutritional aspects of exercise. *Clin Sports Med.* 1999; 469–718

4. Nagle FJ, Bassett DR Jr. Energy metabolism in exercise. In: Hickson JF Jr, Wolinsky I, eds. *Nutrition in Exercise and Sport.* Boca Raton, FL: CRC Press Inc; 1989:87–105

5. Pate TD, Brunn JC. Fundamentals of carbohydrate metabolism. In: Hickson JF Jr, Wolinsky I, eds. *Nutrition in Exercise and Sport.* Boca Raton, FL: CRC Press Inc; 1989:37–49

6. Hickson JF Jr, Wolinsky I. Human protein intake and metabolism in exercise and sport. In: Hickson JF Jr, Wolinsky I, eds. *Nutrition in Exercise and Sport.* Boca Raton, FL: CRC Press Inc; 1989:5–35

7. Squire DL. Heat illness: fluid and electrolyte issues for pediatric and adolescent athletes. *Pediatr Clin North Am.* 1990;37:1085–1109

8. Raunikar RA, Sabio H. Anemia in the adolescent athlete. *Am J Dis Child.* 1992; 146:1201–1205

9. Maughan RJ, Fenn CE, Gleeson M, Leiper JB. Metabolic and circulatory responses to the ingestion of glucose polymer and glucose/electrolyte solutions during exercise in man. *Eur J Appl Physiol Occup Physiol.* 1987;56:356–362

10. Brownell KD, Steen SN, Wilmore JH. Weight regulation practices in athletes: analysis of metabolic and health effects. *Med Sci Sports Exerc.* 1987;19:546–556

11. Landry GL, Primos WA Jr. Anabolic steroid abuse. *Adv Pediatr.* 1990;37:185–205

12. Poortmans J, Francaux M. Adverse effects of creatine supplementation: fact or fiction? *Sports Med.* 2000;30:155–170

13. American Academy of Pediatrics, Committee on Children with Disabilities. Counseling families who choose complementary and alternative medicine for their child with chronic disease or disability. *Pediatrics.* 2001:107:598–601

14. Haschke F. Body composition during adolescence. In: Klish WJ, Kretchmer N, eds. *Body Composition Measurements in Infants and Children: Report of the 98th Ross Conference on Pediatric Research.* Columbus, OH: Ross Laboratories; 1989:76–83

15. American Academy of Pediatrics, Committee on Sports Medicine and Fitness. Medical concerns in the female athlete. *Pediatrics.* 2000;106:610–613

11

Nutrition During Pregnancy

The optimal nutritional support of a mother and her developing fetus begins before conception. This poses a challenge for pediatricians caring for pregnant adolescents. Approximately 1 million teenagers become pregnant in the United States annually. Of these pregnancies, 51% end in live births, 35% end in induced abortion, and 14% result in a miscarriage or stillbirth.[1] Although birth rates have declined in the 1990s, the teenage birth rate in 1996 (54.7 live births/1000) was still higher than the rate in 1980.[2] The pregnant adolescent is more likely to be a member of a poor or low-income family (83%), to be unmarried (72%), and to have an unplanned pregnancy (>90%). One third of adolescents who become parents—mothers as well as fathers—were themselves the product of an adolescent pregnancy.

Adolescent pregnancy is associated with an increased risk of medical complications such as low birth weight, neonatal death, maternal mortality, pregnancy-induced hypertension, and sexually transmitted diseases; the youngest adolescents appear to be at greatest risk.[1] A low prepregnancy body mass index (BMI), low gestational weight gain (GWG), anemia, and a poor-quality diet are related to poor pregnancy outcomes among adolescents. Early prenatal care, including assessment of nutritional status, is of paramount importance for pregnant adolescents. Assessment of nutritional status should identify individuals who are significantly underweight or overweight; conditions such as bulimia, anorexia, pica, hypovitaminosis or hypervitaminosis; and special dietary habits, such as vegetarianism.

Assessment of Nutritional Status

Underweight women are at increased risk for reproductive problems.[3] Not only is fertility compromised, but also the likelihood of premature delivery and intrauterine growth restriction (IUGR) is increased. In addition, the Apgar scores of the offspring are more frequently low. The condition of being underweight is potentially modifiable because it is often related to abusive dieting practices or exercise programs. A woman motivated toward improvement of her body weight-for-height status may achieve her goal within a relatively short period (3 to 6 months).

Overweight women are at greater risk than normal-weight women for an unsatisfactory course or outcome of pregnancy.[4,5] Numerous studies have shown that obese women are at higher risk for antenatal complications, such as gestational diabetes, infertility, hypertension, and pyelonephritis. They are also more likely to experience prolonged labor followed by difficult vaginal delivery, and thus, more frequently deliver by cesarean section. The incidence of adverse perinatal outcomes is likewise higher.

The weight status of a woman planning to become pregnant may be evaluated by her prepregnancy BMI, defined as weight (in kg) divided by height^2 (in m^2)[6] (Table 11.1).

Because of continued linear growth during adolescence, the categories of weight in Table 11.1 are referenced by percentiles. Reference BMI values for females by age for underweight (<25th percentile), normal weight (25th to 85th percentile), at risk for overweight (85th to 95th percentile) and overweight (>95th percentile) are found in Appendix J.

Guidelines for Gestational Weight Gain

Substantial evidence indicates that optimal birth weight is influenced by GWG. Methodologically acceptable studies have been virtually unanimous in reporting a positive relationship between birth weight and GWG. However, maternal prepregnancy BMI is a strong effect modifier of this relationship. A number of studies have demonstrated an increased risk for intrauterine growth retardation (IUGR) with low total gain.[7-9] Others have observed a specific risk associated with low gain during the second trimester[10,11] and/or the third trimester of pregnancy[12,13] (Table 11.2). On the other hand, the increased risk for large-for-gestational-age infants is associated with excessive GWG in very obese

Table 11.1.
Classification of Adult Maternal Prepregnancy Body Mass Index (BMI)*

Classification	BMI
Underweight	<19.8
Normal weight	19.8–26.0
Overweight	>26–29
Obese	>29

*Institute of Medicine and Food and Nutrition Board, 1990.[6]

Table 11.2.

Relative Risk of Intrauterine Growth Retardation Based on Low Trimester Weight Gain in Women With Low, Normal, or High Body Mass Index (BMI)*

	Low BMI	Normal BMI	High BMI
Low weight gain			
First trimester	0.88 (0.50–1.57)	1.31 (0.88–1.95)	1.02 (0.50–2.08)
Second trimester	2.68 (1.46–4.94)	1.92 (1.29–2.87)	1.88 (1.03–3.43)
Third trimester	2.07 (1.22–3.51)	2.12 (1.48–3.04)	1.53 (0.86–2.74)

*Low weight gain was defined as <0.1 kg/wk, <0.3 kg/wk, and <0.3 kg/wk in the first, second, and third trimesters, respectively. Strauss, 1999.[13]

Table 11.3.

High Birth Weight Associated With Excessive Gestational Weight Gain in Obese Women*

	Gestational Weight Gain Range				
	Loss (n=51)	1–7 kg (n=153)	7–12 kg (n=146)	12–16 kg (n=97)	>16 kg (n=80)
Mean birth weight (g)	3302	3192	3337	3506	3453
Small for gestational age (SGA)†	2 (4.0%)	6 (3.9%)	8 (5.6%)	3 (3.1%)	3 (3.8%)
Large for gestational age (LGA)†	6 (12.0 %)	18 (11.8%)	27 (18.8%)	25 (25.8%)	19 (23.8%)

*Bianco, 1998.[14]
†Data as n (%).

(BMI >35) women (Table 11.3).[14] Obese women are more likely to have pregnancy complications of diabetes, hypertension, preeclampsia, arrest of labor, fetal distress, and cesarean delivery. The recognized relationship between GWG and birth weight underlies the 1990 Institute of Medicine (IOM)[6] recommendations for weight gain, based on prepregnancy BMI. Weight gains associated with optimal birth weights and least neonatal morbidity were determined. Recommended ranges for GWG by prepregnancy BMI are shown in Table 11.4.

There is concern that excessive GWG contributes to the rising incidence of obesity among women in the United States. In the past 2 decades, the mean GWG in the US population, as well as the prevalence of overweight women, has increased. Using the cutoff of BMI >25, 45 million women (50%) are classified as overweight. The latest statistics show the greatest increases in women of reproductive ages.[15]

Table 11.4.
Recommended Total Gestational Weight Gain (GWG) Ranges for Pregnant Women by Prepregnancy Body Mass Index (BMI)*

Prepregnancy BMI Category	GWG (kg)	GWG (lb)
Underweight (BMI <19.8)	12.5–18	28–40
Normal weight (BMI 19.8–26.0)	11.5–16	25–35
Overweight (BMI 26–29)	7–11.5	15–25
Obese (BMI >29)	at least 6	at least 15

*Institute of Medicine and Food and Nutrition Board, 1990.[6]

An increasing secular trend in GWG is evident among American women. Gestational weight gain increased from about 9 kg in the 1940s through 1960s to 12 to 14 kg in the 1970s through 1990s.[6] For the majority of women, postpartum weight retention at 6 to 18 months' postpartum is 1 to 2 kg over preconceptional weight.[16,17] However, pregnancy substantially increases weight in a subset of women. Childbearing results in long-term weight gain, but it is unknown if weight gain is caused by pregnancy itself or changes in behaviors and activities related to child rearing.

Studies show that approximately 50% of women receive no advice or inappropriate advice regarding GWG. A large survey of American women revealed that 27% received no medical advice regarding GWG.[18] Among those who received advice, 14% were advised to gain less than recommended, while 22% were advised to gain more than recommended. The odds of being advised to gain more than recommended were higher in the high BMI group, which raises concerns because overweight women are already at risk of obesity and of delivering high-birth-weight infants. In addition, African American women in the survey were more likely than white women to have been advised to gain less than recommended, which also raises concerns because African American women are at greater risk of delivering low-birth-weight infants, and gaining less can increase this risk. Survey findings showed that the advice given and the target weight were strongly associated with actual gain, and no advice was associated with gaining outside IOM recommendations. These findings indicate that greater efforts are needed to improve medical advice about GWG.

During the period of 1990 to 1996, GWG was studied in populations participating in the Special Supplemental Nutrition Program for Women, Infants, and Children (WIC) in Indiana, Kansas, Massachusetts, Minnesota, and

Nebraska.[19] The findings indicated that 34% of the WIC participants gained within, 22% to 23% gained less, and 42% to 43% gained more than the IOM guidelines. Excessively high GWG was observed in young, primiparous, and overweight women. The IOM recommendations apparently have had an impact on reducing inadequate GWG among WIC participants, but closer attention should be paid to preventing excessive gain.

Nutrient Needs During Pregnancy

Energy

Energy requirements during pregnancy increase because of increases in basal and activity energy expenditure, and energy deposition in the newly acquired fetal and maternal tissues. Obligatory energy needs of the fetus, uterus, placenta, and mammary gland have been estimated to comprise only 15% of the total requirement; the remainder supports energy needs for maintenance, work, and maternal fat deposition.

Basal energy expenditure increases during pregnancy because of the metabolic contribution of the uterus and fetus, and increased work of the heart, lungs, and kidney. The increased basal metabolic rate (BMR) is one of the major components of the increased energy requirement during pregnancy.[20] Variation in energy expenditure among individuals is largely due to differences in fat-free mass (FFM), which, in pregnancy, is composed of the expanded plasma, high-energy-requiring fetal and uterine tissues, and moderate-energy-requiring skeletal muscle mass.[20] In late pregnancy, approximately one half of the increment in basal energy expenditure can be attributed to the fetus.[20] Basal metabolic rate of pregnant women has been measured longitudinally in a number of studies using a Douglas bag, ventilated hood, or whole-body respiration calorimeter.[21–25] Cumulative changes in BMR throughout pregnancy ranged from 29 636 to 50 300 kcal. This amounts to 106 to 180 kcal/d.

Until late gestation, the gross energy cost of standardized non–weight-bearing activity does not significantly change. In the last month of pregnancy, the gross energy cost of cycling was increased on the order of 10%.[26] The energy cost of standardized weight-bearing activities such as treadmill walking was unchanged until 25 weeks of gestation, after which it increased by 19%.[26] Standardized protocols, however, do not allow for behavioral changes in pace and intensity of physical activity, which may occur and conserve energy during pregnancy. The doubly labeled water method has been employed in 4 studies of well-nourished, pregnant women to measure free-living total energy expenditure (TEE).[22,27-29] Total energy expenditure increased from ~2200 to 2400 kcal/d before pregnancy to 2700 kcal/d in the third trimester. In British and Swedish women, the activity energy expenditure decreased in the 36th week of gestation, but this decrease was not observed in American women.

Gestational weight gain includes the products of conception (fetus, placenta, and amniotic fluid), and accretion of maternal tissues (uterus, breasts, blood, extracellular fluid, and adipose tissue). The energy cost of deposition can be calculated from the amount of protein and fat deposited. Hytten[20] made theoretical calculations based on a weight gain of 12.5 kg of which 3.8 kg is fat and 925 g is protein, and a birth weight of 3.4 kg (Table 11.5). The energy cost of pregnancy was calculated from the energy deposition, plus the energy cost of maintaining maternal and fetal tissues. The cumulative total gain of 85 000 kcal was divided by gestational duration to yield an increment of ~300 kcal/d.

Fat gains associated with weight gains within the IOM-recommended ranges were measured in 200 women using a 4-component body composition model (Table 11.6).[30] The total energy deposition between 14 and 37+ weeks of gestation was calculated based on an assumed protein deposition of 925 g protein, and energy equivalences of 5.65 kcal/g protein and 9.25 kcal/g fat. Mean fat gain in normal-weight women concurred with Hytten's theoretical model.

Based on Hytten's theoretical model, the 1989 recommended dietary allowance (RDA) for energy during pregnancy was set at an additional 300 kcal/d during the second and third trimesters.[21]

Table 11.5.
Energy Cost of Pregnancy*

	Gestational Weeks				Cumulative Total (kcal)
	0–10	10–20	20–30	30–40	
	Energy Equivalence (kcal/d)				
Protein	3.6	10.3	26.7	34.2	5186
Fat	55.6	235.6	207.6	31.3	36 329
Oxygen consumption	44.8	99.0	148.2	227.2	35 717
Total net energy	104.0	344.9	382.5	292.7	77 234
Metabolizable energy (+10%)	114	379	421	322	84 957

*Hytten, 1991.[20]

Table 11.6.
Energy Deposition During Pregnancy Measured by a 4-Component Body Composition Model*

Prepregnancy Body Mass Index (BMI) Category	Recommended Gestational Weight Gain (kg)	Actual Gestational Weight Gain (kg)	Fat Gain (kg)	Energy Deposition (kcal)
Underweight (BMI <19.8)	12.5–18	12.6	6.0	60 726
Normal (BMI 19.8–26.0)	11.5–16	12.1	3.8	40 376
High (BMI >26.0–29.0)	7–11.5	9.1	2.8	31 126
Obese (BMI >29.0)	6	6.9	−0.6	−324

*Lederman, 1997.[30]

Protein

Protein requirements increase during pregnancy because of the increase in protein turnover and protein deposition in the fetus, uterus, expanded maternal blood volume, mammary glands, and skeletal muscle.[6] The amount of protein accretion is estimated to be 925 g protein.[20] Whole-body protein turnover, measured by leucine and glycine kinetics, is augmented in the second and third trimesters compared with first-trimester and pregravid rates.[31-33] Because of the competition between maternal needs and fetal growth, protein requirements are higher in growing, pregnant adolescents.[34]

Sufficient dietary protein is needed to support the growth of maternal and fetal tissues. Accounting for individual variation (+30%) and the efficiency of protein utilization (70%), an additional 1.3, 6.1, and 10.7 g/d is required during the first, second, and third trimesters. The 1989 RDA for pregnant women is an additional 10 g/d throughout pregnancy.[21]

Iron

Iron functions in the body as an integral part of many proteins, including hemoglobin. About two thirds of the iron in the body is in hemoglobin, and the remainder in other heme-proteins (myoglobin, cytochromes), iron-sulfur enzymes (flavoproteins), and storage and transport vehicles (ferritin, transferrin). Insufficient dietary iron during pregnancy can result in iron-deficiency anemia. Epidemiological evidence demonstrates that maternal anemia is associated with higher mortality, premature delivery, low birth weight, and increased perinatal infant mortality.[35] High hemoglobin levels at delivery also are associated with adverse outcomes of prematurity, low birth weight, and fetal death. The high hemoglobin levels are a result of decreased plasma volume, due to maternal hypertension and eclampsia. While fetal needs take precedence over mother's iron needs, infants born to mothers with severe anemia have lower iron stores. Maternal anemia may also limit the infant's iron stores through premature delivery and low birth weight.

Iron needs increase during pregnancy, even though menstruation does not occur and intestinal absorption of this mineral is enhanced. Dietary iron requirement during pregnancy covers basal losses, deposition in fetal and maternal tissues, and expansion of hemoglobin.[35] Basal losses are estimated to be 250 mg over the 280 days of pregnancy. Approximately 315 mg of iron are deposited in fetal and placental tissues and 500 mg in the expansion of hemoglobin. Accounting for individual variability and an efficiency of absorption of 25%, the RDA was set at 27 mg/d.[35] This can be supplied by the diet if substantial effort is made to consume iron-rich foods. Unfortunately, this challenge can be substantial for women who wish to moderate their intake of red meat or otherwise choose a diet with limited iron sources. The median iron intake of pregnant women in the United States is 15 mg/d, which would indicate a need for supplementation. The IOM recommended that pregnant women receive an oral iron supplement of 30 mg/d during the second and third trimesters of pregnancy.[6] Most prenatal vitamin and mineral supplements supply this recommended level of iron in the form of ferrous salts.

When therapeutic levels of iron (>30 mg/d) are given to treat anemia, supplementation with approximately 15 mg of zinc and 2 mg of copper is recommended because the iron may interfere with the absorption and utilization of those trace elements.[6]

Calcium

Calcium is required not only for bone mineralization, but also for vascular contraction and vasodilation, muscle contraction, nerve transmission, and glandular secretion. During pregnancy, the fetus accretes approximately 25 to 30 g of calcium, with maximum accretion rates in the third trimester. Changes in maternal calcium homeostasis provide for fetal accretion of calcium.[36] Calcium absorption and urinary calcium excretion increase by approximately twofold in pregnant women. Bone resorption as well as bone formation are elevated during pregnancy, as reflected in the 50% to 200% rise in bone turnover markers. Total serum calcium decreases, with a slight rise at term. These changes in calcium homeostasis are mediated in part by the increase in calcitropic hormone 1,25-dihydroxyvitamin D. The major physiological adaptation to meet the increased calcium requirement of pregnancy is the increased efficiency of calcium absorption.

The effect of pregnancy on maternal bone mineral status has been studied in only a few prospective studies, and the results are conflicting.[36] Some have reported increases in bone mineral in the total body and cortical bone; others have reported decreases in bone mineral in sites rich in trabecular bone, whereas others have observed no changes at all.

Dietary calcium intake does not appear to affect bone mineral changes during pregnancy.[37] Although studies are limited, maternal calcium supplementation appears to have little effect on pregnancy-induced changes in calcium and bone metabolism in well-nourished women.

The effect of calcium supplementation in reducing the incidence of pregnancy-induced hypertension remains controversial. A meta-analysis of 14 randomized trials involving 2459 women showed significant reductions in systolic and diastolic blood pressure, and the odds ratio for preeclampsia in women receiving calcium supplement (1500 to 2000 mg) compared to placebo was 0.38.[38] The US Trial of Calcium for Preeclampsia Prevention (CPEP), involving 4589 nulliparous pregnant women on a calcium supplement of 2000 mg/d, did not reduce the incidence of preeclampsia or raised blood pressure.[39] In contrast, a randomized trial in Australia demonstrated a beneficial effect of calcium supplementation (1800 mg/d) on the incidence of preeclampsia.[40] Although no definite recommendation can be made based on these conflicting results, it does appear that some women at risk for preeclampsia may benefit from calcium supplementation. Further studies are needed to identify these susceptible individuals. A beneficial effect of calcium supplementation (2000 mg/d) on the incidence of preterm delivery and low birth weight was seen in a randomized trial involving 189 adolescents[41] and should be confirmed with further studies.

Because of the adaptive maternal responses to fetal calcium needs, it was concluded that there is no need for increased calcium intake, provided dietary calcium intake is adequate for maximizing bone accretion in the nonpregnant state. The recommended intake or adequate intake (AI) for pregnant women is 1300 mg/d calcium for ages 14 to 18 years and 1000 mg/d calcium for ages 19 to 50 years.

Zinc

Zinc is essential for structural integrity of proteins and regulation of gene expression. The additional zinc requirement during pregnancy reflects zinc accretion in newly synthesized maternal and fetal tissues. Changes in intestinal zinc absorption appear to be the primary homeostatic adjustment in zinc metabolism to meet the increased demand for zinc, but this has been technically difficult to prove in women.[42] Zinc deficiency in experimental animals limits fetal growth and, if severe, causes teratogenic anomalies. In humans, teratogenic effects have been observed in pregnancies of women with untreated acrodermatitis enteropathica. Maternal zinc deficiency in animals and humans has been associated with infertility, hypertension, prolonged labor, intrapartum hemorrhage, preterm delivery, IUGR, and embryonic or fetal death, although reports have been inconsistent.[35,42]

Randomized, controlled intervention trials of supplemental zinc yield equivocal results, in part because of issues of subject compliance, sample size, indicators of zinc status, and control for confounding variables.[42] Of 12 trials, 6 showed no effect of the supplement; 2 demonstrated an improvement in fetal growth; 4 showed a reduction in delivery complications, pregnancy-induced hypertension, preterm delivery, or IUGR. Zinc supplementation increased birth weight, head circumference, and gestational age in black women whose plasma zinc concentration was below the median for their population at 20 weeks of gestation.[43]

Based on maternal and fetal zinc accumulation of 2.7 mg/d[44] and a fractional absorption of 27%,[45] the RDA for zinc during pregnancy was set at 13 mg/d for adolescents 14 to 18 years and at 11 mg/d for women. Factors that interfere with zinc absorption (eg, high dietary phytate, fiber and calcium, high doses of supplemental iron, gastrointestinal diseases), or placental transport of zinc (eg, smoking, alcohol abuse, and an acute stress response to stress or infection) can cause a secondary zinc deficiency. Pregnant women with these conditions may benefit from a zinc supplement providing ~25 mg/d.[42]

Iodine

Iodine is an essential constituent of the thyroid hormones thyroxine and triiodothyronine, which regulate essential enzymatic and metabolic processes. Iodine deficiency results in delayed growth and development, mental retardation, hypothyroidism, goiter, and cretinism. Goiter is the earliest clinical manifestation of iodine deficiency during pregnancy. Serum thyroglobin and thyroid stimulating hormone (TSH) also increase.

The daily accumulation of iodine by the newborn is estimated to be 75 μg/d with close to 100% daily turnover.[35] From studies conducted in iodine-deficient areas it is estimated that 160 μg/d prevented goiter in pregnant women. Accounting for individual variability, the RDA for pregnancy was set at 220 μg/d to prevent goiter in most pregnant women.[35]

Vitamins

Vitamin A

Vitamin A is essential for normal vision, gene expression, reproduction, embryonic development, growth, and immune function. Vitamin A deficiency in pregnancy is associated with preterm birth, IUGR, and decreased birth weight.[6]

The RDA during pregnancy of 750 μg/d for girls 14 to 18 years and 770 μg/d for women 19 to 50 years is based on the accumulation of vitamin A in the fetal liver and on the assumption that the liver contains half the body's vitamin A when liver stores are low and a 70% efficiency of absorption.[35] Although most fetal vitamin A is accumulated in the last trimester, it can be stored in the mother's liver and later mobilized for fetal and maternal needs. Therefore, the recommended increment in vitamin A intake is for the entire pregnancy.

Excessive consumption of vitamin A appears to be teratogenic.[46] Adverse drug reaction reports filed with the Food and Drug Administration confirm that circumstances of excessive exposure to vitamin A during pregnancy may interfere with normal embryonic development. The critical period appears to be the first trimester of pregnancy. Birth defects are related to the cranial neural crest cells such as craniofacial malformations and abnormalities of the central nervous system, except neural tube defects (NTD). The hazardous level of vitamin A intake likely varies from one woman to another; concern should begin when the daily intake of vitamin A (through foods or supplements) exceeds the tolerable upper limit (UL) for adults set at 3000 μg/d.[35]

Folate

Folate functions as a coenzyme in single-carbon transfer reactions involved in nucleic and amino acid metabolism. The term folate includes synthetic folic acid in fortified foods and dietary supplements and naturally occurring forms in food. Since January 1998, all enriched cereal-grain products in the United States have been fortified to contain 140 μg/100 g to achieve a projected mean increase of 100 μg of folic acid/d in the US population.[47] Because of differences in bioavailability of food folate and synthetic folic acid, the dietary folate equivalent (DFE) is used to convert synthetic folic acid to a quantity equivalent to the amount in food: 1 μg DFE is equal to 1 μg of food folate, which is equal to 0.5 μg of folic acid on an empty stomach or 0.6 μg of folic acid with a meal.

Because of the marked increase in single-carbon transfer reactions, including those associated with nucleotide synthesis and thus cell division in maternal and fetal tissues, folate requirements increase during pregnancy. The increase in cell division is seen in the fetus, placenta, red blood cell expansion, uterus, and mammary gland. Folate is actively transferred to the fetus; cord blood concentrations of folate are higher than maternal blood concentrations. Inadequate dietary folate and low serum folate are associated with poor pregnancy outcomes.[48] Inadequate folate intake can eventually result in megaloblastic anemia.

The current RDA for folate during pregnancy was based on population-based studies and a controlled metabolic study.[49] It was apparent that low dietary folate plus 100 μg/d of supplemental folate was inadequate to maintain normal folate status in a significant number of pregnant women. Therefore, the RDA was set at 300 μg/d or 600 μg/d of dietary folate equivalents. Based on population and clinical studies, this amount is sufficient to maintain normal folate status in 97% to 98% of pregnant women.

The IOM recommendation for women capable of becoming pregnant is to take 400 μg/d of folate from fortified foods and/or a supplement, as well as food folate from a varied diet.[49] (The RDA for all other women is 400 μg/d of dietary folate equivalents). This preventive measure is based on evidence that a >50% reduction in risk for NTD was observed for women who took a folate supplement of 360 to 800 μg/d in addition to dietary folate of 200 to 300 μg/d. A larger dose of folate (4000 μg/d) beginning at least 1 month before conception and continuing through the first trimester has been recommended to prevent recurrence of NTD by the US Centers for Disease Control and Prevention (CDC)[50] and endorsed by the American Academy of Pediatrics (AAP).[51] Women should be advised not to attempt to achieve the 4000 μg dose from over-the-counter or prescription multivitamin preparations because of the risk of ingesting harmful levels of other vitamins. Also, the patient should understand that folate supplementation did not prevent all NTD in clinical trials, and, therefore, prenatal NTD testing should still be considered.

Vitamin C

Vitamin C functions as an antioxidant and cofactor for enzymes involved in the biosynthesis of collagen, carnitine, and neurotransmitters. Plasma concentrations of vitamin C decrease with the progression of pregnancy, probably because of hemodilution.[52] The placenta takes up the oxidized form of ascorbic acid and delivers the reduced form to the fetus.[53] Vitamin C deficiency is associated with increased risk of infections, premature rupture of membranes, premature birth, and eclampsia.[54] The fetus is subject to maternal status, as evidenced by lower amniotic fluid concentrations of vitamin C in pregnant smokers than nonsmokers.[55]

The RDA for vitamin C is increased by 10 mg/d to allow for adequate fetal transfer. Higher amounts are recommended for women who use illicit drugs, cigarettes, alcohol, and aspirin regularly. Although there is no firm evidence of vitamin C toxicity during pregnancy, megadoses can result in elevated concentrations in the fetus, with possible induction of fetal hemolysis and oxidative damage in preterm infants.[54]

Vitamin E

Vitamin E functions as an antioxidant that prevents propagation of lipid peroxidation. Plasma concentrations of vitamin E increase during pregnancy along with total lipids. Placental transfer of vitamin E appears to be relatively constant throughout pregnancy.[56] Neither vitamin E deficiency nor toxicity has been reported in pregnant women. There is no evidence that maternal supplementation prevents hemolytic anemia in preterm infants. The RDA for pregnancy is assumed to be same as that of nonpregnant women.[54]

Vitamin Supplementation

A varied diet based on the Food Pyramid[57] can meet all vitamin and nutrient needs associated with pregnancy; however, women whose dietary practices seem to be less than satisfactory may benefit from a prenatal vitamin supplement.[6] Special circumstances in which specific supplements are recommended include the following:

- Vitamin D: 10 μg (400 IU) daily for complete vegetarians (those who consume no animal products) and others with a low intake of vitamin D-fortified milk; vitamin D status is a special concern for women at northern latitudes in winter and for others with minimal exposure to sunlight and thus at risk for reduced synthesis of vitamin D in the skin.
- Vitamin B_{12}: 20 μg daily for complete vegetarians.
- Vitamin B_6: Supplements of vitamin B_6 may prevent nausea and vomiting in early pregnancy because vitamin B_6 catalyzes a number of reactions involving neurotransmitter production.[58,59] In 1991, results of a randomized, double-blind, placebo-controlled study were reported in which vitamin B_6 supplementation was evaluated for its effect on nausea and vomiting in early pregnancy.[60] Results indicated that women with mild to

moderate nausea did not benefit from vitamin B$_6$ supplementation. However, women with severe nausea and vomiting showed a substantial reduction in their symptoms. Therefore, some benefit may be derived from vitamin B$_6$ supplementation for women with problematic nausea and vomiting during early pregnancy.

Alcohol

Consumption of alcohol adversely affects fetal development. Fetal alcohol syndrome is estimated to occur in approximately 1 to 2 infants per 1000 live births in the United States.[61] More moderate drinkers may produce offspring with fetal alcohol effects[62]; such women also demonstrate a higher rate of spontaneous abortion, abruptio placentae, and low-birth-weight delivery. All women planning for conception should be advised to avoid consumption of alcoholic beverages. Women with a known addiction to alcohol should be strongly encouraged to enroll in a treatment program and practice contraception if treatment is unsuccessful. Rehabilitation of women who are addicted to alcohol after conception may not prevent adverse embryonic development, but it may positively affect the growth of the fetus.

Caffeine

The effect of caffeine on the course and outcome of pregnancy is still controversial. Research using animals indicates that excessive levels of caffeine intake increase the incidence of congenital malformations; the effects of consuming smaller quantities (eg, 3 to 5 cups of coffee per day) have not been satisfactorily studied. Human observational data suggest that excessive caffeine intake is associated with an increased risk of miscarriage, even accounting for concurrent smoking. Thus, common sense should prevail, and women considering pregnancy could legitimately be advised to use caffeine in moderation if they choose to use it at all.[63]

Aspartame

Since the approval of aspartame for use in carbonated beverages in 1983, the safety of the sweetener in the diets of pregnant women has been debated. Major concern has been voiced about the added phenylalanine load because high circulating levels of phenylalanine (as seen in women with poorly controlled PKU) are known to damage the fetal brain.[64] However, individuals who do not have PKU have plenty of phenylalanine hydroxylase activity in the liver to prevent any substantial and sustained rise in the serum phenylalanine level after consuming aspartame-rich beverages or foods. Because no data exist to suggest that use of aspartame-containing products is associated with adverse pregnancy outcome, directing women to avoid this alternative sweetener seems unreasonable.

Metabolic Disorders

Discussing existing metabolic disorders may be critical to the health of both mother and infant. Examples of disorders in which early intervention is effective are maternal phenylketonuria (PKU) and insulin-dependent diabetes mellitus. Metabolic control of both diseases involves conscientious dietary manipulation well before the critical period of embryonic development. In the case of the woman with PKU, restriction of dietary phenylalanine is mandatory, while satisfying the protein and other nutrient requirements of mother and fetus; evidence indicates that the IQ of the offspring is inversely related to the maternal serum phenylalanine concentration during pregnancy.[64] The woman with insulin-dependent diabetes mellitus must control blood glucose levels through careful food selection and scheduled meal timing in concert with the administration of insulin. By so doing, the risk of spontaneous abortion and congenital defects in the offspring can be markedly reduced.[65,66]

Gestational diabetes mellitus (GDM) is defined as "carbohydrate intolerance of variable severity with onset or first recognition during the present pregnancy."[67] Gestational diabetes mellitus is a heterogeneous disorder in which age, obesity, and genetic background contribute to the severity of the disease. Women with GDM are at risk for later development of non–insulin-dependent diabetes mellitus (NIDDM). Only a 1.6% incidence of islet-cell antibodies is found using a specific monoclonal antibody in women with GDM.[68] In the management of women with GDM, treatment modalities aimed at improving insulin sensitivity may be useful. Changes in diet, exercise, and achievement of desirable GWG should be encouraged to improve insulin sensitivity. Self-monitoring of glucose, daily checking of urinary ketones, and exercise to enhance insulin sensitivity are integral components of many programs for women with GDM. Insulin therapy is initiated if fasting blood glucose exceeds target blood glucose values.

Guidelines for the daily energy intake to support a desirable GWG have been provided for women with GDM. The American College of Obstetricians and Gynecologists (ACOG) recommends energy intakes of 35 to 40, 30, 24, and 12 to 15 kcal/kg present weight for women whose current pregnancy weights are <80, 80 to 120, 120 to 150, and >150% of ideal body weight, respectively.[67] The American Diabetes Association (ADA) has published similar guidelines.[69] Based on 24-hour measurements of total energy expenditure in women with GDM,[70] recommendations of energy intakes ≤ 25 kcal·kg^{-1}·d^{-1} would be unlikely to cover the free-living daily energy expenditure of these overweight women.

Caloric restriction has resulted in improved glycemic control in obese women with GDM.[71,72] With the calorie-restricted diets, the incidence of macrosomia was 6%, versus 23% in untreated controls. Knopp[71] studied obese women with GDM who were prescribed diets of 2400 kcal/d, 1600 to 1800 kcal/d (33% reduction), or 1200 kcal/d (50% reduction). Glycemic control improved on both calorie-restricted diets, but ketonuria increased twofold to threefold on the 50% calorie reduction. Potentially deleterious effects of ketonemia on fetal development and subsequent infant intellectual performance warrant avoidance of ketonemia.[73] IQ was inversely correlated with plasma levels of β-hydroxybutyrate and fatty acids, but not with levels of acetonuria in the third trimester.[73] While maternal weight gain and fetal macrosomia may be reduced, the safety of calorie restriction in the management of GDM has not been established and thus, it is not recommended by ACOG.[67]

Specific recommendations for diet composition have not been made for women with GDM. The ADA states that the percentage of carbohydrate is dependent on individual eating habits and the effect on blood glucose, and the percentage of fat depends on assessment and treatment goals.[69] This position acknowledges the need for individualization of dietary treatment. Several programs have successfully used diets composed of 40% to 50% carbohydrate, 20% protein, and 30% to 40% fat.[74] The lower carbohydrate blunts the postprandial hyperglycemia. In one study, diet-controlled patients with GDM were randomly assigned to a low-carbohydrate diet (<42%) or a high-carbohydrate diet (45% to 50%).[75] Carbohydrate restriction improved glycemic control, decreased the insulin requirement, decreased the incidence of large-for-gestational-age infants, and decreased cesarean deliveries for cephalopelvic disproportion and macrosomia. Exercise has also been shown to improve glycemic control.[76,77] Preventive measures should be aimed at improving insulin sensitivity in women predisposed to GDM.

Additional Dietary and Lifestyle Concerns

Food Cravings and Aversions

Most women change their diets during the course of pregnancy. Some changes are based on medical advice, others on folk medical beliefs, and others on changes in preference and appetite that may be idiosyncratic or culturally patterned. The health care professional should be aware that culturally sanctioned changes in diet might affect a woman's willingness to follow prescribed dietary regimens.

The most commonly avoided foods during pregnancy are also excellent sources of animal protein: milk, meats, pork, and liver. Cravings and aversions are powerful urges toward or away from foods, including foods about which women experience no unusual attitudes outside of pregnancy. The most commonly reported craved foods are sweets and dairy products. The most commonly reported aversions are alcohol, caffeinated drinks, and meats. However, cravings and aversions are not limited to any particular foods or food groups.[78] Pica may result in lead toxicity to mother and fetus if lead-containing paint is ingested.

The nutritional significance of these food-related behaviors is difficult to evaluate. Available information has often been collected in an anecdotal or uncontrolled manner. Thus, limited detailed information exists about dietary alterations that appear to be detrimental. As a result, quantifying the nutritional effect of restrictive beliefs, avoidances, cravings, and aversions is difficult. The nutritional importance of such practices cannot be assessed without reference to the rest of the woman's diet. Overall, however, most cravings result in decreased intake of alcohol, caffeine, and animal protein. Cravings and aversions are not necessarily deleterious.[78]

Herbal Teas

Pregnant women should be discouraged from unlimited consumption of herbal teas because the composition and safety of most of them is unknown. Rather than seek approval from the US Food and Drug Administration, most manufacturers of herbal tea preparations stopped marketing the mixtures as medicine and simply list the ingredients on the label.[79]

Because of the lack of safety testing, pregnant women should be cautious of herbal tea mixtures. They should be advised to choose only products in filtered tea bags and, to avoid displacing more nutritious beverages, to limit herbal tea consumption to two 8-oz servings per day.

Food Additives and Contaminants

The teratogenicity of specific common food additives would be a major concern if the US Food and Drug Administration did not require animal testing of new additives for their potential to cause birth defects. Some food contaminants are recognized as harmful to a developing fetus. Examples include heavy metals, chlorinated dioxin derivatives, and the fungal toxin aflatoxin. By law, no chemical that is found to be a carcinogen in humans or animals can be used as a food additive. There are no reports of birth defects from food additives used in commercial food products in the United States. Non-commercial foods, however, such as fish caught in polluted waters, can have high levels of mercury and other chemicals toxic to the fetus (see Chapter 52). States in which this is a problem have advisories about sport fish consumption, and the pregnant woman should read these with care. While government and industry undertake significant efforts to control contamination of food and water, they cannot eliminate all risks of exposure during pregnancy.

Exercise During Pregnancy

In the absence of medical or obstetric complications, pregnant women who engage in a moderate level of physical activity can maintain cardiovascular and muscular fitness throughout pregnancy.[80] Because of the physiological changes in the pregnant woman, some physical activities are not recommendable. Contraindications to exercise include pregnancy-induced hypertension, premature rupture of membranes, preterm labor, incompetent cervix/cerclage, persistent bleeding, and IUGR. Women with complications, such as chronic hypertension or active thyroid, or cardiac, vascular, or pulmonary disease, should be evaluated to determine if exercise is advisable. The American College of Obstetricians and Gynecologists issued the following guidelines for exercise during pregnancy[80]:

1. Women can continue to exercise and receive benefit from mild to moderate exercise routines, preferably performed regularly (at least 3 times per week).
2. Exercise in the supine position should be avoided.
3. Women should stop exercising when fatigued and not exercise to exhaustion.
4. Exercise involving the potential for even mild abdominal trauma should be avoided.
5. Pregnant women who exercise should augment heat dissipation through adequate hydration, appropriate clothing, and optimal environment.

The effect of vigorous exercise on the pregnant woman and the fetus has been the source of considerable debate. Physical fitness enthusiasts have championed maintenance of vigorous activity during pregnancy, while others have urged caution. A series of well-conducted studies of the effects of vigorous exercise on pregnancy outcome[81–84] concluded that very active women were no more likely to have a spontaneous abortion than were more sedentary women, and they seemed to have fewer difficulties during labor and delivery; however, their infants were smaller. The longer-term consequences of smaller size on later health and well-being of the neonate are unknown. Until more data are available, pregnant women should be advised to exercise moderately during the third trimester.

References

1. American Academy of Pediatrics, Committee on Adolescence. Adolescent pregnancy—current trends and issues: 1998. *Pediatrics.* 1999;103:516–520
2. Ventura SJ, Mathews TJ, Curtin SC. Declines in teenage birth rates, 1991–97: national and state patterns. *Natl Vital Stat Rep.* 1998;47:1–7
3. Garbaciak JA Jr, Richter M, Miller S. Maternal weight and pregnancy complications. *Obstet Gynecol.* 1985;152:238–245
4. Kleigman RM, Gross T. Perinatal problems of the obese mother and her infant. *Obstet Gynecol.* 1985;66:299–306
5. Kleigman R, Gross T, Morton S, Dunnington R. Intrauterine growth and postmeal fasting metabolism in infants of obese mother. *J Pediatr.* 1984;104:601–607
6. Institute of Medicine and Food and Nutrition Board. *Nutrition During Pregnancy.* Washington DC: National Academy Press; 1990
7. Lechtig A, Habicht JP, Delgado H, Klein RE, Yarbrough C, Martorell R. Effect of food supplementation during pregnancy on birthweight. *Pediatrics.* 1975;56: 508–520
8. Kramer MS. Determinants of low birth weight: methodological assessment and meta-analysis. *Bull World Health Organ.* 1987;65:663–737
9. Naeye RL. Teenaged and preteenaged pregnancies: consequences of the fetal maternal competition for nutrients. *Pediatrics.* 1981;67:146–150
10. Abrams B, Selvin S. Maternal weight gain pattern and birth weight. *Obstet Gynecol.* 1995;86:163–169
11. Hickey CA, Cliver SP, McNeal SF, Hoffman HJ, Godenberg RL. Prenatal weight gain patterns and birth weight among nonobese black and white women. *Obstet Gynecol.* 1996;88:490–496
12. Scholl TO, Hediger ML, Ances IG, Belsky DH, Salmon RW. Weight gain during pregnancy in adolescence: predictive ability of early weight gain. *Obstet Gynecol.* 1990;75:948–953

13. Strauss RS, Dietz WH. Low maternal weight gain in the second or third trimester increases the risk for intrauterine growth retardation. *J Nutr.* 1999;129:988–993

14. Bianco AT, Smilen SW, Davis Y, Lopez S, Lapinski R, Lockwood CJ. Pregnancy outcome and weight gain recommendations for the morbidly obese woman. *Obstet Gynecol.* 1998;91:97–102

15. Kuczmarski RJ, Flegal KM, Campbell SM, Johnson CL. Increasing prevalence of overweight among US adults. The National Health and Nutrition Examination Surveys, 1960 to 1991. *JAMA.* 1994;272:205–211

16. Greene GW, Smiciklas-Wright H, Scholl T, Karp RJ. Postpartum weight change: how much of the weight gained in pregnancy will be lost after delivery? *Obstet Gynecol.* 1988;71:701–707

17. Gunderson E, Abrams B. Epidemiology of gestational weight gain and body weight changes after pregnancy. *Epidemiol Rev.* 2000;22:261–274

18. Cogswell ME, Scanlon KS, Fein SB, Schieve LA. Medically advised, mother's personal target, and actual weight gain during pregnancy. *Obstet Gynecol.* 1999;94:616–622

19. Schieve LA, Cogswell ME, Scanlon KS. Trends in pregnancy weight gain within and outside ranges recommended by the IOM in a WIC population. *Matern Child Health J.* 1998;2:111–116

20. Hytten FE. Weight gain in pregnancy. In: Hytten FE, Chamberlain G, eds. *Clinical Physiology in Obstetrics.* Oxford, UK: Blackwell Scientific Publications; 1991:173–203

21. National Research Council FNB. *Recommended Dietary Allowances.* Washington, DC: National Academy Press; 1989

22. Goldberg GR, Prentice AM, Coward WA, et al. Longitudinal assessment of energy expenditure in pregnancy by the doubly labeled water method. *Am J Clin Nutr.* 1993;57:494–505

23. Forsum E, Sadurskis A, Wager J. Resting metabolic rate and body composition of healthy Swedish women during pregnancy. *Am J Clin Nutr.* 1988;47:942–947

24. Spaaij CJK. *The Efficiency of Energy Metabolism During Pregnancy and Lactation in Well-Nourished Dutch Women* [dissertation]. The Netherlands: University of Wageningen; 1993

25. van Raaij JM, Vermaat-Miedema SH, Schonk CM, Peek ME, Hautvast JG. Energy requirements of pregnancy in The Netherlands. *Lancet.* 1987;2:953–955

26. Prentice AM, Spaaij CJ, Goldberg GR, et al. Energy requirements of pregnant and lactating women. *Eur J Clin Nutr.* 1996;50:S82–S111

27. Forsum E, Kabir N, Sadurskis A, Westerterp K. Total energy expenditure of healthy Swedish women during pregnancy and lactation. *Am J Clin Nutr.* 1992;56:334–342

28. Goldberg GR, Prentice AM, Coward WA, et al. Longitudinal assessment of the components of energy balance in well-nourished lactating women. *Am J Clin Nutr.* 1991;54:788–798

29. Kopp-Hoolihan LE, Van Loan MD, Wong WW, King JC. Longitudinal assessment of energy balance in well-nourished, pregnant women. *Am J Clin Nutr.* 1999;69:697–704

30. Lederman SA, Paxton A, Heymsfield SB, Wang J, Thornton J, Pierson RN Jr. Body fat and water changes during pregnancy in women with different body weight and weight gain. *Obstet Gynecol.* 1997;90:483–488

31. Thompson GN, Halliday D. Protein turnover in pregnancy. *Eur J Clin Nutr.* 1992;46:411–417

32. Jackson AA. Measurement of protein turnover during pregnancy. *Hum Nutr Clin Nutr.* 1987;41:497–498

33. Fitch W, King JC. Protein turnover and 3-methylhistidine excretion in non-pregnant, pregnant and gestational diabetic women. *Hum Nutri Clin Nutr.* 1987;41:327–339

34. Scholl TO, Hediger ML, Ances IG. Maternal growth during pregnancy and decreased infant birth weight. *Am J Clin Nutr.* 1990;51:790–793

35. Institute of Medicine. Vitamin A. In: *Dietary Intakes for Vitamin A, Vitamin K, Arsenic, Boron, Chromium, Copper, Iodine, Iron, Manganese, Molybdenum, Nickel, Silicon, Vanadium, and Zinc.* National Academy Press; 2001:65–126

36. Prentice A. Calcium in pregnancy and lactation. *Annu Rev Nutr.* 2000;20:249–272

37. Institute of Medicine Food and Nutrition Board. Dietary reference intakes for calcium, phosphorus, magnesium, vitamin D, and fluoride. 1997

38. Bucher HC, Guyatt GH, Cook RJ, et al. Effect of calcium supplementation on pregnancy-induced hypertension and preeclampsia. A meta-analysis of randomized controlled trials. *JAMA.* 1996;275:1113–1117

39. Levine RJ, Hauth JC, Curet LB, et al. Trial of calcium to prevent preeclampsia. *N Engl J Med.* 1997;337:69–76

40. Crowther CA, Hiller JE, Pridmore B, et al. Calcium supplementation in nulliparous women for the prevention of pregnancy-induced hypertension, preeclampsia and preterm birth: an Australian randomized trial. *Aust N Z J Obstet Gynaecol.* 1999;39:12–18

41. Villar J, Repke J, Belizan JM, Pareja G. Calcium supplementation reduces blood pressure during pregnancy: results of a randomized controlled clinical trial. *Obstet Gynecol.* 1987;70:317–322

42. King JC. Determinants of maternal zinc status during pregnancy. *Am J Clin Nutr.* 2000;71:1334S–1343S

43. Goldenberg RL, Tamura T, Neggers Y, et al. The effect of zinc supplementation on pregnancy outcome. *JAMA.* 1995;274:463–468

44. Swanson CA, King JC. Zinc and pregnancy outcome. *Am J Clin Nutr.* 1987; 46:763–771

45. Fung EB, Ritchie LD, Woodhouse LR, Roehl R, King JC. Zinc absorption in women during pregnancy and lactation: a longitudinal study. *Am J Clin Nutr.* 1997;66:80–88

46. Rosa F, Wilk AL, Kelsey FO. Teratogen update: vitamin A congeners. *Teratology.* 1986;33:355–364

47. Food and Drug Administration. Food standards: amendment of standards of identity for enriched grain products to require addition of folic acid; final rule. *Fed Regist.* 1996;61:21

48. Scholl TO, Hediger ML, Shall JI, Khoo CS, Fischer RL. Dietary and serum folate: their influence on the outcome of pregnancy. *Am J Clin Nutr.* 1996;63:520–525

49. Institute of Medicine: Thiamin. In: Panel on Folate—Other B Vitamins and Choline, eds. *Dietary Reference Intakes for Thiamin, Riboflavin, Niacin, Vitamin B$_6$, Folate, Vitamin B$_{12}$, Pantothenic Acid, Biotin, and Choline.* Washington, DC: National Academy Press; 1998:58–86

50. Centers for Disease Control and Prevention. Use of folic acid for prevention of spina bifida and other neural tube defects: 1983–1991. *MMWR Morb Mortal Wkly Rep.* 1991;40:513–516

51. American Academy of Pediatrics, Committee on Genetics. Folic acid for the prevention of neural tube defects. *Pediatrics.* 1999;104:325–327

52. Morse EH, Clark RP, Keyser DE, Merrow SB, Bee DE. Comparison of the nutritional status of pregnant adolescents with adult pregnant women. I. Biochemical findings. *Am J Clin Nutr.* 1975;28:1000–1013

53. Choi JL, Rose RC. Transport and metabolism of ascorbic acid in human placenta. *Am J Physiol.* 1989;257:C110–C113

54. Institute of Medicine. Vitamin C. In: Panel on Dietary Antioxidants and Related Compounds, eds. *Dietary Reference Intakes for Vitamin C, Vitamin E, Selenium, and Carotenoids.* Washington, DC: 2000;95–185

55. Barrett B, Gunter E, Jenkins J, Wang M. Ascorbic acid concentration in amniotic fluid in late pregnancy. *Biol Neonate.* 1991;60:333–335

56. Abbasi S, Ludomirski A, Bhutani VK, Weiner S, Johnson L. Maternal and fetal plasma vitamin E to total lipid ratio and fetal RBC antioxidant function during gestational development. *J Am Coll Nutr.* 1990;9:314–319

57. United States Department of Agriculture. *The Food Guide Pyramid.* Washington, DC: United States Department of Agriculture; 1994

58. Schuster K, Bailey LB, Dimperio D, Mahan CS. Morning sickness and vitamin B$_6$ status of pregnant women. *Hum Nutr Clin Nutr.* 1985;39:75–79

59. Schuster K, Bailey LB, Mahan CS. Effect of maternal pyridoxine X HCl supplementation on the vitamin B-6 status of mother and infant and on pregnancy outcome. *J Nutr.* 1984;114:977–988

60. Sahakian V, Rouse D, Sipes S, Rose N, Niebyl J. Vitamin B$_6$ is effective therapy for nausea and vomiting of pregnancy: a randomized double-blind placebo-controlled study. *Obstet Gynecol.* 1991;78:33–36

61. Abel EL, Sokol RJ. Incidence of fetal alcohol syndrome and economic impact of FAS-related anomalies. *Drug Alcohol Depend.* 1987;19:51–70

62. Little RE, Wendt JK. The effects of maternal drinking in the reproductive period: an epidemiologic review. *J Subst Abuse Treat.* 1991;3:187–204

63. Worthington-Roberts BS. *Nutrition in Pregnancy and Lactation.* 5th ed. St Louis, MO: Mosby; 1993

64. Levy HL, Waisbren SE. Effects of untreated maternal phenylketonuria and hyperphenylalaninemia on the fetus. *N Engl J Med.* 1983;309:1269–1274

65. Fuhrmann K, Reiher H, Semmler K, Fischer F, Fischer M, Glockner E. Prevention of congenital malformations in infants of insulin-dependent diabetic mothers. *Diabetes Care.* 1983;6:219–223

66. Mills JL, Simpson JL, Driscoll SG, et al. Incidence of spontaneous abortion among normal women and insulin-dependent diabetic women whose pregnancies are identified within 21 days of conception. *N Engl J Med.* 1988;319:1617–1623

67. ACOG Technical Bulletin. Diabetes and pregnancy. *Int J Gynaecol Obstet.* 1995; 48:331–339

68. Catalano PM, Tyzbir ED, Sims EA. Incidence and significance of islet cell antibodies in women with previous gestational diabetes. *Diabetes Care.* 1990; 13:478–482

69. Fagen C, King JD, Erick M. Nutrition management in women with gestational diabetes mellitus: a review by ADA's Diabetes Care and Education Dietetic Practice Group. *J Am Diet Assoc.* 1995;95:460–467

70. Butte NF. Carbohydrate and lipid metabolism in pregnancy: normal compared with gestational diabetes mellitus. *Am J Clin Nutr.* 2000;71:1256S–1261S

71. Knopp RH, Magee MS, Raisys V, Benedetti T. Metabolic effects of hypocaloric diets in management of gestational diabetes. *Diabetes.* 1991;40:165–171

72. Magee MS, Knopp RH, Benedetti TJ. Metabolic effects of a 1200-kcal diet in obese pregnant women with gestational diabetes. *Diabetes.* 1990;39:234–240

73. Rizzo T, Metzger BE, Burns WJ, Burns K. Correlations between antepartum maternal metabolism and intelligence of offspring. *N Engl J Med.* 1991;325:911–916

74. Miller EH. Metabolic management of diabetes in pregnancy. *Semin Perinatol.* 1994;18:414–431

75. Major CA, Henry MJ, De Veciana M, Morgan MA. The effects of carbohydrate restriction in patients with diet-controlled gestational diabetes. *Obstet Gynecol.* 1998;91:600–604

76. Jovanovic-Peterson L, Peterson CM. Exercise and the nutritional management of diabetes during pregnancy. *Obstet Gynecol Clin North Am.* 1996;23:75–86

77. Bung P, Artal R, Khodiguian N, Kjos S. Exercise in gestational diabetes. An optional therapeutic approach? *Diabetes.* 1991;40:182–185

78. National Research Council Food and Nutrition Board. *Alternative Dietary Practices and Nutritional Abuses in Pregnancy.* Washington, DC: National Academy Press; 1982

79. Larkin T. Herbs are often more toxic than magical. In: *FDA Consumer.* Washington, DC: Department of Health and Human Services; 1983

80. American College of Obstetrics and Gynecology. Exercise during pregnancy and the postpartum period. *ACOG Tech Bull.* 1994;189:1–5

81. Clapp JF III, Dickstein S. Endurance exercise and pregnancy outcome. *Med Sci Sports Exerc.* 1984;16:556–562

82. Clapp JF III. The effects of maternal exercise on early pregnancy outcome. *Am J Obstet Gynecol.* 1989;161:1453–1457

83. Clapp JF III. The course of labor after endurance exercise during pregnancy. *Am J Obstet Gynecol.* 1990;163:1799–1805

84. American College of Obstetrics and Gynecology. *Exercise During Pregnancy and the Postnatal Period.* Washington, DC: American College of Obstetrics and Gynecology; 1985

12

Nutritional Aspects of Vegetarian Diets

As the popularity of vegetarian diets has increased dramatically during the last few decades, many parents encourage their children to join them in these eating patterns.[1] Today, approximately 7% of Americans consider themselves vegetarians, less than 1% are lacto-ovo vegetarians who abstain from all meat, fish, and poultry flesh, and perhaps 0.1% are vegan vegetarians who eat no animal foods at all.[2]

People vary in what they mean when they refer to themselves as vegetarians. Vegetarians and nonvegetarians differ in their eating practices and often also in larger belief systems, living habits (eg, vegetarian lifestyles), and values (eg, vegetarianism).[3] Some individuals are actually semi-vegetarians who simply limit their consumption of meat in favor of a plant-based diet and emphasize meatless meals. Others emphasize a plant-based lacto-ovo vegetarian diet that includes varying amounts of animal foods, usually milk and eggs, and sometimes fish, with avoidance of flesh foods (red meat and poultry). Still others eat an exclusively plant diet (a vegan diet) with no animal foods at all. Additional dietary alterations such as exclusions of processed foods, nonorganic foods, or foods produced through biotechnology sometimes accompany these patterns. Each of these eating styles has different implications on the nutrition and health of children and adolescents; therefore, it is important for the nutrition counselor to probe to determine which groups of foods are actually consumed and which are avoided and the degree of conviction and adherence to the dietary pattern so as to provide appropriate recommendations.

Parents choose vegetarian diets for many reasons. The primary reason is real or perceived health benefits. However, other motivations may also be present. Economic reasons alone are usually not involved because, in the United States, a wide variety of both plant and animal foods are widely available and inexpensive. However, some immigrants from developing countries (eg, mainland China, India, Pakistan, and Southeast Asia) may maintain vegetarian eating patterns from tradition, habit, and religious beliefs, coupled with lack of money to purchase more expensive foods of animal origin. As the economic circumstances of these groups improve, the intake of foods of animal origin often increases.[4] Other reasons for eating vegetarian diets include concerns about the risks of omnivorous diets. These are engendered in part by negative publicity about bacterial food-borne disease in animal foods and on milk from cows treated with bovine somatotropin (BST). Recent reports of "mad cow disease" (bovine spongiform encephalopathy) and hoof-and-mouth disease in European cattle and confusion about their implications for humans have also generated alarm, although neither of these diseases has been reported in this country. Ecological reasons involving views that the environmental impact of meat and poultry production is an inefficient use of the planet's resources motivate others.[5,6] Some have religious (eg, Seventh-Day Adventists, some Hindus and Buddhists) or philosophical beliefs (macrobiotics, transcendental meditators, anthroposophists, some yogic groups) that encourage various types of vegetarian diets and/or other food avoidances in their followers. A small but unknown proportion of persons with deeply held personal convictions regard themselves as "ethical vegetarians." They have adopted vegetarianism as the major organizing principle of life, and this value system affects many aspects of their lives.[7] These beliefs are manifested not only by consumption of a vegan diet but also by avoidance of animal products such as honey, leather, wool, or silk; opposition to the slaughter of animals for food; opposition to the inhumane treatment of animals; deeply held beliefs about animal rights; nonviolence toward animals; and other matters. In childhood and adolescence, this can sometimes present with a spontaneous aversion to eating animal products.

The extent and degree of animal food restriction does not always predict either the extent of other food avoidances or the divergences in lifestyle and philosophical beliefs from nonvegetarians, although there is some correspondence. Generally vegetarians with the most restrictive diets have the largest number of reasons for their eating styles, and their dietary patterns are most closely interwoven into their philosophical and belief systems.

Many vegetarian dietary patterns exist, and their health consequences vary. The most common pattern is avoidance of red meat, sometimes called semi vegetarianism. Lacto-ovo vegetarians usually avoid meat, poultry, fish, and seafood. Vegans avoid all animal foods. Avoidance of some or all animal foods is sometimes coupled with other dietary restrictions, such as eating only "natural," "organic," or "unprocessed foods," or avoidance of alcohol or of vitamin-mineral supplements. Foods rarely eaten by omnivores such as soy milk, tofu, meat analogues and other soy products, nuts, nut butters, and many varieties of fruits and vegetables enhance dietary variety. As with any dietary pattern, the degree of adherence to vegetarian patterns varies, and thus, overall nutrient intake differs from one vegetarian to the next. Most dietary patterns can be accommodated while fulfilling nutrient needs with appropriate dietary planning based on scientific principles of sound nutrition. Most vegetarian parents welcome such advice. However, when goals are so zealously pursued and nutrition principles are ignored, the health consequences can be unfortunate, especially for infants and young children.[8]

Over the centuries, many cultural, ethnic, and religious groups have consumed traditional vegetarian diets and remained in good health.[9] Some aspects of vegetarian diets are beneficial. These diets are in accord with the current nutritional emphasis on plant-based diets and dietary guidelines, including a lower intake of saturated fat and cholesterol, higher intakes of fiber and of polyunsaturated and monounsaturated fats, and moderation in food energy. Vegetarian diets tend to be higher than animal food-based diets in thiamin, vitamin C, beta-carotene and other caratenoids, vitamin E, and phytochemicals that may have health benefits. All-cause mortality in adults on vegetarian diets may not be lower, but differences in specific causes of death (such as smoking-related cancers) do seem to differ, although these may reflect lifestyle as well as dietary factors. Vegetarians often have a lower prevalence of several conditions including hypertension,[10] hyperlipidemia, coronary artery disease,[11,12] cancer,[13] obesity,[14] and cholelithiasis.[15]

The American Dietetic Association, the Food and Nutrition Board of the National Research Council, the National Institute of Nutrition (Canada), and the British Dietetic Association all consider vegetarian diets a viable alternative, if well devised.[16-19] However, certain components of the diet may be in short supply and require special attention in meal planning.[20] These concerns are more pronounced for children because of their proportionately greater need for nutrients during growth and development. New or atypical vegetarian diets that have risen in popularity within the last several decades in this country include yogic, transcendental meditation, macrobiotic, fruitarian, anthroposophic, and Rastafarian dietary patterns. The effects of some of the newer vegetarian dietary patterns are not yet clear, particularly in rapidly growing infants, children, and adolescents, pregnant and lactating women, and chronically ill children, all of whose nutrient needs may be especially high.[21]

In their most rigorous forms, the macrobiotic, fruitarian, and Rastafarian diets are extremely restrictive. Macrobiotic diets originally involved a series of progressively restricted regimens with food choices based on perceived meta-physical properties rather than on scientifically valid nutrition principles. Although regimens are currently less restrictive, these diets are still not satisfactory for children at weaning.[22] Rastafarians follow dietary practices similar to vegans, but avoid salt-preserved foods, additives, and alcohol. Fruitarian diets consist largely of fruits, often eaten raw, but nuts, honey, and olive oil are allowed. "Living foods" diets consist of the foods found in the fruitarian diet along with fresh vegetables and cereals, and special health foods, such as wheat grass or carrot juice. On such regimens, risks of iron deficiency anemia, rickets, megaloblastic anemia due to vitamin B_{12} deficiency, and protein calorie malnutrition may arise, although, fortunately, these are rare.

Vegetarian diets are often only one manifestation of the lifestyles of groups advocating vegetarianism. Some parents who choose certain vegetarian eating patterns for their children also have other nontraditional health care beliefs or practices. These may include questioning the need for vaccinations, reliance on homeopathy, and the avoidance of all animal products (eg, honey, leather, and wool). Other practices, such as extended breastfeeding, not smoking, a physically active lifestyle, and avoidance of alcohol, cigarettes, and addictive drugs have positive health implications.

Areas of Concern for Children

Sound Patterns
Sound vegetarian diets provide a food pattern that is adequate but not excessive in energy, protein, fat, minerals, vitamins, water, and fiber. They incorporate dietary variety and diversity, particularly in fruits, vegetables, nuts, legumes, and meat analogues. They meet the needs of the infant or child for growth and development, are age-appropriate, and fulfill any other special health needs that have dietary implications for the individual child. They are coupled with sound anticipatory health and dietary guidance and ongoing growth and health monitoring.[23] In contrast, unsound vegetarian regimens lack these characteristics. In addition, they may be coupled with unwillingness to seek or follow medical advice to prevent or cure common medical conditions.[8]

General
Children exhibit good growth and thrive on most lacto-ovo vegetarian and vegan diets when they are well planned and supplemented appropriately.[23–25] The growth of children of Seventh-Day Adventists and other lacto-ovo vegetarians was indistinguishable from that of omnivores in several recent studies.[26]

Growth delays have occasionally been encountered in children fed severely restricted diets (primarily macrobiotic, Rastafarian, and fruitarian forms).[16,18] Periods of rapid growth during infancy and childhood, especially stages that involve dietary changes, are of special concern among vegan and macrobiotic children. Their parents sometimes feed them inappropriately, particularly during the weaning period, which usually occurs between 6 and 18 months of age.[27,28] By the time children are able to obtain food by themselves at around school age, the growth of vegetarian and nonvegetarians in Western countries becomes more alike. Few differences have been found in the timing of puberty or completed adult growth today. Moreover, little effect is evident on IQ, assuming the vegetarian diet is nutritionally adequate.[29] Also, although Indian and Pakistani children of vegetarian families who have recently emigrated to Western countries are still shorter than their omnivorous peers, they are taller than their counterparts living in their native country.[30]

Energy

Vegan diets are relatively low in caloric density, and while this poses little problem for older individuals, for vegan infants, weanlings, and small children, energy intakes may be too low. During infancy and weaning, the amount of food needed to meet energy needs on vegan diets may be beyond gastric capacity, unless the child is fed frequently. Concentrated sources of calories that are acceptable for older infants and children include oils, nuts, nut butters, and fruit juices.[31]

Protein

Despite the low caloric density of strict vegetarian diets, especially if weaning from the breast occurs relatively early (ie, before 4 to 6 months), food intakes are usually sufficient to support protein needs. Some plant sources of protein are limited in one or more amino acids, and thus the efficiency of protein utilization is decreased. However, this is only likely to be a problem if very restrictive diets are fed that consist of a single plant protein, and this is rarely the case in developed countries. In developing countries, where a single carbohydrate staple is often the weaning food and provides a predominance of calories, consumption of a small amount of foods of animal origin has been shown to improve growth rates, independent of calorie or protein intake.[32] Mixtures of several plant proteins (eg, legumes, cereals, nuts and seeds, fruits, and other vegetables) promote good nutritional status, especially if small amounts of animal protein are eaten.[33] Soy-based commercial infant formulas, which are supplemented with methionine, promote normal growth in term infants. Adequate calorie intakes are vital so that protein is used efficiently rather than being metabolized for energy.[33]

The 5 major food sources of plant protein are legumes, cereals, nuts and seeds, fruits, and other vegetables. Each of these has nutritional advantages and disadvantages. For example, legumes and cereals provide relatively large amounts of quality protein, but they must be cooked or processed to enhance their palatability and to remove substances that decrease digestibility, such as tough skins, amylase inhibitors, lectins, and tannins. Protein quantity, quality, and digestibility are all of potential concern, especially when vegan-vegetarian diets are used during infancy. Then the proportion of essential amino acids needed per unit of body weight is double that required by adults. Lysine is lower in all plant foods than in animal foods. The levels of sulfur-containing amino acids, methionine and cysteine, are lower in legumes and fruits. The level of the essential amino acid, threonine, is lower in cereals, and tryptophan content tends to be lower in fruits than it is in most animal foods. Fortunately, certain plant proteins (or plant and animal proteins) complement each other so when eaten together or separately, they meet the requirements of the child for all amino acids.[33] Therefore, if parents feed diets that are adequate in food energy and select a variety of plant foods with proteins that complement each other, vegetarian children should receive adequate nutrients to grow and thrive.

Fat

If dietary fat intakes of vegetarian children over the age of 2 years are between 25% and 35% of calories, even if they are lower than those of omnivores, effects on growth appear to be small.[34–37] However, when dietary fat is below approximately 15% of calories, special care must be taken to ensure that recommended intakes of essential fatty acids are met. At least 3% of energy should be from linoleic acid (ω-3 fatty acid), and 1% from linolenic acid (ω-6 fatty acid). Linoleic acid is found in seeds nuts and grains. α-linolenic acid is found in the green leaves of plants, in phytoplankton and algae, in certain seeds, and in nuts and legumes, such as flax, canola, walnuts, hazelnuts, and soy. These can be converted into more highly unsaturated fatty acids, arachidonic acid, eicosapentaenoic acid (EPA), and docosahexaenoic acid (DHA). Arachidonic acid is found in animal foods such as meat, poultry, and eggs. Eicosapentaenoic acid and DHA are largely found in fish and seafood. Arachidonic acid and EPA serve as precursors for the eicosanoids. Tentative recommended intakes for these polyunsaturated fatty acids range from 3% to

10% of total energy intakes. Vegan-vegetarians have no direct sources of the long-chain ω-3 fatty acids EPA and DHA in their diets, and thus must convert α-linolenic acid to them. There is concern that pregnant women who are vegans, or macrobiotics who consume little or no fish or other animal foods, may not obtain enough of these fatty acids, especially during pregnancy and in early infancy. Risks are thought to be especially high if the infants are premature and their capacity to desaturate α-linolenic acid to DHA is limited. Such individuals may need DHA supplements, either from fish oils or from cultured microalgae. However, such supplements should only be dispensed under a physician's direction because they are also potent anticoagulants.

Vitamins

Vitamin B$_{12}$

Vitamin B$_{12}$ is found only in foods of animal origin, as a metabolite derived from bacterial synthesis, or in foods to which the vitamin has been added during fortification. Therefore, vegans are at potential risk of vitamin B$_{12}$ deficiency unless a vitamin B$_{12}$ supplement or fortified foods containing sufficient amounts of B$_{12}$ are consumed. Individuals who consume vegan diets should use a vitamin B$_{12}$ supplement or sufficient amounts of foods fortified with synthetic vitamin B$_{12}$. Vegan mothers who are marginally deficient in vitamin B$_{12}$ produce milk that is low in the nutrient. The infants of such mothers should be given some source of supplementary vitamin B$_{12}$ because vitamin B$_{12}$ deficiency has been reported in these infants.[38] Lacto-ovo vegetarians usually obtain enough vitamin B$_{12}$ from the animal foods they eat to meet daily requirements. Some appropriate sources of vitamin B$_{12}$ for vegans are vitamin B$_{12}$ supplements, yeast grown on a vitamin B$_{12}$-enriched medium, vitamin B$_{12}$-fortified soy and nut beverages, soy formulas specifically intended to support the nutritional requirements of infants or children, and vitamin B$_{12}$-fortified cereals. Inappropriate sources include food and water contaminated with vitamin B$_{12}$-producing bacteria because of poor hygiene, foods such as spirulina, kombu, tempeh, and miso, that do not provide a form of B$_{12}$ that humans can use and that may compete with biologically active B$_{12}$ for absorption, and seaweed, which varies in its vitamin B$_{12}$ content by the quantity of plankton it contains.[39]

Usually many years are required for vitamin B$_{12}$ deficiency to develop in a healthy adult who eats a diet devoid of the vitamin because body stores of the vitamin are considerable.[40] However, individuals raised as vegans or near vegans from birth lack these stores. Of special concern in infants is that the glial cells in the brain may be depleted of B_{12} before megaloblastic anemia develops, and permanent neurologic damage may result. Among vegetarians who have a very high intake of folic acid, the anemia may never develop.[41] Therefore, all vegan infants, children, and adolescents should receive vitamin B_{12} supplements.[40]

Riboflavin

Riboflavin has occasionally been deficient in severely restricted macrobiotic diets, but it is not a problem in other forms of vegetarianism.

Vitamin D

Vitamin D intake is often low in vegan diets because the foods in which it occurs naturally, such as liver, fatty ocean fish, egg yolks, and butter, and those to which it has been added, such as fortified soy milk and cow milk, are not included. Because vitamin D status in humans is affected by sunlight exposure, clinical vitamin D deficiency is relatively rare except in the very northern latitudes. However, sunscreens decrease endogenous synthesis.[42] In the United States, fluid cow milk, skim milk powder, and margarine are fortified with vitamin D. Lacto-ovo vegetarian children consume liberal amounts of fortified cow milk, and their vitamin D status is usually adequate. Supplementation of vitamin D is indicated for breastfed infants, young children living in very northern latitudes, or those with inadequate sunlight exposure eating a vegan diet. Acceptable sources of vitamin D include cod liver oil, menhaden oil, and vitamin/mineral supplements that contain vitamin D. Not all soy drinks are fortified with vitamin D; therefore, those providing the vitamin should be chosen.

Folic Acid

Usually vegetarians who consume high amounts of vegetables and fruits as well as other plant foods have adequate intakes of folic acid. However, those who consume vegetables that are usually braised or fried at high temperature, and who rarely drink fruits juices or eat grain products fortified with folic acid, may be at risk. Additionally, post-menarchal adolescent girls who are capable of becoming pregnant should consume 400 μg of folic acid as a supplement or in fortified foods in addition to usual food sources of the nutrient.[43]

Minerals

Iron

Iron is vital at all ages, but even more of the nutrient is needed during infant growth, the adolescent growth spurt, and pregnancy. The iron nutritional status of vegetarian infants and children varies. Iron deficiency is by far the most common of the micronutrient deficiencies exhibited by vegetarian children. It is particularly common in children consuming vegan diets,[44] because vegan diets exclude heme iron sources such as meat, poultry, and fish, which are highly bioavailable and often contain nonheme iron sources from plant foods that are lower in bioavailability. Inhibitors of nonheme iron absorption include dietary fiber, phytates (in whole grains and legumes), and tannins and other polyphenols (in tea, coffee, and other plant foods). Iron deficiency is less prevalent among lacto-ovo vegetarians.[44–47] The presence of enhancers of iron bioavailability, such as ascorbic, citric, and other organic acids, varies in vegetarian diets.[48] It is the balance between all of these factors and the overall amount of iron consumed that determines the vegetarian's iron nutritional status.[48,49] Because vegetarian diets vary in these respects, so too may iron bioavailability.[50,51] Iron absorption can be enhanced by selecting plant foods high in iron or routinely fortified with iron such as iron-fortified breakfast cereals, iron-fortified grain products, dried beans and peas, foods high in ascorbic acid, or iron supplements. At times of very high requirements, such as during adolescent pregnancy, supplements are required for those following a vegetarian diet as well as for most omnivorous women, especially adolescents, because it is difficult to consume enough iron to meet requirements through diet alone.[45–47]

Calcium

In the United States, milk and milk products provide most of the calcium in the diets of infants and children.[52] The high intake of milk and dairy products by lacto vegetarians and lacto-ovo vegetarians makes the risk of inadequate calcium nutrition unlikely.[26] If milk is not consumed or is consumed only in small amounts, calcium intakes may be a problem. Vegan children have more problems meeting calcium requirements.[53] Although the calcium content of breast milk is unaffected by vegan or vegetarian diets, once such infants have been weaned, their intake of calcium is often half or less of the recommended level. The latest dietary reference intakes (DRIs) for adolescents and young adults are increased from previous values, and there is increasing recognition of the need for adequate calcium intake during puberty and later adolescence to achieve peak bone mass.[54] Rich sources of calcium include milk and milk products; calcium-fortified soy products; calcium-fortified cereals and orange juice; dark leafy green vegetables, such as chard, broccoli, kale, dandelion, and mustard greens; nuts, such as almonds; fish, such as sardines with bones; calcium-set tofu; and calcium supplements. However, the number or size of the servings required to meet Adequate Intakes of calcium is very high from some of these sources and, therefore, care is needed in meal planning.[54,55] If vitamin D intake is adequate, an increased absorption of calcium may partly offset a decreased dietary intake. Thus, supplemental calcium is warranted when needs are very high if the diet is low in calcium (eg, the macrobiotic or vegan diet), or when vitamin D intake is marginal.[54–58]

Zinc

Approximately half of the zinc in American diets comes from meat, poultry, and fish.[52] Foods such as red meat contain large amounts of zinc and protein, which enhances zinc bioavailability. Human milk contains zinc in a bioavailable form, but it does not contain enough zinc for infants older than 7 months, so breastfed infants of this age should consume foods containing zinc. The bioavailability of relatively rich plant sources of zinc from whole grain cereals, soy, beans, lentils, peas, and nuts tends to be low, because most of them also contain large amounts of phytate and fiber, which inhibit zinc absorption.[59] In lacto-ovo vegetarians, zinc absorption is approximately one third less than in omnivores.[60] The requirement for zinc may be as much as 50% greater among strict vegetarians.[48] Vegetarian diets also tend to be lower in this mineral than are omnivorous diets. When daily requirements for zinc are increased, as they are in infants and children, the risk of suboptimal zinc nutritional status is increased because the ability to increase zinc absorption is limited.[61] Because the presence of inhibitors is highest in vegan diets, vegans are at special risk. Despite this, zinc supplementation is not recommended because clinical signs of deficiency are rare among vegetarians. Good plant sources of zinc are yeast-fermented whole grain breads (the phytic acid content is reduced) and zinc-fortified infant and adult cereals.

Other Dietary Components

Fiber

The American Academy of Pediatrics recommends that dietary fiber intake not exceed 0.5 g/kg/d in children. The American Health Foundation recently suggested a rule of thumb that conforms closely to these recommendations:

"Age plus 5" g fiber per day, to apply to all children older than 2 years up to the adult recommendations. The intake of vegan children sometimes is 3 or more times higher than that level. In very small children, the sheer bulk and low energy density of such a high-fiber diet may make consumption of sufficient energy difficult for the child and may inhibit absorption of some minerals. The sieving or mashing of cereals, pulses, and vegetables that are fed to infants can increase their digestibility, and partial replacement of whole-grain cereals with more highly refined cereals that are lower in fiber can further increase energy intakes and decrease bulk if this is a problem in small children. Lacto-ovo vegetarian children usually consume adequate but not excessive amounts of dietary fiber.

Carnitine and Taurine

Carnitine and taurine levels in the serum are decreased in lacto-ovo vegetarian and vegan diets; however, the functional significance of the serum levels of these substances is not apparent, and, therefore, supplementation does not appear to be warranted.[62,63]

Age-Related Considerations

Because it is the parents or caretakers who largely determine what vegetarian infants and children eat, their behavior is critical. When adolescents embark upon vegetarian diets on their own, they as well as their parents may need dietary counseling, particularly if they adopt vegan vegetarian diets. Special food guides for vegetarians help health professionals and families ensure dietary adequacy and balance.[64–66]

Infants

Infants older than 6 months are potentially at the greatest risk for overt deficiency states related to inappropriate restrictions of the diet, although deficiencies of vitamins B_{12} and essential fatty acids may appear earlier.[67,68] Infants are particularly vulnerable during the weaning period if fed a macrobiotic diet and may experience psychomotor delay in some instances.[69,70] Attempting to anticipate these problems for vegetarian families and explain the principles of providing calorically dense foods at the time of weaning is important so the increased bulk of vegetarian diets does not interfere with adequate consumption of energy, protein, and other nutrients. Appropriate use of these guidelines has led to adequate nutritional status for most vegetarian groups.

Toddlers

As is true for infants, toddlers are unable to tolerate a bulky diet, so meal plans must include foods of high caloric density. If animal products are not used, plant foods such as pureed nuts, olives, dates, and avocados may be useful calorically dense foods. Because toddlers often prefer a limited variety of foods, the caregiver must encourage as wide a variety as possible.

Older Children and Adolescents

Older children and adolescents eating vegetarian diets are at less risk for growth failure than are younger children, especially if they are lacto-ovo vegetarians, but iron and calcium are still of concern.[71-73] Iron, calcium, and vitamins B_{12} and D are of particular concern among strongly adherent vegan-vegetarian adolescents who do not consume nutrient supplements.[74] As adolescents become more responsible for their own food choices, they must understand some basic principles of food selection. Adolescents who adopt vegetarian eating habits without adequate nutrition knowledge and combine them with schemes to achieve weight loss are most vulnerable to malnutrition and growth failure.

Principles of Management by Diet Group

Partial or Semi-vegetarians

These diets do not pose a threat to children and may actually provide intakes more in keeping with current dietary recommendations.[75]

Lacto Vegetarians or Lacto-Ovo Vegetarians

The presence of a modest amount of dairy products and eggs in the diet allows for completely adequate nutrient intake to meet needs and sustain growth, with the possible exception of iron.[25,76] The dietary principles for this type of vegetarian eating are similar to the guidelines for the general population. Children consuming these diets have normal growth and development, and overt nutrient deficiencies are rare.[8,21]

Pure Vegetarians and Vegans

The most worrisome nutritional risk for pure vegetarians is that of vitamin B_{12} deficiency. Vitamin B_{12} can be supplied through fortified milks, in cereal preparations that contain vitamin B_{12}, or possibly as a separate nutritional supplement if this is acceptable to the parents. Vitamin B_{12} supplementation for vegan mothers may be an important preventive measure against vitamin B_{12} deficiency in nursing infants. A wide variety of food sources is important to provide adequate complementary proteins. Supplementary vitamin D and consumption of green leafy vegetables and fortified soy milk for calcium is advisable. Iron intake may need to be supplemented, particularly in infants and in women during their childbearing years.[76] Zinc intake should be assessed in young children as well. Vegetarian meal guides are available to assist with education.[64–66]

Atypical or New Vegetarians

The macrobiotic dietary pattern presents a special challenge because foods are taken or avoided based on their perceived spiritual or metaphysical properties rather than their nutrient content.[58] Most families are willing to discuss the need for nutrients for their children. By adjusting to a lower-level macrobiotic diet, achievement of acceptable nutrient intake may be possible. Special problems may arise if, at the age of weaning, infants are given homemade human milk substitutes in place of infant formulas or porridges. One such compound, known as kokkoh, is prepared by mixing dry ingredients composed of 30% brown rice, 30% sesame seeds, 20% sweet brown rice, 10% aduki beans, and the remaining 10% of equal parts of soybeans, wheat, and oats. Water is blended with the dry ingredients to form a dilute 10:1 mixture.[58] The resulting milk substitute contains ingredients that have relatively high-quality protein, but, because of the dilution, may contain only 20% to 50% of the calories found in proprietary formulas or breast milk. This means that an infant would need to consume 40 to 70 oz/d to meet energy requirements. Attempts at making milk substitutes using almonds or soybeans with added honey or brown sugar have resulted in formulas that are also extremely dilute. The predictable outcome of feeding this type of "formula," coupled with macrobiotic diet practices, is inadequate weight gain and growth, occasionally coupled with specific nutrient deficiencies, such as vitamin D, iron, and vitamin B_{12}.[55]

Conclusion

Vegetarian diets can be consumed in a healthful manner.[77] Identification of the dietary restrictions of an individual vegetarian is important to make recommendations specific to the nutrients that may be deficient in the diet. Appropriate education for the families who pursue a vegetarian lifestyle is probably the best insurance that the child will receive adequate intake of nutrients to achieve the full potential for growth and development. There are excellent guides for doing so today.[78,79]

References

1. Smith J, Dwyer JT. Vegetarian diets for children. In: Dershewitz RA. *Ambulatory Pediatric Care*. 3rd ed. Philadelphia, PA and New York, NY: Lippincott Raven Publishers; 1998:106–112

2. Dwyer JT. Convergence of plant-rich and plant-only diets. *Am J Clin Nutr*. 1999;70:620S–622S

3. Abrams HL. Vegetarianism: another view. *The Cambridge World History of Food*. Cambridge, England: Kiple, Kriemhild C, Cambridge University Press; 2000;2:1564–1573

4. Campbell TC, Janshi C. Diet and chronic degenerative diseases: perspectives from China. *Am J Clin Nutr*. 1994;59(suppl):1153S–1161S

5. Gussow JD. Ecology and vegetarian considerations: does environmental responsibility demand elimination of livestock? *Am J Clin Nutr*. 1994;59(suppl):1110S–1116S

6. Amato PR, Partridge SA. *The New Vegetarians: Promoting Health and Protecting Life*. New York, NY: Plenum Press; 1989

7. Dwyer JT, Loew FM. Nutritional risks of vegan diets to women and children: are they preventable? *J Agric Environ Ethics*. 1994;7:87–109

8. Jacobs C, Dwyer JT. Vegetarian children: appropriate and inappropriate diets. *Am J Clin Nutr*. 1988;48:811–818

9. Frentzel-Beyme R, Claude J, Eilber U. Mortality among German vegetarians: first results after five years of follow-up. *Nutr Cancer*. 1988;11:117–126

10. Beilin LJ. Vegetarian and other complex diets, fats, fiber and hypertension. *Am J Clin Nutr*. 1994;59(suppl):1130S–1135S

11. Fraser GE. Diet and coronary heart disease: beyond dietary fats and low-density-lipoprotein cholesterol. *Am J Clin Nutr*. 1994;59(suppl):1117S–1123S

12. Resnicow K, Barone J, Enle A, et al. Diet and serum lipids in vegan vegetarians: a model for risk reduction. *J Am Diet Assoc*. 1991:91:447–453

13. Mills PK, Beeson WL, Phillips RL, Fraser GE. Cancer incidence among Californian Seventh Day Adventists 1976–1982. *Am J Clin Nutr*. 1994;59(suppl):1136S–1142S

14. Levin N, Rattan J, Gilat T. Energy intake and body weight in ovo-lacto vegetarians. *J Clin Gastroenterol*. 1986;8:451–453

15. Pixley F, Wilson D, McPherson K, Mann J. Effect of vegetarianism on development of gall stones in women. *BMJ*. 1985;291:11–12

16. Havala S, Dwyer J. Position of the American Dietetic Association: vegetarian diets. *J Am Diet Assoc*. 1993;93:1317–1319

17. Committee on Diet and Health. Dietary intake and nutritional status: trends and assessment. In: *Diet and Health: Implications for Reducing Chronic Disease Risk*. Washington, DC: National Academy Press; 1989:76–77

18. British Dietetic Association. Dietary guidelines: vegetarian diet position paper (UK). *Int J Veg Nutr*. 1997;1:106–114

19. National Institute of Nutrition (Canada). Risks and benefits of vegetarian diets. *Nutr Today*. 1990;Mar/Apr:27–29

20. Dwyer JT. Vegetarianism for women. In: Krummel D, Kris-Etherton PM, eds. *Nutrition in Women's Health*. Gaithersburg, MD: Aspen Publishers Inc; 1996:232–262

21. Dwyer JT. Nutritional implications of vegetarianism for children. In: Suskind RM, Suskind LL, eds. *Pediatric Nutrition*. New York, NY: Raven Press; 1992:181–190

22. Dagnelie PC, van Staveren WA, Verschuren SA, Hautvast JG. Nutritional status of infants on macrobiotic diets aged 4 to 18 months and matched omnivorous control infants: a population-based mixed-longitudinal study, I: weaning pattern, energy, and nutrient intake. *Eur J Clin Nutr*. 1989;43:311–323

23. Dwyer JT. Vegetarian diets for infants and young children. *Pediatr Basics*. 1994;70:11–16

24. O'Connell JM, Dibley J, Sierra J, Wallace B, Marks JS, Yip R. Growth of vegetarian children: the Farm Study. *Pediatrics*. 1989;84:475–481

25. Hackett A, Nathan I, Burgess L. Is vegetarian diet adequate for children? *Nutr Health*. 1998;12:189–195

26. Tayter MS, Stanek KL. Anthropometric and dietary assessment of omnivore and lacto-ovo-vegetarian children. *J Am Diet Assoc*. 1989;89(suppl):1661–1663

27. Miller DR, Specker BL, Ho ML, Norman EJ. Vitamin B_{12} status in a macrobiotic community. *Am J Clin Nutr*. 1991;153:524–529

28. Dagnelie PC, van Staveren WA. Macrobiotic nutrition and child health: results of a population-based mixed-longitudinal cohort study in The Netherlands. *Am J Clin Nutr*. 1994;59(suppl):1187S–1196S

29. Dwyer JT, Miller LG, Arduino NL, et al. Mental age and IQ of predominantly vegetarian children. *J Am Diet Assoc*. 1980;76:142–147

30. Warrington S, Storey DM. Comparative studies on Asian and Caucasian children, I: growth. *Eur J Clin Nutr*. 1988;42:61–67

31. Dietz WH, Dwyer JT. Nutritional implications of vegetarianism for children. In: Suskind RM, ed. *Textbook of Pediatric Nutrition*. New York, NY: Raven Press; 1981:179–188

32. Allen LH, Backstrand JR, Stanek EJ, et al. The interactive effects of dietary quality on the growth and attained size of young Mexican children. *Am J Clin Nutr*. 1992;56:353–364

33. Young VR, Pellett PL. Plant proteins in relation to human protein and amino acid nutrition. *Am J Clin Nutr*. 1994;59(suppl):1203S–1212S

34. Vobecky JS, Vobecky J, Normand L. Risk and benefit of low fat intake in childhood. *Ann Nutr Metab*. 1995;39:124–133

35. Boulton TJ, Magarey AM. Effects of differences in dietary fat on growth, energy and nutrient intake from infancy to eight years of age. *Acta Paediatr*. 1995;84:146–150

36. Kaplan RM, Toshima MT. Does a reduced fat diet cause retardation in child growth? *Prev Med*. 1992;21:33–52

37. Attwood CR. Low-fat diets for children: practicality and safety. *Am J Cardiol*. 1998; 82:77T–79T

38. Specker BL. Nutritional concerns of lactating women consuming vegetarian diets. *Am J Clin Nutr.* 1994;59(suppl):1182S–1186S

39. Specker BL, Miller D, Norman EJ, et al. Increased urinary methylmalonic acid excretion in breast-fed infants of vegetarian mothers and identification of an acceptable dietary source of vitamin B_{12}. *Am J Clin Nutr.* 1988;47:89–92

40. Herbert V. Vitamin B_{12}: plant sources, requirements and assay. *Am J Clin Nutr.* 1988;48(suppl):852–858

41. Herbert V. Staging B_{12} (cobalamin) status in vegetarians. *Am J Clin Nutr.* 1994; 59(suppl):1213S–1222S

42. Matsuoka LY, Ide L, Wortsman J, MacLaughlin JA, Holick MF. Sunscreens suppress cutaneous vitamin D3 synthesis. *J Clin Endocrinol Metab.* 1987;64:1165–1168

43. Standing Committee on the Scientific Evaluation of Dietary Reference Intakes and its Panel on Folate, Other B Vitamins and Choline, Food and Nutrition Board, Institute of Medicine Dietary Reference Intakes for Thiamin, Riboflavin, Niacin, Vitamin B_6, Folate, Vitamin B_{12}, Pantothenic Acid, Biotin, and Choline. Washington, DC: National Academy Press; 1998

44. Nathan I, Hackett AF, Kirby S. The dietary intake of a group of vegetarian children aged 7–11 years compared with matched omnivores. *Br J Nutr.* 1996;75:533–544

45. McEndree LS, Kies CV, Fox HM. Iron intake and iron nutritional status of lacto-ovo vegetarian and omnivore students eating in a lacto-ovo-vegetarian food service. *Nutr Rep Int.* 1983;27:199–206

46. Donovan UM, Gibson RS. Iron and zinc status of young women aged 14 to 19 years consuming vegetarian and omnivorous diets. *J Am Coll Nutr.* 1995;14:463–472

47. Ball MJ, Bartlett MA. Dietary intake and iron status of Australian vegetarian women. *Am J Clin Nutr.* 1999;70:343–358

48. Institute of Medicine. Dietary Reference Intakes for Vitamin A, Vitamin K, Boron, Arsenic, Chromium, Copper, Iodine, Iron, Manganese, Molybdenum, Nickel, Silicon, Vanadiun, and Zinc. Washington, DC: National Academy Press; 2001

49. Beard JL, Campbell TC, Chen J. Iron nutrition in the Cornell-China diet cancer survey. *J Clin Nutr.* 1988;47;771. Abstract

50. Bindra GS, Gibson RS. Iron status of predominantly lacto-ovo vegetarian East Indian immigrants to Canada: a model approach. *Am J Clin Nutr.* 1986;44:643–652

51. Hunt JR, Roughead ZK. Adaptation of iron absorption in men consuming diets with high or low iron bioavailability. *Am J Clin Nutr.* 2000;71:94–102

52. Subar AF, Krebs-Smith SM, Cook A, Kahle LL. Dietary sources of nutrients among US adults, 1989 to 1991. *J Am Diet Assoc.* 1998;98:537–547

53. Weaver CM, Plawecki KL. Dietary calcium: adequacy of a vegetarian diet. *Am J Clin Nutr.* 1994;59(suppl):1238S–1241S

54. Standing Committee on the Scientific Evaluation of Dietary Reference Intakes, Food and Nutrition Board, Institute of Medicine Dietary Reference Intakes for Calcium, Phosphorus, Magnesium, Vitamin D and Fluoride. Washington, DC: National Academy Press; 1997

55. Weaver CM, Proulx WR, Heaney R. Choices for achieving adequate dietary calcium with a vegetarian diet. *Am J Clin Nutr.* 1999;70:543S–548S

56. Miller GD, Jarvis JK, McBean LD. *Handbook of Dairy Foods and Nutrition.* 2nd ed. Boca Raton, FL: CRC Press; 1999

57. Dwyer JT, Dietz WH Jr, Hass G, Suskind R. Risk of nutritional rickets among vegetarian children. *Am J Dis Child.* 1979;133:134–140

58. Dwyer JT. Macrobiotic diets. In: Caballero B, Trugo L, Finglas P. *Encyclopedia of Food Sciences and Nutrition.* London, England: Academic Press; in press

59. Harland BF, Oberleas D. Phytate in foods. *World Rev Nutr Diet.* 1987;52:235–259

60. Hunt JR, Matthys LA, Johnson LK. Zinc absorption, mineral balance and blood lipids in women consuming controlled lactoovovegetarian and omnivorous diets for 8 weeks. *Am J Clin Nutr.* 1998;67:421–430

61. Gibson RS. Content and bioavailability of trace elements in vegetarian diets. *Am J Clin Nutr.* 1994;59(suppl):1223S–1232S

62. Lombard KA, Olson AL, Nelson SE, Rebouche CJ. Carnitine status of lacto-ovo vegetarians and strict vegetarian adults and children. *Am J Clin Nutr.* 1989;50:301–306

63. Laidlaw SA, Shultz TD, Cecchino JT, Kopple JD. Plasma and urine taurine levels in vegans. *Am J Clin Nutr.* 1988;47:660–663

64. Haddad EH. Development of a vegetarian food guide. *Am J Clin Nutr.* 1994; 59(suppl):1248S–1254S

65. Haddad EH. Meeting the RDAs with a vegetarian diet. *Topics Clin Nutr.* 1995; 10:7–16

66. Haddad EH, Sabate J, Whitten CG. Vegetarian food guide pyramid: a conceptual framework. *Am J Clin Nutr.* 1999:70(suppl):615S–619S

67. Sanders TA, Reddy S. Vegetarian diets and children. *Am J Clin Nutr.* 1994;59(suppl): 1176S–1181S

68. Sanders TA. Essential fatty acid requirements of vegetarians in pregnancy, lactation and infancy. *Am J Clin Nutr.* 1999;70:555S–559S

69. Sanders TA. Vegetarian diets and children. *Pediatr Clin North Am.* 1995;42:955–965

70. Dagnelie PC, Vergote FJ, van Staveren WA, et al. High prevalence of rickets in infants on macrobiotic diets. *Am J Clin Nutr.* 1990;51:202–208

71. Sabate J, Lindsted KD, Harris RD, Sanchez A. Attained height of lacto-ovo vegetarian children and adolescents. *Eur J Clin Nutr.* 1991;45:51–58

72. Hebbelinck M, Clarys P, De Malsche A. Growth, development and physical fitness of Flemish vegetarian children, adolescents, and young adults. *Am J Clin Nutr.* 1999; 70:579S–585S

73. Krajcovicova-Kulackova M, Simoncic R, Bederova A, Grancicova E, Magalova T. Influence of vegetarian and mixed nutrition on selected haematological and biochemical parameters in children. *Nahrung.* 1997;41:311–314

74. Worsley A, Skrzypiec G. Teenage vegetarianism: prevalence, social and cognitive contexts. *Appetite.* 1998;30:151–170

75. Thane CW, Bates CJ. Dietary intakes and nutrient status of vegetarian preschool children from a British national survey. *J Hum Nutr Diet*. 2000;13:149–162

76. Johnston PA. Nutritional implications of vegetarian diets. In: Shils ME, Olson JA, Shike M, Ross AC. *Modern Nutrition in Health and Disease*. 9th ed. Baltimore, MD: Williams and Wilkins; 1999:1755–1768

77. Messina VK, Burke KI. Position of the American Dietetic Association: vegetarian diets. *J Am Diet Assoc*. 1997;97:1317–1321

78. Mangels R. Nutrition. In: Wasserman D, ed. *Simply Vegan*. 2nd ed. Baltimore, MD: Vegetarian Resource Group; 1995

79. Messina M, Messina V. *The Dietitian's Guide to Vegetarian Diets*. Gaithersburg, MD: Aspen; 1996:511

13

Fast Foods, Organic Foods, and Fad Diets

The extent to which so-called fast foods are a factor influencing the diet or nutritional status of an individual depends on several variables: the nutritive quality of the particular menu item, the portion size of the item, the availability of these options, the customer's selection of menu items to constitute a meal, the frequency with which those meals are eaten, and the amounts consumed. Depending on how they are used, these choices can be beneficial or deleterious to overall eating patterns. The popularity of fast-food establishments is evident in the 1 of every 10 food dollars spent on fast foods; the total yearly fast foods sales exceed $34 billion.[1] In the past few decades, the popularity of eating meals outside the home has risen. For most families, the primary reason for choosing a fast food is convenience. In addition, deep discounting, "value meals," and super-sized portions have meant that more foods and beverages are available at a low price. Thus, fast food establishments provide convenience and taste, at lower cost than that of most traditional restaurants.

The variety of fast-food establishments and the frequency of changes within the industry make placement of definitive values on the nutritive quality of all fast foods difficult; however, a number of studies have provided information from which some general conclusions about the nutritive value of fast foods can be drawn (Appendix Q). Several fast-food chains have moved toward providing more choices, including healthier choices in their stores.[2] Widely divergent intakes can be consumed, depending on choice. However, the availability of fast foods in locations such as a la carte lines, vending machines and stores in schools, recreational facilities, and other places where children congregate has risen and marketing efforts have intensified. Sales of so-called "competitive foods" (ie, foods sold other than those in the National School Lunch and Breakfast Program) that are high in calories and low in nutrient density in schools have generated concerns about their nutritional value and aggressive promotional techniques. These marketing techniques include, in some instances, exclusive rights to stock vending machines and other outlets only with certain brands, and gifts or rewards to schools based on the volume of products sold.[3]

Studies of fast-food meals and beverages consumed during the 1970s revealed that the nutrient density of these meals was low relative to energy.[4] Many prepared fast-food items were also relatively high in fat, sugar, and sodium. These trends continue today. For example, a slice of the "Cheesecake Factory's" carrot cake is equivalent in saturated fat and calories to 3 McDonald's Quarter Pounders (84 g total fat, 23 g of saturated fat, 1560 calories).[5]

Over the past decade, energy intakes of Americans, and of children in particular, have increased, primarily because of increased carbohydrate consumption.[5] Over the same period, despite the increases in calorie and carbohydrate intakes that were coupled with a slight decrease in protein intake, children's intakes of most vitamins and minerals did not change much. Their fiber intake increased, and their cholesterol intake decreased. They consumed fewer milk products, especially high-fat milk products and meat and meat substitutes, but more vegetables and grain products, sodas, fruit, and fruit-flavored drinks.[6] These trends in choices may be responsible for the decline in fat and calcium consumption and slight increases in fiber evident in some groups of children. Among children and adolescents, much of their increased energy intake has been attributed to increased consumption of non-diet soft drinks and other sweetened beverages like fruitades.[7-9] Consumption of sweetened milk desserts, including ice cream, has also increased. At the same time there appears to have been a displacement of milk consumption by other beverages, including sweetened beverages. Between 1977 and 1994, milk consumption declined 24% among boys and 32% among girls 6 to 11 years of age.[8] One recent national study showed that while calorie intakes of children aged 2 to 17 years increased, intakes of micronutrients other than iron did not increase and calcium intakes decreased.[7] Children consuming large amounts of non-diet soft drinks had lower intakes of several nutrients such as folate, vitamin A, and calcium—all nutrients that have been identified as "shortfall" or problem nutrients among children of these ages, as well as other nutrients such as riboflavin, vitamin C, and phosphorus.[10] The general tendency for the provision of a high amount of calories and the low-nutrient density in the standard portion size of many fast foods and beverages could be magnified when fast foods are used for children, especially since portion sizes of many items have expanded. A single meal of cheeseburger, french fries, and a cola drink could provide up to 36% of the caloric needs of a 6-year-old child, according to the recommended dietary allowances, but not their proportionate share of calcium or many other nutrients. The new recommendations for calcium intakes of children and adolescents to achieve maximal retention of body calcium have increased for adolescents compared with earlier recommendations (800 mg/d, prepubertal children; 1200 to 1500 mg/d, 9- to 18-year-olds).[11] Unless low-fat milk and milk products or other foods high in calcium are selected, the daily recommendation for calcium by children entering an age range when a high intake of calcium is required might not be met when they are eating frequently at a fast-food restaurant. The problem also exists in other eating locations. In a study of children's beverage intakes at luncheon, on average, only children who drank milk at the meal achieved the recommended intake for calcium for the day.[12] Intakes of soft drinks are negatively related to intakes of milk.[10,13,14]

Fast foods are not alone in being high in calories. Studies of school meals several years ago also revealed higher than desirable levels of fat, saturated fat, cholesterol, and sodium, although they did supply considerable amounts of most vitamins and minerals.[15] Efforts have been made to bring these meals in line with recommendations of health experts, and school lunches today are often lower in fat and sodium than in the past.[16]

The nutrients in short supply in fast-food meals can be obtained by balancing them with foods such as beans, dark-green leafy vegetables, yellow vegetables, and a variety of fresh fruits to compensate for the fiber, iron, and folic acid shortfalls in many fast-food meals. Fiber and vitamin-mineral fortified cereals, whole-grain breads, nuts, and seeds provide a variety of nutrients and fiber.

Although fast foods available today still provide relatively large amounts of calories, fat, saturated fat, sugars, cholesterol, and sodium in many meals, many more choices are available. Most of the major chains now provide at least a few menu choices that conform more closely to the Dietary Guidelines for Americans.[17] In general, hamburgers (regular size without the fixings or those with vegetable-protein fillers), grilled and charbroiled chicken (without the skin and sandwiches made without mayonnaise), and salads with low-fat or reduced-calorie dressings are good choices. For beverages, low-fat milk, fortified soy milk, and fruit juices are good options.[18,19]

When serving sizes of foods and beverages are very large, they can be shared if calories are of concern. Many fast-food chains now make nutrition information available on their menu items, and consumers who use this can make choices that are consistent with good nutrition.

Deli sandwiches are also very popular in many fast-food restaurants, and these also vary in their nutrient content. Some choices (such as turkey or roast beef with mustard and no oil or dressing on the bread) provide less than 30% of their calories from fat and no more than 20% of the recommended levels of total and saturated fat, but they provide a substantial amount of sodium.[20]

Some strategies to make such deli choices more healthful are: (1) order extra bread, particularly whole grain, which is higher in fiber; (2) ask the person who is making the sandwich to split up the filling portions between 2 sandwiches instead of 1 to dilute higher-calorie, higher-fat fillings, such as chicken and tuna salad; (3) add low-fat extras, such as lettuce, tomato, onions, mustard, and ketchup; (4) avoid adding mayonnaise, butter, or cheese toppings; and (5) use fat-free or low-calorie dressings.

Salad and other fast-food bars are convenient and popular options, but they are not necessarily low in calories.[21] Good salad bar choices are vegetables, with only small amounts of high-calorie items such as olives, avocado, cheese, bacon bits, meats, and high-fat dressings.[8]

In addition to nutritive quality, item selection, and portion size, frequency is the fourth major variable in determining the effect that fast-food dining has on the nutritional status of an individual. The National Restaurant Association indicates that 79% of the families in the United States are in the "eating-away-from-home market," with the average family studied eating out more than 4 times a week. Other statistics indicate that individuals 17 years or younger visit fast-food restaurants more often than any other restaurant type—about 2 meals a week.[22] Although children and adolescents patronize fast-food restaurants frequently, the frequency of fast-food dining can be offset with complementary foods lower in fat, saturated fat, and sodium at home, school, or in other types of eating establishments. With the exception of the fast-food industry's "shake" (substitute milk shake), no appreciable differences exist in the nutrient quality of raw materials used in fast-food items and their prepared-at-home equivalents. Again, the nutritional quality of a fast-food meal depends in large part on the selection of menu items and their preparation. Excesses or deficiencies should be compensated for at other meals. The US Department of Agriculture (USDA) Food Guide Pyramid is a suitable guide for food selection for older children, and the new USDA Food Guide Pyramid for Young Children under 6 years of age (see Appendix M) is helpful in planning menus for younger children.[23-26] Children with special dietary problems, such as diabetes, who wish to eat fast foods and snacks can be accommodated with dietary planning.[27]

The fast-food industry continues to grow for a number of reasons, one being convenience. Not only do fast foods continue to grow in popularity, but the sports and nutrition bar industry is also expanding, perhaps in part because the label "nutrition bars" may lead people to think that they are all healthy choices. This is not always the case. Refer to Appendix P for nutrition information of popular nutrition and sports bars sold today.

Organic Foods

The terms organic, natural, and health foods have different meanings. Organic foods are plant products grown in soil enriched with humus and compost on which no pesticides, herbicides, or synthetic fertilizers have been used, or they are meat and dairy products from animals raised on natural feeds and not treated with drugs, such as hormones or antibiotics. In 1997, the USDA published a proposed rule for regulation of organic food that would create a definition of what constitutes organic food so that consumers would be certain of what they are buying. The process has been fraught with problems because there is disagreement about exactly what the definition should entail.

Natural foods are those made from ingredients of plant or animal origin that are altered as little as possible and contain no synthetic or artificial ingredients or additives.

Nutritional Aspects

The nutritional value of foods that reach the consumer depends not only on the composition of the raw materials, but also on various changes that occur during processing, storage, and distribution.[28] Nutrient losses occur regardless of whether the food is processed commercially or at home or is stored in an unprocessed state.[29] Variations in the nutrient content of raw foods affect the content of vitamins and minerals in the final food product as much as, and sometimes more than, the processing itself. For example, carrots may vary 100-fold in their concentration of carotene (provitamin A), and samples of fresh tomato juice have shown 16-fold differences in vitamin C content. The raw foods being produced today are not significantly different in terms of vitamin content from those produced 2 or more decades ago. Most food preservation techniques used today minimize the loss of nutritive value of foods and are safe and well standardized.

No chemical or functional test differentiates organically grown and organically processed food from similar commercial products. However, the species or variety may be different, and taste, color, or other sensory characteristics may vary accordingly. Long-term studies have failed to show the nutritional superiority of organically grown crops compared with those grown under standard agricultural conditions with chemical fertilizers. If the soil is deficient in nutrients, crop yields, rather than the nutritional quality of the plant, will be primarily affected.

Other concerns about agricultural practices and food processing procedures may have more validity (eg, residual hormones and antibiotics in meat and pesticide residues in dairy, fruit, and vegetable products). Ongoing monitoring and surveillance systems are important. Each of these issues is complicated, unresolved, and beyond the scope of this handbook. Organically grown foods may cost more than their nonorganically grown counterparts.

Health Foods

Health food is a general term that is often used to include natural and organic foods or other conventional foods that have been subjected to less processing than usual (such as unhydrogenated nut butters and whole-grain flours), as well as items such as brewer's yeast, pumpkin seeds, wheat germ, and herbal teas that are often viewed as especially efficacious by some consumers.

Enthusiasts suggest that "health foods are safer, more nutritious, and superior." No scientific evidence supports such assumptions.[30] Indeed, the lack of control of materials on the shelves of health food stores has raised questions about the safety of some of the available foods, and some health foods may actually contain contaminants.[31] Food purchased in health food stores is of particular concern for low-income families who may need to sacrifice other important items in the budget to afford health foods. There is no compelling evidence that the high cost of health foods results in concomitant benefit to the consumer. For example, a recent review of the evidence from clinical trials of various food supplements that were being marketed to enhance athletic prowess concluded that no published scientific evidence existed to support the promotional claims for two fifths of the 19 products reviewed, and documented human clinical trials were available to support promotional claims for only one fifth of the products. The remaining products had some scientific documentation to support promotional claims, but in most instances the products were marketed in what was judged a misleading manner.[32] Occasionally, a health food such as γ-hydroxybutyrate, which is available in health food markets and is promoted as a food supplement for body builders, has been found to cause adverse effects, including coma and seizures.[33,34]

Those who are enthusiastic about natural foods may overlook the positive benefits of fortified and enriched foods that can help ensure that nutritional status is satisfactory.[35] Iron-fortified infant formulas and infant cereals have been popular in this country for many years. Since 1998, grain products have been fortified with folic acid in the United States in response to growing evidence that diets deficient in folic acid were associated with neural tube defects. Because whole grains are not fortified with folic acid but have other nutritional advantages, it is important to include a variety of grain products in the diet. A variety of foods and beverages are now fortified with calcium, and for those who cannot tolerate or who do not wish to consume milk, they offer healthful alternative sources of this mineral. At the same time, because most of the problems with American diets today are those of macronutrient excesses rather than micronutrient deficiencies, fortified foods should not be regarded as cure-alls.[36] The place of fat substitutes in the diets of children is under debate.[37–39]

Functional Foods (see also Chapter 53)

"Functional foods" or "neutraceuticals" are a new category of substances that are considered as foods or parts of food and that claim to provide medical or health benefits, including the prevention and treatment of disease. In addition to vitamins, they include naturally occurring ingredients such as garlic, ginseng and other herbal products, phytochemicals extracted from plants, and soluble and insoluble fibers. The current US market for such products, including vitamins and other supplements, is about $3 billion,[40] and these products will likely continue to be advertised and marketed aggressively.

Bioengineered Foods (see also Chapter 53)

This category includes a number of different foods and ingredients. Types of corn, soybeans, and canola have been genetically modified to enhance their resistance to pests and herbicides and are now widely available on the market. The genetic engineering processes employed are similar to those used in producing pharmaceutical products such as human insulin and recombinant erythropoietin. The main advantage of these food products is that decreased amounts of chemical pesticides and herbicides are used in their production while crop yields are maintained or improved. Cows that have been treated with another recombinant product, bovine somatotrophin (BST), produce higher milk yields. These products have the same nutritional value, safety, and price as their non-modified counterparts.[41] All products on the market in the United States have undergone rigorous scientific assessment for safety, including reviews to ensure that they lack allergenicity,[42,43] and there are no confirmed cases of allergic reactions to these products. Currently, regulations are being considered for labeling of such products and for further institutionalizing safety testing by the Food and Drug Administration.

Fat and sugar replacers encompass a variety of different ingredients. Table 13.1 describes those currently approved as safe and in use in the United States. Although these ingredients are safe, their efficacy in causing weight loss or enhancing weight maintenance still remains to be proven.

Table 13.1A–E.
Sugar Alternatives and Fat Replacers Available in the United States

Table 13.1A.

High-intensity noncaloric sweeteners	Comments
Acesufame K (acesulfame potassium) Sunett food ingredient (Hoechst Food Ingredients), and in tabletop sweeteners Sweet One and Swiss Sweet	Potassium amount is not sufficient to cause concern in persons with diabetes. 50 mg in packet of sweetener, 40 mg in 12-oz can of soft drink. Often blended with aspartame in products. A new product that is an acesulfame K-aspartame combination at the molecular level known as Twinsweet has recently been introduced.
Aspartame (Nutrasweet, Monsanto)	35-mg packet of sweetener, 200 mg in 12-oz can of soft drink. Contains phenylalanine, and a warning alert that the product contains phenylalanine is required in the United States so that those with phenylketonuria can avoid it.
Sucralose (Splenda) (McNeil Specialty Products, Tate and Lyle)	5 mg per packet of sweetener, approximately 70 mg per 12-oz can of soft drink. No effect on insulin secretion, glucose or fructose absorption; bulk and heat stability provides useful functional qualities in baked goods.
Saccharin	5 mg per packet of sweetener, 70 mg in 12-oz can of soft drink. Some consumers can detect bitter taste. Saccharin aspartame blends used.
Cyclamate (Abbott)	Banned in United States in 1970, still approved in several other countries. Often used in blends with saccharine.
Altitamme (Pfizer)	Not yet approved in the United States.
Polyols (Sugar Alcohols); trade names include Lycasin, Hystar, Neosor, Litesse, StaLite	Found in certain plants, but most are manufactured from monosaccharides, disaccharides, or polysaccharides in various forms for use as food ingredients. Provide from 1 to 4 cal/g, depending on product. Less sweet than sugar. Listed on label as sorbitol, maltitol syrup, polydextrose, specific sugar names, hydrogenated starch hydrolysate, hydrogenated glucose syrup. The taste is similar to sucrose, and they have no aftertaste, but are less sweet than sugar, provide a sweet taste, and provide bulk to food. Generally incompletely absorbed so provide approximately 1 versus 4 cal/g and have lower glycemic effects than nutritive sweeteners or bulking agents (Schiweck and Ziesenitz 1996). Ingredient does not elevate blood glucose and insulin levels. When polyols are used between meals in products such as cough drops, candy, or other between-meal snacks, they have an advantage over sugar-containing between-meal products in that their glycemic response is less. They may be useful alternatives for handling blood glucose fluctuations between meals. If consumed as part of

Table 13.1A. *(continued)*

High-intensity non-caloric sweeteners	Comments
	a meal, the effects are less apparent because other foods buffer or dilute the differences in glycemic response. They are also lower in calories. However, consumption of these sugar replacers is presently quite low so that the net effect on energy intakes is not likely to be large. Consumption of very high amounts may cause gastric discomfort, including bloating, osmotic diarrhea, and abdominal cramps. The products do not help restore blood glucose levels when a person is hypoglycemic.
Isomalt	Provides 2 cal/g and used in candies, cough drops, and other products. Decreased glycemic and insulin response for confectionery products consumed as snacks.
Lactitol	
Maltitol	
Mannitol	Requires label warning when consumption reaches 20 g: "Excess consumption may have a laxative effect."
Sorbitol	Does not contribute to sorbitol pathway; ingested sorbitol not available after metabolism by liver. Requires label warnings when consumption of food reaches 50 g: "Excess consumption may have a laxative effect."
Xylitol	
HSH (hydrogenated starch hydrolysate) mixtures	

Table 13.1B.

Natural sweeteners	Naturally occurring in plants that are incompletely absorbed with lower calories (2 cal/g) and lower glycemic effects than other nutritive sweeteners.
Steviodose	Not approved in United States at present.
Glycyrrhizin	Used as licorice flavoring but not approved for use as a low-calorie sweetener. In very large amounts, may increase blood pressure.

Table 13.1C.

Carbohydrate-based fat replacers	Provide carbohydrate, which increases carbohydrate and may or may not be bioavailable.
Carbohydrate polymers: Maltrin, Lycadex, Paselli Excell, Stelar, N-Oil, Sta-Slim, Oatrim	Derived from cereals, grains, and starches, hold up to 3 times their weight in water. Provide 1 kcal/g when hydrated, and varying amounts of carbohydrate. Label ingredient statement may include these terms: maltodextrin, corn syrup solid, hydrolyzed corn-starch, starch, modified food starch, polydextrose.
Hydrocolloids (gums, gels, and fibers); brand names include: Slendid, Viscarin, Sactarin, Gelcarin, Fibrex, Avicel, Novagel, Rohodigel, Uniguar, Pycol, Jaquar	Some ordinary ingredients like pectin, bran fiber, applesauce, and pureed prunes are high in these substances. Depending on hydra-tion, the hydrocolloids provide 0–0.5 kcal/g. Label ingredient statement may include these terms: pectin, carrageenan, sugar beet fiber or powder, cellulose gel, locust bean gum, xanthan gum, guar gum.

Table 13.1D.

Protein-based fat replac-ers; brand names include Simplesse, K Blazer, Lite, Diry Low, Veri-lo	Microparticulated egg white and milk protein, whey protein con-centrate. Provide 1.3 kcal/g or more in products they are used in. Not possible to use in cooking.

Table 13.1E.

Fat-based fat replacers	
Sucrose polyester (olestra) Olean, Procter and Gamble	Sucrose polyester that cannot be hydrolyzed by gastrointestinal enzymes; provides 1.3 kcal/g. Currently, label advisory statement is required to alert consumers to possible abdominal cramping and loose stools.
Salatrim (short- and long-chain acid triglyc-eride molecules)	Modified triglycerides providing properties of natural fat but reduced energy value; energy value varies from 5 to 9 kcal/kg, depending on the composition of the fatty acids.
Caprenin	Composed of poorly absorbed fatty acids and thus provide 5 kcal/g.
Trailblaer	Composed of poorly absorbed fatty acids and thus provide 5 kcal/g.

Fad Diets (see also Chapter 33)

Fad diets are popular diets that recommend unusual and sometimes inadequate or unbalanced dietary patterns without a scientific rationale. Those intended for weight reduction promise very rapid losses of several pounds a week over a short time. Because obesity is such a pervasive and difficult-to-treat problem, many adults experiment with these regimens, and some feed them to their children. Evidence-based research based on controlled randomized clinical trials of the effectiveness of reducing diets in reducing excessive fatness at 1 and 5 years is the standard against which such diets should be judged. These are lacking for most fad diets used by adults, and, as a recent review of popular diets concluded, "there is [sic] no good data on children and adolescents."[44] Virtually no evidence is available about their efficacy and safety in children, making such regimens a poor choice for children with weight control problems. Fad diets that, in addition, go against usual expert recommendations for child nutrition are of particular concern. Children and adolescents who need to lose weight should not do so without the supervision of a physician. The most appropriate therapies include an increased emphasis on all forms of physical activity, including vigorous exercise, psychological and social support, and a moderate fat (20% to 30% of total energy), balanced diet with a caloric deficit of approximately 500 calories or less, so that weight losses of a pound a week or less are achieved. The best results are achieved when the entire family eats a similar dietary pattern. (See also Chapter 33.)

Reducing Diets

Atkins and Other High-Fat, Low-Carbohydrate Diets

The Atkins diet is a high-fat, low-carbohydrate (<100 g carbohydrate), high-protein diet. The diet in its various forms[45,46] features carbohydrate restriction and is ketogenic; it is also high in fat (55% to 65% of calories) and relatively high in protein. Other popular diets of the same type are Protein Power[47] and Life without Bread. Similar diets have been criticized by the American Medical Association as inappropriate for adults because they are ketogenic and are also inappropriate for children.[48]

Sears Diet (Zone Diet)

The Zone Diet is based on the proposal that a specific balance of protein and carbohydrates in the diet create a "zone" for weight loss at which fat release is maximal and the burning of carbohydrates is also maximized.[49] The diet emphasizes protein, especially meat, and breads and cereals. It is low in fruits.

Protein is adequate but calories range from about 1200 to 1700 cal/d. These restrictive diets do not support the nutritional needs of growing children.

Carbohydrate Addict's Diet

This is a low carbohydrate diet. The authors[50] contend that some people are genetically predisposed to be carbohydrate addicts and to overeat if they are given too many of them. This diet is low in carbohydrate and in the bread and grains group, and as such is not appropriate for children or adolescents.

Ornish, Pritikin, and Other Very Low-Fat Diets

Another group of diets that are not appropriate for children are low-fat (11% to 19% of calories) or very low-fat diets (<10% of calories). The Ornish diet in its most rigorous version is very low in fat (<10% of calories).[51,52] The Ornish program has positive effects in adults with clinically evident coronary disease who are able to adhere to the very rigorous, low-fat, semi-vegetarian diet and other lifestyle changes.[53] However, for children, diets so low in fat and limited in other food groups are too restrictive to support normal growth and do not provide an eating pattern that teaches appropriate food choices after weight is lost. Another group of low-fat diets are those advocated by Pritikin[54–56]; these diets are also low in fat and have similar disadvantages for children.

Very Low-Calorie Diets

Very low-calorie diets (VLCDs) are diets that provide less than 800 and often less than 500 cal/d. These calorie levels are below needs for maintaining a normal resting metabolic rate in most children and adults, and, therefore, they create a state of semi-starvation. This is of particular concern when such diets are used in children. The diets are ketogenic and most dieters are in negative fluid balance while they are on them.[57,58] Because energy allocated is so low, without very careful medical supervision, linear growth may be stunted. Most of the calories are from protein, and carbohydrate is often severely limited to less than 100 g/d; therefore, they are ketogenic. Upon restoration of water balance with refeeding or nonadherence, there is a very rapid weight rebound.

Very low-calorie diets may be self-defeating. As energy deficits increase, so too do the homeostatic mechanisms that regulate food intake. Resting metabolic rates fall by as much as 15% in total starvation, and energy expenditure during physical activity also falls, with the end result being that the energy deficit is less than anticipated. Very low-calorie diets lead to dramatic shifts in fluid and electrolyte balances and may cause lethargy, light-headedness, dizziness, weakness, feeling faint on standing, and exercise intolerance. The dieter may become dehydrated, especially if the diet is very low in carbohydrates and is ketogenic. The VLCD must be supplemented with nutrients to avoid clinically significant electrolyte imbalances and nutrient deficiencies, such as iron and calcium inadequacy.[59] The risk of side effects, compromised metabolism, and other problems is such that VLCDs should be medically supervised, with frequent monitoring. If the VLCD is unsupervised, lean body mass and linear growth in children and adolescents may decrease, and changes in cardiac function may occur. In addition, anemia, constipation, hair loss, and, in adolescents, menstrual irregularity, may result.

Total Fasting

Total fasting or starvation (no food intake at all) is a drastic and inappropriate weight loss strategy for children and adolescents who are growing.[59] It causes nutrient deficiency and very large losses in lean body mass and a drastic lowering of resting metabolic rate (15% or more), as well as decreased voluntary physical activity and intolerance to exercise. Once glycogen stores are depleted, the carbon skeletons of the glucogenic amino acids derived from protein catabolism are used to synthesize glucose to maintain blood sugar. Fasting is appealing initially because the glycogen depletion and protein catabolism cause saluresis, kaliuresis, and diuresis. Partial or intermittent fasts are totally inappropriate for children and adolescents.

Recommendations on Fad Diets

The popularity of fad diets has followed a cycle over a period of several decades.[60] Obviously, if the promises of their proponents were realized, one of these eating patterns would long ago have dominated the field. In reality, the evidence is that none of them appears to be efficacious in adults or children. A better option is to rely on more modest caloric deficits and an eating pattern that promotes healthful lifelong nutrition.[61]

Conclusion

Sensible advice on nutrition in language suitable for parents and older children is available from authoritative sources.[61] Most individuals who adhere to unusual dietary practices, except for balanced vegetarianism or organically grown foods, are aware that their ideas are not in the mainstream of medical and nutritional opinion. Some individuals adopt these diets as an expression of disillusionment with medicine or the "establishment." Physicians and other health professionals should be prepared to encounter strong resistance if they attempt to reverse unusual dietary practices. Parents are likely to resist the suggestion of major dietary changes; therefore, focusing on the features of the diet that are of the most potential harm to their children may be the best approach. However, even with the more extreme dietary practices, serious harm can usually be prevented by striving for dietary variety and balance and working within the value system or philosophy of the group or individual.

References

1. Heald FP. Fast food and snack food: beneficial or deleterious. *J Adolesc Health.* 1992;13:380–383
2. Burklow J, Aubertin A. Fast food chains move toward healthier choices. *J Natl Cancer Inst.* 1991;83:325–326
3. Kramer JL, Dwyer JT, Hoelscher DM, Nicklas T, Johnson R, Shutz GK. Schools, food and eating at the millennium: implications for school food services. *J Am Diet Assoc.* Submitted
4. How nutritious are fast food meals? *Consum Rep.* 1975;40:278
5. Food and Nutrition Service. US Department of Agriculture. *Nutr Week.* 2001;31:1
6. Anand RS, Basiotis PP. Is total fat consumption really decreasing? *Nutrition Insights.* Washington, DC: US Department of Agriculture, Center for Nutrition Policy and Promotion; 1998
7. US Department of Agriculture, Food and Nutrition Service, Office of Analysis, Nutrition and Evaluation. *Changes in Children's Diets: 1989–1991 to 1994–1996.* CN 01 CD2 by Phil Gleason and Carol Suitor, Project Officer Ed Herzog. Alexandria, VA: US Department of Agriculture; 2001
8. Morton JF, Guthrie JF. Changes in children's total fat intakes and their food group sources of fat, 1989–91 vs 1994–95: implications for diet quality. *Fam Econ Nutr Rev.* 1998;11:44–57
9. Borrud L, Enns CW, Mickle S. What we eat: USDA surveys food consumption changes. *Commun Nutr Inst.* 1997;27:4–5
10. Tippett KS, Cleveland LE. How current diets stack up: comparison with dietary guidelines. In: Frazao E, ed. *America's Eating Habits: Changes and Consequences.* United States Department of Agriculture, Economic Research Service, Agriculture Information Bulletin Number 750. 1999:51–70
11. Harnack L, Stang J, Story M. Soft drink consumption among US children and adolescents: nutritional consequences. *J Am Diet Assoc.* 1999;99:436–441
12. Institute of Medicine. *Dietary Reference Intakes for Calcium, Phosphorus, Magnesium, Vitamin D and Fluoride.* Washington, DC: National Academy Press; 1997
13. Johnson RK, Panely C, Wang MQ. The association between noon beverage consumption and the diet quality of school age children. *J Child Nutr Manag.* 1998;22:95–100
14. Guenther PM. Beverages in the diets of American teenagers. *J Am Diet Assoc.* 1986;86:493–499

15. Skinner JD, Carruth BR, Moran J, Houck K, Coletta F. Fruit juice intake is not related to children's growth. *Pediatrics.* 1999;103:58–64

16. Burghardt JA, Devaney BL. *The School Nutrition Dietary Assessment Study: Summary of Findings.* Princeton, NJ: USDA, Food and Nutrition Service, Office of Analysis and Evaluation; 1993

17. US Department of Agriculture and US Department of Health and Human Services. *Dietary Guidelines for Americans.* Washington, DC: US Department of Agriculture; 2000

18. Think fast. *Nutr Action Healthletter.* 1995;22:13–14

19. A pickle. *Nutr Action Healthletter.* 1995;22:12

20. Sandwich tips. *Nutr Action Healthletter.* 1995;22:3

21. Garceau AO, Dwyer JT, Nicklas TA, et al. Do food bars measure up? Nutrient profiles of food bars vs traditional school lunches in the CATCH. *Fam Econ Nutr Rev.* 1997;10:18–28

22. Dalis GT. Effective health instruction: both a science and an art. *J Health Educ.* 1994;25:289–298

23. US Department of Agriculture, Center for Nutrition Policy and Promotion. *Tips for Using the Food Guide Pyramid for Young Children 2 to 6 Years Old.* Program Aid 1647. Washington, DC: US Department of Agriculture; 1999

24. Marcoe KL. Technical research for the food guide pyramid for young children. *Fam Econ Nutr Rev.* 1999;12:18–32

25. Tarone C. Consumer research: food guide pyramid for young children. *Fam Econ Nutr Rev.* 1999;12:33–44

26. US Department of Agriculture, Center for Nutrition Policy and Promotion. *USDA Food Guide Pyramid Home and Garden Bulletin.* Washington, DC: 252 US Government Printing Office; 1996. Available at: http://www.usda.gov/fcs/cnpp.htm

27. Loghmani E, Rickard KA. Alternative snack system for children and teenagers with diabetes mellitus. *J Am Diet Assoc.* 1994;94:1145–1148

28. Senauer B, Asp E, Kinsey J. *Food Trends and the Changing Consumer.* St Paul, MN: Eagan Press; 1991

29. Erdman JW Jr, Poneros-Schneier AG. Factors affecting nutritive value in processed foods. In: Shils ME, Olson JA, Shike M, eds. *Modern Nutrition in Health and Disease.* 8th ed. Philadelphia, PA: Lea and Febiger; 1994:1569–1578

30. Barrett S, Herbert V. Fads, frauds, and quackery. In: Shils ME, Olson JA, Shike M, eds. *Modern Nutrition in Health and Disease.* 8th ed. Philadelphia, PA: Lea and Febiger; 1994:1526–1532

31. Williams AW, Erdman J. Food processing: nutrition safety and quality balances. In: Shils ME, Olson JA, Shike M, Ross K. *Modern Nutrition in Health and Disease.* 9th ed. Philadelphia, PA: Lippincott Williams & Wilkins; 1999:1813–1822

32. Hathcock JH, Rader JI. Food additives, contaminants, and natural toxins. In: Shils ME, Olson JA, Shike M, eds. *Modern Nutrition in Health and Disease.* 8th ed. Philadelphia, PA: Lea and Febiger; 1994:1593–1610

33. Barron RL, Vanscoy GJ. Natural products and the athlete: facts and folklore. *Ann Pharmacother*. 1993;27:607–615

34. Dyer JE. Gamma-hydroxybutyrate: a health-food product producing coma and seizurelike activity. *Am J Emerg Med*. 1991;9:321–324

35. Clydesdale FM. Fortified vs natural foods: the debate continues. *J Am Diet Assoc*. 1994;94;1252

36. Gussow JD, Akabas S. Are we really fixing up the food supply? *J Am Diet Assoc*. 1994;93:1300–1304

37. Bergholz CM. Olestra and potential role of a nonabsorbable lipid in the diets of children. *Ann N Y Acad Sci*. 1991;623:356–368

38. Black DM, Knauer SL. The legal implications of dietary fats: risks of cardiovascular disease and the duty of food manufacturers. *J Nutr*. 1991;121:578–582

39. Warshaw HS, Powers MA. Ingredients that replace fat: their role in today's foods and challenges in educating people with diabetes. *Diabetes Educ*. 1993;19:419–430

40. Ouellett J. Mainstream nutraceuticals. Food Additives 95: Chemical and Marketing Reporter. May 29, 1995

41. Mackey MA and Santerre CR. Biotechnology and our food supply. *Nutr Today*. 35:120–128

42. Metcalfe DD, Astwood JD, Townsend R, Sampson HA, Taylor SL, Fuchs RL. Assessment of the allergenic potential of foods derived from genetically engineered crop plants. *Crit Rev Food Sci Nutr*. 1996;36(suppl):S165–S186

43. Food and Agriculture Organization. Biotechnology and food safety: report of a joint FAO/WHO consultation. Rome, Italy: FAP; 1996. Food and Nutrition Paper 61

44. Freedman MR. Popular diets: a scientific review. *Int J Obesity*. In press

45. Atkins RC. *Dr Atkins' New Diet Revolution*. New York, NY: Avon Books, Inc; 1992

46. Atkins RC. *Dr Atkins' Diet Revolution*. New York, NY: David McKay Publishers; 1972

47. Eades MR, Eades MD. *Protein Power*. New York, NY: Bantam Books; 1996

48. Council on Foods and Nutrition, American Medical Association. A critique of low carbohydrate, ketogenic weight reduction regimens: A review of Dr Atkins' Diet Revolution. *JAMA*. 1973;224:1415–1419

49. Sears B. *The Zone*. New York, NY: Harper Collins; 1995

50. Heller R, Heller R. *Carbohydrate Addict's Diet*. New York, NY: Penguin Books; 1991

51. Ornish D. *Eat More, Weigh Less*. New York, NY: Harper Paperbacks; 1993

52. Ornish D. *Dr Dean Ornish's Program for Reversing Heart Disease*. New York, NY: Ballantine Books; 1990

53. Ornish D. Avoiding revascularization with lifestyle changes: the Multicenter Lifestyle Demonstration Project. *Am J Cardiol*. 1998;82:72T–76T

54. Pritikin R. *The New Pritikin Program*. New York, NY: Simon and Schuster, Inc; 1990

55. Pritikin R. *The Pritikin Weight Loss Breakthrough*. New York, NY: Signet; 1999

56. Pritikin R. *The Pritikin Principle*. Alexandria, VA: Time Life Books; 2000

57. Van Itallie TB, Yang MU. Current concepts in nutrition: diet and weight loss. *N Engl J Med*. 1977;297:1158–1160

58. National Institutes of Health. *Clinical Guidelines on the Identification, Evaluation and Treatment of Overweight and Obesity in Adults: the Evidence Report.* Bethesda, MD: National Heart, Lung, and Blood Institute; 1998

59. Konnikoff R, Dwyer J. Popular diets and other treatments of obesity. In: Heffner TG, Lockwood DH. *Obesity: Pathology and Therapy.* New York, NY: Springer; 2000

60. Allara L. The return of the high-protein, low carbohydrate diet: weighing the risks. *Nutr Clin Pract.* 2000;15:26–29

61. Woteki CE, Thomas PR, eds. *Eat For Life: The Food and Nutrition Board's Guide to Reducing Your Risk of Chronic Disease.* Washington, DC: National Academy Press; 1992

This material is based upon work supported by the US Department of Agriculture, under agreement No. 58–1950–9–001. Any opinions, findings, conclusions, or recommendations expressed in this publication are those of the author and do not necessarily reflect the views of the US Department of Agriculture.

III
Micronutrients and Macronutrients

14

Protein

Dietary protein provides the amino acids required for the synthesis of body proteins and other nitrogenous compounds with important functional roles, such as glutathione, heme, creatine, taurine, nucleotides, and some neurotransmitters. Amino acids can exist as various stereoisomers in nature. Only the L-amino acids are biologically active and can be incorporated into proteins. Body proteins also can be catabolized and serve as an energy source when energy intake, in particular carbohydrate intake, is inadequate.

Dietary protein digestion begins in the stomach through the activity of pepsin in the presence of hydrochloric acid. In the young infant, pepsin and acid production are low, but this does not appear to limit the digestibility of protein. Protein digestion continues in the presence of pancreatic enzymes in the duodenum and the enzymes in the brush border of the jejunum and proximal ileum. Some of these enzymes, such as enterokinase, also have low activity during the newborn period, but the low activity does not appear to limit protein digestion. Digestion results in the hydrolysis of proteins to oligopeptides and amino acids that are absorbed. Oligopeptides are hydrolyzed to amino acids by enzymes in the cells of the intestinal epithelium. Protein that escapes digestion in the small intestine can be broken down by bacteria in the colon and the resulting ammonia can be absorbed and incorporated into amino acids.

Absorbed amino acids are first transported from the intestine to the liver and then enter the general amino acid pool of the body in the plasma and exchange with tissue pools. In the growing organism, an influx of amino acids to the tissues from the diet rapidly stimulates protein synthesis. This contrasts with the response observed in adults, where protein consumption primarily reduces protein breakdown and has only minimal effects on protein synthesis. Dietary amino acids consumed in excess of the body's needs cannot be stored. The nitrogen component of amino acids is converted to urea, and the remaining ketoacids are used directly for energy production or converted to glucose and fat when energy intake is adequate. Therefore, blood urea nitrogen is a good indicator of recent protein intake when hydration and renal function are normal. The stimulation of protein synthesis by the influx of amino acids from the diet, together with the body's inability to store excess dietary amino acids, are primary reasons for the recommendation that, in infants and children, the daily protein requirement should be consumed over several meals at intervals throughout the day.

Body proteins and the other nitrogenous compounds are continuously degraded and resynthesized. Several times more endogenous protein is turned over every day than is usually consumed. The rate of turnover can be rapid, as in bone marrow and in gastrointestinal mucosa, or it can be slow, as in muscle and collagen. Protein turnover also changes with age; it is highest during early life when tissues are maturing and their growth rates are at their highest. The amino acids released from the breakdown of endogenous proteins are recycled, but this process is not completely efficient. Amino acids that are not reused are catabolized or lost in urine, feces, sweat, desquamated skin, hair, and nails. These losses create an obligatory requirement for dietary amino acids, in addition to any requirement for the net accretion of body protein. This obligatory fraction constitutes the maintenance needs of the organism and, once growth has ceased, represents an individual's entire protein requirement.

Amino acids are usually categorized into 3 groups: essential, conditionally essential, and nonessential. The amino acids that adults cannot synthesize are regarded as essential amino acids and must be provided by the diet; they include leucine, isoleucine, valine, threonine, methionine, phenylalanine, tryptophan, lysine, and histidine. Cysteine and tyrosine are considered essential amino acids for the preterm and young term infant because of the immaturity of the enzyme activities necessary for their synthesis.

Conditionally essential amino acids and other nutrients are those that ordinarily can be synthesized, but an exogenous source is required under certain circumstances. Taurine, carnitine, and glycine are in this category. Taurine and carnitine can be synthesized by the body and are present in a mixed diet containing proteins of animal origin. The rates of synthesis in infants fed by total parenteral nutrition or receiving synthetic formulas devoid of these amino acids may be insufficient to meet all of their needs. Glycine is required for the synthesis of creatine, porphyrins, glutathione, nucleotides, and bile salts; therefore, the requirement for this amino acid during times of rapid growth is relatively high. Because the metabolic pathways for the synthesis of glycine are immature in early life and glycine is present in relatively small amounts in milk, glycine may be a conditionally essential amino acid for the preterm and young term infant.

The body can normally synthesize several amino acids, although they may be essential for individuals with certain diseases. Arginine is essential in patients with defects of the urea cycle. Cysteine may be essential in patients with hepatic disease or homocystinuria. Tyrosine is essential for persons with phenylketonuria and may be required for patients with hepatic disease. Glutamine is the preferred fuel for rapidly dividing cells, such as enterocytes and lymphocytes. Thus, during times of critical stress, such as after surgical procedures, nonsurgical trauma, or sepsis, or in patients with gastrointestinal mucosal injury, large amounts of glutamine are synthesized by the skeletal muscle from the amino acids of skeletal muscle proteins.

To sustain normal growth after the requirements for essential amino acids have been met, the additional dietary nitrogen required must be provided as nonessential amino acids. The body can synthesize 9 nonessential amino acids: alanine, arginine, glycine, serine, glutamine, aspartic acid, glutamic acid, asparagine, and proline.

Recommended Dietary Allowance for Protein

The recommended dietary allowance (RDA) for protein is the amount of protein in a normal diet that meets the nutrient needs of most healthy people (Appendix C).[1–4] It considers 3 factors:

1. *The average physiologic requirement for absorbed protein according to gender, age, and reproductive status for females.* The physiologic requirement is defined as the lowest level of protein intake needed to replace losses from the body when energy intake is in balance (maintenance requirement). In growing individuals and pregnant and lactating women, the protein requirement also includes the protein required for tissue accretion and milk production at a level associated with good health. The need for growth decreases from approximately 65% of total intake at birth to 5% at 5 years of age and accounts largely for the reduction with age in protein requirements (Table 14.1).

2. *The digestibility and amino acid pattern of proteins in the diet (ie, protein quality).* Proteins from different dietary sources vary in these characteristics, and, thus, the extent to which they deviate from the ideal must be considered.[2]

3. *The individual variability in protein needs.* Whereas the requirement is derived for individuals, the RDA applies to groups of individuals and,

Table 14.1.
Contribution of Maintenance and Growth to Protein Needs of Infants and Children[4]

Age	Protein Gain (g/[kg·d^{-1}])	Intake		Maintenance
		Growth		
		(% of total)		
0–1 month	1.00	64		36
1–3 months	0.57	50		50
3–6 months	0.30	35		65
6–12 months	0.18	24		76
1–2 years	0.11	16		84
2–5 years	0.07	11		89

therefore, must consider the variability in the requirements among groups of similar individuals. Thus, the average requirement is increased by 2 standard deviations (approximately 25%) to encompass 98% of individuals within a given group.[2,4]

Protein requirements and balance data are frequently expressed by nitrogen content, which constitutes approximately 16% of the weight of a protein. Thus, a factor of 6.25 is used to convert grams of nitrogen to grams of protein.

Methods for Determining Protein Requirements

Protein Quantity

Protein needs have been estimated using various approaches.[1–4] During the first 6 months of life, the average intake of breastfed infants has been used to define the protein requirements. Provided energy needs are met, the quantity and quality of protein provided by human milk are assumed to be sufficient to support optimal growth. Various approaches, including measurements of nitrogen balance at a variety of nitrogen intakes, the factorial method, studies using nonradioactive, stable-isotope tracer techniques, and biochemical measurements (such as plasma amino acid profiles, the concentration of various plasma proteins, and urea concentrations), have been used to evaluate the protein needs of older infants, children, and adolescents.

Maintenance protein requirements are derived from nitrogen balance studies. This method involves determination of the difference between the intake and excretion of nitrogen (in urine, feces, sweat, and minor losses via other routes) for 1 to 3 weeks, or longer. Several different levels of a quality protein source, such as milk or egg, are usually tested at a constant and adequate energy intake. From the relationship between intake and retention (intake minus excretion), the amount of nitrogen required for maintenance (zero balance) is extrapolated.

Total protein requirements of infants and children older than 6 months of age have been determined using a modified factorial method. To the maintenance requirements defined by nitrogen balance, additional amounts of protein that would be sufficient to support appropriate body protein gains have been added. The mean rate of protein gain during growth has been estimated from the expected daily rate of weight gain at the National Center for Health Statistics (NCHS) 50th percentile and the nitrogen concentration in the body. The body composition data used are those of Fomon, et al[5]; these and the NCHS data are based primarily on studies of formula-fed infants.

Protein Quality

The recommended intakes for protein are for sources of protein that are highly digestible (greater than 95%) and that contain essential amino acids in amounts that closely meet human needs. These properties apply to animal proteins, such as egg protein, milk protein, meat, and fish, whereas vegetable proteins often have a lower digestibility (70% to 80%) and often provide inadequate amounts of lysine or the sulphur amino acids (for examples, see Table 14.2).[2,3] Although plant proteins are generally of a lower quality than proteins of animal origin, equivalent amino acid patterns can be achieved by mixing plant proteins from different sources. Processing of foods can also increase or decrease the digestibility of dietary proteins. Thus, to apply the recommendations for protein intake to mixed diets containing protein sources other than animal-based foods, it is necessary to adjust for the protein digestibility and correct for the adequacy of the amino acid composition of the food.

A pattern of requirements for amino acids that must be provided by dietary protein is derived by dividing the essential amino acid requirement by the recommended allowance of an ideal protein for a given age group. Thus, an ideal protein is one containing all the essential amino acids in amounts sufficient to meet requirements without any excess. For infants to 1 year of age, the amino acid pattern of human milk proteins is considered the ideal. Thus, provided the protein requirement is met with milk, the amino acid intake will be appropriate. However, once the protein source in the diet becomes more varied, the amino acid pattern requires more detailed consideration. Slightly different

Table 14.2.

Mean Values for Digestibility and Amino Acid Scores of Various Protein Sources in a Typical US Mixed Diet

Protein source	Digestibility*		Amino acid score†	
	True	Relative	Preschool child	School-aged child
Whole egg (hen)	97	100	109 (trp)	133 (trp)
Cow milk, cheese	95	100	127 (trp)	155 (s)
Meat, fish	94	100	100 (trp)	122 (trp)
Peanut butter	95	90	62 (lys)	82 (lys)
Maize	85	89	48 (lys)	64 (lys)
Rice, polished	88	93	62 (lys)	82 (lys)
Wheat, whole	86	90	48 (lys)	64 (lys)
Wheat, refined	96	101	38 (lys)	50 (lys)
Beans	78	82	100 (S)	114 (S)
Soy protein isolate	86	90	108 (S)	123 (S)
US mixed diet	96	101	109 (trp)	113 (trp)

*True digestibility (%) = $\dfrac{\text{Nitrogen intake} - (\text{Fecal nitrogen on test protein} - \text{Fecal nitrogen on nonprotein diet}) \times 100}{\text{Nitrogen intake}}$

Relative digestibility is the digestibility of the protein relative to that of a reference protein, such as milk or egg. A factor of 6.25 is used to convert nitrogen to protein. Data taken from Reference 2.

†The amino acid score for various protein sources was derived using the amino acid requirement pattern for preschool and school-aged children in Reference 2. The amino acid composition of the protein sources was obtained from the USDA Nutrient Database for Standard Reference, Release 14 (July 2001). Value shown is for the most limiting amino acid; Trp, tryptophan; lys, lysine; S, cysteine + methionine. Values of more than 100 indicate that the protein source contains relatively more of that amino acid than the reference protein.

patterns are currently recommended for 2- to 6-year-olds and 6- to 13-year-olds. The adult pattern applies to adolescents older than 13 years. Requirements for the essential amino acids decrease more rapidly with age than do requirements for total nitrogen. This change with age reflects a greater need of essential amino acids for growth, whereas maintenance places a heavier demand on nonessential amino acids. Given the higher requirement of essential amino acids as well as the conditionally essential nature of certain other amino acids, the quality of proteins is more critical in infants and small children than it is in older children and adults. Nonetheless, because the composition and content of essential amino acids in human milk is probably in excess of an infant's true needs, using the amino acid pattern of breast milk as a basis for evaluating the adequacy of weaning diets may be overly stringent. In general, diets with an essential amino acid content and pattern that meet the needs of infants and younger children will also be adequate for older children and adolescents, whereas the converse may not be true.

To adjust for the amino acid composition of a protein source, the amino acid score is calculated, which is determined by the amino acid that will be the most limiting for a specific age group:

$$\text{Amino acid score} = \frac{\text{mg of amino acid in 1 g of food protein}}{\text{mg of amino acid in reference pattern}} \times 100$$

Only 4 essential amino acids are likely to affect the quality of a food protein: lysine, the sulfur amino acids (methionine + cysteine), threonine, and tryptophan. Examples of the amino acid score for various protein sources if they were the only protein source in the diet of a preschool or school-aged child are shown in Table 14.2. In the formulation of special purpose diets in clinical practice, the scoring patterns for all essential amino acids should be considered.

Protein Requirements

Because of the differences in the quality of proteins available in the diet and other factors such as age, gender, activity levels, and methodological limitations, confidence in the recommendations for protein and amino acid intakes for individuals or populations is limited. Recommendations are needed to guide the design of diets and the content of educational programs in nutrition and for planning specific intervention programs.

Infants[4,6]

One nutritional statement that can be made with confidence is that the ideal food for full-term infants is human milk. It is the lowest in protein content of any species and contains only 0.8 to 0.9 g/dL true protein and 0.2 to 0.3 g/dL of nonprotein nitrogen compounds. The protein composition of human milk, in which the whey proteins rather than the caseins are the dominant protein constituents, is exceptional because of its high cysteine content and high cysteine/methionine ratio (Appendix A). The nonprotein nitrogen component of human milk also contains substantial quantities of taurine, which is virtually absent from cow's milk but is added to commercially prepared infant formulas.

The relatively low protein content of human milk implies that these proteins have a high nutritional quality and are digested and absorbed efficiently. The same increments of growth are obtained with the low protein intake of human milk as are observed with the higher protein intake of various commercial infant formulas. Thus, a 4-kg, full-term infant ingesting 800 mL/d of human milk receives about 7.2 g protein plus 1.6 g/d of the protein equivalents of nonprotein nitrogen compounds. This is about 1.8 g/kg/d of high-quality protein and 0.4 g/kg/d nonprotein nitrogen, of which approximately 46% is utilizable. This protein intake appears to satisfy the infant's requirements for maintenance and growth without an amino acid or solute excess. The total protein equivalent of 1.5 g/dL in the commercial infant formulas available in the United States (Appendix E) provides a margin of safety for the less abundant sulfur-containing proteins. Some commercial infant formulas have a whey protein-to-casein ratio similar to that of human milk. Although the specific proteins of bovine whey differ considerably from those of human whey, the amino acid composition of these "humanized" formulas is closer to that of human milk proteins than are formulas with the whey protein-to-casein ratio of bovine milk.

Despite their growth and the decreasing protein content of human milk during lactation, breastfed infants only show a small, compensatory increase in the volume of milk they consume during the first 6 months of life. Protein intakes, therefore, decrease during this time and are lower than the requirement derived by the factorial approach, which uses the intake data and weight gain patterns of formula-fed infants. The rate of weight gain of breastfed infants falls off more rapidly than that of formula-fed infants after 3 to 4 months of age, and, thus, the adequacy of human milk as the sole source of protein after this age is frequently questioned.[6] However, despite the differences in protein intake, there are no apparent differences in length gain and no association between weight gain and protein intake to suggest that protein is limiting in the older breastfed infant.[7] The differences in weight gain have been attributed to higher rates of fat accretion in formula-fed infants. Measurements of the composition of weight gain of infants fed by different modalities are needed to resolve this issue. Irrespective of these uncertainties, studies that have compared morbidity and developmental indices of infants up to 1 year of age living in healthy environments have identified no relationship between these functional parameters and protein intake.[4,7]

A revision to the current recommendations for the protein intake of young infants is being considered currently.[4] The revisions being considered are based on the following: (a) the use of updated intake data for breastfed infants, which is somewhat lower than those previously used; (b) the recognition that, if the breastfed infant is to be the model, intake is likely to be greater than the requirement after 3 to 4 months of age; (c) maintenance needs are probably lower than previously assumed; and (d) there is yet a paucity of information to determine if the requirements of non-breastfed infants differ from those of breastfed infants.

Children

During the preschool and school-age years, a continuing but slow decline in protein needs relative to weight is evident. Current protein allowances have been derived from estimates of the average requirements by the factorial method and by assuming that the variability of protein needs among individual children is the same as that of other age groups. On the basis of more information, the appropriateness of these recommendations is being reevaluated.[4] The primary assumptions being reconsidered include the value for maintenance protein needs, which is likely to be from 10% to 20% lower than currently assumed; and the adjustments for the day-to-day variability in growth rate within an individual.

There are few data on the amino acid requirement of children and adolescents. The best available data were obtained from one study of preschool children.[4] Because growth contributes to only a small proportion of total needs after the first year of life (Table 14.1), it has been suggested that, until there is additional information, this amino acid pattern for preschool children should be used to estimate the requirement for all pediatric age groups except infants.

Food consumption surveys in the United States have established that the amino acid patterns and digestibility of proteins in foods commonly consumed is uniform from 1 year of age on and that no adjustment to the RDA is required for individuals consuming a typical US diet.[3] However, appropriate corrections must be made if a diet of lower quality than any acceptable reference protein is customarily consumed.[2]

Adolescents

Few data are available on the protein requirements of adolescents specifically. Values have been estimated using the factorial approach, with estimates of the maintenance needs interpolated from the values for infants and adults. Recommendations do not emphasize the growth spurt because it is small relative to body size. However, the RDA for adolescent males between 15 and 18 years (0.9 g/kg/d) is slightly higher than that for adolescent females (0.8 g/kg/d) of the same age. There have been no further developments in identifying any specific amino acid needs for adolescents, and the same recommendations as for children have been adopted.

Factors Affecting Dietary Protein Requirements

Dietary requirements for protein are affected by a variety of factors, including gender, age, growth, pregnancy, lactation, illness, the adequacy of other nutrients in the diet, and, possibly, genetic variation. In various ways, these factors influence the maintenance needs of the organism and the efficiency with which amino acids can be used for growth. The primary factor that influences protein requirements is energy intake. All balance measurements and recommendations are based on the assumption that energy needs are adequately met. When energy intake is inadequate, proteins are catabolized for the provision of energy, effectively increasing protein requirements.

Protein requirements for pregnancy and lactation are increased to meet the need for maternal and fetal tissue deposition and milk protein production.[1-3] It has not been definitively established whether adolescent mothers have different needs from adult mothers.

Infections and stressful stimuli, such as severe thermal or physical injury, are among factors that increase individual protein and amino acid needs. In these conditions, maintenance needs are increased because of increased rates of protein and amino acid catabolism and increased losses, such as those that occur with burns. Despite the clear-cut evidence for a greater protein need during periods of infection and stress, exact recommendations are not available. On the basis of some studies, a reasonable estimate is a 20% to 30% increase in total protein after an infection (30% to 50% in the case of severe prolonged diarrhea) and during the recovery period, which is 2 to 3 times longer than the duration of the illness.[8]

Although athletic activity and heavy physical work increase energy needs, it is not clear whether the need for protein is also increased once the energy needs are met. Athletes undertaking intense exercise appear to require 1 to 1.5 g/kg/d to remain in nitrogen balance.[9] Provided individuals consume a well-balanced diet (in which approximately 15% of the total energy content is made up of proteins), the increased food consumption that usually accompanies the increased energy needs of physical activity ensures that protein intake also is increased. Thus, any increased needs will be met without the need for specific supplements or a change in the composition of the diet. Increased protein intake in itself will not increase skeletal muscle protein deposition.

Protein requirements are increased in infants and children undergoing catch-up growth.[2,4] The additional amount of protein that must be supplied depends on the desired rate and composition of weight gain. Approximately 0.23 g of dietary protein is needed for every extra gram of tissue deposited; this assumes that 16% of tissue deposited is protein and that the efficiency of conversion of dietary protein to body protein is 70%. Along with the additional protein, energy must also be supplemented to support catch-up growth. The level of energy supplementation that is needed varies depending on whether the child is wasted or not. Weight gain in a wasted child will have a larger proportion of fat, which carries a greater energy cost than an equivalent weight of lean body tissue. However, when refeeding malnourished children by supplementing with both protein and energy, careful consideration must also be given the overall protein-energy ratio of the diet because it will influence the composition of the tissues deposited. Because children who are very wasted are often stunted, foods with high protein-energy ratios are preferable, as they will minimize the likelihood of excessive fat deposition. Catch-up growth also increases the requirements for micronutrients, such as zinc, magnesium, iron, and copper. Thus, the intake of these nutrients must be increased to maximize the efficiency with which the protein is utilized.

Effects of Insufficient and Excessive Protein Intake

Protein-energy malnutrition encompasses a wide spectrum of conditions, with kwashiorkor, the result of a greater deficiency of protein than energy intake, at one end of the spectrum, and marasmus, resulting primarily from an inadequate energy intake, at the other. Especially in kwashiorkor, the condition is often precipitated by the development of conditions that increase the child's protein needs, such as an infection or trauma. A marginally adequate diet (as weaning diets often can be in less developed countries) does not meet these increased needs. Although protein-energy malnutrition is observed even in industrialized countries, such as the United States, the cause is usually associated with the presence of clinical conditions that decrease food intake or impair the digestion or absorption of food.

The effects of too much dietary protein have not been studied extensively. Multinational studies have shown a correlation between protein intake and the prevalence of atherosclerosis and accelerating glomerulosclerosis, but a causal relationship has not been established. Extremely high protein intakes increase obligatory fluid loss, and, if the fluid is not adequately replaced, dehydration can occur; this can be a concern in warmer climates, especially when activity levels are high. High intakes of protein, especially casein, by small infants can result in acidosis, aminoacidemia, and cylinduria. Studies in adults show that high protein intakes lead to hypercalciuria and even a negative calcium balance. This is of particular concern during adolescence when significant bone mineralization is still occurring.

References

1. Pellett PL. Protein requirements in humans. *Am J Clin Nutr*. 1990;51:723–737
2. FAO/WHO/UNU Expert Consultation. *Energy and Protein Requirements*. WHO Technical Bulletin #724. Geneva, Switzerland: World Health Organization; 1985
3. Food and Nutrition Board, National Research Council. *Recommended Dietary Allowances*. 10th ed. Washington, DC: National Academy Press; 1989:52–77
4. Dewey KG, Beaton G, Fjeld C, Lonnerdal B, Reeds P. Protein requirements of infants and children. *Eur J Clin Nutr*. 1996;50(suppl):S119–S147
5. Fomon SJ, Haschke F, Ziegler EE, Nelson R. Body composition of reference children from birth to age 10 years. *Am J Clin Nutr*. 1982;35:1169–1175
6. Fomon SJ. Protein. In: *Nutrition of Normal Infants*. St Louis, MO: Mosby-Year Book, Inc; 1993:121–146
7. Dewey KG, Heinig MJ, Nommsen LA, Lonnerdal B. Adequacy of energy intake among breast-fed infants in the DARLING study: relationships to growth velocity, morbidity, and activity levels. *J Pediatr*. 1991;119:538–547
8. Scrimshaw NS. Effect of infection on nutritional status. *Proc Natl Sci Counc Repub China B*. 1992;16:46–64
9. Lemon PW, Proctor DN. Protein intake and athletic performance. *Sports Med*. 1991;12:313–325

15

Energy

Definitions

Energy is defined as the capacity to do work or to produce a change in matter. Applied to nutrition, energy refers mainly to the chemical energy derived from foods, principally from oxidative metabolism of the macronutrients fat, carbohydrate, and protein. Energy is required for all the biochemical and physiologic functions that sustain life (eg, respiration, circulation, maintenance of electrochemical gradients across cell membranes, and maintenance of body temperature), as well as for growth and physical activity.[1,2] Inadequate intake of energy inevitably has adverse consequences, even if other nutrient requirements are met.

Although in a strict sense, energy is not a nutrient (ie, fat, carbohydrate, and protein are the substances ingested), it is useful to think in terms of the energy requirement of an individual, which an international working group defined as "that level of energy intake from food which will balance energy expenditure when the individual has a body size and composition, and level of physical activity, consistent with long-term good health; and which will allow for the maintenance of economically necessary and socially desirable physical activity. In children and pregnant or lactating women the energy requirement includes the energy needs associated with the deposition of tissues or secretion of milk at rates consistent with good health."[3] In the United States, the kilocalorie has been the most widely used unit of energy in nutrition; however, as use of the International System of Units (SI units) becomes more widespread, energy expressed in terms of kilojoules will become more common (1 kcal = 4.184 kilojoules).

In any individual, energy partitioning can be described by the following relationship: Energy Intake = Energy Excretion + Energy Expenditure + Energy Storage.[4,5] Most clinical problems involving energy balance can be approached by systematic evaluation of the terms in this equation. *Digestible energy* refers to gross energy intake minus energy lost in the feces. *Metabolizable energy* is gross energy intake minus energy excreted in feces and urine and is the value used for food labeling. Inadequate energy intake may be a consequence of insufficient provision of appropriate food by the child's caretakers or may be due to problems inherent to the child (eg, neurologic, behavior, or certain gastrointestinal disorders). Fecal excretion of fat usually accounts for most of the energy excretion, although in some instances, carbohydrate and nitrogenous losses also may be clinically important. Clinically significant increased energy excretion most commonly is secondary to intestinal, pancreatic, or hepatobiliary disorders that result in macronutrient maldigestion and/or malabsorption. In some situations (eg, diabetes mellitus, ketosis), energy losses in urine may be significant.

Energy expenditure includes energy expended for basal metabolic requirements, the thermic effect of food ingestion, energy expended for activity, and energy expended for thermoregulation.[5] Resting energy expenditure (REE) is the energy expended by a person at rest in a thermoneutral environment (ie, an environmental temperature at which the metabolic rate and, therefore, oxygen consumption are at a minimum). Basal metabolic rate (BMR) is energy expenditure under standard conditions (ie, after a 12- to 18-hour fast, awake, but quietly lying down [in early morning on awakening], in a thermoneutral environment, bodily and mentally at rest). The BMR reflects energy required for vital body processes during physical, emotional, and digestive rest, and usually differs from the REE by less than 10%. Important factors that affect energy expenditure at rest include age, body size and composition, and the presence of disease (eg, infection, fever, or trauma).

Thermogenesis refers to increases in energy expenditure above the REE that are not due to physical activity, including the effects of food intake, cold exposure, thermogenic agents, and psychological influences. The *thermic effect of feeding* (TEF), or *specific dynamic action*, is the increase in energy expenditure resulting from ingestion of food; it constitutes 5% to 10% of energy ingested. The TEF is due mainly to the obligatory metabolic costs of processing a meal, which include nutrient digestion, absorption, transport, and storage. The remaining facultative TEF is the component of the TEF not accounted for by known energy costs that may be related to stimulation of the sympathetic nervous system, increased futile cycle activity (net hydrolysis of adenosine triphosphate and the generation of heat via a cycle of phosphorylation and dephosphorylation catalyzed by enzymes that normally function in separate pathways), cell membrane pump activity, or changes in hormonal status. Energy required to maintain body temperature depends on environmental temperature. Little additional energy is needed between environmental temperatures of 20°C and 30°C. Outside these limits, an additional 5% to 10% of total energy may be necessary to maintain body temperature. The thermoneutral temperature range is higher for neonates, particularly for those born prematurely.

Energy expenditure is determined in several ways, most commonly by indirect calorimetry, in which oxygen consumption and carbon dioxide production are measured. The respiratory quotient is the ratio of carbon dioxide production to oxygen consumption and varies depending on substrate utilization (ie, the relative contributions of carbohydrate, fat, and protein catabolism to total expenditure). The respiratory quotient for fat is 0.7; for protein, 0.85; for carbohydrate, 1.0; and for lipogenesis (conversion of carbohydrate to stored fat), greater than 1. The ingestion or administration of a high percentage of calories as carbohydrate may cause difficulties for children with respiratory insufficiency because excess carbon dioxide is produced. This is especially true if the energy intake from carbohydrate exceeds the energy expenditure.

In addition to actual measurement of energy expenditure, a number of formulas, tables, and nomograms have been developed to estimate the REE of infants, children, and adults based on such factors as weight, height, age, gender, and body surface area. A method of estimating BMR based on weight, age, and gender is given in Table 15.1. The values listed in Appendix C are estimates of the average requirements for various age groups. The potential fallibility of such estimates in individual instances, particularly in disease states, should not be forgotten. Recent research suggests that several commonly used equations for predicting energy expenditure tend to overestimate the REE in healthy infants and underestimate the REE in infants with cystic fibrosis.[6]

Table 15.1.
Food and Agriculture Organization and World Health Organization Equations for Predicting Basal Metabolic Rate From Body Weight*

Males		Females	
Age, y	Basal Metabolic Rate, kcal/d	Age, y	Basal Metabolic Rate, kcal/d
0–3	$60.7 \times wt - 54$	0–3	$61.0 \times wt - 51$
3–10	$22.7 \times wt + 495$	3–10	$22.5 \times wt + 499$
10–18	$17.5 \times wt + 651$	10–18	$12.2 \times wt + 746$
18–30	$15.3 \times wt + 679$	18–30	$14.7 \times wt + 496$

*Body weight in kilograms; wt indicates weight. Adapted with permission from the World Health Organization. *Energy and Protein Requirements.* Geneva, Switzerland: WHO; 1985.

Requirements

Any estimate of total energy requirements must consider energy expenditure due to physical activity, as well as the energy cost of growth; the latter is important in energy balance primarily during infancy. Estimates for energy expenditure for physical activities vary. Examples of energy expenditure while performing various activities are given in Chapter 10. During infancy, the energy cost of growth is about 5 kcal/g of new tissue. After 1 year, as growth slows, the energy needed for growth represents about 1% of the total energy intake and ranges from 8.7 to 12 kcal/g gained depending on the composition of the tissue accreted. Factorial estimates of energy requirements for infants from 1 to 6 months of age are given in Figure 15.1.[5] Significantly lower mean energy intakes of healthy breastfed infants in this age group have been recorded by some investigators,[5,7] and it has been suggested that current recommendations for energy intake during the first 2 years of life overestimate actual requirements.[8]

Although food intake is the result of complex interactions among central nervous regulating regions (mainly hypothalamic) and peripheral neural (ie, vagal) and humoral (eg, gut peptides and insulin) signals and environmental factors, energy balance at all ages is regulated with a fair degree of precision.

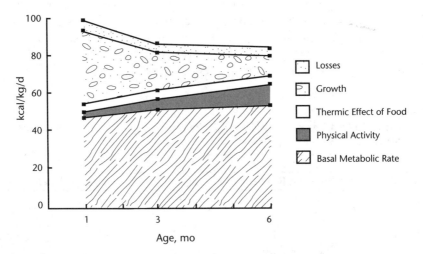

Figure 15.1. Nutritional requirements of normal infants. From Waterlow JC. Basic concepts in the determination of nutritional requirements of normal infants. In: Tsang RC, Nichols BL, eds. *Nutrition During Infancy.* Philadelphia, PA: Hanley and Belfus, Inc; 1988:6.

This is reflected in the observation that most infants and children grow in regular fashion, and many adults maintain stable body weight for long periods. Infants appear to eat to satisfy energy needs and will compensate for low-food energy density and poor digestibility by increasing food intake.[4] Observations of young children fed ad libitum while recovering from malnutrition showed that their voracious appetites abated as they approached normal weight for height.[9] Despite the usual balancing of energy intake against energy expenditure and energy needs for growth,[10] obesity (see Chapter 33), a consequence of long-term energy intake in excess of energy requirements, has become alarmingly prevalent among children in the United States.

The average diet of individuals in the United States supplies 12% to 15% of calories from protein. The remainder of calories are derived from carbohydrate, fat, and alcohol; the latter accounts for as much as 10% of the total calories in adults. Although an appropriate balance of total calories and protein is required for adequate growth, especially in response to malnutrition, the importance of energy intake is underscored by the observations that the speed of recovery from severe infantile malnutrition is more closely related to energy than to protein intake[11] and that pregnancy outcomes can be improved as much by additional calories as by protein supplements.[12] Many common pathologic entities may alter energy requirements, interfere with nutrient availability, or affect substrate utilization. Provision of adequate energy may be especially important in certain clinical settings, particularly if a patient's ability to regulate intake is impaired. During infancy, childhood, and adolescence, if energy intake is adequate for energy excretion and energy expenditure, adequate energy should be available for sufficient energy storage. The growth rate, in fact, serves as a good "bioassay" for the adequacy of energy intake. Careful consideration of the factors affecting energy balance (ie, energy intake, energy excretion, energy expenditure, and energy storage) can often clarify seemingly complex clinical problems.

References

1. Food and Nutrition Board, National Research Council. *Recommended Dietary Allowances*. 10th ed. Washington, DC: National Academy Press; 1989
2. Pellett PL. Food energy requirements in humans. *Am J Clin Nutr*. 1990;51:711–722
3. FAO/WHO/UNU Expert Consultation. *Energy and Protein Requirements*. WHO Technical Bulletin #724. Geneva, Switzerland: World Health Organization; 1985
4. Fomon SJ. *Nutrition of Normal Infants*. St Louis, MO: Mosby-Year Book, Inc; 1993
5. Tsang RC, Nichols BL. *Nutrition During Infancy*. Philadelphia, PA: Hanley and Belfus, Inc; 1988

6. Thomson MA, Bucolo S, Quirk P, Shepherd RW. Measured versus predicted resting energy expenditure in infants: a need for reappraisal. *J Pediatr*. 1995;126:21–27

7. Butte NF, Wong WW, Garza C, et al. Energy requirements of breast-fed infants. *J Am Coll Nutr*. 1991;10:190–195

8. Butte NF, Wong WW, Hopkinson JM, Heinz CJ, Mehta NR, Smith EO. Energy requirements derived from total energy expenditure and energy deposition during the first 2 y of life. *Am J Clin Nutr*. 2000;72:1558–1569

9. Ashworth A. Growth rates in children recovering from protein-calorie malnutrition. *Br J Nutr*. 1969;23:834–845

10. Forbes GB, Brown MR. Energy need for weight maintenance in human beings: effect of body size and composition. *J Am Diet Assoc*. 1989;89:499–502

11. Waterlow JC. The rate of recovery of malnourished infants in relation to the protein and calorie levels of the diet. *J Trop Pediatr*. 1961;7:16–28

12. Lechtig A, Delgado H, Lasky R, et al. Maternal nutrition and fetal growth in developing countries. *Am J Dis Child*. 1975;129:553–556

16
Carbohydrate and Dietary Fiber

Carbohydrate provides 50% to 60% of the calories consumed by the average American. Although relatively little carbohydrate is needed in the diet, carbohydrate spares protein and fat being metabolized for calories. The principal dietary carbohydrates are sugars and starches. Sugars include monosaccharides (eg, glucose, galactose, and fructose) and disaccharides (eg, lactose, sucrose, maltose, and trehalose). Starches are the storage carbohydrates of plants and consist of sugars (eg, glucose) linked together.

Digestion of Disaccharides and Starches
Lactose and sucrose are hydrolyzed to monosaccharides via lactase and sucrase, respectively (Figure 16.1). Lactase activity increases substantially during the third trimester whereas sucrase activity by the onset of the last trimester is already at levels found at birth.[1,2] Starch digestion is more complex. The production of amylase by the pancreas increases to mature levels during the first year of life.[3] Salivary, and more likely mucosal enzymes (glucoamylase, sucrase, isomaltase) are responsible for starch digestion in young infants.[4,5] Pancreatic and salivary amylase hydrolyze the interior α-1,4 bonds (Figure 16.1). Glucoamylase sequentially cleaves α-1,4 bonds from the nonreducing end of the molecule (Figure 16.1).[6] It is most active against starches between 5 and 9 glucose residues in length.[6] Isomaltase and sucrase also have some activity in this regard. Isomaltase is primarily responsible for cleaving the α-1,6 bonds.

Absorption of Monosaccharides
The end products of disaccharide and starch digestion are monosaccharides. These are absorbed in the small intestine (Figure 16.1). The transport of monosaccharides into and out of the intestinal epithelial cell is accomplished via transporters (Figure 16.1).[7] GLUT 1 actively transports glucose and galactose across the brush border whereas GLUT 5 is responsible for passive absorption of fructose. GLUT 2 releases the sugars across the basolateral membrane of the enterocyte. Carbohydrates that are not absorbed in the small intestine are fermented by colonic bacteria and converted to short-chain fatty acids, which are, in turn, absorbed by the colon.[8]

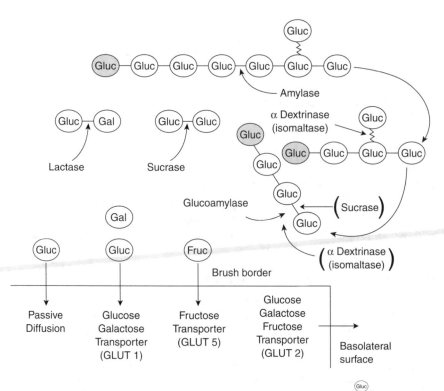

Figure 16.1. Pancreatic and salivary amylase hydrolyze interior α-1,4 bonds 2. ⊖̣. Glucoamylase sequentially cleaves α-1,4 bonds from the nonreducing end of the molecule. The reducing end is designated: ⊖. Isomaltase and sucrase also have some activity in this regard. Isomaltase is primarily responsible for cleaving the α-1,6 bonds (2 ⊖̣). Lactose and sucrose are hydrolyzed by their respective hydrolases. The monosaccharides are transported across the epithelial surface by various active or passive means and then extruded across the basolateral membrane.

Metabolism of Glucose

Dietary carbohydrates are converted to glucose in the liver. It is the most abundant carbohydrate. The majority of glucose is metabolized for energy.[9] Quantitatively, the brain is the largest user of glucose as an energy source. There are few data that allow the limits of carbohydrate intake to be defined.[9] Amino acids and glycerol from lipids can be converted to glucose. However, in the case of amino acids, this potentially shunts substrate away from protein synthesis. Glucose synthesis from both amino acids and glycerol is not very metabolically efficient. Estimates of minimum glucose requirements based on cerebral glucose utilization are shown in Table 16.1.

The upper limits of glucose requirements should be defined by that amount that defines a minimal need for fat and protein and maximum glucose oxidation rates (Table 16.2).[9]

These are theoretical limits as they presume the minimal intake of protein and fat with glucose providing essentially all energy needs. However, doing so can be associated with adverse effects.

Table 16.1.
Estimates of Glucose Consumption by the Brain*

	Body Weight	Brain Weight	Glucose Consumption		
	(kg)	(g)	$(mg \cdot kg^{-1} \cdot min^{-1})$	$(g \cdot kg^{-1} \cdot d^{-1})$	(g/d)
Newborn	3.2	399	6.0	11.5	37
1 y	10	997	7.0	10.1	101
5 y	19	1266	4.7	6.8	129
Adolescent	50	1360	1.9	2.7	135
Adult	70	1400	1.0	1.4	98

*Adapted from reference 9.

Table 16.2.
Upper Limit of Carbohydrate Intake for Infants and Children*[†]

Age	Total Energy Expenditure[‡] $(kcal \cdot kg^{-1} \cdot d^{-1})$	Carbohydrate Equivalent[§] $(g \cdot kg^{-1} \cdot d^{-1})$
Newborn	73	19
1–3 y	85	22
4–6 y	68	18
12–13 y	55	14
18–19 y	44	12
Adult	35	9

*Adapted from reference 9.
[†]Upper limit should be determined by the minimal need for protein and fat obtained. Therefore, the described upper limits here are theoretical maximal to meet all the energy needs.
[‡]Average of data for boys and girls. Estimate based on double-labeled water method.
[§]Carbohydrate equivalent = TEE/3.8, assuming each gram of carbohydrate yields 3.8 kcal.

Glucose that is not immediately oxidized can be polymerized to form glycogen. Present data suggest that in the human newborn, gluconeogenesis appears soon after birth and contributes 30% to 70% to glucose produced.[10] As noted above, the majority of glucose is used by the central nervous system. Storage and mobilization of glycogen are under the hormonal control of insulin and glucagon (see Chapters 30 and 31). During periods of fasting, the liver and kidney can mobilize glucose from glycogen. If fasting is prolonged, hepatic glycogen stores will be drained in a few hours and gluconeogenesis from lactate, alanine, glycerol, and glutamine must be stimulated to maintain euglycemia.[11] The newborn infant has about 34 g of glycogen, only 6 g of which is in the liver and is accumulated during the last weeks of fetal life. Hepatic glycogen is totally depleted during the first few days postnatally and then re-accumulates. Carbohydrate-free diets lead to ketosis, as does fasting. Ketosis occurs when carbohydrate intake drops below about 10% of total calories. It occurs more readily in children than in adults during fasting or when extremely low-carbohydrate diets are consumed. Low-carbohydrate diets and low-carbohydrate, high-fat diets (the ketogenic diet) have been used in the treatment of epilepsy and as a diagnostic test for ketotic hypoglycemia.

In addition to glycogen stores in the liver and skeletal muscle, the body contains carbohydrate in many different forms. These include mucopolysaccharides (structural carbohydrates that are important constituents of connective and collagenous tissues) and components of nucleic acids, glycoproteins, glycolipids, and various hormones and enzymes.

Recently, abnormalities in these structural carbohydrates have been associated with specific symptoms or disorders. Genetic defects in glycoprotein metabolism usually result in neurologic symptoms. However, defects in glycoprotein biosynthesis (the carbohydrate-deficient glycoprotein syndromes) also present with hypoglycemia, protein-losing enteropathy, and hepatic pathology.[12] In these conditions, the N-glycosylation pathway is affected resulting in alterations in the number or structure of sugar chains on the proteins. The diagnosis often can be made via isoelectric focusing of transferrin.[12]

Lactose

Lactose is present in almost all mammalian milks and is the major carbohydrate consumed by young infants.[13] However, at an early age, infants in the United States are fed a variety of other carbohydrates, including sucrose, natural and modified starches, starch hydrolysates, and small amounts of monosaccharides and indigestible carbohydrate (eg, fiber). Lactase, an enzyme on the brush border of the enterocyte in the small intestine, hydrolyzes the disaccharide, lactose, into the monosaccharides, glucose and galactose.

Although a congenital form of lactase deficiency exists (also termed primary lactase deficiency) it is extremely rare. It manifests at birth in the presence of a lactose-containing diet. Much more commonly, lactase activity begins to decline in a genetically programmed fashion so that, by adulthood, in many ethnic groups it is low.[14] The highest prevalence of low lactase activity is found in the Far East. The prevalence in the United States varies according to ethnicity. In whites, it is approximately 15% to 25%; in African Americans, it is approximately 80%; in Hispanics, approximately 53%; and in Asians, approximately 90%.[14] The age at which lactase activity begins to decline also is related to ethnicity. In the United States, the decline usually begins to occur around 3 to 7 years of age; ethnic groups with a higher prevalence of lactase typically have an earlier decline. People with low lactase activity often do not manifest symptoms of lactose intolerance, such as flatulence, bloating, abdominal pain, nausea, and diarrhea.[15] (See also Chapter 1.) In fact, most people with low lactase activity can tolerate some lactose intake, particularly when it is part of a meal.

Symptoms of lactase intolerance are caused by lactose that escapes digestion in the small intestine and passes into the colon where it is fermented by enteric bacteria, forming organic acids, hydrogen, carbon monoxide, and methane.[16] The gases may cause bloating and pain, and the unabsorbed sugar and acids may cause an increase in osmotic pressure, which may result in osmotic diarrhea. Lactose malabsorption may be detected by an increase in expired breath hydrogen after lactose ingestion.[17] As noted previously, however, the likelihood of developing symptoms depends on the amount of residual lactase activity, the amount of lactose ingested, and the composition of the meal.

Lactase activity also can be diminished secondary to mucosal injury in the small intestine (also termed secondary lactase deficiency). This occurs most commonly in infants with viral gastroenteritis. It is a consequence of damage to the intestinal villi and resolves with resolution of the illness. In the otherwise healthy infant, the lactase deficiency may not be clinically significant. For example, most infants with rotavirus are not lactose intolerant.[18]

However, infants who have had inadequate weight gain or prolonged diarrhea may have clinical lactose intolerance until the illness resolves. Using a lactose-free formula until the infant recovers from diarrhea may be beneficial.[19]

The intolerance usually lasts 1 to 2 weeks except in severe cases. Carbohydrate malabsorption (including that from lactose) is detected by testing the pH of the stool by using nitrazine paper (pH <5.5 indicates carbohydrate fermentation due to malabsorption) and testing for glucose (based on copper reduction) using the same products used to test for glucose in the urine. The glucose derives from the breakdown of lactose by the colonic flora. It is important to test the watery part of the stool, as the formed part of the stool is likely to give a false-negative result. This test can be used to detect the presence of other sugars such as sucrose and starches as the bacteria will degrade some proportion of these sugars to glucose. Detectable carbohydrate malabsorption should be treated to reduce fluid losses due to osmotic diarrhea with the consequent risks of dehydration and acidosis.

Very preterm (<32 weeks) infants may be a special case in which lactose intolerance may be clinically significant. Preterm infants do not digest lactose as well as other sugars such as glucose polymers.[20] Recent studies suggest that the feeding of formula containing lactose as the sole carbohydrate to very preterm infants may be associated with an increased risk of feeding intolerance and that the risk of feeding intolerance is inversely related to lactase activity.[21,22] It has not yet been determined whether this is true for human milk.

Starches

As noted above, starches are the storage carbohydrate of plants consisting of amylose (a linear 1,4-glucan) and amylopectin (a 1,4-glucan with [1–6] branch points). Starches that contain 10 or more sugars linked glycosidically in branched or unbranched chains are arbitrarily termed polysaccharides. The larger the starch, the less osmotically active it is.

Corn syrup is a generic term for products derived from cornstarch by hydrolysis with acid or enzymes. These products are classified according to their chemical-reducing power relative to glucose, which has a dextrose equivalent (DE) of 100%. The DE of corn syrups ranges from less than 20% to more than 95%. A low-DE corn syrup is somewhat hydrolyzed and is, therefore, more like starch than a high-DE corn syrup. Glucose polymers (or maltodextrins) is another term for corn syrup that has been hydrolyzed to (usually) a high-DE carbohydrate. They often are added to formulas to provide additional calories without greatly increasing the osmolality of the feeding. Approximately 20% to 25% of infants in the United States are fed lactose-free soy isolate formulas containing sucrose or corn syrup solids or a combination of both as the carbohydrate source(s).

Modified food starches possess certain technical properties, such as altered viscosity and "mouth feel," freeze-thaw stability, gel clarity, and stability in acid products. Caloric availability of modified food starches is similar to unmodified starches in studies using animals. Modified food starches appear to be safe and reasonably well digested by human infants although concern has been raised about the long-term implications of their feeding.[23,24] Many powdered special formulas and strained foods contain modified corn or tapioca starches. Special formulas may provide approximately 15% of the total calories in the form of modified starch, which is used to facilitate suspension of insoluble nutrients during feeding. The amount of modified starch in a few commercial infant desserts may amount to as much as 45% of the total content of the solids.

Fiber

Fiber is defined as the endogenous components of plant materials in the diet that are resistant to digestion by enzymes produced by humans.[25,26] Fiber is also called bulk or roughage. Fiber is composed predominantly of nonstarch polysaccharides and nonpolysaccharides (mainly lignins). Nonstarch polysaccharides include cellulose and noncellulosic polysaccharides (eg, hemicelluloses, pectins, gums, and mucilages). This definition excludes other substances in the plant materials such as phytates, cutins, saponins, lectins, proteins, waxes, silicon, and other organic constituents. Fibers are present in the cell walls of all plants.

Fiber also is classified as soluble (some hemicelluloses, pectins, gums, and mucilages) or insoluble (most hemicelluloses, celluloses, and lignins). Soluble fiber, found in beans, fruits, psyllium, and oat products, dissolves in water. Soluble fiber is metabolized in the colon, and to a lesser extent in the small intestine, by the enzymatic action of anaerobic bacteria. Soluble fibers have been shown to increase stool size moderately, to slow the rate of intestinal transit, gastric emptying, and glucose absorption, and to decrease serum cholesterol (see following text).[27] Insoluble fiber, found in whole-grain products and vegetables, does not dissolve. It consists of nondigestible polysaccharide and lignins. The intestinal flora does not significantly metabolize insoluble fibers (found in large amounts in bran cereals such as wheat or rice). Insoluble fibers significantly increase fecal bulk, decrease intestinal transit time, delay glucose absorption, and slow down the process of starch hydrolysis.[27]

Crude fiber refers to the residue left after strong acid and base hydrolysis of plant material. This process dissolves pectin, gums, mucilages, and most of the

Table 16.3.
Dietary Fiber and Related Compounds*

Nonstarch polysaccharides
  Celluloses
  Noncelluloses: hemicelluloses, pectins, gums, mucilages
  Nonpolysaccharides: lignins
Classification based on solubility
  Soluble (highly fermented): pectins, gums, mucilages, and some hemicelluloses
  Insoluble (poorly fermented): celluloses, lignins, and most hemicelluloses
Minor components
  Phytates, cutins, saponins, lectins, protein, waxes, silicon
Related components
  Resistant starch and protein
  Lignins

*Adapted from reference 26.

hemicellulose. Thus, crude fiber is mainly a measure of cellulose and lignin and tends to underestimate the total amount of fiber in the food. Most food composition tables give only crude fiber values. Appendix V lists the fiber content of common foods. It has been estimated in adults that 5% to 10% of dietary starch reaches the colon ("resistant starch").[28] Young infants have a limited ability to digest starches such as those in cereal.[29–31] Dietary fiber and related compounds are summarized in Table 16.3.

The current interest in fiber was stimulated in part by the suggestion that fiber could help prevent certain diseases common in the United States such as cancer of the colon, irritable bowel syndrome, constipation, obesity, and coronary heart disease. Epidemiologic studies noted that Africans in rural areas where the fiber intake was high rarely had these diseases. However, as urban migration has increased, the adoption of Western habits and dietary patterns has coincided with the increased incidence of Western diseases. A high-fiber diet increases fecal bulk, produces softer and more frequent stools, and speeds transit through the intestine.

A number of hypotheses have been put forth how increased dietary fiber could reduce the risk of colorectal carcinoma. These include dilution of potential carcinogens, reduced colon contact time with carcinogens because of fiber-induced faster transit, and inhibition of tumor cell lines.[26] Initial review of the data suggested a protective effect in some populations although not in others.[26] Recent studies call into question the efficacy of fiber in preventing recurrence of colorectal cancer.[32]

Increasing fiber intake has been used as a treatment in children with recurrent abdominal pain.[33] In a double-blind study, supplementation with corn fiber was associated with a 50% decrease in the frequency of abdominal pain.[33] Because of its ability to hold water, increasing fiber intake reduces the risk of constipation. It has been estimated that 5 to 7 g/d are needed to facilitate normal stooling in children.[34]

Obesity is less prevalent in populations that consume most carbohydrate as complex carbohydrate and have a high fiber intake. The lower energy density of this type of diet may increase satiety. However, in many cultures in which this type of diet is common, the total energy intake is low by Western standards. Given the increasing prevalence of childhood obesity in the United States, there is interest on the role of fiber in reducing the risk of obesity.[35] There are several explanations for the role of fiber in preventing obesity but none have been unequivocally proven. These include effects on (1) reducing food intake because of earlier satiety achieved with a larger volume in the stomach and intestine but reduced caloric density compared with a high-fat diet as well as slower gastric emptying, (2) reducing absorption of carbohydrate and protein (but not fat) related to faster small intestinal transit, and (3) flattening the insulin response curve to carbohydrate, thereby reducing the appetite stimulating effects of insulin.[35]

Interpretation of the potential relationship between fiber intake and the development of obesity in children is problematic because of a lack of data and limitations on the interpretation of the available data. For example, fiber and carbohydrate intake in one study were not separated from one another.[35] There is some preliminary evidence that fiber supplementation may aid in weight reduction for children with obesity.[35,36] Clearly, more work is needed in this area.

Atherosclerosis has its origins in childhood. Fatty streaks begin in the coronary arteries at about the age of 10 years and in the abdominal aorta at 2 years.[37,38] Given that studies suggest a direct correlation between the percent of calories from saturated fat and cholesterol in the children's diets and their blood cholesterol levels, the potential effects of fiber on reducing blood lipids and thereby the risk of heart disease are of great interest.[37]

The lipid-lowering effect is seen with soluble fiber but not with the insoluble form (see Table 16.3). A review of the current data strongly suggests that the addition of soluble fiber to a Step 1 lipid-lowering diet can reduce further certain fractions of blood lipids and/or increase serum high-density lipoprotein (HDL).[37] The degree of reduction, the fraction of lipid that is reduced, and the effect on serum HDL may depend on the type of soluble fiber used. Supplementation with psyllium appeared to decrease serum LDL and increase HDL in 48 children aged 2 to 11 years with moderate hypercholesterolemia.[37,39]

Objections have been made to an increased fiber intake for children. One of the concerns has been that fiber may compromise intake of other nutrients. In young infants, it has been shown that addition of cereal in the amounts used to treat gastroesophageal reflux decreases total daily formula.[40] On the other hand, the addition of a soy polysaccharide to infant formula does not appear to affect intake in infants with diarrhea.[40]

Another concern is that fiber supplementation will affect the absorption of nutrients, particularly micronutrients. Some plant foods contain phytate (inositol hexaphosphate), which serves as the storage form of phosphorus for plants and may form insoluble compounds with minerals, such as calcium, iron, copper, magnesium, and zinc, rendering them unavailable for normal absorption and metabolism.[41] Although phytate is destroyed in the process of leavening in the making of bread, it remains intact in many foods, such as legumes and grains. Consumption of primarily plant-based diets is considered to be a major etiologic factor for mineral deficiencies on a global basis.

Although it is possible that children on high-fiber diets may have a deficiency of these minerals, especially in situations in which mineral intake is low, children in the United States on a varied complete dietary regimen are unlikely to have mineral deficiencies, irrespective of fiber intake.[41] Some foods, such as spinach, rhubarb, and chards, also contain oxalic acid, which interferes with absorption of iron and calcium, especially in individuals on high-fiber diets.[41] A review of the data suggests that addition of fiber to an otherwise normal omnivorous diet for a child in the United States does not adversely affect micronutrient status including that of iron.[41] This has recently been confirmed by a study in adolescents using dietary recall to evaluate fiber intake.[42]

It has been recommended that, during age 6 to 12 months, whole cereals, green vegetables, and legumes are introduced gradually increasing to 5 g/d by the first year.[43] With the introduction of solid foods into the diet of the older child, whole-grain cereals, breads, fruits, and vegetables should be included. Recommendations for providing increased fiber to children are given in Appendix V.

The American Health Foundation has set forth a suggested guideline for the recommended amount of fiber in a child's diet.[44] The recommendation suggested that children older than 2 years take in an amount of fiber approximately equivalent to the child's age plus 5 g/d. A safe range was believed to be up to age plus 10 g/d.[44] This "age plus 5" guideline results in a gradual increase of fiber intake over time, with 17-year-olds eating 22 g/d. The amount recommended for an older adolescent is also within the range recommended by the National Cancer Institute.[41] These recommendations were endorsed by a conference that was held on dietary fiber in childhood.[45] However, a diet that emphasizes high-fiber, low-calorie foods to the exclusion of the other common food groups is not recommended for children.

References

1. Weaver LT, Laker MF, Nelson R. Neonatal intestinal lactase activity. *Arch Dis Child.* 1986;61:896–899
2. Antonowicz I, Chang SK, Grand RJ. Development and distribution of lysosomal enzymes and disaccharidases in human fetal intestine. *Gastroenterology.* 1974; 67:51–58
3. Hadorn B, Zoppi G, Shmerling DH, Prader A, McIntyre I, Anderson CM. Quantitative assessment of exocrine pancreatic function in infants and children. *J Pediatr.* 1968;73:39–50
4. Raul F, Lacroix B, Aprahamian M. Longitudinal distribution of brush border hydrolases and morphological maturation in the intestine of the preterm infant. *Early Hum Dev.* 1986;13:225–234
5. Shulman RJ, Kerzner B, Sloan HR, et al. Absorption and oxidation of glucose polymers of different lengths in young infants. *Pediatr Res.* 1986;20:740–743
6. Eggermont E. The hydrolysis of naturally occurring alpha glucosides by the human intestinal mucosa. *Eur J Biochem.* 1969;9:483–487
7. Ferraris RP, Diamond J. Regulation of intestinal sugar transport. *Physiol Rev.* 1997; 77:257–302
8. Cummings JH, Macfarlane GT. Colonic microflora: nutrition and health. *Nutrition.* 1997;13:476–478
9. Kalhan SC, Kilic I. Carbohydrate as nutrient in the infant and child: range of acceptable intake. *Eur J Clin Nutr.* 1999;53:S94–S100
10. Kalhan S, Parimi P. Gluconeogenesis in the fetus and neonate. *Semin Perinatol.* 2000;24:94–106
11. Halliday D, Bodamer OA. Measurement of glucose turnover—implications for the study of inborn errors of metabolism. *Eur J Pediatr.* 1997;156:S35–S38
12. Freeze HH. Disorders in protein glycosylation and potential therapy: tip of an iceberg? *J Pediatr.* 1998;133:593–600

13. American Academy of Pediatrics, Committee on Nutrition. Practical significance of lactose intolerance in children: supplement. *Pediatrics.* 1990;86:643–644
14. Sahi T. Genetics and epidemiology of adult-type hypolactasia. *Scand J Gastroenterol Suppl.* 1994;202:7–20
15. Carroccio A, Montalto G, Cavera G, Notarbatolo. A Lactose intolerance and self-reported milk intolerance: relationship with lactose maldigestion and nutrient intake. Lactase Deficiency Study Group. *J Am Coll Nutr.* 1998;17:631–636
16. American Academy of Pediatrics, Committee on Nutrition. The practical significance of lactose intolerance in children. *Pediatrics.* 1978;62:240–245
17. Strocchi A, Corazza G, Ellis CJ, Gasbarrini G, Levitt MD. Detection of malabsorption of low doses of carbohydrate: accuracy of various breath H2 criteria. *Gastroenterology.* 1993;105:1404–1410
18. Rings EH, Grand RJ, Buller HA. Lactose intolerance and lactase deficiency in children. *Curr Opin Pediatr.* 1994;6:562–567
19. Caballero B, Solomons NW. Lactose-reduced formulas for the treatment of persistent diarrhea. *Pediatrics.* 1990;86:645–646
20. Shulman RJ, Feste A, Ou C. Absorption of lactose, glucose polymers, or combination in premature infants. *J Pediatr.* 1995;127:626–631
21. Griffin MP, Hansen JW. Can the elimination of lactose from formula improve feeding tolerance in premature infants? *J Pediatr.* 1999;135:587–592
22. Shulman RJ, Schanler RJ, Lau C, Heitkemper M, Ou CN, Smith EO. Early feeding, feeding tolerance, and lactase activity in preterm infants. *J Pediatr.* 1998;133: 645–649
23. Filer LJ Jr. Modified food starch—an update. *J Am Diet Assoc.* 1988;88:342–344
24. Lanciers S, Mehta DI, Blecker U, Lebenthal E. Modified food starches in baby foods. *Indian J Pediatr.* 1998;65:541–546
25. Asp NG. Definition and analysis of dietary fibre. *Scand J Gastroenterol Suppl.* 1987;129:16–20
26. AGA Technical Review: Impact of Dietary Fiber on Colon Cancer Occurrence. *Gastroenterology.* 2000;118:1235–1257
27. Southgate DAT. Dietary fibre and the diseases of affluence. In: Dobbins J, ed. *A Balanced Diet?* London, England. Springer-Verlag; 1988:117–141
28. Stephen AM, Haddad AC, Phillips SF. Passage of carbohydrate into the colon: direct measurements in humans. *Gastroenterology.* 1983;85:589–595
29. Shulman RJ, Wong WW, Irving CS, Nichols BL, Klein PD. Utilization of dietary cereal by young infants. *J Pediatr.* 1983;103:23–28
30. Shulman RJ, Boutton TW, Klein PD. Impact of dietary cereal on nutrient absorption and fecal nitrogen loss in formula-fed infants. *J Pediatr.* 1991;118:39–43
31. Shulman RJ, Gannon N, Reeds PJ. Cereal feeding and its impact on the nitrogen economy of the infant. *Am J Clin Nutr.* 1995;62:969–972
32. Alberts DS, Martinez ME, Roe DJ, et al. Lack of effect of a high-fiber cereal supplement on the recurrence of colorectal adenomas. Phoenix Colon Cancer Prevention Physicians' Network. *N Engl J Med.* 2000;342:1156–1162

33. Feldman W, McGrath P, Hodgson C, Ritter H, Shipman RT. The use of dietary fiber in the management of simple, childhood, idiopathic, recurrent abdominal pain. Results in a prospective, double-blind, randomized, controlled trial. *Am J Dis Child.* 1985;139:1216–1218

34. Anderson JW, Smith BM, Gustafson NJ. Health benefits and practical aspects of high fiber diets. *Am J Clin Nutr.* 1994;59:1242S–1247S

35. Kimm SY. The role of dietary fiber in the development and treatment of childhood obesity. *Pediatrics.* 1995;96:1010–1014

36. Gropper SS, Acosta PB. The therapeutic effect of fiber in treating obesity. *J Am Coll Nutr.* 1987;6:533–535

37. Kwiterovich PO Jr. The role of fiber in the treatment of hypercholesterolemia in children and adolescents. *Pediatrics.* 1995;96:1005–1009

38. Strong JP, McGill HC Jr. The natural history of coronary atherosclerosis. *Am J Pathol.* 1969;9:251–266

39. Williams CL, Spark A, Haley N, Axelrad C, Strobino B. Effectiveness of a psyllium-enriched step I diet in hypercholesterolemic children. *Circulation.* 1991;84:II-6

40. Vanderhoof JA, Murray ND, Paule CL, Ostrom KM. Use of soy fiber in acute diarrhea in infants and toddlers. *Clin Pediatr (Phila).* 1997;36:135–139

41. Williams CL, Bollella M. Is a high-fiber diet safe for children? *Pediatrics.* 1995;96:1014–1019

42. Nickels TA, Myers L, O'Neil C, Gustafson N. Impact of dietary fat and fiber intake on nutrient intake of adolescents. *Pediatrics.* 2000;105:E21

43. Agostoni C, Riva E, Giovannini M. Dietary fiber in weaning foods of young children. *Pediatrics.* 1995;96:1002–1005

44. Williams CL, Bollella M, Wynder EL. A new recommendation for dietary fiber in childhood. *Pediatrics.* 1995;96:985–988

45. American Academy of Pediatrics. A summary of conference recommendations on dietary fiber in childhood. Conference on Dietary Fiber in Childhood, New York, May 24, 1994. *Pediatrics.* 1995;96:1023–1028

17

Fats and Fatty Acids

General Considerations

The absolute fat requirement of the human species is the amount of essential fatty acids needed to maintain optimal fatty acid composition of all tissues and normal eicosanoid (prostaglandins, prostacyclins) synthesis. At most, this requirement is no more than about 5% of an adequate energy intake. However, fat accounts for approximately 50% of the nonprotein energy content of both human milk and currently available infant formulas. This is thought to be necessary to ensure that total energy intake is adequate to support growth and optimal utilization of dietary protein. In theory, the energy supplied by fat could be supplied by carbohydrate from which all fatty acids except the essential ones can be synthesized, but, in practice, it is difficult to ensure an adequate energy intake without a fat intake considerably in excess of the requirement for essential fatty acids. In part, this is because the osmolality of such a diet containing simple carbohydrates (eg, mono and disaccharides) will be sufficiently high to produce diarrhea and such a diet containing more complex carbohydrates may not be fully digestible, particularly during early infancy. Moreover, metabolic efficiency is greater if nonprotein energy is provided as a mixture of fat and carbohydrate rather than predominately carbohydrate. This is because approximately 25% of the energy content of carbohydrate that is converted to fatty acids is consumed in the process of lipogenesis. Fat also facilitates the absorption, transport, and delivery of fat-soluble vitamins and, in addition, is an important satiety factor. Considering these issues, participants in a recent workshop concluded that the lower limit of fat intake that can be recommended is at least 15% of total energy intake but that a more practical recommendation is in the range of 30% of energy intake.[1] These issues are important in consideration of the age at which a prudent (ie, lower fat) diet to reduce the risks of cardiovascular disease is recommended (see Chapter 45).

Dietary Fats

Triglycerides account for the largest proportion of dietary fat. Structurally, these have 3 fatty acid molecules esterified to a molecule of glycerol. They usually contain at least 2, often 3, different fatty acids. Other dietary fats include phospholipids, free fatty acids, monoglycerides, and diglycerides, as well as sterols and other non-saponifiable compounds. Together, these account for less than 2% of most dietary fats, including the fat of human milk and infant formulas.

Naturally occurring fatty acids generally contain from 4 to 26 carbon atoms. Some of these are saturated (ie, no double bonds in the carbon chain), some are monounsaturated (ie, 1 double bond) and some are polyunsaturated (ie, 2 or more double bonds). All have common names but, by general convention, are identified by their number of carbon atoms, their number of double bonds, and the site of the first double bond from the terminal methyl group of the molecule. For example, palmitic acid, a saturated, 16-carbon fatty acid, is designated 16:0. Similarly, oleic acid, an 18-carbon, monounsaturated fatty acid with the single double bond located between the ninth and tenth carbon from the methyl terminal, is designated 18:1ω9. Linoleic acid is designated 18:2ω6, indicating that it is an 18-carbon fatty acid with 2 double bonds, the first between the sixth and seventh carbon from the methyl terminal. The common names as well as the shorthand numerical designations of a number of common fatty acids are shown in Table 17.1.

Table 17.1.
Common Names and Numerical Nomenclature of Selected Fatty Acids

Common Name	Numerical Nomenclature
Caprylic Acid	8:0
Capric Acid	10:0
Lauric Acid	12:0
Myristic Acid	14:0
Palmitic Acid	16:0
Stearic Acid	18:0
Oleic Acid	18:1ω9*
Linoleic Acid	18:2ω6*
Arachidonic Acid	20:4ω6
Linolenic Acid[†]	18:3ω3*
Eicosapentaenoic Acid	20:5ω3
Docosahexaenoic Acid	22:6ω3

*ω9, ω6, and ω3 are used interchangeably with n-9, n-6, and n-3.
[†]Usually designated α-linolenic acid to distinguish it from 18:3ω6 or γ-linolenic acid.

Unsaturated fatty acids are folded at the site of each double bond; in this configuration they are said to be in the *cis* form. During processing, the molecules may become unfolded transforming them to *trans*-fatty acids, which have been implicated as a factor in development of atherosclerosis. In general, the amount of trans-fatty acids in infant formulas and foods is low; however, some processed foods (eg, margarines) may have a higher content. The trans-fatty acid content of human milk also is reasonably low unless the mother's diet is high in trans-fatty acids.

Fat Digestion, Absorption, Transport, and Metabolism

At birth, the infant must adjust from using carbohydrate as the major energy source to using a mixture of carbohydrate and fat. Hence, some aspects of fat digestion and metabolism are not fully developed, even at term. However, most term infants have sufficient fat digestive capacity to adjust satisfactorily. The limitations of fat digestion are somewhat more serious in the preterm infant but there is little evidence that these infants have significant limitations beyond the first few weeks of life.

Fat digestion begins in the stomach where lingual lipase hydrolyzes short- and medium-chain fatty acids from triglycerides and gastric lipase hydrolyzes long- as well as medium- and short-chain fatty acids.[2] The intragastric release of fatty acids with formation of monoglycerides delays gastric emptying and also facilitates emulsification of fat in the intestine. Further, some of the released short- and medium-chain fatty acids can be absorbed directly from the stomach.[3] Upon entry into the duodenum, the monoglycerides and free fatty acids stimulate release of a number of enteric hormones; among these is cholecystokinin, which stimulates contraction of the gall bladder and secretion of pancreatic enzymes.[4] Lingual and gastric lipases are largely inactivated in the duodenum and fat digestion continues through the action of pancreatic lipase and colipase that may be somewhat limited during the first several weeks of life. Like lingual and gastric lipase, pancreatic lipase hydrolyzes triglycerides into free fatty acids and a monoglyceride.

Human milk contains 2 additional lipases—lipoprotein lipase and bile salt-stimulated lipase. The former is essential for formation of milk lipid in the mammary gland but plays little role in intestinal fat digestion.[5] The latter is present in much larger amounts. It is stable at a pH as low as 3.5 if bile salts are present and it is not affected by intestinal proteolytic enzymes.[6] However, it is heat labile and, hence, is inactivated by pasteurization. Bile salt-stimulated lipase hydrolyzes triglyceride molecules into free fatty acids and glycerol rather than into free fatty acids and a monoglyceride. In theory, the bile salt-stimulated lipase of human milk can substitute for limited pancreatic lipase[7]; however, this does not appear to be of great importance to fat digestion of most infants. On the other hand, since bile salt-stimulated lipase is much more effective than pancreatic lipase in hydrolyzing esters of vitamin A, the primary form of this vitamin in human milk and most other foods, it may be important for optimal vitamin A absorption.[6]

The bile acids released by contraction of the gall bladder help emulsify the intestinal contents, thereby facilitating triglyceride hydrolysis and fat absorption. They are released primarily as salts of taurine or glycine and, hence, have both a water-soluble and a lipid-soluble portion. Alone, bile salts are poor emulsifiers, but, in combination with monoglycerides, fatty acids, and phospholipids, they are quite effective. Thus, the fat hydrolysis that occurs in the stomach is an important adjunct to intestinal fat digestion.

The rate of synthesis of bile salts by newborn infants is less than that of adults and the bile salt pool of newborns is only about one fourth that of adults.[8] However, an intraduodenal concentration of bile salts below 2 to 5 mM, the critical concentration required for the formation of micelles, is unusual.[9] Bile salts are actively reabsorbed in the distal ilium, transported back to the liver and eventually reappear in bile.[10] This entrohepatic circulation occurs approximately 6 times daily with loss of only about 5% of the bile salts with each circulation.[11]

The monoglycerides and diglycerides and long-chain fatty acids resulting from lipolysis as well as phospholipids, cholesterol, and fat-soluble vitamins are insoluble in water but are solubilized by physicochemical combination with bile salts to form micelles.[11] Because of their amphiphilic nature, bile salts aggregate with their hydrophobic region to the interior, or core, of the micelle and their hydrophilic region to the exterior. The components of the micelle are transferred into the enteric mucosal cell where long-chain fatty acids and monoglycerides are re-esterified into triglycerides and subsequently combined with protein, phospholipid, and cholesterol to form chylomicrons or very low-density lipoproteins. In this form, they enter the intestinal lymphatics, then the thoracic duct and, finally, the peripheral circulation.

Medium-chain triglycerides can be absorbed into the enteric cells without being hydrolyzed.[11] However, they also are rapidly hydrolyzed in the duodenum and, since the released medium-chain fatty acids are relatively soluble in the aqueous phase of the intestinal lumen, they can be absorbed without being incorporated into micelles. This makes them particularly useful in treatment of infants and children with a variety of pancreatic, hepatic, biliary, and/or intestinal disorders.

In general, long-chain unsaturated fatty acids are absorbed more readily than long-chain saturated fatty acids. The ease of absorption of palmitic acid (16:0) is further related to its position in the triglyceride molecule.[12] The 2-monoglyceride of palmitic acid is well absorbed, but free palmitic acid released from the terminal positions of the triglyceride molecule is not. The palmitic acid content of human milk is esterified primarily to the 2-position of glycerol, which probably accounts for its better absorption from human milk than from formulas containing butterfat.[13-15] Synthetic fats that contain palmitic acid primarily in the 2-position are available,[16] but, as yet, have not been used extensively in infant formula.

In the circulation, chylomicrons acquire a specialized apoprotein from high-density lipoproteins.[11] This enables the triglycerides of the chylomicron to be hydrolyzed by lipoprotein lipase, the major enzyme responsible for intravascular hydrolysis of chylomicrons and very low-density lipoproteins.[17] Lipoprotein lipase is synthesized in most tissues and the flow of fatty acids to tissues reflects its activity on the tissue's capillary bed. Levels of lipoprotein lipase are somewhat low in preterm and small-for-gestational-age infants,[18] but this does not appear to impose major difficulties except, perhaps, intolerance of intravenously administered lipid emulsions.

The phospholipid and most of the apoproteins remaining after hydrolysis of chylomicron triglyceride are transferred to high-density lipoprotein and the remainder of the apoproteins are transferred to other lipoprotein particles. This reduces the chylomicron to a fraction of its original mass, resulting in a chylomicron remnant that is removed from the circulation by specialized hepatic receptors.

Essential Fatty Acids

Fatty acids with double bonds in the ω6 and ω3 positions cannot be synthesized endogenously by the human species.[19] Therefore, specific ω3 and ω6 fatty acids or their precursors with double bonds at these positions, (ie, linoleic acid [LA; 18:2ω6] and α-linolenic acid [ALA; 18:3ω3]) must be provided in the diet. The precursor fatty acids are metabolized by the same series of desaturases and elongases to longer-chain, more unsaturated fatty acids,[20] referred to col-

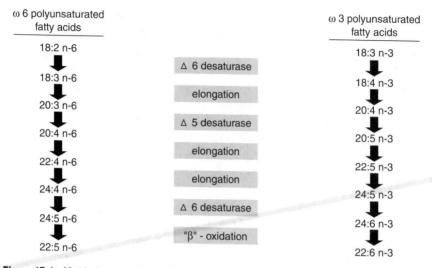

Figure 17.1. Metabolism of ω6 and ω3 Fatty Acids

lectively as long-chain polyunsaturated fatty acids (LC-PUFAs). This pathway is outlined in Figure 17.1. Important metabolites of 18:2ω6 and 18:3ω3 include 18:3ω6 (ω linolenic acid [GLA]), 20:3ω6 (dihomogamma linolenic acid [DHLA]), 20:4ω6 (arachidonic acid [AA]), 20:5ω3 (eicosapentaenoic acid [EPA]), and 22:6ω3 (docosahexaenoic acid [DHA]).

Linoleic acid and ALA are present in many vegetable oils (see Table 17.2). In vivo, they are found in storage lipids, cell membrane phospholipids, intracellular cholesterol esters and plasma lipids. The longer-chain, more unsaturated fatty acids synthesized from these precursors, in contrast, are found primarily in specific cell membrane phospholipids. Dihomogamma linolenic acid, AA, and EPA are immediate precursors of eicosanoids,[19,21] each being converted to a different series with different biological activities and/or functions.

The same series of desaturases and elongases that catalyse desaturation and elongation of ω6 and ω3 fatty acids also catalyse desaturation and elongation of ω9 fatty acids. The substrate preference of these enzymes is ω3, ω6, and, finally, ω9.[20] Thus, competition between the ω9 fatty acids and either the ω6 or ω3 fatty acids is rarely an issue but if the concentrations of LA and/or ALA are low, as occurs in deficiency states, oleic acid (18:1ω9) is readily desaturated and elongated to eicosatrienoic acid (20:3ω9). The ratio of this fatty acid to 20:4ω6 (ie, the triene-tetraene ratio) is a useful diagnostic index of ω6 fatty acid deficiency.

Table 17.2.
Fatty Acid Composition of Common Vegetable Oils*

Fatty Acid	Canola	Corn	Coconut	Palm Olein	Safflower†	Soy	High Oleic Sunflower
6:0–12:0	–	0.1	62.1	0.2	–	–	–
14.0	–	0.1	18.1	1.0	0.1	0.1	–
16:0	4.0	12.1	8.9	39.8	6.8	11.2	3.7
18:0	2.0	2.4	2.7	4.4	2.4	0.4	5.4
18:1	55.0	32.1	6.4	42.5	12.5	22.0	81.3
18:2	26.0	50.9	1.6	11.2	76.8	53.8	9.0
18:3	10.0	0.9	–	0.2	0.1	7.5	–
Other	2.0	1.0	–	<1.6	<1.0	<1.0	<1.0

* Percent of total fatty acids (g/100 g).
† High oleic safflower oil: ~77% 18:1 and 12.5% 18:2.

This ratio usually is <0.1. A ratio of >0.4 is usually cited as indicative of deficiency,[22] but an even lower value (eg, >0.2) might be more reasonable. In the few documented cases of isolated 18:3ω3 deficiency in which it was measured (see following text), the triene-tetraene ratio was not elevated.

Linoleic acid (18:2 ω6) has been recognized as an essential nutrient for the human species for almost 75 years.[23,24] The most common symptoms of deficiency are poor growth and scaly skin lesions. These are usually preceded by an increase in the triene-tetraene ratio of plasma lipids. It is now clear that ALA (18:3ω3) also is an essential nutrient. In animals, deficiency of this fatty acid results in visual and neurologic abnormalities.[25–28] Neurologic abnormalities also were observed in a human infant who had been maintained for several weeks on a parenteral nutrition regimen lacking ALA,[29] and in elderly nursing home residents who were receiving intragastric feedings of an elemental formula with no ALA.[30]

Although symptoms related to deficiency of the 2 series of fatty acids seem to differ, many studies on which the description of ω6 fatty acid deficiency are based employed a fat-free or very low-fat diet rather than a diet deficient in only 18:2ω6. Thus, there may be some overlap in the symptoms of LA and ALA deficiency. Linoleic acid or AA can correct the clinical symptoms of ω6 fatty acid deficiency; ALA, EPA, or DHA can correct those related to ALA deficiency. Thus, it is not clear whether LA and ALA serve specific functions other than as precursors of LC-PUFA.

Linoleic acid usually comprises between 8% and 20% of the total fatty acid content of human milk and ALA usually comprises between 0.5% and 1%.[31] Human milk also contains small amounts of a number of longer-chain, more unsaturated metabolites of both fatty acids, primarily AA ($20:4\omega6$) and DHA ($22:6\omega3$). Maternal diet has a marked impact on the concentration of all fatty acids in human milk. The concentration of DHA in the milk of women consuming a typical North American diet is generally in the range of 0.1% to 0.3% of total fatty acids and the level of AA ranges from 0.4% to 0.6%.[31] The milk of vegetarian women contains less DHA[32] and that of women whose dietary fish consumption is high or who take DHA supplements is higher.[33-35] The AA content of human milk is less variable and appears to be less dependent on maternal AA intake, perhaps reflecting the relatively high LA intake of most populations.

Corn, coconut, safflower, and soy oils as well as high-oleic safflower and sunflower oils and palm olein oil are commonly used in the manufacture of infant formulas (see Table 17.2). All except coconut oil contain adequate amounts of LA, but only soybean oil contains an appreciable amount of ALA (6% to 9% of total fatty acids). Canola oil, a component of many formulas available outside the United States, contains somewhat less LA and more ALA. Until recently, little emphasis was placed on the ALA content of infant formulas and many with virtually no ALA were available as recently as a decade ago. Current recommendations specify minimal intakes of LA ranging from 2.7% to 8% of total fat and maximum intakes ranging from 21% to 35% of total fatty acids.[36,37] The most recent recommendations for the minimum and maximum contents of ALA in term infant formulas are 1.75% and 4% of total fatty acids, respectively.[37] To maintain a reasonable balance between the 2 fatty acids, it is recommended that the LA-ALA ratio be between 5:6 and 15:16.[36,37] The term and preterm infant formulas currently available in the United States contain approximately 20% of total fatty acids as LA and approximately 2% as ALA; hence, their LA-ALA ratios are ~10.

Long-Chain Polyunsaturated Fatty Acids

Long-chain polyunsaturated fatty acids are fatty acids with a chain length of more than 18 carbons and 2 or more double bonds. Those of primary interest for infant nutrition are AA and DHA, the plasma and erythrocyte lipid contents of which are higher in breastfed than formula-fed infants.[38-41] Since human milk contains these fatty acids but formulas do not, the lower content of these fatty acids in plasma lipids of formula-fed infants has been interpreted to indicate that the infant cannot synthesize enough of these fatty acids to meet ongoing needs. Concurrent observations of better cognitive function of breastfed versus formula-fed infants[42–45] focused attention on the possibility that the lower cognitive function of formula-fed infants might be related to inadequate LC-PUFA intake.

This possibility is supported by the facts that AA and DHA are the major ω6 and ω3 fatty acids of neural tissues[46–48] and DHA is a major component of retinal photoreceptor membranes.[48] Further, the major supply of these fatty acids to the fetus during development is from maternal plasma.[49,50] Thus, the need for these fatty acids by the preterm infant who is born during the third trimester of pregnancy and, therefore, receives a limited supply of LC-PUFA prior to birth is thought to be greater than that of the term infant. However, the rates of accumulation of these fatty acids in the developing central nervous system change minimally between mid-gestation and 1 year of age.[48]

Based on postmortem studies,[51–53] the cerebral content of DHA, but not AA, is minimally but significantly lower in formula-fed term infants. However, the DHA content of the retina does not differ between breastfed and formula-fed infants,[53] perhaps because the content of this fatty acid in retina reaches adult levels at approximately term, whereas adult levels in cerebrum are not reached until much later.[48] In one of the postmortem studies, the cerebral DHA content of formula-fed infants reflected the ALA content of the formula that the infant received before death.[52] This is consistent with data showing that ALA intakes less than 0.7% of total energy result in low brain levels of DHA in piglets[54] and studies in infants showing a positive relationship between ALA intake and rates of DHA synthesis.[55]

Both term and preterm infants can convert LA to AA, and ALA to DHA.[55–60] This was established by studies in which the precursor fatty acids labeled with stable isotopes of either carbon (^{13}C) or hydrogen (^{2}H) were administered to the infant and blood levels of the labeled fatty acids as well as labeled metabolites of each were measured by gas chromatography/mass spectroscopy (see Figure 17.1). The studies of Sauerwald et al[55,59] and Uauy et al[60] suggest that the overall ability of preterm infants to convert LA and ALA to LC-PUFA is at least as good as that of term infants. On the other hand, there is considerable variability in conversion among both preterm and term infants fed the same formula. Moreover, since measurements of enrichment have been limited to plasma, which represents only a small fraction of the body pool of both the precursor and product fatty acids and may not be representative of fatty acid pools of other tissues, the amount of LC-PUFA that either preterm or term infants can synthesize is not known.

The higher DHA content of plasma lipids of breastfed infants and infants fed formulas supplemented with LC-PUFA versus infants fed unsupplemented formulas, including those with a relatively high ALA content[38–41,61–63] suggests that the amounts of LC-PUFA formed endogenously are less than the amounts provided by human milk or supplemented formulas. However, the extent to which the concentration of individual LC-PUFA in plasma reflects the content of these fatty acids in tissues, particularly the brain, is not known.

In this regard, animal studies show that the content of LC-PUFA in plasma is much less highly correlated with the content of these fatty acids in brain than with the content in erythrocytes and liver.[64] In contrast, the postmortem studies in human infants show a statistically significant correlation between the plasma and brain contents of DHA.[53] However, this correlation is reasonably weak and the correlation between the content of this fatty acid in plasma and the contents of other tissues was not reported. Studies in isolated cell systems have shown that precursors of DHA are transferred from plasma to astrocytes where they are converted to DHA, which is subsequently transferred to neurons.[65,66] Whether this pathway for direct synthesis of DHA within the central nervous system occurs in vivo is not known.

Although not definitive, the studies discussed support the possibility that failure to provide preformed LC-PUFA during early infancy, and perhaps longer, may compromise visual and central nervous system development. Thus, a number of studies have been conducted over the past decade to determine if there are differences in visual acuity and neurodevelopmental indices between breastfed and formula-fed infants as well as between infants fed LC-PUFA-supplemented formulas and unsupplemented formulas. Since human milk contains a number of factors other than LC-PUFA that might result in better visual acuity or neurodevelopmental indices, studies of breastfed versus formula-fed infants are difficult to interpret. Hence, the discussions that follow are based solely on studies of infants fed supplemented versus unsupplemented formulas.

LC-PUFA Intake and Visual Function. Early studies in rodents established the importance of ω3 fatty acids for normal retinal function[25,28] and subsequent studies confirmed this for primates.[26,27] More recently, studies have focused on the effect of ω3 fatty acids on retinal function and/or overall visual function of human infants. A difference in focus of the animal versus the human studies is that the abnormal retinal/visual function of ω3 fatty acid-deficient animals clearly was produced by an inadequate intake of ALA, whereas studies in infants have focused primarily on the effects of DHA intake on retinal and/or visual function. These studies have been conducted in both term and preterm infants and have used both behavior- and electrophysiologic-based methods for assessing visual function.

Meta-analyses of data from all studies in term as well as preterm infants have been reported.[67,68] The meta-analysis of data from randomized studies in term infants using behavior-based tests of visual acuity showed an advantage of DHA-supplemented versus unsupplemented formula of 0.32 ± 0.09 octaves at 2 months of age but no advantage at other ages. Meta-analysis of data from studies using electrophysiologic-based tests showed no statistically significant advantages of supplementation at any age. A recently reported study,[69] which was not included in the meta-analysis, showed no advantages of DHA (0.14% of total fatty acids) plus AA (0.46% of total fatty acids) supplementation on visual function as assessed by the Teller Acuity Card procedure, visual evoked potentials and electroretinograms at 2, 4, 6, or 12 months of age. Whether inclusion of these additional data in the meta-analysis will change the conclusions is not clear.

The meta-analysis of data from randomized studies in preterm infants showed an advantage of DHA-supplemented versus unsupplemented formulas on both behavior-based and electrophysiologic-based measurements of visual acuity.[68] With behavior-based tests, DHA-supplemented formula resulted in an advantage of 0.47 ± 0.14 octaves at 2 months of age and an advantage of 0.28 ± 0.08 octaves at 4 months of age, but no advantage at other ages. With electrophysiologic-based measurements, there was an advantage of DHA supplementation of 0.83 ± 0.20 octaves at 4 months of age but not at other ages. The most recent randomized controlled trial in preterm infants[70] showed no advantage of AA and DHA supplementation (0.42% and 0.26% of total fatty acids, respectively, from birth to term and then 0.42% and 0.16%, respectively, through the first year of life) on visual acuity as assessed by acuity cards at 2, 4, or 6 months of age, but an advantage of supplementation on acuity as assessed by swept parameter visual-evoked potentials in a subgroup of infants at 6- but not at 4-months post-term. Inclusion of these new data in the meta-analysis is unlikely to change the overall conclusions.

LC-PUFA Intake and Cognitive/Behavioral Development. Arachidonic acid and DHA, the predominant ω6 and ω3 fatty acids of the central nervous system, are present primarily in non-myelin membranes such as cortical synaptic terminals.[19] Accretion occurs during the brain growth spurt from the beginning of the third trimester of gestation until approximately 2 years of age.[46–48] Because of this and the possibility that endogenous synthesis of AA and DHA may not be sufficient to provide the amounts needed for normal rates of brain accretion, there has been considerable interest in the importance of AA and DHA intake for normal cognitive/behavioral development.

Studies addressing the cognitive/behavioral development of infants fed DHA-supplemented versus unsupplemented formulas have used both the Bayley Scales of Infant Development and the Fagan Test of Infant Intelligence (FTII). The Bayley Scales provide indices of both mental (MDI) and psychomotor development (PDI). They have been used for years and are considered the "gold standard" for assessing global abilities of infants from birth to approximately 3 years of age. However, the relationship between either the MDI or the PDI and later cognitive and/or psychomotor function is poor, particularly for "normal" or low-risk infants.[71] The FTII assesses novelty preference.[72] In this test, the infant is shown a single stimulus (usually a face) for a standardized period of time based on age followed by this stimulus plus a novel one. If the infant has "learned" the original stimulus prior to the novelty test, the typical response is to look selectively toward the novel versus the "familiar" image. Scores on this test during infancy are somewhat more predictive of later cognitive function than the Bayley MDI; however, the internal consistency (reproducibility) of the test is relatively poor.[73] Look duration during the familiarization and the paired comparison phases of the test also has been shown to be a modest predictor of both concurrent performance on tasks and later intelligence[73]; shorter look durations during the familiarization phase predict better concurrent as well as later cognitive performance.

One or both of these tests has been used in studies of LC-PUFA supplementation of both term and preterm infants. Some of these have shown advantages of LC-PUFA supplementation and some have not. The studies in term infants were reviewed by the Life Sciences Research Organization (LSRO) Expert Panel on Assessment of Nutrient Requirements for Term Infant Formulas.[37] As a group, they were criticized by consultants to the Panel for including too few infants, failing to control adequately for confounding factors, failing to assess function at multiple times, failing to examine individual differences in development, and failing to follow the infants for a sufficiently long period. For example, none of the studies cited in the report included data beyond 1 year of age.

Four recently published randomized trials in term infants[69,74-76] illustrate some of the difficulties of assessing the impact of LC-PUFA supplementation on infant development. One of these[74] compared a formula supplemented with both AA and DHA (0.3% and 0.32% of total fatty acids, respectively, from purified egg yolk phospholipid and triglyceride fractions) and an unsupplemented formula, both fed for the first 6 months of life. The mean Bayley MDIs of the supplemented group (n=125), the control group (n=125) and a breastfed reference group (n=104) were 95.5 ± 1.2 (SE), 94.5 ± 1.2 and 96.0 ± 1.0, respectively, at 18 months of age. Mean Bayley PDIs of the 3 groups, respectively, were 96.4 ± 0.9, 95 ± 0.8, and 94.4 ± 1.20. There obviously were no statistically significant differences among groups.

Another of these studies[75] included a breastfed reference group (n=46) as well as groups fed a control formula (no LC-PUFA, n=21), a formula supplemented with only DHA (0.35% of total fatty acids as tuna oil; n=23), and a formula supplemented with both DHA and AA (0.34% of total fatty acids as each from egg yolk phospholipid; n=24). The formulas were fed through 12 months of age, at which time neither the MDI nor the PDI differed among groups. Scores of the 3 formula groups also did not differ at 24 months of age.

Yet another recently published study[76] included 3 formula-fed groups, all fed the assigned formula through 4 months of age: A control group (no LC-PUFA; n=20); a group fed a DHA-supplemented formula (0.35% of total fatty acids as a triglyceride derived from unicellular organisms (n=17); and a group fed a formula supplemented with both DHA and AA (0.36% and 0.72% of total fatty acids, respectively, as triglycerides from unicellular organisms; n=19). In this study, the mean Bayley MDI of the group fed the formula supplemented with DHA and AA was 7.3 points higher than that of the control group at 18 months of age (105.6 ± 11.8; SD) versus 98.3 ± 8.2; p<0.05) and 3.2 points higher than that of the DHA-supplemented group (102.4 ± 7.5; NS). Bayley PDIs of the 3 groups did not differ.

The most recently reported study[69] included reference groups of breastfed infants (n=165) weaned to formulas with or without AA and DHA (0.46% and 0.14% of total fatty acids, respectively) as well as groups fed a control formula (n=77) or 1 of 2 formulas with the same contents of AA and DHA from either egg triglyceride (n=80) or a combination of fish and fungal oil (n=82) for the first year of life. There were no differences among groups in visual acuity (discussed previously), information processing (FTII), general development (Bayley Scales of Infant Development), language development (MacArthur

Communicative Development Inventories), or temperament (Infant Behavior Questionaire).

Reasons for the discrepant results among these studies (and others) are not clear. Possibilities include different LC-PUFA sources, different durations of treatment, different amounts of AA, and/or different ratios of AA/DHA. There also were some differences in the LA and ALA contents of the control and experimental formulas; the LA-ALA ratios ranged from 8.5 to 16. In addition, the studies were conducted on 3 different continents—Europe,[74] Australia,[75] North America.[69,70] The variance in Bayley MDI and PDI scores also varied among studies and it may be noteworthy that the variance was smallest in the study that showed a statistically significant difference in Bayley MDI scores between infants who received a formula supplemented with DHA and AA and those who received an unsupplemented formula.

Even fewer studies are available in preterm infants fed supplemented versus unsupplemented formulas, and these are subject to the same criticisms as those in term infants. However, the available data, including those from a recently reported large and comprehensive study,[70] suggest that preterm infants are more likely to benefit from supplementation than term infants. In the latest study, infants weighing between 750 and 1800 g at birth were assigned randomly, before initiation of enteral feeding, to receive 1 of 3 formulas until term—A control formula (n=144); a formula with AA and DHA (0.46% and 0.26% of total fatty acids, respectively, as a combination of fish and fungal oils; n=140); or a formula with the same amounts of AA and DHA from a combination of egg yolk triglyceride and fish oil (n=143). From term through 12 months of age, the AA and DHA contents of the formulas were 0.42% and 0.16% of total fatty acids, respectively, from the same sources. Infants fed human milk exclusively through term served as a reference group. The effects of the supplemented formulas on visual acuity are previously described. Scores on the Fagan Test of Novelty Preference were higher at 6 months in the group supplemented with the combination of egg yolk triglyceride and fish oil than in the control group or the group supplemented with fish and fungal oils. There were no differences among groups at 9 months of age. There was no difference among groups in Bayley MDI at 12 months of age, but the Bayley PDI of infants who weighed <1250 g at birth was higher in the group assigned to the fish and fungal oil supplement than in the control group. The Bayley PDI of the group supplemented with egg yolk triglyceride and fish oil was not different from either the control or the other supplemented group. If twins and infants from Spanish-speaking families were excluded, supplemented infants had better vocabulary comprehension at 14 months' corrected age than the control group; however, without these exclusions, there was no difference in vocabulary comprehension among groups.

Sources for LC-PUFA Supplementation. Available sources for LC-PUFA supplementation include egg yolk lipid, phospholipid, and triglyceride, all of which contain ω6 as well as ω3 LC-PUFA, fish oils, and oils produced by single cell organisms (ie, microalgal and fungal oils). Aside from the possible effect of fish oil on growth of infants (see following text), few untoward effects of the available supplements have been noted. In vitro and animal studies of toxicity also have revealed little toxicity of any of these sources. In fact, the Food and Drug Administration has recently accepted the conclusion of a manufacturer of single cell oils that their products are GRAS (generally regarded as safe) sources of ARA and DHA for addition to formulas intended for normal infants.[77]

Adverse Effects of Long-Chain Polyunsaturated Fatty Acids. The observation in the early 1990s that preterm infants supplemented with fish oil (0.3% of total fatty acids as EPA and 0.2% as DHA) weighed less or had a lower weight-for-length at various times during the first year of life than infants assigned to an unsupplemented formula[78] has generated considerable concern. In this study, weight at 12 months' corrected age was correlated with plasma phospholipid AA content at various times during the first year of life,[79] (ie, the better the AA status, the higher the weight at 12 months' corrected age. Interestingly, a smaller study in which preterm infants were supplemented with more of the same (or similar) fish oil did not show differences in growth between supplemented and unsupplemented infants.[63] However, the duration of this study may not have been sufficient to permit detection of weight differences. A less marked effect on growth also was observed by Carlson et al[80] in preterm infants fed a formula supplemented with low-EPA fish oil versus an unsupplemented formula. In this study, there was no correlation between AA status and growth but there was a correlation between weights at some ages and the plasma phospholipid ratio of AA-DHA. Ryan et al[81] observed lower rates of growth in preterm male, but not female, infants fed a formula supplemented with the same low-EPA fish oil (0.2% of total fatty acid as DHA) versus a control formula from shortly before hospital discharge until 59 weeks' postmenstrual age (PMA). In this study, plasma phospholipid AA content of the infants assigned to the supplemented formula was lower through 59 weeks' PMA, but there was no correlation between plasma phospholipid

AA content and any aspect of growth. Rather, rates of increase in weight and length of male infants were inversely correlated with plasma phospholipid DHA content. A lower weight at 4 months of age also was observed in term infants fed formulas with a LA-ALA ratio of ~4 versus ~40 during this time; weight at 4 months of age was correlated with plasma phospholipid AA.[82]

In contrast to these observations of an apparent adverse effect of ω3 fatty acids on growth, Diersen-Schade et al[83] observed no difference in growth of preterm infants fed a DHA-supplemented (0.34% of fat as an algal oil) versus a control formula for at least 28 days prior to hospital discharge and followed until 57 weeks' PMA, and somewhat better growth than observed in either of these groups in a third group fed a formula supplemented with both DHA (0.33% of fat as an algal oil) and AA (0.6% of fat as a fungal oil). Other studies have shown no effect of LC-PUFA supplementation on growth.[70,84–86]

The reason(s) for the apparent effects of ω3 fatty acids on growth is not clear. Reasons that have been suggested include inhibition of desaturation and elongation of LA to AA by the ω3 fatty acids and/or inhibition of eicosanoid synthesis from AA by the intake of preformed EPA or endogenous synthesis of EPA from a moderately high intake of ALA. Regardless of the reason(s), it is important to note that the mean rates of increase in both weight and length of infants supplemented with ω3 fatty acids differ only minimally from the mean rates of increase in weight and length of normal term infants of the same ages.[87] Equally important, no study in which DHA supplementation was accompanied by AA supplementation has shown an adverse effect on any aspect of growth of either term or preterm infants.

In addition to concerns about adverse effects of ω3 fatty acids on growth, a number of theoretical concerns related to the known biological effects of ω6 and ω3 LC-PUFA must be considered.[88] Among these is the possibility that supplementation with highly unsaturated oils will increase the likelihood of oxidant damage. This is because peroxidation occurs at the site of double bonds making membranes with unsaturated fatty acids more vulnerable to oxidant damage. Thus, it is possible that LC-PUFA supplementation will increase the incidence of conditions thought to be related to oxidant damage (eg, necrotizing enterocolitis, bronchopulmonary dysplasia, retrolental fibroplasia). There also is concern that unbalanced supplementation with ω3 and/or ω6 LC-PUFA will result in altered eicosanoid metabolism with potential effects on a variety of physiological mechanisms (eg, blood clotting, infection). Further, more polyunsaturated fatty acids in muscle cell membranes has been related to enhanced insulin sensitivity[89–91] and specific LC-PUFA have been shown to inhibit as well as enhance transcription of a variety of genes.[92] There are few data to either support or allay these theoretical concerns with respect to the small amounts of LC-PUFA likely to be added to infant formulas.

Three recently reported, relatively large, randomized, controlled, double-blind studies in preterm infants[70,83,85] have shown no difference in the incidence of bronchopulmonary dysplasia, necrotizing enterocolitis, or other neonatal conditions between infants receiving supplements of either DHA or both AA and DHA from a variety of sources (single cell oils; low-EPA fish oil; egg yolk triglyceride) and infants receiving unsupplemented formula. Further, as discussed above, no difference in growth was observed. Together, these studies included more than 750 infants assigned to supplemented or unsupplemented formulas. Thus, despite the relative absence of definitive data concerning the validity of a number of the specific theoretical safety concerns related to the known biological effects of LC-PUFA, the fact that supplementation of formulas with the amounts of DHA and AA used in the studies of preterm infants cited above did not result in a greater incidence of conditions thought to be related etiologically to the theoretical concerns suggests that the amounts of the sources of LC-PUFA used in these studies are safe.

Supplementation of Infant Formulas With LC-PUFA

The American Academy of Pediatrics has no official position on supplementation of term or preterm infant formulas with LC-PUFA. The LSRO Expert Panel on Assessment of Nutrient Requirements of Term Infant Formulas recommended neither a minimum nor maximum content of either AA or DHA.[37] The LSRO Panel specified a maximum amount of AA and DHA for preterm infant formulas but did not specify a minimum amount of either fatty acid.[93] In contrast, regulatory and advisory groups from other countries recommend that infant formulas, particularly those intended for preterm infants, be supplemented with these 2 fatty acids[36,94–96] and such formulas are available in most areas other than the United States. The evidence for efficacy of supplementing term infant formulas with these fatty acids is only minimally, if at all, different from that available to the LSRO term formula Panel. In contrast, the evidence for efficacy of supplementation of preterm formulas is more convincing. Few studies in preterm infants have failed to document at least transient advantages of supplementation on visual acuity, and many studies suggest that there are advantages with respect to level of general development. Moreover, many of the safety concerns expressed earlier seem to have been resolved, or appear to be less urgent. Most notably, no recent study in which formulas were supplemented with both AA and DHA has shown an adverse effect on growth. Moreover, it now seems clear that supplementation with DHA alone or DHA plus AA does not result in a higher incidence of conditions such as necrotizing enterocolitis, retrolental fibroplasia, and bronchopulmonary dysplasia that, theoretically, might increase if these bioactive compounds were added to formulas. Thus with the GRAS designation of one type of supplementation product for use as a source of AA and DHA,[77] infant formula manufacturers in the United States can add these oils to the formulas if they satisfy the regulations of the Infant Formula Act.

References

1. Bier DM, Brosnan JT, Flatt RW, et al. Report of the IDECG Working Group on lower and upper limits of carbohydrate and fat intake. *Eur J Clin Nutr.* 1999; 53:S177–S178

2. Hamosh M. A review. Fat digestion in the newborn: role of lingual lipase and pre-duodenal digestion. *Pediatr Res.* 1979;13:615–622

3. Faber J, Goldstein R, Blondheim O, et al. Absorption of medium chain triglycerides in the stomach of the human infant. *J Pediatr Gastroenterol Nutr.* 1988;7:189–195

4. Linscheer WG, Vergroesen AJ. Lipids. In: Shils ME, Young VR, eds. *Modern Nutrition in Health and Disease.* 7th ed. Philadelphia, PA: Lea & Febiger; 1988:72–107

5. Hernell O, Olivecrona T. Human milk lipases. I. Serum-stimulated lipase. *J Lipid Res.* 1974;15:367–374

6. Hernell O, Blackberg L, Fredrikzon B. et al. Bile salt stimulated lipase in human milk and lipid digestion during the neonatal period. In: Lebenthal E, ed. *Textbook of Gastroenterology and Nutrition in Infancy.* New York, NY: Raven Press; 1981:465–471

7. Hernell O. Human milk lipases. III. Physiological implications of the bile salt-stimulated lipase. *Eur J Clin Invest.* 1975;5:267–272

8. Watkins JB, Ingall D, Szczepanik P, et al. Bile salt metabolism in the newborn: Measurement of pool size and synthesis by stable isotope technique. *N Engl J Med.* 1972;288:431–434

9. Watkins JB. Lipid digestion and absorption. *Pediatrics.* 1985;75(suppl):151–156

10. Hofmann AF, Roda A. Physicochemical properties of bile acids and their relationship to biological properties: an overview of the problem. *J Lipid Res.* 1984;25: 1477–1489

11. Gray GM. Mechanisms of digestion and absorption of food. In: Sleisenger MH, Fordtran JS, eds. *Gastrointestinal Disease. Pathophysiology, Diagnosis, Management.* 3rd ed. Philadelphia, PA: W.B. Saunders; 1983:844–858

12. Filer LJ Jr, Mattson FH, Fomon SJ. Triglyceride configuration and fat absorption by the human infant. *J Nutr.* 1969;99:293–298

13. Carnielli VP, Luijendijk IHT, van Beek RHT, et al. Effect of dietary triacylglycerol fatty acid positional distribution on plasma lipid classes and their fatty acid composition in preterm infants. *Am J Clin Nutr.* 1995;62:776–781

14. Carnielli VP, Luijendijk IHT, van Goudoever JB, et al. Feeding premature newborn infants palmitic acid in amounts and stereoisomeric position similar to that of human milk: effects on fat and mineral balance. *Am J Clin Nutr.* 1995;61:1037–1042

15. Carnielli VP, Luijendijk IHT, van Goudoever, JB, et al. Structural position and amount of palmitic acid in infant formulas: effects on fat, fatty acid, and mineral balance. *J Pediatr Gastroenterol Nutr.* 1996;23:553–560

16. Lucas A, Quinlan P, Abrams S, et al. Randomised controlled trial of a synthetic triglyceride milk formula for preterm infants. *Arch Dis Child.* 1997;77:F178–F184

17. Bensadoun A. Lipoprotein lipase. *Annu Rev Nutr.* 1991;11:217–237

18. Griffin EA, Bryan MH, Angel A. Variations in intralipid tolerance in newborn infants. *Pediatr Res.* 1983;17:478–481

19. Innis SM. Essential fatty acids in growth and development. *Prog Lipid Res.* 1991; 30:39–103

20. Holman RT. Nutritional and biochemical evidences of acyl interaction with respect to essential polyunsaturated fatty acids. *Prog Lipid Res.* 1986;25:29–39

21. Oliw E, Gramström E, Änggärd E. The prostaglandins and essential fatty acids. In: Pace-Asciak C, Gramström E, eds. *Prostaglandins and Related Substances.* Amsterdam, The Netherlands: Elsevier; 1983:1–19

22. Holman RT. The ratio of trienoic: tetraenoic acids in tissue lipids as a measure of essential fatty acid requirement. *J Nutr.* 1960;70:405–410

23. Burr GO, Burr MM. A new deficiency disease produced by the rigid exclusion of fat from the diet. *J Biol Chem.* 1929;82:345–367

24. Hansen AE, Steward RA, Hughes G, et al. The relation of linoleic acid to infant feeding, a review. *Acta Paediatr.* 1962;51(suppl 137):1–41

25. Benolken RM, Anderson RE, Wheeler TG. Membrane fatty acids associated with the electrical response in visual excitation. *Science.* 1973;182:1253–1254

26. Neuringer M, Connor WE, Van Petten C, et al. Dietary omega-3 fatty acid deficiency and visual loss in infant Rhesus monkeys. *J Clin Invest.* 1984;73:272–276

27. Neuringer M, Connor WE, Lin DS, et al. Biochemical and functional effects of prenatal and postnatal ω3 fatty acid deficiency on retina and brain in Rhesus monkeys. *Proc Natl Acad Sci U S A.* 1986;83:4021–4025

28. Wheeler TG, Benolken RM. Visual membranes: specificity of fatty acid precursors for the electrical response to illumination. *Science.* 1975;188:1312–1314

29. Holman RT, Johnson SB, Hatch RF. A case of human linolenic acid deficiency involving neurological abnormalities. *Am J Clin Nutr.* 1982;35:617–623

30. Bjerve KS, Fischer S, Alme K. Alpha-linolenic acid deficiency in man: effect of ethyl linolenate on plasma and erythrocyte fatty acid composition and biosynthesis of prostanoids. *Am J Clin Nutr.* 1987;46:570–576

31. Jensen RG. Lipids in human milk. *Lipids.* 1999;34:1243–1271

32. Sanders TAB, Reddy S. The influence of a vegetarian diet on the fatty acid composition of human milk and the essential fatty acid status of the infant. *J Pediatr.* 1992; 120:S71–S77

33. Henderson RA, Jensen RG, Lammi-Keefe CJ, et al. Effect of fish oil on the fatty acid composition of human milk and maternal and infant erythrocytes. *Lipids.* 1992; 27:863–869

34. Makrides M, Neumann MA, Gibson RA. Effect of maternal docosahexaenoic acid (DHA) supplementation on breast milk composition. *Eur J Clin Nutr.* 1996;50: 352–357

35. Jensen CL, Maude M, Anderson RE, Heird WC. Effect of docosahexaenoic acid supplementation of lactating women on milk total lipid, and maternal and infant plasma phospholipid fatty acids. *Am J Clin Nutr.* 2000;71(suppl):292S–299S

36. ESPGAN Committee on Nutrition. Comment on the content and composition of lipids in infant formulas. *Acta Paediatr.* 1991;80:887–896

37. Raiten DJ, Talbot JM, Waters JH. LSRO Report: Assessment of nutrient requirements for infant formulas. *J Nutr.* 1998;128:2059S–2293S

38. Carlson SE, Rhodes PG, Ferguson MG. Docosahexaenoic acid status of preterm infants at birth and following feeding with human milk or formula. *Am J Clin Nutr.* 1986;44:798–804

39. Innis SM, Akrabawi SS, Diersen-Schade DA, et al. Visual acuity and blood lipids in term infants fed human milk or formulae. *Lipids.* 1997;32:63–72

40. Jorgensen MH, Hernell O, Lund P, et al. Visual acuity and erythrocyte docosahexaenoic acid status in breast-fed and formula-fed term infants during the first four months of life. *Lipids.* 1996;31:99–105

41. Ponder DL, Innis SM, Benson JD, et al. Docosahexaenoic acid status of term infants fed breast milk or infant formula containing soy oil or corn oil. *Pediatr Res.* 1992; 32:683–688

42. Lucas A, Morley R, Cole TJ, et al. Early diet in preterm babies and developmental status at 18 months. *Lancet.* 1990;335:1477–1481

43. Lucas A, Morley R, Cole TJ. Randomised trial of early diet in preterm babies and later intelligence quotient. *BMJ.* 1998;317:1481–1487

44. Morrow-Tlucak M, Haude RH, Ernhart CB. Breastfeeding and cognitive development in the first 2 years of life. *Soc Sci Med.* 1988;26:635–639

45. Rogan WJ, Gladen BC. Breastfeeding and cognitive development. *Early Hum Dev.* 1993;31:181–193

46. Clandinin MT, Chappell JE, Leong S, et al. Intrauterine fatty acid accretion rates in human brain: implications for fatty acid requirements. *Early Hum Dev.* 1980;4: 121–129

47. Clandinin MT, Chappell JE, Leong S, et al. Extrauterine fatty acid accretion in infant brain: implications for fatty acid requirements. *Early Hum Dev.* 1980;4:131–138

48. Martinez M. Tissue levels of polyunsaturated fatty acids during early human development. *J Pediatr.* 1992;120:S129–S138

49. Berghaus TM, Demmelmair H, Koletzko B. Fatty acid composition of lipid classes in maternal and cord plasma at birth. *Eur J Pediatr.* 1998;157:763–768

50. Dutta-Roy AK. Transport mechanisms for long-chain polyunsaturated fatty acids in the human placenta. *Am J Clin Nutr.* 2000;71:315S–322S

51. Farquharson J, Cockburn F, Patrick WA, et al. Infant cerebral cortex phospholipid fatty acid composition and diet. *Lancet.* 1992;340:810–813

52. Jamieson EC, Abbasi KA, Cockburn F, et al. Effect of diet on term infant cerebral cortex fatty acid composition. *World Rev Nutr Diet.* 1994;75:139–141

53. Makrides M, Neumann MA, Byard RW, et al. Fatty acid composition of brain, retina, and erythrocytes in breast- and formula-fed infants. *Am J Clin Nutr.* 1994; 60:189–194

54. Arbuckle LD, MacKinnon MJ, Innis SM. Formula 18:2 (n-6) and 18:3 (n-3) content and ratio influence long-chain polyunsaturated fatty acids in the developing piglet liver and central nervous system. *J Nutr.* 1994;124:289–298

55. Sauerwald TU, Hachey DL, Jensen CL, et al. Effect of dietary α-linolenic acid intake on incorporation of docosahexaenoic and arachidonic acids into plasma phospholipids of term infants. *Lipids.* 1996;31:S131–S135

56. Carnielli VP, Wattimena DJ, Luijendijk IH, et al. The very low birth weight premature infant is capable of synthesizing arachidonic and docosahexaenoic acids from linoleic and linolenic acids. *Pediatr Res.* 1996;40:169–174

57. Demmelmair H, von Schenck U, Behrendt E, et al. Estimation of arachidonic acid synthesis in full term neonates using natural variation of ^{13}C content. *J Pediatr Gastroenterol Nutr.* 1995;21:31–36

58. Salem Jr N, Wegher B, Mena P, et al. Arachidonic and docosahexaenoic acids are biosynthesized from their 18-carbon precursors in human infants. *Proc Natl Acad Sci U S A.* 1996;93:49–54

49. Sauerwald TU, Hachey DL, Jensen CL, et al. Intermediates in endogenous synthesis of C22:6ω3 and C20:4ω6 by term and preterm infants. *Pediatr Res.* 1997;41:183–187

60. Uauy R, Mena P, Wegher B, et al. Long chain polyunsaturated fatty acid formation in neonates: Effect of gestational age and intrauterine growth. *Pediatr Res.* 2000; 47:127–135

61. Carlson SE, Cooke RJ, Rhodes PG, et al. Long-term feeding of formulas high in linolenic acid and marine oil to very low birth weight infants: phospholipid fatty acids. *Pediatr Res.* 1991;30:404–412

62. Uauy RD, Birch DG, Birch EE, et al. Effect of dietary omega-3 fatty acids on retinal function of very-low-birth-weight neonates. *Pediatr Res.* 1990;28:485–492

63. Uauy RD, Hoffman DR, Birch EE, Birch DG, Jameson DM, Tyson JE. Safety and efficacy of omega-3 fatty acids in the nutrition of very-low-birth-weight infants: soy oil and marine oil supplementation of formula. *J Pediatr.* 1994;124:612–620

64. Rioux FM, Innis SM, Dyer R, et al. Diet-induced changes in liver and bile but not brain fatty acids can be predicted from differences in plasma phospholipid fatty acids in formula and milk fed piglets. *J Nutr.* 1997;127:370–377

65. Moore SA, Yoder E, Murphy S, et al. Astrocytes, not neurons, produce docosa-hexaenoic acid (22:6ω3) and arachidonic acid (20:4ω6). *J Neurochem.* 1991; 56:518–524

66. Moore SA. Cerebral endothelium and astrocytes cooperate in supplying docosa-hexaenoic acid to neurons. *Adv Exp Med Biol.* 1993;331:229–233

67. SanGiovanni JP, Berkey CS, Dwyer JT, Colditz GA. Dietary essential fatty acids, long-chain polyunsaturated fatty acids, and visual resolution acuity in healthy full-term infants: a systematic review. *Early Hum Dev.* 2000;57:165–188

68. SanGiovanni JP, Parra-Cabrera S, Colditz GA, et al. Meta-analysis of dietary essen-tial fatty acids and long-chain polyunsaturated fatty acids as they relate to visual res-olution acuity in healthy preterm infants. *Pediatrics.* 2000;105:1292–1298

69. Auestad N, Halter R, Halla RT, et al. Growth and development in term infants fed long-chain polyunsaturated fatty acids: A double-masked, randomized, parallel, prospective, multivariate study. *Pediatrics.* 2001;108:372–381

70. O'Connor DL, Hall R, Adamkin D, et al. Growth and development in preterm infants fed long-chain polyunsaturated fatty acids: A prospective, randomized con-trolled trial. *Pediatrics.* 2001;108:359–371

71. McCall RB, Mash CW. Long-chain polyunsaturated fatty acids and the measure-ment and prediction of intelligence (IQ). In: Dobbing J, ed. *Developing Brain and Behaviour.* London, England: Academic Press; 1997:295–338

72. Fagan JF III, Singer LT. Infant recognition memory as a measure of intelligence. *Adv Infancy Res.* 1983;2:31–78

73. Colombo J. Individual differences in infant cognition: Methods, measures, and models. In: Dobbing J, ed. *Developing Brain and Behaviour.* London, England: Academic Press; 1997:295–338

74. Lucas A, Morley R. Efficacy and safety of long-chain polyunsaturated fatty acid sup-plementation of infant-formula milk: a randomised trial. *Lancet.* 1999;354: 1948–1954

75. Makrides M, Neumann MA, Simmer K, et al. A critical appraisal of the role of dietary long-chain polyunsaturated fatty acids on neural indices of term infants: a randomized, controlled trial. *Pediatrics.* 2000;105:32–38

76. Birch EE, Garfield S, Hoffman DR, et al. A randomized controlled trial of early dietary supply of long-chain polyunsaturated fatty acids and mental development in term infants. *Dev Med Child Neurol.* 2000;42:174–181

77. FDA. GRAS status of DHASCO and ARASCO. Food and Drug Administration, Office of Premarket Approval. http://www.cfsan.fda.gov/~/rd/foodadd.html

78. Carlson SE, Cooke RJ, Werkman SH, et al. First year growth of preterm infants fed standard compared to marine oil n-3 supplemented formula. *Lipids.* 1992;27: 901–907

79. Carlson SE, Werkman SH, Peeples JM, et al. Arachidonic acid status correlates with first year growth in preterm infants. *Proc Natl Acad Sci U S A.* 1993;90:1073–1077

80. Carlson SE, Werkman SH, Tolley EA. Effect of long-chain n-3 fatty acid supplementation on visual acuity and growth of preterm infants with and without bronchopulmonary dysplasia. *Am J Clin Nutr*. 1996;63:687–689

81. Ryan AS, Montalto MB, Groh-Wargo S, et al. Effect of DHA-containing formula on growth of preterm infants to 59 weeks postmenstrual age. *Am J Hum Biol*. 1999; 11:457–487

82. Jensen CL, Prager TC, Fraley JK, et al. Effect of dietary linoleic/alpha-linolenic acid ratio on growth and visual function of term infants. *J Pediatr*. 1997;131:200–209

83. Diersen-Schade DA, Hansen JW, Harris CL, et al. Docosahexaenoic acid plus arachidonic acid enhance preterm infant growth. In: Riemersma RA, Armstrong R, Kelly RW, Wilson R, eds. *Essential Fatty Acids and Eicosanoids: Invited Papers from the Fourth International Congress*. Champaign, IL: AOCS Press; 1998:123–127

84. Foreman-vonDrongelen MMHP, van Houwelingen AC, Kester ADM, et al. Influence of feeding artificial formulas containing docosahexaenoic and arachidonic acids on the postnatal long-chain polyunsaturated fatty acid status of healthy preterm infants. *Br J Nutr*. 1996;76:649–667

85. Vanderhoof J, Gross S, Hegyi T. Evaluation of a long-chain polyunsaturated fatty acid supplemented formula on growth tolerance, and plasma lipids in preterm infants up to 48 weeks postconceptional age. *J Pediatr Gastroenterol Nutr*. 1999;29:318–326

86. Vanderhoof J, Gross S, Hegyi T, for the Multicenter Study Group. A multicenter long-term safety and efficacy trial of preterm formula supplemented with long-chain polyunsaturated fatty acids. *J Pediatr Gastroenterol Nutr*. 2000;31:121–127

87. Fomon SJ, Nelson SE. Size and Growth. In: Fomon SJ, ed. *Nutrition of Normal Infants*. St Louis, MO: Mosby-Year Book, Inc; 1993:36–84

88. Heird WC. Biological effects and safety issues related to long-chain polyunsaturated fatty acids in infants. *Lipids*. 1999;34:207–214

89. Borkman M, Storlien LH, Pan DA, et al. The relationship between insulin sensitivity and the fatty-acid composition of skeletal muscle phospholipids. *N Engl J Med*. 1993;328:238–244

90. Pan DA, Hylbert AJ, Storlien LH. Dietary fats, membrane phospholipids and obesity. *J Nutr*. 1994;124:1555–1565

91. Storlien LH, Jenkins AB, Chisholm DJ, et al. Influence of dietary fat composition on development of insulin resistance in rats: relationship to muscle triglyceride and ω3 fatty acids in muscle phospholipid. *Diabetes*. 1991;40:280–289

92. Clarke SD, Jump DB. Polyunsaturated fatty acid regulation of hepatic gene transcription. *J Nutr*. 1996;126(suppl):1105–1109

93. Life Sciences Research Office, American Society for Nutritional Sciences for the Center for Food Safety and Applied Nutrition, Food and Drug Administration, Department of Health and Human Services, Washington, DC 20204 under Contract No. 223-92-2185. Assessment of Nutrient Requirements for Infant Formulas. *J Nutr*. 1998;128(suppl 11S)

94. ISSFAL Board statement: Recommendations for the essential fatty acid require-ments for infant formulas. *ISSFAL Newsletter.* 1994;4–5

95. British Nutrition Foundation Task Force on Unsaturated Fatty Acids. Unsaturated fatty acids and early development. In: *Unsaturated Fatty Acids: Nutritional and Physiological Significance.* London, England: Chapman & Hall; 1992;63–67

96. Food and Agriculture Organization/World Health Organization. Lipids in early development. In: *Fats and Oils in Human Nutrition: report of a joint expert consulta-tion.* Rome, Italy: FAO/WHO; 1994;49–55

18

Calcium, Phosphorus, and Magnesium

Basic Physiology

The minerals calcium, magnesium, and phosphorus participate in many of the body's most important functions. These elements play prominent roles in energy processes and transport of metabolites in a host of molecular biochemical reactions. In addition, calcium and phosphorus constitute the principal components of the skeleton in the form of hydroxyapatite $Ca_{10}(PO_4)_6(OH)_2$. Magnesium, a cell constituent, catalyzes many necessary metabolic functions and transmission systems. Thus, these elements are essential nutrients for life processes and for forming the mineral skeleton.[1-3]

Phosphorus is abundantly available from virtually all animal and vegetable sources. Calcium sources include milk and other dairy products, animal bones and, in lesser amounts, a number of vegetables (Appendix N, Table N-2). In addition, calcium is widely found in fortified food products such as breakfast cereals and fruit juices. Magnesium, like phosphorus, is abundant in animal and plant cells. Together, these 3 elements constitute 98% of body minerals by weight. Bone accounts for 99% of the calcium, 80% of the phosphorus, and 60% of the magnesium. Magnesium is taken up by the hydroxyapatite, as are virtually all biological cations in a dynamic state.[1-4]

Regulation: Calcium and Phosphorus

Both calcium and phosphorus appear in the serum and extracellular fluid in low concentrations. The calcium level is closely controlled in a narrow range of 2.13 to 2.63 mmol/L (8.5 to 10.5 mg/dL). About half of the calcium in the serum is bound to albumin at normal levels of the latter; the remainder is ionized. The ionized fraction is the physiologically active portion, and, in health, the concentration is constant. At an acid pH, the ionized fraction increases. If hypoalbuminemia should occur, the calcium concentration decreases, but the ionized portion remains undisturbed. The phosphorus concentration varies and is age dependent. In infants, the normal range is 1.6 to 2.4 mmol/L (5.0 to 7.5 mg/dL); in older children, 1.3 to 1.78 mmol/L (4 to 5.5 mg/dL); and in adults, 0.8 to 1.6 mmol/L (2.5 to 4.5 mg/dL).[4]

Factors that regulate calcium metabolism include the mucosa of the upper small intestine, parathyroid hormone, calcitonin, vitamin D, the kidney, and bone. The gastrointestinal tract regulates calcium absorption; a portion of the calcium is absorbed by passive diffusion and a portion of it is actively transported. Parathyroid hormone enhances serum calcium primarily by releasing calcium from bone. The concentration of ionized calcium in the fluid perfusing the parathyroid gland is a major determinant of the rate of synthesis and release of this hormone. Calcitonin, a hormone elaborated by the parafollicular cells of the thyroid, inhibits bone reabsorption.[4-6]

Vitamin D facilitates transcellular calcium intestinal absorption. To achieve this effect, it must undergo sequential hydroxylation in the liver to calcidiol and in the kidney to the final product, calcitriol (1,25 dihyroxyvitamin D).[7] Calcidiol (25-hydroxyvitamin D) represents the primary storage form of vitamin D. Anticonvulsant drugs, such as phenobarbital and phenytoin, can interfere with vitamin D hydroxylation and metabolism, increasing the daily requirement. The reservoir of calcium in bone also serves a regulatory function, because a portion of bone calcium exchanges readily with the calcium of extracellular fluid. The physical forces of muscle tension and gravity help preserve skeletal integrity.

The regulation of phosphorus metabolism is less well understood. Phosphorus is absorbed efficiently in the small intestine. It is filtered and reabsorbed in the kidney. Parathyroid hormone inhibits its reabsorption. Phosphorus absorption is also inhibited by aluminum-containing antacids. A significant aspect of phosphorus regulation is by renal excretion.

Regulation: Magnesium

Only a small fraction of total body magnesium is present in serum. The normal serum total magnesium concentration is 0.75 to 1.15 mmol/L (1.5 to 2.3 mEq/L). Approximately half of this magnesium is protein-bound, principally to albumin. While magnesium depletion is likely, although not always, to be associated with hypomagnesemia, the latter is more likely to reflect a disturbance of magnesium metabolism. Measurement of intracellular (eg, skeletal muscle) magnesium concentration may provide more information on magnesium nutritional status but is not feasible in clinical practice.

Magnesium appears to be absorbed principally in the ileum by 3 mechanisms—passive diffusion, "solvent drag," and, probably, by active transport. Absorption of magnesium is inversely related to intake. Absorption is probably very minimally affected by vitamin D; absorption is also affected by high intake of calcium, phosphorus, and phytate. Magnesium homeostasis is maintained partly by control of intestinal absorption, but also by control of renal excretion.

Parathyroid hormone decreases renal reabsorption of filtered magnesium. Release of parathyroid hormone is modestly suppressed by increased concentrations of magnesium in extracellular fluid, an action that may be mediated by an increase in calcium in the cytosol of parathyroid cells. Conversely, acute (but not chronic) hypomagnesemia stimulates the release of parathyroid hormone.[8–12]

Transient neonatal hypomagnesemia has been observed most often in association with hypocalcemia and hyperphosphatemia and has become uncommon after reduction of phosphorus concentrations in infant formulas. Transient neonatal hypomagnesemia is more common in infants with intrauterine growth retardation and infants of mothers with diabetes, hypophosphatemia, or hyperparathyroidism. Magnesium supplements may be required for these infants. Rarely, severe hypomagnesemia associated with convulsions occurs in early infancy as a result of a genetically determined disorder. This disorder probably results in defective intestinal absorption of magnesium. Long-term magnesium supplementation is necessary.[10]

Requirements: Calcium

The specific requirements for calcium intake by full-term infants, children, and adolescents have been extensively reviewed in recent years.[8,13] The most current recommendations are shown in Appendix C.

The American Academy of Pediatrics has affirmed the findings of these panels in a policy statement published in 1999.[14] The recommendations of the Food and Nutrition board of the National Academy of Sciences[8] represent the more complete and more recent evaluation of dietary recommendations and should be the primary guidelines used.[14] For infants under age 6 months fed cow milk-based formulas, the 1997 Food and Nutrition Board Guideline should be followed. **It states that a calcium intake of 315 mg/d leads to comparable calcium retention as would be achieved by breastfed infants and should represent an adequate intake for these infants. This value is similar to the recommendations of the Life Sciences Research Office (LSRO) report, published in 1998, which recommended a minimum calcium concentration of 50 mg/100 kcal for infant's fed cow milk-based formula.**

Multiple approaches are used to assess mineral requirements in children. They include the following: (1) measurement of calcium balance in persons with various levels of calcium intake; (2) measurement of bone mineral content, by dual-energy x-ray absorptiometry or other techniques, in groups of children before and after calcium supplementation; and (3) epidemiological studies relating bone mass or fracture risk in adults with childhood calcium intake. Calcium requirements are affected substantially by genetic variability and other dietary constituents. The interactions of these factors make it impossible to identify a single unique number for the calcium "requirement" for all children.[15]

The calcium balance technique consists of measuring the effects of any given calcium intake on the net retention of calcium by the body. This approach has been the most commonly used to estimate requirement for minerals. Its usefulness is based on the rationale that virtually all retained calcium must be used, especially by children, to enhance bone mineralization. It, therefore, is reasonable to expect that the dietary intake that leads to the greatest level of calcium retention is the intake that will lead to the greatest benefit for promoting skeletal mineralization and decreasing the ultimate risk of osteoporosis.[16–18]

The substantial limitations involved in obtaining and interpreting data about calcium balance are well known. These include substantial technical problems with measuring calcium excretion and the difficulty obtaining dietary intake control in children. These problems have been partly overcome by the development of stable isotopic methods to assess calcium absorption and excretion.[18] Nevertheless, more data are needed to establish the "optimal" level of calcium retention at different ages and the effects of development on calcium balance.

A major advance in the field during the last 25 years has been the development and improvement of methods to measure total body and regional bone mineral content by using various bone density techniques. Currently, the technique used in many studies is dual-energy x-ray absorptiometry. This technique can rapidly measure the bone mineral content and bone mineral density of the entire skeleton or of regional sites with a virtually negligible level of radiation exposure. Furthermore, recent enhancements in the precision of the technique have made it particularly suitable for assessing the effects of calcium supplementation on bone mass in children of all ages.[19,20]

Preterm Infants

Inadequate mineral intake in preterm infants places them at risk for the condition called osteopenia of prematurity. This is a condition in which the bone mineral content of a premature infant is significantly decreased relative to the expected level of mineralization for a fetus or infant of comparable size or gestational age. It is a common problem in infants less than 1000 g birth weight who have low intakes of calcium and phosphorus. The frequency of osteopenia is increased in infants who are born at less than 28 weeks' gestation, who require long-term parenteral nutrition, or who require medications such as diuretics, which may affect mineral metabolism.[21]

The presence of osteopenia can be assessed by direct radiologic evaluation. Increased lucency of the cortical bone with or without epiphyseal changes is characteristic of significant osteopenia. Although the presence of a fracture can be the presenting sign of osteopenia of prematurity, most infants with decreased bone mineralization, including some with severe rickets, do not have fractures.

The accretion of calcium and phosphorus rise exponentially during the third trimester in utero. Human milk is relatively low in calcium and phosphorus relative to the in utero accretion rates of these minerals. Although minerals are well absorbed from human milk (60% to 70%), the net retention of calcium and phosphorus is far below the in utero rates and leads to the development of undermineralized bones. Supplementary calcium and phosphorus are needed to sustain optimal calcium balance. Currently, several commercial mineral supplements (for human milk-fed infants) and formulas are marketed for use by premature infants (see Appendix H). Use of these products has led to net calcium retention comparable to that achieved in utero.[22,23]

In small premature infants fed by parenteral nutrition, the danger of calcium-phosphorus precipitation in the solution limits the amount of these minerals that can be administered intravenously. As a result, prenatal retention rates of calcium and phosphorus are not achieved.[24] After hospitalization, there may be benefits to providing formula-fed premature infants formulas with higher calcium concentrations than those of routine cow milk-based formulas. These formulas recently have been made available for use after discharge from the hospital (see Appendix H, Table H-1). The optimal concentrations and length of time needed for such formulas are unknown.

Full-term Infants and Children

The optimal primary nutritional source during the first year of life is human milk. No available evidence shows that exceeding the amount of calcium retained by the exclusively breastfed full-term infant during the first 6 months of life or the amount retained by the human milk-fed infant supplemented with solid foods during the second 6 months of life is beneficial to achieving long-term increases in bone mineralization. Due to the possibility of diminished absorption of calcium from infant formulas relative to human milk, it has been deemed prudent to increase the concentration of calcium in all infant formulas relative to human milk to ensure comparable levels of calcium retention. Relatively greater concentrations are found in specialized formulas, such as soy formulas and casein hydrolysates, to account for the potential lower bioavailability of the calcium from these formulas relative to cow milk-based formula.[10] Although variations exist in the amount of calcium absorbed by infants from different formulas, there is no evidence at present that these differences lead to clinically significant differences in bone mass in infancy or later in life. Longer-term studies are needed to evaluate these issues. Studies comparing the bone mineral content of full-term infants during the first year of life have generally found a slightly greater value for those fed infant formulas than those fed human milk.[25] However, it is uncertain if this difference is maintained later in childhood.

Few data are available about the calcium requirements of children before puberty. Calcium retention is relatively low in toddlers and slowly increases as puberty approaches. The benefits of high levels of intake in this age group are uncertain. High levels of calcium intake may negatively affect other minerals, especially iron. As these minerals are important for growth and development and may be marginal in toddlers and preschool children, more data about the risks and benefits of high calcium intake are needed before it can be recommended prior to puberty. However, recent data have not identified a harmful effect in children on iron absorption or status of increasing calcium intake.[26,27]

Perhaps of most importance in this age group is the development of eating patterns that will be associated with adequate calcium intake later in life. As such, it is important that families learn to identify the calcium content of foods based on the food label and incorporate this information into their food-buying habits.

Preadolescents and Adolescents

The majority of research in children about calcium requirements has been directed toward 9- to 18-year-olds. The efficiency of calcium absorption is increased during puberty, and the majority of bone formation occurs during this period. Data from balance studies suggest that, for most healthy children in this age range, the maximal net calcium balance (plateau) is achieved with intakes between 1200 and 1500 mg/d. That is, at intake levels above this, almost all of the additional calcium is excreted and not used. At intakes below that level, the skeleton may not receive as much calcium as it can use, and peak bone mass may not be achieved.[14–20] Virtually all the data used to establish this intake level are from white children; minimal data are available for other ethnic groups.

Numerous controlled trials have found an increase in the bone mineral content in children in this age group who have received calcium supplementation.[8,14,28] However, the available data suggest that if calcium is supplemented only for relatively short periods (ie, 1 to 2 years), there may not be long-term benefits to establishing and maintaining a maximum peak bone mass.[29] This emphasizes the importance of diet in achieving adequate calcium intake and in establishing dietary patterns with a calcium intake near recommended levels throughout childhood and adolescence.

In addition to calcium intake, exercise is an important aspect of achieving maximal peak bone mass. There is evidence that childhood and adolescence may represent an important period for achieving long-lasting skeletal benefits from regular exercise. Recent data support the possibility that a low bone mass may be a contributing factor to some fractures in children.[30]

Adolescent Pregnancy and Lactation

At birth, the fetus contains approximately 30 g of calcium. This represents approximately 2.5% of typical maternal body calcium stores.[10] Evidence suggests that, in adult women, much of this 30 g comes from increases in dietary calcium absorption during pregnancy.[31] Specific studies in groups of adolescents have not been performed to identify their ability to increase calcium absorption during pregnancy.

During lactation, a period of 6 months of exclusive breastfeeding would lead to an additional 45 g of calcium secreted by the mother. Although some of this is accounted for by decreased urinary calcium excretion during lactation, there is extensive evidence demonstrating a loss of maternal bone calcium during lactation.[32,33] In adults, however, bone remineralization occurs post-weaning and neither pregnancy nor lactation is associated with persistent bone loss. Because of recent data demonstrating that calcium supplementation is not effective in preventing lactation-associated bone loss or enhancing post-weaning bone mass recovery,[32] recent dietary recommendations do not suggest increases in calcium for healthy adult women who are pregnant or lactating above the 1000 mg/d recommended for non-lactating adult women. Similarly, the recommendations do not suggest increased intake above the age-appropriate maximum for adolescents (1300 mg/d) who are pregnant, or lactation either.[8]

At the present time, the available evidence supports the position that the benefits to breastfeeding greatly outweigh any demonstrated risks to adolescents in terms of achieving either optimal growth or peak bone mass. No available data suggest that calcium intakes above the recommended amounts are beneficial to pregnant or lactating adolescents. However, it should be noted that these recommended intake levels are far above those typical of the diet of most adolescents.

The American Academy of Pediatrics Recommends the Following:

1. Pediatricians should actively support the goal of achieving calcium intakes in children and adolescents comparable to those in recently recommended guidelines. The prevention of future osteoporosis, as well as the possibility of a decreased risk of childhood and adolescent fractures, should be discussed as potential benefits to achieving these goals. Currently, relatively few children and adolescents achieve dietary calcium intake goals.

2. To emphasize the importance of calcium nutriture, pediatricians should consider including the following questions about dietary calcium intake.
   What do you drink, either white or chocolate milk, with your meals?
   Do you drink milk with meals, snacks, or cereal or any other time during the day?
   Do you eat cheese, yogurt, or other dietary products such as cottage cheese?
   Do you eat any of the following: broccoli, tofu, oranges, or legumes (dried beans and peas?)
   Do you take any mineral or vitamin supplements?
   Do you drink calcium-fortified juices or eat any calcium-fortified foods?

3. For children and adolescents whose calcium intake seems deficient, specific information about the sources of dietary calcium should be provided. Adolescents may need to be reminded that low-fat dairy products, including skim milk and low-fat yogurts, are good sources of calcium that are not high in fat.

Phosphorous Requirements

As with calcium, the recommended intake for phosphorus for infants was based on usual dietary intakes of breastfed infants. These values are 100 mg/d from ages 0 to 6 months and 275 mg/d from ages 7 through 12 months. The higher value in older infants reflects the considerable contribution of solid foods to usual phosphorus intakes of these infants. There are few data on which to base estimates of phosphorus requirements for older children. Dietary guidelines[14] used a factorial approach based on limited estimates of phosphorus absorption, excretion, and accretion to determine average requirements. An allotment of an additional 20% was provided to calculate the RDA. Using this method, values of 460 mg/d for children ages 1 through 3, and 500 mg/d for children ages 4 through 8 were derived. These values are well below typical intakes for children of these ages.

For adolescents, both the factorial method and estimates of intake needed to maintain typical serum phosphorus were used to determine intake guidelines. A value of 1250 mg/d was calculated for boys and girls ages 9 through 18 years. This value is much closer to typical intake values for adolescents and reflects the rapid bone and muscle growth during this time period.

Magnesium Requirements

Commercial cow milk-based infant formulas are generally higher in magnesium concentration (40 to 50 mg/L) than human milk. Soy-based formulas may have even higher levels of magnesium (50 to 80 mg/L).[8,10] In a large series of studies, Fomon and Nelson[10] reported approximately 40% net absorption of magnesium in infants fed soy- or milk-based formulas with a net retention (based on total intake of 53 to 59 mg/d) of 9 to 10 mg/d.[10]

Few metabolic balance studies have been done for magnesium in children, especially those between ages 1 and 8 years. Based on balance studies, it appears that a magnesium intake of 5 mg/kg/d should lead to positive magnesium balances in most children. It should be noted that a substantial number of adolescents might be in negative magnesium balance when receiving typical diets.[18]

Current dietary guidelines for infants are based on the intakes of human milk-fed infants. The recommended intakes are 30 mg/d for infants in the first 6 months of life and 75 mg/d from ages 7 through 12 months. For older children, intake recommendations are based on an average requirement of 5 mg/kg with an allotment for the RDA of an additional 20%. Using average weight for age data, this leads to an RDA of 80 mg/d for ages 1 through 3 years, 130 mg/d for ages 4 through 8 years, and 240 mg/d for ages 9 through 13 years. For adolescents ages 14 through 18 years, slightly greater average intakes are needed (5.3 mg/kg/d) to account for increased pubertal magnesium needs. Differences in average weights of boys and girls were used to calculate RDAs of 410 mg/d for boys and 360 mg/d for girls.

Because of efficient homeostatic mechanisms, especially renal conservation of magnesium, low dietary magnesium alone does not usually cause clinically apparent magnesium deficiency. Magnesium deficiency is, however, quite common in young children with protein-energy malnutrition, especially when accompanied by gastroenteritis. Muscle magnesium is depressed, but serum magnesium may be normal. Hypomagnesemia sometimes occurs in malabsorption syndromes, and magnesium depletion may develop in subjects with severe diarrhea. Convulsions are the most clearly documented feature of hypomagnesemia with or without total body magnesium deficiency in infants and young children. Neuropsychiatric disorders are well documented in magnesium-depleted adults. Hypocalcemia associated with magnesium deficiency may be the result of defective synthesis or release of parathyroid hormone. Hypokalemia also occurs secondary to magnesium deficiency.[34]

Numerous conditions may be related to subacute magnesium deficiency, however. For example, recent evidence has also linked magnesium deficiency with insulin resistance and worsening diabetic regulation. Increased blood pressure, migraines, and inadequate bone mineralization may also be linked to habitually low magnesium intake, although data for these relationships continue to be incomplete.[8]

Dietary Sources: Calcium and Phosphorus

The calcium-phosphorus weight ratio varies widely in foods, from a high of 2.8:1 in green vegetables to a low of 0.06:1 in meat. The ratio for human milk is 2:1, for cow milk it is 1.2:1, and for commercial infant formulas it is usually intermediate between these values. The high phosphorus content of cow milk, and sometimes of infant formulas, with their lower calcium-phosphorus ratio, is one factor in the pathogenesis of neonatal tetany, a situation rarely, if ever, encountered in the breastfed infant. Phosphorus is widely distributed in animal proteins, vegetables, cereals, and soft drinks. Insufficient intake is uncommon in most children receiving a typical mixed diet. There is concern about excess intake, especially from carbonated soda beverages. However, the impact of this phosphorus intake on mineral health remains uncertain.[8]

The gap between the recommended calcium intakes and the typical intakes of children and adolescents is substantial. A list of foods relatively high in calcium is given in Appendix N, Table N-2. Most adolescents, especially females, have calcium intakes below the recommended levels (see Appendix C). Preoccupation with being thin is common in this age group, especially among females, as is the misconception that all dairy foods are fattening. Many children and adolescents are unaware that low-fat milk contains at least as much calcium as whole milk.

Knowledge of dietary calcium sources is a first step toward increasing the intake of calcium-rich foods. The largest source of dietary calcium for most persons is milk and other dairy products. Most vegetables contain calcium, although at low density. Therefore, relatively large servings are needed to equal the total intake achieved with typical servings of dairy products. The bioavailability of calcium from vegetables is generally high. An exception is spinach, which is high in oxalate, making the calcium virtually non-bioavailable. Several products have been introduced that are fortified with calcium. These products, most notably orange juice, are fortified to achieve a calcium concentration similar to that of milk. Breakfast foods also are frequently fortified with minerals, including calcium.

Several alternatives exist for children with lactose intolerance. Lactose intolerance is more common in African Americans, Mexican Americans, and Asian Pacific Islanders than in whites. Many children with lactose intolerance can drink small amounts of milk without discomfort. Other alternatives include the use of other dairy products, such as solid cheeses and yogurt, which may be better tolerated than milk. Lactose-free and low-lactose milks are available. Increasing the intake of nondairy products, such as vegetables, may be helpful, as may the use of calcium-supplemented foods.

Dietary Sources: Magnesium

Most foods contain useful amounts of magnesium. Quantities in infant formulas range from 40 to 70 mg/L (3.3 to 5.8 mEq/L). Whole grains, beans, and legumes are good sources. As magnesium is a component of chlorophyll, green leafy vegetables are high in magnesium. Other dietary sources include milk, eggs, and meat. Depending on its "hardness," water may also significantly contribute to dietary magnesium intake.

References

1. Cohn SH, Vaswani A, Zanzi I, Aloia JF, Roginsky MS, Ellis KJ. Changes in body chemical composition with age measured by total-body neutron activation. *Metabolism.* 1976;25:85–95
2. Widdowson EM, Spray CM. Chemical development in utero. *Arch Dis Child.* 1951; 26:205–214
3. Widdowson EM, McCance RA, Spray CM. The chemical composition of the human body. *Clin Sci (Lond).* 1951;10:113–125
4. Broadus AE. Physiological functions of calcium, magnesium, and phosphorus and mineral ion balance. In: Favus MJ, ed. *Primer on the Metabolic Bone Diseases and Disorders of Mineral Metabolism.* 2nd ed. New York, NY: Raven Press; 1993:41–46
5. Salle BL, Delvin EE, Lapillonne A, Bishop NJ, Glorieux FH. Perinatal metabolism of vitamin D. *Am J Clin Nutr.* 2000;71:1317S–1324S

6. Bronner F, Pansu D. Nutritional aspects of calcium absorption. *J Nutr.* 1999; 129:9–12

7. Kim Y, Linkswiler HM. Effect of level of protein intake on calcium metabolism and on parathyroid and renal function in the adult human male. *J Nutr.* 1979;109: 1399–1404

8. Institute of Medicine, Food and Nutrition Board: Dietary Reference Intakes for Calcium, Phosphorus, Magnesium, Vitamin D, and Fluoride. Washington, DC: National Academy Press; 1997

9. Hardwick LL, Jones MR, Brautbar N, Lee DB. Magnesium absorption: mechanisms and the influence of vitamin D, calcium, and phosphate. *J Nutr.* 1991;121:13–23

10. Fomon SJ, Nelson SE. *Calcium, Phosphorus, Magnesium, and Sulfur: Nutrition of Normal Infants.* St Louis, MO: Mosby-Year Book, Inc; 1993:192–218

11. Shils ME. Magnesium in health and disease. *Annu Rev Nutr.* 1988;8:429–460

12. Yamamoto T, Kabata H, Yagi R, Takashima M, Itokawa Y. Primary hypomagnesemia with secondary hypocalcemia: report of a case and review of the world literature. *Magnesium.* 1985;4:153–164

13. National Institutes of Health Consensus Conference. Optimal Calcium Intake. *JAMA.* 1994;272:1942–1948

14. American Academy of Pediatrics, Committee on Nutrition. Calcium requirements of infants, children, and adolescents. *Pediatrics.* 1999;104:1152–1157

15. Miller GD, Weaver CM. Required versus optimal intakes: a look at calcium. *J Nutr.* 1994;124:1404S–1405S

16. Jackman LA, Millane SS, Martin BR, et al. Calcium retention in relation to calcium intake and postmenarcheal age in adolescent females. *Am J Clin Nutr.* 1997;66: 327–333

17. Abrams SA, Stuff JE. Calcium metabolism in girls: current dietary intakes lead to low rates of calcium absorption and retention during puberty. *Am J Clin Nutr.* 1994;60:739–743

18. Abrams SA, Grusak MA, Stuff J, O'Brien KO. Calcium and magnesium balance in 9–14-y-old children. *Am J Clin Nutr.* 1997;66:1172–1177

19. Ellis KJ, Abrams SA, Wong WW. Body composition in a young multiethnic female population. *Am J Clin Nutr.* 1997;65:724–731

20. Christiansen C, Rodbro P, Nielsen CT. Bone mineral content and estimated total body calcium in normal children and adolescents. *Scand J Clin Lab Invest.* 1975; 35:507–510

21. Atkinson SA. Human milk feeding of the micropremie. *Clin Perinatol.* 2000;27: 235–247

22. Schanler RJ, Abrams SA. Postnatal attainment of intrauterine macromineral accretion rates in low birth weight infants fed fortified human milk? *J Pediatr.* 1995; 126:441–447

23. Abrams SA, Esteban NV, Vieira NE, Yergey AL. Dual tracer stable isotopic assessment of calcium absorption and endogenous fecal excretion in low birth weight infants. *Pediatr Res.* 1991;29:615–618

24. Prestridge LL, Schanler RJ, Shulman RJ, Burns PA, Laine LL. Effect of parenteral calcium and phosphorus therapy on mineral retention and bone mineral content in very low birth weight infants. *J Pediatr.* 1993;122;761–768

25. Specker BL, Beck A, Kalkwarf H, Ho M. Randomized trial of varying mineral intake on total body bone mineral accretion during the first year of life. *Pediatrics.* 1997;99:E12

26. Ames SK, Gorham BM, Abrams SA. Effects of high versus low calcium intake on calcium absorption and incorporation of iron by red blood cells in small children. *Am J Clin Nutr.* 1999;70:44–48

27. Ilich-Ernst JZ, McKenna AA, Badenhop NE, et al. Iron status, menarche, and calcium supplementation in adolescent girls. *Am J Clin Nutr.* 1998;68:880–887

28. Lloyd T, Andon MB, Rollings N, et al. Calcium supplementation and bone mineral density in adolescent girls. *JAMA.* 1993;270:841–844

29. Lee WT, Leung SS, Leung DM, Cheng JC. A follow-up study on the effects of calcium-supplement withdrawal and puberty on bone acquisition of children. *Am J Clin Nutr.* 1996;64:71–77

30. Goulding A, Cannan R, Williams SM, Gold EJ, Taylor RW, Lewis-Barned NJ. Bone mineral density in girls with forearm fractures. *J Bone Miner Res.* 1998;13:143–148

31. Heaney RP, Skillman TG. Calcium metabolism in normal human pregnancy. *J Clin Endocrinol Metab.* 1971;33: 661–670

32. Kalkwarf HJ, Specker BL, Bianchi DC, Ranz J, Ho M. The effect of calcium supplements on bone density during lactation and after weaning. *N Engl J Med.* 1997;337:523–528

33. Kalkwarf HJ, Specker BL. Bone mineral loss during lactation and recovery after weaning. *Obstet Gynecol.* 1995;86:26–32

34. Rude RK. Magnesium deficiency: a cause of heterogeneous disease in humans. *J Bone Miner Res.* 1998;13:749–758

19

Iron Deficiency

Iron deficiency is the most common nutritional deficiency in the United States, affecting mainly older infants, young children, and women of childbearing age. Preterm infants, growth-retarded infants, and infants of mothers with diabetes are born with low iron stores and are therefore at risk for early iron deficiency. Young children are the most susceptible to iron deficiency as a result of an increased iron requirement related to rapid growth during the first 2 years of life and a relatively low iron content in most infant diets when iron is not added by supplementation or fortification. On the basis of the third National Health and Nutrition Examination Survey (NHANES III, 1989–1994) results, 9% of children younger than 3 years have evidence of iron deficiency based on iron biochemistry tests, and a third of them are also anemic.[1] Children 3 to 11 years old are at less risk for iron deficiency until the rapid growth period that occurs during puberty. Adolescent females are at greater risk for iron deficiency because of blood lost through menstruation. Adolescent athletes also have a higher rate of iron deficiency.

During the past 2 decades, significant improvements have been made in the iron nutritional status of infants and young children in the United States. Several studies have demonstrated a significant reduction in the prevalence of anemia.[2] Concurrent with the decline in the prevalence of childhood anemia among younger children, changes were made in infant feeding patterns, including increased dietary iron content or iron bioavailability. Other changes included an increase in breastfeeding and the use of iron-fortified formula with a concomitant reduction in the use of whole milk and low-iron formula during the first year of life. The American Academy of Pediatrics (AAP) statement on Iron Fortification of Infant Formulas recommends discontinuing manufacturing of low-iron formulas and that infant formulas be fortified with 4.0 to 12 mg/L of iron.[3] This encouraging trend of improved iron status related to better dietary practices during infancy underscores the importance of primary prevention for the control of childhood iron deficiency.

One consequence of the lower prevalence of iron deficiency anemia is the limited ability to use anemia as a screening indicator for iron deficiency. Because iron deficiency is becoming a less common cause of anemia in general, the presence of anemia is increasingly a poorer predictor for iron deficiency. Therefore, approaches to maintain optimal childhood iron nutrition should continue the emphasis on primary prevention with sound iron nutrition during infancy and selective use of anemia testing for the subset of children whose background indicates a greater risk for iron deficiency.[2,4] These subsets include premature infants, intrauterine growth-retarded infants, breastfed infants greater than 6 months old not receiving iron supplementation, infants fed low-iron formula, and children living at or below the poverty level.

Consequences of Iron Deficiency

The most well-known consequence of iron deficiency is anemia. However, unless severe (hemoglobin, <8 g/dL), anemia in itself does not constitute a grave threat to health. Rather, it is an indicator of the severity of iron deficiency. The majority of infants in negative iron balance have iron deficiency without anemia (characterized by low-serum ferritin concentrations reflecting low iron stores). A smaller percentage has the more advanced finding of iron deficiency anemia. It is important to recognize that anemia represents the most severe end of the iron deficiency spectrum since iron is prioritized to the red blood cells at the expense of all other tissues, including the brain. The limitation of screening for iron deficiency by routine hemoglobin testing is that by the time anemia is diagnosed, the neurologic consequences have already occurred.

Among the major consequences of iron deficiency that have been studied, the evidence that significant iron deficiency adversely affects child development and behavior is of greatest concern. There are now 40 studies that have investigated the adverse effect of early iron deficiency on neurodevelopmental outcome.[5] Both cognitive and motor deficits have been documented.[5,6] The developmental deficits, to some extent, can be corrected with iron treatment.[7] However, evidence also showed that some deficits were not reversible with iron treatment.[8] The threat of irreversible developmental delay due to a temporary nutritional deficiency emphasizes the importance of prevention. It is the tissue-level iron deficiency that likely results in the neurobehavioral consequences.

Another health consequence of iron deficiency is enhanced lead absorption. Animal and human studies have demonstrated that gastrointestinal absorption of lead increases with the severity of iron deficiency.[9] Clinical and epidemiologic studies also demonstrate an association between an elevated blood lead level and iron deficiency.[10] Because childhood lead poisoning is a well-documented cause of neurologic and developmental deficits, iron deficiency appears to contribute to this problem directly and indirectly though increased absorption of lead.

Iron Metabolism and Factors Affecting Iron Balance

Iron in the body exists in 2 major forms: functional and stored. Most of the functional iron is in the form of heme iron as hemoglobin and myoglobin. A number of important enzymes, including those controlling cellular respiration, dopamine synthesis, and CNS myelination, require iron, even though these account for less than 1% of the total body iron. The stored iron in the form of ferritin and hemosiderin accumulates when a positive iron balance exists; stored iron can be mobilized to meet iron requirements when intake is low. Factors that affect iron stores, intake, and loss will determine iron status and the risk for iron deficiency.

Iron Stores

Infants are born with an endowment of iron stores. The amount of iron in storage is proportional to birth weight or size. On average, the iron stores in an appropriate-for-gestational-age full-term infant can meet the infant's iron requirement until 4 to 6 months of age.[11] For this reason, anemia screening for iron deficiency before 4 to 6 months is of little value. Because preterm and low-birth-weight infants are born with much less stored iron and because they experience a greater rate of growth during infancy, their iron stores become depleted much earlier than those of full-term infants, often by 2 to 3 months of age. Therefore, low-birth-weight and preterm infants are more vulnerable to iron deficiency. Twenty-six percent to 86% of preterm infants <1500 g birth weight are at risk for iron deficiency if fed a diet containing less than 2 mg/kg/d of iron. After the exhaustion of iron stores up to 24 months of age, maintaining substantial iron stores, even when iron intake is adequate, is difficult because of the increased iron required for rapid growth. During this period, a low or depleted iron store per se, as reflected by low serum ferritin, does not meet the definition of iron deficiency anemia, but does classify the child as iron deficient. After the liver iron stores are depleted, as reflected by a ferritin concentration below the fifth percentile for age, iron-related physiologic functions are compromised. After 2 years of age, as growth velocity is reduced to a lower baseline, iron stores start to accumulate, and the risk for iron deficiency declines.

Iron Intake and Factors Affecting Iron Absorption

An adult man absorbs about 1 mg/d of iron, an amount equivalent to iron losses through desquamation of intestinal and skin cells. Infants between 4 and 12 months of age, on average, absorb almost as much: 0.8 mg/d. However, in contrast to the adult, three fourths of this amount is needed for growth and one fourth is needed to replace losses. The dietary source of iron strongly influences the efficiency of its absorption. The amount of iron absorption from a variety of foods ranges from less than 1% to more than 50% in the case of human milk. Foods of vegetable origin are at the lower end of the range, dairy products are in the middle, and meat is at the upper end. About 4% of the iron in fortified infant formulas is absorbed, and about 10% of the small amount of iron in unfortified formulas or whole milk is absorbed. The content of iron in breast milk is comparable to that of unmodified cow milk (ie, not iron-fortified formula), but 50% of the iron in breast milk can be absorbed. Therefore, breast milk is a better source of iron than nonfortified formula or cow milk. However, the better absorption efficiency of breast milk does not entirely compensate for the relatively low iron content. By about 6 months of age, term breastfed infants require an additional source of iron in their diets to meet their iron requirement. Infants born prematurely and/or with lower birth weights, or those with rapid growth in the early months of life or with some medical conditions, may benefit from an additional source before 6 months. Because milk-based diets make up most of the energy consumed during the first year of life, the iron content of various milk products and their absorption efficiency is a strong predictor of iron nutrition status.[12] For practical purposes, infants who consume primarily iron-fortified formula have about an 8% risk for iron deficiency and less than 1% risk for iron deficiency anemia. Those consuming nonfortified formula or whole cow milk have a 30% to 40% risk of iron deficiency by 9 to 12 months. Infants who are exclusively breastfed have a 20% risk of iron deficiency by 9 to 12 months of age.

In the United States, major nonmilk sources of iron in the infant diet are iron-fortified cereal and meats. The absorption of reduced iron of small particle size, used to fortify infant cereals, is estimated to be about 4%. Meat is a good source of iron because most iron is in the form of heme iron that has an absorption efficiency of 10% to 20%, 2 to 3 times of that for nonheme iron (2% to 7%). Nonheme iron found in plant foods and fortified food products is less well absorbed, and the absorption is strongly influenced by the other foods ingested at the same meal. Ascorbic acid and an unknown component of meat are among the most potent enhancers of nonheme iron absorption. Tea, bran, and milk tend to inhibit nonheme iron absorption from the meal with which they are consumed. Normally, the diet contains 5 to 20 times the amount of iron absorbed.

Iron Loss

The normal turnover of intestinal mucosa with some blood loss can be regarded as physiologic, and this blood loss is considered in the daily requirement. For the same reason, normal menstrual blood loss is an obligatory or physiologic loss. The most common reason for abnormal blood loss in infants and younger children is the sensitivity of some children to the protein in cow milk, resulting in increased gastrointestinal occult blood loss.[13] For this reason, consumption of whole cow milk carries 2 risk factors for iron deficiency during infancy—low iron content and increased fecal blood loss in some infants. In some tropical countries, hookworm infection is a major cause of gastrointestinal blood loss, but this is not a problem in the United States. Gastrointestinal disorders, such as peptic ulcer disease and inflammatory bowel disease, can obviously cause increased blood loss and, therefore, iron loss.

Assessment of Iron Status

A number of laboratory tests can be used to assess iron nutritional status, including serum ferritin, free erythrocyte protoporphyrin, zinc protoporphyrin/heme ratio, transferrin saturation, transferrin receptors, and hemoglobin or hematocrit. These tests reflect different aspects of iron metabolism and together can characterize the iron nutritional status as a spectrum from overload to severe deficiency. The earliest finding when iron intake does not match iron requirements is a decrease in serum ferritin, which, under most circumstances, reflects reduced liver iron stores. Intervention at that time most likely prevents any physiologic consequences of iron deficiency, including anemia. However, the serum ferritin concentration is not a widely available test and factors other than low iron stores, such as an inflammatory process, can alter the value. For these reasons, the Centers for Disease Control and Prevention (CDC) does not advocate its use as a general screening tool for iron deficiency in spite of its advantage of early detection compared with hemoglobin screening.[14] After the ferritin concentration has decreased, evidence of pre-anemic disordered erythropoiesis occurs with increases in serum transferrin and protoporphyrin concentrations. Again, these assessments are not currently designed for large-scale population screening but can be used to assess the iron status of specific at-risk patients. The CDC and the AAP currently recommend periodic assessment of hemoglobin or hematocrit as a screening tool for iron deficiency although anemia represents the most severe end of the iron deficiency spectrum. Figure 19.1 details the spectrum of iron status in relation to the major tests available for clinical application.

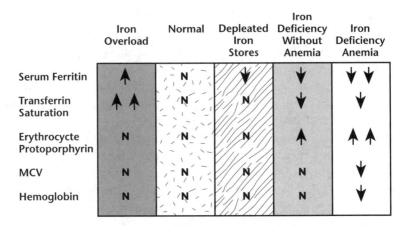

	Iron Overload	Normal	Depleted Iron Stores	Iron Deficiency Without Anemia	Iron Deficiency Anemia
Serum Ferritin	↑	N	↓	↓	↓↓
Transferrin Saturation	↑↑	N	N	↓	↓
Erythrocyte Protoporphyrin	N	N	N	↑	↑↑
MCV	N	N	N	N	↓
Hemoglobin	N	N	N	N	↓

Figure 19.1. The spectrum of iron status in relation to the major tests available for clinical application. MCV indicates mean corpuscular volume; ↑, increased; ↑↑, markedly increased; ↓, decreased; ↓↓, markedly decreased; and N, normal.

Screening for Iron Deficiency

Although a number of biochemical tests can be used to define iron deficiency, for practical purposes, anemia screening, using hemoglobin or hematocrit, is the main approach in a general pediatric setting. Anemia is defined as a hemoglobin or hematocrit level below the fifth percentile of an age- and gender-specific US representative sample after excluding persons with biochemical evidence of iron deficiency (Table 19.1). On the basis of this definition, even in a population free of iron deficiency, about 5% of the children would be expected to meet the criteria for anemia. This type of baseline or statistical anemia among healthy children becomes a substantial source of false-positive cases of iron deficiency when iron deficiency anemia is uncommon. The other assessments listed previously or a trial response to iron supplementation can be used as adjunctive evidence to confirm or rule out iron deficiency. Beyond iron deficiency, a number of other common causes of mild anemia exist. Among younger children, current and recent infection can cause mild anemia. Among African American and certain Asian American populations, mild hereditary anemia, such as thalassemia traits, can play a role. A common reason for suspecting mild anemia is the imprecision of hemoglobin determination related to capillary blood sampling or the accuracy of the instrument. For this reason, confirmation of anemia by a second test or by venous puncture can eliminate many false-positive results. Table 19.2 summarizes some of the common

Table 19.1.

Estimated Normal Mean Values and Lower Limits of Normal (Fifth Percentile) for Hemoglobin and Hematocrit*

| Age, y | Hemoglobin, g/dL | | Hematocrit, % | |
	Mean	Lower Limit	Mean	Lower Limit
0.5–1.9	12.3	11.0	35.9	32.9
2.0–4.9	12.5	11.1	36.3	33.0
5.0–7.9	12.8	11.5	37.2	34.5
8.0–11.9	13.2	11.9	38.4	35.4
Female				
12.0–14.9	13.4	11.8	39.0	35.7
15.0–17.9	13.5	12.0	39.0	35.9
≥18	13.5	12.0	39.0	35.7
Male				
12.0–14.9	14.0	12.5	40.5	37.3
15.0–17.9	14.8	13.3	43.0	39.7
≥18	15.3	13.5	44.5	39.9

*All data are based on venous blood samples after excluding individuals with laboratory evidence of iron deficiency or inflammatory disease. Adapted from Yip R, et al. Age-related changes in laboratory values used in the diagnosis of anemia and iron deficiency. *Am J Clin Nutr.* 1984;39:427–436; and Centers for Disease Control and Prevention. CDC criteria for anemia in children and childbearing-aged women. *MMWR Morb Mortal Wkly Rep.* 1989;38:400–404 and reference 14.

Table 19.2.

Major Causes of Anemia or Reasons for Low Hemoglobin or Hematocrit Values*

True Anemia
Iron deficiency
Anemia related to recent or current infections
Hereditary defects in red blood cell production or hemoglobinopathies Thalassemia trait, sickle cell trait, glucose-6-phosphate dehydrogenase deficiency
Chronic illness or inflammatory conditions
False Anemia
Technical anemia: result of inadequate testing instrument or inadequate capillary blood sampling
Statistical anemia or normal variation: the criteria for anemia are set at a level at which some healthy children can be classified as anemic

*Adapted from Yip R. Changing characteristics of iron nutritional status in the United States. In: Filer LJ, ed. *Dietary Iron: Birth to Two Years.* New York, NY: Raven Press; 1989 reasons for anemia. Evidence is increasing that African American children and adults have lower hemoglobin values than do their white counterparts and that this difference is not due to differences in iron status.[15] For this reason, if the purpose of anemia screening is to detect children with the likelihood of iron deficiency, the hemoglobin cutoff value for African American children can be adjusted downward by 0.3 g/dL of hemoglobin or 1% of hematocrit to achieve a comparable screening performance for iron deficiency.

In recent years, a simplified outpatient laboratory method to measure erythrocyte protoporphyrin, the hematoflorameter method, has been used for screening for childhood lead poisoning. Because most children with elevated erythrocyte protoporphyrin have iron deficiency, this simplified test can also be used for screening for iron deficiency, although the lack of ubiquity of the hematoflorameter currently keeps it from replacing hemoglobin as the screening tool. An advantage of the method is that it is likely elevated in iron deficiency before anemia is present.[16] Only a minority of children with elevated erythrocyte protoporphyrin actually have elevated blood lead levels. The screening cutoff for erythrocyte protoporphyrin is 35 μg/dL of whole blood or 3.0 μg/g of hemoglobin. Blood lead testing programs use erythrocyte protoporphyrin as a screening test for lead poisoning; however, this test is still useful for screening for iron deficiency.

Diagnosis of Iron Deficiency

Anemia screening enables the identification of children who are at risk for iron deficiency. However, because anemia is not specific for iron deficiency, only a presumptive diagnosis can be made. Two approaches can be used to diagnose iron deficiency when a child has anemia. One approach is to use the hemoglobin response to oral iron treatment as a diagnosis of iron deficiency. An increase of the hemoglobin level by 1.0 g/dL or more by the 1-month follow-up is a positive response. The other approach is the application of one or more of the iron-related tests for biochemical evidence of iron deficiency. Among the multiple tests that can be used, serum ferritin appears to be the best confirmatory test. A low serum ferritin level (<15 μg/L) is the most specific laboratory finding for iron deficiency. If a child with anemia does not experience a substantial hemoglobin response after 1 month of oral iron treatment, the laboratory evaluation for iron deficiency is also indicated. Beyond biochemical tests such as serum ferritin, a complete blood cell count is also helpful. The mean corpuscular volume (MCV), red blood cell (RBC) count, and red blood cell distribution width (RDW) can provide valuable clues for differentiating iron deficiency from other forms of microcytic anemia or other types of anemia.[17]

Specific Recommendations

Because dietary intake during infancy is a strong determinant of iron status for older infants and younger children, the specific recommendations emphasize the role of a dietary approach for the primary prevention of iron deficiency in younger children. The epidemiologic evidence indicates that secondary prevention through anemia screening and treatment is of limited value among children who had a sound infant diet and can best be used for children who are at higher risk for iron deficiency.[2,4,14]

Dietary Recommendations for Infants and Children Younger Than 3 Years

Breastfed Infants

1. Full-term appropriate-for-gestational-age breastfed infants need a supplemental source of iron starting at 4 to 6 months of age (approximately 1 mg/kg/d) preferably from complementary foods. Iron-fortified infant cereal and/or meats are a good source of iron for initial introduction of an iron-containing food. An average of 2 servings ($^1/_2$ oz or 15 g of dry cereal per serving) is needed to meet the daily iron requirement.
2. If a full-term breastfed infant is unable to consume sufficient iron from dietary sources after 6 months of age, elemental iron, 1 mg/kg/d, should be used.
3. For breastfed preterm or low-birth-weight infants, an oral iron supplement (elemental iron) in the form of drops once a day at 2 mg/kg/d starting at 1 month should be given until 12 months of age. The dose of iron (1 mg/kg) in a vitamin preparation with iron is not likely to provide sufficient iron for the preterm breastfed infant.
4. For all infants younger than 12 months, only iron-fortified formula (10 to 12 mg/L) should be used for weaning or supplementing breast milk.

Formula-Fed Infants

1. For full-term and preterm infants, only iron-fortified formula should be used during the first year of life regardless of the age when infant formula is started. All soy-based formulas are iron fortified to 12 mg/L. Current preterm infant and preterm discharge formulas also contain 12 mg/L of iron and thus supply approximately 1.8 mg/kg/d to the average preterm

infant consuming 150 cc/kg/d of formula. This dose is less than the recommended 2 to 4 mg of iron/kg/d. Therefore, formula-fed preterm infants may benefit from an additional 1 mg/kg/d, which can be administered as either iron drops or in a vitamin preparation with iron.

2. No common medical indication exists for the use of a low-iron formula. The AAP has recommended the discontinuation of the manufacture of low-iron formula and that all infant formulas contain at least 4 mg/L of iron. Although some believe that iron-fortified formula increases gastrointestinal symptoms, no scientific evidence supports this belief, so using non-iron-fortified formula for healthy infants is not justified.

Solid Foods

The specific recommendations related to solid foods are more crucial for breast-fed infants than for formula-fed infants to ensure adequate iron nutrition.

1. Introduce iron-fortified infant cereal or meat between 4 and 6 months of age or when the child is developmentally ready (able to sit up and swallow such food).*

2. The iron content of selected foods is listed in Appendix N, Table N-2.

Milk

1. Avoid the use of regular cow, goat, or soy milk for the milk-based part of the diet before 12 months of age.

2. For young children, avoid excessive milk intake, which can displace the desire for food items with greater iron content. A milk intake of 24 oz/d is sufficient to meet the daily calcium requirement of children 1 to 5 years old.

Young Children

Iron deficiency and iron deficiency anemia continue to be a problem into the second postnatal year with an incidence of about 10%.[18-20] The cause of this high incidence is unknown, but may relate to the large numbers of infants born with low iron stores (infants of diabetic mothers, intrauterine growth-retarded infants and premature infants); or to those with low dietary intake of iron in the first postnatal year (breastfed infants, infants fed low-iron formula,

---

*There is a difference of opinion among AAP experts on this matter. The Committee on Nutrition acknowledges that the Section on Breastfeeding recommends exclusive breastfeeding for at least 6 months.

and infants switched to cow milk before 12 months of age). The rate is unacceptably high for public health purposes and reasonable attempts should be made to reduce it. It may be prudent to supplement high-risk children with iron in the form of a daily vitamin with iron during the second year, especially if the child does not have a source of meat-based iron in the diet.

Screening and Treatment of Iron Deficiency Anemia

Anemia Screening

Two options are available. The universal screening option is for communities and populations in which a significant level of iron deficiency anemia exists or for infants whose diet puts them at risk for iron deficiency. Selective screening is for communities or practices with low rates of anemia (5% or less) and generally good infant dietary practices related to iron nutrition. Selective screening is also targeted at the subset of children who have a less than satisfactory diet, for example, early introduction of cow milk or use of low-iron formula, or who have particular medical risks, such as prematurity or low birth weight.

Option 1: *Universal Screening.* Initial measurement of hemoglobin or hematocrit for all full-term infants between 9 and 12 months of age and a second screening 6 months after the initial screening at 15 to 18 months.

Option 2: *Selective Screening.* Same schedule as universal screening except that only infants and children deemed to be at risk are screened. Infants at risk include preterm infants, low-birth-weight infants, infants not receiving iron-fortified formula, and breastfed infants older than 6 months who are not consuming a diet with adequate iron content.

Note: Anemia screening before 6 months of age is of little value for the detection of iron deficiency because iron stores are adequate for most infants except the preterm infant. In the preterm infant, iron stores at birth are sufficient for 2 to 3 months postnatally. Although no official recommendations exist for screening for iron status in preterm infants, it may be prudent to screen these infants at approximately 4 months. The highest risk group appears to be infants born prior to 32 weeks' gestation who were not transfused, or who received recombinant erythropoietin, and were subsequently not supplemented with iron. After 2 years of age, routine screening is not indicated because few children in the United States have iron deficiency anemia after this time. For children at risk for iron deficiency because of special health needs, a low-iron diet (eg, nonmeat diet), or environmental factors (eg, poverty or limited access to food), annual screening for anemia can be considered between 2 and 5 years of age.

Treatment and Follow-up

1. Anemia (low hemoglobin or hematocrit measurement) based on capillary blood sampling should be confirmed by subsequent measurement of hemoglobin and hematocrit. After confirmation of anemia, the presumptive iron deficiency anemia can be treated with oral (elemental) iron, 3 to 6 mg/kg/d, for 4 weeks.

2. Repeat the hemoglobin or hematocrit measurement in 4 weeks. An increase of the hemoglobin level of more than 1 g/dL or of the hematocrit value of more than 3% confirms iron deficiency anemia. Continue iron treatment for another 2 months and recheck the measurements. Assess the hemoglobin level or hematocrit value about 6 months after successful treatment.

3. If the hemoglobin level or hematocrit value does not increase after 4 weeks of iron treatment, further laboratory evaluation is indicated. This recommendation assumes that the child is not ill, because illness, such as upper respiratory tract infection, otitis, and diarrhea, can cause a significant reduction in the hemoglobin level and hematocrit value. Two suggested tests are as follows:

   - Red blood cell indices by electronic blood counter: a low MCV ($<$70 fL) and RBC count ($<4.0 \times 10^{12}$/L) suggest iron deficiency, and a low MCV ($<$70 fL) and relatively high RBC count ($>4.8 \times 10^{12}$/L) suggest hereditary anemia, such as thalassemia trait; RDW more than 17 suggests iron deficiency; a normal RDW is consistent with thalassemia trait.

   - Serum ferritin: a serum ferritin below 15 μg/L confirms iron deficiency. A value equal to or higher than 15 μg/L suggests that a cause other than iron deficiency is more likely responsible for the anemia.

Recommendations for School-aged Children

Preadolescent school-aged children are at less risk for iron deficiency in the United States unless their diet is very restricted. For this reason, routine anemia screening may not be necessary. Selective anemia screening is indicated for children who consume a strict vegetarian diet and are not receiving an iron supplement.

Adolescents

Adolescent males are at risk near the peak growth period when iron stores may not meet the demand of rapid growth. However, the iron deficiency anemia generally corrects itself after the growth spurt. For adolescent females, menstrual blood loss increases the risk of iron deficiency. For this reason, anemia screening of adolescent females is indicated.

1. *Male*—Screen for anemia during routine physical examination during the peak growth period.
2. *Female*—Screen for anemia during all routine physical examinations.

Treatment and Follow-up for Anemia

As with younger children, an oral iron trial for 4 weeks should be performed. If substantial increases in the hemoglobin level or hematocrit value are not seen, laboratory evaluation is indicated.

References

1. Looker AC, Dallman PR, Carroll MD, Gunter EW, Johnson CL. Prevalence of iron deficiency in the United States. *JAMA*. 1997;277:973–976
2. Dallman PR, Yip R. Changing characteristics of childhood anemia. *J Pediatr*. 1989;114:161–164
3. American Academy of Pediatrics, Committee on Nutrition. Iron fortification of infant formulas. *Pediatrics*. 1999;104:119–123
4. Earl R, Woteki CE, eds. *Iron Deficiency Anemia: Recommended Guidelines for Prevention, Detection and Management Among U.S. Children and Women of Childbearing Age*. Washington, DC: National Academy Press; 1993
5. Nokes C, van den Bosch C, Bundy DAP. *The Eeffects of Iron Deficiency and Anemia on Mental and Motor Performance, Educational Achievement and Behavior in Children: A Report of the International Nutritional Anemia Consultative Group*. Washington, DC: INACG; 1998
6. Lozoff B. Behavioral alterations in iron deficiency. *Adv Pediatr*. 1988;35:331–359
7. Idjradinata P, Pollitt E. Reversal of developmental delays in iron-deficient anemic infants treated with iron. *Lancet*. 1993;341:1–4
8. Lozoff B, Jimenez E, Hagen J, Mollen E, Wolf AW. Poorer behavioral and developmental outcome more than 10 years after treatment for iron deficiency in infancy. *Pediatrics*. 2000;105:E51
9. Watson WS, Hume R, Moore MR. Oral absorption of lead and iron. *Lancet*. 1980;2:236–237
10. Centers for Disease Control. *Preventing Lead Poisoning in Young Children: A Statement by the Centers for Disease Control*. Atlanta, GA: Centers for Disease Control; 1985. Report No. 99–2230
11. Dallman PR, Siimes MA, Stekel A. Iron deficiency in infancy and childhood. *Am J Clin Nutr*. 1980;33:86–118
12. Pizarro F, Yip R, Dallman PR, Olivares M, Hertrampf E, Walter T. Iron status with different infant feeding regimens: relevance to screening and prevention of iron deficiency. *J Pediatr*. 1991;118:687–692

13. Ziegler EE, Fomon SJ, Nelson SE, et al. Cow milk feeding in infancy: further observations on blood loss from the gastrointestinal tract. *J Pediatr*. 1990;116:11–18

14. Center for Disease Control and Prevention. Recommendations for preventing and controlling iron deficiency in the United States. *MMWR Morb Mortal Wkly Rep*. 1998;47(RR-3):1–36

15. Johnson-Spear MA, Yip R. Hemoglobin difference between black and white women with comparable iron status: justification for race-specific anemia criteria. *Am J Clin Nutr*. 1994;60:117–121

16. Yip R, Schwartz S, Deinard AS. Screening for iron deficiency with erythrocyte protoporphyrin test. *Pediatrics*. 1983;72:214–219

17. Glader BE. Screening for anemia and erythrocyte disorders in children. *Pediatrics*. 1986;78:368–369

18. Eden AN, Mir MA. Iron deficiency in 1- to-3-year old children. A pediatric failure? *Arch Pediatr Adolesc Med*. 1997;151:986–988

19. Brugnara C, Zurakowski D, Dficanzio J, Boyd T, Platt O. Reticulocyte hemoglobin content to diagnose iron deficiency anemia in children. *JAMA*. 1999;281:2225–2230

20. Bogen DL, Duggan AK, Dover GJ, Wilson MH. Screening for iron deficiency by dietary history in a high-risk population. *Pediatrics*. 2000;105:1254–1259

20
Trace Elements

An element is considered to be a trace element when it constitutes less than 0.01% of total body weight. Trace elements are essential to metabolic processes because they are components of many enzyme systems and act as integral components of metalloenzymes or cofactors for enzymes activated by metal ions. Trace element deficiencies have been reported in humans and can be deleterious to health, growth, and development. Because effects of deficiency are frequently most severe during periods of rapid growth, trace element deficiencies are of special concern to pediatricians. Thirteen trace elements are believed to be nutritionally important for higher animals. These trace elements, in order of importance to children, are iron, zinc, copper, fluoride, iodine, selenium, manganese, chromium, cobalt, molybdenum, nickel, silicon, and vanadium. All these trace elements are discussed in this chapter except iron and fluoride, which are discussed in Chapters 19 and 48.

The Food and Nutrition Board of the Institute of Medicine, National Academy of Sciences, has recently established Dietary Reference Intakes (DRIs) for humans for zinc, copper, manganese, chromium, iodine, molybdenum, and selenium, which is a framework containing 4 sets of standards: Estimated Average Requirements (EARs), Recommended Dietary Allowances (RDAs), Adequate Intakes (AIs), and Tolerable Upper Intake Levels (Upper Levels or ULs).[1] The RDA is the nutrient intake that is sufficient to meet the needs for nearly all individuals (~97%) in an age and gender group. The RDAs (or, if not yet established, the AIs) of the major trace minerals discussed in this chapter are shown in Table 20.1 (see also Appendix C). The table also summarizes biochemical actions, effects of deficiency, effects of excess, and food sources of the trace elements.

Zinc

Zinc is an essential cofactor for many enzymes with a multitude of functions.[2] These enzymes are involved in nucleic acid and protein metabolism. In many species, including humans, zinc deficiency has limited growth prenatally and in

Table 20.1.
Trace Elements

Name/Normal Serum Values	Biochemical Action	Effects of Deficiency	Effects of Excess	Recommended Dietary Allowance (RDA) or Adequate Intake*	Food Sources
Zinc (Zn)/ 0.75–1.20 mg/L or 11.5–18.5 μmol/L	Components of many enzymes and transcription factors	Anorexia, hypogeusia, retarded growth, delayed sexual maturation, impaired wound healing, skin lesions	Few toxic effects; may aggravate marginal copper deficiency	Infants, 0–6 mo 2 mg/d* 7–12 mo 3 mg/d Children, 1–3 y 3 mg/d 4–8 y 5 mg/d Males, 9–13 y 8 mg/d 14–18 y 11 mg/d Females, 9–13 y 8 mg/d 14–18 y 9 mg/d	Oysters, liver, meat, cheese, legumes, whole grains
Copper (Cu)/ 1.10–1.45 mg/L or 11–22 μmol/L	Constituent of ceruloplasmin; component of key metalloenzymes; role in connective tissue biosynthesis	Sideroblastic anemia, retarded growth, osteoporosis, neutropenia, decreased pigmentation	Few toxic effects; Wilson disease, liver dysfunction	Infants, 0–6 mo 0.20 mg/d* 7–12 mo 0.22 mg/d* Children, 1–3 y 0.34 mg/d 4–8 y 0.44 mg/d Adolescents, 9–13 y 0.70 mg/d 14–18 y 0.89 mg/d	Shellfish, meat, legumes, nuts, cheese

Table 20.1.
Trace Elements (continued)

Name/Normal Serum Values	Biochemical Action	Effects of Deficiency	Effects of Excess	Recommended Dietary Allowance (RDA) or Adequate Intake*	Food Sources
Manganese (Mn)† 4–12 µg/L or 73–210 µmol/L	Activator of metal-enzyme complexes important for synthesis of polysaccharides and glycoproteins; constituent of pyruvate carboxylase and Mn-superoxide dismutase	Human, not documented; animals, growth retardation, ataxia of newborn, bone abnormalities, reduced fertility	Few toxic effects; neurologic manifestations from industrial contamination and in long-term TPN	Infants, 0–6 mo 0.003 mg/d* 7–12 mo 0.6 mg/d* Children, 1–3 y 1.2 mg/d* 4–8 y 1.5 mg/d* Males, 9–13 y 1.9 mg/d* 14–18 y 2.2 mg/d* Females, 9–13 y 1.6 mg/d* 14–18 y 1.6 mg/d*	Nuts, whole grains, tea
Selenium (Se)/ 30–75 µg/L or 0.35–1.00 µmol/L	Component of enzymes: glutathione peroxidase and deiodinase	Humans, cardiomyopathy; animals, hepatic necrosis, muscular dystrophy, exudative diathesis, pancreatic fibrosis	Irritation of mucous membranes (nose, eyes, upper respiratory tract), pallor, irritability, indigestion	Infants, 0–6 mo 15 µg/d* 7–12 mo 20 µg/d* Children, 1–3 y 20 µg/d* 4–8 y 30 µg/d* Adolescents, 9–13 y 40 µg/d* 14–18 y 55 µg/d*	Seafood, meat, whole grains

Table 20.1.
Trace Elements *(continued)*

Name/Normal Serum Values	Biochemical Action	Effects of Deficiency	Effects of Excess	Recommended Dietary Allowance (RDA) or Adequate Intake*	Food Sources
Chromium (Cr)	Required for maintenance of normal glucose metabolism; potentiates the action of insulin	Humans, impairment of glucose utilization; animals, impaired growth, disturbances of carbohydrate, protein, and lipid metabolism	Few toxic effects; humans, not well documented; animals, growth retardation, hepatic and kidney damage	Infants, 0–6 mo 0.2 $\mu g/d$* 7–12 mo 5.5 $\mu g/d$* Children, 1–3 y 11 $\mu g/d$* 4–8 y 15 $\mu g/d$* Males, 9–13 y 25 $\mu g/d$* 14–18 y 35 $\mu g/d$* Females, 9–13 y 21 $\mu g/d$* 14–18 y 24 $\mu g/d$*	Meat, cheese, whole grains, brewer's yeast
Cobalt (Co)	Component of vitamin B_{12}	Humans, unknown; animals, anemia, growth retardation	Few toxic effects; polycythemia, myocardial degeneration	Not established	Green leafy vegetables

Table 20.1.
Trace Elements *(continued)*

Name/Normal Serum Values	Biochemical Action	Effects of Deficiency	Effects of Excess	Recommended Dietary Allowance (RDA) or Adequate Intake*	Food Sources
Molybdenum (Mo)	Component of enzymes involved in production of uric acid (xanthine oxidase) and in oxidation of aldehydes and sulfides	Humans, unknown; animals: growth retardation, anorexia	Humans, gout-like syndrome, antagonist of copper	Infants, 0–6 mo 2 µg/d* 7–12 mo 3 µg/d* Children, 1–3 y 17 µg/d 4–8 y 22 µg/d Adolescents, 9–13 y 34 µg/d 14–18 y 43 µg/d	Meats, grains, legumes
Iodine (I)	Component of thyroid hormones (T₃, T₄)	Goiter, impaired mental function, delayed development	"Toxic goiter"	Infants, 0–6 mo 110 µg/d* 7–12 mo 130 µg/d* Children, 1–3 y 90 µg/d 4–8 y 90 µg/d Adolescents, 9–13 y 120 µg/d 14–18 y 150 µg/d	Iodized salt, dairy products, saltwater fish, seafood

*For healthy breastfed infants, the AI is the mean intake.
†Whole blood.

infants and children. The exact mechanism behind the decreased growth is not known, but zinc is an integral part of DNA and RNA polymerase, several transcription factors (in so-called zinc-fingers), and enzymes involved in energy metabolism, all possibly contributing to lower cellular activity during zinc deficiency. Cells and tissues that are turning over rapidly are first affected; the immune system, the intestinal mucosa, and the skin are impaired early during zinc deficiency.

Severe zinc deficiency in infants and children is characterized by acrodermatitis, gastrointestinal discomfort (diarrhea), and slow growth.[3] An autosomal recessive genetic disorder of zinc metabolism, acrodermatitis enteropathica, causes severe zinc deficiency by decreased cellular retention of zinc.[3] The signs are similar to those of dietary zinc deficiency, and the patients require daily zinc supplements for alleviation of all symptoms. In children, the proper daily dose may be difficult to determine, particularly during periods of rapid growth, and there is a risk of excessive doses causing copper deficiency.[4] Recovery from zinc deficiency is rapid after introduction of oral zinc; the violent dermatitis is often in complete remission within 4 to 5 days. Mild zinc deficiency in infants was first described by Walravens and Hambidge, who found slower than normal growth in male formula-fed infants[5] and lower plasma zinc levels[6] than in breastfed infants. Fortification of the formula to a zinc level of 5.8 mg/L led to normal growth. Several recent studies have shown a positive effect of zinc supplements on the growth of infants and children,[7,8] but others fail to show an effect.[9] Zinc status at baseline, dose given, growth rate, infections, compliance, etc, may be factors affecting the outcome. Whether the growth impairment in children with suboptimal zinc status is due to effects on hormonal mediators of growth, reduced appetite and food intake, or more frequent infections is not yet known.

Zinc status is often evaluated by measurement of the plasma or serum zinc level. However, neither is a sensitive indicator and can be affected by infection, stress, growth rate, and other factors.[10] Hair zinc level is sometimes used, but it is difficult to analyze and may be affected by factors other than zinc status.[11] When a zinc deficiency is suspected, a zinc supplementation trial (usually 1 mg/kg/d) may provide a response.[12] The supplement can be administered as a solution of zinc acetate (30 mg of zinc acetate in 5 mL of water). Infants with cystic fibrosis have been shown to have low plasma zinc concentrations and abnormal zinc homeostasis[13] and may therefore have a higher requirement for zinc.

Zinc absorption from breast milk has been shown to be high as compared with cow milk-based formula or cow milk.[14] Indirect support for this was obtained from the observation that infants with acrodermatitis enteropathica were symptom free while breastfed but not when fed formula, even when the zinc concentrations were similar. The higher bioavailability of zinc from breast milk may be because zinc is loosely bound to citrate and serum albumin in breast milk[15] but tightly bound to casein in cow milk and milk formula. Citrate-bound zinc is readily absorbed, and the limited digestive capacity of neonates may be sufficient to release zinc from serum albumin but possibly inadequate for complete digestion of casein, resulting in unabsorbed zinc.[16] Zinc absorption from soy formula and infant cereals is even lower than from milk formula, most likely because of the high phytate content of these diets.[14,17] Phytic acid contains several negative charges and can bind divalent cations like zinc, iron, and calcium. Because humans cannot digest phytate to any significant degree, fecal zinc losses will increase. Since removal of phytate increases zinc absorption considerably,[18] efforts are being made to reduce the phytate content of staple foods (corn, rice, barley) by fermentation, precipitation, phytase treatment or genetic selection.[19] However, such products are not yet commercially available.

Zinc intake from breast milk varies during lactation as the breast milk zinc content decreases, but is usually around 0.5 to 1.0 mg/d. Infant formulas are usually fortified with zinc to a level higher than that of breast milk (to compensate for lower bioavailability). Thus, intake is usually around 3 to 5 mg/d (or 1 mg/kg/d). Lower zinc intakes may be adequate for healthy term infants because zinc concentrations as low as 1.1 mg/L do not cause zinc deficiency.[20] However, the safety margin may not be high; some women produce breast milk with a lower than normal level of zinc, and this has been shown to cause overt zinc deficiency.[21] This is of particular concern in preterm infants because their rapid growth increases their zinc requirement. In preterm infants, deficiency due to low milk content of zinc can be precipitated quickly. The cause of the lower than normal milk zinc levels is unknown, but maternal zinc supplementation does not increase the content of zinc in the milk. Recently, several novel zinc transporters were found in the mammary gland and the small intestine.[22–25] Factors regulating these transporters (ZnT-1,2,3,4; Zip1) are still poorly characterized, but zinc intake has an effect by up- or down-regulating their expression. It can be expected that further knowledge of these transporters may help explain both regulation of milk zinc, homeostatic regulation of zinc absorption and, possibly, the defect in acrodermatitis enteropathica.

The high level of iron fortification used in most formulas was implicated to have a negative effect on zinc absorption.[26] However, this concern may be unfounded because an iron-zinc ratio found in infant formula does not appear to affect zinc absorption.[27] Decreases in the iron level do not seem to affect zinc status either.[28] However, when oral supplements are given, iron is likely to partially inhibit zinc absorption,[27] which should be considered when determining the appropriate dose and ratio of iron to zinc.

During the second 6 months of life, zinc requirements remain relatively high, and the amount of zinc provided from breast milk may be inadequate.[29] The concentration of zinc in breast milk is about 2 to 3 mg/L during early lactation, but by 6 months postpartum, levels are usually only ~0.5 mg/L.[30] The quantity of zinc provided from breast milk may be too low to meet the requirement; however, another likely reason for the beneficial effect of zinc supplements on growth of these infants[29] may be that phytate-containing weaning foods reduce the bioavailability of zinc from breast milk.[31] It is apparent that zinc intake is a limiting factor during recovery from malnutrition and during rapid catch-up growth after stunting.[32] This was considered when new recommendations for complementary foods were issued by the World Health Organization/United Nations Children's Fund.[33]

Zinc is vitally important for proper immune function,[34] but also for mucosal integrity, which may explain the positive effects of zinc supplements that have been observed on acute and chronic diarrhea,[35-37] and other diseases.[38-40] Recently, zinc has also been shown to have a positive affect on activity of preschool children[41] and on cognition and development,[42,43] which is possibly due to the involvement of zinc in neuropsychological development.[44]

The RDA for zinc for older infants (7 to 12 months) and toddlers (1 to 3 years) is 3 mg/d. Infants who are exclusively breastfed ingest only about 0.4 to 0.6 mg of zinc per day at 6 months of age without signs of zinc deficiency.[45] We still know little about the infant's capacity to homeostatically regulate zinc metabolism, but novel zinc transporters that are affected by zinc intake and zinc status have been found in the small intestine. Stable isotope experiments in infants suggest that zinc absorption is increased and fecal losses decreased when zinc intake is low.[46] It is obvious that zinc intakes of infants and children often are low, which emphasizes the need for zinc-containing foods such as meats and possibly some zinc-fortified cereals.

Copper

Copper is an essential trace element and functions as a cofactor in several physiologically important enzymes such as lysyl oxidase, elastase, monoamine oxidases, cytochrome oxidase, ceruloplasmin, and superoxide dismutase.[47,48] Lysyl oxidase and elastase are involved in connective tissue synthesis and collagen cross-linking, cytochrome oxidase in the electron transport system and energy metabolism, and ceruloplasmin (ferroxidase) in iron metabolism, and superoxide dismutase is an antioxidant and scavenger of free radicals. The signs of copper deficiency can all be related to impaired activities of these enzymes.[49]

The copper intake of infants is usually low because breast milk contains only 0.2 to 0.4 mg copper/L,[30] and infant formulas are usually fortified to a similar level (0.4 to 0.6 mg/L). This level of copper intake appears adequate in healthy term infants because copper deficiency is rare.[3] In fact, even formula that had not been fortified with copper and only contained 0.08 mg/L resulted in adequate copper status.[50] The World Health Organization has set the minimum recommended intake for infants[51] at 60 μg/kg/d and the new RDA for Cu is 200 μg/d.[1]

Risks for copper deficiency include low stores in the liver of premature infants, rapid growth rate, malabsorption syndromes and increased copper losses, but the deficiency is usually not precipitated unless the dietary intake of copper also is low.[48,52] Preterm infants have substantially lower hepatic stores of copper (which mainly accumulate during the third trimester); these prenatal stores are normally used during neonatal life by being incorporated into ceruloplasmin and exported into the blood stream, causing an early rise in serum copper and ceruloplasmin.[53] Thus, many of the first case reports of copper deficiency were about preterm infants that had been fed low copper diets (usually cow milk) for prolonged periods. Copper deficiency has also been found in malnourished infants and children.[54] Signs of copper deficiency include neutropenia, microcytic anemia (which does not respond to iron supplementation), bone abnormalities, skin disorders, and depigmentation of skin and hair.[3,49] The immune system is affected, reflected by decreased phagocytic capacity of neutrophils and impaired cell immunity.[52,55] The anemia is caused by the low levels of ceruloplasmin, or, as it more correctly should be called, ferroxidase. This enzyme is needed in several steps leading to the incorporation of iron into hemoglobin. Patients with the recently discovered genetic defect "aceruloplasminemia" have normal copper status, but have pronounced iron deficiency anemia.[56] When treated with copper (2 to 3 mg of copper sulfate as 1% solution daily or infusion), recovery of infants or children with copper deficiency is usually rapid. Clinical parameters that are used to assess copper status include serum copper and ceruloplasmin, hair copper, and erythrocyte superoxide dismutase.[49] In infants older than 1 or 2 months, serum copper levels lower than 0.5 μg/mL or ceruloplasmin levels lower than 15 μg/100 mL should be considered abnormally low. However, serum copper and ceruloplasmin are not very responsive to marginal copper deficiency and are affected by other conditions, such as infection, which may raise levels. The level of hair copper also has limited value because it may be affected by external factors.[11] The erythrocyte level of superoxide dismutase has been suggested as a good indicator of long-term copper status,[57] but the measurement has not reached routine clinical use.

Stable isotope studies in preterm infants,[58] balance studies in term infants,[59] and radioisotope studies in experimental animals[60] demonstrate higher bioavailability of copper from breast milk than from cow's milk formula and cow milk. Copper in human milk seems to be bound to serum albumin, while casein binds most copper in cow milk.[15] Copper bioavailability from soy formula and infant cereals appears to be even lower, although phytate present in these products does not seem to have the same strong inhibitory effect on the absorption of copper as found for zinc absorption.[61] Dietary factors known to affect copper absorption negatively include high levels of ascorbic acid, zinc, iron, and cysteine. However, levels of these nutrients used in infant diets are moderate and usually exert no pronounced effects on copper absorption.[62] Some types of heat processing of infant formula, however, may have a negative effect on copper absorption,[63] possibly by formation of unabsorbable complexes.

Our knowledge about copper absorption and homeostasis has been very limited, but several novel copper transporters (ATP7A, ATP7B, Ctr1) were discovered recently,[48] which may help us understand normal copper metabolism better, as well as genetic disorders of copper metabolism.

An x-linked recessive genetic disorder of copper metabolism, Menkes syndrome, usually is manifested soon after birth and is characterized by pallor, anemia, steely hair, and a progressive degeneration of the brain.[64] The patients become copper deficient at a very young age and aggressive treatment with copper should be used, but the long-term outcome for these patients is not good.[65] The gene was identified by work on mouse models of Menkes syndrome,[66] and the defective protein is a P-type ATPase, ATP7A or MNK protein, which is involved in cellular copper metabolism, particularly the export of copper out of the cell.[67,68] Thus, copper is blocked in the enterocyte and little copper is transported into the systemic circulation, resulting in severe copper deficiency.

Wilson disease is another autosomal recessive genetic disorder of copper metabolism that results in toxic effects of copper. In patients with Wilson disease, excessive amounts of copper are accumulated in the body, particularly in liver and brain, and clinical symptoms include liver cirrhosis, eye lesions (Kayser-Fleisher ring), kidney malfunction, and neurological problems.[69] Despite very high levels of copper in the liver, serum copper and ceruloplasmin are low. Treatment has included a variety of chelating agents (eg, penicillamine and triethylenetetramine), oral treatment with large doses of zinc to reduce copper absorption,[70] and hepatic transplantation for advanced cases. This disorder of copper metabolism has also been shown to be due to a defective transporter, in this case ATP7B or the WD protein.[71] Copper absorption per se does not appear to be dysregulated in these patients; rather tissue copper metabolism, particularly in the liver, is affected, causing excessive cellular accumulation of copper.[69] The outcome for these patients under treatment is usually good, but continuous monitoring of copper, zinc, and iron status is needed.

Acute copper toxicity is rare and is usually due to the consumption of contaminated foods or beverages, or accidental or deliberate ingestion of large quantities of copper salts.[72] Symptoms include nausea, vomiting, and diarrhea. Chronic toxicity is also rare, but appears to appear in geographic clusters. Indian childhood cirrhosis has been reported in families that were consuming milk boiled or stored in brass or copper containers.[73] Children consuming such milk may consume up to 1 mg/kg/d, which is enough to explain the observed liver damage. In the Austrian Tyrol, infants and children were reported to have died from liver cirrhosis due to high chronic copper intake.[74,75] In these cases, inheritance followed the typical pattern of a mendelian recessive trait, suggesting that these individuals were particularly sensitive to copper exposure. This was supported by the observation that many children were found that had no liver damage, but had received similar levels of copper. Sporadic cases have been reported in other areas, and some of these cases have occurred in consanguineous marriages.[76] Cases were much more frequent in boys, and a genetic origin is possible. Whether a genetic disorder of copper metabolism is present in the patients with liver cirrhosis is not known, but should be explored in the light of the new findings of copper transporters in humans.

After weaning, cereals and other foods provide more copper than does milk, and copper intake increases rapidly. Studies on older infants and children[77] indicate that copper intake at this age meets the requirements for growth and maintenance. While there has been some concern that drinking water may be excessively high in copper in some areas, either due to the environment (copper mining areas) or to copper pipes, infants fed formula at the current maximum copper level according to WHO, 2 mg/L, exhibited no negative signs after 6 months of exposure.[78]

Manganese

The essentiality of manganese in humans has not been fully established, although it has been determined for most other species. Manganese is a necessary cofactor for some enzymes like arginase, glutamate-ammonia ligase, manganese superoxide dismutase, and pyruvate carboxylase. Several other enzymes contain manganese, but research has shown that magnesium ions can replace manganese with maintained enzyme activity.[79] It is possible that manganese deficiency does not occur in infants and children and that, instead, concern should be directed toward toxic effects of manganese (or overload).

The concentration of manganese in breast milk is very low, only 4 to 8 μg/L.[80] Most of this manganese is bound to the major iron-binding protein in breast milk (ie, lactoferrin).[81] Cow milk and cow milk formula are about 10 times higher in manganese concentration (30 to 60 μg/L), while soy formula is about 50 to 75 times higher in manganese than is breast milk.[82] Although in the past some formulas were fortified with manganese, and, in some cases, were quite high in manganese,[83] the present levels of manganese in cow milk formula and soy formula reflect the natural levels of manganese in the protein sources used.

Although manganese absorption from human milk appears high compared with that from cow milk formula and soy formula,[84] there is little regulation of manganese uptake at young ages, and absorption is strongly correlated to dietary intake.[85] Thus, the body burden of absorbed and retained manganese will be much larger in infants fed cow milk-based formula or, in particular, soy formula than in breastfed infants.[82] This is reflected in higher whole blood manganese concentrations in formula-fed infants.[86] Manganese status is difficult to assess because of the very low levels of manganese in biological tissues and fluids; blood levels are only 10 μg/L, and serum concentrations are around 1 μg/L,[83] making analysis impossible for most laboratories. Because few of the manganese-dependent enzymes are found in blood, they have no value in the evaluation of manganese status.

Balance studies in infants show that breastfed infants accumulate little manganese, while formula-fed infants are in positive balance.[59] Little is known about the threshold for development of toxic effects of manganese, but because manganese absorption is high at young ages,[85,87] the possibility should be considered in appropriate circumstances. For example, manganese absorption increases substantially during iron deficiency,[82] which is not uncommon in children. Another concern is the recent interest in adding manganese compounds to gasoline (as an antiknock agent), which would further increase the environmental exposure to this element.

Toxic effects of manganese in human adults are manifested by central nervous system dysfunction, such as lack of coordination and balance, mental confusion, and muscle cramps.[79] The major site for the toxic effects of manganese is the extrapyramidal part of the brain, and several symptoms resemble those of Parkinson's disease. Even if the toxic effects usually are not precipitated in infants and children, an excessive intake of manganese may impair iron absorption.[88] Children receiving long-term parenteral nutrition, however, may be at risk of excessive manganese exposure as these solutions frequently are high in manganese.[89] In such patients, cholestatic disease and nervous system disorders have been associated with high blood concentrations of manganese. The normal homeostatic mechanisms of the liver and gut are bypassed in these patients leading to hypermanganesemia, and a reduction in the manganese concentration of parenteral nutrition solutions has been advocated.[90] Bile is involved in this excretion, which explains the finding of elevated plasma manganese in children with biliary obstruction.[91]

Weaning diets are usually good sources of manganese, and manganese intake increases dramatically after weaning. However, mechanisms for manganese excretion appear to become more efficient at this age, and the body may retain only a small fraction of absorbed manganese.

Selenium

The essentiality of selenium in human nutrition was discovered recently, although selenium deficiency in animals had been known for quite some time. In a province of China, Keshan, a cardiomyopathy of unknown etiology led to high mortality in children.[92] Because the pathologic changes of Keshan disease had similarities to the signs of selenium deficiency in cattle, and the soil was found to be low in selenium, a large study evaluated the effects of selenium fortification of salt. Mortality decreased significantly and selenium fortification has been used since. However, other factors may have contributed to the cause of Keshan disease because Keshan disease is not evident in other areas with similarly low intakes of selenium. It has been suggested that the low selenium environment puts evolutionary pressure on normally harmless viruses (such as Coxsackie virus) causing them to mutate, which makes them pathogenic.[93] Evidence for such mutations in Coxsackie that can cause cardiomyopathy has been obtained at the molecular level, but it is not yet clear if this was a major contributing factor to Keshan disease. Selenium deficiency has been found in children receiving long-term total parenteral nutrition solutions that were not supplemented.[94] Signs of deficiency include macrocytosis and loss of skin and hair pigmentation.

Selenium in the diet is strongly affected by local conditions; soil and water selenium levels affect plant selenium levels and the levels in grazing animals and their milk.[95] Similarly, selenium in breast milk is affected by maternal selenium intake.[96] Thus, the selenium intake of infants and children is affected by the geographic location. Some areas of the United States have high levels of selenium, while other areas have considerably lower levels. The raw material used for formulas, such as skim milk powder, whey protein, and soy protein isolate, strongly affects the selenium content of formula.

Selenium is an integral and necessary part of a limited number of proteins, such as selenium-dependent glutathione peroxidase, selenoprotein P in serum, and deiodinase. In these proteins, selenium is specifically incorporated into the proteins as selenocysteine, because of a unique transfer RNA using a specific serine codon.[97] Thus, the number of selenocysteine residues in each protein is tightly regulated. Selenium can also be incorporated nonspecifically into methionine. Our diet consists of organic selenium (largely selenomethionine) and inorganic selenium in the form of selenite and selenate. Knowledge is limited about the metabolism of these different forms of selenium in humans, but they appear to metabolize quite differently.[95,98]

Glutathione peroxidase participates in the antioxidant defense and helps to scavenge free radicals that may cause tissue damage. Several forms of selenium-dependent and selenium-independent glutathione peroxidase exist.[97] The selenium-dependent glutathione peroxidase found in serum and erythrocytes has been used to assess selenium status. However, the situation is complicated because they are different gene products and, therefore, are regulated differently. To date, the level of serum glutathione peroxidase, which usually is closely correlated with the level of serum selenium, has been used as an indicator of short-term selenium status, while erythrocyte glutathione peroxidase has been used as an indicator of long-term status. The serum selenium level is also used frequently to assess selenium status.

The selenium concentration of breast milk has been shown to be as low as 3 μg/L in some areas of China, while levels in other low selenium areas, such as Finland and New Zealand, are around 10 μg/L.[95] Selenium levels in breast milk from women in the United States vary, but are usually around 15 μg/L.[99] A lower level of selenium was shown in formula-fed infants than in breastfed infants in several studies.[99,100] Formulas that are not fortified with selenium often contain considerably lower selenium levels (2 to 6 μg/L) than the level in breast milk. Furthermore, the bioavailability of selenium in breast milk, which is mostly in protein-bound form,[101] seems higher than that of selenium-fortified formula. A study in which the selenium status of formula-fed infants was lower than the level in breastfed infants, even though the formula was fortified with selenium to a level higher than that of breast milk, supports this.[100] At least part of the difference in selenium bioavailability may be related to the form of selenium in the diet; selenite or selenate (ie, inorganic selenium) is used in formula, while most selenium in breast milk is protein-bound (organic selenium). A difference in utilization of selenium given in different forms was shown in a study in which lactating women were given selenium supplements. Yeast selenium (ie, organic selenium) resulted in higher selenium levels in breast milk than when selenite was given.[96] These differences were also manifested in the selenium status of their breastfed infants.

Soy formula often provides even less selenium than does cow milk formula. Again, this depends on the soy protein source used, but several commercial soy formulas have been reported to contain only 2 to 6 μg selenium per liter.[102,103] Selenium fortification of soy formula has therefore recently been implemented. Both selenite[102] and selenate[103] have been studied; the latter form is possibly better absorbed. The level of fortification has been chosen to provide the infant with an amount equal to the RDA of 15 to 20 μg/kg/d for infants from birth to 6 months of age. Another factor to consider is the selenium status of infants at birth. Markedly different levels of plasma selenium in infants in Finland and the United States may explain why increases after birth were seen in one study[55] but not in another.[104]

Tissue selenium and plasma selenium concentrations are lower in preterm infants than in term infants.[105] A selenium intake of at least 1 μg/kg/d is recommended to achieve intrauterine tissue accretion. However, evaluation of the selenium status of preterm infants is difficult. When preterm infants were fed breast milk (containing 24 μg/L selenium) or formula with or without selenium fortification (34.8 and 7.8 μg/L selenium, respectively), no differences were found in plasma selenium, erythrocyte selenium, or glutathione peroxidase.[105] However, all these infants may have had suboptimal selenium status and selenium may have been quickly removed from the circulation and incorporated into newly synthesized tissue. A recent study in the United States shows that selenium fortification of formula improves selenium status of preterm infants,[106] possibly because the infants were not as selenium deprived as in the other study. A stable isotope study in premature infants showed that selenite in formula was absorbed to about 70% and that most of this was retained.[107] It is also possible that synthesis of selenoproteins, such as glutathione peroxidase and selenoprotein P that transport selenium in plasma, is immature in these infants. The low plasma glutathione peroxidase levels of infants fed preterm formula without selenium fortification decreased with age in infants in New Zealand, which may be due to a combination of low status at birth and a low dietary supply of selenium.[108] Concern was raised about possibly impaired antioxidant defenses because preterm infants are at risk of oxidative diseases, such as bronchopulmonary dysplasia and retinopathy of prematurity.

Iodine

The primary biological role of iodine is in the synthesis of thyroid hormones. Iodine is readily absorbed and is rapidly taken up by the thyroid gland, but also by other tissues. Excess iodine is excreted via the urine, and urinary iodine is often used as an indicator of iodine status. Although iodine deficiency is one of the most common nutrient deficiencies worldwide, it is highly uncommon among infants and children in the United States. Common use of iodine in baked goods and in dairy cattle management, together with iodination of table salt, makes the dietary iodine intake of the US population more than sufficient to meet the requirements.

The RDA of iodine for infants up to 6 months of age is 110 μg/d and from 6 to 12 months of age, 130 μg/d. The concentration of iodine in breast milk depends on maternal intake and therefore varies, but values of 50 to 60 μg/L were found in a multicenter study.[109] The iodine concentration in breast milk of women in the United States seems higher, with a mean value of 130 μg/L[110]; maternal dietary intake strongly influences the iodine concentration.[111] Cow milk is a rich source of iodine, and milk-based infant formula is therefore a good source of iodine. Soy formula usually contains about 70 to 100 μg/L. Thus, it is evident that formula-fed and breastfed infants will receive adequate quantities of iodine. Children in the United States will get an ample supply of iodine from salt, dairy products, and baked goods. For areas that are not reached by iodine fortification, low-dose oral iodized oil has been developed for children.[112]

It has recently been found that goitrous children with iron deficiency anemia do not respond to iodine supplementation,[113] suggesting that iron may be important for some vital step in iodine metabolism. Oral iron supplementation of such children led to a significantly improved response to iodine supplementation.[114] Whether low iron status in US children can impair iodine status without precipitating goiter is not yet known.

Other Trace Elements

Chromium functions as a cofactor for insulin. Chromium deficiency is characterized by impaired growth and longevity and by impaired glucose, lipid, and protein metabolism in experimental animals. However, chromium deficiency in infants is most likely rare and has only been reported associated with protein-calorie malnutrition. Depletion of chromium also may occur during prolonged parenteral alimentation. The only reliable indicator of chromium deficiency is the demonstration of a beneficial effect of chromium supplementation.

Cobalt is considered essential for humans only because it is a component of the vitamin B_{12} molecule. Cobalt deficiency has never been demonstrated in humans or laboratory animals, and the requirement for cobalt is considered minute.

The biochemical functions of molybdenum are in the synthesis and function of xanthine oxidase, aldehyde oxidase, and sulfite oxidase. Molybdenum deficiency has not been reported under any natural conditions in humans, but it has recently been suggested that low-birth-weight infants may not meet their molybdenum requirement, particularly when receiving parenteral nutrition.[115]

Arsenic, nickel, silicon, and vanadium are other trace elements considered as possibly nutritionally important. Human deficiency states have not been demonstrated, and dietary requirements have not been set because of insufficient experience.

Aluminum, although poorly absorbed, can accumulate in patients with renal insufficiency, and this accumulation has been associated with osteomalacia and encephalopathy. Care should be taken when administering aluminum-containing antacids to children with renal insufficiency. Although some soy formulas contain elevated aluminum levels, it is most likely poorly absorbed and has not been associated with negative consequences.[116]

The American Academy of Pediatrics Recommends the following:

1. Aluminum-containing phosphate binders should not be administered to infants and children who have renal failure.
2. Continued efforts should be made to reduce the levels of aluminum in products that are added to intravenous solutions that are used for premature infants and infants and children with renal failure.
3. Continued efforts should be made to reduce the aluminum content of all formulas used for infants, but especially soy formulas and formulas tailored specifically for pre-mature infants.
4. In infants at risk for aluminum toxicity (eg, an infant with renal failure or who was born prematurely), attention should be paid to the aluminum content of the water used in reconstitution of infant formulas.

Note: These recommendations do not indicate an exclusive course of treatment or procedure to be followed. Variations, taking into account individual circumstances, may be appropriate.

Pediatrics. 1996;97:413–415

References

1. Institute of Medicine. *Dietary Reference Intakes for Vitamin A, Vitamin K, Arsenic, Boron, Chromium, Copper, Iodine, Iron, Manganese, Molybdenum, Nickel, Silicon, Vanadium, and Zinc.* Washington, DC: National Academy Press; 2001:155–398
2. Prasad AS. Clinical and biochemical spectrum of zinc deficiency in human subjects. In: Prasad AS, ed. *Clinical, Biochemical, and Nutritional Aspects of Trace Elements.* New York, NY: Alan R Liss, Inc; 1982;3:62
3. Walravens PA. Nutritional importance of copper and zinc in neonates and infants. *Clin Chem.* 1980;26:185–189
4. Sandström B, Cederblad Å, Lindblad BS, Lönnerdal B. Acrodermatitis enteropathica, zinc metabolism, copper status and immune function. *Arch Pediatr Adolesc Med.* 1994;148:980–985
5. Walravens PA, Hambidge KM. Growth of infants fed a zinc supplemented formula. *Am J Clin Nutr.* 1976;29:1114–1121
6. Hambidge KM, Walravens PA, Casey CE, Brown RM, Bender C. Plasma zinc concentrations of breast-fed infants. *J Pediatr.* 1979;94:607–608
7. Ruz M, Castillo-Duran C, Lara X, et al. A 14-mo zinc-supplementation trial in apparently healthy Chilean preschool children. *Pediatrics.* 1997;66:1406–1413
8. Rivera JA, Ruel MT, Santizo MC, et al. Zinc supplementation improves the growth of stunted rural Guatemalan infants. *J Nutr.* 1998;128:556–562
9. Brown KH, Peerson JM, Allen LH. Effect of zinc supplementation on children's growth: a meta-analysis of intervention trials. *Bibl Nutr Dieta.* 1998;54:76–83
10. Brown KH. Effect of infections on plasma zinc concentration and implications for zinc status in low-income populations. *Am J Clin Nutr.* 1998;68:S425–S429
11. Hambidge KM. Hair analyses: worthless for vitamins, limited for minerals. *Am J Clin Nutr.* 1982;36:943–949

12. Hotz C, Brown KH. Identifying populations at risk of zinc deficiency: the use of supplementation trials. *Nutr Rev*. 2001;59:80–84
13. Krebs NF, Westcott JE, Arnold TD, et al. Abnormalities in zinc homeostasis in young infants with cystic fibrosis. *Pediatr Res*. 2000;48:256–261
14. Sandström B, Cederblad Å, Lönnerdal B. Zinc absorption from human milk, cow's milk, and infant formulas. *Am J Dis Child*. 1983;137:726–729
15. Lönnerdal B, Hoffman B, Hurley LS. Zinc and copper binding proteins in human milk. *Am J Clin Nutr*. 1982;36:1170–1176
16. Lönnerdal B. Dietary factors influencing zinc absorption. *J Nutr*. 2000;130:1378S–1383S
17. Lönnerdal B, Cederblad Å, Davidsson L, Sandström B. The effect of individual components of soy formula and cow's milk formula on zinc bioavailability. *Am J Clin Nutr*. 1984;40:1064–1070
18. Lönnerdal B, Bell JG, Hendrickx AG, Burns RA, Keen CL. Effect of phytate removal on zinc absorption from soy formula. *Am J Clin Nutr*. 1988;48:1301–1306
19. Gibson RS, Yeudall F, Drost N, Mtitimuni B, Cullinan T. Dietary interventions to prevent zinc deficiency. *Am J Clin Nutr*. 1998;68:484S–487S
20. Krebs NF, Reidinger C, Robertson AD, Hambidge KM. Growth and intakes of energy and zinc in infants fed human milk. *J Pediatr*. 1994;124:32–39
21. Atkinson SA, Whelan D, Whyte RK, Lonnerdal B. Abnormal zinc content in human milk. *Am J Dis Child*. 1989;143:608–611
22. Palmiter RD, Findley SD. Cloning and functional characterization of a mammalian zinc transporter that confers resistance to zinc. *EMBO J*. 1995;14:639–649
23. Palmiter RD, Cole TB, Findley SD. ZnT-2, a mammalian protein that confers resistance to zinc by facilitating vesicular sequestration. *EMBO J*. 1996;15:1784–1791
24. McMahon RJ, Cousins RJ. Mammalian zinc transporters. *J Nutr*. 1998;128:667–670
25. Gaither LA, Eide DJ. The human ZIP1 transporter mediates zinc uptake in human K562 erythroleukemia cells. *J Biol Chem*. 2001;276:22258–22264
26. Solomons NW, Jacob RA. Studies on the bioavailability of zinc in humans: effects of heme and nonheme iron on the absorption of zinc. *Am J Clin Nutr*. 1981;34:475–482
27. Sandström B, Davidsson L, Cederblad Å, Lönnerdal B. Oral iron, dietary ligands and zinc absorption. *J Nutr*. 1985;115:411–414
28. Yip R, Reeves JD, Lönnerdal B, Keen CL, Dallman PR. Does iron supplementation compromise zinc nutrition in healthy infants? *Am J Clin Nutr*. 1985;42:683–687
29. Walravens PA, Chakar A, Mokni R, Denise J, Lemonnier D. Zinc supplements in breastfed infants. *Lancet*. 1992;340:683–685
30. Krebs NF, Reidinger CJ, Hartley S, Robertson AD, Hambidge KM. Zinc supplementation during lactation: Effects on maternal status and milk zinc concentrations. *Am J Clin Nutr*. 1995; 61: 1030–1036

31. Bell JG, Keen CL, Lönnerdal B. Effect of infant cereals on zinc and copper absorption during weaning. *Am J Dis Child.* 1987;141:1128–1132

32. Castillo-Duran C, Heresi G, Fisberg M, Uauy R. Controlled trial of zinc supplementation during recovery from malnutrition: effects on growth and immune function. *Am J Clin Nutr.* 1987;45:602–608

33. Brown KH. WHO/UNICEF review on complementary feeding and suggestions for future research: WHO/UNICEF guidelines on complementary feeding. *Pediatrics.* 2000;106:S1290–S1291

34. Shankar AH, Prasad AS. Zinc and immune function: the biological basis of altered resistance to infection. *Am J Clin Nutr.* 1998;68:447S–463S

35. Sazawal S, Black RE, Bhan MK, et al. Efficacy of zinc supplementation in reducing the incidence and prevalence of acute diarrhea—a community-based, double-blind, controlled trial. *Am J Clin Nutr.* 1997;66:413–418

36. Ruel MT, Rivera JA, Santizo, MC, et al. Impact of zinc supplementation on morbidity from diarrhea and respiratory infections among rural Guatemalan children. *Pediatrics.* 1997;99:808–813

37. Bhutta ZA, Bird SM, Black RE, et al. Zinc Investigators Collaborative Group. Therapeutic effects of oral zinc in acute and persistent diarrhea in children in developing countries: pooled analysis of randomized controlled trials. *Am J Clin Nutr.* 2000;72:1516–1522

38. Sazawal S, Black RE, Jalla S, et al. Zinc supplementation reduces the incidence of acute lower respiratory infections in infants and preschool children: a double-blind, controlled trial. *Pediatrics.* 1998;102:1–5

39. Black RE. Therapeutic and preventive effects of zinc on serious childhood infectious diseases in developing countries. *Am J Clin Nutr.* 1998;68:476S–479S

40. Bhutta ZA, Black RE, Brown KH, et al. Zinc Investigators Collaborative Group. Prevention of diarrhea and pneumonia by zinc supplementation in children in developing countries: Pooled analysis of randomized controlled trials. *J Pediatr.* 1999;135:689–697

41. Sazawal S, Bentley P, Black RE, et al. Effect of zinc supplementation on observed activity in low socioeconomic Indian preschool children. *Pediatrics.* 1996;98:1132–1137

42. Sandstead HH, Penland JG, Alcock NW, et al. Effects of repletion with zinc and other micronutrients repletion on neuropsychological performance and growth of Chinese children. *Am J Clin Nutr.* 1997;16:268–272

43. Castillo-Duran C, Perales CG, Hertrampf ED, et al. Effect of zinc supplementation on development and growth of Chilean infants. *J Pediatr.* 2001;138:229–235

44. Frederickson CJ, Suh SW, Frederickson CJ, et al. Importance of zinc in the central nervous system: the zinc-containing neuron. *J Nutr.* 2000;130:S1471–S1483

45. Krebs NF, Hambidge KM. Zinc requirements and zinc intakes of breast-fed infants. *Am J Clin Nutr.* 1986;43:288–292

46. Ziegler EE, Serfass RE, Nelson SE, et al. Effect of low zinc intake on absorption and excretion of zinc by infants studied with 70Zn as extrinsic tag. *J Nutr.* 1989;119: 1647–1653

47. Cousins RJ. Absorption, transport, and hepatic metabolism of copper and zinc: special reference to metallothionein and ceruloplasmin. *Physiol Rev.* 1985;65: 238–309

48. Olivares M, Araya M, Uauy R. Copper homeostasis in infant nutrition: deficit and excess. *J Pediatr Gastroenterol Nutr.* 2000;31:102–111

49. Milne DB. Copper intake and assessment of copper status. *Am J Clin Nutr.* 1998; 67:1041S–1045S

50. Salmenperä L, Siimes MA, Näntö V, Perheentupa J. Copper supplementation: failure to increase plasma copper and ceruloplasmin concentrations in healthy infants. *Am J Clin Nutr.* 1989;50:843–847

51. Salim S, Farquharson J, Arneil GC, et al. Dietary copper intake in artificially fed infants. *Arch Dis Child.* 1986;61:1068–1075

52. Lönnerdal B. Copper nutrition during infancy and childhood. *Am J Clin Nutr.* 1998;67:1046S–1053S

53. Salmenperä L, Perheentupa J, Pakarinen P, Siimes MA. Cu nutrition in infants during prolonged exclusive breast-feeding: low intake but rising serum concentrations of Cu and ceruloplasmin. *Am J Clin Nutr.* 1986;43:251–257

54. Graham GG, Cordano A. Copper depletion and deficiency in the malnourished infant. *Johns Hopkins Med J.* 1969;124:139–150

55. Percival SS. Copper and immunity. *Am J Clin Nutr.* 1998;67:1064S–1068S

56. Harris ZL, Takahashi Y, Miyajima H, Serizawa M, MacGillivray RT, Gitlin JD. Aceruloplasminemia: molecular characterization of this disorder of iron metabolism. *Proc Natl Acad Sci U S A.* 1995;92:2539–2543

57. Uauy R, Castillo-Duran D, Fisberg M, Fernandez N, Valenzuela A. Red cell superoxide dismutase activity as an index of human copper nutrition. *J Nutr.* 1985;115: 1650–1655

58. Ehrenkranz RA, Gettner PA, Nelli CM, et al. Zinc and copper nutritional studies in very low birth weight infants: comparison of stable isotopic extrinsic tag and chemical balance methods. *Pediatr Res.* 1989;26:298–307

59. Dörner K, Dziadzka S, Hohn A, et al. Longitudinal manganese and copper balances in young infants and preterm infants fed on breast-milk and adapted cow's milk formulas. *Br J Nutr.* 1989;61:559–572

60. Lönnerdal B, Bell JG, Keen CL. Copper absorption from human milk, cow's milk and infant formulas using a suckling rat model. *Am J Clin Nutr.* 1985;42:836–844

61. Lönnerdal B, Jayawickrama L, Lien EL. Effect of reducing the phytate content and of partially hydrolyzing the protein in soy formula on zinc and copper absorption and status in infant rhesus monkeys and rat pups. *Am J Clin Nutr.* 1999;69:490–496

62. Stack T, Aggett PJ, Aitken E, Lloyd DJ. Routine L-ascorbic acid supplementation does not alter iron, copper, and zinc balance in low birthweight infants fed a cow's milk formula. *J Pediatr Gastroenterol Nutr.* 1990;10:351–356

63. Lönnerdal B, Kelleher SL, Lien EL. Extent of thermal processing of infant formula affects copper status in infant rhesus monkeys. *Am J Clin Nutr.* 2001;73:914–919

64. Danks DM, Campbell PE, Stevens BJ, Mayne V, Cartwright E. Menkes's kinky hair syndrome: an inherited defect in copper absorption with widespread effects. *Pediatrics.* 1972;50:188–201

65. Kaler SG. Diagnosis and therapy of Menkes syndrome, a genetic form of copper deficiency. *Am J Clin Nutr.* 1998;67:1029S–1034S

66. Mercer JF, Livingston J, Hall B, et al. Isolation of a partial candidate gene for Menkes disease by positional cloning. *Nat Genet.* 1993;3:20–25

67. Camakaris J, Petris MJ, Bailey L, et al. Gene amplification of the Menkes (MNK; ATP7A) P-type ATPase gene of CHO cells is associated with copper resistance and enhanced copper efflux. *Hum Mol Genet.* 1995;4:2117–2123

68. Yamaguchi Y, Heiny ME, Suzuki M, Gitlin JD. Biochemical characterization and intracellular localization of the Menkes disease protein. *Proc Natl Acad Sci U S A.* 1996;93:14030–14035

69. Danks DM. Disorders of copper transport. In: Scriver CL, Beaudet AL, Sly WS, Valle D, eds. *The Metabolic and Molecular Bases of Inherited Disease.* New York, NY: McGraw-Hill, 1995:2211–2235

70. Brewer GJ, Hill GM, Prasad AS, Cossack ZT, Rabbani P. Oral zinc therapy for Wilson's disease. *Ann Intern Med.* 1983;99:314–319

71. Petrukhin K, Lutsenko S, Chernov I, Ross BM, Kaplan JH, Gilliam TC. Characterization of the Wilson disease gene encoding a P-type copper transporting ATPase: genomic organization, alternative splicing, and structure/function predictions. *Hum Mol Genet.* 1994;3:1647–1656

72. Pizarro F, Olivares M, Uauy R, Contreras P, Rebelo A, Gidi V. Acute gastrointestinal effects of graded levels of copper in drinking water. *Environ Health Perspect.* 1999; 107:117–121

73. Tanner MS, Kantarjian AH, Bhave SA, Pandit AN. Early introduction of copper-contaminated animal milk feeds as a possible cause of Indian childhood cirrhosis. *Lancet.* 1983;2:992–995

74. Müller T, Feichtinger H, Berger H, Müller W. Endemic Tyrolean infantile cirrhosis: an ecogenetic disorder. *Lancet.* 1996;347:877–880

75. Müller T, Müller W, Feichtinger H. Idiopathic copper toxicosis. *Am J Clin Nutr.* 1998;67:1082S–1086S

76. Müller-Höcker J, Meyer U, Wiebecke B, et al. Copper storage disease of the liver and chronic dietary copper intoxication in two further German infants mimicking Indian childhood cirrhosis. *Pathol Res Pract.* 1988;183:39–45

77. Sorenson AW, Butrum RR. Zinc and copper in infant diets. *J Am Diet Assoc.* 1983;83:291–297

78. Olivares M, Pizarro, Speisky H, et al. Copper in infant nutrition: safety of World Health Organization provisional guideline value for copper content of drinking water. *J Pediatr Gastroenterol Nutr.* 1998;26:251–257
79. Mena I. Manganese. In: Bronner F, Coburn JW, eds. *Disorders of Mineral Metabolism.* Orlando, FL: Academic Press Inc; 1981;1:233–270
80. Vuori E. A longitudinal study of manganese in human milk. *Acta Paediatr Scand.* 1979;68:571–573
81. Lönnerdal B, Keen CL, Hurley LS. Manganese binding proteins in human and cow's milk. *Am J Clin Nutr.* 1985;41:550–559
82. Lönnerdal B. Manganese nutrition of infants. In: Klimis-Tavantzis DJ, ed. *Manganese in Health and Disease.* Boca Raton, FL: CRC Press Inc; 1994:175
83. Stastny D, Vogel RS, Picciano MF. Manganese intake and serum manganese concentration of human milk-fed and formula-fed infants. *Am J Clin Nutr.* 1984; 39:872–878
84. Davidsson L, Cederblad Å, Lönnerdal B, Sandström B. Manganese absorption from human milk, cow's milk and infant formulas in humans. *Am J Dis Child.* 1989;143:823–827
85. Keen CL, Bell JG, Lönnerdal B. The effect of age on manganese uptake and retention from milk and infant formulas in rats. *J Nutr.* 1986;116:395–402
86. Hatano S, Aihara K, Nishi Y, Usui T. Trace elements (copper, zinc, manganese, and selenium) in plasma and erythrocytes in relation to dietary intake during infancy. *J Pediatr Gastroenterol Nutr.* 1985;4:87–92
87. Ballatori N, Miles E, Clarkson TW. Homeostatic control of manganese excretion in the neonatal rat. *Am J Physiol.* 1987;252:R842–R847
88. Rossander-Hulten L, Brune M, Sandström B, Lönnerdal B, Hallberg L. Competitive inhibition of iron absorption by manganese and zinc in humans. *Am J Clin Nutr.* 1991;54:152–156
89. Dickerson RN. Manganese intoxication and parenteral nutrition. *Nutrition.* 2001; 17:689–693
90. Fell JM, Reynolds AP, Meadows N, et al. Manganese toxicity in children receiving long-term parenteral nutrition. *Lancet.* 1996;347(9010):1218–1221
91. Bayliss EA, Hambidge KM, Sokol RJ, et al. Hepatic concentrations of zinc, copper and manganese in infants with extrahepatic biliary atresia. *J Trace Elem Med Biol.* 1995;9:40–43
92. Keshan Disease Research Group of the Chinese Academy of Medical Sciences, Beijing. Observations on effect of sodium selenite in prevention of Keshan disease. *Chin Med J (Engl).* 1979;92:471–476
93. Nelson HK, Shi Q, Van Dael P, et al. Host nutritional status as a driving force for influenza virus. *FASEB J.* 2001;15:U488–U499
94. Vinton NE, Dahlstrom KA, Strobel CT, Ament ME. Macrocytosis and pseudoalbinism: manifestations of selenium deficiency. *J Pediatr.* 1987;111:711–717
95. Litov RE, Combs GF Jr. Selenium in pediatric nutrition. *Pediatrics.* 1991;87: 339–351

96. Kumpulainen J, Salmenperä L, Siimes MA, Koivstoinen P, Perheentupa J. Selenium status of exclusively breast-fed infants as influenced by maternal organic or inorganic selenium supplementation. *Am J Clin Nutr.* 1985;42:829–835

97. Sunde RA. Molecular biology of selenoproteins. *Annu Rev Nutr.* 1990;10:451–474

98. Thomson CD, Robinson MF. Urinary and fecal excretion and absorption of a large supplement of selenium: superiority of selenate over selenite. *Am J Clin Nutr.* 1986;44:659–663

99. Smith AM, Picciano MF, Milner JA. Selenium intakes and status of human milk and formula fed infants. *Am J Clin Nutr.* 1982;35:521–526

100. Kumpulainen J, Salmenpera L, Siimes MA, Koivistoinen P, Lehto J, Perheentupa J. Formula feeding results in lower selenium status than breast-feeding or selenium-supplemented formula feeding: a longitudinal study. *Am J Clin Nutr.* 1987;45:49–53

101. Milner JA, Sherman L, Picciano MF. Distribution of selenium in human milk. *Am J Clin Nutr.* 1987;45:617–624

102. Johnson CE, Smith AM, Chan GM, Moyer-Mileur LJ. Selenium status of term infants fed human milk or selenite-supplemented soy formula. *J Pediatr.* 1993; 122:739–741

103. Smith AM, Chen LW, Thomas MR. Selenate fortification improves selenium status of term infants fed soy formula. *Am J Clin Nutr.* 1995;61:44–47

104. Litov RE, Sickles VS, Chan GM, Hargett IR, Cordano A. Selenium status in term infants fed human milk or infant formula with or without added selenium. *Nutr Res.* 1989;9:585–596

105. Smith AM, Chan GM, Moyer-Mileur LJ, Johnson CE, Gardner BR. Selenium status of preterm infants fed human milk, preterm formula, or selenium-supplemented preterm formula. *J Pediatr.* 1991;119:429–433

106. Tyrala EE, Borschel MW, Jacobs JR. selenate fortification of infant formulas improves the selenium status of preterm infants. *Am J Clin Nutr.* 1996;64:860–865

107. Ehrenkranz RA, Gettner PA, Nelli CM, et al. Selenium absorption and retention by very-low-birth-weight infants: studies with the extrinsic stable isotope tag 74Se. *J Pediatr Gastroenterol Nutr.* 1991;13:125–133

108. Sluis KB, Darlow BA, George PM, Mogridge N, Dolamore BA, Winterbourn CC. Selenium and glutathione peroxidase levels in premature infants in a low selenium community (Christchurch, New Zealand). *Pediatr Res.* 1992;32:189–194

109. Parr RM, DeMaeyer EM, Lyengar VG, et al. Minor and trace elements in human milk from Guatemala, Hungary, Nigeria, Philippines, Sweden and Zaire. *Biol Trace Elem Res.* 1991;29:51–75

110. Bruhn JC, Franke AA. Iodine in human milk. *J Dairy Sci.* 1983;66:1396–1398

111. Gushurst CA, Mueller JA, Green JA, Sedor F. Breast milk iodide: reassessment in the 1980s. *Pediatrics.* 1984;73:354–357

112. Zimmermann M, Adou P, Torresani T, et al. Low dose oral iodized oil for control of iodine deficiency in children. *Br J Nutr.* 2000;84:139–141

113. Zimmermann M, Adou P, Torresani T, et al. Persistence of goiter despite oral iodine supplementation in goitrous children with iron deficiency anemia in Cote d'Ivoire. *Am J Clin Nutr.* 2000;71:88–93

114. Zimmermann M, Adou P, Torresani T, et al. Iron supplementation in goitrous, iron-deficient children improves their response to oral iodized oil. *Eur J Endocrinol.* 2000;142:217–223

115. Friel JK, MacDonald AC, Mercer CN, et al. Molybdenum requirements in low-birth-weight infants receiving parenteral and enteral nutrition. *JPEN J Parenter Enteral Nutr.* 199;23:155–159

116. Litov RE, Sickles VS, Chan GM, Springer MA, Cordano A. Plasma aluminum measurements in term infants fed human milk or a soy-based infant formula. *Pediatrics.* 1989;84:1105–1107

21

Vitamins

Introduction

Vitamins are essential components of cofactors in a wide range of metabolic reactions. These functions are summarized in Table 21.1. Supplemental vitamins are expensive and probably unnecessary for the healthy child older than 1 year who consumes a varied diet. Milk from a well-nourished mother contains sufficient vitamins for the young healthy term infant except for vitamin K and vitamin D. All standard commercial infant formulas contain vitamins in quantities sufficient to meet the recommended dietary allowances (RDAs) if the infant consumes 750 mL of formula. Evaporated milk and pasteurized whole cow milk contain added vitamin D and sufficient vitamin A and most water-soluble vitamins except vitamin C (unless added by the processor).

Recently, the Standing Committee on the Scientific Evaluation of Dietary Reference Intakes of the Food and Nutrition Board, Institute of Medicine, National Academy of Sciences, has undertaken a comprehensive expansion of the RDA periodic reports into a set of 4 nutrient-based values known as Dietary Reference Intakes (DRIs). Dietary reference intakes of vitamins are given in Appendix C.[1] These reference values include the Estimated Average Requirement (EAR), RDA, Adequate Intake (AI), and the Tolerable Upper Intake Level (UL). If sufficient scientific evidence is not available to calculate an RDA, a reference intake called an AI is provided instead. Recommended dietary allowances and AIs are levels of intake recommended for individuals. They should reduce the risk of developing a condition that is associated with the nutrient in question that has a negative functional outcome. The DRIs apply to the apparently healthy general population. They are based on nutrient balance studies, the nutrient intakes of breastfed infants and healthy adults, biochemical measurement of tissue saturation or molecular function, and extrapolation from animal models. Unfortunately, only limited data are available on vitamin requirements in infants and children because of ethical, cost, and time concerns. Meeting the recommended intakes for the nutrients would not necessarily provide enough for individuals who are already malnourished, nor would

Table 21.1.
Vitamins: Summary Table*

Name	Characteristics	Biochemical Action	Effects of Deficiency	Effects of Excess	Food Sources
		WATER-SOLUBLE VITAMINS			
Biotin (no RDA established)	Water soluble; synthesized by intestinal bacteria; deficiency only with large intake of raw egg white (avidin irreversibly binds) or during TPN	Coenzyme: acetyl CoA carboxylase, other carboxylases	Seborrheic dermatitis, anorexia, nausea, pallor, alopecia, myalgias, paresthesias	Unknown	Liver, egg yolk, Soybeans, milk, Meat
Cyanocobalamin (vitamin B_{12})	Slightly soluble in water, heat stable only at neutral pH, light sensitive; absorption (in ileum) depends on gastric intrinsic factor; CoA a part of the molecule	Coenzyme component; red blood cell maturation; central nervous system metabolism; methyl-malonyl-CoA mutase	Pernicious anemia; neurologic deterioration, methyl-Malonicacidemia	Unknown	Animal foods only: meat, fish, poultry, cheese, milk, eggs, vitamin B_{12}-fortified soy milk
Folacin group of compounds containing pteridine ring, and P-aminobenzoic and glutamic acids	Slightly soluble in water, light sensitive, heat stable; ascorbic acid involved in inter conversions; interference from oral contraceptives, antiepileptic drugs, alcohol	Tetrahydrofolic acid is the active form; synthesis of purines, pyrimidines, methylation reactions, one carbon acceptor	Megaloblastic anemia, impaired cellular immunity, irritability, paranoid behavior, neural tube defects in fetus of pregnant women	Masking of B_{12} deficiency symptoms in patients with pernicious anemia not receiving cyanocobalamin	Yeast, liver, leafy green vegetables, oranges, cantaloupe, seeds, fortified breads and cereals (grains)

Table 21.1.
Vitamins: Summary Table* (continued)

Name	Characteristics	Biochemical Action	Effects of Deficiency	Effects of Excess	Food Sources
WATER-SOLUBLE VITAMINS					
Niacin (nicotinic acid, amide) (vitamin B_3)	Water soluble, heat and light stable; availability from corn enhanced by alkali; synthesized in the body from tryptophan (60:1), some by intestinal bacteria	Component of coenzymes I and II (NAD, NADP), many enzymatic reactions	Pellagra: dermatitis, diarrhea, dementia	Nicotinic acid (not the amide): flushing, pruritis, liver abnormalities, hyperuricemia, decreased LDL and increased HDL cholesterol	Milk, eggs, poultry, meat, fish, whole grains, enriched cereals and grains
Pantothenic acid	Water soluble, heat stable	Component of CoA; many enzymatic reactions	Observed only with use of antagonists; depression, fatigue, hypotension, muscle weakness, abdominal pain	Unknown	Organ meats, yeast, egg yolk, fresh vegetables, whole grains, legumes
Pyridoxine (vitamin B_6) also pyridoxal, pyridoxamine	Water soluble, heat and light labile; interference from isoniazid; pyridoxal is the active form	Cofactor for many enzymes, (eg, transaminases, decarboxylases)	Irritability, depression, dermatitis, glossitis, cheilosis, peripheral neuritis; in infants, irritability, convulsions, microcytic anemia	Neuropathy, photosensitivity	Liver, meat, whole grains, legumes, potatoes

341

Table 21.1.
Vitamins: Summary Table* (continued)

Name	Characteristics	Biochemical Action	Effects of Deficiency	Effects of Excess	Food Sources
		WATER-SOLUBLE VITAMINS			
Riboflavin (vitamin B_{12})	Water soluble, light labile, heat stable; synthesis by intestinal bacteria	Oxidation reduction, cofactor for many enzymes, synthesis of FMN and FAD	Pure riboflavin deficiency rare, photophobia, cheilosis, glossitis, corneal vascularization, poor growth	Unknown	Meat, dairy products, eggs, green vegetables, whole grains, enriched breads and cereals
Thiamine (vitamin B_1)	Water soluble, heat labile; absorption impaired by alcohol; requirements a function of carbohydrate intake	Coenzyme for decarboxylation, other reactions as thiamine pyrophosphate	Beriberi: neuritis, edema, cardiac failure, hoarseness, anorexia, restlessness, aphonia	Unknown	Enriched cereals and breads, lean pork, whole grains, legumes, in small amounts in most nutritious foods
Ascorbic acid (vitamin C)	Water soluble, easily oxidized, especially in presence of copper, iron, high pH; absorption by simple diffusion	Reversible reductant: functions in folacin metabolism, collagen biosynthesis, iron absorption and transport, tyrosine metabolism, neurotransmitter, carnitine synthesis	Osmotic diarrhea, bleeding gums, perifollicular hemorrhage, frank scurvy	Massive doses predispose to kidney stones; nausea, abdominal pain; rebound scurvy when massive doses stopped	Papaya, citrus fruits, tomatoes, cabbage, potatoes, cantaloupe, strawberries

Table 21.1.
Vitamins: Summary Table* *(continued)*

Name	Characteristics	Biochemical Action	Effects of Deficiency	Effects of Excess	Food Sources
		FAT-SOLUBLE VITAMINS			
Vitamin A (retinol) 1 μg retinol = 3.31 IU	Light sensitive, fat soluble, heat stable; bile necessary for absorption; specific plasma binding protein; stored in liver	Component of photorhodopsin; integrity of epithelial tissues, bone cell, and immune function	Night blindness, xerophthalmia, keratomalacia, poor bone growth, impaired resistance to infection, follicular hyperkeratosis	Hyperostosis, hepatomegaly, Hepatic fibrosis alopecia, increased cerebrospinal fluid pressure	Fortified milk, liver, egg, cheese, yellow fruits and vegetables (carotenoid precursors)
Carotenoids (primarily carotene = 1/12 activity of retinol)	Fat soluble converted to retinol in liver and intestinal mucosa; absorptive efficiency decreases with increased doses			Carotenemia	Dark green vegetables, yellow fruits and vegetables, tomato
Vitamin D (D$_2$, activated calciferol; D$_3$, activated dehydrocholesterol) 1 μg = 40 IU	Fat soluble D$_2$ from plant sources or fortification; D$_3$ from action of ultraviolet light on skin, animal sources, or fortification; hydroxylated sequentially in liver and kidney to form 1,25-dihydroxy-chole-calciferol, the active compound; regulated by dietary calcium, PTH; now called a pro hormone; anti-epileptic drugs interfere with metabolism	Maintains serum calcium via intestinal and bone effects; regulates synthesis of calcium-binding protein in intestinal epithelial cells, increasing calcium and phosphorus absorption; enhances mobilization of calcium and phosphorus from bone during deprivation	Rickets, osteomalacia, anti-epileptic drugs interfere with metabolism	Hypercalcemia, azotemia, poor growth, vomiting, nephrocalcinosis	Fortified milk fish, liver, egg yolk

Table 21.1.
Vitamins: Summary Table* *(continued)*

Name	Characteristics	Biochemical Action	Effects of Deficiency	Effects of Excess	Food Sources
FAT-SOLUBLE VITAMINS					
Vitamin E (1 IU=1 mg D 1 α-tocopheryl acetate); 8 compounds with biological activity, the most active being naturally occurring α-tocopherol 1.49 IU=1 mg	Fat soluble, heat labile; stored in adipose tissue, transported with lipoproteins; absorption depends on pancreatic juice and bile (iron may interfere); tocopherol transport protein in liver regulates plasma levels; requirement increased by intake of large amounts of polyunsaturated fats	Free radical scavenger, antioxidant, role in red blood cell fragility; stabilizes biological membranes; prevents peroxidation of unsaturated fatty acids	Hemolytic anemia in premature infants; fat malabsorption causes deficiency: hyporeflexia, and spinocerebellar and retinal degeneration; familial isolated vitamin E deficiency	Bleeding, impaired leukocyte function	Sardines, green and leafy vegetables, vegetable oils, wheat germ, whole grains, butter, liver, egg yolk
Vitamin K (napthoquinones)	Light sensitive, fat soluble; bile necessary for absorption; synthesis by intestinal bacteria; antagonized by coumarin, salicylates, some antibiotics	Blood coagulation: factors II, VII, IX, X, Proteins C, S, K dependent bone proteins, and matrix Gla protein	Primary deficiency Rare; hemorrhagic Manifestations, possible effect on bone mineral density	Water-soluble analogs only: hyperbilirubinemia, hemolysis	Cow milk, green leafy vegetables, pork, liver

*CoA indicates coenzyme A; TPN, total parenteral nutrition; NAD, nicotinamide adenine dinucleotide; NADP, nicotinamide-adenine dinucleotide phosphate; LDL, low-density lipoprotein; HDL, high-density lipoprotein; FMN, flavin mononucleotide; FAD, flavin adenine dinucleotide; and PTH, parathyroid hormone. Adapted from Shils ME, Olson JA, Shike M, eds. *Modern Nutrition in Health and Disease.* Philadelphia, PA: Lea and Febiger; 1994:247–448; and Forbes GB. Nutrition. In: Hoekelman RA, Blatman S, Freidman SB, Nelson NM, Seidel HM, eds. *Primary Pediatric Care.* St Louis, MO: CV Mosby; 1987:160–164.

they be adequate for certain disease states marked by increased nutritional requirements.

Vitamin preparations available in the United States for infants and children younger than 4 years are in accord with Food and Drug Administration (FDA) regulations.[2] These regulations (designed to minimize misuse) cover the minimum and maximum levels allowed or required in multivitamin and multimineral supplements for infants and children younger than 4 years and for pregnant or lactating women. Preparations for older children and adults are not subject to FDA regulations, and this may increase the likelihood of the development of toxic effects from these preparations.

Vitamin and mineral products on the market for infants and children consist primarily of the following:

1. Liquid drop preparations, for infants, that contain vitamins A, D, and C, with or without iron; or vitamins A, D, C, and E, thiamine, riboflavin, niacin, and vitamin B_6, with or without iron.
2. Chewable tablets, for young children, that contain vitamins A, D, and C, with or without iron; or vitamins A, D, E, and C, thiamine, folic acid, riboflavin, niacin, vitamin B_6, and vitamin B_{12}, with or without iron. Infants and children who are ill or receive certain medications may require supplements of specific vitamins. Extra allowances are suggested for pregnant and lactating women. The widespread consumption of supplemental products is fostered by a combination of advertising pressure and concern about dietary adequacy. Many individuals regard vitamin and mineral supplements as a reliable method of ensuring that real or imagined dietary shortcomings are corrected. A vitamin pill containing the RDA given to the child daily, although unnecessary, probably does no harm. Like all medications, these should be safely stored.

Fat-Soluble Vitamins

Intestinal absorption of the fat-soluble vitamins (A, D, E, and K) is strongly dependent on adequate secretion of pancreatic enzymes and of bile acids from the liver into the intestinal lumen. In addition, vitamin A and vitamin E esters require hydrolysis prior to intestinal absorption by an intestinal esterase that is bile acid dependent. Therefore, each of these vitamins may be poorly absorbed if any phase of fat digestion, absorption, or transport is interrupted. Recently, the Institute of Medicine of the National Academy of Sciences has published new DRIs for vitamins A, E, and K (see Appendix C) and each are described in the following text.

Vitamin A

The term vitamin A refers to retinol and derivatives that have the same β-ionone ring and qualitatively similar biologic activities. The principal vitamin A compounds—retinol, retinal (retinaldehyde), retinoic acid, and retinyl esters—differ in the terminal C-15 group at the end of the side chain. The functions of vitamin A are maintenance of proper vision, epithelial cell integrity, and regulation of glycoprotein synthesis and cell differentiation.

Vitamin A is present in the diet as retinyl esters derived almost exclusively from animal sources (liver and fish liver oils, dairy products, kidney, and eggs) and provitamin A carotenoids (mainly β-carotene) that are distributed widely in green and yellow vegetables. The recent report by the Institute of Medicine of the National Academy of Sciences suggests that carotene-rich fruits and vegetables (carrots, sweet potatoes, broccoli) provide the body with half as much vitamin A as previously thought. Vitamin A activity is expressed as retinol activity equivalents (RAE; 1 μg of all-trans-retinol = 1 RAE = 3.3 IU vitamin A activity; 1 μg of all-trans-retinol = 12 μg of all-trans-β-carotene = 24 μg of other provitamin A carotenoids). The AI for infants is 400 μg RAE for ages 0 to 6 months and 500 μg RAE for ages 7 to 12 months. The RDA is 300 μg RAE for children aged 1 to 3 years, 400 μg RAE for children aged 4 to 8 years, and 600 to 900 μg RAE for older children and adults. Human milk, cow milk, and commercial infant formulas are excellent sources of vitamin A. Vitamin A status is monitored by serum retinol and retinol-binding protein (RBP) concentrations.

Vitamin A deficiency occurs in children not given vitamin A and in those with fat malabsorption. Deficiency may lead to xerophthalmia, keratomalacia, and irreversible damage to the cornea, as well as night blindness and pigmentary retinopathy. Deficiency may also increase morbidity and mortality from various infections, such as measles. Administration of the vitamin may be life-saving in children with chronic deficiency and malnutrition.[3] Additionally, routine supplementation with vitamin A during early childhood has decreased visual complications as well as overall childhood mortality in developing countries.[4] While vitamin A supplementation during measles infection has been demonstrated to decrease overall morbidity, the role of supplementation in other infectious diseases is less clear. In several studies, vitamin A supplementation made no difference in clinical symptoms in non-measles infections (pneumonia, RSV, infectious diarrhea),[5–8] and in several instances, actually worsened clinical symptoms.[9,10]

Claims that extremely high doses of vitamin A (7500 to 15000 μg RAE/d) improve visual acuity in those who work in bright or dim light are unsubstantiated. Large doses of vitamin A are also used for the treatment of acne and to prevent infection. As little as 6000 μg RAE daily can produce serious toxic effects in children. Vitamin A toxicity is manifested by anorexia, increased intracranial pressure (vomiting and headaches), painful bone lesions, precocious bone growth, desquamative dermatitis, and hepatotoxicity.[11–13] To monitor for vitamin A toxicity during high-dose vitamin A therapy, serum retinyl esters, normally not present, should be monitored. Plasma levels of retinol and RBP are not reliable means of detecting vitamin A toxicity.[13,14] Caffey warned that the hazards of vitamin A poisoning from the routine prophylactic use of concentrates of vitamins A and D to well-fed healthy infants and children in the United States are considerably greater than the hazards of vitamin A deficiency in healthy infants and children not fed vitamin concentrates.[15] Toxic effects of vitamin A were found in young children who were fed large amounts of chicken liver, which contains 90 μg RAE vitamin A/g,[16] for 1 month or longer. Vitamin A excess, including vitamin A derivatives such as retinoic acid, are teratogenic; teenagers who may become pregnant should be informed of the dangers of vitamin A or derivatives used in the treatment of acne.[17]

Vitamin D

Vitamin D (calciferol) refers to 2 secosteroids, vitamin D_2 (ergocalciferol) and vitamin D_3 (cholecalciferol). Vitamin D_2 is derived from plants and fungi, and is added to vitamin D-supplemented cow milk. Vitamin D_3 is synthesized in the skin from 7-dehydrocholesterol upon exposure to sunlight. Vitamins D_2 and D_3 are considered prohormones and subsequently undergo 25-hydroxylation in the liver to form 25-hydroxy vitamin D (25 OH-D, calcidiol), which is the major circulating form of vitamin D. From the liver, 25 OH-D is transported to the kidney for hydroxylation to form the biologically active hormone 1,25 dihydroxyvitamin D (1,25,OH2-D, calcitriol). Calcitriol is the biologically active form of vitamin D, which stimulates intestinal absorption of calcium and phosphorous, renal reabsorption of filtered calcium, and the mobilization of calcium and phosphorous from bone. Vitamin D is, therefore, essential for bone formation and mineral homeostasis.

Vitamin D is synthesized in the skin by the action of ultraviolet light on a cholesterol precursor (the most effective wavelengths are in the range of 290 to 315 nm); therefore, the requirement for dietary vitamin D depends on the amount of exposure to sunlight. The actual requirement for vitamin D in the absence of sunlight is unknown. The AI is 200 IU (5.0 μg cholecalciferol) in infants, children, and adults. The vitamin D content of human milk is low (22 IU/L), and rickets can occur in deeply pigmented breastfed infants or in those with inadequate exposure to sunlight. Consequently, vitamin D supplementation at 200 IU/d is recommended for breastfed infants. Most formulas contain 1.5 μg (62 IU) of vitamin D per 100 calories, or 10 μg/L, as do cow milk and evaporated milks. This is double the estimated requirement for full-term infants. Vitamin D status is monitored by serum 25-OH vitamin D concentration, serum calcium, phosphorous, and alkaline phosphatase.

The primary manifestations of vitamin D deficiency are related to the effects on calcium metabolism. Hypocalcemia, hypophosphatemia, tetany, osteomalacia, and rickets are the most common clinical features. Deficiency occurs in those with fat malabsorption and may occur in infants not exposed to sunlight who have an inadequate dietary intake of vitamin D. The best estimate for adequate exposure to sunlight for white infants is 30 minutes per week clothed only in a diaper, or 2 hours per week fully clothed with no hat.[18]

No evidence supports the claim that vitamin D, in amounts much greater than the RDA of 10 μg daily, leads to improved bone mineralization. The AI provides an ample margin of safety even without exposure to sunlight. The principal manifestations of vitamin D intoxication are hypercalcemia leading to depression of the central nervous system and ectopic calcification, and hypercalciuria leading to nephrocalcinosis and nephrolithiasis. Overuse of vitamin D in Britain and Europe, with intakes between 70 and 100 μg daily, is believed to be related to the idiopathic hypercalcemia of infants, which was seen frequently during and after World War II.

Vitamin E
There are 4 major forms (I, δ, Δ, and K) of tocopherol and tocotrienols, the 2 main forms of vitamin E. α-tocopherol has the highest biologic activity, and is the predominant form in foodstuffs with the exception of soy oil that contains high levels of gamma tocopherol. The major function of vitamin E is its role as an antioxidant, protecting cell membrane polyunsaturated fatty acids, thiol-rich proteins, and nucleic acids from oxidant damage initiated by free-radical reactions. Vitamin E is essential for the maintenance of structure and function of the human nervous system, retina, and skeletal muscle.

<hr>

American Academy of Pediatrics recommendations:

To prevent rickets and vitamin D deficiency in healthy infants and children and acknowledging that adequate sunlight exposure is difficult to determine, we reaffirm the adequate intake of 200 IU/d of vitamin D by the National Academy of Sciences[4] and recommend a supplement of 200 IU/d for the following:

1. All breastfed infants unless they are weaned to at least 500 mL per day of vitamin D-fortified formula or milk.
2. All nonbreastfed infants who are ingesting less than 500 mL per day of vitamin D-fortified formula or milk.
3. Children and adolescents who do not get regular sunlight exposure, do not ingest at least 500 mL per day of vitamin D-fortified milk, or do not take a daily multivitamin supplement containing at least 200 IU of vitamin D.

<hr>

The common dietary sources of vitamin E are the oil-containing grains, plants, and vegetables. The AI for infants aged 0 to 6 months is 4 mg (9.3 μmol)/d of α-tocopherol and for infants aged 7 to 12 months is 5 mg (11.6 μmol)/d of α-tocopherol (~0.6 mg/kg). The RDA for children aged 1 to 3 years is 6 mg (13.9 μmol), 4 to 8 years is 7 mg (16.3 μmol), and 9 to 18 years is 11 to 15 mg (25.6–34.9 μmol)/d of α-tocopherol. The RDA for adults is 15 mg (34.9 μmol)/d of α-tocopherol (1 mg d-α-tocopherol = 1 tocopherol equivalent [TE]; 1 mg dL-α-tocopheryl acetate = 1 International Unit [IU]). Vitamin E status is monitored by serum α-tocopherol concentrations and serum α-tocopherol:total lipid ratios.

The wide distribution of vitamin E in vegetable oils and cereal grains makes deficiency in humans from developed countries unlikely. Vitamin E supplements are necessary for those with malabsorption (eg, pancreatic insufficiency or cystic fibrosis), biliary atresia and other biliary tract disorders, cirrhosis, and lipid transport disorders. Uncorrected vitamin E deficiency during childhood leads to a chronologic sequence of progressive neurologic symptoms including, truncal and limb ataxia, hyporeflexia, depressed vibratory and position sensation, impairment in balance and coordination, peripheral neuropathy, proximal muscle weakness, ophthalmoplegia, and retinal dysfunction.[19] Significant cognitive and behavioral abnormalities have been described in association with prolonged vitamin E deficiency. The neurologic lesions may be irreversible to a substantial degree if vitamin E deficiency remains untreated. Congenital deficiency of the hepatic tocopherol transport protein also results in vitamin E deficiency and ataxia, despite normal absorption of vitamin E.[20] Deficiency of vitamin E has also been associated with hemolytic anemia in premature infants fed a diet high in polyunsaturated fatty acids.[21]

Vitamin E may lower the risk of retinopathy of prematurity. Vitamin E supplementation prevents severe neuropathy in infants with biliary atresia and other forms of chronic cholestatic liver disease, and it prevents muscle weakness in children with cystic fibrosis.[19] Little or no basis exists for the claim that high dietary intakes of vitamin E prolong life, increase sexual potency, and prevent conditions such as mental retardation and cancer. However, recent evidence suggests that vitamin E supplementation in adults may play a role in the prevention of cardiovascular disease.[22] Vitamin E toxicity is rare. Normal adults appear to tolerate oral doses of 100 to 800 mg/d without clinical signs or biochemical evidence of toxicity.[23] In several studies, adults who received very large doses of vitamin E (>1000 to 1500 IU/d) in conjunction with warfarin therapy had a significantly prolonged prothrombin time (PT) beyond that expected from the warfarin alone.[24,25] In addition, large parenteral doses of vitamin E in preterm infants, resulting in extremely high serum vitamin E levels (>40 to 50 μg/mL), were associated with an increased incidence of bacterial and fungal sepsis, presumably due to inhibition of neutrophil function.[26]

Vitamin K

Vitamin K belongs to the family of 2 methyl-1,4 naphthoquinones and exists as 3 forms.[27] Phylloquinone (vitamin K_1) is obtained from leafy vegetables, soybean oil, fruits, seeds, and cow milk. Menaquinone (vitamin K_2), which has 60% of the activity of vitamin K_1 is synthesized by intestinal bacteria. Menadione (vitamin K_3) is not a natural form but is synthesized chemically, and has better water solubility than the 2 natural forms. Vitamin K is necessary for the posttranslational carboxylation of glutamic acid residues of the vitamin K-dependent coagulation proteins (Factors II, VII, IX, and X, protein C, and protein S). Carboxylation allows these proteins to bind calcium, thus leading to activation of the clotting factors.[28] Other proteins undergoing this carboxylation of glutamic acid residues include osteocalcin, which is involved in bone mineralization.

The newborn infant is usually given vitamin K soon after birth for prophylaxis against hemorrhagic disease of the newborn. Vitamin K should be given as a single intramuscular dose of 0.5 to 1 mg, or as an oral dose of 1 to 2 mg administered at birth, 1 to 2 weeks and 4 weeks of age.[29] Vitamin K is present in most cow milk formulas, and the bottle-fed infant ordinarily does not need added vitamin K. The AI for infants is 2 μg/d of phylloquinone or menaquinone for the first 6 months and 2.5 μg/d for the second 6 months. Adequate intake for older children is 30 μg/d for ages 1 to 3 years, 55 μg/d ages 4 to 8 years, and 60 to 75 μg/d for older children and adolescents. Vitamin K status is monitored by PT and proteins-induced-in-vitamin K absence II (PIVKA II) analysis. In 1990, Golding et al[30] reported a study of a 1970 birth cohort in Britain in which they noted an unexpected association between childhood cancer and pethidine given in labor and the neonatal administration of vitamin K. Subsequently, they reported in a retrospective, case-controlled study a significant association between intramuscular vitamin K and cancer when compared with no vitamin K or oral vitamin K.[31] Draper and Stiller[32] have questioned this study based on other data from Great Britain and have called for large cohort studies. The American Academy of Pediatrics formed a Vitamin K Ad Hoc Task Force to study this area in greater detail.[29] The task force found no convincing links between vitamin K administration and childhood cancer. Indeed, if intramuscular vitamin K doubles the incidence of childhood leukemia, a sharp increase should have been observed after 1961, which was not the case. Golding et al suggest that sister chromatid exchanges (SCEs) induced by vitamin K may be responsible for the increased incidence of cancer observed in their study.[33] However, in a study of human infants, no differences in SCEs were observed in those who received vitamin K versus those who did not. Based on these observations, the task force continues to recommend the routine administration of vitamin K to newborns (see box).

The American Academy of Pediatrics recommends the following concerning the administration of vitamin K to newborns:

Since parenteral vitamin K prevents a life-threatening disease of the newborn and the risks of cancer are unproven and unlikely, the American Academy of Pediatrics* recommends:

1. Vitamin K$_1$ should be given to all newborns as a single, intramuscular dose of 0.5 to 1 mg.[29]
2. Further research on the efficacy, safety, and bioavailability of oral formulations of vitamin K is warranted.
3. An oral dosage form is not currently available in the United States but ought to be developed and licensed. If an appropriate oral form is developed and licensed in the United States, it should be given at birth (2.0 mg) and should be administered again at 1 to 2 weeks and at 4 weeks of age to breastfed infants. If diarrhea occurs in an exclusively breastfed infant, the dose should be repeated.
4. The conflicting data of Golding et al[30] and Draper and Stiller[32] and the data from the United States[29] suggest that additional cohort studies are unlikely to be helpful.

*American Academy of Pediatrics. Controversies concerning vitamin K and the newborn. *Pediatrics.* 1993;91:1001–1003

Water-Soluble Vitamins

Deficiencies of the water-soluble vitamins are rare in formula-fed infants and in breastfed infants of mothers consuming varied diets. Most children and adolescents, if eating a diet consisting of fruits, vegetables, animal protein sources, cereals or bread, and dairy products, consume sufficient water-soluble vitamins to meet daily allowances, particularly after the rapid growth periods. In fact, many water-soluble vitamin deficiency states in infancy and childhood are a result of inborn errors of metabolism and not dietary deficiencies. The B vitamins are essential for carbohydrate, protein, and fat metabolism, oxidation-reduction reactions, transamination and decarboxylation, glycolysis, and blood formation (see Table 21.1). Given their involvement in the metabolism of all the macronutrients, the DRIs for the B vitamins are based on total caloric intake (see Appendix C). The basis for requirements for the remaining water-soluble vitamins are discussed in each relevant subsection of this chapter.

Rapid simple and reliable high-performance liquid chromatographic techniques now exist for the measurement of water-soluble vitamins in infant formula[34] and in multivitamin pharmaceutical formulations.[35] These techniques are more sensitive and specific than the calorimetric, fluorometric, spectrophotometric, and titrimetric techniques employed previously. It can be expected that application of these techniques, which allow simultaneous assessment of multiple water-soluble vitamins, to analysis of dietary water-soluble vitamins, will continue to enhance our ability to assess requirements and deficiency states in various pediatric populations. Another methodology that has now been shown to be a fairly simple and reliable means of assessing water-soluble vitamin intake is the food frequency questionnaire. An 84-item food frequency questionnaire was used in children aged 1 to 5 years[36] with correlations of 0.5 or more between the questionnaire and 24-hour dietary recalls for water-soluble vitamins, including vitamins C, B_1, B_2, B_6, niacin, and folate. Thus application of both the newer analytical techniques as well as this simple inexpensive clinical tool should prove useful for both research and policy development.

Water-soluble vitamin intake has been studied in several groups of children and adolescents within the last few years. For example, 2-year-old children on cow milk-restricted diets were shown to have decreased intake of riboflavin and niacin compared with cow milk consumers.[37] On the other hand, adolescents following current nutrition recommendation to consume a low-fat diet (<30% of total energy intake) were shown to have a greater likelihood of inadequate vitamin B_{12} intake compared with high-fat consumers.[38] Adolescents taking a diet high in fiber (>20 g/d) had a greater likelihood of adequate intake of vitamins B$_6$, B$_{12}$, niacin, thiamin, riboflavin, and folacin. Not surprisingly, children and adolescents who eat dinner with their family regularly had substantially higher intakes of vitamins B$_6$, B$_{12}$, C, and folate.[39] It is known that physical activity stresses metabolic pathways that depend on thiamine, riboflavin, and vitamin B$_6$[40]; on the other hand, adolescent athletes in some parts of the world take large amounts of water-soluble vitamin supplements.[41] Systematic studies of water-soluble vitamin status in adolescent athletes in the United States have not been done. Children with metabolic diseases such as phenylketonuria treated with special diets may be at risk for deficiencies of multiple water-soluble vitamins,[42] and children and adolescents with malabsorption conditions such as Crohn's disease are also known to be at risk for water-soluble vitamin deficiency.[43]

Thiamin (Vitamin B$_1$)

Although severe thiamin deficiency is rare in developed countries, the incidence of moderate thiamin deficiency may be underestimated in certain groups, including infants and children.[44] Pediatric age-specific reference ranges for total, phosphorylated, and nonphosphorylated thiamin have been determined in whole blood and also in cerebrospinal fluid,[45] given the increasing evidence that thiamin may serve as a neurotransmitter.[46] Whole-blood thiamin decreases from birth until 12 months of age, primarily due to a decrease in phosphorylated thiamin, the biologically active form. The cerebrospinal fluid thiamin decreases until age 15 months, due initially to a decrease in non-phosphorylated thiamin. Therefore, studies of thiamin status in infancy should use age-dependent norms.

Wernicke encephalopathy is a manifestation of severe thiamin deficiency characterized by a triad of ophthalmoplegia, ataxia, and mental confusion, and is extremely rare in children. In a report of 30 cases of the syndrome in children, many of whom had underlying malignancy, 42% of the children were diagnosed at autopsy, suggesting that this potentially reversible syndrome is underdiagnosed in children.[47] Reversible brain magnetic resonance imaging changes in a child with the syndrome have been reported.[48] The shortfall of intravenous multivitamins that occurred in the late 1990s resulted in several cases of Wernicke encephalopathy in children as well as in adults. Since intravenous thiamin is available and can readily reverse the neurologic abnormalities, prompt diagnosis is important.[49] Reversal of the symptoms associated with pyruvate dehydrogenase complex deficiency by administration of high-dose thiamin and sodium dichloroacetate has been reported.[50]

Riboflavin (Vitamin B₂)

Milk either from human or cow is the principal source of riboflavin for infants and at least one third of the DRI for US adults is thought to be supplied by milk and dairy products.[51] Thus, accurate assessment of the riboflavin content of both human and cow milk is important. Recently developed techniques involving acid-phenol extractions followed by high-performance liquid chromatography have shown that the content of riboflavin and other flavins in both human[52] and cow milk[53] is higher than reported in earlier studies where no correction for the internal fluorescence quenching of flavin adenine dinucleotide was made. The erythrocyte glutathione reductase activation test has demonstrated subclinical riboflavin deficiency in 35% of solely breastfed Indian infants.[54] Although the functional significance of riboflavin deficiency in young subjects is not clear, there are suggestions that psychomotor abnormalities can occur in affected patients.[55]

Niacin (Vitamin B₃)

Pellagra is the dermatological disease associated with severe niacin deficiency. In the United States during the 1930s and 1940s, at a time of decreased food availability and variety, pellagra was sufficiently common that the US food supply was fortified with niacin. This practice was designed to restore nutrients lost through grain milling and has played a significant role in elimination of pellagra in the United States.[56] High-dose niacin has been effective in treating adults with primary hyperlipidemia; administration results in significant decreases in both LDL cholesterol and apolipoprotein B, as well as significant increases of high-density lipoprotein cholesterol[57]; pediatric trials have not been reported.

Pyridoxine (Vitamin B₆)

Pyridoxine appears to be critically important for the developing brain and pyridoxine-responsive seizures occur primarily in the very young. The prevalence of pyridoxine-dependent seizures and other forms of pyridoxine responsive seizures in the UK and Ireland has been reported at 1/687 000.[58] Over one third of the reported cases had atypical presentations and a trial of pyridoxine was, therefore, recommended for all cases of early onset intractable seizures or status epilepticus. Pyridoxine-dependent seizures are the result of a metabolic defect of K cystathionase, not a dietary deficiency of pyridoxine. Congenital sideroblastic anemia is a relatively rare disease that has been shown to be caused by missense mutations in the Δ-aminolevulinic acid synthase gene. An 8-month-old male infant with profound anemia secondary to this disorder responded to 50 mg/d of oral pyridoxine.[59]

Andon et al[60] measured dietary intake of total and glycosylated vitamin B_6 in unsupplemented lactating women and their infants and found intake to be adequate; infant plasma pyridoxal 5'-phosphate concentrations were in the normal range as were the infants' length and weight measurements. Maternal intake of glycosylated vitamin B_6 had little effect on maternal plasma pyridoxal 5'-phosphate. In contrast, Kang-Yoon et al[61] showed that supplementation of maternal or infant diet with vitamin B_6 resulted in increased plasma pyridoxal 5'-phosphate concentrations in their breastfed term infants. The concentration of vitamin B_6 in both breast milk of mothers of preterm infants and preterm infant plasma was low and did not increase with maternal supplementation. Thus, the question of whether or not to supplement the diet of breastfed infants and/or of the maternal diet with vitamin B_6 remains unsettled.

Plasma pyridoxal 5'-phosphate declines with infant age and does not correlate with diet after age 1 month in one study[62] or age 5 years in another.[63] Driskell et al[64] utilized a functional assay for pyridoxine (coenzyme stimulation of erythrocyte alanine aminotransferase activities) as well as dietary intakes of the vitamin to assess vitamin B_6 status in southern adolescent girls; approximately half of the girls consumed inadequate amounts and had coenzyme stimulation values indicative of marginal or deficient status.

Cobalamin (Vitamin B_{12})

Higher concentrations of cobalamin are found in colostrum compared with values for the third month of lactation. There are, however, no significant differences in cobalamin and its binding protein between breasts, fore and hindmilk, and morning, afternoon, and evening samples; thus, representative samples of breast milk for cobalamin analysis can be obtained for population studies irrespective of time of day or moment within the feed.[65]

Breastfed infants of strict vegan mothers are at risk for vitamin B_{12} deficiency. Maternal vitamin B_{12} deficiency has also been associated with neural-tube defects.[66] Breast milk vitamin B_{12} is inversely related to the length of time on a vegetarian diet and infant urinary methymalonic acid is inversely related to milk vitamin B_{12} concentrations.[67] The 1989 RDA for vitamin B_{12} of 221 pmol/d for infants was close to the intake below which infant urinary methylmalonic acid excretion is increased, suggesting that RDA provided little margin of safety.[67] Plasma methymalonic acid and total homocysteine are useful indicators of functional cobalamin deficiency in infants on macrobiotic diets[68] and administration.

Administration of oral or intramuscular vitamin B_{12} normalized urinary values of methylmalonic acid in infants with vitamin B_{12} deficiency.[69] Interestingly, one mother modified her diet in a manner consistent with the vegetarian philosophy by increasing the consumption of sea vegetables and fermented foods, thought to be rich in vitamin B_{12}. Although the fermented food (tempeh) was low in vitamin B_{12}, the sea vegetables wakame and kombu contained high amounts. Within 2 months of consistent maternal consumption of these vegetables, the urinary methylmalonic acid of her breastfed infant normalized. Severe neurologic abnormalities can result from infantile vitamin B_{12} deficiency secondary to a maternal vegan diet[70] and have even been reported in 1 of a set of monozygous twins.[71] Abnormalities can often, but not always, be reversed by administration of parenteral or oral vitamin B_{12}. Megaloblastic anemia secondary to vitamin B_{12} deficiency in children consuming alternative diets has also been reported.[72]

Recently, 2 novel causes of vitamin B_{12} deficiency have been described in adults. Prolonged administration of proton-pump inhibitors resulting in long-term acid suppression[73] and *Helicobacter pylori*-induced gastritis.[74] Although both prolonged administration of proton pump inhibitors and *H pylori* infection are not rare in children and adolescents, there are no reports of vitamin B_{12} status in such subjects. Patients with phenylketonuria on an unrestricted or relaxed diet are at risk for vitamin B_{12} deficiency.[75] There are a number of vitamin B_{12} responsive inborn errors of metabolism, including transcobalamin II deficiency.[76]

Folate

As with the other water-soluble vitamins, there have been methodologic advances for determination of total folate content and derivatives in human milk (the basis of determination of nutrient requirement for infants) that should allow more accurate determination of these requirements. The microbiological protocols for determination of total folate and the pteroylpolyglutamate content of human milk that do not use folate conjugase and do not release folate from binding proteins will seriously underestimate milk folate values.[77] Total serum homocysteine is increased in the presence of folate deficiency in neonates.[78] Supplemental folate, taken alone or added to food, is better absorbed than folate that is a normal constituent in a food. Cereals, grains, and breads are now fortified with folate.

In contrast to most of the other water-soluble vitamins, potentially inadequate intake of folate in children is not rare. In one study of white preschool children aged 2 to 5 years of middle-and upper-socioeconomic status, the mean folate intake was consistently below recommended amounts.[79] Foods most commonly eaten were fruit drinks, carbonated beverages, 2% milk, and french fries. Picciano et al[80] also noted that folate intakes at 12 months were 79% of recommended amounts, with an increase to 100% by 18 months. There have been fairly dramatic changes in US adolescent food choices over the last 30 years with increased consumption of soft drinks and non-citrus juices. The intake of fruits and vegetables is below the recommended 5 servings per day, and intakes of folate by girls have consistently been below recommended amounts.[81] Adolescents with low folate intake have exhibited higher mean diastolic blood pressures compared with those with a high folate intake.[82]

5,10–Methylenetetrahydrofolate reductase is involved in folate metabolism. It is located on chromosome 1, and 2 common alleles have been described: C677T and A1298C. C677T homozygosity in infants is associated with a moderately increased risk for spina bifida.[83] Maternal C677T homozygosity appears to be a moderate risk factor for spina bifida in the fetus as well. There are some data to suggest that the risk of spina bifida in subjects with C677T homozygosity may depend on the subject's nutritional folate status, and it can be anticipated that much more will be learned about nutrient-gene interaction in this area in the next decade. The prevalence of the C677T allele may be doubled in children who had a stroke compared to controls of the same age group.[84] Those who had a stroke also had hyperhomocysteinemia. Homocysteine values and serum folate were inversely related in the children who had a stroke as well. Thus, systematic studies are indicated to determine if folate supplementation of children with this polymorphism would prevent recurrent stroke.

Folate supplementation has been shown to reduce methotrexate toxicity in children with juvenile arthritis, without affecting the clinical efficacy of the drug.[85] Hyperhomocysteinemia has also been observed in children treated with sodium valproate and carbamazepine for epilepsy; serum folate was decreased in children with high plasma levels of homocysteine.[86] The significance of these findings is unclear. Methylenetetrahydrofolate reductase deficiency has been described in 4 siblings; clinical manifestations included retarded psychomotor development, poor social contact, and seizures. Folate levels in serum and red cells were low.[87]

Vitamin C

In the recent DRIs recommended by the Panel on Dietary Antioxidants and Related Compounds of the Institute of Medicine, the RDA for vitamin C for adults was established on the basis of the vitamin C intake to maintain near-maximal neutrophil concentration with minimal urinary excretion of ascorbate.[88] Since similar data in infants was not available, the AI for vitamin C in infants was based on mean vitamin C intake of breastfed infants. Recommended dietary allowances for children and adolescents were estimated on the basis of relative body weight.

The intake of vitamin C by school-aged children has been studied extensively in the 1994–1996 Continuing Survey of Food Intakes by Individuals. Among 7- to 12-year-olds, 12% of boys and 13% of girls had mean vitamin C intakes that were less than 30 mg/d.[89] Among 13- to 18-year-olds, 14% of boys and 20% of girls had low vitamin C intakes. Children with low vitamin C intake tended to have greater energy-adjusted intakes of fat and saturated fat. Children with desirable vitamin C intakes consumed more high-vitamin C fruit juice, high-vitamin C-containing vegetables and whole milk, and more citrus fruits than children with low vitamin C intake. In a group of children receiving long-term dialysis, dietary intake of vitamin C (and in fact all water-soluble vitamins) was <100% of RDA in most[90]; supplementation was necessary to reach the RDA.

Other

Information on human needs for pantothenic acid is limited. In one survey, 49% of female adolescents and 25% of the male adolescents consumed less than 4 mg/d, the amount recommended by the Food and Nutrition Board.[91] However, average blood levels for both groups were in a normal range. Deficiency symptoms have not been characterized.

Clinical biotin deficiency is characterized by hypotonia and severe exfoliative dermatitis. To date, symptomatic deficiency has been described only in infants given total parenteral nutrition that was free of biotin and in children given undercooked eggs containing large amounts of avidin, a biotin-binding protein. However, children given long-term anticonvulsant therapy exhibit impaired biotin status.[92]

Conclusion

Some vitamin-dependency states are the result of inborn errors of metabolism in which pharmacologic doses of vitamins may ameliorate signs of disease. These states have been described for thiamin, pyridoxine, folic acid, vitamin B_{12}, biotin, niacin, riboflavin, and vitamin C. The genetic polymorphisms responsible for some of these diseases have been delineated. In the era of the human genome project, it can be predicted that many more such diseases will be delineated in the future. Thus, to restate, supplemental vitamins are probably unnecessary for the healthy child over age 1 year who consumes a varied diet. Some at-risk children may benefit from supplemental multivitamin preparations providing the RDA. Groups at particular nutritional risk include the following:

1. Infants with malabsorption and liver disease.
2. Children and adolescents from deprived families or children who experience parental neglect or abuse.
3. Children and adolescents with anorexia or inadequate and capricious appetites or who consume fad diets.
4. Children with chronic disease (eg, cystic fibrosis, inflammatory bowel disease, renal or liver disease).
5. Children participating in dietary regimens to manage obesity.
6. Pregnant teenagers. Iron and folic acids are needed by these young women, but uncertainty about overall nutritional status in those considered at special nutritional risk warrants use of a multivitamin-multimineral supplement. The nutritional needs during pregnancy are more fully discussed in Chapter 11.

References

1. Dietary Reference Intakes: Recommended Intakes for Individuals, Food and Nutrition Board The National Academies of Sciences, see www.nap.edu
2. Dietary Supplement Health and Education Act (DSHEA), Public Law 103–417, Oct. 25, 1994
3. Rahmathullah L, Underwood BA, Thulasiraj RD, et al. Reduced mortality among children in Southern India receiving a small weekly dose of vitamin A. *N Engl J Med.* 1990;323:929–935
4. Underwood BA, Arthur P. The contribution of vitamin A to public health. *FASEB J.* 1996;10:1040–1048

5. Kjolhede CL, Chew FJ, Gadomski AM, Marroquin DP. Clinical trial of vitamin A as adjuvant treatment for lower respiratory tract infections. *J Pediatr.* 1995;126: 807–812

6. Quinlan K, Hayani K. Vitamin A and respiratory syncytial virus infection. *Arch Pediatr Adolesc Med.* 1996;150:25–30

7. Bresee J, Fischer M, Dowel S, et al. Vitamin A therapy for children with respiratory syncytial virus infection: a multicenter trial in the United States. *Pediatr Infect Dis J.* 1996;15:777–782

8. Henning B, Stewart K, Zaman K, Alam AN, Brown KH, Black RE. Lack of therapeutic efficacy of vitamin A for non-cholera, watery diarrhea in Bangladeshi children. *Eur J Clin Nutr.* 1992;46:437–443

9. Stephensen C, Franchi L, Hernandez H, Campos M, Gilman R, Alvarez J. Adverse effects of high-dose vitamin A supplements in children hospitalized with pneumonia. *Pediatrics.* 1998;101:E3

10. Fawzi W, Mbise R, Fataki M, et al. Vitamin A supplementation and severity of pneumonia in children admitted to the hospital in Dares Salaam, Tanzania. *Am J Clin Nutr.* 1998;68:187–192

11. Rubin E, Florman AL, Degnan T, Diaz J. Hepatic injury in chronic hypervitaminosis. *Am J Dis Child.* 1970;119:132–138

12. Lippe B, Hensen L, Mendoza G, Finerman M, Welch M. Chronic vitamin A intoxication. *Am J Dis Child.* 1981;135:634–636

13. Mobarhan S, Russell RM, Underwood BA, et al. Evaluation of the RDR test for vitamin A nutriture in cirrhotics. *Am J Clin Nutr.* 1981;34:2264–2270

14. Smith FR, Goodman DS. Vitamin A transport in human vitamin A toxicity. *N Engl J Med.* 1976;294:805–808

15. Caffey J. Chronic poisoning due to excess vitamin A: description of the clinical and roentgen manifestations in seven infants and young children. *Pediatrics.* 1950;5: 672–688

16. Mahoney CP, Margolis MT, Knauss TA, Labbe RF. Chronic vitamin A intoxication in infants fed chicken liver. *Pediatrics.* 1980;65:893–897

17. Lammer EJ, Chen DT, Hoar RM, et al. Retinoic acid embryopathy. *N Engl J Med.* 1985;313:837–841

18. Specker BL, Valanis B, Hertzberg V, Edwards N, Tsang RL. Sunshine exposure and serum 25 hydroxyvitamin D concentrations in exclusively breast-fed infants. *J Pediatr.* 1985;107:372–376

19. Sokol RJ. Vitamin E and neurologic deficits. *Adv Pediatr.* 1990;37:119–148

20. Traber MG, Sokol RJ, Burton GW, et al. Impaired ability of patients with familial isolated vitamin E deficiency to incorporate alpha-tocopherol into lipoproteins secreted by the liver. *J Clin Invest.* 1990; 85:397–407

21. Oski FA, Barness LA. Vitamin E deficiency: a primarily unrecognized cause of hemolytic anemia in the premature infant. *J Pediatr.* 1967;70:211–220

22. Pryor WA. Vitamin E and heart disease: basic science to clinical intervention trials. *Free Radical Biol Med.* 2000;28:141–164

23. Farrell PM, Bieri JG. Megavitamin E supplementation in man. *Am J Clin Nutr.* 1975;28:1381–1386

24. Corrigan JJ, Marcus Fl. Coagulopathy associated with vitamin E ingestion. *JAMA.* 1974;1230:1300–1301

25. Corrigan JJ. The effect of vitamin E on warfarin-induced vitamin K deficiency. *Ann NY Acad Sci.* 1982;393:361–368

26. Johnson L, Bowen FW, Abbasi S, et al. Relationship of prolonged pharmacologic serum levels of vitamin E to incidence of sepsis and necrotizing enterocolitis in infants with birth weights of 1500 grams or less. *Pediatrics.* 1985;75:619–638

27. Olson RE. The function and metabolism of vitamin K. *Annu Rev Nutr.* 1984;4:281–337

28. Suttie JW. Vitamin K responsive hemorrhagic disease of infancy. *J Pediatr Gastroenterol Nutr.* 1990;11:4–6

29. American Academy of Pediatrics. Controversies concerning vitamin K and the newborn. *Pediatrics.* 2003;112:191–192

30. Golding J, Paterson M, Kinlen LJ. Factors associated with childhood cancer in a national cohort study. *Br J Cancer.* 1990;62:304–308

31. Golding J, Greenwood R, Birminham K, Mott M. Childhood cancer, intramuscular vitamin K, and pethidine given during labour. *BMJ.* 1992;305:341–346

32. Draper GJ, Stiller CA. Intramuscular vitamin K and childhood cancer. *BMJ.* 1992;305:709

33. Cornelissen EM, Smeets D, Merkx G, De Abreu R, Kollee L, Monnens L. Analysis of chromosome aberrations and sister chromatid exchanges in peripheral blood lymphocytes of newborns after Vitamin K prophylaxis at birth. *Pediatr Res.* 1991;30: 550–553

34. Albala-Hurtado S, Novella-Rodriguez S, Veciana-Nogues MT, Marine-Font A. Determination of vitamins A and E in infant milk formulae by high-performance liquid chromatography. *J Chromatogr A.* 1997;778:243–246

35. Moreno P, Salvado V. Determination of eight water- and fat-soluble vitamins in multi-vitamin pharmaceutical formulations by high-performance liquid chromatography. *J Chromatogr A.* 2000;870:207–215

36. Blum RE, Wei EK, Rockett HR, et al. Validation of a food frequency questionnaire in Native American and Caucasian children 1 to 5 years of age. *Matern Child Health J.* 1999;3:167–172

37. Henriksen C, Eggesbo M, Halvorsen R, Botten G. Nutrient intake among two-year-old children on cow milk-restricted diets. *Acta Paediatr.* 2000;89:272–278

38. Nicklas TA, Myers L, O'Neil C, Gustafson N. Impact of dietary fat and fiber intake on nutrient intake of adolescents. *Pediatrics.* 2000;105:E21

39. Gillman MW, Rifas-Shiman SL, Frazier AL, et al. Family dinner and diet quality among older children and adolescents. *Arch Fam Med.* 2000;9:235–240

40. Manore MM. Effect of physical activity on thiamine, riboflavin, and vitamin B-6 requirements. *Am J Clin Nutr.* 2000;72(suppl 2):598S–606S

41. Kim SH, Keen CL. Patterns of vitamin/mineral supplement usage by adolescents attending athletic high schools in Korea. *Int J Sport Nutr Exerc Metab.* 1999;9: 391–405

42. Schulz B, Bremer HJ. Nutrient intake and food consumption of adolescents and young adults with phenylketonuria. *Acta Paediatr.* 1995;84:743–748

43. Kuroki F, Iida M, Tominaga M, Matsumoto T, Hirakawa K, Sugiyama S, Fujishima M. Multiple vitamin status in Crohn's disease. Correlation with disease activity. *Dig Dis Sci.* 1993:1614–1618

44. Hass RH. Thiamin and the brain. *Annu Rev Nutr.* 1988;8:483–515

45. Wyatt DT, Nelson D, Hillman RE. Age-dependent changes in thiamin concentrations in whole blood and cerebrospinal fluid in infants and children. *Am J Clin Nutr.* 1991;53:530–536

46. Butterworth RF. Neurotransmitter function in thiamine-deficiency encephalopathy. *Neurochem Int.* 1982;4:449–464

47. Vasconcelos MM, Silva KP, Vidal G, Silva AF, Domingues RC, Berditchevsky CR. Early diagnosis of pediatric Wernicke's encephalopathy. *Pediatr Neurol.* 1999;20: 289–294

48. Sparacia G, Banco A, Lagalla R. Reversible MRI abnormalities in an unusual paediatric presentation of Wernicke's encephalopathy. *Pediatr Radiol.* 1999;29: 581–584

49. Hahn JS, Berquist W, Alcorn DM, Chamberlain L, Bass D. Wernicke encephalopathy and beriberi during total parenteral nutrition attributable to multivitamin infusion shortage. *Pediatrics.* 1998;101:E10

50. Naito E, Ito M, Yokota I, et al. Concomitant administration of sodium dichloroacetate and thiamine in West syndrome caused by thiamine-responsive pyruvate dehydrogenase complex deficiency. *J Neurosci.* 1999;171:56–59

51. Block G, Dresser CM, Hartman AH, Carroll MD. Nutrient sources in the American diet: quantitative data from the NHANES survey. *Am J Epidemiol.* 1985;122:13–26

52. Roughhead AK and McCormick DB. Flavin composition of human milk. *Am J Clin Nutr.* 1990;52:854–857

53. Roughead ZK, McCormick DB. Qualitative and quantitative assessment of flavins in cow milk. *J Nutr.* 1990;120:382–388

54. Bamji MS, Chowdhury N, Ramalakshmi BA, Jacob CM. Enzymatic evaluation of riboflavin status of infants. *Eur J Clin Nutr.* 1991;45:309–313

55. Prasad AP, Bamji MS, Lakshmi AV, Satyanarayana K. Functional impact of riboflavin supplementation in urban school children. *Nutr Res.* 1990;10:275–281

56. Park YK, Sempos CT, Barton CN, Vanderveen JE, Yetley EA. Effectiveness of food fortification in the United States: the case of pellagra. *Am J Public Health.* 2000; 90:727–738

57. Goldberg A, Alagona P Jr, Capuzzi DM, et al. Multiple-dose efficacy and safety of an extended-release form of niacin in the management of hyperlipidemia. *Am J Cardiol.* 2000;85:1100–1105

58. Baxter P. Epidemiology of pyridoxine dependent and pyridoxine responsive seizures in the UK. *Arch Dis Child.* 1999;81:431–433

59. Kudo K, Ito M, Horibe K, Iwase K, Kojima S. [An infant case of sideroblastic anemia that responded to oral pyridoxine]. *Rinsho Ketsueki.* 1999;40:667–672

60. Andon MB, Reynolds RD, Moser-Veillon PB, Howard MP. Dietary intake of total and glycosylated vitamin B-6 and the vitamin B-6 nutritional status of unsupplemented lactating women and their infants. *Am J Clin Nutr.* 1989;50:1050–1058

61. Kang-Yoon SA, Kirksey A, Giacoia GP, West KD. Vitamin B-6 adequacy in neonatal nutrition: associations with preterm delivery, type of feeding, and vitamin B-6 supplementation. *Am J Clin Nutr.* 1995;62:932–942

62. Borschel MW, Kirksey A, Hannemann RE. Effects of vitamin B6 intake on nutriture and growth of young infants. *Am J Clin Nutr.* 1986;43:7–15

63. Heiskanen K, Kallio M, Salmenpera L, Siimes MA, Ruokonen I, Perheentupa J. Vitamin B-6 status during childhood: tracking from 2 months to 11 years of age. *J Nutr.* 1995;125:2985–2992

64. Driskell JA, Clark AJ, Moak SW. Longitudinal assessment of vitamin B-6 status in southern adolescent girls. *J Am Diet Assoc.* 1987;87:307–310

65. Trugo NM, Sardinha F. Cobalamin and cobalamin-binding capacity in human milk. *Nutr Research.* 1994;14:23–33

66. Steen MT, Boddie AM, Fisher AJ, et al. Neural-tube defects are associated with low concentrations of cobalamin (vitamin B12) in amniotic fluid. *Prenat Diagn.* 1998;18:545–555

67. Specker BL, Black A, Allen L, Morrow F. Vitamin B-12: low milk concentrations are related to low serum concentrations in vegetarian women and to methylmalonic aciduria in their infants. *Am J Clin Nutr.* 1990;52:1073–1076

68. Schneede J, Dagnelie PC, van Staveren WA, Vollset SE, Refsum H, Ueland PM. Methylmalonic acid and homocysteine in plasma as indicators of functional cobalamin deficiency in infants on macrobiotic diets. *Pediatr Res.* 1994;36:194–201

69. Specker BL, Miller D, Norman EJ, Greene H, Hayes KC. Increased urinary methylmalonic acid excretion in breast-fed infants of vegetarian mothers and identification of an acceptable dietary source of vitamin B-12. *Am J Clin Nutr.* 1988;47:89–92

70. Kuhne T, Bubl R, Baumgartner R. Maternal vegan diet causing a serious infantile neurological disorder due to vitamin B12 deficiency. *Eur J Pediatr.* 1991;150:205–208

71. Gambon RC, Lentze MJ, Rossi E. Megaloblastic anaemia in one of monozygous twins breastfed by their vegetarian mother. *Eur J Pediatr.* 1986;145:570–571

72. Dagnelie PC, van Staveren WA, Hautvast JG. Stunting and nutrient deficiencies in children on alternative diets. *Acta Paediatr Scand Suppl.* 1991;374:111–118

73. Laine L, Ahnen D, McClain C, Solcia E, Walsh JH. Review article: potential gastrointestinal effects of long-term acid suppression with proton pump inhibitors. *Aliment Pharmacol Ther.* 2000;14:651–668

74. Kaptan K, Beyan C, Ural AU, et al. Helicobacter pylori—is it a novel causative agent in Vitamin B12 deficiency? *Arch Intern Med.* 2000;160:1349–1353

75. Robinson M, White FJ, Cleary MA, Wraith E, Lam WK, Walter JH. Increased risk of vitamin B12 deficiency in patients with phenylketonuria on an unrestricted or relaxed diet. *J Pediatr.* 2000;136:545–547

76. Bibi H, Gelman-Kohan Z, Baumgartner ER, Rosenblatt DS. Transcobalamin II deficiency with methylmalonic aciduria in three sisters. *J Inherit Metab Dis.* 1999;22: 765–772

77. O'Connor DL, Tamura T, Picciano MF. Pteroylpolyglutamates in human milk. *Am J Clin Nutr.* 1991;53:930–934

78. Minet JC, Bisse E, Aebischer CP, Beil A, Wieland H, Lutschg J. Assessment of vitamin B-12, folate, and vitamin B-6 status and relation to sulfur amino acid metabolism in neonates. *Am J Clin Nutr.* 2000;72:751–757

79. Skinner JD, Carruth BR, Houck KS, et al. Longitudinal study of nutrient and food intakes of white preschool children aged 24 to 60 months. *J Am Diet Assoc.* 1999; 99:1514–1521

80. Picciano MF, Smiciklas-Wright H, Birch LL, Mitchell DC, Murray-Kolb L, McConahy KL. Nutritional guidance is needed during dietary transition in early childhood. *Pediatrics.* 2000;106:109–914

81. Cavadini C, Siega-Riz AM, Popkin BM. US adolescent food intake trends from 1965 to 1996. *Arch Dis Child.* 2000;83:18–24

82. Falkner B, Sherif K, Michel S, Kushner H. Dietary nutrients and blood pressure in urban minority adolescents at risk for hypertension. *Arch Pediatr Adolesc Med.* 2000;154:918–922

83. Botto LD, Yang Q. 5,10-Methylenetetrahydrofolate reductase gene variants and congenital anomalies: a HuGE review. *Am J Epidemiol.* 2000;151:862–877

84. Cardo E, Monros E, Colome C, et al. Children with stroke: polymorphism of the MTHFR gene, mild hyperhomocysteinemia, and vitamin status. *J Child Neurol.* 2000;15:295–298

85. Ravelli A, Migliavacca D, Viola S, Ruperto N, Pistorio A, Martini A. Efficacy of folinic acid in reducing methotrexate toxicity in juvenile idiopathic arthritis. *Clin Exp Rheumatol.* 1999;17:625–627

86. Verrotti A, Pascarella R, Trotta D, Giuva T, Morgese G, Chiarelli F. Hyperhomocysteinemia in children treated with sodium valproate and carbamazepine. *Epilepsy Res.* 2000;41:253–257

87. Tonetti C, Burtscher A, Bories D, Tulliez M, Zittoun J. Methylenetetrahydrofolate reductase deficiency in four siblings: a clinical, biochemical, and molecular study of the family. *Am J Med Genet.* 2000;91:363–367

88. *Dietary Reference Intakes for Vitamin C, Vitamin E, Selenium, and Carotenoids.* Washington, DC: National Academy Press; 2000:95–185

89. Hampl JS, Taylor CA, Johnston CS. Intakes of vitamin C, vegetables and fruits: which schoolchildren are at risk? *J Am Coll Nutr.* 1999;18:582–590

90. Pereira AM, Hamani N, Nogueira PC, Carvalhaes JT. Oral vitamin intake in children receiving long-term dialysis. *J Ren Nutr.* 2000;10:24–29

91. Eissenstat BR, Wyse BW, Hansen RG. Pantothenic acid status of adolescents. *Am J Clin Nutr.* 1986;44:931–937

92. Krause KH, Bonjour JP, Berlit P, Kynast G, Schmidt-Gauk H, Schellenberg B. Effect of long-term treatment with antiepileptic drugs on the vitamin status. *Drug Nutr Interact.* 1988:5;317–343

IV
Nutrient Delivery Systems

22

Parenteral Nutrition

Clinical experience has demonstrated the value of optimal nutritional status in resisting the effects of trauma and disease and in improving the response to medical and surgical therapy. The metabolic demands of rapid growth and the low nutritional reserves in infancy make the potential benefit of good nutrition to critically ill pediatric patients even greater. Details concerning the physiologic effects, techniques for administration, and efficacy of parenteral nutrition (PN) have been discussed previously.[1,2]

Several gastrointestinal and medical problems arise in infants that preclude or severely limit the use of the intestine for nutritional support. Since the first successful use of total parenteral nutrition (TPN) in a malnourished infant in 1944, its use has become a common practice. Premature infants with severe respiratory disease, congenital anomalies of the gastrointestinal tract, or inflammatory disease of the intestinal mucosa (eg, necrotizing enterocolitis) are frequent candidates for this form of nutritional support. Older infants with intractable diarrhea, short-bowel syndrome, or severe malnutrition have been successfully rehabilitated with parenteral feedings. Extensive body surface burns, malignancies (especially after bone marrow transplantation), cardiac failure, and renal failure are examples of extraintestinal disorders in which PN has been useful. Specific formulations and procedures are available for such situations in adults,[3] but each of these regimens must be specifically tailored for infants and children.

In certain settings, particularly in larger hospitals with seriously ill patients who require PN, a nutrition support team is beneficial in providing optimal care. An interdisciplinary team consisting of medical, nursing, dietary, pharmaceutical, and surgical staff with expertise in PN provides invaluable consultative services, helps to decrease costs, and potentially shortens the length of hospital stays and occurrence of complications associated with PN.

Catheters

Parenteral nutrition can be administered through peripheral veins using standard peripheral intravenous catheters and solutions with an osmolarity of 300 to 900 mOsm/L. When solutions of higher osmolarity are used, larger veins with a high blood flow must be used to avoid sclerosis and inflammation of the wall of the vein. Several commercially available central venous catheters can be used when long-term access is needed. Strict asepsis is mandatory during catheter placement. Peripheral PN regimens maintain existing body composition and are a reasonable choice for a normally nourished infant or child without significant fluid restrictions who is likely to tolerate an adequate enteral regimen in less than 2 weeks. Use of central PN can result in normal and catch-up growth and is a more reasonable choice for infants or older children, regardless of their initial nutritional status, who will be intolerant of enteral feedings for longer than 2 weeks.

The central vein catheters are made of a flexible material, such as silicone elastomer or polyurethane. Anesthesia is usually required for their placement in the subclavian or internal jugular vein, from which they are advanced to the junction of the superior vena cava and the right atrium. Some of these catheters can be introduced percutaneously into the subclavian vein. The more flexible catheters (eg, Hickman and Broviac) can be introduced through a hollow needle, or they can be placed by incising the skin and subcutaneous tissue to expose the vein. For long-term use, a subcutaneous tunnel can be created to provide some protection from the migration of skin bacteria into the vein. A subcutaneous tunnel is not created for a temporary catheter. Some catheters are impregnated with silver salts to prevent infection at the site of insertion of the catheter. A recent randomized controlled trial and meta-analysis indicated that central venous catheters impregnated with an antiseptic combination of chlorhexidine and silver sulfadiazine are efficacious in reducing the incidence of catheter-related bloodstream infection (CR-BSI). Subsequently, these catheters have been shown to decrease the incidence of CR-BSI and death and provide significant savings in cost.[4] Other special catheters and infusion ports are available. The placement of polymeric silicone (Silastic) catheters in the preterm infant has a lower incidence of vein perforation and thrombosis than the use of stiffer catheters. Occasionally, when jugular or subclavian sites are unavailable, veins that course toward the inferior vena cava, such as the inferior epigastric veins, can be used. Peripherally inserted central catheters (PICCs) are becoming increasingly popular as an alternative for patients needing intermediate to long-term access.[5] Regardless of the site, roentgenographic confirmation of the intravascular placement of the catheter is mandatory before PN solutions are infused.

A number of complications directly related to the catheter may occur. Malposition of a central venous catheter outside the vein, with infusion of hypertonic solutions into the pleural or pericardial space, may be life threatening. A rapid decrease in serum glucose level or the acute onset of circulatory or respiratory compromise should signal this complication. Hemorrhage, associated with erosion of central veins or of the wall of the right atrium, has been reported. Pneumothorax and brachial plexus injuries may complicate the placement of percutaneous subclavian line insertion in infants and small children. Air embolus may occur, but air-eliminating filters and properly secured tubing junctions help prevent this complication. Catheter emboli have occurred from the rupture of silicone elastomer catheters perfused under a high pressure or from the tips of polyethylene catheters sheared off when the catheter was withdrawn through the hub of the needle used to insert it. Thrombophlebitis may be observed in peripheral veins receiving hypertonic solutions. Skin slough is a rare but serious complication of extravasation of the parenteral solution into the interstitial space, particularly if the solution is of high osmolality or contains calcium. Hyaluronidase (Wydase) is injected locally by the subcutaneous or intradermal route for suspected and known extravasations caused by dextrose, TPN, calcium solutions, aminophylline, and nafcillin to prevent possible tissue damage from the extravasation. Best results occur if the hyaluronidase is administered within the first few minutes to 1 hour after the extravasation is recognized.

Catheter-related sepsis is a major complication of an indwelling central venous catheter. Fever alone is not an indication for removal of a PN catheter. Other sources of infection should be sought; if none are found, removal of the catheter should be considered. Some episodes of sepsis may be treated with the catheter in place. Fungal sepsis almost always necessitates removal of the catheter. Signs of sepsis in the neonate include lethargy, hyperbilirubinemia, temperature instability, and nutrient intolerance (eg, hyperglycemia or hypertriglyceridemia, in response to previously tolerated glucose and lipid loads). Careful placement of the central catheter and strict adherence to established guidelines for catheter care and maintenance considerably decrease the incidence of catheter-related complications.[6] Catheter occlusion may be caused by a clot or thrombus, fat deposition, calcium-phosphorus precipitation, or drug precipitation. Many hospitals have standard protocols to deal with each type of occlusion—infusing 70% ethanol for fat deposition, 0.1N hydrochloric acid for calcium-phosphorus precipitation, and 0.1N HCl or 0.1N NaOH for medication precipitates.[7] For years, urokinase was widely used to treat catheter thrombosis. Urokinase has been removed from the market after inspections of the urokinase-manufacturing facilities revealed a significant risk of infectious agent contamination. Currently, Alteplase (t-PA) is recommended for catheter-related thrombosis; it has been proven to be an effective and well-tolerated alternative to urokinase.[8]

Metabolic complications caused by the composition and administration of the infusate are discussed in the next section. A schedule for monitoring PN is shown in Table 22.1.

Composition of Solutions for Infants and Children

For the preterm neonate, a nonprotein energy intake of 100 kcal/kg/d with a concomitant protein intake of 3 g/kg/d allows weight gain approximating the intrauterine growth rate. Greater energy intake may lead to greater weight gain, but the additional weight gain will likely be mostly fat deposition. The aforementioned recommendations are based on the landmark study by Zlotkin et al.[9] Heird[10] recommended that an infant who weighs less than 10 kg receive 90 to 120 kcal/kg/d and 2.5 to 3.0 g/kg/d of protein. Outside of the

Table 22.1.

Suggested Clinical and Laboratory Monitoring Schedule During Total Parenteral Nutrition in the Hospitalized Patient*

Variable Monitored	Initial Period[†]	Later Period[‡]
Serum electrolytes (and carbon dioxide)	3–4 times/wk	Weekly
Serum urea nitrogen	3 times/wk	Weekly
Serum calcium, magnesium, phosphorous	3 times/wk	Weekly
Serum glucose	§	§
Serum protein (electrophoresis or albumin/globulin prealbumin/transferrin)	Weekly	Weekly
Liver function studies	Weekly	Weekly
Hematocrit	Weekly	Weekly
Urine glucose	Daily	Daily
Clinical observations (eg, activity, temperature)	Daily	Daily
Blood cell count and differential count	As indicated	As indicated
Cultures	As indicated	As indicated
Serum triglyceride	4 hours after an increase in dose	Weekly

*Schedule may vary with age and underlying medical condition of the patient.
[†]Initial period is the period before full glucose, protein, and lipid intake is achieved or any period of metabolic instability.
[‡]Later period is the period during which patient is in a metabolic steady state.
§Blood glucose should be monitored closely during a period of glucosuria and for 2 to 3 days after cessation of parenteral nutrition to determine the degree of hypoglycemia. In the latter instance, frequent determination of blood glucose levels in fingertip venous blood constitutes adequate screening. After a month or more of receiving total parenteral nutrition, measurements can be made once a week or less frequently.

intensive care nursery, few studies like that of Zlotkin et al[9] have been performed. The consensus from the literature about parenteral requirements by age is shown in Table 22.2.[11]

Table 22.2.
Components of Maintenance Parenteral Nutrition in Infants and Children*

Base Components	Weight		
	<10 kg	10–20 kg	>20 kg
Fluid	100–150 mL/kg	1000 mL + 50 mL/kg >10 kg	1500 mL + 20 mL/kg >20 kg
Calories, kcal/kg[†] Dextrose, g/kg (3.4 kcal/g)	80–130 10–30	60–90 8–28	30–75 5–20
Protein, g/kg[†] (1 g protein = 0.16 g nitrogen)	1.5–3	1–2.5	0.8–2.0
Fat, g/kg	0.5–4	1–3	1–3
Additive	**Infants and Toddlers**	**Children**	**Adolescents**
Sodium	2–4 mEq/kg	2–4 mEq/kg	60–150 mEq
Potassium	2–4 mEq/kg	2–4 mEq/kg	70–180 mEq
Chloride	2–4 mEq/kg	2–4 mEq/kg	60–150 mEq
Magnesium (125 mg/mEq)	0.25–1 mEq/kg	0.25–1 mEq/kg	8–32 mEq
Calcium[‡] (20 mg/mEq)	0.45–4 mEq/kg	0.45–3.15 mEq/kg	10–40 mEq
Phosphorus (31 mg/mmol)	0.5–2 mmol/kg	0.5–2 mmol/kg	9–30 mmol/kg
Heparin (optional)	0.5–1 U/mL	0.5–1 U/mL	0.5–1 U/mL
Trace Elements	0.2 mL/kg (Pediatric Trace Elements)[§]	0.2 mL/kg (Pediatric Trace Elements)[§]	(Adult Trace Elements) 5 mL[§ǁ]
Selenium (maximum 30 μg/d)	2 μg/kg	2 μg/kg	2 μg/kg
Molybdenum (maximum 5 μg/d)	0.25 μg/kg	0.25 μg/kg	0.25 μg/kg
Adult multivitamin (maximum 10 mL/d)[¶]	NA	NA	10 mL[#]
Pediatric multivitamin (maximum 5 mL/d)[¶]	<2.5 kg 2 mL	2.5–40 kg 5 mL	>40 kg NA

* See Chapter 2 for preterm infants. IU indicates International Units; and NA, not applicable.
† Ideal weight (50th percentile for length or height.
‡ If given as calcium gluconate: 1 mL of a 10% solution of calcium gluconate provides 9.3 mg of elemental calcium.
§ See Table 20.2a. If patient receives parenteral nutrition for more than 30 days with no significant enteral intake, the addition of trace elements is advisable.
ǁ Omit copper and manganese in patients with obstructive jaundice; omit selenium, chromium, and molybdenum in patients with renal dysfunction. Maximum Pediatric Trace Elements: 5 mL/d.
¶ See Table 20.2b.
# Add 200 μg Vitamin K (phytonadione).

Table 22.2a.
Parenteral Trace Element Solutions

Ingredient	Adult Trace/mL	Pediatric Trace/mL
Zinc	1 mg	1 mg
Copper	0.4 mg	0.1 mg
Manganese	100 μg	25 μg
Chromium	4 μg	1 μg

Table 22.2b.
Parenteral Vitamin Solutions

Ingredient	Adult MVI/10 mL*	Pediatric MVI/5 mL*
Vitamin A	0.99 mg (3300 IU)	0.7 mg (2300 IU)
Vitamin D	5 μg (200 IU)	10 μg (400 IU)
Vitamin E	10 mg (10 IU)	7 mg (7 IU)
Vitamin B$_1$	3 mg	1.2 mg
Vitamin B$_2$	3.6 mg	1.4 mg
Vitamin B$_6$	4 mg	1 mg
Niacin	40 mg	17 mg
Dexpanthenol	15 mg	5 mg
Folic acid	400 μg	140 μg
Vitamin B$_{12}$	5 μg	1 μg
Biotin	60 μg	20 μg
Ascorbic acid	100 mg	80 mg
Vitamin K$_1$	...	200 μg

*Armour Pharmaceutical Co. (among others).

Carbohydrate

Glucose (dextrose), fructose, galactose, sorbitol, glycerol, and ethanol all have
been used as sources of carbohydrate calories in infants. The small amount of
glycerol present in lipid emulsions contributes to carbohydrate calories. The
other carbohydrate sources have no advantage over glucose and can produce
serious complications in preterm infants.

The quantity of infused glucose that preterm infants tolerate varies.
Infusing glucose at 5 mg/kg/min and advancing gradually to 15 mg/kg/min
over several days may reduce intolerance. This is best accomplished by increasing the concentration of glucose in the solution while keeping the volume of
infusate constant at between 80 and 150 mL/kg/d, depending on the infant's

fluid requirements. Gradual increases of 2.5% to 5% dextrose per day are usually well tolerated. The consequences of acute intolerance to glucose are serum hyperosmolarity and osmotic diuresis, which can be avoided by careful monitoring. Hypoglycemia is usually related to the sudden cessation of the PN solution. In adult postsurgical patients, an increase in the glucose infusion rate from 4 to 7 mg/kg/min is associated with an increased rate of glucose oxidation; at higher infusion rates, fat is synthesized from the glucose without a further increase in oxidation.[12] Higher glucose loads delivered by solutions containing more than 25% dextrose at 150 mL/kg/d (>26 mg/kg/min) may not be beneficial to infants and may contribute to the fatty infiltration of the liver.

Insulin should not be routinely added to the solution because of unpredictable responses to this hormone in infants.[13] Several recent studies have shown that continuous insulin infusion by pump is beneficial for extremely low-birth-weight infants, resulting in an increase in nonprotein energy intake and in significant increases in weight gain. Serious concerns about the use of insulin in the neonate include the following: (1) Suppression of muscle proteolysis may not be desirable (glutamine released is an important substrate for intestinal epithelial cells and the immune system); (2) The composition of the weight gain (especially protein accretion) in these infants is not clearly understood; (3) Would increased glucose utilization deprive the brain of this important substrate?; and (4) Will the increased glucose taken up by the cells be efficiently oxidized or be converted to fat? Further study of the effects of insulin in infants is suggested before it is recommended for routine use.[2]

Protein

Current solutions supply nitrogen requirements as crystalline amino acids. Infants have demonstrated adequate growth with this source of protein. Commercial preparations are available as concentrated 3.5% to 15% mixtures of crystalline amino acids that can be diluted to meet the nutritional requirements of infants at different ages. Some newer amino acid solutions (eg, TrophAmine and Aminosyn PF) have been especially formulated to meet the special requirements of neonates. These solutions contain taurine, tyrosine, histidine, aspartic acid, and glutamic acid, all of which are found in human milk. They contain lower concentrations of methionine, glycine, and phenylalanine than are found in amino acid solutions intended for older patients. The plasma amino acid profile of infants receiving these solutions for nutritional maintenance is similar to that of breastfed infants. In addition, greater weight gain and positive nitrogen balance are achieved by infants receiving these formulations than by infants receiving standard adult amino acid solutions. These solutions may reduce the incidence of PN-induced cholestasis in neonates who receive PN for long periods.[14,15] Two preliminary studies demonstrate a significant lower incidence of cholestasis with TrophAmine compared to Aminosyn PF.[16,17]

The commercial solutions do not contain cysteine, although separate preparations of cysteine can be added to the solutions. Cysteine must be added during compounding because it converts to its dimeric form and precipitates over time in solution. Cysteine may be an essential amino acid in infants with low activity of hepatic cystathionine γ-lyase, which converts methionine to cysteine. Taurine, which is formed from cysteine and is present in human milk, may also be important in preterm infants. Albumin at a dose of 0.5 to 1.0 g/kg/d may be administered to PN patients who are hypoalbuminemic from nonnutritive causes. Such infusions are for oncotic, **never** nutritive benefits, since albumin has a long half-life and is not useful nutritionally. Albumin should be infused separately via a "Y" connector and not placed in the PN solution since (1) albumin is a blood product and should not be hung for more than 8 hours, (2) recent concerns exist about flocculation of albumin in PN solutions, and (3) albumin in PN solutions increases the risk of sepsis.[2,18] Because albumin contains a significant amount of aluminum, caution should be exercised with the routine use of exogenous albumin in PN for neonates (see Chapter 20).

No commercially available PN amino acid solution currently contains glutamine (primarily because of its short shelf life when placed in solution). Glutamine is a primary fuel for enterocytes, lymphocytes, and macrophages and is a precursor for nucleotide synthesis and glutathione, an important antioxidant. Glutamine supplementation may be of value to very-low-birth-weight infants and pediatric patients with short-bowel syndrome.[19] A small randomized trial conducted by Lacey and colleagues showed no adverse effects of parenteral glutamine supplementation in premature infants.[20] In the <800 g subgroup, they also found that infants receiving glutamine required fewer days on parenteral nutrition (13 vs 21 days), had shorter length of time to full enteral feeds (8 vs 14 days), and needed less time on the ventilator (38 vs 47 days). In addition, the <800 g subgroup who received glutamine supplementation had a significantly higher lymphocyte count and fewer infants with episodes of neutropenia versus the control infants. No significant toxicities were seen in infants who received 20% of their protein intake as glutamine. A large multicenter randomized clinical trial of parenteral glutamine supplementation in very-low-birth-weight infants is also currently underway.

Despite the recognized potential deficiencies, infants have tolerated the available solutions and have grown well while using them. Most metabolic complications related to amino acids, such as azotemia and acidosis, have occurred when infants received more than 4 g of protein equivalent per kilogram per day and from earlier TPN preparations. Complications are rarely encountered with the recommended intake of 1.5 to 3 g of protein equivalent per kilogram per day. Hyperammonemia, seen with earlier solutions, now rarely occurs because of the increased amounts of arginine and decreased quantities of glycine in the formulations. Thus, routine monitoring of blood ammonia levels in patients receiving PN is no longer necessary. Hyperchloremic metabolic acidosis, another problem noted with earlier crystalline amino acid solutions, has been ameliorated by the substitution of acetate for chloride in the salts of lysine and the use of basic salts of histidine.

Lipids

The composition, use, and complications of intravenous fat emulsions have been discussed previously.[2,21] They are a concentrated source of energy, provide essential fatty acids, and are iso-osmolar. When lipid and amino acid-glucose solutions are infused simultaneously into the same vein, the patient receives a higher energy and lower osmolar solution (which helps spare peripheral veins) than with a glucose and amino acid solution alone. The use of "Y" connector tubing after the in-line filter (Micropore) to infuse lipids simultaneously with, but separately from, the amino acid-glucose solution has greatly improved the effectiveness of peripheral intravenous nutrition and increased substantially its use in nutritional support.

Some centers are using a 3-in-1 solution (also called a total nutrient admixture) in which the lipid emulsion is mixed with the amino acid-glucose solution and administered through a single line. This method of delivery has certain advantages: (1) simplified administration, which may prove to be a cost savings; (2) less manipulation of the delivery system (reduced opportunity for contamination); (3) lessened loss of vitamin A; and (4) continuous infusion of all nutrients. One retrospective study of 3-in-1 solutions in infants found such use safe, efficacious, and cost-effective for infants younger than 1 year.[22] If these infusates are administered without an in-line filter, the presence of lipid in the infusate will obscure any visual precipitation that may occur on removal from refrigeration (4°C) and warming before or during administration. However, a 1.2-Tm in-line filter is available that can be used with lipids. The use of 3-in-1 solutions in low-birth-weight infants may compromise efforts to maximize calcium and phosphate intakes to meet their high requirements. The addition of lipid emulsion to the amino acid-glucose solution increases the pH of the solution, which may result in a decrease in solubility of calcium and phosphorus, and, therefore, a lower concentration of these nutrients is available to the infant. On April 18, 1994, a safety alert was issued by the Food and Drug Administration about 3-in-1 solutions because one institution reported 2 deaths and 2 cases of respiratory distress using such solutions. The solutions may have contained a precipitate of calcium phosphate. Autopsies revealed diffuse microvascular pulmonary emboli containing calcium phosphate.[2] However, the precipitates were caused by improper preparation of the solution, and 3-in-1 solutions are widely and safely used in pediatrics. Iron is not compatible with 3-in-1 solutions. This is particularly a problem for home TPN, because 3-in-1 formulations simplify administration and patients who receive long-term TPN are most likely to need iron supplementation.[18]

The requirement for I-linoleic acid (an essential fatty acid) can be achieved by supplying 0.5 to 1 g/kg body weight per day of intravenous lipid. Small amounts of I-linolenic acid should be included, perhaps one tenth the amount of linoleic acid. Preterm infants younger than 32 weeks of gestation may be unable to clear lipid doses in excess of 2 g/kg/d. Nephelometry results and visual inspection of serum for turbidity correlate well with serum chylomicron concentration but not well with triglyceride or free fatty acid concentrations; therefore, serum lipid monitoring is required. Serum triglyceride levels can be performed by microtechnique by most laboratories, which allows for frequent triglyceride monitoring as the intravenous lipid doses are advanced (Table 22.1). Continuous infusion of up to 3 g/kg body weight per day of intravenous lipid should minimize the chance of lipid intolerance. Under certain circumstances (eg, sepsis), the lowest dose that meets essential fatty acid requirements should be used to avoid potential complications.

Twenty percent intravenous fat is cleared more efficiently than 10% fat emulsions and is the preparation of choice. The phospholipid-triglyceride ratio is 0.12 in 10% intravenous fat and 0.06 in 20% intravenous fat. Phospholipid is believed to inhibit lipoprotein lipase, the main enzyme for intravenous fat clearance; therefore, using a fat emulsion with the lowest ratio of phospholipid to triglyceride (eg, 20% fat emulsions) is preferable. Recently, concerns have been raised about the safety of using fat emulsions during the first week of life in the premature infant.[23] Toxic lipid peroxidation products in the fat emulsions may lead to the development of chronic lung disease, and ambient and phototherapy light increases this lipid oxidation.[24] Data to date are conflicting but disturbing. No available PN solutions contain carnitine, which is required for the optimal metabolism of fatty acids. Infants have a poorly developed capacity to synthesize and store carnitine. Some experts do recommend supplementation (2.4 to 10 mg/kg/d in preterm and term infants),[25,26] but the lack of carnitine in PN formulations has not been associated with any clinical deficiency syndrome and the results of clinical studies of its addition to PN formulations have been contradictory.

Vitamins, Minerals, and Trace Elements

Vitamins, minerals, and trace elements must be supplied in parenteral solutions. Metabolic complications have been described for deficiencies and excesses of some of these nutrients. Intravenous dose requirements are not fully known. Guidelines from an expert panel[27] for multivitamin and trace element preparations for parenteral use are shown in Tables 22.3 and 22.4. A higher, more physiologic calcium-phosphorus ratio of 1.7:1 by weight (1.3:1 by molar ratio, similar to the fetal mineral accretion ratio) allows for the highest absolute

Table 22.3.
Suggested Daily Intakes of Parenteral Vitamins in Infants and Children

Vitamin	Term Infants and Children ≥2.5 kg	Infants <2.5 kg*
Lipid soluble†		
A, µg	700	280
E, mg	7	2.80
K, µg	200	80
D, (IU)‡	400	160
Water soluble		
Ascorbic acid, mg	80	32
Thiamine, mg	1.2	0.48
Riboflavin, mg	1.4	0.56
Pyridoxine, mg	1.0	0.40
Niacin, mg	17	6.80
Pantothenate, mg	5	2
Biotin, µg	20	8
Folic acid, µg	140	56
Vitamin B$_{12}$, µg	1	0.40

*Dose/kg body weight/d for preterm infants, not to exceed daily dose for term (≥2.5 kg) infants.
†700 µg retinol equivalents = 2300 IU; 7 mg α-tocopherol = 7 IU; 10 µg vitamin D = 400 IU.
‡Recent data indicate that 40 IU/kg/d of vitamin D (maximum of 400 IU/d) is adequate for term and preterm infants. The higher dose of 160 IU/kg/d has not been associated with complications and maintains blood levels within the reference range for term infants fed orally. This dosage, therefore, appears acceptable until further studies using the lower dose formulation indicate its superiority.

Table 22.4.
Suggested Parenteral Intakes of Trace Minerals in Infants and Children

Element	Preterm, μg/kg/d	Term, μg/kg/d	Children, μg/kg/d (maximum, μg/d)
Zinc*	400	250 <3 mo	50 (5000)
		100 >3 mo	
Copper†	20	20	20 (300)
Selenium‡	2	2	2 (30)
Chromium‡	0.20	0.20	0.20 (5.0)
Manganese†	1	1	1 (50)
Molybdenum‡§	0.25	0.25	0.25 (5.0)
Iodide	1	1	1 (1.0)

* When total parenteral nutrition is supplemental only or is limited to less than 4 weeks, only zinc need be added. Thereafter, addition of the remaining elements is advisable.

† Omit in patients with obstructive jaundice. (Manganese and copper are excreted primarily in bile.)

‡ Omit in patients with renal dysfunction.

§ Available concentrations of molybdenum and manganese are such that dilution of the manufacturer's product may be necessary. Neotrace (Lyphomed Co, Rosemont, IL) contains a higher ratio of manganese to zinc than suggested in this table (ie, zinc, 1.5 mg and manganese, 25 μg in each milliliter).

retention of both minerals. This ratio provides 76 mg/kg/d of elemental calcium and 45 mg/kg/d of phosphorus.[28] Dunham et al[29] have generated calcium and phosphorus precipitation curves for PN using TrophAmine (its low pH allows for the maximum possible calcium and phosphorous in solution) to help pharmacists and clinicians avoid compounding TPN solutions that will precipitate (Figure 22.1). Different precipitation curves for PN should be used if Aminosyn PF is used or cysteine is added to the base amino acid solution. Precipitation information can also be found in the package inserts of the amino acid solutions.

Vitamin A supplementation for VLBW infants has been used to decrease the risk of BPD.[30,31] This must be delivered intramuscularly, not in PN solutions and is discussed in Chapter 2.

A number of substances commonly administered intravenously, including calcium and phosphorus salts and albumin, have high levels of aluminum. Premature infants receiving intravenous fluid therapy may accumulate aluminum and show evidence of aluminum toxicity.[32] Calcium gluconate can contribute up to 80% of the total aluminum load from PN. The Food and Drug Administration has proposed labeling requirements concerning aluminum contents on PN additives, establishing an upper limit permitted in

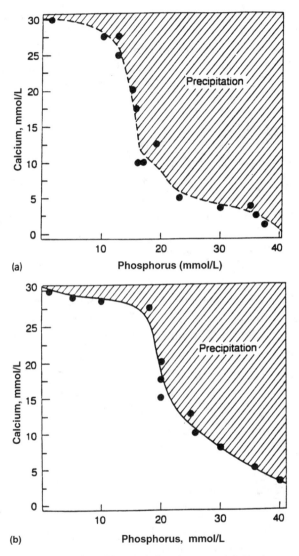

(a)

(b)

Figure 22.1. Ninetieth percentile for calcium and phosphorus precipitation in neonatal total parenteral nutrition solutions containing (a) 1% or (b) 2% amino acids. The measured calcium solubility after 24 hours is greater than 90% on the left side of the 90th percentile curve and less than 90% on the right side. Reproduced with permission from Dunham et al.[29]

PN additives and has suggested that manufacturers develop validated assay methods.[33] Bishop and others demonstrated developmental delay in premature infants on PN solutions receiving aluminum 45 μg/kg/d.[34] Aluminum intake should be determined in children at high risk for toxicity: preterm infants, infants or children with impaired renal function, and patients on prolonged PN.[2]

Ordering Parenteral Nutrition

Preprinted PN order sheets (Figure 22.2) save time for the house staff and pharmacy personnel. In addition, the order sheet helps to avoid errors of omission, ensuring that all necessary nutrients are ordered. The order sheet provides the necessary input for specific PN computer programs. Required data for some of these programs include the patient's weight (in kg), total fluid intake for the day (mL/kg/d), the amount of fat emulsion (g/kg/d), fat concentration (10% or 20%), fluid volumes contributed by other parenteral solutions or enteral feedings, desired protein intake via amino acids (g/kg/d), and the percentage concentration of dextrose. The doses of trace elements, vitamins, and electrolytes are ordered in amounts per day or amounts per kilogram per day. The computer performs all necessary calculations. Protocol recommendations are provided in the right-hand column of the order sheet for reference.

The output of the computer program includes:

1. Total parenteral nutrition and fat emulsion bottle labels
2. Mixing instructions for the pharmacy with calcium phosphate precipitation curve data
3. A detailed nutritional summary including calories, nitrogen ratio, kcal/kg/d, and the percentage of total calories to be given as fat

---

The American Academy of Pediatrics recommends the following:

1. Aluminum-containing phosphate binders should not be administered to infants and children with renal failure.
2. Continued efforts should be made to reduce the levels of aluminum in products that are added to intravenous solutions that are used for premature infants and infants and children with renal failure.
3. Continued efforts should be made to reduce the aluminum content of all formulas used for infants, but especially soy formulas and formulas tailored specifically for premature infants.
4. In infants at risk for aluminum toxicity (renal failure and prematurity), attention should be paid to the aluminum content of the water used in reconstitution of infant formulas.

PARENTERAL NUTRITION

(addressograph stamp)

A. Please send TPN orders to the Pharmacy before 11:00 A.M. DAILY.

B. Order all additives on a 24-hour basis: i.e., mEq/kg/day, mM/kg/day, mL/day, mL/kg/day

PERIPHERAL _____ or CENTRAL _____ TPN LINE (check one)   Today's DATE _____

DUE DATE _____ TIME DUE_____ (AM PM)   Today's WEIGHT _____ kg

(month/day/year)

TOTAL FLUID INTAKE (mL/kg/day)_____ Next Bottle # _____

AMOUNT OF FAT EMULSION (g/kg/day) _____ Fat Concentration 10% 20% (check one)

How many IV or IA lines exist which will not be used for TPN? _____

	Line		Line
Enter flow rates (mL/hr):	(1) _____ and % NaCl:	(1) _____	
	(2) _____ (e.g., 0.45%)	(2) _____	
	(3) _____	(3) _____	

If taking enteral feeds, complete the following section (check one):

_____1. Total fluids administered as parenteral and advancing enteral, i.e., "TPN + PO." (Additives are distributed assuming that the total fluids will be given parenterally)

_____2. Total fluids administered as parenteral and fixed enteral. (Additives are distributed in parenteral fluids only; ignores electrolyte content of enteral fluids)

Enter Amount _____(mls),   Frequency: q _____hrs,   Calories/mL_____,   Product Name _____

Enter AMINO ACIDS (g/kg/day)†   Enter DEXTROSE CONCENTRATION   %

TODAY'S ADDITIVES			PROTOCOL RECOMMENDATION
TRACE ELEMENTS AND VITAMINS:			
1. PEDIATRIC TRACE ELEMENTS	_____	mL/kg/day	0.2 mL/kg/day (weight <20 kg)
2. ADULT TRACE ELEMENTS	_____	mL/day	5 mL/day (weight >20 kg)
3. ZINC (additional)	_____	µg/kg/day	200 µg/kg/day Preemies Only
4. PEDIATRIC M.V.	_____	mL/day	2 mL/kg/day infants < 2.5 kg
	_____	mL/day	5 mL/day infants > 2.5 kg and children up to 11 years of age
5. ADULT M.V.I. - 12 (or generic)	_____	mL/day	10 mL/day children > 11 yrs. of age
6. VITAMIN K	_____	mg/day	0.5 mg/day children > 11 yrs. of age
ELECTROLYTES AND MINERALS:			
1. PHOSPHATE*	_____	nM/kg/day	0.5-2 mM/kg/day
2. SODIUM	_____	mEq/kg/day	2.4 mEq/kg/day (Sodium from other IVs is included)
3. POTASSIUM	_____	mEq/kg/day	2-3 mEq/kg/day
4. ACETATE	_____	mEq/kg/day	1-4 mEq/kg/day
5. MAGNESIUM	_____	mEq/kg/day	0.25-0.5 mEq/kg/day
6. CALCIUM GLUCONATE	_____	mg/kg/day	50-500 mg/kg/day
7. HEPARIN	_____	Units/mL	0.5-1 Unit/mL
8. INSULIN	_____	Units/liter	
9. OTHER (specify)	_____		
10. OTHER (specify)	_____		

* NOTE: Balance of anions will be provided as chloride.

† Each 0.5 g/kg/day of Amino Acid provides either 0.47 mEq/kg/day of Acetate (TrophAmine) or 0.74 mEq/kg/day of Acetate (Aminosyn).

_____RN _____MD

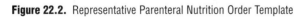

Figure 22.2. Representative Parenteral Nutrition Order Template

Gastrointestinal and Hepatic Effects of Parenteral Nutrition

Hepatic disease is the major complication of PN. When the liver is examined histologically, cholestasis, hepatocellular necrosis, and, in advanced cases, cirrhosis may be found.[35] The hepatic response to TPN depends on the age of the patient. A cholestatic response predominates in infants; steatosis and steatohepatitis develop in older children and adults. In either case, end-stage liver disease may result. Biliary sludge and cholelithiasis occur in both groups. In infants, the first clinical indication of PN-induced injury is mild hepatomegaly followed by biochemical evidence of cholestasis. The first biochemical abnormality is an increase in serum bile salts followed by an increase in conjugated bilirubin concentration. These changes may develop any time after 2 to 3 weeks of TPN. Serum alkaline phosphatase and transaminases increase days to weeks later. Steatosis is the result of excess caloric infusions, usually in the form of glucose.[36]

Enteral starvation is a critical factor in the pathogenesis of TPN-related hepatic disease. The most severe hepatic pathologic changes are noted in the patients with the poorest enteral intake. Significantly less serious hepatic disease is being documented in recent years because of more appropriate amino acids (especially for neonates) and the earlier initiation of enteral feeding (stimulating bile flow and increasing secretion of gastrointestinal hormones). In all patients receiving PN, enteral feedings should be initiated as soon as possible, even if only in minimal amounts (trophic feedings) to minimize the risk of hepatic dysfunction.

Less is known about the long-term effects of TPN on the stomach, pancreas, and small bowel. Studies in animals have documented decreased pancreatic secretion and intestinal mucosal atrophy, which are reversible on resumption of enteric feeding. A few studies in humans suggest that exocrine pancreatic secretion and gastric parietal cell mass are decreased and that the small intestine atrophies during TPN, although the observed changes are minor. Amino acids infused intravenously stimulate gastric acid secretion, but much less than if these solutions are infused into the stomach. These gastrointestinal effects disappear over a variable period after return to enteral nutrition. Although similar studies have not been done in preterm infants, clinical experience suggests that enteric function in premature infants also returns to normal with time.

Compatibilities

The approach to interrupting PN therapy for drug administration differs from institution to institution and should be carefully discussed with pharmacy staff and the institution's PN committee. Acyclovir, amphotericin B, metronidazole, and trimethoprim-sulfamethoxazole cannot be given with the PN solution. They may be given in 10% dextrose with the PN turned off. Bicarbonate also should not be given with the PN solution. Cimetidine and ranitidine are compatible with PN solutions. Information about the compatibility of individual drugs with PN is available in the pharmacy of all major hospitals.

Transition to Enteral Feedings

Initiation of enteral feedings should begin as soon as the gastrointestinal tract is functional. Initially, enteral feedings may supplement PN. Parenteral nutrition should not be discontinued until the patient tolerates enteral feedings well enough to meet nutritional requirements. The central catheter may be kept in place until the patient tolerates full enteral feedings. Enteral feedings provide less risk of infection, are less expensive, are associated with fewer metabolic abnormalities, and facilitate recovery of intestinal morphology and enzymes. See Chapter 23 for further details.

Conclusion

The nutritional requirements of young infants, preterm and full-term, can be met better by recognizing their limitations in absorption and digestion. When gastrointestinal disease is superimposed on an immature digestive system, special nutrition support is needed to maintain adequate growth. This support can be given with parenteral or specialized enteral feeding techniques and formulations. Because parenteral solutions can provide complete nutrition support, they may be used for extended periods.

Recommendations for use include the following:

1. Careful catheter placement and confirmation of position by roentgenogram; strict adherence to aseptic techniques and established guidelines of catheter care; and laboratory and clinical monitoring of patients for intolerance to components of the PN solution.
2. Protein in the form of crystalline amino acids at a rate of 1.5 to 3 g/kg/d. The concentration of glucose should be advanced methodically to ensure

Table 22.5.
Parenteral Nutrition Advancing Guidelines

		Dextrose	Fat g/kg/d	Amino Acids g/kg/d
Premature Infant	Initial	4–6 mg/kg/min	0.5	1.5–2.0†
	Advance*	1–2 mg/kg/min	05	0.5-1.0
Term Neonate	Initial	5%	0.5-1.0	1.5
	Advance*	2.5%	0.5	0.5-1.0
Older Infant/ Children	Initial	10%	1.0	1.5
	Advance*	5%	0.5-1.0	1.0
Adolescent and Older	Initial	10%	1.0	1.5
	Advance*	5%-10%	1.0	1.0

* Rate of advancement may be limited by metabolic tolerance (eg, hyperglycemia, hypertriglyceridemia, azotemia).

† When given parenteral glucose alone, an infant will lose 1% of body protein stores per day.[37] A number of studies over the past 12 years indicate that most preterm infants will tolerate 1.5 to 2 g/kg/d of parenteral amino acid intake on the first day of life.[38]

tolerance. Essential fatty acid requirements can be met by infusing 0.5 to 1 g/kg/d of intravenous lipid. The continuous infusion (over 24 hours) of up to 3 g/kg/d of intravenous lipid should maximize tolerance. Vitamins, minerals, and trace elements are essential nutrients and should be contained in PN solutions. See Table 22.5 for suggested advancing guidelines for the macronutrients.

3. The transition to enteral nutrition beginning as soon as possible with continuation of PN until full nutritional support is achieved via the gastrointestinal tract.

4. Continuous monitoring of nutritional status to ensure the adequacy of nutritional support. A nutrition support team with expertise in PN helps provide optimal care, decrease costs and complications, and, potentially, shorten the length of hospitalization.

References

1. American Academy Pediatrics, Committee on Nutrition. Commentary on parenteral nutrition. *Pediatrics.* 1983;71:547–552

2. Mascarenhas MR, Kerner JA Jr, Stallings VA. Parenteral and enteral nutrition. In: Walker WA, Durie PR, Hamilton JR, Walker-Smith JA, Watkins JB, eds. *Pediatric Gastrointestinal Disease.* 3rd ed. Toronto, Canada: B.C. Decker, Inc; 2000;1705–1752

3. Fischer JE. *Total Parenteral Nutrition.* 2nd ed. Boston, MA: Little Brown & Co Inc; 1991

4. Veenstra DL, Saint S, Sullivan SD. Cost effectiveness of antiseptic-impregnated central venous catheters for the prevention of catheter-related bloodstream infection. *JAMA*. 1999;282:554–560

5. Loughran SC, Borzatta M. Peripherally inserted central catheters: a report of 2506 catheter days. *JPEN J Parenter Enteral Nutr*. 1995;19:133–136

6. Maki DG, ed. *Improving Catheter Site Care*. London, England: Royal Society of Medicine Services Limited; 1991

7. Garcia MG, Poole RL, Rubin GD, Kerner JA Jr. Successful use of repeated ethanol injections to clear a central venous catheter occlusion after Urokinase failure. *J Pediatr Pharm Pract*. 1999;4:152–156

8. Haire WD, Herbst SL. Use of Alteplase (t-PA) for the management of thrombotic catheter dysfunction: guidelines from a concensus conference of the National Association of Vascular Access Networks (NAVAN). *Nutr Clin Pract*. 2000;15:265–275

9. Zlotkin SH, Bryan MH, Anderson GH. Intravenous nitrogen and energy intakes required to duplicate in utero nitrogen accretion in prematurely born human infants. *J Pediatr*. 1981;99:115–120

10. Heird WC. Justification for intravenous feeding. In: Yu VYH, MacMahon RA, eds. *Intravenous Feeding of the Neonate*. New York, NY: Edward Arnold; 1992:166–175

11. Chan DS. Recommended daily allowance of maintenance parenteral nutrition in infants and children. *Am J Health Syst Pharm*. 1995;52:651–653

12. Wolfe RR, Allsop JR, Burke JF. Glucose metabolism in man: responses to intravenous glucose infusion. *Metabolism*. 1979;28:210–220

13. Bresson JL, Narcy P, Putet G, Ricour C, Sachs C, Rey J. Energy substrate utilization in infants receiving total parenteral nutrition with different glucose to fat ratios. *Pediatr Res*. 1989;25:645–648

14. Heird WC, Dell RB, Helms RA, et al. Amino acid mixture designed to maintain normal plasma amino acid patterns in infants and children requiring parenteral nutrition. *Pediatrics*. 1987;80:401–408

15. Heird WC, Hay W, Helms RA, Storm MC, Kashyap S, Dell RB. Pediatric parenteral amino acid mixtures in low birth weight infants. *Pediatrics*. 1988;81:41–50

16. Ernst K, Gaylord M, Burnette T, et al. Aminosyn PF associated with doubled incidence of neonatal cholestasis (Abstract). *Pediatr Res* (supplement). 2000;47:286A

17. Cloney DB, Bouthillier MJ, Staublin SA, et al. Total parenteral nutrition–associated cholestasis in neonates receiving two different pediatric amino acid formulations (Abstract). *Pharmacotherapy*. 1996:16:66

18. Acra SA, Rollins C. Principles and guidelines for parenteral nutrition in children. *Pediatric Ann*. 1999;28:113–120

19. LeLeiko NS, Walsh MJ. The role of glutamine, short chain fatty acids, and nucleotides in intestinal adaptation to gastrointestinal disease. *Pediatr Clin North Am*. 1996;43:451–469

20. Lacey JM, Crouch JB, Benfell K, et al. The effects of glutamine supplemented parenteral nutrition in premature infants. *JPEN J Parenter Enteral Nutr.* 1996; 20:74–80

21. American Academy of Pediatrics, Committee on Nutrition. Use of intravenous fat emulsions in pediatric patients. *Pediatrics.* 1981;68:738–743

22. Rollins CJ, Elsberry VA, Pollack KA, Pollack PF, Udall JN Jr. Three-in-one parenteral nutrition: a safe and economical method of nutritional support for infants *JPEN J Parenter Enteral Nutr.* 1990;14:290–294

23. Sosenko IR. Intravenous lipids and the management of chronic lung injury: helpful or harmful? *Semin Neonatal Nutr Metab.* 1995;3:3–5

24. Neuzil J, Darlow BA, Inder TE, Sluis KB, Winterbourn CC, Stocker R. Oxidation of parenteral lipid emulsion by ambient and phototherapy lights: potential toxicity of routine parenteral feeding. *J Pediatr.* 1995;126:785–790

25. Koo WK, Cepeda EE. Parenteral nutrition in neonates. In: Rombeau JL, Rolandelli RH, eds. *Clinical Nutrition: Parenteral Nutrition.* 3rd ed. Philadelphia, PA: W.B. Saunders Co; 2001;463–475

26. Falcone RA Jr, Warner BW. Pediatric parenteral nutrition. In: Rombeau JL, Rolandelli, RH, eds. *Clinical Nutrition: Parenteral Nutrition.* 3rd ed. Philadelphia, PA: W.B. Saunders Co; 2001;476–496

27. Greene HL, Hambidge KM, Schanler R, Tsang RC. Guidelines for the use of vitamins, trace elements, calcium, magnesium and phosphorous in infants and children receiving total parenteral nutrition: report of the Subcommittee of Pediatric Parenteral Nutrient Requirements from the Committee on Clinical Practice Issues of the American Society for Clinical Nutrition. *Am J Clin Nutr.* 1988;48:1324–1342

28. Pelegano JF, Rowe JC, Carey DE, et al. Effect of calcium/phosphorous ratio on mineral retention in parenterally fed premature infants. *J Pediatr Gastroenterol Nutr.* 1991;12:351–355

29. Dunham B, Marcuard S, Khazanie PG, Meade G, Craft T, Nichols K. The solubility of calcium and phosphorus in neonatal total parenteral nutrition solutions. *JPEN J Parenter Enteral Nutr.* 1991;15:608–611

30. Hazinski TA. Vitamin A treatment for the infant at risk for bronchopulmonary dysplasia. *NeoReviews.* 2000;1:e11–e15

31. Tyson JE, Wright LL, Oh W, et al. Vitamin A supplementation for extremely-low-birth-weight infants. *N Engl J Med.* 1999;340:1962–1968

32. American Academy of Pediatrics Committee on Nutrition. Aluminum toxicity in infants and children. *Pediatrics.* 1996;97:413–416

33. Klein GL, Leichtner AM, Heyman MB: Aluminum in large and small volume parenterals used in total parenteral nutrition: response to the food and drug administration notice of proposed rule by the North American Society for Pediatric Gastroenterology and Nutrition. *J Pediatr Gastroenterol Nutr.* 1998;27:457–460

34. Bishop NJ and others: Aluminum neurotoxicity in preterm infants receiving intravenous-feeding solutions. *N Engl J Med.* 1997; 36:1557–1562

35. Whitington PF. Cholestasis associated with total parenteral nutrition in infants. *Hepatology.* 1985;5:693–696
36. Quigley EM, Marsh MN, Shaffer JL, Markin RS. Hepatobiliary complications of total parenteral nutrition. *Gastroenterology.* 1993;104:286–301
37. Heird WC. The importance of early nutritional management of low-birthweight infants. *Pediatr Rev.* 1999;20:e43–e44
38. Thureen PJ. Early aggressive nutrition in the neonate. *Pediatr Rev.* 1999;20:e45–e55

23

Enteral Nutrition Support

Pediatric patients unable to be adequately fed orally may be given enteral tube feedings for nutritional management. Commonly used enteral tube feeding routes include nasogastric, gastrostomy, nasojejunal, gastrojejunal, and jejunostomy. As with all pediatric patients, the nutritional goal should be the provision of nutrients appropriate to the child's metabolic and physiologic requirements and to promote growth and development. Although enteral and parenteral routes can be used to provide nutritional support to pediatric patients, enteral nutritional support is preferred for a number of reasons. Enteral feedings provide nutrients more physiologically, are more economical, and are easier and safer to administer than parenteral nutrition. In addition, they pose fewer metabolic and infectious complications and better support the integrity of the barrier function of the gastrointestinal tract. Enteral nutrition also can provide a more complete range of nutrients, including glutamine, long-chain polyunsaturated fatty acids, short-chain fatty acids, and fiber. Finally, enteral feedings provide a trophic effect on the gut by promoting pancreatic and biliary secretions as well as endocrine, paracrine, and neural factors that help promote the physiologic and immunologic integrity of the gastrointestinal (GI) tract.

Indications for Enteral Tube Feedings: Management of Nutrition-Related Disorders

Prematurity
A feeding method for preterm infants should be individualized to gestational age, birth weight, and medical status. Preterm infants present a unique nutritional challenge due to their GI immaturity, limited fluid tolerance, high nutrient requirements, limited renal function, and predisposition to specific metabolic and clinical complications, such as hypoglycemia and necrotizing enterocolitis. Because the coordination of sucking and swallowing appears at approximately 34 weeks of gestation, intragastric or jejunal feedings are often used before this time. These techniques may be useful beyond 34 weeks in selected infants who are unable to achieve and/or tolerate adequate oral feed-

Table 23.1.
Conditions Under Which Enteral Tube Feeding May Be Warranted*

Prematurity
Cardiorespiratory illness
Chronic lung disease
Cystic fibrosis
Congenital heart disease
Gastrointestinal disease and dysfunction
Inflammatory bowel disease
Short-bowel syndrome
Biliary atresia
Gastroesophageal reflux
Protracted diarrhea of infancy
Chronic nonspecific diarrhea
Renal disease
Hypermetabolic states
Burn injury
Severe trauma or closed head injury
Cancer
Neurologic disease or cerebral palsy

*Modified from: Sutphen, et al. *Enteral Nutrition in Pediatric Gastrointestinal Disease.* 2nd ed. Walker, et al, eds. St Louis, MO: Mosby-Year-Book, Inc; 1996.

ings. Recent studies in preterm infants suggest that minimal enteral feedings (2 to 8 mL/kg/d) administered soon after birth promote a GI hormonal response and, thus, mediate intestinal adaptation.[1] These small-volume, hypocaloric enteral feedings, in conjunction with parenteral nutrition, are used to prime the gut and are thought to promote maturation of GI motor patterns, increase general growth and feeding tolerance, and encourage earlier progression to full enteral feedings and discharge from the hospital. For further information about feeding the preterm infant, see Chapter 2.

Cardiorespiratory Illness
Infants and children with cardiac and pulmonary disease often require enteral nutritional support during acute exacerbations of their primary disease, as well as for nutritional rehabilitation of chronic secondary malnutrition. The etiology of growth failure in patients with neonatal chronic lung disease is

unclear but may be related to prolonged hypoxia, hypercapnia, increased oxygen dependency, elevated metabolic rates, inefficient suck and swallow mechanisms, poor appetite, decreased intake, and recurrent emesis with decreased gastric motility. Children with cystic fibrosis (CF) (see also Chapter 46) also have elevated energy needs and poor intake, which results from their lung disease, malabsorption, chronic infection, debilitation, and fatigue. Nocturnal nasogastric (NG) feedings using elemental or intact nutrient formulas supplemented with pancreatic enzymes have been promoted for use with children and adolescents in whom conservative nutritional supplement measures have failed. Short-term NG feedings have resulted in increased caloric intake and significant weight gain for patients with CF, but long-term effectiveness may be limited by noncompliance. Gastrostomy feedings are more appropriate when long-term gastric infusions are required.

Infants with congenital heart disease (see also Chapter 45) are also at significant nutritional risk. Growth failure resulting from inadequate intake and elevated energy expenditure may be caused by labored and rapid respiration, increased metabolic needs, reduced peripheral blood flow, tissue hypoxia, impaired absorption, and protein-losing enteropathy. Due to their elevated nutritional needs and limited fluid tolerance, these infants often require high caloric density formulas achieved through formula concentration (Appendix E, Table E-4). Concentration beyond 24 kcal/oz, while not absolutely contraindicated, may not allow enough free water for excretion of the renal osmotic load. When necessary, additional calories can be provided through carbohydrate (eg, Polycose) or fat supplementation (eg, Microlipid). Infants with CHD often experience prolonged gastric emptying times that may result in early satiety or promote gastroesophageal reflux (GER).[2] Continuous nocturnal NG feedings or 24-hour enteral feedings of infants with CHD may result in significant catch-up growth.

Gastrointestinal Disease and Dysfunction

Pediatric patients with acute and chronic gastrointestinal disease and dysfunction often benefit from enteral feeding regimens. (See also Chapter 44.) Growth failure in children with Crohn's disease is multifactorial in origin but is most often related to inadequate nutrient intake. Elemental diets administered orally and nasogastrically have been demonstrated to produce a clinically significant improvement in nutritional status. Clinical remission of Crohn's disease of the small bowel by the use of elemental diets alone has been reported, but this effect remains controversial.[3]

The nutritional management for short-bowel syndrome involves the initial use of total parenteral nutrition (TPN). The period of transition to complete enteral feedings may take weeks to years depending on the length of intestinal resection. If the ileocecal valve is preserved, the outcome is vastly improved. Important considerations for provision of adequate enteral feedings include method of administration, volume, osmolality, and nutrient quality (polymeric vs elemental). Polymeric nutrients are usually not well tolerated in the initial stages of the enteral feeding progression, whereas glucose and glucose polymers, medium-chain triglycerides (MCTs), and hydrolyzed protein and dipeptides, which require less digestion, are more easily tolerated.[4] Long-term parenteral nutrition for infants with short-bowel syndrome often leads to hepatic disease, including TPN-associated cholestasis, which is a significant cause of morbidity in infants and children with short-bowel syndrome. Enteral nutrition seems to decrease the incidence and severity of hepatic disease in this situation. Cyclic (10 to 12 hours) TPN with continuous and intermittent enteral feedings and promoting oral intake as tolerated are usually the most successful strategies.[5]

Several other illnesses affecting GI function and nutritional status can be managed successfully with enteral tube feedings. Infants with biliary atresia frequently experience reduced intake associated with hepatic disease and infection. Nutritional support with continuous NG feedings using a semi or elemental formula rich in MCTs can promote energy and nitrogen balance in preparation for and after hepatic transplantation. Once the clinical condition of the infant or child is stable after transplantation, transition to an intact nutrient formula or an oral diet should be made. Infants with GER and growth failure in whom conservative therapy (eg, thickened feedings and upright positioning) and pharmacologic management have failed may benefit from continuous NG feedings with improved intake, reduction or cessation of vomiting, and catch-up growth.[6] Children with chronic nonspecific or protracted diarrhea and malnutrition can also benefit from continuous enteral tube feedings.

Postoperative Malnutrition
Enteral feeding for the postoperative pediatric patient has improved in recent years because of improvements in enteral feeding products, equipment, and techniques. Postoperative feeding via the gut plays a multifactorial role in reducing sepsis and enhancing immune function. Clinical studies have demonstrated that GI function can be adequately maintained with improved nitrogen

balance and nutritional status in the postsurgical trauma patient. Postsurgical pediatric patients may be treated with oral, enteral, or parenteral nutrition or a combination of these depending on the affected portion of the GI tract and the extent of the operative procedure.

Renal Disease

Chronic renal failure in infants and children commonly results in growth failure and developmental delay, particularly in patients with congenital renal disease early in life.[7] The cause of growth failure is thought to be related to protein-energy malnutrition, renal osteodystrophy, chronic metabolic acidosis, and endocrine dysfunction. Despite aggressive medical management and specialized high caloric density formulas, inadequate growth and development often persist. Early nutritional intervention and dialysis can result in improved growth and development. Supplemental tube feedings over a period of 8 to 12 hours in patients with renal insufficiency may lead to catch-up growth.

Hypermetabolic States

Hypermetabolic states, such as cancer, head trauma, burn injury, human immunodeficiency virus (HIV) infection, or acquired immunodeficiency syndrome (AIDS) (see Chapter 39), often require specialized nutritional support. Patients with advanced cancer (see Chapter 42) who are at high nutritional risk and who have minimal GI symptoms and adequate platelet counts may be enterally fed via nocturnal or 24-hour NG or gastrostomy feedings depending on the extent of oral intake.[7,8] Enteral nutrition support is the preferred method for the nutritional support of children with uncomplicated severe head injuries who have protein and caloric requirements equivalent to those of severely burned patients.[9] Metabolic effects associated with burn wounds that can lead to malnutrition include accelerated rate of energy expenditure, increased urine and wound nitrogen losses, and abnormal protein and glucose metabolism.

Neurologic Disease or Impairment

The specific nutritional requirements and feeding approach for neurologically impaired children are highly variable and depend on the degree of impairment, oral motor function, mobility, and muscular tone. Children with Down syndrome, Prader-Willi syndrome, or myelomeningocele have decreased energy needs, growth rates, and motor activity compared with healthy children.[10] Children with cerebral palsy, however, are generally underweight for height and may have increased energy needs, particularly if they have severe contractures or choreoathetoid movements. Patients who are severely affected often require high caloric density enteral feedings and may be treated with a combination of continuous nocturnal gastrostomy feedings and intermittent bolus feedings during the day when oral intake is inadequate. Important considerations for the enteral feeding of these patients include method of feeding, risk of aspiration, formula caloric density, osmolality and fiber content, fluid intake, and effect of enteral feeding therapy on current and future oral-motor function and intake. A fundoplication may be indicated to diminish the risk of aspiration. The nutritional goals for feeding the child with devastating neurologic disease may be less than those predicted by standard growth charts. Excessive intake may place the child at risk for aspiration. Obesity can compromise neuromuscular and respiratory function. The concerns of primary caregivers about lifting heavy children must also be considered.

Fluid balance is important in the pediatric patient who is tube fed because several metabolic complications can be related to inadequate intake. Children with neurodevelopmental disease, like infants in general, may not be able to communicate thirst. Fluid requirements can be calculated by estimating normal water requirements adjusted for specific disease-related factors. Special consideration must be given to monitoring the fluid balance of children receiving high-calorie, high-protein formulas and children with excess water loss due to emesis, diarrhea, fever, or polyuria.[11]

Enteral Formula Selection for Children Aged 1 to 10 Years

Formula selections for children younger than 1 year are discussed in Chapter 4. Until recently, adult formulas had been used for the enteral nutrition support of children older than 1 year because a tube-feeding formula for young children had not been available. The primary disadvantages of using adult tube-feeding formulas for young children are the elevated renal solute load and insufficient vitamin and mineral levels. Dilution of the formulas to reduce the renal solute load results in further reduction of the vitamin and mineral concentration.

A variety of formulas are now available to meet the specialized nutritional needs of the 1- to 10-year-old child (Pediasure [Ross Laboratories], Peptamen Jr [Clintec], Nutren Jr [Clintec], Kindercal [Mead Johnson], Vivonex Pediatric [Sandoz], Neocate One + [SHS North America]). These products can be used for enteral tube feedings and as an oral supplement. The energy distribution of protein, carbohydrate, and fat is between that of infant and adult formulas (Appendix O). The vitamin and mineral concentrations in 950 to 2000 mL of formula meet or exceed 100% of the recommended dietary allowances (RDAs) for children 1 to 10 years of age. At a caloric density of 1 kcal/mL, the formulas are useful for children with increased metabolic needs or for those with fluid restrictions. The 1 kcal/mL caloric density permits some flexibility in dilution; 1100 mL of 24 Kcal/oz formula meets 100% of the RDAs. Children 10 years or older or those with highly specialized nutrient and metabolic needs can generally be adequately fed adult formulas.

Standard Hospital Tube-Feeding Formulas

Standard tube-feeding formulas (Appendix O) have various properties that permit their use and tolerance by the nutritionally compromised patient. These standard formulas are polymeric, consisting of mixtures of protein isolates, oligosaccharides, vegetable oil, MCTs, and added vitamins and minerals. They can be further subdivided into categories based on their osmolality and nutrient composition and density. These formulas, most of which are lactose free and low residue, vary in osmolality from 300 to 650 mOsm/kg and in caloric density from 1.0 to 2.0 kcal/mL. Isotonic formulas Osmolite (Ross Laboratories) and Isocal (Mead Johnson), which contain MCT oil, are often useful for persons with a history of delayed gastric emptying, dumping syndrome, or osmotic diarrhea. Because of their low osmolality, caloric density, and moderate protein content, these isotonic tube feedings are the formulas of choice for general use with pediatric patients older than 7 years. The low osmolality permits their use for bolus intragastric and transpyloric continuous feedings. Children with significant fluid restriction may require vitamin and mineral supplementation. Tube-feeding formulas with added fiber, such as Jevity (Ross Laboratories), range in osmolality from 300 to 480 mOsm/kg and are often useful in the management of patients with chronic constipation and diarrhea.

Although high-calorie, high-nitrogen, hypertonic formulations are often well tolerated by adults with elevated metabolic needs, they are usually not tolerated by children and often lead to diarrhea, emesis, abdominal distention, and delayed gastric emptying. Children and adolescents with markedly elevated calorie and protein requirements due to severe trauma or burn injury are best managed with high-nitrogen formulations such as Perative (20.5% protein, Ross Laboratories) and Nutren 1.5 (16% protein, Clintec). Because of the elevated protein levels in these formulas, however, hydration status must be closely monitored in children.

Elemental Formulas

Elemental formulas with predigested nutrients can be used for the nutritional support of pediatric patients with short-bowel syndrome, pancreatic insufficiency, inflammatory bowel disease, or other severe malabsorptive conditions (Appendices G and O). Elemental formulas may also be used in the enteral nutrition support of patients with CF, although the use of intact protein formulas with appropriate pancreatic enzyme administration may be just as effective. Nitrogen is more rapidly and effectively absorbed in both the healthy and compromised bowel in the form of dipeptides and tripeptides than from free amino acids; therefore, emphasis in elemental product formulation is on the use of peptide formulas with supplemental free essential amino acids. Fats in these formulas are typically provided from a blend of medium-chain and long-chain triglycerides, which provide the essential fatty acids. Recent data suggest that the amino acid, glutamine, may be important for maintenance of the integrity of the intestinal mucosa. Before considering newer products fortified with glutamine, however, consideration of intact whole protein foods as a less expensive and more palatable alternative is prudent.

Specialized formulas have been designed for the nutritional support of patients with specific diseases such as hepatic encephalopathy, renal failure, trauma, AIDS, and sepsis. Significant expense is often associated with these specialty products, however, and clinicians should assess their clinical efficacy as demonstrated in the medical literature before prescribing them.

Oral Supplements

Various flavored milk-based and polymeric formulas may be used as oral supplements for pediatric patients. Milk-based formulas are of moderate residue and high osmolality owing to the high lactose content. High-calorie and protein concentrations also may not be tolerated by the nutritionally compromised patient when taken in large volumes; therefore, consuming them in small frequent sips is often recommended. The constant supervision required to enforce frequent intake can be a source of considerable family conflict. Oral supplements mixed with milk, such as Carnation Instant Breakfast (Clintec), are often better accepted by children than are the lactose-free commercial supplements. Flavored polymeric formulas that contain intact proteins, long-chain fatty acids, and simple carbohydrates are usually marketed as oral supplements because of their palatability. These products, which have osmolarities ranging from 450 to 600 mOsm/kg, are often not sufficiently palatable for long-term voluntary supplementation for children. Some examples of milk-based and polymeric oral supplements include Sustacal (Mead Johnson), Shake-Up Plus (Minute Maid Food Service Group, Houston, Tex), Ensure Plus (Ross Laboratories), and Resource Plus (Sandoz).

It may be preferable to use commonly available energy-dense foods and supplements to increase energy intake. These have the advantage of improved taste and lower cost. Plus, the child may see siblings consuming similar foods and be encouraged by example.

Blenderized Formulas

Commercially available blenderized diets consist of beef, eggs, milk, cereal, fruits and vegetables, and vegetable oils. These formulas, which contain a moderate to high level of residue, have osmolalities ranging from 300 to 435 mOsm/kg. Blenderized feedings are beneficial for chronically ill patients

Table 23.2.
Increasing the Nutrient Density of Foods

- Use cream, whole milk, or evaporated whole milk instead of water for baking whenever possible.
- Use liberal portions of butter, margarine, oil, and cheeses on vegetables and breads and in soups and hot cereals. Add sauces and gravies to foods.
- Add sugar, jelly, or honey to toast and cereals. Use fruits canned in heavy syrup, or sweeten fresh fruits with added sugar.
- Add skim milk powder or instant breakfast powder to regular whole milk for use as a beverage or for cooking. Add powdered milk to puddings, potatoes, soups, and cooked cereals.
- Use peanut butter (after 3 years of age) or cheese on fruit or crackers. Make finger sandwiches for meals or snacks.

Table 23.3.
Energy and Protein Content of Selected Energy-Dense Foods*

	Energy, kcal	Protein, g
Instant breakfast powder (1 packet)	30	7
Mixed with 1 cup whole milk	280	5
Powdered milk (1 tbsp)	33	3
Evaporated milk (1 tbsp)	25	1
Cheese (1 oz)	100	7
Peanut butter (1 tbsp)	95	4
Butter or margarine (1 tsp)	45	0†

*See also Appendix P.
†Not the "spreads," which have a lot of air and water added and, therefore, are lower in kcal.

who have normal digestive capabilities and require long-term enteral nutrition; however, they may not be well tolerated by the malnourished pediatric patient with compromised gastrointestinal function. Often, these products are expensive. Their high viscosity may predispose to obstruction of pediatric feeding tubes.

Blenderized feedings can be prepared at home from milk, juices, cereals, and baby food. Parents of neurologically impaired children who require long-term nutritional management through a feeding gastrostomy are often interested in learning how to prepare blenderized feedings at home because of the economic and psychosocial advantages. The help of a registered dietitian is important to ensure that adequate free water, macronutrient, and micronutrient concentrations are appropriate with these often eclectic mixtures.

Modular Components

Because of the unique and often elevated nutritional requirements of the enterally fed pediatric patient, modification of enteral formulas with modular components is often necessary. In these clinical situations, standard, specialized, pediatric, or adult formulas may be supplemented with caloric modular components, including carbohydrate, fat, and protein modules. Modular protein products, such as Casec (Mead Johnson) and ProMod (Ross Laboratories), may be used to increase the protein density of the formula. Emulsified fat products, such as Microlipid (Sherwood Medical), may also be added. The addition of glucose polymers, such as Polycose (Ross Laboratories) or Moducal (Mead Johnson), as a supplemental carbohydrate source can also increase the caloric density of the formula. If modular nutrients are added, the final macronutrient composition of the diet must be calculated to avoid single nutrient deficiency. Instant breakfast powder, powdered milk, and evaporated milk may also be used to increase the caloric density of whole milk (see Appendix O).

Tube Feeding

When the requirement for enteral nutritional support has been established, the optimal route of delivering nutrients must be determined. Many practitioners recommend the placement of nasogastric or nasoduodenal feeding tubes when the estimated course of therapy will not exceed 3 months (5F or 6F tubes are usually adequate). These tubes should be changed from one nostril to the other every 1 to 3 weeks to decrease associated sinus and ear disease. Extra care should be taken to avoid airway compromise during upper respiratory infections. Tube placement should be verified after episodes of emesis before restarting feedings. If the risk of aspiration is not significant, gastric feedings are preferable owing to ease of management. Tubes made of polyurethane and silicone rubber are soft and pliable and may be left in place for indefinite periods. Polyvinyl chloride tubes become stiff and nonpliable when left in place for more than a few days; however, they are useful for intestinal decompression or short-term feeding. They should be changed every 2 to 3 days to avoid skin necrosis or intestinal perforation.

Some feeding tubes made of polyurethane or silicone rubber have a tungsten or mercury weight at the tip that makes them useful for duodenal or jejunal feedings. Placement of transpyloric tubes can be greatly facilitated by the use of an intravenous prokinetic drug, such as metoclopramide. Children who require long-term tube feeding are candidates for placement of a gastrostomy tube. Gastroesophageal reflux, which may occur in neurologically impaired children or healthy infants after gastrostomy tube placement, may necessitate an operative antireflux procedure (eg, Nissen fundoplication).[12] Although the procedure is effective in reducing GER, postoperative complications can be troublesome. Intractable retching episodes, dumping syndrome, continued problems with swallowing, impaired esophageal emptying, slow feeding, and gas bloating have all been reported. Controversy exists over the necessity of an antireflux procedure in neurologically impaired children who require a feeding gastrostomy. A trial of NG feedings to determine whether they are well tolerated without significant GER before the placement of the gastrostomy can help the clinician determine the need for a simultaneous Nissen fundoplication. Documented pulmonary disease associated with GER is also an indication for a Nissen fundoplication when a gastrostomy is performed.

A common problem with all gastrostomies is migration of the tube through the ostomy site. Ultimately, the tip of the catheter contacts the pylorus where it occasionally induces retching as it passes in and out of the gastric outlet. These problems may be minimized by firmly attaching the tube and placing a mark on the tube to detect inward migration. When a urinary catheter is used as a temporary gastrostomy tube, migration (due to lack of an effective external bolster) remains a common problem.

The gastrostomy button is a feeding device that can be used to form an effective one-way valve at the gastrostomy site. The button fits flush with the skin and attaches to commercial feeding tubes that lock onto the button in a variety of ways. Gastrostomy buttons are less likely to migrate through the pylorus and cause retching and are also less prone to accidental removal.

Buttons may be placed in gastrostomies after the site has matured by healing for several weeks.

To overcome problems related to gastric emptying and frequent GER, transpyloric feedings offer potential benefit. Feeding jejunostomies can be placed through existing gastrostomies. If a modified (eg, urinary catheter) tube is used to convert a gastrostomy to a jejunostomy, extreme care must be exercised to be certain that retching or emesis has not moved the tip of the tube into the esophagus. Retrograde continuous delivery of formula into the esophagus presents an extreme risk for aspiration. Nasal transpyloric tubes may be easily displaced and are uncomfortable as a long-term approach to enteral nutritional support. Often the emesis that occurs in patients with gastric emptying problems predisposes them to dislodged feeding jejunostomies. Operative feeding jejunostomies overcome these difficulties and may be indicated for a select few patients. Patients with feeding jejunostomies generally do not tolerate large bolus feeding over short intervals without experiencing dumping syndrome.

The transition from enteral feeding to full oral feeding can be prolonged. If infants and children are completely deprived of oral feeding during critical maturation phases, difficulties are common when oral feedings are resumed.[13] Reinstituting oral feedings in children who have been fed by means of a gastrostomy tube can evoke a resistant response, such as gagging, choking, or vomiting. To preserve oral motor function during prolonged tube feedings, offering oral intake whenever possible is important. This may require interrupting the infusion to allow a sufficient amount of hunger to develop to facilitate oral intake. Generally, this takes at least 3 hours. Speech pathologists and occupational therapists can help provide oral motor stimulation exercises for such children.

Continuous Versus Intermittent Feeding

Two methods are used for delivery of enteral feedings. Intermittent bolus feedings deliver the formula over a period similar to that for an oral feeding (ie, 10 to 20 minutes). This technique is simple, requires minimal supplies, and may facilitate the transition to home care. Intolerance of this method is indicated by gastric residuals, malabsorption, dumping syndrome, aspiration, or persistent regurgitation. When intermittent bolus feeding is not tolerated, continuous infusion is an alternative. Continuous enteral feeding is administered by infusion pump and has been used successfully when bolus feeding has failed. Continuous feeding may be particularly beneficial when used for patients with impaired absorption, such as chronic diarrhea or short-bowel syndrome. Also, lack of gastric distention may decrease postcibal GER.[14]

References

1. Meetze W, Valentine C, McGuigan JE, Conlon M, Sacks N, Neu J. Gastrointestinal priming prior to full enteral nutrition in very low birth weight infants. *J Pediatr Gastroenterol Nutr.* 1992;15:163–170

2. Cavell B. Effect of feeding an infant formula with high energy density on gastric emptying in infants with congenital heart disease. *Acta Paediatr Scand.* 1981; 70:513–516

3. Bernstein CN, Shanahan F. Braving the elementals in Crohn's disease. *Gastroenterology.* 1992;103:1363–1364

4. Vanderhoof JA, Langnas AN, Pinch LW, Thompson JS, Kaufman SS. Short bowel syndrome. *J Pediatr Gastroenterol Nutr.* 1992;14:359–370

5. Weber TR, Tracy T Jr, Connors RH. Short bowel syndrome in children: quality of life in an era of improved survival. *Arch Surg.* 1991;126:841–846

6. Ferry GD, Selby M, Pietro TJ. Clinical response to short-term nasogastric feeding in infants with gastroesophageal reflux and growth failure. *J Pediatr Gastroenterol Nutr.* 1983;2:57–61

7. ASPEN Board of Directors. Guidelines for the use of parenteral and enteral nutrition in adult and pediatric patients. *JPEN J Parenter Enteral Nutr.* 1993;17: 1SA–52SA

8. Rickard KA, Grosfeld JL, Coates TD, Weetman R, Baehner RL. Advances in nutrition care of children with neoplastic diseases: a review of treatment, research, and application. *J Am Diet Assoc.* 1986;86:1666–1676

9. Stool SE. Nutritional management after severe head injury in children. *Nutr Support Serv.* 1983;3:21–23

10. Cloud HH. Developmental disabilities. In: Queen PM, Lang CE, eds. *Handbook of Pediatric Nutrition.* Gaithersburg, MD: ASPEN Publishers Inc; 1993:400–421

11. Vanlandingham S, Simpson S, Daniel P, Newmark SR. Metabolic abnormalities in patients supported with enteral tube feeding. *JPEN J Parenter Enteral Nutr.* 1981:5:322–324

12. Albanese CT, Towbin RB, Ulman I, Lewis J, Smith SD. Percutaneous gastrojejunostomy versus Nissen fundoplication for enteral feeding of the neurologically impaired child with gastroesophageal reflux. *J Pediatr.* 1993;123:371–375

13. Illingworth RS, Lister J. The critical or sensitive period, with special reference to certain feeding problems in infants and children. *J Pediatr.* 1964;65:839–848

14. Sutphen JL, Dillard VL. Effect of feeding volume on early postcibal gastroesophageal reflux in infants. *J Pediatr Gastroenterol Nutr.* 1988;7:185–188

V
Nutrition in Acute and Chronic Illness

24

Assessment of Nutritional Status

Assessment of nutritional status is the primary step in the evaluation of all children whose growth differs from the norm and should be an integral part of the evaluation and management of all children with acute and chronic disease.[1] During a prolonged hospital stay, nutritional disturbances can occur, particularly when oral intake is suspended or limited. This chapter discusses nutritional assessment methods and their practical application. For most patients, a dietary history, physical examination, and longitudinal changes in height, weight, and body mass index (BMI) are sufficient to assess nutritional status.

Assessment by History

Because an assumption cannot be made that all children eat normally, a detailed diet history is important. Children on a strict vegetarian diet may ingest inadequate amounts of protein, vitamin B_{12}, iron, or pyridoxine if their meals are not properly planned. Adolescents often skip meals, and athletic children may not ingest adequate calories, or they may become involved in sport fad diets. Older children and adolescents may attempt weight loss by starvation, or anorexia nervosa or bulimia may develop. On the other hand, children may be snacking continuously, eating large amounts of sugar-containing beverages, and have sedentary behavior, all of which leads to obesity.

The most accurate method of dietary assessment is a 3- to 5-day diet diary to account for most of the daily variation in diet and eliminate the subjectiveness of diet recall records. Dietary analysis is best done by a registered dietitian. Some medications can cause nutritional disturbances (Appendix I).

Clinical Assessment

Careful inspection of the patient remains a valid method of nutritional assessment.[2] Obesity and wasting are obvious, although they need to be confirmed by growth charts. Observation is a useful screening test for gross changes in body composition. Edema, dehydration, excess or inadequate subcutaneous fat, and increase or decrease of the muscle mass can be detected. Some of the

Table 24.1.
Signs and Symptoms of Vitamin Deficiency or Excess (See Also Chapter 21)

Vitamin	Deficiency	Excess
A	Night blindness, xerophthalmia, keratomalacia, follicular hyperkeratosis	Scaly skin, bone pain, pseudotumor cerebri, hepatomegaly
C	Scurvy: capillary hemorrhage of gingiva, skin, bone, poor wound healing	"Rebound" deficiency after high intake
D	Rickets, osteomalacia	Constipation, renal stones, myositis ossiferous, hypercalcemia
E	Hemolysis (in premature infant), peripheral neuropathy	Suppresses hematologic response to iron in anemia
K	Bruising, bleeding	Jaundice
Thiamine	Beriberi: cardiomyopathy, peripheral neuropathy, and encephalopathy	None known
Riboflavin	Cheilosis, glossitis, angular stomatitis	None known
Niacin	Pellagra: dementia, diarrhea, and dermatitis	Flushing
Pyridoxine	Seizures, anemia, irritability	Neuropathy
Biotin	Dermatitis, alopecia, muscle pain	None known
Folate	Macrocytic anemia, stomatitis paresthesia, glossitis, neural tube defects of fetus	None known
B_{12}	Megaloblastic anemia, neuropathy, paresthesia, glossitis	None known

findings of vitamin and mineral deficiencies are listed in Tables 24.1 and 24.2. Deficiency of any trace substance can result in growth failure. The clinical signs and symptoms of specific vitamin or mineral deficiencies or toxic effects are usually not pathognomonic.

Anthropometry

Anthropometric measurements can assess growth cross-sectionally or longitudinally. If children are measured once, their growth status for age can be assessed by comparing this measurement with the appropriate reference chart. If children are measured more than once, growth velocity data are obtained that can be more valuable because they reflect change. The intervals between measurements that are necessary to develop meaningful incremental data are listed in Table 24.3. Particular care should be taken to use appropriate equipment and techniques for measuring stature/length and weight. This can significantly improve the assessments that need to be performed before evaluating aspects of body composition, such as body fatness.

Table 24.2.
Signs and Symptoms of Mineral Deficiency or Excess

Mineral	Deficiency	Excess
Aluminum	None known	Central nervous system disorder
Boron	Calcification abnormalities	None known
Calcium	Osteomalacia, tetany	Constipation, heart block, vomiting
Chloride	Alkalosis	Acidosis
Chromium	Diabetes (in animals)	None known
Cobalt	Vitamin B_{12} deficiency	Cardiomyopathy
Copper	Anemia, neutropenia, osteoporosis, neuropathy, depigmentation of hair and skin	Cirrhosis, central nervous system effects, Fanconi nephropathy, corneal pigmentation
Fluoride	Caries	Fluorosis
Iodine	Goiter, cretinism	Goiter
Iron	Anemia, behavioral abnormalities	Hemosiderosis
Lead	None known	Encephalopathy, neuropathy, stippled red blood cells
Magnesium	Hypocalcemia, hypokalemia, tremor, weakness, arrhythmia	Weakness, sedation, hypotension, nausea, vomiting
Molybdenum	Growth retardation (in animals)	None known
Phosphorus	Rickets, neuropathy	Calcium deficiency
Potassium	Muscle weakness, cardiac abnormalities	Heart block
Selenium	Cardiomyopathy, anemia, myositis	Nail and hair changes, garlic odor
Sodium	Hypotension	Edema
Sulfur	Growth failure	None known
Zinc	Growth failure, dermatitis, hypogeusia, hypogonadism, alopecia, impaired wound healing	Gastroenteritis

Table 24.3.
Minimal Time Intervals to Detect Changes in Growth Velocity

Measurement	Interval
Weight	7 d
Length	4 wk
Stature	8 wk
Head circumference	7 d, infants 4 wk, up to 4 years of age
Midarm circumference	4 wk

Length or Stature

Length or stature is the most useful indicator of growth status. Unfortunately, in infants and small children, it is also the most difficult measurement to obtain accurately. In infants and children younger than 2 years, recumbent length is measured. Two people are required to accomplish this measurement. The measuring table or board should consist of a fixed headboard, a movable footboard, and a rule attached at one side. One of the measurers should hold the crown of the infant's head against the headboard so the external auditory meatus and the lower margin of the eye orbit are aligned perpendicular to the table. The second measurer grips both ankles of the infant with one hand and positions the heels firmly against the footboard, which is manipulated with the other hand. The knees, which are slightly flexed, are then pressed down on the table with the lateral edge of the hand. The recumbent length should be recorded to the nearest 0.1 cm (according to the National Center for Health Statistics [NCHS]/Centers for Disease Control and Prevention [CDC] recommendations).

Stature, or standing height, is measured in children older than 2 years. Several apparatuses are available that can be affixed to a wall. Measurements are made with the child's feet bare. The child should stand erect with the heels, buttocks, shoulders, and head all touching the measuring board. The feet should be positioned at a 90-degree angle. The child's axis of vision should be horizontal, with the child looking ahead and the external auditory meatus and lower margin of the orbit aligned horizontally. Children should be told to make themselves "as tall as possible with their heels on the ground." The head projection of the measuring apparatus is then slid down firmly onto the crown of the head and the stature is recorded to the nearest 0.1 cm.

Reference values for length, stature, and growth velocity are shown in Appendix J.[3–6] Reference values for length and stature are also available for children with Down syndrome (Appendix J) or many other conditions. Premature infants can be compared with reference values derived from intrauterine lengths for various gestational ages as shown in Appendix K. The reference charts used should be appropriate for the population segment.

When possible, the parents' stature should be obtained to determine the influence of genetics on growth (Appendix L). If only one parent is available, the maternal stature is more valuable for comparison.

Weight

Various types of apparatuses, such as infant scales, beam-balance scales, and readout scales, are available to measure body weight. The type used needs to be regularly calibrated to maintain accuracy. Weight should always be recorded as nude weight. If the subject is not weighed nude, then the estimated weight of the clothing should be subtracted from the total weight. Reference values for body weight are included in Appendix J, as are reference values for children with Down syndrome. Weight reference values for premature infants are shown in Appendix K.

Weight for Height

The ratio of actual weight to the ideal weight for height (usually referred to as *weight for height*) can be used to differentiate stunted growth from wasting and is independent of age. Stunting is caused by genetic or endocrine abnormalities or more often by chronic malnutrition and/or chronic illness and results in a child who is small for age but has a body weight proportional to the length. Wasting results from acute or subacute nutritional deprivation and by acute medical conditions such as diarrhea. In this condition, body weight is depleted out of proportion to length, making the weight-for-height ratio low. The current internationally accepted index is the weight-for-height z-score or the percentile based on the NCHS/CDC growth reference. Reference values that reflect the normal distribution of weight in relation to height for healthy prepubescent children are shown in Appendix J.

Body Mass Index (BMI)

Body mass index (weight/height^2) is the best indicator of adiposity in children as well as the adolescent (Appendix J). To calculate BMI, divide the weight in kg by the square of the height in meters (kg/m^2). It can also be calculated by dividing the weight in pounds by the height in inches squared, and multiplied by 703 (lbs/in 2×703). Body mass index is an important tool to determine overweight in children. By consensus, any child higher than the 85th percentile is at risk for overweight, and higher than the 95th percentile is considered at risk for obesity. All children followed by a physician should have their BMI calculated periodically. If the child begins to cross percentile lines on the BMI chart, the family can be counseled early about prevention of obesity.

Head Circumference

Head circumference is a useful measurement until about 3 years of age, when head growth slows. It must be measured with a narrow and nonstretchable measuring tape. To obtain an accurate measurement, the tape must cross the forehead just above the supraorbital ridges, passing around the head at the same level on both sides to the occiput. It is then moved up or down slightly to obtain the maximum circumference. The tape should have sufficient tension to press the hair against the skull. Normal reference values from birth to 3 years are shown in Appendix J. Reference values for premature infants are shown in Appendix K.

Midarm Circumference

The midupper arm circumference is an indicator of muscle growth in all ages. The left arm is usually measured by convention. The tape to be used should be the same as that used to measure the head circumference. A point is marked midway between the acromion (shoulder) and the olecranon (elbow) on the vertical axis of the upper arm with the arm bent at a right angle and between the lateral and medial surface of the arm. The child should then stand or sit with the arm hanging loose at the side. The tape is passed around the arm at the level marked and is tightened so it touches but does not compress the skin or alter the contour of the arm. Because the arm on cross section is not an exact circle, some difficulty is usually met in ensuring that the tape touches the arm on the medial surface. To accomplish this, the middle finger of the examiner's left hand can be used to gently press the tape to the skin. Normal reference values are available for children 1 year and older and are shown in Appendix L.[7]

Midarm Circumference-to-Head Circumference Ratio

The ratio of midarm circumference to head circumference was developed by Kanawati and McLaren[8] as a method to estimate nutritional status when the proper apparatus for measuring weight or height is not available, although this is rarely the case in clinical practice today. The midarm circumference is substantially influenced by subcutaneous fat and, therefore, fluctuates with total body weight. The head circumference in an infant and young child parallels the child's linear growth. Therefore, the midarm-to-head circumference ratio varies directly with the weight-for-height ratio and can be used as a substitute until head growth slows at about 3 years of age. A ratio greater than 0.31 is considered normal, and a ratio less than 0.25 indicates severe malnutrition. Various degrees of undernutrition lie between.

Nutritional Assessment Through the Measurement of Body Composition

The major form of stored energy in the body is fat. A small amount of carbohydrate in the form of glycogen is present, but this can be depleted after only 1 or 2 days of starvation. Protein can also be used for energy, but all protein in the body is present only as functional tissue, so its use results in a decrease in the functional body mass. Because fat is used preferentially by the body as an energy source during starvation or periods of metabolic stress, the accurate measurement of this body compartment would be the ideal method to assess a child's nutritional status. Longitudinal measurements would allow estimates of nutritional sufficiency during periods of recovery from disease. Many methods of measurement of the fat and fat-free compartments of the body exist; however, most are not applicable to the child because they are too inaccurate or too cumbersome for use in children.[9] New methods that offer easy measurement of fat and fat-free mass have been developed.[10,11] If these methods prove practical, they will enhance the accuracy of surveillance of the nutritional status of the hospitalized child. Table 24.4 shows the average amount of lean body mass and body fat in non-obese healthy individuals from birth to age 22 years.

Table 24.4.
Lean Body Mass and Body Fat*

Age[†]	Males			Females		
	LBM, kg	Fat, kg	% Fat	LBM, kg	Fat, kg	% Fat
Birth	3.06	0.49	14	2.83	.49	15
6 mo	6.0	2.0	25	5.3	1.9	26
12 mo	7.9	2.3	22	7.0	2.2	24
2 y	10.1	2.5	20	9.5	2.4	20
4 y	14.0	2.7	16	13.2	2.8	18
6 y	17.9	2.8	14	16.3	3.2	16
8 y	22.0	3.3	13	20.5	4.3	17
10 y	27.1	4.3	14	26.2	6.4	20
12 y	34	8	19	32	10	24
14 y	45	10	18	38	13	25
16 y	57	9	14	42	13	24
18 y	61	9	13	43	13	23
20 y	62	9	13	43	14	25
22 y	62	10	14	43	14	25

*From the American Academy of Pediatrics, Committee on Nutrition. *Pediatric Nutrition Handbook.* 2nd ed. Elk Grove Village, IL: American Academy of Pediatrics; 1985:346. Data are given as normative means. LBM indicates lean body mass.
†At nearest birthday.

Fat-Fold Measurements

The most frequently used method to estimate body fatness in the hospitalized patient is the skin fat-fold measurement. This method is limited because of 2 assumptions: (1) that the subcutaneous fat mantle reflects the total amount of fat in the body, and (2) that the measurement sites selected represent the average thickness of the entire mantle. Neither assumption is true. Two studies of humans address the first assumption. Forbes et al[12] showed that only 42% of the total body fat of a full-term neonate resides in the subcutaneous compartment. Moore et al[13] found the value to be 32% in an adult woman. The second assumption can be discredited simply by observing the regional variation of subcutaneous fat among individual persons.

In the infant and young child, the use of skin fat-fold measurements as an index of total body fat has not been fully validated by an alternative method.[14] Accurately and reproducibly measuring a skin fat fold is difficult and in edematous or obese individuals, perhaps impossible. These problems limit the usefulness of this measurement as a tool for nutritional assessment. It is sometimes useful, however, for the longitudinal assessment of a patient's response to nutritional therapy. The calipers recommended for fat-fold measurements include the Holtain caliper (Pfister Imports, Carlstadt, NJ) and the Lange caliper (Cambridge Instruments, Silver Spring, MD). All measurements are taken on the left side of the child. The most frequent sites of skinfold measurements are the triceps and the suprailiac crest. The level for the triceps skinfold is the same level of the upper arm as marked for a circumference measurement (midway between the acromion and the olecranon with the arm bent at a right angle). With the arm dropped and hanging loosely, the skinfold is lifted away from the underlying muscle fascia with a sweeping motion of the fingers with the observer gripping the "neck" of the fold between middle finger and thumb. The skinfold caliper is then applied to the fold. The point of measurement for the suprailiac skinfold is 1 cm above and 2 cm medial to the anterior superior iliac spine. This position is best palpated with the subject standing facing the observer and is marked with a pen. The skinfold is picked up as a vertical skinfold and the caliper applied below the fingers.[7,15]

Hydrodensitometry

The oldest method of estimating the relative proportion of lean and fat in the human body is densitometry, which was introduced in 1942 by Albert Behnke.[16] This method uses the Archimedes principle to determine the density of a person by dividing the actual weight by the amount of weight lost when the person is completely submerged in water. Because the density of fat and the lean compartments of the body are assumed to be constants, calculation of the proportion of each is possible when the density of the whole body is known. This method is widely used to measure body fat in adults. Its use in children, however, is limited because young children cannot be submerged under water. Even in older children, the method is limited by the change in density of lean body mass during maturation, thus, invalidating one of the basic assumptions of the method.[17] In the hospitalized patient, this method is useless because neither sick children nor adults can be submerged in water even if problems such as intravenous lines and dressings could be managed. Newer methods using this principle with air rather than water displacement are being developed; however, no data exist to determine their practicality.

Total Body Potassium

Another method that has become a standard for the measurement of lean body mass and body fat is the measurement of total body potassium.[18,19] This method is based on the fixed proportion (0.0118%) of the radioactive isotope, ^{40}K, contained in the naturally occurring potassium ^{39}K. In determining lean body mass, the subject is placed in a specially designed scintillation chamber and the number of radioactive emissions from ^{40}K is recorded during a 30- to 60-minute period. Total body potassium is then calculated from the amount of ^{40}K present. Because potassium resides in a relatively fixed concentration only in the lean body mass and not in fat, an estimate of the total amount of lean body mass can be derived. Fat can then be calculated by the subtraction of lean body mass from total body weight. This technique is noninvasive, but has several limitations, particularly for the hospitalized patient. The counting time is long and requires isolation in a special chamber, which may not be possible for a child or a person who is seriously ill. Few machines have sufficient sensitivity to measure infants or small children who have little lean body and relatively fewer radioactive disintegrations per unit of time than do adults.

Total Body Water

Because neutral fat does not bind water, the measurement of total body water offers a means for estimating the nonfat compartment of the body.[20] This can be accomplished in a fairly noninvasive manner by oral administration of water labeled with a known amount of radioactive tritium (^{3}H) or the stable isotopes, deuterium (^{2}H) or oxygen 18. Total body water then can be estimated by determining the dilution of the isotope within a body fluid, such as serum, urine, or saliva, after a suitable period of equilibration. Because the water content of lean body mass is relatively constant, this compartment can be esti-mated. Although this method is simple, its application to clinical problems is limited because the assays for deuterium and oxygen 18 are cumbersome, and radioactive tritium is not suitable for use in children. A basic methodological problem also exists because the water content of lean body mass changes with age and may also vary slightly among people of the same age. Isotopes of hydrogen also appear to exchange with nonaqueous hydrogen, resulting in an overestimation of body water content. Oxygen 18 does not seem to have the same problem, but it is expensive.

Neutron Activation

Many elements can be made radioactive by bombarding them with neutrons. The neutron-activation method of total body analysis uses this principle by activating the body with a known amount of neutron energy and counting the induced radioactivity in a whole-body counting chamber. A given dose of neu-trons will generate a known amount of activity within a defined mass of sub-stance. The total activity will, therefore, reflect the total mass of the substance. A particular element can be identified by the characteristic energy of the elec-tromagnetic radiation it emits. This method can be used to determine the amount of a number of elements in the body, including calcium, sodium, chlo-rine, phosphorus, magnesium, and nitrogen. Total body nitrogen can be used to estimate lean body mass. This method should allow a much better understand-ing of human body composition through its use as a research tool; however, its clinical use is limited by the great expense of a neutron-activation facility. Also, although the radiation exposure by this method is small (approximately 30 mrad), any radiation exposure limits its use in children.

Photon and X-ray Absorptiometry

Abnormalities in bone mineralization as a complication of prematurity or dis-ease (such as renal or hepatic disease) are being recognized with increasing fre-quency. The traditional method to assess this parameter has been radiologic, but radiographs are not a sensitive indicator of bone density. The development of photon absorptiometry and, more recently, x-ray absorptiometry may pro-vide tools for the assessment of this parameter. In this technique, the bone is scanned transversely by a low-energy photon beam generated by ^{125}I or an x-ray beam, and the transmission is monitored by a scintillation detector. The change in transmission of the beam as it is moved across the bone is a function of the bone density in the region. Evidence exists that the bone density of the distal radius can be related to the total skeletal mass, at least in adults. Dual photon or x-ray absorptiometry of the spine provides an index of the density of trabecular bone, and total body scans can generate an estimate of total body calcium. Total body scans can also give an estimate of fat mass since fat also has differential absorption of x-rays relative to lean body mass. Even though this method of determining percent body fat is not as accurate as other methods, the noninvasive methodology and the relative inexpense of the apparatus has made this a relatively popular tool.

Bioelectrical Impedance Analysis

Bioelectrical impedance analysis [21-24] has become somewhat popular as a research tool. This method is based on the principle that a weak electrical current passes through the body by way of the lean compartment rather than through fat. The impedance to electrical flow is directly proportional to the amount of lean tissue present. This method has been validated with hydrodensitometry and total body water measurement by isotope dilution in adults. It is noninvasive, portable, and relatively inexpensive; however, it appears to be imprecise. Small changes in body water, such as normal diurnal variation, appear to make significant differences in the estimate of lean body mass. Placement of the electrodes (on the wrist and ankle) that inject and record the electrical current is critical. As a result, the standard error of the estimate is rather high (2 kg to 2.5 kg in adults). Bioelectrical impedance analysis has not yet been accurately applied to infants. The changing water content and distribution of the lean body mass of growing children should cause the impedance to change progressively with age, making this method extremely difficult to calibrate for children.

Total Body Electrical Conductivity

A recently developed electrical method that is very useful in the clinical setting is total body electrical conductivity (TOBEC),[25-27] which is based on the principle that organisms placed in an electromagnetic field perturb the field. The degree of perturbation depends on the amount of volume of distribution of electrolytes present within the body. Electrolytes reside exclusively in the lean body mass, thus allowing estimation of this body compartment. Fat is then estimated by subtracting lean body mass from total body weight. This method is safe. The total energy dissipated in a subject measured is at least 100 times less than what has been established as a safety standard for exposure to electromagnetic energy. The instrument consists of a hollow chamber, open at both ends, the walls of which contain transducer coils that generate the appropriate electromagnetic field. To obtain a reading, the subject is passed through the chamber and current is applied for less than 1 minute in the machine for older children and adults, and approximately 1 second in the machine for infants. The machine for infants has been calibrated against the fat-free mass of infant miniature pigs as determined by chemical analysis. The machine for older children and adults has been calibrated against hydrodensitometry, total body water measurement by isotope dilution, and total body potassium measurement. The standard error of the estimate of lean body mass for this method is around 70 g for infants and 930 g for adults. The TOBEC method allows rapid, safe, noninvasive, and accurate determination of body composition. Its major limitation is its lack of portability and the cost of the instrument.

Laboratory Assessment

The initial laboratory assessment of nutritional status includes the measurement of hematologic status and protein nutrition. The absence of anemia may not exclude nutritional deficiencies, such as iron, folate, and vitamin B_{12} deficiency. Red blood cell size is valuable in the differential diagnosis of anemias. The total serum protein determination is interpretable only if the globulins can be assumed to be normal. Albumin is a better measure of protein nutrition than serum globulins because its biological half-life is shorter. A low concentration occurs when albumin is lost from the body in large amounts, as in nephrosis, exudative enteropathy, burns, or surgical drains. The so-called visceral proteins synthesized by the liver (such as retinol binding protein with a half-life of 12 hours, transthyretin [prealbumin] with a half-life of 1.9 days, and transferrin with a half-life of 8 days) have shorter half-lives than does albumin, and their levels are better indicators of protein status than is the serum albumin level. Serum levels of essential amino acids may be lower than those of nonessential amino acids, and 3-methyl histidine excretion is increased during states of protein insufficiency. Other abnormalities of protein depletion include a decreased creatinine level and decreased hydroxyproline excretion. Values for protein status may or may not reflect the degree of nutritional deficiency. In simple starvation (marasmus), a tendency to maintain the circulatory pool of visceral proteins at the expense of somatic protein is evident. The blood urea nitrogen level tends to decrease during starvation; however, in patients in whom water intake is restricted, such as those with anorexia nervosa, the serum value may be elevated.

The serum sodium concentration is frequently decreased in malnutrition as the result of dilution because total body water is physiologically increased during starvation. This value is seldom lower than 133 mEq/L, however. The dilution effect can also be seen with hematologic parameters such as hematocrit and hemoglobin. Immunologic abnormalities, such as loss of delayed hypersensitivity, fewer T lymphocytes, and changes in lymphocyte response to in vitro stimulation by phytohemagglutinin are sometimes helpful clinical measurements of nutritional status.

Assays of specific nutrients can be helpful in the assessment of the nutritional status of an individual, but their usefulness is limited by their wide variation within normal groups and the lack of easy availability of many of the vitamin assays. Normal values for some of these biochemical measurements are shown in Table 24.5. Other vitamins, such as biotin and niacin, as well as essential fatty acids can be measured. These measurements are seldom clinically indicated. Assessment of the levels of minerals, such as calcium, magnesium, phosphorus, iodine, copper, and selenium, is readily available in most laboratories and sometimes is important to measure as part of the nutritional assessment.

Table 24.5.
Normal Values: Biochemical Measurement of Specific Nutritional Parameters

Test	Normal Value	Exceptions
Protein		
Blood		
Serum albumin, g/dL	3.7–5.5	Infant, 2.9–5.5
Retinol binding protein, mg/dL	1.3–9.9	Children <9 y, 1–7.8
Blood urea nitrogen, mg/dL	7–22	
Thyroxine binding protein, mg/dL	20–50	
Transferrin, mg/dL	170–440	
Fibronectin, mg/dL	30–40	
Prealbumin, mg/dL	17–42	Premature infant, 4–14; term infant, 4–20; 6- to 12-mo-old child, 8–24; 1- to 6-y-old child, 17–30
Urine		
Creatinine/height index	>0.9	…
3-methyl histidine, μmol/kg	3.2±0.6 male	
	2.1±0.4 female	
	4.2±1.3 neonate	
3-methyl histidine, μmol/g creatinine	126±32 male	
	92±23 female	
Hydroxyproline index	253±78 neonate	
	>2	

Table 24.5.
Normal Values: Biochemical Measurement of Specific Nutritional Parameters *(continued)*

Test	Normal Value	Exceptions
Vitamin A Plasma retinol, μg/dL	20–72	Infant, 13–50
Vitamin D 25-OH-D$_3$, μg/L 1-25-OH-D$_3$, μg/L	2–30 15–60	† ...
Riboflavin Red blood cell glutathione reductase stimulation, %	<20	...
Vitamin B$_6$ Red blood cell transaminases, Plasma pyridoxal phosphate, Xanthurenic acid excretion	Feasible and useful in all age groups, but not readily available and not practical in children <9 y	...
Folic acid Serum folate, ng/mL Red blood cell folate, ng/mL	>6 >160	...
Vitamin K Prothrombin time, sec	11–15	...
Vitamin E Plasma alphatocopherol, mg/dL Red blood cell hemolysis test, %	0.7–10 10	Preterm infant, 0.5–3.5
Vitamin C Plasma level, mg/dL Leukocyte level, mg/100 cells	0.2–2.0 Difficult to perform on children because of sample requirements	...
Thiamine Red blood cell transketolase stimulation, %	<15	...
Vitamin B$_{12}$ Serum vitamin B$_{12}$, pg/mL Absorption test	200–900 Excretion of more than 7.5% of ingested labeled vitamin B$_{12}$	...
Iron Hematocrit, %	39	Neonate, 31; infant, 33; child and menstruating females, 36

Table 24.5.
Normal Values: Biochemical Measurement of Specific Nutritional Parameters *(continued)*

Test	Normal Value	Exceptions
Iron *(continued)*		
Hemoglobin, μg/dL	14	Neonate, 11; infant, 12; child and menstruating females, 13
Serum ferritin, ng/mL	>15	Neonate, <60
Serum iron, μg/dL	>60	Neonate, >30; infant, >40; child <4 y, >50
Serum total iron binding capacity, μg/dL	350–400	
Serum transferrin saturation, %	>16	Infant, >12; child <9 y, >14–15
Serum transferrin, mg/dL		
Erythrocyte protoporphyrin, μg/dL red blood cells	170–250 <70	Neonate, <80; infant, <75
Zinc		
Serum level, μg/dL	60–120	…
Erythrocyte level	Erythrocytes contain approximately 10 times more zinc than does plasma	
Phosphorus		
Serum phosphate, mg/dL	2.9–5.6	Newborn, 4.0–8.0; 1-y-old child, 3.8–6.2; 2- to 5-y-old child, 3.5–6.8
Calcium		
Serum total calcium, mg/dL	8.5–10.5	Preterm infant, 6–10; term infant, 7–12; child, 8–10.5
Serum ionized calcium, mg/dL	4.48–4.92	
Magnesium		
Serum magnesium, mEq/L	1.5–2.0	…

References

1. Fomon SJ. *Nutritional Disorders of Children: Prevention, Screening, and Followup.* Rockville, MD: Department of Health and Human Services; 1977. US Dept of Health Education and Welfare publication (HSA) 77–5104

2. Baker JP, Detsky AS, Wesson DE, et al. Nutritional assessment: a comparison of clinical judgment and objective measurements. *N Engl J Med.* 1982;306:969–972

3. Hamill PV, Drizd TA, Johnson CL, Reed RB, Roche AF, Moore WM. Physical growth: National Center for Health Statistics percentiles. *Am J Clin Nutr.* 1979;32:607–629

4. Roche AF, Himes JH. Incremental growth charts. *Am J Clin Nutr.* 1980;33: 2041–2052

5. Tanner JM, Davies PS. Clinical longitudinal standards for height and height velocity for North American children. *J Pediatr.* 1985;107:317–329

6. Himes JH, Roche AF, Thissen D, Moore WM. Parent-specific adjustments for evaluation of recumbent length and stature of children. *Pediatrics.* 1985;75:304–313

7. Frisancho AR. New norms for upper limb fat and muscle areas for assessment of nutritional status. *Am J Clin Nutr.* 1981;34:2540–2545

8. Kanawati AA, McLaren DS. Assessment of marginal malnutrition. *Nature.* 1970; 228:573–575

9. Kagan BM, Stanincova V, Felix NS, Hodgman J, Kalman D. Body composition of premature infants: relation to nutrition. *Am J Clin Nutr.* 1972;25:1153–1164

10. Lohman TG. Research progress in validation of laboratory methods of assessing body composition. *Med Sci Sports Exerc.* 1984;16:596–605

11. Lohman TG. Applicability of body composition techniques and constants for children and youths. *Exerc Sport Sci Rev.* 1986;14:325–357

12. Forbes RM, Cooper AR, Mitchell HH. Composition of the adult human body as determined by chemical analysis. *J Biol Chem.* 1953;203:359–366

13. Moore FD, Lister J, Boyden CM, Ball MR, Sullivan N, Dagher FJ. The skeleton as a feature of body composition. Values predicted by isotope dilution and observed by cadaver dissection in an adult female. *Hum Biol.* 1968;40:135–188

14. Infant body composition by skinfold measurements. *Nutr Rev.* 1975;33:7–9

15. Karlberg P, Engstrom I, Lichtenstein H, Svennberg I. The development of children in a Swedish urban community. A prospective longitudinal study. III. Physical growth during the first three years of life. *Acta Paediatr Scand Suppl.* 1968;187:48–66

16. Lohman TG. Skinfolds and body density and their relation to body fatness: a review. *Hum Biol.* 1981;53:181–225

17. Forbes GB. Body composition in adolescence. *Prog Clin Biol Res.* 1981;61:55–72

18. Forbes GB, Schultz F, Cafarelli C, Amirhakimi GH. Effects of body size on potassium–40 measurement in the whole body counter (tilt-chair technique). *Health Phys.* 1968;15:435–442

19. Remenchik AP, Miller CE, Kessler WV. *Body Composition Estimates Derived From Potassium Measurements.* Argonne, IL: Argonne National Laboratory; 1968:73–90. US Atomic Energy Commission publication ANL-7461

20. Lukaski HC, Johnson PE. A simple inexpensive method of determining total body water using a tracer dose of D_2O and infrared absorption of biological fluids. *Am J Clin Nutr.* 1985;41:363–370

21. Katch FI, Solomon RT, Shayevitz M, Shayevitz B. Validity of bioelectrical impedance to estimate body composition in cardiac and pulmonary patients. *Am J Clin Nutr.* 1986;43:972–973

22. Lukaski HC, Bolonchuk WW, Hall CB, Siders WA. Validation of tetrapolar bioelectrical impedance method to assess human body composition. *J Appl Physiol*. 1986;60:1327–1332
23. Lukaski HC, Johnson PE, Bolonchuk WW, Lykken GI. Assessment of fat-free mass using bioelectrical impedance measurements of the human body. *Am J Clin Nutr*. 1985;41:810–817
24. Rinke WJ. Electrical impedance: a new technique to assess human body composition. *Mil Med*. 1986;151:338–341
25. Cochran WJ, Klish WJ, Wong WW, Klein PD. Total body electrical conductivity used to determine body composition in infants. *Pediatr Res*. 1986;20:561–564
26. Fiorotto ML, Cochran WJ, Funk RC, Sheng HP, Klish WJ. Total body electrical conductivity measurements: effects of body composition and geometry. *Am J Physiol*. 1987;252:R794–R800
27. Fiorotto ML, Klish WJ. Total body electrical conductivity measurements in the neonate. *Clin Perinatol*. 1991;18:611–627

25

Pediatric Feeding and Swallowing Disorders

Because pediatric swallowing dysfunction may result in substantial morbidity, timely recognition and treatment is essential. Swallowing is a complex sequence of motor events requiring coordination of muscles in the oral cavity, pharynx, larynx, and esophagus. Intact sensation from areas of the mouth, pharynx, and larynx is essential to normal swallowing because initiation of swallowing and protection of the airway rely on adequate sensory input to the swallowing control centers in the brain. Anatomic defects of the oropharynx, larynx, or esophagus, as well as disease processes that alter motor or sensory function, may lead to swallowing abnormalities.[1–2]

Swallowing develops early and has been reported in fetuses as early as 12 to 14 weeks' gestation. Near term, a fetus swallows an estimated half of the total volume of amniotic fluid per day. Swallowing is generally described in 3 phases—oral, pharyngeal, and esophageal. Changes occur in these phases during the progression of normal development.[3–7] Therefore, swallowing problems in children can be either congenital or acquired. Dysfunction in the oral phase of swallowing with children is often characterized as a "feeding" problem, unless the problem compromises the safety of the swallow. Feeding problems can be developmental in nature where there is a delay in acquiring developmental feeding skills such as mature sucking, chewing, or cup drinking.[8]

Common Conditions Associated With Swallowing Disorders

The prevalence of swallowing disorders in the general pediatric population is largely unknown; however, it is quite common among certain pediatric disease states. The causes of dysphagia are numerous (Table 25.1). Dysphagia among children and adults with neuromuscular disease has been well documented.[9–13] The problem may be in the muscles, nerves, neuromuscular junction, or the central nervous system.[14] Central nervous system disease is a frequent cause of pediatric dysphagia. Of all children with cerebral palsy, 27% to 40% are believed to have a swallowing abnormality.[11,12] Also, behavioral components are often interwoven with biological or organic causes related to feeding and swallowing problems and can be difficult to distinguish as separate etiologies.[15,16] Burklow and colleagues[16] found that 80% of their study cohort (n = 103) presented with behavioral and biological components to their feeding disorders and, thus, they proposed a biobehavioral classification system of pediatric feeding issues. Other common etiologies of pediatric dysphagia or swallowing dysfunction include cardiorespiratory, metabolic, and anatomical problems.[2,16,17]

Finally, anatomic abnormalities leading to dysphagia may be congenital or acquired and located in the nasopharynx, oral cavity, oropharynx, larynx, or esophagus. Cleft lip and cleft palate represent some of the more common anatomic defects that interfere with swallowing. The incidence is believed to lie between 0.8 and 2.7 cases per 1000 live births.[18] Other anomalies associated with dysphagia include tracheoesophageal fistula (TEF) and type III–IV laryngeal clefts. These are generally identified and surgically corrected at birth to prevent aspiration. In addition, choanal atresia, subglottic stenosis, and tracheomalacia or laryngomalacia can lend to respiratory problems that compromise coordination of respiration with swallowing.

Table 25.1.
Conditions Commonly Associated With Swallowing Disorders[2,13,19]

Local anatomical abnormality (congenital and acquired)
Nasal and nasopharyngeal
Choanal atresia
Tumors
Oral cavity and oropharynx
Cleft lip or cleft palate
Micrognathia
Macroglossia, microglossia
Inflammation of mouth and pharynx
Traumatic and caustic lesions
Pharyngeal obstruction
Adenotonsillar hypertrophy
Poor dentition
Ankyloglossia
Laryngeal
Laryngeal stenosis, webs
Laryngeal clefts
Laryngomalacia
Vocal cord paralysis (unilateral and bilateral)

Table 25.1.
Conditions Commonly Associated With Swallowing Disorders[2,13,19] *(continued)*

Tracheal
Tracheoesophageal fistula
Tracheotomy
Tracheomalacia
Esophageal
Congenital anomalies
Caustic burn
Infection
Strictures, webs
Esophageal dysmotility
Esophagitis
Foreign body
Miscellaneous
Craniofacial syndromes
Chromosomal defects
Neuromuscular abnormalities
Central nervous system
Brain damage secondary to anoxia, trauma, metabolic disease, vascular accidents, hydrocephalus, seizures, infections
Chiari malformations
Mental retardation
Cerebral palsy
Mobius syndrome, poliomyelitis
Cranial nerve palsy (V, VII, IX, X, XI, XII)
Spinal muscular atrophy
Huntington's chorea
Brain stem glioma
Peripheral nervous system
Traumatic
Congenital
Miscellaneous
Prematurity
Delayed maturation
Pseudophagia
Post-Nissan syndrome

*Adapted from Weiss,[13] Kramer,[19] Kosco, et al.[2]

Consequences of Dysphagia

Pediatric dysphagia may result in any of the following problems: (1) unsuccessful feeding leading to malnutrition; (2) behavioral feeding problems, including refusal of food, expulsion of food, and disruptive mealtime behaviors; (3) drooling; and (4) respiratory compromise linked to aspiration, including apnea and bradycardia, hypoxemia, laryngospasms, bronchiolar obstruction, coughing, choking, chronic noisy breathing, recurrent wheezing, recurrent pneumonia, and chemical pneumonitis.[9,19–28]

These consequences of pediatric feeding problems can be motor-based and/or sensory-based problems. Motor-based dysphagia during the oral stage of swallowing can involve difficulty moving the food from the front to the back of the mouth before swallowing. For example, children with low muscle tone may have weak or uncoordinated tongue movements resulting in prolonged mealtimes or even choking with liquids because food spills in the airway before the swallow has been initiated; or perhaps they have difficulty chewing because of weak chewing muscles. Dysphagia can also occur during the pharyngeal stage of swallowing while the larynx is elevating, the vocal cords are closing to protect the airway, and the pharyngeal muscles are moving in a wave-like motion to move food into the esophagus. Vocal cord paralysis, especially bilateral paralysis, is an important cause of dysphagia and choking disorders. Low muscle tone can also impact the muscles in the pharynx (pharyngeal constrictors) creating weak peristalsis; and solid foods may be more difficult to clear from the throat. Medical problems that impact the respiratory system (eg, bronchopulmonary dysplasia (BPD); laryngomalacia or tracheomalacia) can also disrupt swallowing coordination and create risks of choking or even aspiration. These motor-based swallowing problems can lead to serious medical compromise and may warrant further radiological assessment because of concern for aspiration, with imaging techniques that examine the oral/pharyngeal stages of swallowing. Signs that may indicate a **motor-based** swallowing problem include the following[29]:

- Greater difficulty with liquids, especially water or juice
- Difficulty with chewing; prolonged mealtimes
- Coughing or choking during or immediately after eating
- A gurgly vocal quality after eating
- Respiratory compromise, including pneumonia

In contrast to motor-based swallowing problems, difficulties with eating can also stem from dysfunction with the sensory system. This includes difficulty integrating sensory information related to the taste and texture of food. It is not uncommon to find sensory-based feeding problems when there is a history of reflux, slow gastric emptying, and sensitivity to touch. Children with reflux to the level of the pharynx can develop reduced sensitivity in the hypopharynx from inflammation and can result in laryngeal penetration. A common feeding history may include difficulty transitioning to textured foods, gagging, and vomiting either at the smell of foods or when the food is placed on the tongue. These children may also present with additional sensory problems such as sensitivity to touch, loud noises, and light. Parent reports may include not tolerating going barefoot on the carpet or grass; preferring not to be "messy" while eating; and dislike of tags in their clothing or seams in their socks. The following red flags for **sensory-based** problems related to feeding include the following[29]:

- No problems with taking liquids
- Gag on foods that require chewing
- Will separate textures from smooth food and pocket them or spit them out

Recognition of Pediatric Dysphagia

Dysphagia is usually indicated by a history of unsuccessful feeding (eg, gagging or vomiting during feeding, nasopharyngeal regurgitation, malnutrition, or failure to thrive); or a history of aspiration, evidenced by choking or coughing during feeding, recurrent pneumonia, or upper respiratory tract infections.[2,22,30] Children who drool and have behavioral feeding problems, have experienced long-term deprivation of oral feeding as infants, or have abnormal posture (eg, hyperextension of the neck with scapular retraction and shoulder girdle elevation) are also at risk for swallowing abnormalities.[22,31] Dysphagia should also be suspected in children who have diseases that have been associated with swallowing dysfunction.

A comprehensive history and physical examination are important in the evaluation of the child with dysphagia; during this evaluation, emphasis should be placed on the feeding history and neurological, pulmonary, and gastrointestinal function (Table 25.2). If a risk for aspiration or oropharyngeal stage dysfunction is suspected, then a videofluoroscopic examination is indicated to further assess the swallow function and safety for oral eating. This examination is generally conducted by a speech-language pathologist in conjunction with a pediatric radiologist. If concerns arise related to feeding and growth, a referral should be made to a multidisciplinary feeding team.[33] Core members of such a team usually include a speech-language pathologist or an occupational thera-

Table 25.2.
History and Examination of a Child With Dysphagia*

Feeding and swallowing history
Sucking ability
Ability to chew
Method of feeding
Body position during feeding
Gagging, choking, or coughing before, during, or after swallowing (adenotonsillar hypertrophy)
Drooling
Time required to feed
Consistency of foods tolerated
Food refusal, food expulsion, or disruptive mealtime behaviors
Neurological evaluation
Birth history
Apgar scores
Prolonged hypoxia
Polyhydramnios
Traumatic delivery
Intubation and problems related to intubation
Paucity of fetal movements
Prolonged labor
Developmental history
Family history of neuromuscular disorders
Dystonia or dyskinesia
Cerebral palsy or other specific diagnosis
Cognitive or physical impairment
Epilepsy
Developmental delay
Physical examination
Ophthalmoplegia
Facial and tongue movement (ankyloglossia)
Spasticity or hypotonia
Gag reflex (hyperreflexia or hyporeflexia)
Jaw jerk
Visual acuity
Speech (hoarseness, suggesting vocal cord paralysis)
Aversive behavior (extensor dystonia)

Table 25.2.
History and Examination of a Child With Dysphagia* *(continued)*

Respiratory evaluation
History
Respiratory symptoms (eg, wheezing, coughing, choking, or noisy breathing)
Recurrent bronchitis or pneumonia
Apnea
Physical examination
Weak respiratory muscles
Wheezing
Gastrointestinal evaluation
History
Regurgitation
Vomiting
Unexplained irritability
Nasopharyngeal reflux
Failure to thrive
Ingestion of foreign body or caustic substance
Peptic esophagitis
Physical examination
Oral cavity for structural abnormalities
Height and weight

*Adapted from Couriel et al.[32]

pist, nurse, dietitian, and perhaps a gastroenterologist, developmental pediatrician, or a physical therapist. Table 25.3 provides referral guidelines for further evaluation of feeding and swallowing problems.

Clinical Evaluation

Clinical evaluation of pediatric feeding and swallowing involves assessment of how effectively the child performs the oral, pharyngeal, and esophageal phases of swallowing, along with several other factors.[34,35] The child's feeding history is important to the clinical evaluation. Elements of the history include the following: (1) how the child received nutrients and fluids, (2) the duration of non-oral nutrition, and (3) the child's ability to swallow effectively when first given oral feedings. Children who have been ill and have been fed by alternative methods have often not had normal oral experiences and, therefore, may not seek oral input.

Table 25.3.
Referral Guidelines for Feeding and Swallowing Problems

Primary Care Visit
Concerns with feeding
• Falling off growth curve
• Refusing bottle/food
• Gagging on textured food
• Not progressing with age-appropriate diet
• Behind in age-expected feeding skills
• Prolonged time to complete a meal
• Developmental delays
• Gastrointestinal/respiratory/neurological/cardiac medical history
• Taking liquids fine but choking on solids
–Consider referral to pediatric feeding team
Concerns with swallowing safety
• Choking on liquids
• Fevers; congested breathing or other signs of respiratory infection
• Does better with solid foods
• Neurological involvement (abnormal muscle tone)
• Poor head control
• Anatomical anomaly interfering with swallowing (repaired tracheosophageal fistula; cleft palate; laryngeal/tracheal stenosis; laryngeal cleft)
• Wet vocal quality immediately after eating or during eating
–Consider referral for videofluoroscopic (modified barium swallow) study with a speech-language pathologist

Once the medical status, medication use, and feeding history of the child have been ascertained, examination of the oral-peripheral structures is performed. Assessment of the strength and movement of the structures, if possible, in addition to identification of the presence or absence of normal oral reflexes is part of this examination. Assessment of the child's respiratory status is also important in this examination. Audible respiration may indicate a developing respiratory infection or difficulty in managing secretions. Once liquid or food is given to the child, changes in respiratory behavior can indicate certain types of problems (eg, poor coordination of swallowing and breathing and airway protection problems). The strength of the cry is a measure of respiratory capabilities and laryngeal function, both of which can affect feeding performance. The child's ability to maintain a certain posture provides information about the stability of the trunk, head, and neck. Observing how the child manages oral secretions provides information about swallowing function, airway protection, and oral-motor control.

The evaluation includes direct observation of the child with liquid and food to determine whether the child is capable of oral ingestion. Evaluation of the oral phase in infants involves noting the timeliness with which sucking is initiated after presentation of a stimulus, strength and coordination of the suck, and lip seal and the ability to maintain the bolus orally. In addition, performance is observed over many suck-swallow cycles to determine whether fatigue causes changes in function. In older infants and children, the ability to manipulate and posteriorly transport a pureed bolus is observed, as is the chewing adequacy for solid foods. Oral clearance is assessed by checking the mouth for pocketing in the cheeks and residue on the tongue and palate, particularly after the child seems to have finished chewing and swallowing.

In older children, evaluation of the pharyngeal phase of the swallow is done by externally palpating the thyroid cartilage of the larynx. Elevation of this cartilage occurs during the swallow and judgments about the timing of swallow initiation and the amounts of laryngeal excursion are made. Because this palpation usually cannot be done in infants, close observation of the neck and listening for the sounds of swallowing must suffice. Cervical auscultation with a stethoscope is another method of screening swallow function during a feeding evaluation to assess for gross episodes of aspiration.[36] Coughing and problems with respiration during and after the swallow are signs that airway protection may be inadequate. Changes in phonation after the swallow should also be noted (eg, wet gurgling voice or cry), as should the number of swallows required to clear a bolus, since vocal cord paralysis may be responsible for these findings. When sucking is in a continuous pattern in infants, swallowing should be coordinated with the pattern.

Asking the parent to feed the child so any differences in feeding performance can be noted, particularly if reported problems were not observed, is often helpful. Feeding styles vary, and different feeding styles (eg, positioning, rate, and verbalization during the feeding) and different feeders may affect performance in some children. Observing the independent feeding behavior of children who feed themselves is also important. Finally, if the cause of the problem is clear, and changes, such as the feeding position or utensil or the rate of feeding, are indicated, the changes should be attempted to evaluate their effectiveness.

When problems with the pharyngeal or esophageal phase of the swallow are noted and the reason is unclear, radiographic or instrumental evaluation is indicated.

Instrumental and Radiographic Evaluation of Dysphagia

Videofluoroscopy (VFS), or modified barium swallow, is the current procedure of choice for the assessment of children with swallowing disorders. The study is generally done under the direction of a radiologist and a speech pathologist. A patient is usually given 2 swallows each of at least 3 barium-labeled food consistencies. During a swallow, the oral cavity, pharynx, and cervical esophagus are visualized first in the lateral view to assess aspiration; an anter-posterior view is later taken to study symmetry. Therapeutic techniques may be evaluated at this time to monitor their effectiveness. The study is videotaped for later review.[37] In the detection of aspiration,[30,38] a pharyngeal phase-swallowing abnormality defined as the passage of food below the true vocal cords, VFS has proved superior to bedside clinical assessment[8,37] and has also effectively determined which patients are at risk for pneumonia.[10,30] Other radiological methods to evaluate dysphagia include ultrasonography and scintigraphy.[39–42] Ultrasound is a noninvasive approach that provides information regarding tongue, hyoid, and soft palate movement during swallowing but does not allow direct viewing of aspiration or penetration.

Pharyngeal Manometry

Pharyngeal manometry is the best method for evaluating pharyngeal and esophageal motor function. Manometry requires the transnasal insertion of a catheter housing a series of intraluminal pressure transducers.[43] In the evaluation of dysphagia, it is best used as a complementary diagnostic procedure to endoscopy, VFS, or electromyography.[44–47] In children, manometry has been used mainly to investigate gastroesophageal reflux, esophageal motor, and pharyngeal motor disorders.

Fiberoptic Endoscopic Evaluation of Swallowing

Instrumental evaluation of dysphagia includes fiberoptic endoscopic evaluation of swallowing. It has been used primarily in the evaluation of adults for whom VFS is unsuitable but the use is now increasing with the pediatric population. An endoscope is passed transnasally through the nasopharynx and hypopharynx and positioned just above the false vocal folds. This technique is particularly useful to directly assess laryngeal function for adduction and airway protection. Other indications for use include assessment of possible anatomic contributing factors, assessment of pharyngeal or laryngeal sensitivity, and a risk for aspiration of even minute amounts of material.[48] Other reported advantages include detection of pooling in the pharynx and training the child to use compensatory swallowing techniques. The age of the child is a factor for tolerance of the procedure.[48,49]

Treatment

Treatment of pediatric feeding and swallowing disorders varies greatly depending on the symptoms, the cause of the problem, and the child's feeding history. However, treatment can generally be categorized into 5 areas—positioning, oral sensory normalization, modification of food consistency, adaptive feeding devices, and oral feeding exercises.[50,51]

Positioning during feeding is very important. Eating is naturally a flexor-biased activity, but an overall balance in body tone is needed. Therefore, children with deviations in muscle tone, as in cerebral palsy, require special attention to positioning for feeding.[52] A child who has difficulty eating (eg, frequent coughing during meals) when poorly positioned can often swallow safely if properly positioned. For older children, sitting upright with knees bent and feet stabilized is best. The tray of a high chair provides elbow stability for the child with limited trunk control. For a child with inadequate oral control but normal swallow initiation, a more reclined position may be helpful because the liquid bolus has less chance to spill out through the lips. Conversely, a more upright position reduces the chance that a bolus will spill prematurely into the pharynx of a child who has delayed swallow initiation. In addition to positioning during feeding, positioning after a feeding is also important; less risk is posed to the airway in the child with gastroesophageal reflux when the child is positioned upright during feeding.

Oral sensory normalization is used to treat the child with oral hypersensitivity. Hypersensitivity generally results from a lack of normal oral experiences or negative oral experiences. Oral hypersensitivity can relate to touch, taste, or texture. Some children tolerate food in the anterior part of the mouth but gag when it moves to the posterior oral cavity. Other children display refusal behaviors, gag, or vomit when food, toys, or any object approaches the perioral area. A gradual desensitization program therefore is necessary. Once desensitized to touch, the child must be desensitized to food. Often the desensitization steps must be repeated several times as the child learns to tolerate new foods or flavors, textures, and consistencies. A gradual but consistent program is necessary for children with substantial hypersensitivity and aversion to foods.

In addition, building on foods, flavors, or textures the child tolerates is an important step in getting started.

Modification of food consistencies is another treatment strategy.[8] In general, thinner consistencies (eg, thin liquids) are indicated for children with problems with bolus transport and children who are weak or fatigue easily. Thicker consistencies (eg, purees and soft solids) are indicated when oral containment of the bolus, poor tongue control, delayed swallow initiation, or decreased laryngeal closure during the swallow is the problem. In some children, marked differences in performance and swallow safety can be seen with different food consistencies. Difficulty with a particular food consistency does not necessarily mean that elimination from the diet is necessary, but the child may need adaptations in one of the other treatment categories to eat foods of the particular consistency safely and effectively.

Special feeding devices are commonly used in treating the child with dysphagia. Feeding devices range from adaptive positioning seats to special feeding utensils, cups, bottles, and nipples.[51] New Visions is one resource Web site for feeding equipment for children (www.new-vis.com). Infants with difficulty sucking can show very different performance with different nipples. Infants with delayed swallow initiation may require a nipple with a slower flow rate. Infants with a weak suck but intact swallow initiation benefit from a nipple with a faster flow rate or a softer nipple that will expend less energy during sucking.

Behavioral approaches that can be helpful include following the child's lead, feeding the child when hunger signs begin, gaining the child's attention but not over arousing, and watching for the child's signals for satiation.[53] Also some general rules to follow may include a regular mealtime schedule, a neutral atmosphere with avoidance of force feeding, offering small portions with solids first and fluids last. Goals of behavioral approaches may include increasing desired behavior with reinforcement and decreasing maladaptive behaviors with a variety of methods (eg, extinction or time out). For example, mixing a non-preferred food with a preferred food, altering textures, or not attending to inappropriate behaviors.[15] Arvedson[15] also discusses techniques such as shaping, prompting, and modeling.

Weaning from non-oral feedings should be a slow and gradual process.[54] Children who have received chronic tube feedings often miss critical transition periods for eating, such as beginning solid foods. Subsequently, these children can demonstrate significant oral aversion to eating, especially textured foods. A methodical process to wean from tube feedings is required for children who meet the appropriate criteria.[55,56] One method is to first transition patients on continuous feedings to bolus feedings. Next, offer food by mouth before each daytime bolus feed to simulate a mealtime schedule. The eventual plan is to eliminate nighttime tube feeds. As the child consumes more calories by mouth, then the tube feedings can be decreased accordingly. This process will be most successful when done in conjunction with an oral sensory treatment program.

Oral *feeding exercises* can help to facilitate normal oral motor movement patterns needed for feeding. For example, stroking the cheek facilitates sucking, and using a pacifier provides resistance to suction achieved by the infant. Older children can practice bolus manipulation and tongue movement with real food or nonfood items. Another exercise used with older children is the "effortful swallow" that involves producing a strong swallow resulting in more forceful pharyngeal contractions. Thermal stimulation can be used to provide added sensory input to the anterior faucial pillars (palatoglossus muscle), which is where the swallow is believed to be triggered.

Nutrition—The process to achieve adequate sensory receptivity and oral motor function to accept sufficient nutrition and age-appropriate foods can be a prolonged process. To achieve a normal eating pattern in the interim, parents are encouraged to maintain mealtime routines when possible, not to have the child "grazing" on food continuously, and to provide a high-calorie diet to reduce episodes of forced feeding to meet calorie intake goals. Nutritional supplements can provide an entire meal for children who are averse to solid foods. An evaluation by a dietician is critical when determining the child's calorie needs and the optimal nutrition plan to meet those needs.[57] For those children with a gastrostomy (G-tube), enteral feeds can also assuage mealtime pressures for parents. Calorie needs that are not met at mealtimes can be given later by G-tube until the child is ready to begin weaning from the tube feedings.

Most health care professionals who treat patients with dysphagia believe that the best exercise for swallowing is swallowing. Therefore, the goal for all children with dysphagia is safe eating, even if only in small amounts. Factors such as parental involvement, the child's behavior, schedules of non-oral feedings, respiratory health, and overall medical status all help determine the progress a child makes in response to treatment. Because some children have no positive feeding history, eating is not necessarily pleasurable. Therefore, motivation is also important.[58]

Treatment can be simple for some children with dysphagia, but it can be gradual and lengthy for others. Treatment is generally most successful when all involved health care professionals (eg, physicians, nurses, dietitians, speech-language pathologists, and occupational therapists) work as a team and coordinate recommendations and treatments. Families and professionals can find additional resource information from the Carolina Pediatric Dysphagia Web site with written as well as interactive information provided (www.feeding.com).

Feeding Infants With Craniofacial Anomalies

Infants with cleft palate require a special feeding device because they are unable to suck normally. In the absence of other neurological problems, infants with cleft palate generally have appropriate sucking motions of the lips, tongue, cheeks, and jaw, but, because of the cleft, they cannot achieve the negative pressure necessary for creating suction. Although they may be able to compress some fluid from a nipple, by gumming or "munching," this alone is not an effective means of fluid expression. A variety of commercial bottles and nipples are available (eg, Haberman feeder [Medela, Inc., McHenry, IL] and Pigeon bottle [Galtak Houseware, Ltd, Markham Ontario, Canada]). The Haberman allows the person feeding to squeeze fluid from the nipple into the infant's mouth in controlled amounts. Squeezing the fluid eliminates the need for suction, and the infant with a cleft palate can continue to produce sucking motions and swallows in coordination. Placing the infant in a semi-reclined position while feeding can reduce nasal regurgitation. Although open communication exists between the oral and nasal cavities with an unrepaired cleft, the nipple is placed far enough back in the mouth so gravity and movements of the tongue generally transport the liquid bolus to the pharynx without substantial loss of fluid into the nasal cavity.

An infant with a cleft palate can breastfeed and obtain small amounts of milk by compression. However, because the infant with a cleft palate cannot create sufficient negative pressure for adequate suction, supplementation with a special feeder is necessary. To maintain adequate milk supply, the mother can pump her breasts and store the milk for use with the special feeder. In some cases, it may be appropriate to allow the infant to breastfeed 5 to 10 minutes before bottle-feeding. The purpose would be to stimulate the mother's breast milk supply as well as a pleasurable time for mother-infant interaction. When airway management is a problem, as is often the case in Pierre Robin syndrome and a cleft palate, positioning a baby at the breast for optimal airway patency and for minimal fluid loss into the nasal cavity is more difficult than it is using a special bottle. Consequently, breastfeeding, even in minimal amounts, is generally not encouraged except for infants with a cleft lip only. Another option for children with severe palatal clefts is an oral obturator that is fitted to cover the cleft opening and normalize intra-oral pressure for sucking.[59] This can be cumbersome as it must be regularly altered to fit the changing size of the palate.

Infants with micrognathia and subsequent retracted tongue positioning benefit from positional and equipment modifications. For example, sitting the baby more upright and bringing the jaw manually forward during bottle-feeding or breastfeeding, or using an L-shaped bottle. Stimulation to the tongue prior to feeding to establish a more forward tongue position can also facilitate a more efficient sucking pattern.

Efficacy of Rehabilitative Dysphagia Management
Improvement in swallowing after rehabilitative dysphagia management has been demonstrated in children.[8,9,29,35,50,59] Documented improvements in feeding and swallowing include better spoon-feeding, biting, and chewing; increased caloric intake and rate of weight gain; reduced coughing, choking, and feeding avoidance behaviors; improved pharyngeal transit times; decreased aspirate amount; and decreased number of swallows required to clear the oropharynx.[9,52,60,61]

Conclusion
Dysphagia is commonly associated with certain pediatric disorders and can result in substantial morbidity. The timely identification of pediatric swallowing disorders is important for initiating evaluation and treatment when indicated. This can prevent or reduce future medical and/or nutritional compromise for the at-risk child.

References
1. Derkay CS, Schecter GL. Anatomy and physiology of pediatric swallowing disorders. *Otolaryngol Clin North Am.* 1998;31:397–404
2. Kosko JR, Moser JD, Erhart N, Tunkel DE. Differential diagnosis of dysphagia in children. *Otolaryngol Clin North Am.* 1998;31:435–451
3. Bosma JF. Postnatal ontogeny of performances of the pharynx, larynx, and mouth. *Am Rev Respir Dis.* 1985;131:S10–S15
4. Humphrey T. Some correlations between the appearance of human fetal reflexes and the development of the nervous system. *Prog Brain Res.* 1964;4:93–135
5. Hooker D. Fetal reflexes and instinctual processes. *Psychosom Med.* 1942;4:199–205
6. Ianniruberto A, Tajani E. Ultrasonographic study of fetal movements. *Semin Perinatol.* 1981;5:175–181
7. Diamant NE. Development of esophageal function. *Am Rev Respir Dis.* 1985;131: S29–S32
8. Arvedson JC, Brodsky L. *Pediatric Swallowing and Feeding: Assessment and Management.* San Diego, CA: Singular Publishing; 1993

9. Griggs CA, Jones PM, Lee RE. Videofluoroscopic investigation of feeding disorders of children with multiple handicap. *Dev Med Child Neurol.* 1989;31:303–308

10. Taniguchi MH, Moyer RS. Assessment of risk factors for pneumonia in dysphagic children: significance of videofluoroscopic swallowing evaluation. *Dev Med Child Neurol.* 1994;36:495–502

11. Waterman ET, Koltai PJ, Downey JC, Cacace AT. Swallowing disorders in a population of children with cerebral palsy. *Int J Pediatr Otorhinolaryngol.* 1992;24: 63–71

12. Love RJ, Hagerman EL, Taimi EG. Speech performance, dysphagia and oral reflexes in cerebral palsy. *J Speech Hear Disord.* 1980;45:59–75

13. Weiss MH. Dysphagia in infants and children. *Otolaryngol Clin North Am.* 1998;21: 727–735

14. Manikam R, Perman JA. Pediatric feeding disorders. *J Clin Gastroenterol.* 2000;30: 34–46

15. Arvedson JC. Behavioral issues and implications with pediatric feeding disorders. *Semin Speech Lang.* 1997;18:51–70

16. Burklow KA, Phelps AN, Schultz JR, McConnell K, Rudolph C. Classifying complex pediatric feeding disorders. *J Pediatr Gastroenterol Nutr.* 1998;27:143–147

17. Arvedson JC. Dysphagia in pediatric patients with neurologic damage. *Semin Neurol.* 1996;16:371–386

18. Vanderas AP. Incidence of cleft lip, cleft palate, and cleft lip and palate among races: a review. *Cleft Palate Craniofac J.* 1987;24:216–225

19. Kramer SS. Special swallowing problems in children. *Gastrointest Radiol.* 1985;10: 241–250

20. Christensen JR. Developmental approach to pediatric neurogenic dysphagia. *Dysphagia.* 1989;3:131–134

21. Rogers BT, Arvedson J, Msall M, Demerath RR. Hypoxemia during oral feeding of children with severe cerebral palsy. *Dev Med Child Neurol.* 1993;35:3–10

22. Lespargot A, Langevin MF, Muller S, Guillemont S. Swallowing disturbances associated with drooling in cerebral-palsied children. *Dev Med Child Neurol.* 1993;35:298–304

23. Gadol CL, Joshi VV, Lee EY. Bronchiolar obstruction associated with repeated aspiration of vegetable material in two children with cerebral palsy. *Pediatr Pulmonol.* 1987;3:437–439

24. Shapiro BK, Green P, Krick J, Allen D, Capute AJ. Growth of severely impaired children: neurological versus nutritional factors. *Dev Med Child Neurol.* 1986;28: 729–733

25. Faubion WA, Zein NN. Gastroesophageal reflux in infants and children. *Mayo Clin Proc.* 1998;73:166–173

26. Maarsingh EJ, Hoekstra MO, Derkx HH, van Aalderen WM. Gastroesophageal reflux in infants with wheezing. *Pediatr Pulmonol.* 2000;29:480–482

27. Tsou VM, Bishop PR. Gastroesophageal reflux in children. *Otolaryngol Clin North Am.* 1998;31:419–434

28. Vijayarantnam V, Lin CH, Simpson P, Tolia V. Lack of significant proximal esophageal acid reflux in infants presenting with respiratory symptoms. *Pediatr Pulmonol.* 1999;27: 231–235

29. Palmer MM, Heyman MB. Assessment and treatment of sensory-versus motor-based feeding problems in very young children. *Infants Young Child.* 1993;6:67–73

30. Friedman B, Frazier JB. Deep laryngeal penetration as a predictor of aspiration. *Dysphagia.* 2000;15:153–158

31. Tuchman DN. Cough, choke, sputter: the evaluation of the child with dysfunctional swallowing. *Dysphagia.* 1989;3:111–116

32. Couriel JM, Bisset R, Miller R, Thomas A, Clarke M. Assessment of feeding problems in neurodevelopmental handicap: a team approach. *Arch Dis Child.* 1993;69: 609–613

33. Lefton-Greif MA, Arvedson JC. Pediatric feeding/swallowing teams. *Semin Speech Lang.* 1997;18:5–12

34. Darrow DH, Harley CM. Evaluation of swallowing disorders in children. *Otolaryngol Clin North Am.* 1998;31:405–418

35. Newman LA. Optimal care patterns in pediatric patients with dysphagia. *Semin Speech Lang.* 2000;21:281–291

36. Vice FL, Bamford O, Heinz JM, Bosma JF. Correlation of cervical auscultation with physiological recording during suckle-feeding in newborn infants. *Dev Med Child Neurol.* 1995;37:167–179

37. Arvedson JC, Lefton-Grief MA. *Pediatric Videofluourscopic Swallow Studies: A Professional Manual With Caregiver Guidelines.* San Antonio, TX: Communication Skill Builders/Psychological Corp; 1998

38. Arvedson JC, Rogers B, Buck G, Smart P, Msall M. Silent aspiration prominent in children with dysphagia. *Int J Pediatr Otorhinolaryngol.* 1994;28:173–181

39. Weber F, Woolridge MW, Baum JD. An ultrasonographic study of the organisation of sucking and swallowing by newborn infants. *Dev Med Child Neurol.* 1986;28:19–24

40. Guillet J, Basse-Cathalinat B, Christophe E, Ducassou D, Blanquet P, Wynchank S. Routine studies of swallowed radionuclide transit in paediatrics: experience with 400 patients. *Eur J Nucl Med.* 1984;9:86–90

41. Muz J, Mathog RH, Rosen R, Miller PR, Borrero G. Detection and quantification of laryngotracheopulmonary aspiration with scintigraphy. *Laryngoscope.* 1987;97: 1180–1185

42. Yang WT, Loveday EJ, Metrewell C, Sullivan PB. Ultrasound assessment of swallowing in malnourished disabled children. *Br J Radiology.* 1997;70:992–994

43. Sonies BC. Instrumental procedures for dysphagia diagnosis. *Semin Speech Lang.* 1991;12:185–198

44. Feussner H, Kauer W, Siewert JR. The place of esophageal manometry in the diagnosis of dysphagia. *Dysphagia.* 1993;8:98–104

45. Elidan J, Shochina M, Gonen B, Gay I. Manometry and electromyography of the pharyngeal muscles in patients with dysphagia. *Arch Otolaryngol Head Neck Surg.* 1990;116:910–913

46. Palmer JB. Electromyography of the muscles of oropharyngeal swallowing: basic concepts. *Dysphagia.* 1989;3:192–198

47. Elidan J, Gonen B, Shochiana M, Gay I. Electromyography of the inferior constrictor and cricopharyngeal muscles during swallowing. *Ann Otol Rhinol Laryngol.* 1990;99:466–469

48. Hartnick CJ, Hartley BE, Miller C, Willging JP. Pediatric fiberoptic endoscopic evaluation of swallowing. *Ann Otol Rhinol Laryngol.* 2000;109:996–999

49. Leder SB, Karas DE. Fiberoptic endoscopic evaluation of swallowing in the pediatric population. *Laryngoscope.* 2000;110:1132–1136

50. Jaffe MB. Feeding at-risk infants and toddlers. *Top Lang Disord.* 1989;10:13–25

51. Morris SE, Klein MD. *Prefeeding Skills: A Comprehensive Resource for Mealtime Development.* Tucson, AZ: Therapy Skill Builders; 2000

52. Larnert G, Ekberg O. Positioning improves the oral and pharyngeal swallowing function in children with cerebral palsy. *Acta Paediatr.* 1995;84:689–692

53. Satter E. Feeding dynamics: helping children to eat well. *J Pediatr Health Care.* 1995;9:178–184

54. Palmer MM. Weaning from gastrostomy tube feeding: commentary on oral aversion. *Pediatr Nurs.* 1995;24:475–478

55. Blackman JA, Nelson CL. Reinstituting oral feedings in children fed by gastrostomy tube. *Clin Pediatr (Phila).* 1985;24:434–438

56. Dell'Olio J, Hollenstein J, Dwyer J. Noah grows up: transitioning problems from special feeding routes to oral intake. *Nutr Rev.* 2000;58:118–128

57. Kovar AJ. Nutrition assessment and management in pediatric dysphagia. *Semin Speech Lang.* 1997;18:39–49

58. Satter E. *How to Get Your Kid to Eat … But Not Too Much.* Palo Alto, CA: Bull Publishing; 1987

59. Reisberg DJ. Dental and prosthodontic care for patients with cleft or craniofacial conditions. *Cleft Palate Craniofac J.* 2000;37:534–537

60. Gisel EG. Oral-motor skills following sensorimotor intervention in the moderately eating-impaired child with cerebral palsy. *Dysphagia.* 1994;9:180–192

61. Weiss MH. Dysphagia in infants and children. *Otolaryngol Clin North Am.* 1988;21:727–735

26

Failure to Thrive (Pediatric Undernutrition)

Definition of Terms

Malnourished children have been described as "failing to thrive" since at least the 19th century, but the term has still escaped a valid and reliable definition.[1] "Undernutrition" has been proposed as a preferable term, but failure to thrive continues to be used commonly in medical parlance. Quantitative criteria should therefore be employed in making the diagnosis. Commonly used criteria include children whose

(1) Weight (or weight for height) is less than 2 standard deviations below the mean for sex and age.
and/or

(2) Weight curve has crossed more than 2 percentile lines on the National Center for Health Statistics (NCHS) growth charts after having achieved a previously stable pattern.

Alternative wordings of the first criterion include "less than the third percentile" or "a weight for age (or weight for height) Z score less than –2.0." Z scores are standard deviation scores that express anthropometric data normalizing for age and sex, and can be calculated with software available from the Centers for Disease Control and Prevention (CDC) (www.cdc.gov/epiinfo). Z scores allow more precision in describing anthropometric status than does the customary placement "near" or "below" a certain percentile curve, and are recommended when expressing nutritional parameters of groups of subjects.

The second criterion underscores the fact that weight loss or even lack of normal growth during infancy and childhood is abnormal. What constitutes a "stable pattern" can be open to discussion, although one group defined the baseline percentile as the maximum achieved between 4 and 8 weeks of age, since weight at this point was found to correlate more strongly with weight at age 12 months than did birthweight.[2]

Anthropometric assessment of nutritional status can also be categorized to help determine chronicity of nutritional deprivation. Although some authors recommend using weight alone as a screening criterion,[3] a weight for age cutoff is nonspecific, since patients included can be either well-proportioned and just constitutionally small or truly undernourished. A classic distinction between acute malnutrition ("wasting," or low weight for height) and chronic malnutrition ("stunting," or low height for age) was proposed by Waterlow and has been widely adopted (Table 26.1).

An important caution should be noted when a subject's height faltering is used to call attention to nutritional status. Genetic and constitutional causes of short stature need to be ruled out before implicating chronic malnutrition as the cause of poor height growth; elicitation of family history and interpretation of growth parameters in light of mid-parental height can be helpful in this regard. In addition, children should not be expected to grow exactly along a centile line. Most growth curves are mathematical averages based on large numbers of children (ie, cross-sectional curves) and not growth lines along which individual children should be expected to grow (ie, longitudinal).[4] Perhaps 30% of healthy, full-term, white infants cross one percentile line and 23% cross 2 lines as they move from birth to age 2 years.[4] These fluctuations in length percentiles are a normal phenomenon in infant growth and, especially in the face of normal weight gain, should not prompt evaluation for nutritional disease.

Accurate measurements of weight, length, age, and, in children less than age 3, head circumference, are required for the diagnosis of undernutrition to be made. These data should be obtained and plotted on appropriate graphs (see Appendix J). Compared with earlier growth curves, the 2000 NCHS reference curves better reflect the racial/ethnic composition of the United States, and also include more infants who were breastfed. The inclusion of the third as well as the fifth percentile line also allows better assessment of undernutrition,

Table 26.1.
Classification of Protein-Calorie Malnutrition*

	Acute malnutrition (weight for height) (% of median)	Chronic malnutrition (height for age) (% of median)
Normal	>90	>95
Mild	80–90	90–95
Moderate	70–80	85–90
Severe	<70	<85

*Waterlow criteria for categorizing type and chronicity of malnutrition. Abnormalities of weight for height are termed wasting and those of height for age are called stunting. Adapted from Waterlow JC. Classification and definition of protein-calorie malnutrition. *Br Med J.* 1972;3:566–569.

since the third percentile more closely approximates a Z score of –2.0. Infants with a history of premature birth should have their chronological age corrected by gestational age until age 24 months for weight measurements, 40 months for length, and 18 months for head circumference. Infants and children should be weighed with minimal clothing on scales accurate to at least 100 g (infants 0 to 2 years nude with a dry diaper; 2 years to adult, no shoes, light clothes, empty pockets). Infants' lengths should be measured supine on a length board until age 2 years, after which time they should be measured standing using a stadiometer. One person in the office should ideally be designated as solely responsible for weighing and measuring patients. Detailed summaries of anthropometric techniques have been published.[5]

Medical Risk Factors for Malnutrition

Table 26.2 lists several common medical and psychosocial risk factors for the development of failure to thrive. Almost all chronic medical conditions

Table 26.2.
Risk Factors for the Development of Failure to Thrive*

Infant characteristics
- Any chronic medical condition resulting in:
  - Inadequate intake (eg, swallowing dysfunction, central nervous system depression, or any condition resulting in anorexia)
  - Increased metabolic rate (eg, bronchopulmonary dysplasia, congenital heart disease, fevers)
  - Maldigestion or malabsorption (eg, AIDS, cystic fibrosis, short gut, inflammatory bowel disease, celiac disease)
- Premature birth (especially intrauterine growth retardation)
- Developmental delay
- Congenital anomalies
- Intrauterine toxin exposure (eg, alcohol)
- Plumbism and/or anemia

Family characteristics
- Poverty
- Unusual health and nutrition beliefs
- Social isolation
- Disordered feeding techniques
- Substance abuse or other psychopathology (including Munchausen syndrome by proxy)
- Violence or abuse

*From Duggan C: Failure to Thrive: Malnutrition in the Pediatric Outpatient Setting. In: Walker WA, Watkins JB. *Nutrition in Pediatrics: Basic Science and Clinical Applications.* Hamilton, Ontario: BC Decker Inc; 1996.

in a child can result in poor weight gain through a number of factors. These include decreased energy intake (anorexia, food withholding, altered mental status), increased caloric requirements (fever, infections), and/or inefficient utilization of ingested calories (maldigestion, malabsorption). Nutritional recommendations for specific disease states are found elsewhere in this manual.

An important medical risk factor for undernutrition in childhood is premature birth. There are myriad potential complications of prematurity that can lead to malnutrition, including chronic lung disease, necrotizing enterocolitis and intestinal resection, developmental delay, and sensorineural abnormalities. In addition, behavioral abnormalities of some premature infants (including irritability and oral aversion) can predispose to poor postnatal growth. The infant who is small for gestational age is a special case among premature infants, since prenatal factors have already exerted a deleterious effect on somatic growth. The reasons for in utero growth failure include both genetic problems (such as chromosomal aberrations) and environmental influences (such as maternal smoking, malnutrition, or exposure to drugs or other toxins). The former group of patients tends to have symmetric growth retardation (in which weight, height, and head circumference are equivalently depressed) and, therefore, are less likely to respond to nutritional supplementation with catch-up growth. Conversely, asymmetrically growth-retarded infants (whose weight is disproportionately low) have more truly suffered in utero malnutrition and can, therefore, be expected to achieve better growth after birth.[6]

The child with neurologic disease is also at special risk for poor growth. Anthropometric evaluation of children with spastic cerebral palsy can be difficult due to contractures or scoliosis, and interpretation of growth should be done in light of the growth potential of any known diagnosis (eg, Down syndrome). Many children with developmental delay are short for their age, and, although stunting due to chronic malnutrition is a possible cause, genetic programming due to the underlying condition can also be an etiology. Because of these difficulties in correctly measuring and interpreting linear growth, emphasis should instead be placed on obtaining adequate weight for height as a measure of good nutrition. Measures of arm circumference and/or triceps skinfold can serve as supplementary measures of anthropometric status. Reference growth curves for children with several genetic syndromes are available on the Internet.

Children born with congenital anomalies are also at nutritional risk. For example, infants born with cleft lips and/or palates may have significant oral-motor dysfunction requiring special nipples and feeding instructions. The occurrence of some congenital anomalies may represent a part of a genetic syndrome of which short stature is a component. As with the child who is developmentally delayed, weight for height is the best anthropometric assessment of nutritional status in these patients.

A final medical risk factor for poor growth is lead intoxication.[7] High blood lead levels probably correlate with poor nutrition based on the fact that a high-fat, low-iron diet promotes lead absorption from the intestine; what is less clear is to what extent the anorexia and other behavioral problems seen with iron deficiency and/or lead poisoning are contributing factors to malnutrition.

Psychosocial Risk Factors for Malnutrition

In the United States, the majority of factors that predispose to poor growth are not attributable solely to medical characteristics of the child, but are more social in origin. The "transactional model" of failure to thrive[8] emphasizes the interrelationships between medical, behavioral, and developmental characteristics of the infant or child on one hand, and the familial, psychosocial, and economic environment of the child's caretakers on the other. For instance, many of the medical risk factors (eg, prematurity, lead poisoning) have obvious socioeconomic correlates. Similarly, it is often noted that infants with failure to thrive are perceived by their families as having temperaments that make them difficult to nurture; problems with attachment, self-regulation, sleeping patterns, and affection are attributed to them. Some infant feeding patterns have also been associated with subsequent failure to thrive.[9] Of all the social risk factors, poverty is the most pervasive among children seen for growth failure. Frank and Zeisel reported that 13% of their patients are homeless, and note that inadequate medical care can exacerbate the tendency of acute illnesses to lead to poor growth.[8]

Other psychosocial risk factors for failure to thrive include unusual health and nutrition beliefs of the family, including a fear of obesity or cardiovascular disease.[10] Such concerns can lead to suboptimal energy intake, or a diet low in fat, resulting in poor growth. Parental beliefs about multiple food allergies have also been associated with undernutrition.[11] Another dietary practice that can lead to poor nutrition, especially in the toddler age range, is excessive intake of fruit juices. Juices can displace more energy-dense items from the diet.

Reduction of juice intake was associated with improved weight gain in a series of 8 children who were referred for evaluation of growth failure,[12] emphasizing the key role of dietary evaluation in these patients.

Parenting skills (especially feeding skills), life stresses, and social isolation are also factors that likely contribute to growth failure. In one series, 66% of mothers of infants with growth failure reported having been abused as children themselves, compared to 26% of controls from a similar socioeconomic group.[13] A series of children diagnosed with Munchausen syndrome by proxy reported that 29% had been diagnosed with failure to thrive, and 17% of their siblings had had either non-accidental injury, neglect, inappropriate medication administration, or failure to thrive.[14] These reports all underscore the fact that infants with growth failure may represent a flag for serious social and psychological problems in the family.

Approach to the Patient With Failure to Thrive

Evaluation of a child with growth failure must include a thorough history and physical examination, since the diagnostic benefits of additional laboratory tests are minimal. Simple, noninvasive efforts should be made to screen for possible underlying medical problems, and the identification of psychosocial issues that may be afflicting the family should be done concurrently. Since many children with poor growth suffer from behavioral and developmental problems as well as social and economic disadvantage, a multidisciplinary approach has been advocated as an effective method of diagnosis and therapy.[15,16] Evaluation by a social worker, behavioral specialist, and/or psychologist should supplement the primary medical and nutritional evaluation.

In the medical assessment, important historical points to consider (Table 26.3) include maternal history (especially use of drugs, possible congenital infections, maternal nutrition, and health during pregnancy), labor, delivery, and neonatal events. The child's general medical history should also be explored, especially with regard to intercurrent illnesses, medication use, and immunization history. Acute infections can worsen nutritional status by the increased metabolic demands of fever and stress response, as well as by reducing caloric intake through anorexia. At the same time, a history of recurrent or unusual infections should increase the clinician's suspicion for the presence of an immunodeficiency, including Acquired Immunodeficiency Syndrome (AIDS).

The growth history should be reviewed by careful plotting of growth points on the NCHS/CDC 2000 curves. Dietary history should include a qualitative

Table 26.3.
Historical Evaluation of Infants and Children With Growth Failure*

Prenatal
General obstetrical history
Recurrent miscarriages
Was the pregnancy planned?
Use of medications, drugs, or cigarettes
Labor, delivery, and neonatal events
Neonatal asphyxia or Apgar scores
Prematurity
Small for gestational age
Birth weight and length
Congenital malformations or infections
Maternal bonding at birth
Length of hospitalization
Breastfeeding support
Feeding difficulties as neonate
Medical history of child
Regular physician
Immunizations
Development
Medical or surgical illnesses
Frequent infections
Growth history
Plot previous points
Nutrition history
Feeding behavior and environment
Perceived sensitivities or allergies to foods
Quantitative assessment of intake (3-day diet record, 24-hour food recall)
Social history
Age and occupation of parents
Who feeds the child?
Life stresses (loss of job, divorce, death in family)
Social and economic supports (Special Supplemental Nutrition Program for Women, Infants, and Children; Aid for Families with Dependent Children)

Table 26.3.
Historical Evaluation of Infants and Children With Growth Failure* (*continued*)

Perception of growth failure as a problem
History of violence or abuse by or of caretaker
Review of systems/clues to organic disease
Anorexia
Change in mental status
Dysphagia
Stooling pattern and consistency
Vomiting or gastroesophageal reflux
Recurrent fevers
Dysuria, urinary frequency
Activity level, ability to keep up with peers

*From Duggan C. Failure to Thrive: Malnutrition in the Pediatric Outpatient Setting. In: Walker WA, Watkins JB, eds. *Nutrition in Pediatrics: Basic Science and Clinical Applications.* Hamilton, Ontario: BC Decker Inc; 1996.

assessment of feeding behavior and organization of the household at mealtimes, as well as a quantitative measure of caloric intake. Intake data are most easily obtained by 24-hour food recall, but a more reliable and valid assessment is a prospective collection of food consumed over 3 to 5 days. The child's activity level, feeding history, perceived food allergies, and presence of dietary restrictions should be assessed.

Family history should include growth parameters of siblings as well as stature of parents. Average of maternal and paternal heights can be calculated to derive a mid-parental height; comparison with published values can be done to predict adult stature. A social history that documents the caretakers' economic status is crucial to help guide diagnostic and therapeutic efforts. Any use of alternative or complementary medicines should be documented.

Screening for organic disease should also include a thorough review of systems. Questions about gastrointestinal function (dysphagia, vomiting, abdominal pain, bloating, diarrhea) are especially important.

The physical examination of a child with malnutrition should be comprehensive and findings therein can implicate both organic and socioeconomic causes. The importance of accurate anthropometric measurements cannot be overemphasized. Indeed, the pattern of growth failure itself is often indicative of whether genetic or environmental factors are to blame; genetically small children often maintain normal weight for height, have proportionately low weights, lengths, and head circumferences, and can grow parallel to but lower than the fifth percentile curve. Alternatively, children with inadequate energy intake or malabsorption fall off their weight curves first, followed by length, followed by head circumference. They will, therefore, acutely show a deficit of weight for length, and then more chronically a deficit of height for age. An assessment of maternal-child interaction, such as physical proximity, verbalization towards each other, and eye contact is a critical aspect of the physical examination. Evidence of child neglect should be sought by paying attention to general hygiene, oral health, and presence of diaper dermatitis. The possibility of organic disease can be evaluated by examination of all major organ systems. Table 26.4 gives a summary of possible findings on physical examination in children with growth failure that should prompt further evaluation for underlying medical problems.

Unfortunately, the extensive differential diagnosis engendered by undernutrition can lead to excessive diagnostic testing. Sills succinctly showed the lack of utility of many laboratory tests in children with poor growth, especially given the psychosocial etiology of most cases.[17] In 185 children less than 3 years old admitted for evaluation of failure to thrive, only 36 of 2607 laboratory tests performed (1.4%) were helpful in making a diagnosis, and all of these 36 positive results were suspected on clinical grounds. It has also been pointed out[18] that weight gain or loss in the hospital may not distinguish between organic and psychosocial causes of poor growth, so hospitalization should be avoided except in extreme cases (Table 26.4). Thus, a good history and physical examination are effective screening tools for the presence of organic disease, and laboratory testing should be minimized. Examples can include complete blood count, blood urea nitrogen, albumin, alkaline phosphatase, erythrocyte sedimentation rate, lead level, and urinalysis; by no means is it necessary for all patients undergoing evaluation to be so tested.

Treatment of Growth Failure

Treatment of malnutrition in children is obviously determined by the etiology of any underlying pathology. Obviously, if a medical illness is diagnosed via physical examination and subsequent laboratory evaluation, treatment of this underlying problem should proceed. Alternatively, if inadequate energy intake is the etiology of the poor growth, primary nutritional therapy should be the treatment of choice. The pace and aggressiveness of nutritional repletion should be dictated by the degree of malnutrition. Indications for hospital admission include: (1) anthropometric evidence of severe acute malnutrition, (2) evidence

Table 26.4.
Physical Examination of Infants and Children With Growth Failure*

	Abnormality	Considerations
Vital signs	Hypotension	Adrenal or thyroid insufficiency
	Hypertension	Renal disease
	Tachypnea/tachycardia	Increased metabolic demands
Skin	Pallor	Anemia
	Poor hygiene	Neglect
	Ecchymoses	Abuse
	Candidiasis	Immunodeficiency
	Eczema	Allergic disease
	Erythema nodusom	Ulcerative colitis Vasculitis
HEENT	Hair loss	Stress
	Chronic otitis media	Immunodeficiency Structural orofacial defect
	Cataracts	Congenital infections Galactosemia
	Papilledema	Increased intracranial pressure
	Uveitis	Vasculitis
	Aphthous stomatitis	Crohn's disease
	Delayed tooth eruption	Delayed bone age
	Milk bottle caries	Neglect
	Thyroid enlargement	Thyroid disease
Chest	Wheezes	Cystic fibrosis Asthma
Cardiovascular	Murmur	Congenital malformations
Abdomen	Distension, hyperactive bowel sounds	Malabsorption
	Hepatosplenomegaly	Liver disease Glycogen storage Tumor
Genitourinary	Anomalies	Associated endocrinopathies
	Diaper rashes	Diarrhea Neglect

Table 26.4.
Physical Examination of Infants and Children With Growth Failure* *(continued)*

	Abnormality	Considerations
Rectum	Fistulae	Crohn's disease
	Empty ampulla	Hirschsprung's disease
Extremities	Edema	Hypoalbuminemia
	Loss of muscle mass	Chronic malnutrition
	Clubbing	Chronic lung disease
Nervous System	Abnormal deep tendon reflexes	Cerebral palsy
	Developmental delay	Altered caloric intake or requirements
	Cranial nerve palsy	Dysphagia
Behavior and Temperament	Uncooperative	Difficult to feed

*Adapted from Collins J, Mezey AP. Failure to thrive. In: Shelov SP, Mezey AP, Edelman CM, Barnett HL, eds. *Primary Care Pediatrics*. Norwalk, CT: Appleton-Century-Crofts; 1984:327–329.

of child abuse or neglect, (3) significant dehydration, (4) psychosis or drug addiction of caretaker, or (5) failure of outpatient management to achieve weight gain.

In mild malnutrition, therapy should center on ways to increase oral caloric intake. Commonly, dietary supplementation with high-calorie foods and food additives are recommended to increase macronutrient intake. Infants may respond well to increasing the caloric density of their formula, whereas the use of sour cream, butter, peanut butter, and cheese as dietary additives are helpful for older children. For micronutrients, routine supplementation with a zinc- and iron-containing multivitamin is probably prudent, with the need for further iron therapy determined by laboratory values. Appetites stimulants such as cyproheptadine may be useful, but have no proven long-term benefit.

In addition to nutritional therapy, social evaluation to assess family dynamics and economic situation (eg, eligibility for state and federal assistance) should be performed. Home nursing visits can also be enlightening in this regard, and have been associated with better outcomes.[19] Weekly outpatient and/or home visits should occur to document adequate weight gain and compliance with dietary management. Behavioral modification should center on improving feeding techniques, reducing between meal snacking or grazing, and eliminating television during mealtimes. Table 26.5 recounts a helpful schema in which 3

Table 26.5.
Classification of Feeding Disorders in Infants and Children With Growth Failure*

Disorder Type	Age of Onset	Associated Medical Conditions	Features of Infants	Features of Caretakers	Treatment
Homeostasis	0–2 months	Limited experience with oral feeds (eg, respiratory distress)	Excitable Irritable Passive	Anxious Depressed Over- or understimulates infant	Pacifier during nasogastric feeds Occupational therapy re: suck and swallow
Attachment	2–6 months	Prolonged hospitalization or separation from mother Developmental delay	Sad Hypervigilant Arches or resists when picked up	Detached Depressed Holds infant loosely	Emotional nurturance Developmental stimulation Education of caretaker re: needs of infant
Individuation or Separation	6 months–3 years	Any condition which limits or restricts food intake (eg, diabetes, celiac disease)	Refuses food Defiant Plays with food	Frustrated Doesn't allow infant to self-feed	

*Adapted from Chatoor I, Dickson L, Schaefer S, Egan J. A Developmental Classification of Feeding Disorders Associated with Failure to Thrive: Diagnosis and Treatment. In: Drotar D, ed. *New Directions in Failure to Thrive: Implications for Research and Practice.* New York, NY: Plenum Press; 1985.

developmental stages of feeding disorders are described, with typical features of affected infants and caretakers.

A general guideline for caloric requirements for infants with poor growth is as follows:

$$\text{kcal per kg required} = \frac{\text{RDA for age (kcal/kg)} \times \text{Ideal weight for height}}{\text{Actual weight}}$$

where ideal weight for height is the median weight for the patient's height (as read from the NCHS weight for height curves).

For example, a 3-month-old boy with a weight of 3.6 kg and length of 57 cm has the following anthropometric measures: weight for age Z score −2.50, height for age Z score −1.55, weight for height Z score −2.11. In addition, assessment via the Waterlow classification shows that he has moderate acute malnutrition (weight for height = 74% of the median) and mild chronic malnutrition (height for age = 93% of the median). Since his recommended dietary allowance (RDA) for calories is 108 kcal/kg/d, and his ideal weight for length is 4.8 kg, his estimated caloric requirement for catch-up growth is (108 × 4.8)/3.6 = 144 cal/kg/d. Similarly, since his RDA for protein is 2.2 g/kg/d, his protein requirement for catch-up growth is closer to (2.2 × 4.8)/3.6 = 2.9 g/kg/d.

Any calculations used to judge energy and protein requirements are merely estimates, and the sufficiency of any diet is proven by the occurrence of subsequent weight and, eventually, height gain. These parameters should be measured and charted graphically to allow assessment of the dietary intervention.

Prognosis

The relationship between malnutrition in early infancy and subsequent intellectual and behavioral performance has been investigated widely. Studies from developing countries have clearly shown that children who were admitted early in life with protein-energy malnutrition had subsequently lower intellectual performance on standardized tests. Many of these studies, however, have been confounded by social and economic factors that may also bear upon ultimate intellectual function. Studies have supported the concept that appropriate psychosocial stimulation is important for cognitive development both early and later[20] in the child's life. A large case-control study of 7- to 9-year-old children from an industrial economy who had had poor weight gain as infants confirmed continued lower attainments in weight, height, and head circumference but not significant difference in IQ.[21] Emerging data have also linked food insecurity and hunger with behavioral and school problems even in the absence of undernutrition.[22]

References

1. Stickler GB. 'Failure to thrive' or the failure to define. *Pediatrics.* 1984;74:559
2. Edwards AG, Halse PC, Parkin JM, Waterston AJ. Recognising failure to thrive in early childhood. *Arch Dis Child.* 1990;65:1263–1265
3. Raynor P, Rudolf MC. Anthropometric indices of failure to thrive. *Arch Dis Child.* 2000;82:364–365
4. Smith DW, Truog W, Rogers JE, et al. Shifting linear growth during infancy: illustration of genetic factors in growth from fetal life through infancy. *J Pediatr.* 1976;89: 225–230
5. Jelliffe DB, Patrice EF. *Community Nutritional Assessment: With Special Reference to Less Technically Developed Countries.* New York, NY: Oxford University Press; 1989
6. Villar J, Smeriglio V, Martorell R, Brown CH, Klein RE. Heterogeneous growth and mental development of intrauterine growth-retarded infants during the first 3 years of life. *Pediatrics.* 1984;74:783–791
7. Bithoney WG. Elevated lead levels in children with nonorganic failure to thrive. *Pediatrics.* 1986;78:891–895
8. Frank DA, Zeisel SH. Failure to thrive. *Pediatr Clin North Am.* 1988;35:1187–1206
9. Wright C, Birks E. Risk factors for failure to thrive: a population-based survey. *Child Care Health Dev.* 2000;26:5–16
10. Pugliese MT, Weyman-Daum M, Moses N, Lifshitz F. Parental health beliefs as a cause of nonorganic failure to thrive. *Pediatrics.* 1987;80:175–182
11. Roesler TA, Barry PC, Bock SA. Factitious food allergy and failure to thrive. *Arch Pediatr Adolesc Med.* 1994;148:1150–1155
12. Smith MM, Lifshitz F. Excess fruit juice consumption as a contributing factor in nonorganic failure to thrive. *Pediatrics.* 1994;93:438–443
13. Weston JA, Colloton M, Halsey S, et al. A legacy of violence in nonorganic failure to thrive. *Child Abuse Negl.* 1993;17:709–714
14. Bools CN, Neale BA, Meadow SR. Co-morbidity associated with fabricated illness (Munchausen syndrome by proxy). *Arch Dis Child.* 1992;67:77–79
15. Peterson KE, Washington J, Rathbun JM. Team management of failure to thrive. *J Am Diet Assoc.* 1984;84:810–815
16. Bithoney WG, McJunkin J, Michalek J, Snyder J, Egan H, Epstein D. The effect of a multidisciplinary team approach on weight gain in nonorganic failure-to-thrive children. *J Dev Behav Pediatr.* 1991;12:254–258
17. Sills RH. Failure to thrive. The role of clinical and laboratory evaluation. *Am J Dis Child.* 1978;132:967–969
18. Berwick DM, Levy JC, Kleinerman R. Failure to thrive: diagnostic yield of hospitalisation. *Arch Dis Child.* 1982;57:347–351
19. Wright CM, Callum J, Birks E, Jarvis S. Effect of community based management in failure to thrive: randomized controlled trial. *Br Med J.* 1998;317:571–574

20. Grantham-McGregor SM, Walker SP, Chang SM, Powell CA. Effects of early child-hood supplementation with and without stimulation on later development in stunted Jamaican children. *Am J Clin Nutr.* 1997;66:247–253

21. Drewett RF, Corbett SS, Wright CM. Cognitive and educational attainments at school age of children who failed to thrive in infancy: a population-based study. *J Child Psychol Psychiatry.* 1999;40:551–561

22. Kleinman RE, Murphy JM, Little M, et al. Hunger in children in the United States: potential behavioral and emotional correlates. *Pediatrics.* 1998;101:E3

27

Chronic Diarrheal Disease

Introduction and Pathophysiology

Chronic diarrhea remains a significant concern even as improved management of acute diarrheal disease is achieved. Indeed, aggressive oral rehydration programs have reduced the frequency of hospitalization and death from acute diarrhea, but have not yet demonstrated any influence on the morbidity and mortality from chronic diarrhea in developing countries. Chronic or persistent diarrhea still accounts for 30% to 40% of diarrhea-associated deaths worldwide.

Persistent diarrhea is defined by the World Health Organization as "diarrheal episodes of presumed infectious etiology that begin acutely but last at least 14 days."[1] To the physician, diarrhea is best defined on the basis of volume rather than frequency or consistency. Thus, diarrhea in infants and toddlers is defined as a volume of more than 10 g of stool/kg/24 h, while, in older children, a volume of more than 200 g/d is used.[2] To the parents, it is one more dirty diaper than they wish to change each day.

The etiologies of chronic diarrhea can be divided by pathophysiology into 4, often overlapping, mechanisms. The first is osmotic diarrhea secondary to the failure to absorb a solute that creates an osmotic load in the distal bowel producing increased fluid losses. This can result from either congenital or acquired disease and is most evident in the failure to absorb a carbohydrate, such as lactose. Excessive carbohydrate intake, as seen with juices in early childhood, also contributes to this form of diarrhea.[3] By definition, the diarrhea ceases with elimination of the offending solute from the diet.

The second form, secretory diarrhea, occurs when there is a net secretion of electrolyte and fluid from the intestine, relative to the degree of absorption. This includes disorders such as congenital chloridorrhea and neural crest tumors. This form of diarrhea persists even with cessation of oral intake.

The third form of diarrhea results from pure motility or dysmotility. Children with this form usually have intact absorptive ability even in the face of rapid transit. The most common forms of dysmotility in childhood include toddler's or chronic nonspecific diarrhea and the childhood forms of irritable bowel syndrome.

The fourth pathophysiologic form of diarrhea is inflammatory diarrhea. This often encompasses components of all of the prior 3 forms as well. The etiologies range from acute viral enteritis to chronic villus or colonic inflammation from celiac disease to inflammatory bowel diseases. Increased enteric loss of protein, mucus, and blood may also be noted in the stool.

Evaluation of the Infant and Child With Persistent Diarrhea

History and Physical Examination

The initial step is to define with the family the extent of diarrhea using criteria such as frequency, volume, duration, character, and relation to dietary content. A prospective 3- to 5-day history of dietary intake, stool pattern, and associated symptoms is very helpful.

Historical features, including family history, cultural factors in feeding, travel, and preschool exposures, will be helpful.

The physical examination begins with documenting growth parameters of weight, height, and head circumference, ideally on the standardized growth chart relative to the child's prior growth parameters. More complete anthropometric evaluation is also valuable. The examination will focus on evidence of chronic disease, features of nutrient deficiency such as rickets (Vitamin D) or hypotonia (Vitamin E), abdominal distension with loss of sub-cutaneous tissue (celiac), and must include the rectal examination (factitious diarrhea from encopresis or inflammatory diarrhea from aganglionosis).

Examination of Stool Sample

Confirmation of the diagnosis of persistent diarrhea requires evaluation of a fresh stool sample.[4] This begins with the macroscopic inspection of consistency and color. The presence or absence of occult blood is confirmed. The presence of significant numbers of polymorphonuclear cells is determined by mixing a drop of methylene blue with the stool and examining under a coverslip. The presence of large numbers of polys is expected with invasive bacterial disease and inflammatory colitis, and is an argument against viral or malabsorptive diarrheas. Techniques for analysis of the stool for malabsorbed fat using Sudan black stains are available in clinical laboratories but are too cumbersome and dependent on experience in interpretation for routine office use.

As noted previously, the presence of unabsorbed carbohydrate in the stoolis a major component of osmotic and small-bowel inflammatory diarrhea. Unless bacterial fermentation in the large bowel has converted the malabsorbed carbohydrate to organic acids, these sugars can be detected by reagent tablets (eg, Clinitest) for reducing sugars or test-tape analysis for glucose. Breastfed healthy infants will often have a trace of reducing sugar in the stool. Sucrose is not a reducing sugar and thus infants malabsorbing from a sucrose-containing formula will require the stool sample to be hydrolyzed by 0.1N hydrochloric acid and heat before testing.

In patients with high-volume ostomy losses, it is often helpful to analyze the ostomy output for volume, osmolality, and electrolyte content. This allows documentation of true electrolyte needs and the osmolar impact of malabsorbed sugar in the feedings. Children with hypoalbuminemia or suspected of having persistent diarrhea complicated by protein-losing enteropathy can have this concern proven by determining the fecal content of I-1-antitrypsin, a large molecular weight serum protein marker of increased mucosal permeability to protein.

To exclude ongoing infection as a contributing factor to persistent diarrhea, it is appropriate to culture the stool for enteric pathogens and analyze for parasites, including *Giardia* and *Cryptosporidium*. Fecal antigen analysis for *Giardia* antigen is now readily available and sensitive. Persistent or recurrent infection is a hallmark of preschoolers and children with immune deficiencies. While most relevant after antibiotic use, analysis for the toxins of *clostridium difficile* should be done routinely with persistent diarrhea, especially in the presence of fecal polys and/or blood.

For children with diarrhea in the context of failure to thrive or suspected steatorrhea, a formal documentation of quantitative fecal fat should be attempted with the 72-hour fecal fat analysis. This is coupled with a 4-day history of dietary fat intake, which is maximized to be more than 25 g/d in infants and up to more than 100 g/d in school-aged children. The coefficient of fat malabsorption is calculated with more than 5% malabsorption abnormal after early infancy.

Sweat Test

The analysis of sweat sodium and/or chloride by iontophoresis should be performed in all infants and toddlers with growth failure and diarrhea as well as any child with suspected or documented steatorrhea. Fecal elastase concentrations are another way of assessing pancreatic sufficiency after 1 month of age. The test is not effected by oral pancreatic enzyme replacement therapy. Cystic fibrosis is discussed in detail in Chapter 46.

Screening Laboratory Blood Studies

The performance of blood work is individualized by the clinical situation and degree of concern for malabsorption, malnutrition, and inflammatory disease. The routine complete blood count with indices addresses issues of anemia and the status of iron, Vitamin B_{12}, and folate. The platelet count is elevated in Vitamin E deficiency and as an acute phase reactant. Diagnostic alterations of red cell morphology are seen in abetalipoproteinemia. The erythrocyte sedimentation rate and C-reactive protein will usually be elevated with chronic inflammatory bowel disease.

Serum immunoglobulins are measured specifically with special emphasis on IgA. To screen for celiac disease or gluten-sensitive enteropathy, the specific IgA anti-transglutaminase antibody has replaced the role of less specific anti-gliadin antibodies. Of note, IgA anti-transglutaminase antibody tests cannot be interpreted in individuals with IgA deficiency. Low serum albumin and pre-albumin concentrations reflect low dietary protein intake.

To evaluate issues of Vitamin D, the serum calcium, phosphorus, and alkaline phosphatase are determined. When fat-soluble vitamin malabsorption or deficiency is suspected, specific serum levels of 25-OH vitamin D and Vitamin E can be requested. The serum carotene level is less commonly employed as it is heavily dependent on extent of dietary intake.

Though often complicated by issues of gastric emptying, the 1-hour blood d-xylose assay is helpful when issues of reduced small bowel mucosal surface area are in question. After a 6-hour fast, 5 g of d-xylose, a non-digestible pentose sugar, are given orally with a blood analysis of the serum level at 1 hour. A rise of less than 20 mg/dL suggests mucosal villus injury. Older children and teens can also cooperate with timed urine collection for analysis.

Roentgenograms

The value of x-rays for issues of chronic diarrhea are limited. The abdominal flat plate may reveal constipation, dilated blind loops of bowel, or calcifications of the biliary or pancreatic system. Oral contrast studies and computed tomography scans with contrast are routine for the evaluation of inflammatory bowel disease. The role of bone density analysis in childhood is under investigation.

Breath Hydrogen Analysis

The hydrogen breath test, by virtue of its noninvasive nature, has replaced the oral carbohydrate tolerance tests. The test requires a normal enteric bacterial flora so it is not valid after recent antibiotic use. When an oral carbohydrate is given, it is either digested and absorbed normally or it reaches the bacterial flora and is fermented to produce hydrogen gas that is absorbed and excreted in the breath. Analysis of breath hydrogen that reveals a rise of greater than 20 ppm confirms carbohydrate malabsorption or bacterial overgrowth. The test is performed with oral lactose (for lactase deficiency), sucrose (for sucrase-isomaltase deficiency), or glucose (for small-bowel bacterial overgrowth).

Endoscopic Procedures

When persistent diarrhea appears to be related to an inflammatory process of the small bowel or colon, invasive endoscopic visualization of the bowel with biopsy is indicated. Even grossly normal bowel is routinely biopsied as the diagnostic features are often only microscopic. Routine staining may be supplemented by electron microscopy or biochemical analysis of the biopsy.

Differential Diagnosis of Persistent Diarrhea

A review of the many disorders capable of inducing persistent or chronic diarrhea is beyond the scope of this chapter. In Table 27.1, the major conditions are listed as either commonly associated with normal growth or those expected to be complicated by growth failure or failure to thrive. Inappropriate nutritional management of any of these disorders, however, can lead to weight loss and growth failure.[5]

Diarrhea Without Failure to Thrive

Chronic Nonspecific (Toddler's) Diarrhea

This is the most common form of persistent diarrhea in the first 3 years of life.[6] It may begin acutely before 1 year of age, but settles into a pattern of 2 to 5 looser-than-desired stools daily. There is an occasional day with formed stool and there is nearly never stooling during sleep. Multiple dietary manipulations may produce transient improvement, but usually contributes to the problem by removing higher fat nutrients and increasing ingestion of fruit juices. This is especially true with the intake of high sorbitol-containing non-citrus juices such as prune, pear, cherry, or apple (Appendix X).

By definition, these infants are clinically well with normal intestinal digestive and absorptive ability. Toddlers will do best on a normal diet that includes 30% to 40% of calories from fat and less than 8 oz of juice per day. The diarrhea often resolves with the acquisition of successful bowel toilet training, which allows greater duration of rectal retention.

Table 27.1.
Chronic Diarrhea in Childhood

Diarrhea Without Failure to Thrive

Chronic nonspecific (toddler's) diarrhea

Dietary-induced diarrhea

- Excessive juice, tea
- Prolonged low-fat diet
- Disaccharide intolerance: lactose, sucrose

Persistent enteritis

- Parasitic: *Giardia, Strongyloides, Cryptosporidium*
- Immunodeficient: IgA deficiency, HIV
- Small-bowel bacterial overgrowth

Factitious diarrhea

- Laxative abuse
- Encopresis
- Munchausen by proxy

Secretory diarrhea

- Neural crest tumors
- Familial chloride diarrhea

Diarrhea With Failure to Thrive

Pancreatic insufficiency

- Cystic fibrosis
- Shwachman-Diamond syndrome

Disorders of lipid digestion, absorption, or transport

- Primary bile acid (micelle) deficiency
- abetalipoproteinemia
- Intestinal lymphangiectasia
- Chylomicron retention disease

Disorders of the mucosal villus

- Congenital
  - Microvillus inclusion disease
  - Tufting disease
- Reduced mucosal surface area
  - Short-bowel syndrome
  - Malnutrition
  - Ischemic, radiation enteropathy
  - Graft-versus-host disease

Table 27.1.
Chronic Diarrhea in Childhood *(continued)*

- Inflammatory villus injury
  - Postgastroenteritis diarrhea with malabsorption
  - Acute infectious diarrhea
  - Gluten-sensitive enteropathy
  - Dietary protein induced enteropathy: milk, soy, egg, fish
  - Allergic eosinophilic gastroenteropathy
  - Autoimmune enteritis
  - Crohn's disease
  - Blind loop/pseudo-obstruction
  - Whipple enteropathy
  - Intractable diarrhea

Disaccharide Intolerance

The major disaccharide in the child's diet is lactose, the primary sugar of all mammalian milks other than the sea lion. Lactose is both a major calorie source and a facilitator for the intestinal absorption of calcium, magnesium, and manganese. It is digested by an intestinal mucosal brush border oligosaccharidase, lactase, to glucose and galactose. Lactase activity declines, under genetic control, after weaning and is especially sensitive to intestinal mucosal injury. Congenital lactase deficiency is very rare.[7]

As lactase activity declines, dietary lactose is incompletely digested and induces an osmotic secretion of electrolytes and fluid in the distal small bowel. As the lactose reaches the bacterial flora of the distal bowel, it is fermented to hydrogen, methane, and carbon dioxide. This allows the diagnosis by breath hydrogen analysis, as noted above, but also contributes to the child's sense of discomfort from gas and increased flatus. The fermentation of lactose also produces volatile fatty acids that are absorbed across the colonic epithelium as a caloric source.

The treatment of lactose malabsorption is to document the threshold for symptoms by initial elimination then gradual reintroduction of lactose-containing foods. Lactose-reduced milks are now routinely marketed. Two commercial lactase products are also available for oral use prior to ingestion of lactose or for addition to a lactose-containing liquid. These lactases are derived from the yeast (Kluyveromyces lactis) and the fungus (Aspergillus oryzae). A number of probiotics are under investigation, but the commonly marketed *Lactobacillus acidophilus* has minimal lactase activity. While the heating and fermentation of many cheeses reduces lactase content, the inconsistent content of probiotic bacteria in yogurt means most yogurts are high in lactose content. The major risk of lactose-restricted diets is the reduction in dietary calcium intake, particularly in the age group of 9 to 20 where desired daily intakes of 1300 mg of calcium are difficult to achieve.

Infants with diarrhea on sucrose or glucose polymer-containing formulas may have congenital sucrase-isomaltase deficiency. This diagnosis is confirmed by sucrose breath hydrogen testing and sucrase deficiency can be treated with the recent production of a baker's yeast (*Saccharomyces cerevisiae*) processed to a high content of a yeast invertase that cleaves sucrose. In normal children, sucrase-isomaltase activity is near adult levels by age 1 month and is highly resistant to reduction during mucosal injury.[8]

Small-Bowel Bacterial Overgrowth

There is an increasing awareness that bacterial overgrowth contributes to a significant frequency of persistent diarrhea and abdominal discomfort, especially in children under age 2 years.[9] The diagnosis is established by a breath hydrogen test using glucose as the carbohydrate as the glucose will be fermented by the bacteria high in the small bowel before it can be absorbed completely. Treatment is usually with a brief course of antibiotic, often coupled with use of a probiotic.[10]

Diarrhea With Failure to Thrive

Postgastroenteritis Diarrhea With Malabsorption

Protracted diarrhea following an acute episode of infectious diarrhea remains a major concern in both developed and developing countries. In contrast to toddler's diarrhea, the intestinal morphology is not normal, even after the infectious origin has been cleared. Small-bowel biopsies reveal patchy villus atrophy with increased inflammatory infiltrates featuring intraepithelial lymphocytes with increased plasma cells and macrophages in the lamina propria and adherent bacteria on the mucosal surface.[11] Nonspecific absorptive alterations are seen for nutrient in the jejunum and for bile acids in the ileum. Disaccharide intolerance is common, contributing to osmotic diarrhea and increased fluid needs.

While persistent infection requires exclusion, the major determinants of this persistent inflammation include young age, relative malnutrition, and altered immune response.[5] In developing countries, lack of breastfeeding is a major risk factor. The failure to intervene in this concern leads to intractable diarrhea with its attendant high frequency of morbidity and death. The intervention is nutritional, adapted to the enteric ability of the individual child.

Dietary protein intolerance is rarely the limiting factor. While a subgroup will require amino acid-based or elemental diets (see also Chapter 34), most can be managed on traditional home-available diets or mixed protein diets.[5,12] Carbohydrate tolerance is always an issue, but recent studies show that intakes of 1.9 g/kg/d of lactose, from cow milk, providing 30% of calories will be tolerated and have huge cost-saving advantages in the developing world.[13] Breastfeeding is encouraged when possible. With severe enteropathy, both sucrose and monosaccharides may be incompletely absorbed. A modest degree of steatorrhea is commonly seen in these children, the result of increased fecal bile acid excretion from reduced ileal reabsorption. Both macronutrient and micronutrient deficiency may be present from reduced intake and increased fecal loss. Total caloric need for enteric recovery and catch-up growth often exceeds 120 kcal/kg/d.

Enteric feedings are thus encouraged, either by continuous tube feeding or frequent small-volume bolus feedings. Initial caloric intake is attempted at 50 to 75 kcal/kg/d, increasing over 5 to 7 days to 130 to 150 kcal/kg/d. Protein is initiated at 1 to 2 g/kg/d increasing to 3 to 4 g/kg/d as caloric intakes are maximized. The requirement for potassium, calcium, phosphorus, magnesium, and trace minerals is usually increased and must be monitored closely in severely involved children. While renal and cardiac function is usually normal, rapid increases in fluid and electrolytes must be monitored closely. Aggressive refeeding may rarely precipitate acute pancreatitis. Tolerance of normal intakes and clinical improvement are usually noted in 2 to 3 weeks.

Gluten-Sensitive Enteropathy (Celiac Disease)

This enteropathy features severe villus injury and loss of mucosal surface area. It is the result of a T-cell mediated immune response against gluten protein in wheat and related proteins in barley and rye. Involvement of oat proteins remains under active investigation. The protein-induced injury triggers a release of tissue transglutaminase, a highly specific endomysial antigen. The IgA antibody to this transglutaminase is detected in serum of affected children and serves as a highly specific screening test. At this time, the diagnosis is confirmed by small-bowel biopsy, usually obtained by endoscopy rather than by blind capsule techniques used in the past. There is a significant increased frequency of gluten-sensitive enteropathy in children with diabetes, Trisomy 21, and thyroid-related autoimmune disorders.[14] Treatment is with complete elimination of gluten and related barley, rye, and oat protein. Gluten-free foods are now readily marketed and parents are instructed to read labels of processed foods carefully. At this time, a gluten challenge with re-biopsy is advised in the school-aged child to confirm the need for lifelong gluten restriction. Whether serologic testing will replace this need is under investigation.

Short-Bowel Syndrome

Short-bowel syndrome is the consequence of massive small-bowel resection and the resulting unique severe nutritional consequences with loss of mucosal surface area. It is encountered after surgical intervention for necrotizing enterocolitis, midgut volvulus, acute ischemic injury, small-bowel aganglionosis, gastroschisis, and diffuse Crohn's disease of the small bowel. The best prognosis is for children in whom the duodenum, distal ileum, and ileocecal valve can be preserved. Indeed, with preservation of the ileocecal valve, only 10 to 15 cm of residual bowel may be required, while, with loss of the ileocecal valve, more than 75 cm of residual bowel may be required.

In the initial postoperative period, total parenteral nutrition is universally employed. The early initiation of enteral feedings, adapted to the individual residual absorptive ability, maximizes the enteric hormonal stimulation and adaptation of the residual bowel by elongation, hypertrophy, and reduction in peristaltic rate.

The greatest potential for recovery is in infancy. The normal absorptive surface area at birth is approximately 950 cm^2, increasing to 7500 cm^2 in the adult. As noted above, enteral feedings are begun as soon as possible to minimize the enteric atrophic effect of parenteral feeding. The initial feedings offer protein as casein hydrolysate or amino acids, lipid with a combination of medium-chain triglycerides and long-chain triglycerides, and carbohydrate as glucose polymer. As with postgastroenteritis malabsorption, calories are gradually increased by 5 to 15 kcal/kg/d by intragastric infusion to full oral intake.

Inflammatory Bowel Disease

The model of inflammatory diarrhea is Crohn's disease with its unique ability to inflame all levels of the bowel from the mouth to the anus. The nutritional consequences of this can be devastating. The children present with abdominal pain and diarrhea that is minimized by reduced caloric intake. Combined with increased enteric loss of protein, zinc, and blood across the inflamed mucosa, the result is weight loss, reduced growth rate, delayed puberty, and anemia unresponsive to iron alone. This is further complicated by active disease during pubertal demands for growth and utilization of anti-inflammatory and growth-inhibiting corticosteroid therapy.

While the etiology of inflammatory bowel disease is not known, there is a role for enteric nutrition as primary therapy for Crohn's disease.[15,16] The studies to date have been inconsistent with regard to the feeding formulation of elemental versus polymeric proteins and the relative value in the newly diagnosed child versus failure to respond to routine therapy child. There appears to be greater value in the child with small bowel as opposed to exclusively colonic disease.

Regardless of whether nutritional therapy is used as primary or supplemental intervention, all children with inflammatory bowel disease should be assessed at presentation with anthropometric measurements, documentation of growth velocity, and biochemical determinations. To achieve catch-up growth, the inflammatory disease must be controlled, the use of corticosteroid minimized, and the calories increased to more than 150% of the recommended dietary allowance for age.[17] All patients are requested to use oral caloric supplements and some patients will require nocturnal tube feedings to achieve desired caloric intakes.

Micronutrient adequacy must also be addressed. Folic acid deficiency may have developed in more than 50% of involved children with further folic acid supplementation required during treatment with salicylate-based medication. Vitamin B_{12} levels are reduced by ileal disease and/or resection. Mineral deficiencies for iron, zinc, calcium, and magnesium are anticipated and supplemented while trace mineral concerns increase with use of parenteral nutrition. The value of adding antioxidants, glutamine, α fatty acids, growth factors, and short-cain fatty acids remains under investigation.

Due to the chronicity and variable severity of the inflammatory bowel diseases, the child must be regularly reassessed for nutritional deficits. Parents, eager for a quick fix, will often embark on unproven trials of dietary intervention with no idea of the nutritional risk to the child. If the increased nutritional needs of these children are not met, the delayed growth and sexual development produces significant psychological concerns.

References

1. Snyder JD, Merson MH. The magnitude of the global problem of acute diarrhoeal disease: a review of active surveillance data. *Bull World Health Organ.* 1982;60: 605–613

2. Vanderhoof JA. Chronic diarrhea. *Pediatr Rev.* 1998;19:418–422

3. Hyams JS, Etienne NL, Leichter AM, Theuer RC. Carbohydrate malabsorption following fruit juice ingestion in young children. *Pediatrics.* 1988;82:64–68

4. Sondheimer JM. Office stool examination: a practical guide. *Contemp Pediatr.* 1990; 7:63–82

5. Bhutta ZA, Hendricks KM. Nutritional management of persistent diarrhea in childhood: a perspective from the developing world. *J Pediatr Gastroenterol Nutr.* 1996;22:17–37

6. Cohen SA, Hendricks KM, Eastham EJ, Mathis RK, Walker WA. Chronic nonspecific diarrhea. A complication of dietary fat restriction. *Am J Dis Child.* 1979;133: 490–492

7. Saavedra JM, Perman JA. Current concepts in lactose malabsorption and intolerance. *Annu Rev Nutr.* 1989;9:475–502

8. Treem WR. Clinical heterogeneity in congenital sucrase-isomaltase deficiency. *J Pediatr.* 1996;128:727–729

9. de Boissieu D, Chaussain M, Badoual J, Raymond J, Dupont C. Small-bowel bacterial overgrowth in children with chronic diarrhea, abdominal pain, or both. *J Pediatr.* 1996;128:203–207

10. Vanderhoof JA. Probiotics and intestinal inflammatory disorders in infants and children. *J Pediatr Gastroenterol Nutr.* 2000;30(suppl 2):S34–S38

11. Shiner M, Putman M, Nichols VN, Nichols BL. Pathogenesis of small-intestinal mucosal lesions in chronic diarrhea of infancy: I. A light microscopic study. *J Pediatr Gastroenterol Nutr.* 1990;11: 455–463

12. Kleinman RE, Galeano NF, Ghishan F, Lebenthal E, Sutphen J, Ulshen MH. Nutritional management of chronic diarrhea and/or malabsorption. *J Pediatr Gastroenterol Nutr.* 1989;9:407–415

13. Bhatnager S, Bhan MK, Singh KD, Saxena SK, Shariff M. Efficacy of milk-based diets in persistent diarrhea: a randomized, controlled trial. *Pediatrics.* 1996;98: 1122–1126

14. Molberg O, McAdam SN, Solled LM. Role of tissue transglutaminase in celiac disease. *J Pediatr Gastroenterol Nutr.* 2000;30:232–240

15. Ruemmele FM, Roy CC, Levy E, Seidman EG. Nutrition as primary therapy in pediatric Crohn's disease: fact or fantasy? *J Pediatr.* 2000;136:285–291

16. Griffiths AM. Enteral nutrition: the neglected primary therapy of active Crohn's disease. *J Pediatr Gastroenterol Nutr.* 2000;31:3–5

17. Motil KJ, Grand RJ, Davis-Kraft L, Ferlic LL, Smith EO. Growth failure in children with inflammatory bowel disease: a prospective study. *Gastroenterology.* 1993;105: 681–691

28

Oral Therapy for Acute Diarrhea

Diarrheal illness and accompanying acute dehydration, alone or in combination with acute respiratory illness, account for the overwhelming majority of childhood deaths in the world.[1] Reduction of diarrheal illness and death rates through the use of oral rehydration solutions (ORSs) has been targeted by the United Nations Children's Fund (UNICEF) and the World Health Organization (WHO) as one of the major strategies for saving children's lives.[1,2] Because of its simplicity, extreme effectiveness, and low expense, ORS is an ideal treatment for use in the developing world and in industrialized nations.[2,3] Although the death rate from diarrheal illness in the industrialized world is fortunately not high, diarrheal illness still accounts for a substantial proportion of the preventable childhood deaths and a large proportion of the morbidity and the expense associated with pediatric care.[4] For example, in the United States alone, each year roughly $1.5 billion is spent to provide evaluation and care for approximately 16 million episodes of diarrheal illness in children younger than 5 years.[5] In Third World countries, oral rehydration therapy is credited with saving approximately 1 million children's lives each year.[1]

Oral Rehydration Solutions

The physiologic basis of ORS is at the same time simple and extraordinarily elegant. A combination of sodium with simple organic molecules, such as glucose, in the lumen of the small intestine can promote the absorption of water.[6] This system, characterized in the 1960s,[7] is now referred to as the glucose-sodium cotransport system. Molecular details of the system are now reasonably well understood. In the cotransport mechanism, a single molecule of glucose or other simple organic substrate is transported across the luminal membrane of the villus crypt cells of the small intestine.[6] In concert with the transport of a glucose molecule, a sodium molecule is also brought from the luminal side of the membrane to the interior of the cell. This sodium ion is subsequently transferred into the adjacent capillaries and, thus, into the circulation. Water follows the movement of sodium along a concentration gradient, with the net result being absorption of sodium and water. The earliest clinical studies of solutions that take advantage of the cotransport system were performed in patients with diarrhea resulting from cholera.[8] We now know that the glucose-sodium cotransport system remains intact in virtually all kinds of infectious diarrhea. This fact makes oral therapy appropriate for use in any kind of enteric infection in which dehydration is an end result. The other components of ORS include potassium and chloride to replace stool losses and base, usually in the form of citrate, to replace stool losses and to combat acidosis.[6]

Many fluids that have traditionally been recommended for the treatment of diarrhea and dehydration are inappropriate and non-physiologic and may worsen the condition.[3,6] For example, juices such as apple or white grape juice have a high osmolality related to their high sugar content and contain virtually no sodium and very little potassium. Table 28.1 lists the composition of some currently available rehydration solutions. Some of the frequently used inappropriate fluids are listed for comparison. Particular attention should be paid to the osmolality of the fluids. In general, solutions with osmolality lower

Table 28.1.
Composition of Fluids Frequently Used in Oral Rehydration*

Solution	Glucose/ CHO, g/L	Sodium, mEq/L	HCO_3^-, MEq/L	Potassium, mEq/L	Osmolality, mmol/L	CHO/ Sodium
Pedialyte† (Ross Laboratories)	25	45	30	20	250	3.1
Pediatric Electrolyte (NutraMax)	25	45	20	30	250	3.1
KaoLectrolyte (Pharmacia)	20	48	28	20	240	2.4
Rehydralyte‡ (Ross Laboratories)	25	75	30	20	310	1.9
WHO ORS packet‡	20	90	30	20	330	1.2
WHO Hypo-osmolar	15	60	20	30	224	1.4
Cola	126	2	13	0.1	750	1944
Apple juice	125	3	0	32	730	1278
Gatorade	45	20	3	3	330	62.5

*Cola, juice, and Gatorade are shown for comparison only; they are not recommended for use. CHO indicates carbohydrate; HCO_3^-, bicarbonate; and WHO, World Health Organization.
†Mainly for *maintenance* therapy; may be used for *rehydration* therapy in mildly dehydrated patients.
‡Best for rehydration therapy; may be used during the maintenance phase with adequate access to free water in the form of breast milk, formula, or diluted juices.

than serum (approximately 310 mOsm/L) make the most effective ORS if the ratio of glucose to sodium is maintained near 1.[9] Solutions containing less sodium than the standard WHO/UNICEF formulation and having glucose to sodium ratios of about 3 have proven effective in maintaining hydration in non-cholera diarrhea.[3]

Effective ORS has also been made using complex carbohydrates (starches), which do not contribute significantly to the osmotic content of the solution and yield individual glucose molecules at the brush border of the small intestine.[6] This allows the delivery of large numbers of glucose molecules to the cotransport system without causing osmotic diarrhea. Numerous studies have demonstrated that cereal-based ORS can reduce the volume of stools and the duration of diarrheal illness.[10] However, when cereal-based solutions are compared with the combination of glucose-based solutions and the early reinstitution of feeding, the differences between the 2 approaches disappear and, therefore, cereal-based ORS has not replaced the easier-to-prepare glucose ORS.[10,11]

Cereal-based oral rehydration solutions are available that use precooked dry cereal-electrolyte mixes and are safe and effective for the treatment of older infants and young children with diarrhea. Since the data suggest that the reduction in illness severity is approximately equivalent whether a food-based solution is used or a standard glucose-based solution is used in combination with the early return to normal feeding, either approach may be chosen depending largely on personal preference.

Limitations of Oral Rehydration Solutions

The major controversies about the use of ORS have centered on concern for the development of hypernatremia, issues of usage (and taste), and the lack of antidiarrheal properties.[12] Oral rehydration solutions were originally developed to treat the dehydration resulting from cholera, in which stool losses of sodium are substantial. Concerns have been expressed about the risk of hypernatremia with the use of solutions containing 90 mEq/L of sodium in infants and children whose diarrhea results from non-cholera organisms.[2,3] In the presence of mature functioning kidneys, the use of a 90-mEq sodium solution is safe and extremely effective in children with a wide range of initial serum sodium concentrations and is an effective treatment for hypernatremia.[2,3,13] In contrast, when solutions with little sodium, such as juices, sodas, or water (Table 28.1) are used, the risk of hyponatremia is very real.[2,3] Of greater importance than the sodium concentration is the ratio of sodium to glucose (or other cotransport molecule), which should be close to 1.[6]

Although ORS has an impressive record of success, it remains underused, especially in industrialized countries.[12] Refusal of pediatric patients to take ORS is a common complaint of practitioners in North America, but children who are dehydrated rarely refuse ORS because they usually crave salt and water. By recognizing that ORS may not be required in children with mild diarrhea and no dehydration, the problem of refusal could be greatly reduced.[3] Methods to try to increase ORS intake include the use of flavored ORS, which does not alter the composition of fluid and electrolytes but improves taste.[3] These flavored solutions are now the most popular forms of ORS sold in North America. Another effective technique to increase intake is to freeze the ORS in an ice-pop form.

Perhaps the most important limitation of glucose-based ORS is that it does not decrease the volume or duration of diarrheal stools.[2,3,14] Recent studies on finding solutions that can reduce stool output have shown that hypo-osmolar ORS solutions are absorbed more effectively than iso- or hyper-osmolar solutions.[9] Clinical trials in children demonstrate that hypo-osmolar solutions can result in fewer treatment failures and decreased use of intravenous therapy.[15] For this reason, WHO is now recommending the use of 2 solutions: the standard ORS for patients with cholera, and the hypo-osmolar solution for children with non-cholera diarrhea.[15]

Early, Appropriate Feeding

For more than a decade, clinicians have recognized that return to an age-appropriate and healthy diet early in the course of diarrheal illness is superior to the outdated practice of "resting the gut" by providing only clear liquids or dilute milks.[3,6,16] Appropriate feeding is the component of oral therapy that has the potential for the greatest impact on stool volume and duration.[2,3] In addition, the appetite of the infant and child is generally better maintained and intestinal repair can occur.[3]

Successful feeding trials have been carried out using breast milk, dilute or full-strength animal milk or animal milk formulas, dilute and full-strength lactose-free formulas, and mixed diets of staple foods with milk.[3,16,17] Recent data support the use of lactose-containing milks during diarrhea, especially if given with complex carbohydrates.[18] In general, changes to a lactose-free formula should be made only if the stool output increases on a milk-based diet.[3] Semi-solid and solid foods that have proven to be effective in controlled trials include rice, wheat, peas, potatoes, chicken, and eggs.[3,17]

Oral Therapy for Diarrhea

Before embarking on management, it is essential to consider the importance of parent education. Parents should be given a realistic idea of the likely duration of their child's illness. When possible, explaining to the parent that the child's diarrhea is likely to continue, regardless of therapy, for between 3 and 7 days is extremely helpful. Parents who understand that hydration is the primary concern, not the duration of the diarrheal stool, will generally be more comfortable managing the child's illness at home. By emphasizing to the parents that ORS replaces fluid and electrolyte losses and does not stop diarrhea, less disappointment and discouragement should develop. A positive approach to teaching parents includes pointing out the degree of control that the parent retains when the child receives ORS compared with the loss of that control that results when intravenous solutions are used. In addition, pointing out that ORS is less painful and has fewer complications than intravenous therapy is useful. Finally, most parents greatly desire to feed their child, particularly when the child appears to be hungry and thirsty, and this should be encouraged.

The 2 components of effective oral therapy are used together in almost all situations to ensure a favorable outcome. The following management guidelines are based on the severity of the child's condition.[2,3]

Children With Diarrhea and No Dehydration

If no dehydration develops, which is the case in the great majority of diarrhea cases in the United States, continued age-appropriate feeding is the only therapy required.[3] Non-weaned infants should receive breast milk or continued use of the regular formula. The formula does not require dilution if the diarrhea remains mild. If a diluted formula is used, the concentration should be increased rapidly if the diarrhea does not worsen. Weaned infants and children should have their regular nutritionally balanced diet continued, emphasizing complex carbohydrates (such as rice, wheat, and potatoes), meats (especially chicken), and the child's regular milk or formula. Diets high in simple sugars and fats should be avoided.[2] The "BRATT" diet (bananas, rice, applesauce, tea, and toast) should be avoided as it is not a balanced diet and is low in calories.[3]

Children With Mild or Moderate Dehydration

After dehydration is corrected (Table 28.2), appropriate feeding is begun, using the previous guidelines. The most convenient method for carrying out rehydration is to divide the total volume deficit by 4 and aim to deliver this volume of fluid during each of the 4 hours of the rehydration phase. A tea-

Table 28.2.
Fluid Therapy Chart

Degree of Dehydration	Signs	Fluids	Feeding
Mild*	Slightly dry mucous membranes, increased thirst	Oral rehydration solution (ORS), 50–60 mL/kg†	Breastfeeding, undiluted lactose-free formula, full-strength cow milk, or lactose-containing formula
Moderate	Sunken eyes, sunken fontanelle, loss of skin turgor, dry mucous membranes	ORS, 80–100 mL/kg†	Same as above
Severe	Signs of moderate dehydration plus one or more of the following: rapid thready pulse, cyanosis, rapid breathing, delayed capillary refill time, lethargy, coma	Intravenous or intraosseous isotonic fluids (0.9% saline or Ringer's lactate), 40 mL/kg/h until pulse and state of consciousness return to normal, then 50–100 mL/kg of ORS based on remaining degree of dehydration‡	Begin after clinically improved and ORS has begun

*If no signs of dehydration are present, rehydration phase may be omitted. Proceed with maintenance therapy and replacement of ongoing losses.
†First 4 hours, repeat until no signs of dehydration remain. Replace ongoing stool losses and vomitus with oral rehydration solution (ORS), 10 mL/kg for each diarrheal stool and 5 mL/kg for each episode of vomiting.
‡While parenteral access is being sought, nasogastric infusion of ORS may be begun at 30 mL/kg/h, provided airway protective reflexes remain intact.

spoon or 5-mL syringe can be used for the initial administration of fluid, especially if the child is vomiting. The parent is instructed to administer at least 1 teaspoon (5 mL) of solution each minute. Having a clock with a sweep second hand available is useful. While this rate of fluid delivery may appear slow, 5 mL/min results in an hourly intake of 300 mL. In a 10-kg infant, this is equivalent to 30 mL/kg. Children larger than 15 to 20 kg can receive 2 teaspoons, or 10 mL, per minute and achieve a similar volume of fluid intake. In general, this rate of fluid administration is more than adequate to replace the entire calculated volume deficit within a 4-hour period.

During rehydration, the volume of stool and emesis should be carefully recorded and added to the hourly quantity of fluid to be administered. After 1 or 2 hours of successful rehydration using a syringe or teaspoon, most infants and children will be able to take the fluid ad libitum. On rare occasions, a child will not cooperate in taking the solution from a syringe (this is most often the case with toddlers) or may be too exhausted to remain awake during the administration of fluid. In these cases and after carefully establishing that airway protective reflexes are intact, a soft 5F polymeric silicone nasogastric tube may be placed into the lumen of the stomach. The ORS may then be administered via the nasogastric tube at approximately 5 to 10 mL/kg/min. This method has been widely used in the developing world and has also proved quite successful in industrialized countries.

Children With Severe Dehydration

Children with severe dehydration, which is a shock or a near shock-like condition, should be treated as an emergency.[2,3] A large-bore catheter should be used for the infusion of Ringer's lactate, normal saline, or similar solutionand boluses of 20 to 40 mL/kg should be administered until signs of shock resolve. Fluid and electrolyte resuscitation may require more than 1 intravenous site, and the use of alternate access sites including venous cutdown, femoral vein, or interosseous locations may be needed.[12] As the level of consciousness improves, oral rehydration therapy can be instituted. The hydration status must be frequently reassessed to monitor the effectiveness of the therapy. When rehydration is complete, feeding is continued as previously mentioned.

Vomiting

Vomiting, which is commonly associated with acute diarrhea, can make oral therapy more challenging, but almost all children with vomiting can be treated successfully with ORS.[2,3] Correction of fluid and electrolyte deficits by balanced electrolyte ORS can help speed recovery from vomiting. As vomiting decreases, ORS can be given in larger volumes.

A precautionary note must be made about vomiting, which can be evidence of bowel obstruction. For this reason, efforts should be made to eliminate the possible diagnosis of bowel obstruction on a clinical basis before proceeding with ORS. In a patient who may have an obstructive or other acute process, immediate vascular access must be gained, a surgical consultation must be obtained, and the child should be kept without oral fluids or food.

Failure of Therapy

Failure of ORS occurs when the net output over a 4- to 8-hour period exceeds net intake or when clinical indicators of dehydration are worsening rather than improving. Before determining that ORS has failed in a child, a review of the treatment guidelines should be made with the parents or other caregiver. Often treatment failures and unnecessary intravenous line placement can result from lack of understanding or encouragement to staff or parents to continue to administer ORS.

References

1. Claeson M, Merson MH. Global progress in the control of diarrheal diseases. *Pediatr Infect Dis J.* 1990;9:345–355

2. Duggan C, Santosham M, Glass RI. The management of acute diarrhea in children: oral rehydration, maintenance, and nutritional therapy. *MMWR Recomm Rep.* 1992;41(RR-16):1–20

3. American Academy of Provisional Pediatrics Committee on Quality Improvement, Subcommittee on Acute Gastroenteritis. Practice parameter: the management of acute gastroenteritis in young children. *Pediatrics.* 1996;97:424–435

4. Ho MS, Glass RI, Pinsky PF, et al. Diarrheal deaths in American children. Are they preventable? *JAMA.* 1988;260:3281–3285

5. Glass RI, Lew JF, Gangarosa RE, LeBaron CW, Ho MS. Estimates of morbidity and mortality rates for diarrheal diseases in American children. *J Pediatr.* 1991;118: S27–S33

6. Hirschhorn N, Greenough WB III. Progress in oral rehydration therapy. *Sci Am.* 1991; 264:50–56

7. Sladen GE, Dawson AM. Interrelationships between the absorptions of glucose, sodium and water by the normal human jejunum. *Clin Sci.* 1969;36:119–132

8. Hirschhorn N. The treatment of acute diarrhea in children. An historical and physiological perspective. *Am J Clin Nutr.* 1980;33:637–663

9. Thillainayagam AV, Hunt JB, Farthing MJ. Enhancing clinical efficacy of oral rehydration therapy: is low osmolality the key? *Gastroenterology.* 1998;114:197–210

10. Gore SM, Fontaine O, Pierce NF. Impact of rice based oral rehydration solution of stool output and duration of diarrhoea: meta-analysis of 13 clinical trials. *BMJ.* 1992;304:287–291

11. Fayad IM, Hashem M, Duggan C, et al. Comparative efficacy of rice-based and glucose-based oral rehydration salts plus early reintroduction of food. *Lancet.* 1993; 342:772–775

12. Avery ME, Snyder JD. Oral therapy for acute diarrhea. The underused simple solution. *N Engl J Med.* 1990;323:891–894

13. Pizarro D, Posada G, Villavicencio N, Mohs E, Levine MM. Oral rehydration in hypernatremic and hyponatremic diarrheal dehydration. *Am J Dis Child.* 1983;137:730–734

14. ESPGAN Working Group. Recommendations for composition of oral rehydration solutions for the children of Europe. *J Pediatr Gastroenterol Nutr.* 1992;14:113–115

15. CHOICE Study Group. Multicenter, randomized, double-blind clinical trial to evaluate the efficacy and safety of a reduced osmolarity oral rehydration salts solution in children with acute watery diarrhea. *Pediatrics.* 2001;107:613–618

16. Brown KH. Appropriate diets for the rehabilitation of malnourished children in the community setting. *Acta Paediatr Scand Suppl.* 1991;374:151–159

17. Brown KH. Dietary management of acute childhood diarrhea: optimal timing of feeding and appropriate use of milks and mixed diets. *J Pediatr.* 1991;118:S92-S98

18. Brown KH, Peerson JM, Fontaine O. Use of nonhuman milks in the dietary management of young children with acute diarrhea: a meta-analysis of clinical trials. *Pediatrics.* 1994;93:17–27

29

Inborn Errors of Metabolism

Definitions

Metabolism may be defined as the sum of chemical processes through which food is converted into smaller molecules and energy. An inborn error of metabolism (IEM), therefore, may be defined as an inherited defect in the structure or function of a key protein in a metabolic pathway. These diseases involve processes of energy production, the anabolism and catabolism of fats, carbohydrates, or amino acids, the synthesis and degradation of complex macromolecules, transport of substances across cell membranes, and the detoxification of cellular wastes. The spectrum of cardinal features, age of clinically apparent symptoms, morbidity, mortality, and types of currently used therapies vary widely across this diverse group of disorders.

Inheritance

Each individual IEM occurs only rarely with population incidences ranging from 1:2500 births for hemochromatosis to disorders with only a few single case reports. Collectively, the total incidence of inborn errors of metabolism in the population is approximately 1:1000 births. Many inborn errors of metabolism are known or considered to be autosomal recessive diseases due to single gene defects encoded by nuclear DNA. A few inborn errors of metabolism are inherited in an autosomal dominant pattern while small fractions are X-linked disorders, exhibiting a more severe phenotype in hemizygous males than in heterozygous females. Still other inborn errors of metabolism are due to alterations in the mitochondrial DNA and are inherited only through a maternal lineage.

Newborn Screening for Inborn Errors of Metabolism

While a few inborn errors of metabolism, such as fructokinase deficiency (essential fructosuria), do not cause any clinical disease, the vast majority cause organ dysfunction. With some disorders, signs and symptoms may not be present in the immediate neonatal period, although deleterious compounds are accumulating in the brain, other organs, and body fluids. Because recognition of the disease and early institution of therapy can significantly alter the morbidity and mortality of these initially occult disorders, screening tests have been developed. All states currently require neonatal blood screening for phenylketonuria and hypothyroidism, and many states have additional mandated screening for homocystinuria, maple syrup urine disease, galactosemia, biotinidase deficiency, and congenital adrenal hyperplasia. A few states have implemented screening for medium-chain acyl-CoA dehydrogenase deficiency (MCADD) and other organic acidemias using the relatively new technology of tandem mass spectrometry. Recently, the American Academy of Pediatrics (AAP) has published an executive summary addressing key requirements of an effective neonatal screening program and calling for evaluation of new technologies such as tandem mass spectroscopy for possible inclusion in screening programs nationwide.[1] Key elements to a successful screening program are rapid identification of abnormal results, notification of health care professionals, follow-up with a definitive assay, and the existence of an effective treatment to be carried out by a multidisciplinary center specializing in IEM therapy. Patients with abnormal results, especially when the disease in question may have acute manifestations, should be referred promptly to a metabolic disease center that can further evaluate the potential disorder. If the patient is at risk for acute or severe illness, immediate consultation with a metabolic clinician by telephone for diagnosis and treatment options is advised. Precise and early diagnosis is essential so that effective therapies are instituted safely and the family receives proper counseling.

Signs and Symptoms of Inborn Errors of Metabolism

Inborn errors of metabolism should be suspected whenever a newborn infant has an acute catastrophic illness following a period of normal behavior and feeding, or a child of any age has unexplained lethargy or coma, recurrent seizures, persistent or recurrent vomiting, jaundice, failure to thrive, unusual body odor, developmental delay, hyperammonemia, hypoglycemia, metabolic acidosis, or a family history of recurrent illness or unexplained deaths in siblings. The steps and timing of the evaluation are tempered in part by the acuity of the problem and by the presentation. Algorithms for evaluation of patients with these signs and symptoms have been published.[2,3] If an IEM is suspected, early consultation with a metabolic specialist for advice about the appropriate diagnostic evaluation is advised.

Emergent Therapy of Suspected Inborn Errors of Metabolism

Once an IEM is diagnosed, or in the case of infants in an acutely decompensated state, as soon as the suspicion of such a disorder is entertained, therapy should be instituted. After appropriate blood, urine, and cerebrospinal fluid samples have been obtained for diagnostic evaluation but prior to a definitive diagnosis being made, emergent nonspecific therapy should include restriction of dietary protein and fat intake with vigorous administration of intravenous fluids. While this initial approach is not ideal for every known IEM, it is appropriate for the most common inborn errors of metabolism, which are usually the result of urea cycle defects or abnormalities of amino or organic acid metabolism. The key to emergent nonspecific therapy is the reversal of catabolism and the promotion of anabolism. Intravenous fluids should contain at least 10% dextrose and be given at double the usual maintenance rate to provide calories and promote urinary excretion of toxic metabolites. Severe acidosis (pH <7.1) should be treated with sodium bicarbonate infusion. Hyperammonemia, if not immediately responsive to intravenous fluid therapy, should be treated by hemodialysis. Insulin infusion and growth hormone therapy have been used to promote anabolism and to reverse a metabolically decompensated state. Enteral feedings will also promote anabolism and may be safely given if the protein content is restricted to 0.5 gm/kg/d and the fat content to less than 30% of total energy intake.

Once the diagnosis of a specific IEM has been made, therapy should be tailored to the specific disorder. Therapy for inborn errors of metabolism is rapidly evolving, and metabolic clinicians and contemporary medical literature should be consulted for new advances. A well-organized treatment guide for many inborn errors of metabolism has been published.[4] Therapy for any inherited metabolic disease is based on the pathophysiologic effects of the disease. For many inborn errors of metabolism due to a single enzyme defect, disease-associated pathology is caused by accumulation of an immediate or remote precursor of the impaired reaction. The accumulated substrate may have direct toxic effects or may secondarily impair other critical biochemical reactions. For instance, the accumulation of phenylalanine in phenylalanine hydroxylase deficiency is the primary cause of the pathology associated with untreated phenylketonuria (PKU). For other disorders, symptoms may be caused by a deficiency of a critical reaction product. Finally, the substrate of the deficient reaction may be converted to an alternative product via little-used pathways. These secondary metabolites may in themselves be toxic. For example, succinylacetone, a product of alternative metabolism of fumarylacetoacetic acid, accumulates in the disease tyrosinemia type I, inhibits certain steps in heme synthesis, and causes symptoms mimicking porphyria. Disease-specific therapy may, therefore, include attempts to limit the accumulation of substrate, enhance the excretion of toxic substrate or secondary metabolites, restore the supply of an essential product, or inhibit alternative metabolism of the substrate. Other therapeutic approaches may include stabilization of the impaired enzyme to improve residual activity, replacement of deficient enzymatic cofactors, induction of enzyme production or enzyme replacement, or even correcting the defect at the level of the abnormal gene (gene therapy).

Nutritional Therapy Utilizing Synthetic Medical Foods

Manipulation of precursor and limitation of substrates form a major portion of the available therapies for many inborn errors of metabolism. Special diets have been devised to limit the amount of precursor, balancing growth and maintenance requirements of the body[5] with the toxicity of too much or too little substrate. For some disorders, commercially available medical foods can be used as a mainstay of diet therapy (see Table 29.1 and Appendix O). Medical foods are, by design, incomplete nutrition and should be used only under the supervision of a physician. In addition to the commercial synthetic diet components, low-protein foods available from several vendors are used to complete a nutritionally appropriate diet.

Education of the patient and family about the pathophysiology and the dietary therapy of the disorder in question is essential. Families must be taught to measure and mix special medical food powders, prepare meals with special food products, and determine the protein or fat content and serving size of table foods. Systems of food exchanges based on protein and calorie content are very useful in assisting families to provide a varied diet that is compliant with the required dietary restrictions. For some inborn errors of metabolism, families must also be taught to recognize the signs and symptoms of impending metabolic decompensation and to institute emergency procedures including administration of a generally more restrictive "sick" diet (see following text). Education of the family and patient at regular intervals is a critical component to a successful therapy plan.

Other Nutritional Therapies

Some inborn errors of metabolism are or may be vitamin or cofactor dependent. Cofactor supplementation may be an adjunct to therapy with medical foods for some of the inborn errors of metabolism listed in Table 29.1. For other inborn errors of metabolism, cofactor administration may be the mainstay of treatment (see Table 29.2). Cofactor dependency can be determined empirically through controlled trials of vitamin supplementation with monitoring of laboratory studies and clinical response. For some inborn errors of metabolism, such as maple syrup urine disease, cofactor dependency may be

Table 29.1.
Selected Inborn Errors of Metabolism Treated With Commercially Available Medical Foods

Inborn Error of Metabolism	Modify or Restrict	Vitamin or Cofactor Responsive	Other Therapies
Phenylketonuria	Phenylalanine	<1% of cases due to biopterin synthetic defect	Supplemental tyrosine
Tyrosinemia type I	Phenylalanine, tyrosine, methionine	No	NTBC, a 4-hydroxyphenyl-pyruvate dioxygenase inhibitor
Tyrosinemia type II	Phenylalanine, tyrosine	No	
Maple syrup urine disease	Leucine, valine, isoleucine	Some cases are thiamine responsive	
Isovalericacidemia	Leucine	No	Supplemental carnitine and glycine
Methylmalonicacidemia	Isoleucine, valine, methionine, threonine	Some cases due to defect in cobalamin metabolism	Supplemental carnitine
Propionicacidemia	Isoleucine, valine, methionine, threonine	Possible role for biotin	Supplemental carnitine
Homocystinuria	Methionine	50% pyridoxine responsive	Supplemental folate, betaine
Ornithine transcarbamylase deficiency	Protein	No	Supplemental citrulline, benzoate, phenylacetate, phenylbutyrate
Citrullinemia	Protein	No	Supplemental arginine, benzoate, phenylacetate, phenylbutyrate
Glutaric aciduria type I	Lysine, tryptophan	Possible role for riboflavin	Supplemental carnitine

assessed through in vitro assays of enzyme function in the presence and absence of cofactor. The goal of cofactor therapy may be to stabilize a poorly functional enzyme, to overcome a block in cofactor binding, or to correct a block in cofactor metabolism that results in secondary metabolic derangement.

Therapy of other selected inborn errors of metabolism is presented in Table 29.2. As for the inborn errors of metabolism listed in Table 29.1, treatment of several other inborn errors of metabolism is based on dietary avoidance of

Table 29.2.
Therapy of Other Selected Inborn Errors of Metabolism

Inborn Error of Metabolism	Modify or Restrict	Vitamin or Cofactor Responsive	Other Therapies
Biotinidase	None	Biotin	
Familial hypophos-phatemic rickets	None	1,25-dihydroxy-vitamin D	Phosphorus
Acrodermatitis enteropathica	None	Zinc	
Pyruvate dehydroge-nase deficiency	Low-carbohydrate, high-fat diet	Possibly thiamine responsive	Alkali therapy
Galactosemia (transferase deficiency)	Galactose, lactose		Lactose-free infant formula
Glycogen storage diseases	Lactose, fructose, sucrose		Frequent feedings, complex starches, high-protein diet
Fructosemia (fructose-1,6-bisphosphatase or aldolase deficiency)	Fructose		Frequent glucose feedings in bisphosphatase deficiency
Medium-chain acyl-CoA dehydrogenase deficiency (MCADD)	Dietary fat	Riboflavin	Avoid fasting, supplemental carnitine
Cystinosis	None	None	Cysteamine, phosphate, potassium, vitamin D, alkali

substrate, but for these disorders, dietary supplement with synthetic medical food is not required. For instance, the treatment of galactosemia includes avoidance of dietary galactose that is primarily found as lactose (milk sugar) in dairy products. In infancy, this dietary restriction is easy to accomplish as the affected infant may be fed non–lactose-containing soy-based formula. As the child ages, however, avoidance of dairy products, especially in baked goods and processed foods, is more difficult. Parents and patient must be taught to read food labels and to contact manufacturers of prepared foods to determine whether food stuffs contain galactose. They should assume that all new foods contain galactose until proven otherwise and should be encouraged to seek other hidden sources of galactose in over-the-counter and prescription medications.

For some inborn errors of metabolism, the goal of nutritional therapy is to prevent the body's attempt to switch to alternative fuels. In defects of glycogenolysis (glycogen storage diseases), therapy attempts to prevent fasting with its potential for hypoglycemia. Frequent feedings during infancy, overnight enteral tube feedings, and after 1 year of age, the administration of uncooked cornstarch as a slowly released source of glucose are key to the prevention of hypoglycemia and preservation of liver function. In medium-chain acyl-CoA dehydrogenase deficiency (MCADD), the most common disorder of fatty acid oxidation, prevention of fasting eliminates the body's need to metabolize fat for energy, reduces the accumulation of toxic partially oxidized fatty acids, and reduces the risk of hypoglycemia.

Prevention of micronutrient deficiencies is another important aspect of nutritional therapy for inborn errors of metabolism. These deficiencies may be direct effects of certain inborn errors of metabolism or may be a consequence of dietary restrictions. For instance, the elimination of dairy products in low-protein diets or in the therapy of galactosemia increases the risk for calcium deficiency and osteoporosis. The lack of meat in low-protein diets also raises the risk of iron deficiency anemia and vitamin B_{12} deficiency. Zinc and selenium deficiencies are also potential problems in organic acidemias. Severe dietary fat restriction for disorders of fatty acid metabolism or the administration of nutritionally incomplete synthetic medical foods may lead to deficiencies of essential polyunsaturated fatty acids. Multivitamin preparations with minerals should be prescribed to all patients on altered diets who are not receiving most of their nutrition from vitamin-fortified medical foods. All patients on nutritional therapy must be periodically assessed for micronutrient deficiencies.

The successful implementation of a satisfactory diet during a period of relative health does not ensure that the diet is appropriate during periods of metabolic decompensation. Further restriction or even elimination of protein intake and increasing energy intake from other sources are used in many of the organic acidemias and aminoacidopathies during minor illnesses. Such manipulations are designed to compensate for the metabolic stress of illness with the attendant increased energy demands and propensity for muscle catabolism leading to an increased endogenous protein load. Families must be encouraged to contact health care professionals during these minor illnesses because the additionally restricted diet is nutritionally incomplete and may not be adequate to prevent further metabolic derangement. Illnesses that would normally be manageable at home in typical children may trigger the need for hospitalization in patients with inborn errors of metabolism. Intravenous hydration, nutrition, and, in some inborn errors of metabolism, administration of special medications play major roles in correcting the acutely decompensated state.

Other Therapeutic Modalities

Nutritional therapy, although important, is only one modality used for many of the disorders of metabolism. Pharmacologic agents, such as alkali to reduce metabolic acidosis, benzoate and phenylacetate to provide alternative metabolic sinks and to enhance alternative pathways for ammonia excretion in urea cycle disorders, vitamin D and phosphorus supplementation in hypophosphatemic rickets, and cysteamine to enhance cellular cystine release in the lysosomal storage disease cystinosis form another class of therapies.

For a few disorders, enzyme replacement therapies are available. In cystic fibrosis, exogenous digestive enzymes are given as enteral supplements to replace the deficient secretion of the exocrine pancreas. In Gaucher disease, a lysosomal storage disease, repetitive intravenous infusions of purified enzyme is used to reduce gradually the amount of stored glucocerebroside, reversing some of the pathophysiologic changes and improving the quality of life. Similar enzyme replacement strategies are now being developed on a research basis for a variety of lysosomal storage diseases including Pompe's disease, Fabry's disease, and several mucopolysaccharidoses.

Organ transplantation has been attempted in several inborn errors of metabolism. The most common transplanted organs are bone marrow and liver. Bone marrow or stem cell transplantation has been employed in many lysosomal storage disorders, such as the mucopolysaccharidoses, in attempts to provide a tissue that is capable of metabolizing the stored material. The efficacy of this therapy has been limited in disorders associated with accumulation of storage material in brain because of the inability to populate the central nervous system with enzyme-producing cells derived from the bone marrow graft. Liver transplantation has been performed in tyrosinemia type I to prevent hepatocellular carcinoma, a known complication of the disease, and to correct the primary defect. Liver transplantation has also been used successfully to cure urea cycle disorders, organic acidemias such as propionic acidemia, and maple syrup urine disease. Thus, a successful graft may have a profound effect upon the health of an individual with an IEM.

Permanent replacement of the mutant gene with the correct DNA sequence in the somatic cells of an individual with an IEM is a very attractive potential treatment modality for the future. Several research centers around the world are actively investigating gene therapy as a treatment for a wide variety of inborn errors of metabolism. Using contemporary DNA transfer methods, achieving stable, physiologically significant gene expression continues to be the major limiting factor in clinical gene therapy trials. Issues of treatment toxicity using certain gene transfer technologies have also slowed the progress of moving gene therapy from the lab to the clinical bedside. However, recent limited success using gene therapy to treat hemophilia and severe combined immunodeficiency in humans has provided renewed promise that gene therapy may be a viable treatment option for inborn errors of metabolism in the future.

Conclusion

Regardless of the specific therapy plan, successful treatment of inborn errors of metabolism requires a multidisciplinary approach to include the expertise of the metabolic physician, clinic nurse, nutritionist, genetic counselor, and social worker, backed up by a full complement of medical specialists and ancillary services. Education of the family, genetic counseling, and family support are all essential components. Genetic counseling teaches the family about the risks associated with future pregnancies and demystifies the concepts of defective genes being passed from asymptomatic carrier to affected child. The availability and implications of prenatal diagnosis for inborn errors of metabolism are also explained. Heterozygote detection and the ethical issues of sharing that information within a family or with future mates are other issues that may be addressed by counseling. Support for the family needs to ensure availability of coping mechanisms for dealing with a member who may have significant restrictions in developmental capacity or who has extraordinary needs for care. Educational goals include the successful implementation of the diet and the need for immediate intervention during metabolic crises.

Nutritional therapies will continue to be the cornerstone of the treatment for most inborn errors of metabolism in the foreseeable future. The lessons learned with several inborn errors of metabolism, especially phenylketonuria, emphasize the need for lifelong therapy in all these disorders. The necessity of "diet for life" has recently been affirmed by a National Institutes of Health Consensus Development Conference on the treatment of phenylketonuria.[6] This necessity therefore requires a long-term commitment from parents, patient, and health care professionals to implement and maintain the appropriate dietary therapy. The needs of an individual for energy, protein, and cofactors change with age and body mass. Therapeutic diets must be established and reevaluated at regular intervals to allow for the most normal growth and development possible. The adequacy of nutritional therapy must be assessed periodically through combinations of diet-diary review, food-list recollection, anthropometric measurement, and laboratory testing. Cooperation of the patient, family, and the metabolic clinic as a dedicated team throughout the life of the patient is essential for successful treatment of inborn errors of metabolism.

The American Academy of Pediatrics recommends that:

- All foods for special dietary use with accepted benefit for treatment of a medical condition should be reimbursed as a medical expense, provided the costs are over and above usual foods. Individual and family financial barriers to obtaining these foods should be removed.
- All states should enact legislation that would require health insurance policy providers to reimburse all foods for special dietary use with accepted medical benefit recommended by a physician to prevent death and serious disability or to foster normal growth and development.
- All expenses for medical equipment and medical supplies necessary for the delivery of foods for special dietary use should be reimbursed.
- Reimbursement for foods for special dietary use should be mandatory for the following:
  - any medical condition for which specific dietary components or the restriction of specific dietary components is necessary to treat a physical, physiologic, or pathologic condition resulting in inadequate nutrition.
  - an inherited metabolic disorder, including but not limited to disorders of carbohydrate, lipid, amino acid, nitrogen, vitamin and mineral metabolism.
  - a condition resulting in impairment of oral intake that affects normal development and growth.

American Academy of Pediatrics.
Reimbursement for foods for special dietary use.
Pediatrics. 2003;111:1117–1119.

References

1. Newborn screening: a blueprint for the future executive summary: newborn screening task force report. *Pediatrics*. 2000;106:386–388
2. Saudubray J, Charpentier C. Clinical phenotypes: diagnosis/algorithms. In: Scriver CR, Beaudet AL, Sly WS, Valle D, eds. *The Metabolic and Molecular Bases of Inherited Disease*. Vol 1. New York, NY: McGraw-Hill; 2001:1327–1406
3. Gilbert-Barness E, Barness LA. Approach to diagnosis of metabolic disease. In: *Metabolic Diseases: Foundations of Clinical Management, Genetics, and Pathology*. Vol 1. Natick, MA: Eaton Publishing; 2000:1–14
4. Winter S, Buist N. Clinical treatment guide to inborn errors of metabolism. *J Rare Dis*. 1998;IV:18–46
5. Institute of Medicine. *Dietary Reference Intakes: Applications in Dietary Assessment*. Washington, DC: National Academy Press; 2000
6. National Institutes of Health Consensus Development Program. Phenylketonuria, (PKU): screening and management. October 16–18, 2000. Available at: http://consensus.nih.gov/cons/113/113_intro.htm. Accessed March 7, 2003

30

Dietary Management of Diabetes Mellitus in Children

Type 1 Diabetes Mellitus

Introduction

Type 1 diabetes mellitus is a disorder caused by autoimmune destruction of beta cells resulting in hyperglycemia and, with complete absence of insulin, ketoacidosis. Treatment consists of insulin administration, diet, and exercise; teaching the patient to adjust these 3 components of the diabetes regimen is essential to attainment and maintenance of good metabolic control. It is recommended that children with diabetes eat at consistent times to coincide with peak action of the insulin preparation used and to adjust insulin doses based on food intake, physical activity, and blood glucose levels. Children using the insulin pump or insulin glargine have more flexibility in timing of meals, as there are no significant peaks in their insulin regimens. The Diabetes Control and Complications Trial (DCCT), a 5- to 9-year prospective, randomized multicenter trial of 1441 patients with type 1 diabetes mellitus, revealed that intensive therapy, defined as 3 or more insulin injections daily or the insulin pump; 4 or more blood glucose readings per day; frequent contact with the diabetes care team; and education in self-management, was superior to conventional treatment (1 to 2 BG tests daily, 1 to 2 insulin injections daily, quarterly clinic visits) in improving metabolic control. This improvement in metabolic control was associated with reduced onset and progression of microvascular disease.[1] Patients were predominantly young adults, but children aged 13 years and older were included. As the study conclusively showed that any improvement in glycemic control conferred a reduced risk of retinopathy and nephropathy, pediatric endocrinologists have intensified the care of children with diabetes in efforts to improve metabolic control. Subsequently, the United Kingdom Prospective Diabetes Study (UKPDS) of more than 5000 patients with type 2 diabetes mellitus followed prospectively for up to 16 years showed that normalizing blood pressure and serum lipids also reduced the risk of both microvascular and macrovascular disease.[2–4]

Metabolic control is monitored by HbA1C levels, a measure of average glycemia over a 2- to 3-month period and home blood glucose monitoring. It is important to remember, however, that widely fluctuating blood sugar levels may result in reasonable HbA1C values but are not indicative of good metabolic control. Also, a rapid turnover of red blood cells can lead to misleadingly low HbA1C levels. Erratic glucose values most often indicate inconsistent timing and amount of food.

In addition, weight and blood pressure should be checked every 3 months and hypertension aggressively treated. Lipid levels and renal status should be assessed annually; persistent microalbuminuria and hyperlipidemia require treatment and close monitoring.

Insulin

In an individual without diabetes, insulin is secreted into the portal vein in a continuous low-dose basal pattern to inhibit hepatic gluconeogenesis with a sevenfold to tenfold increased amount secreted in response to meals.[5] Insulin regimens have attempted to duplicate these patterns with the use of insulin analogues. By substituting amino acids on the beta chain of the insulin molecule, these insulin analogues have a more rapid onset (15 to 30 minutes) and shorter duration of action (2 to 3 hours) than the previous short-acting Regular insulin and were designed to time the action of each insulin dose to cover the expected rise in blood glucose after ingestion of food. Attempts to mimic basal and postprandial physiologic insulin secretion are made by various combinations of the aforementioned insulin analogues, short-acting Regular, intermediate-acting isophane insulin suspensions (Neutral Protamine Hagedorn [NPH]) or insulin zinc suspensions (Lente) and longer-lasting insulin zinc suspensions (Ultralente). Because a single daily injection is inadequate to cover glucose excursions with the normal pattern of meals and snacks, most children receive 2, 3, or more daily insulin injections, with variable amounts of an insulin analogue and/or Regular insulin mixed with NPH or Lente before breakfast and, commonly, before dinner as well. Many children are also given short-acting insulins before lunch, and many are also splitting their evening dose with short-acting insulin given before dinner and an intermediate-acting insulin given before bed. Studies have shown that there is reduced risk of nocturnal hypoglycemia if an insulin analogue rather than Regular insulin is used for the evening injection.[6] The average daily insulin dose for prepubertal children is about 0.6 to 1.0 U/kg body weight. Increased doses of up to 1.5 U/kg may be needed during puberty because of the insulin resistance caused by elevated growth hormone levels present during that time. Higher reported insulin requirements together with inadequate glycemic control strongly suggest missed injections. Overeating, as evidenced by excessive weight gain, may be another cause of high insulin doses and poor metabolic control.

Insulin glargine, a long-lasting insulin analogue with minimal peak of action, has a duration of action of 24 hours in most children, although younger children may have a shorter-lived effect. It serves as a basal insulin and can be given once a day with short-acting insulin analogues given before meals to cover the glycemic excursion of the meal. Young children may require 2 injections of the glargine insulin. This regimen allows for flexibility in timing of meals and avoids the need for snacks. By obtaining blood glucose levels before and after injection of the rapid-acting insulin analogue, the carbohydrate ratio (number of units of insulin given for a given amount of carbohydrates) and insulin sensitivity (number of units of insulin required to treat hyperglycemia adequately) can be determined. This method of intensive treatment requires at least 4 injections of insulin daily and monitoring of blood glucose before all meals, thus requiring more diabetes management to be done in the school setting. Increasing numbers of children are choosing to use this insulin regimen because of the increased flexibility in lifestyle it confers and ability to tailor administration to amount of food consumed.

Continuous subcutaneous infusion using an insulin pump is becoming increasingly common in the pediatric age group. Children receiving insulin using an insulin pump base their meal insulin bolus on the amount of carbohydrates consumed as well as ambient blood glucose levels. Thus, the bolus is often given after the meal when the actual consumption of carbohydrates is known.

Nutrition Overview

The philosophical approach to the nutrition component of diabetes treatment in children has varied widely from the "free diet," in which intake is unrestricted except for avoidance of foods rich in simple sugars (concentrated sweets), to a system in which all food is measured. The overriding principle, however, is that children with diabetes should eat the same nutritious food that the entire family should eat.

The overall goals of dietary treatment for children with diabetes are the provision of adequate nutrition and balanced calories for (1) normal growth and development, (2) prevention of hyperglycemia and hypoglycemia, (3) achievement of optimal serum lipid levels, and (4) for youth with type 2 diabetes to facilitate changes in eating and physical activity habits that reduce insulin resistance and improve metabolic control.[7] The dietary management of diabetes is one of the most challenging aspects of the diabetes regimen by both patients and physicians. Teaching dietary principles and meal planning is an important part of the education and ongoing care of a child with diabetes and is essential for effective home management.

Optimal glycemic control is achieved only if patients and their families can adequately balance food, insulin, and exercise. Consistent timing, portion sizes, and relative content of food is important for good glycemic control in patients using NPH insulin. The DCCT identified key nutritional behaviors that are associated with significantly improved blood glucose control. These behaviors include adherence to the recommended meal and snack plan, adjustment of insulin dose in response to meal size, adjustment of food or insulin in response to hyperglycemia, and avoidance of overtreatment of hypoglycemia.[8-10] Nutrition counseling, therefore, should emphasize these effective behaviors.

A team consisting of physicians, a nurse educator, a dietitian, and a mental health professional is optimal for effective disease management. Although not all children require the services of a mental health professional, psychological counseling is invaluable for dealing with children who are having difficulty coping with their disease or families who require behavior modification. To provide adequate nutrition, the dietitian must perform a thorough initial assessment of the nutritional needs of the child and the family.

This assessment includes the pattern of growth plotted on a standard growth curve, weight for height, or body mass index (BMI), and pattern of activity and food intake including meals and snacks. The family's living style and pattern of eating should be considered, and, as far as possible, a schedule of meals and snacks should be created to fit the child's usual times of eating and pattern of activity. In addition, the meal plans should take into account food preferences based on the family's ethnicity, religious beliefs, vegetarian eating habits, etc. After diagnosis, several sessions with the dietitian are usually needed for a full nutritional assessment, basic nutrition education, setting goals, and teaching the skills the family will need to plan appropriate meals and snacks. In addition, continued follow-up visits with a thorough review of dietary intake should occur annually and when the following occur:

- Unexplained failure to grow
- Unexplained recurrent hypoglycemia

- Unexplained recurrent hyperglycemia
- Excessive weight gain or loss
- Elevated glycohemoglobin
- Hypertension
- Hyperlipidemia
- Nephropathy
- Pregnancy, lactation

Meal Plans

To allow for changes in growth rate, activity, and development of different food preferences, the meal plans and patient's nutritional knowledge should be reviewed at least twice a year.[9] At each visit, growth increments in height and weight should be plotted on the appropriate standard curves.

The percentages of calories from fat, protein, and carbohydrate recommended for the diabetic meal plan differ from those currently found in the average American diet,[11-13] which tends to be higher in total fat than recommended. The 2001 American Diabetes Association (ADA) Position Statement for Nutrition Recommendations provides dietary guidelines for persons with diabetes.[14] Fat should provide up to 30% of the total calories with no more than one third of this as saturated fat. A protein intake of 10% to 20% of the total calories is recommended. Carbohydrates should contribute the remaining 50% of the total calories; the majority should be provided by sugars, starch, and fiber. These guidelines promote a healthy diet and are identical to those recommended for the population as a whole.[15]

In school, snacks should be provided to cover the peak action of insulin and vigorous activities such as physical education. The older child may manage without a morning snack as long as the lunch break is not late. A less active older child may not need an afternoon snack if dinner is relatively early. More dietary flexibility is gained with more frequent insulin injections and the newer insulin analogues.

Medical Nutrition Therapy Education

The approach to nutrition education is dependent on the education level and motivation of the family. Other factors that need consideration when designing the meal plan are school routines, weekend routines, who does the food shopping, who takes care of the child after school, and whether the family has any formal education in nutrition. Basic Nutrition Education focuses on providing basic information and goal setting in a manner that is simple, easy to under-

Table 30.1.
Nutrition Guidelines

Calories:

The caloric needs of the patient should be sufficient to attain and/or maintain a reasonable body weight in order to support normal growth and development for children and adolescents.
 	
Estimating Needs for Calories in Youth
1. Base calories on nutrition assessment
2. Validate calorie needs
  • Method 1: National Academy of Sciences/Recommended Dietary Allowances guidelines
  • Method 2: 1000 kcal for first year
    – Toddlers between 1 and 3 years, 40 kcal/in length
    – Add 100 kcal/y up to age 11
    – Girls 11 to 15 years, add 100 kcal or less per year after age 10
    – Girls >15 years, calculate as an adult
    – Boys 11 to 15 years, add 200 kcal/y after age 10
    – Boys >15 years, 23 kcal/lb very active
      • 18 kcal/lb usual
      • 16 kcal/lb sedentary
  • Method 3: 1000 kcal for first year
    – Add 125 kcal × age for boys
    – Add 100 kcal × age for girls
    – Up 20% more kcal for activity

Protein:
10% to 20% of calories. Should not exceed recommended dietary allowance for age (0.8 g/kg body weight per day) with evidence of nephropathy.
Fat:

Saturated fat <10% of daily calories, <7% with elevated low-density lipoprotein cholesterol
  Polyunsaturated fat up to 10% of total calories
  Remaining total fat varies with treatment goals
  ~30% for normal weight and normal lipids
  <30% for obesity, elevated low-density lipoprotein cholesterol
  Predominately monounsaturated fat
  Cholesterol <300 mg/d

Carbohydrate:
Difference after protein and fat goals have been met   Percentages varies with treatment goals

Table 30.1.
Nutrition Guidelines *(continued)*

Sweeteners:
Sucrose need not be restricted and must be counted in the meal plan as carbohydrate
Nutritive sweeteners have no advantage over sucrose and must be substituted as carbohydrate
Nonnutritive sweeteners approved by the Food and Drug Administration include saccharin, aspartame, acesulfame potassium, sucralose
Fiber:
20 to 35 g/d
Sodium:
<3000 mg/d
<2400 mg/d with mild to moderate hypertension
Vitamins/Minerals:
Same as general population

Holler HJ, Pators JG. *A Professional Guide to Management and Nutrition Education Resources.* Diabetes Medical Nutrition Therapy. Chicago, IL: The American Dietetic Association; 1998

stand, and adaptable to individual needs. Several excellent publications can help in this endeavor.

Nutrition Intervention

Nutrition intervention is defined as offering structure to the process of meal planning with information on specific nutrition or calorie content. This allows for more individualized meal planning. There are 3 recommended approaches: menu-based, exchange list, and carbohydrate counting.

The exchange list offers a structure on which to base food choices for consistent caloric intake and quantities of carbohydrate, fat, and protein.[16] The foods in each of 6 food groups (ie, starch, fruit, vegetable, milk, meat, and fat) have relatively consistent amounts of carbohydrate, fat, and protein. This approach serves as an excellent educational tool.

Carbohydrate counting has received renewed attention since it was used in the DCCT trials. Patients enjoy the flexibility it provides, and it has become the preferred nutrition intervention for determining insulin dosing at mealtimes. This simple approach focuses on determining the number of grams of carbohydrate in the diet (ie, starch, fruit, starchy vegetables, and milk).[17] The rationale for carbohydrate counting is that postprandial hyperglycemia is largely due to the amount of carbohydrate in a given meal. Meals containing more than the usual amount of carbohydrate can be covered by using extra insulin.

Table 30.2
Resources for Nutrition Education and Intervention

EDUCATION	
General Nutrition:	Dietary Guidelines for Americans Guide to Good Eating Food Guide Pyramid
National Institutes of Health/NIDDK	
Diabetes Nutrition:	First Step in Diabetes Meal Planning Healthy Food Choices Healthy Eating Single-Topic Diabetes Resources
Resources:	
American Diabetes Association, Alexandria, VA, www.diabetes.org	
American Dietetic Association, Chicago, IL, www.eatright.org	
MEDICAL NUTRITION THERAPY INTERVENTION	
Menu-based:	Month of Meals 1, 2, 3, 4, and 5
American Diabetes Association	
Exchange list:	Healthy Food Choices Exchange Lists for Meal Planning
Resources:	
American Diabetes Association, American Dietetic Association Exchange Lists for Meal Planning: Alexandria, VA. The American Diabetes Association and Chicago, IL: American Dietetic Association; 1986.	
Counting:	Carbohydrate Counting Levels 1, 2, and 3 Calorie Counting and Fat Gram Counting
Resource:	
Calorie Counting and Fat gram: American Diabetes Association. American Dietetic Association.	

For example, if a child is going to attend a class party and will eat more carbohydrate than usual, he or she could administer additional rapid-acting insulin to prevent postprandial hyperglycemia. (Table 30.3).

When used in conjunction with postprandial blood glucose monitoring, carbohydrate counting offers patients more freedom to choose the type and amount of food they eat. If the postprandial readings are out of range, patients can choose to (1) increase the dose of insulin analogue for a given carbohydrate consumption, (2) increase exercise, or (3) reduce the amount of carbohydrates at the same meal the next day.

Table 30. 3.
Four-Step Process of Medical Nutrition Therapy: Illustration of Carbohydrate Counting

Step 1: Assessment
Calculate usual eating habits by evaluating 24-hr recall and food history. Determine usual carbohydrate intake for each meal and snack. Evaluate other factors that may affect diabetes and nutritional health (eg, timing of meals,timing and amount of exercise, frequency and treatment of hypoglycemia, dining out). Assess readiness to change.
Step 2: Goal setting
Determine the diet and lifestyle changes patient is willing to make. Determine clinical or metabolic outcomes (target HbA1C, fasting BS target lipids).
Step 3: Intervention
Level 1: Practice identifying carbohydrate foods. Recognize 15-g carbohydrate portion of foods. Demonstrate measuring skills using scale, cups, and spoons. Discuss plan for keeping protein consistent and fat intake low to moderate. Practice label-reading skills to obtain nutrition information. Plan a sample meal.
Level 2: Practice reading food records, blood glucose readings, physical activity to interpret blood glucose patterns. Determine appropriate actions or strategies, including adjustment of carbohydrates to achieve blood glucose goals.
Level 3: Calculate carbohydrate-insulin ratio by dividing the total grams of carbohydrate usually consumed for each meal by the number of units of short-acting insulin taken before that meal. (This is appropriate for patients being treated with insulin pumps or multiple daily injections.)
Demonstrate how both carbohydrate intake and insulin can be adjusted to fine-tune blood glucose levels.
Step 4: Evaluation
Assess effect of intervention by conducting process, outcome, and impact evaluations. Continuously collect data on progress toward behavioral goals and changes in medical status (HbA1cc, weight, blood pressure, lipids) and risk factor reduction (decrease in hypoglycemia, increase in exercise).

Maryniuk MD. *Medical Nutrition Therapy in Diabetes: Clinical Guidelines for Primary Care Physicians.* New York, NY: Dekker; 2000

Carbohydrate counting does not take into account the protein and fat content of meals, making it easy to ignore good nutrition if only carbohydrate counting is emphasized during nutritional counseling. It is essential to discuss the importance of a healthy, well-balanced diet in any discussion of nutrition.

The Nutrition Facts label now available on packaged foods has made the carbohydrate counting approach to nutrition therapy more practical and allows the patient to have more flexibility in food choices. As all carbohydrates are broken down to simple sugars, families are taught to ignore the sugar content per serving. Label reading should concentrate on serving size, calories, and total carbohydrates. "Sugar" is defined as the sum of all monosaccharides and disaccharides contained in a defined serving (glucose, fructose, lactose, and maltose) and added sucrose, high fructose, corn syrup, honey, and fruit juice concentrate. Many times, patients and families will read the sugar content and not total carbohydrate and wonder why their blood sugars are so high after a meal. For example, Fritos have no "sugar" on the label, but contain 29 g of carbohydrate in a serving. The expanded food choices available with carbohydrate counting eliminate the "forbidden food" philosophy of the past. However, serving sizes are very important. A cup of Raisin Bran cereal has 29 g of carbohydrate, whereas a cup of Cheerios has only 13 g. Both serving sizes are the same, but the carbohydrate content is quite different and will have an effect on the postprandial blood sugars.

Glycemic index refers to the degree blood glucose increases following ingestion of a single food. A number of factors influence glycemic responses to food, including the amount of carbohydrate, type of sugar (glucose, fructose, sucrose, lactose), nature of starch (amylase, amylopectin, resistant starch), cooking and food processing (degree of starch gelantinization, particle size, cellular form), food form, and other food components such as fat and natural substances that slow digestion (lectins, phytates, tannins, and starch-protein and starch-lipid combinations). Fasting and preprandial glucose concentrations, the severity of glucose intolerance and second meal, or lente effect of carbohydrate are other factors affecting glycemic response to foods.

Studies in patients with type 1 diabetes and patients with type 2 diabetes show that ingestion of a variety of starches or sucrose, both acutely and for up to 6 weeks, produced no significant difference in glycemic response if the amount of carbohydrate was similar. Therefore, the total amount of carbohydrate in meals and snacks will be more important than the source.[8] The use of the glycemic index is controversial; classification of carbohydrates as "simple" or "complex" is of little use in predicting glycemic index as foods are rarely eaten alone. The glycemic index is influenced by starch structure (amylose vs amylopectin), fiber content, food processing, physical structure of the food, and other macronutrients in the meal.[16,17] Researchers suggest that fat or protein in combination with carbohydrate reduces the postprandial glycemic rise because of delayed food absorption. Thus, although carbohydrates have different glycemic responses, the data reveal no clear benefits from low versus high glycemic index diets consumed by patients with diabetes. More research is needed in this area as a number of studies are limited and results are conflicting.[18,19]

Carbohydrate

For children receiving NPH insulin twice daily, carbohydrate intake should be distributed throughout the day, considering the child's pattern of activity. Consistency in the timing and amount of ingested carbohydrate for each meal and snack allows for a more predictable glycemic response to injected insulin. Children using insulin pumps or glargine insulin have more flexibility in timing and amount of ingested carbohydrate, as rapid-acting insulin given immediately before a meal or carbohydrate-containing snack in a dose dependent on the carbohydrate content of that meal. For a younger child, the distribution of carbohydrates could be as follows: breakfast 20%, mid-morning snack 10%, lunch 20%, mid-afternoon snack 10%, dinner 30%, and bedtime snack 10%.

If the family becomes comfortable knowing which foods are carbohydrates and the effect on the child's blood sugars, the multiple special events in a child's life (school picnics, birthday parties, eating outside the home, holidays) can proceed smoothly with adjustment of insulin dose to cover extra carbohydrate intake. The more the family is able to determine how to maintain glycemic control by knowledge of how to match food choices with adjustments of insulin and activity, the more freedom from restriction the child will have.

Fat

Dietary fat intake requires attention because of the increased risk for cardiovascular disease in persons with diabetes.[20,21] The UKPDS trial showed that a decrease in total or low-density lipoprotein (LDL) cholesterol of 1 mmol/L reduced the risk of any diabetes-related endpoint (myocardial infarction, angina, heart failure, stroke, renal failure, amputation, or retinopathy requiring photocoagulation) by 15% and 18% respectively. An increase in high-density lipoprotein cholesterol of 0.1 mmol/L reduced the risk by 5%. The Bogolusa Heart Study, a long-term longitudinal study of individuals in a small parish in Louisiana, found that 8% of children who died from accident or violence between the ages of 2 and 15 years already had fibrous plaques in their coronary arteries and 50% had fatty streaks in their coronary arteries. The atherosclerotic lesions correlated with triglycerides and LDL and total cholesterol levels.[21] Thus, fat intake and lipid levels must be monitored throughout childhood. For infants and children younger than 2 years, dietary fat should not be restricted. For those older than 2 years, the guidelines from the pediatric panel of the National Cholesterol Education Program (NCEP) should be followed.

No more than 30% of total calories should come from fat and no more than 10% should be saturated fat. Monitoring of blood lipid levels should follow the ADA guidelines, in which it is recommended that total cholesterol and LDL be maintained at levels less than 170 mg/dL and 100 mg/dL, respectively.[22] If total cholesterol is elevated, the diabetes regimen and dietary intake should both be reevaluated. Inadequate metabolic control is the predominant cause of hyperlipidemia in type 1 diabetes. However, if attempts at dietary modification, increase in exercise, and intensification of the diabetes regimen fail to normalize serum lipids, pharmacologic therapy may be indicated. Autoimmune hypothyroidism occurs more commonly in children with diabetes and should be excluded as a cause of an elevated blood cholesterol level.

Protein

Protein consumption by Americans generally exceeds the recommended dietary allowance. Protein intake should be similar to that recommended for the general population (10% to 20% of daily calorie intake). Lower intakes of protein should be considered in patients with overt nephropathy as several small studies have shown that a protein diet of 0.7 g/kg/d slows the rate of fall of glomerular filtration rate (GFR). However, the Modified Diet in a Renal Disease study failed to show a benefit of protein restriction. Only a minority (3%) of patients in that study, however, had diabetes, and none had type 1 disease.[23] Although there is a lack of clear-cut evidence upon which to base a recommendation, the ADA has issued a consensus recommendation that patients with nephropathy be prescribed a protein intake of 0.8 mg/kg/d. It further suggests that when the GFR begins to decline, further restriction of protein to 0.6 mg/kg/d be initiated in selected patients.[24]

- Approximately 50% to 60% of the dietary protein is converted to glucose and released into the bloodstream. This process occurs between 2 to 5 hours following the meal/snack.
- Protein-rich foods include meat, fish, poultry, eggs, peanut butter, cheese, and meat alternatives.
- A protein-rich food is recommended at lunch.

Sweeteners

Sucrose is the most widely used sweetener, but its use had been limited in children with diabetes because of concern it would cause elevated blood glucose levels. Recent studies, however, do not show an adverse effect of usual amounts of dietary sucrose on glycemic control in type 1 or type 2 diabetes.[25] Sucrose is present in many prepared foods and must be counted in the tally of carbohydrates. The nutritive sweeteners, fructose, and other sugars have no significant advantage over sucrose. Recent data suggest that high fructose intake may adversely impact the lipid profile. Sorbitol and other sugar alcohols have lower glycemic response than sucrose but may have a laxative effect when large amounts are ingested. The nonnutritive sweeteners, aspartame, saccharine, and asulfame K, do not affect blood glucose levels and are acceptable alternatives for children with diabetes.

Fiber

The addition of fiber to reduce the glycemic effect of food does not appear to be significant enough to recommend intake beyond that recommended for the general population. The average daily fiber intake among children ranges from 11.2 g (3 to 5 years old) to 14.0 g (6 to 11 years old). These levels have remained unchanged since 1976. Although ideal dietary intake has not been scientifically determined, current recommendations for children older than 2 years is to increase dietary fiber intake to an amount equal to their age in years plus 5 g/d to maximum of age and 10 g until the adult recommendation of 25 to 35 g daily dietary fiber intake recommended in adults. On a Nutrition Facts food label, the grams of fiber are included in the total grams of carbohydrate. On a practical basis, from total carbohydrates, the only time fiber grams need to be subtracted is with cereals containing 5 g or more of insoluble fiber per serving.[26]

In another example, sugar alcohols are also included in the total grams of carbohydrate on the Nutrition Facts panel. Sugar alcohols are calculated as having half the calories (2 kcal/g) of most other carbohydrates (4 kcal/g). Specific sugar alcohol values approved by the FDA include:

- Hydrogenated starch hydrolysate (HSH): 3/g
- Isomalt: 2 g
- Maltilol: 3 g
- Mannitol: 1.6 g
- Sorbitol: 2.6 g
- Xylitol: 2.4 g

Exercise

Children with diabetes are encouraged to exercise regularly. However, to avoid hypoglycemia, families must be taught to monitor blood glucose levels before exercise and to give appropriate snacks based on blood glucose value and intensity of exercise (Table 30.4). Carbohydrate should always be ingested if blood glucose is less than 100 mg/dL before exercise.

Table 30.4.
Sample Nutrition Guidelines for Exercise

Type of Activity	If Blood Sugar Prior to Activity Is:	Then Eat the Following Carbohydrates Before Activity:
Short duration (less than 30 minutes	Less than 100 Greater than 100	15 g carbohydrate No carbohydrate necessary
Moderate duration (1 hour)	Less than 100 100–180 180–240	25–50 g carbohydrates plus protein source 15 g carbohydrate No carbohydrate necessary
Strenuous (1–2 hours)	Less than 100 100–180 180–240	50 g of carbohydrate Plus protein source 15 g carbohydrate
Snack choices for physical activity		
15 g carbohydrates:		One 4-oz juice box 1 c Gatorade 1 sliced orange or apple 1 small box raisins 6 saltines 1 c light yogurt 1/2 c dry cereal
30 g carbohydrates:		1 cereal bar One 8-oz juice box 2 slices bread 1 small bagel
45–50 g carbohydrates plus protein:		1 sports nutrition bar 1 package of 6 cheese or peanut butter sandwich crackers plus 4 oz juice
Protein sources:		Peanut butter Sliced or string cheese Lunch meat Egg Peanuts, walnuts, or almonds

Different Stages for Different Phases

The age and developmental stage of the child should be considered when determining which meal plan to use. It is much easier to design the insulin regimen around the patient's typical lifestyle than it is to change behaviors to match the insulin. Elementary-aged children are more likely to have predictable lifestyles, whereas middle- and high-school adolescents might not. Most pediatric diabetes educators prefer to start with a structured meal plan and later teach a more flexible approach that is dependent on active decision making. Continuous assessment with frequent contact should be made. Changes in growth and development, school routines, seasonal sports, and child care arrangements may necessitate a change in meal plans.

Preschool children often have inconsistent food intake and activity. If the child has eaten poorly or activity is prolonged, small snacks may be offered. Food battles should be avoided and parents may need assistance in developing the skills needed to deal with those instances in which the child will not cooperate. Children who have erratic eating patterns may receive the rapidly acting insulin analogues after the meal to decrease the fear of acute hypoglycemia if the child refuses to eat. The dose of insulin to be given is based on the amount of food consumed.

Children in the early grades of school need constructive supervision of meal and snack times until they are able to understand food groups and select appropriate foods and portion sizes. As adolescents become increasingly independent, education should be geared toward teaching them to take responsibility for label reading and choosing appropriate foods.[3] They should be taught that extra food (eg, pizza parties) can be handled with extra rapid acting insulin. During the early adolescent years, compliance is often challenged by wanting to fit in and be like everybody else, not wanting people to know they have special needs, and not wanting to snack for fear of gaining weight.

Issues of Weight Loss and Weight Gain

Weight loss, poor growth, and delayed sexual maturation in children with type 1 diabetes is most often associated with poor metabolic control. Inadequate insulin dose leads to excessive glycosuria with caloric loss. However, poor weight gain may also be associated with inadequate energy intake because of rigorous adherence to an outgrown meal plan or inappropriate fat restriction in a young child. Delayed linear growth is associated with prolonged inadequate control of diabetes, but hypothyroidism should be excluded.

Eating disorders are more common in adolescents with diabetes mellitus than in the general population.[27,28] Bulimia is most common, and may be associated with deliberate limitation of the insulin dose resulting in weight loss and glycosuria ("insulin purging"), erratic blood glucose levels, diabetes, fluctuating weight, and a very elevated level of glycosylated hemoglobin. Anorexia nervosa, with limitation of food intake and insulin, may manifest as recurrent episodes of severe and unexplained hypoglycemia, with the unstable management of diabetes masked by acceptable glycosylated hemoglobin levels. Clinicians should be aware of the manifestations of eating disorders in adolescents with type 1 diabetes mellitus.

"Overweight" occurs more readily in children with diabetes. Rapid weight gain is normal just after starting treatment for diabetes, but it should slow to a normal rate after the appropriate weight for the child is regained. Children may receive excess insulin if repeated increases in the insulin dose are made in response to hyperglycemia without investigating the cause or modifying the food intake. Increased weight gain was noted during intensified insulin management in young adults during the DCCT study, but weight gain may be controlled by careful attention to dietary management.[29] Many children with a history of low blood sugar gain weight because they eat in an attempt to prevent hypoglycemia. When weight reduction is necessary, the treatment program for a child with diabetes must include closely integrated efforts of the physician, dietitian, diabetes educator, and mental health professional to balance decreased food and insulin needs.

Treatment of Hypoglycemia

Hypoglycemia commonly occurs with decreased food intake or with increased physical activity. The goal of treatment is to achieve rapid normalization of blood sugar without use of excess food and resultant hyperglycemia.

Low blood sugars should initially be treated with simple sugar (juice, glucose tablets). This will be rapidly absorbed and raise the blood glucose level in 10 to 15 minutes. In general, 15 g of carbohydrate will raise the blood glucose approximately 30 mg/dL. The blood glucose should again be checked 10 to 15 minutes after treatment. If the glucose level is less than 80 mg/dL, another 15 g of carbohydrate should be given and blood glucose again checked 15 minutes later. Once the blood glucose is greater than 80 mg/dL, the child should be given 15 g of carbohydrate in a protein snack (Table 30.5) or fed his meal or snack if it is scheduled to be given within 30 to 60 minutes. This regimen

Table 30.5.
Sources of 15 g of Carbohydrate*

Fluids containing 10–15 g carbohydrates:
1 c Gatorade
1 c milk (any kind)
1/2 c fruit juice
1/2 c regular soft drink
Foods containing 10–15 g carbohydrates:
1/2 c regular Jello
1/2 c cooked cereal
1/2 c mashed potatoes
1/2 c regular ice cream
1 popsicle
6 saltines
6 vanilla wafers
3 graham crackers
1 slice bread or toast

*FDA *Diet Manual 2000 Edition Diabetes Mellitus* CI 36.

allows for more rapid correction of hypoglycemia and avoids the overfeeding that usually occurs because of persistence of symptoms despite normalization of blood glucose.

Treatment of Hyperglycemia

The insulin analogues have made treatment of acute hyperglycemia feasible. Administration of an insulin analogue according to a predetermined formula with measurement of blood glucose before and 2 hours after insulin injection will allow for assessment of adequacy of dosing. The post-injection blood glucose should be in the 100 to 150 mg/dL range.

Cow Milk and Type 1 Diabetes

Type 1 diabetes occurs in genetically susceptible individuals as the endpoint of an immunologically mediated attack on pancreatic beta cells. The autoimmune process is thought to be triggered by environmental factors. Once immune destruction of the beta cells has begun, there is release of pancreatic beta cell antigens associated with antibody production to these islet antigens. These antibodies (islet cell antibodies [ICA], insulin autoantibodies [IAA], antibodies to glutamic acid decarboxylase [GAD], and tyrosine decarboxylase [IA-2]) are present for months to several years before clinical onset of disease and have been used to predict disease in both high-risk and low-risk populations. In children especially, the presence of these autoantibodies are predictive of later onset of diabetes. Cow milk protein contains a 17-amino acid fragment of bovine serum albumin (ABBOS), which has structural similarities to an islet autoantigen protein (ICA 69). Because of this structural similarity, some investigators have hypothesized that early introduction of cow milk would result in absorption of the intact protein before gut maturation, thus immunizing the infant and directing an immune response to the islets through molecular mimicry. In both the rat and the mouse model for type 1 diabetes, semi-purified diets composed of simple sugars and hydrolyzed casein routinely retards the development of diabetes.[30] Over the past 17 years, there have been a plethora of articles, mainly case-controlled epidemiological surveys, either supporting or challenging the cow milk hypothesis. The extensive meta analysis of 13 such studies demonstrated a weak but statistically significant association (odds ratio 1.5) between type 1 diabetes and both the shortened period of breastfeeding and cow milk exposure before 3 to 4 months of age.[31] Others found no difference in exposure to milk or foods containing cow milk up to 6 months of age in 18 children who were positive for beta cell autoimmunity compared to children who had no evidence of autoimmunity.[28] Cow milk consumption has been shown to be correlated with type 1 diabetes in some countries, but this is not consistent. Sardinia has the second highest incidence rates of diabetes in Europe, after Finland, yet cow milk ingestion is less than half that in Finland. Sera from patients with childhood and adult onset type 1 diabetes do not have an increased incidence of antibodies to bovine serum albumin (BSA) at diagnosis, and BSA antibodies are not increased in high-risk patients who later developed type 1 diabetes.[32,33] Because of these conflicting data, the relationship between type 1 diabetes and early ingestion of cow milk formula is unclear. Long-term prospective double-blind clinical trials, such as are currently being performed in Finland and Canada, are necessary for resolution of this issue. Current data are too preliminary and not conclusive.

Type 2 Diabetes Mellitus

Since 1979, when type 2 diabetes was first reported in the Pima Indian population, the prevalence of type 2 diabetes in the pediatric age group has increased markedly. In the initial report, 9 of 1000 15- to 24-year-olds had type 2 diabetes. None were reported younger than 15 years of age.[34] By the 1990s, the prevalence of type 2 diabetes in the 15- to 19-year age group had increased to 51 of 1000 with a prevalence rate of 22 of 1000 in the 10- to 14-year-old Pima Indian population. Thirteen of 3000 American children aged 12 to 19 years studied between 1988 and 1994 were identified as having diabetes. This provided a national prevalence estimate for all types of diabetes of 4.1 per 1000 and suggested that approximately 30% of people with diabetes in this age group have type 2 disease.[35] This is comparable to the experience of many pediatric diabetes clinics.

The increased incidence of type 2 diabetes in childhood parallels the increased incidence of obesity. Since 1980, the incidence of type 2 diabetes mellitus has increased by 33% in African Americans and by 11% in white adults. During the same period, overweight has increased from 25% to 48% in adults.[36] Since 1970, the rate of obesity in childhood has doubled with 22% of children being obese in 1990.

The initial problem in children with type 2 diabetes mellitus is insulin resistance. This is influenced by (1) pubertal stage—insulin sensitivity of adolescents in general is approximately 30% lower than that of either pre-adolescents or adults, likely because of increased activity of the growth hormone axis[37]; (2) family history—prepubertal children with a family history of type 2 diabetes are more insulin resistant than prepubertal children without a family history when data are controlled for body mass index[38]; (3) ethnicity—insulin sensitivity is approximately 35% to 40% lower in African American adolescents than in white peers matched for age, gender, weight, and body composition.[39] Native Americans and Mexican Americans are also at high risk; and (4) adiposity—total adiposity explains 55% of the variance in insulin sensitivity.[40] Obese children have hyperinsulinism and a 40% decrease in insulin-stimulated glucose metabolism compared with children who are not obese. The inverse relationship between insulin sensitivity and abdominal fat is greater for visceral than for abdominal subcutaneous fat.[34] The insulin resistance is reflected by elevated fasting insulin levels followed by impaired insulin secretion with inadequate first phase stimulated insulin release resulting in postprandial hyperglycemia. Subsequent blunting of second-phase insulin release causes fasting hyperglycemia.[41] Because pediatric endocrinologists are relative newcomers to dealing with type 2 diabetes mellitus, there are no longitudinal studies on the management of this disease in children. Guidelines have therefore been extrapolated from those for adults.[42] As with type 2 diabetes in adults, the cornerstone of treatment is lifestyle modification, including dietary changes and increased exercise. Implementation of such measures is extremely challenging and requires involvement of the whole family. Longstanding habits and attitudes toward eating and exercise must be recognized and changed. Dietary modifications are most likely to be effective when kept simple and attainable. It is recommended that patients make 2 to 3 basic changes that are not too demanding. Examples include switching from regular to diet soda and decreasing the amount of high-calorie juices and whole milk in the diet. It is important to stress to patients that incremental weight loss could result in significantly improved insulin sensitivity and blood pressure. A reasonable weight loss goal is 3 lbs per month. Increased exercise and a diet with moderate calorie restriction (eg, 500 to 1000 calories below usual daily intake) should be adequate to produce gradual weight loss. Exercise, too, must be easily incorporated into the patient's and family's lifestyle. Physical activity need not involve organized sports. It may involve walking or bicycling to school and using the stairs instead of the elevator. It has been recommended that patients exercise for at least 30 minutes daily. All family members should adopt the same healthy eating patterns and exercise together or individually.

Treatment of type 2 diabetes in children is based on symptoms at diagnosis. Asymptomatic children who are diagnosed following a routine examination or family testing can be treated with non-pharmacologic means. These children are instructed to monitor their blood glucose levels at least twice per day (before breakfast and 2 hours after dinner). If dietary modification and lifestyle changes are unsuccessful in achieving fasting plasma glucose levels of 120 mg/dL and hemoglobin A1C levels of 7% or less, pharmacotherapy is necessary. In addition, monitoring and aggressive treatment of blood pressure and hyperlipidemia, co-morbidities associated with insulin resistance, are an essential part of the care of patients with type 2 diabetes.

Prevention

Although we cannot affect the non-modifiable factors that predispose to type 2 diabetes mellitus (ethnicity, gender, and family history), it is essential that all children and parents be educated about the need for physical activity and healthy diet so that we can improve factors that are modifiable in high-risk children. Lifestyle modification is essential for prevention of type 2 diabetes. The Diabetes Prevention Program showed that exercise of 25 minutes daily for 6 days per week combined with decreased calorie intake was more effective in preventing development of type 2 diabetes in adults with impaired glucose tolerance than use of Metformin. Both were more effective than placebo or routine care. Thus, it is important to involve the entire family in modifying behavior to increase exercise and encourage healthy eating habits as soon as we notice a trend toward overweight on the child's growth curve.[43] If we are unable to curb the increasing incidence of obesity and, thus, of insulin resistance and type 2 diabetes mellitus in children, we will be faced with a tremendous public health problem.

References

1. The Diabetes Control and Complications Trial Research Group. The effect of intensive treatment of diabetes on the development and progression of long-term complications in insulin-dependent diabetes mellitus. *N Engl J Med*. 1993; 329:977–986

2. UK Prospective Diabetes Study Group. Tight blood pressure control and risk of macrovascular and microvascular complication in type 2 diabetes: UKPDS 38. *BMJ*. 1998;317:703–713

3. Cull CA, Mehta Z, Stratton IM, Manley SE, Neil A, Holman RR. Association of lipid levels over time with clinical outcomes in patients with type 2 diabetes in the UKPDS [abstract]. *Diabetes*. 2000;49(suppl):1110

4. Haffner SM, Alexander CM, Cook TJ, et al. Reduced coronary events in simvastatin-treated patients with coronary heart disease and diabetes or impaired fasting glucose levels: subgroup analyses in the Scandinavian Simvastatin Survival Study. *Arch Intern Med*. 1999,59:2661–2667

5. Lebovitz HE. Insulin secretagogues, old and new. *Diabetes Rev*. 1999;7:139–153

6. Ferguson SC, Strachan MWJ, Janes J, Frier BM. Insulin lispro lowers the incidence of severe hypoglycemia, without a detrimental effect on glycemic control, in those individuals with type 1 diabetes at high risk of severe hypoglycemia [abstract]. *Diabetes*. 1999;48(suppl):A526

7. American Diabetes Association Position Statement. Evidence based nutrition principles and recommendations for the treatment and prevention of diabetes and related complications. *Diabetes Care*. 2002;25(suppl):550–560

8. Delahanty LM, Halford BN. The role of diet behaviors in achieving improved glycemic control in intensely treated patients in the Diabetes Control and Complications Trial. *Diabetes Care*. 1993;16:1453–1458

9. Laredo R. Carbohydrate counting for children and adolescents. *Diabetes Spectrum*. 2000;13:150

10. Anderson EJ, Richardson M, Castle G, et al. Nutrition interventions for intensive therapy in the Diabetes Control and Complications Trial. *J Am Diet Assoc*. 1993; 93:768–772

11. Position of the American Dietetic Association: child and adolescent food and nutrition programs. *J Am Diet Assoc*. 1996;96:913–917

12. Wildey MB, Pampalone SZ, Pelletier RL, Zire MM, Elder JP, Sallis JF. Fat and sugar levels are high in snacks purchased from student stores in middle schools. *J Am Diet Assoc*. 2000;100:319–322

13. The obesity epidemic: a mandate for a multidisciplinary approach. *J Am Diet Assoc.* 1998;98:(10 suppl 2):S1–S61

14. American Diabetes Association. Nutrition recommendations and principles for people with diabetes mellitus. *Diabetes Care.* 2001;24:S44–S47

15. US Department of Agriculture. *Nutrition and Your Health: Dietary Guidelines for Americans.* 3rd ed. Washington, DC: US Department of Health and Human Services; 1990

16. American Diabetes Association and American Dietetic Association. *Exchange Lists for Meal Planning.* Alexandria, VA: American Diabetes Association and Chicago, IL: American Dietetic Association; 1986

17. Maryniuk MD. Chapter 15: Medical nutrition therapy in diabetes. In: *Clinical Guidelines for Primary Care Physicians.* New York, NY: Dekker; 2000

18. Morris KL, Zemel MB. Glycemic index, cardiovascular disease, and obesity. *Nutr Rev.* 1999;57:273–276

19. Brand Miller JC, Colagiuri S, Foster-Powell K. The glycemic index is easy and works in practice. *Diabetes Care.* 1997;20:1628–1629

20. Cull CA, Mehta Z, Stratton IM, Manley SE, Neil A, Holman RR. Association of lipid levels over time with clinical outcomes in patients with type 2 diabetes in the UKPDS [abstract]. *Diabetes.* 2000;49(suppl):A267

21. Berenson GS, Srinivasin SR, Weihang B, Newman WP III, Tracy RE, Walligney WA. Association between multiple cardiovascular risk factors and atherosclerosis in children and young adults. *N Engl J Med.* 1998;338:1650–1656

22. American Diabetes Association. Management of dyslipidemia in adults with diabetes. *Diabetes Care.* 2002;25(suppl):574–577

23. Levey AS, Adler S, Caggiula AW, et al. Effects of dietary protein restriction on the progression of advanced renal disease in the Modification of Diet in Renal Disease Study. *Am J Kidney Dis.* 1996;27:652–663

24. American Diabetes Association. Diabetic nephropathy (Position Statement). *Diabetes Care.* 2002;25(suppl):S85–S89

25. American Diabetes Association. Evidence-based nutrition principles and recommendations for the treatment and prevention of diabetes and related complications. *Diabetes Care.* 2002;25(suppl):S50–S60

26. Williams CL. Importance of dietary fiber in childhood. *J Am Diet Assoc.* 1995;95: 1140–1149

27. Rodin GM, Daneman D. Eating disorders and IDDM. A problematic association. *Diabetes Care.* 1992;15:1402–1412

28. Meltzer LJ, Johnson SB, Prine JM, Banks RA, Desrosiers PM, Silverstein JH. Disordered eating, body mass, and glycemic control in adolescents with type I diabetes. *Diabetes Care.* 2001;24:678–682

29. Diabetes Control and Complications Trial Research Group. Weight gain associated with intensive therapy in the Diabetes Control and Complications Trial. *Diabetes Care.* 1988;11:567–573

30. Schatz DA, Maclaren NK. Cow's milk and insulin-dependent diabetes mellitus. Innocent until proven guilty. *JAMA*. 1996;276:647–648

31. Gerstein HC. Cow's milk exposure and type 1 diabetes mellitus. A critical overview of the clinical literature. *Diabetes Care*. 1994;17:13–19

32. Norris JM, Beaty B, Klingensmith G, et al. Lack of association between early exposure to cow's milk protein and beta-cell autoimmunity. *JAMA*. 1996;276:609–614

33. Atkinson MA, Bowman MA, Kao KJ, et al. Lack of immune responsiveness to bovine serum albumin in insulin-dependent diabetes. *N Engl J Med*. 1993;329:1853–1858

34. Savage PJ, Bennett PH, Senter RG, Miller M. High prevalence of diabetes in young Pima Indians: evidence of phenotypic variation in a genetically isolated population. *Diabetes*. 1979;28:937–942

35. Fagot-Campagna A, Pettitt DJ, Engelgau MM, et al. Type 2 diabetes among North American children and adolescents: an epidemiologic review and a public health perspective. *J Pediatr*. 2000;136:664–672

36. Troiano RP, Flegal KM. Overweight children and adolescents: description epidemiology, and demographics. *Pediatrics*. 1998;101:497–504

37. Arslanian SA, Kalhan SC. Correlations between the fatty acid and glucose metabolism. Potential explanation of insulin resistance of puberty. *Diabetes*. 1994;43: 908–914

38. Danadian K, Balasekaran G, Lewy V, Meza MP, Robertson R, Arslanian SA. Insulin sensitivity in African-American children with and without a family history of type 2 diabetes. *Diabetes Care*. 1999; 22:1325–1329

39. Arslanian S. Insulin secretion and sensitivity in healthy African-American vs American white children. *Clin Pediatr (Phila)*. 1998;37:81–88

40. Caprio S, Tamborlane WV. Metabolic impact of obesity in childhood. *Endocrinol Metab Clin North Am*. 1999;28:731–747

41. Martin MM, Martin LA. Obesity, hyperinsulinism, and diabetes mellitus in childhood. *J Pediatr*. 1973;82:192–201

42. Dean H. Treatment of type 2 diabetes in youth: an argument for randomized controlled studies. *Paediatr Child Health*. 1999;4:265–270

43. Knowler WC, Barrett-Connor E, Fowler SE, et al. Reduction in the incidence of type 2 diabetes with lifestyle intervention or metformin. *N Engl J Med*. 2002;346:393–403

31
Hypoglycemia in Infants and Children

Introduction

In healthy individuals, maintenance of a normal plasma glucose concentration depends on a normal endocrine system for integrating and modulating substrate mobilization, interconversion, and utilization; functionally intact enzymes for glycogenolysis, glycogen synthesis, glycolysis, gluconeogenesis, and utilization of other metabolic fuels for oxidation and storage; and an adequate supply of endogenous fat, glycogen, and potential gluconeogenic substrates (eg, amino acids, glycerol, and lactate). Adults are capable of maintaining a near normal blood glucose concentration, even when totally deprived of calories for weeks or, in the case of obese subjects, for months.[1] In contrast, the healthy neonate and young child are less able to meet the obligatory demands for this metabolic fuel and exhibit a progressive fall in the plasma concentration of glucose to hypoglycemic values when they fast for even short periods (24 to 48 hours).[2,3]

Abnormalities in hormone secretion, substrate interconversion, and mobilization of metabolic fuels contribute to abnormalities in glucose production and utilization that ultimately result in hypoglycemia in the pediatric patient. To evaluate and treat the child with hypoglycemia appropriately, the factors that regulate glucose metabolism in adults and the unique aspects of glucose metabolism in infants and young children must be understood.

Unique Aspects of Glucose Homeostasis in Infants and Children

Several aspects of glucose homeostasis are unique to the newborn infant and young child. Throughout gestation, glucose is transported from the maternal circulation across the placenta to meet a substantial proportion of the energy needs of the fetus. Animal studies have demonstrated that fetal hepatic gluconeogenesis is essentially absent, and there is no evidence of fetal glucose production at birth in humans.[4] In animals, the activity of one or more important rate-limiting enzymes (pyruvate carboxylase, phosphoenolpyruvate carboxykinase, glucose-6-phosphatase, and fructose 1,6-diphosphatase) of gluconeogenesis in the fetus is low, does not increase until the perinatal period, and reaches adult levels only after several hours to days of extrauterine life.[5] However, hepatic glucose production and gluconeogenesis are well established within hours of birth, even in very premature infants.[6] During the last 3 to 4 weeks of gestation in humans, hepatic glycogen stores increase, while the enzyme activities for glycogen synthesis and glycogenolysis are present before the accumulation of glycogen during late fetal life.[5]

The interruption of maternal blood flow at birth creates the newborn's first fast with a resultant decrease in the plasma glucose concentration during the first 2 hours of life. This decrease is accompanied by an increase in the plasma concentrations of nonesterified fatty acids (NEFAs) and ketone bodies.[7] By 4 to 6 hours of life, however, the plasma glucose concentration has stabilized or is increasing. Hepatic content of glycogen decreases during the first several days of extrauterine life and is used to facilitate a smooth transition from the continuously fed (intrauterine) to the fasted state (early hours of extrauterine life). Hepatic glycogen content is limited and, within a short period, the fasting neonate depends on gluconeogenesis as the primary mechanism to maintain euglycemia.[6,7]

Of substantial importance in the maintenance of glucose homeostasis in infants and children is the role of fatty acid availability (endogenous stores) for oxidative metabolism. Plasma NEFAs and ketone bodies can be used by a variety of body tissues and, thus, decrease the demands of these tissues for glucose as an energy source. In the case of brain tissue, the tissue with the highest rate of glucose utilization, ketone bodies (eg, hydroxybutyric acid and acetoacetic acid) but not NEFAs, can cross the blood-brain barrier and partially supplant the need for glucose.[1] Although the metabolic response to fasting in children is similar to that in adults, the relatively faster decline in the glucose concentration and increase in the plasma concentration of ketone bodies during brief periods of fasting in children suggest that the relative increase in the glucose requirement in children may result in an acceleration of the normal adaptive mechanism(s) of fasting observed in adults.[3]

The rates of glucose production and utilization increase rapidly over the first 8 to 10 years and then continue to increase more gradually into early adult life (Figure 31.1).[8] On a per kilogram of body weight basis, rates of glucose flux (production and utilization) in adults are 13 μmol/kg/min (2 to 2.5 mg/kg/min) in the postabsorptive state (14-hour fast) and decrease to 9.8 μmol/kg/min (1.8 mg/kg/min) by 30 hours of fasting.[9] The rate of glucose

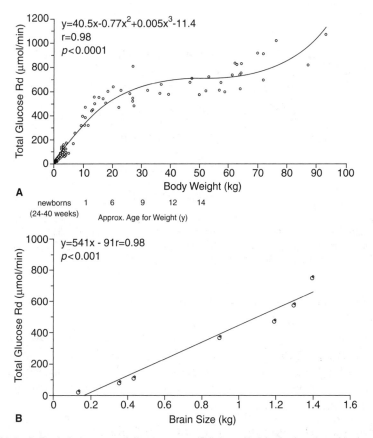

Figure 31.1. A. Total glucose rate of disappearance (Rd) (μmol/min) as a function of body weight from infancy to adulthood (n=141; body weights range from 0.6 to 94 kg). B. Relationship between total glucose Rd (μmol/min) and estimated brain weight from infancy to adulthood (n=141). The data points represent mean values. Reprinted with permission from Haymond MW, Sunehag A. Controlling the sugar bowl. Regulation of glucose homeostasis in children. *Endocrinol Metab Clin North Am.* 1999;28:663–694.

flux in infants and children after 4 to 14 hours of fasting is nearly 3 times higher (35 μmol/kg/min [6 mg/kg/min]) than that of adults and decreases to 23 μmol/kg/min (4 mg/kg/min) after a 30- to 40-hour fast.[9,10] This observation is consistent with the relatively higher proportion of brain mass to body size, which places infants and children at higher risk of hypoglycemia. In the premature and term infant, over 90% of the glucose is used by the brain. Over

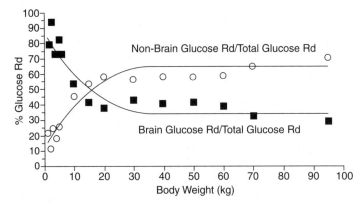

Figure 31.2. Estimated percentage of glucose Rd used by brain and non-brain tissue from infancy to adulthood (n=141). The tissue data points represent the mean values. Reprinted with permission from Haymond MW, Sunehag A. Controlling the sugar bowl. Regulation of glucose homeostasis in children. *Endocrinol Metab Clin North Am.* 1999;28:663–694.

time, this value decreases to ~40 % of glucose turnover in overnight-fasted adults (Figure 31.2).[8]

Although children can mount a greater counter-regulatory hormone response (eg, with cortisol, epinephrine, and glucagon) than adults when their plasma glucose is suddenly decreased,[11] any child or infant who has a quantitative plasma glucose less than 2.2 mmol/L (<40 mg/dL) should be considered hypoglycemic.

Symptoms of Hypoglycemia in Infants and Children

Signs and symptoms of hypoglycemia can be broadly divided into those resulting from neuroglycopenia and those from autonomic response to hypoglycemia.[12] The early symptoms and signs of hypoglycemia are usually autonomic and include sweating, weakness, tachycardia, tremor, and feeling of nervousness and/or hunger. Prolonged hypoglycemia may lead to more signs and symptoms that relate to neuroglycopenia and can include lethargy, irritability, mental confusion, behavior that is out of character, and, in its extreme, seizure and coma. The autonomic symptoms and signs normally occur at a higher blood glucose concentration than do those of neuroglycopenic origin. With repeated or prolonged episodes of hypoglycemia, the threshold for autonomic symptoms decreases to those of the neuroglycopenic symptoms. As a result, the individual develops severe symptoms of hypoglycemia with little or no warning, a condition termed hypoglycemia unawareness. With severe repeated and/or prolonged hypoglycemia, permanent central nervous system damage and occasionally death may result.

These signs and symptoms of hypoglycemia are less obvious or absent in infants and young children; autonomic and neuroglycopenic symptoms are less obvious or absent.[7] The nonspecific signs of hypoglycemia in newborns and young infants may be manifested by irritability, jitteriness, feeding difficulties, lethargy, cyanosis, tachypnea, and/or hypothermia. These signs are not specific for hypoglycemia and are also the early manifestations of a number of other disorders, including septicemia, congenital heart disease, ventricular hemorrhage, and respiratory distress syndrome. Therefore, some health care professionals have recommended that all infants should have their plasma glucose concentration monitored during the early hours of life (2–6 hours) and for longer periods in infants with underlying conditions that place them at high risk for the development of hypoglycemia.[7]

Transient Hypoglycemia of the Newborn

Transient Neonatal Hyperinsulinemia

Transient hyperinsulinemia and hypoglycemia almost exclusively occur in the infant whose mother has diabetes. On the basis of high insulin content and marked β-cell hyperplasia in pancreata from these infants and the rapid disappearance rates of exogenously administered glucose, fetal hyperglycemia and fetal and neonatal hyperinsulinemia have long been implicated as the causes of the hypoglycemia of the infant of a mother with diabetes. The standard of care is to maintain mothers with diabetes mellitus euglycemic throughout their pregnancy. Such practice has decreased late gestational fetal loss, prematurity, and neonatal hypoglycemia. Two additional causes of transient neonatal hypoglycemia resulting from hyperinsulinemia are erythroblastosis fetalis (a disease rarely seen today) and Beckwith-Wiedemann syndrome (characterized by macroglossia, omphalocele, and visceromegaly).[7]

The plasma glucose concentration should be monitored frequently during the first several days of life in all infants at high risk of neonatal hypoglycemia. Early feedings should be initiated if clinically appropriate. Should hypoglycemia occur, parenteral glucose should be administered at a rate sufficient to maintain the plasma glucose concentration in the normal range (3.3 to 5.6 mmol/L [60 to 100 mg/dL]). Glucose should be administered at an initial rate of 6 to 8 mg/kg/min, with stepwise advances of 10% to 15% increments until the plasma glucose concentration stabilizes or a rate of 15 to 20 mg/kg/min is reached. If hypoglycemia recurs and is difficult to control with intravenous glucose, intramuscular cortisone acetate (5 mg/kg/d, every 8 hours) during the first several days of life has been clinically useful in stabilizing the plasma glucose concentration. After stabilization, the parenteral glucose and cortisone acetate can be gradually decreased.[7] If the hypoglycemia recurs or is persistent, consideration should be given to the use of a somatostatin analogue to stabilize the glucose concentration, and a diagnosis of persistent hyperinsulinemic hypoglycemia of infancy (PHHI) should be pursued.

Hypoglycemia in the Small-for-Gestational-Age Infant

Transient neonatal hypoglycemia develops in 40% to 50% of small-for-gestational-age (SGA) infants. Hypoglycemia in the SGA infant is associated with elevated plasma concentrations of lactate and amino acids. This, together with the inability of infants who are SGA to generate a normal glycemic response to oral or intravenous alanine during the first day of life, is consistent with depleted glycogen stores and a defect, albeit transient, in hepatic gluconeogenesis. In addition, decreased fatty acid availability and presumed low rates of ketone body production could result in relatively increased rates of glucose utilization.

Once an infant is determined to be SGA, careful monitoring of the plasma glucose concentration during the first several days of life is indicated. If clinically appropriate, early frequent feedings should be initiated, and should hypoglycemia occur or persist, parenteral glucose and, if necessary, cortisone acetate should be administered. If oral feeding is not possible, parenteral glucose should be initiated to minimize the risk of hypoglycemia.[13]

Other Conditions

Intrauterine exposure to β-adrenergic blockers has been associated with neonatal hypoglycemia. In addition, any of the conditions associated with hypoglycemia of childhood may first manifest during the early hours of life and should be considered in the evaluation of any newborn with profound or recurrent hypoglycemia. In addition, asphyxia and septicemia can be associated with hypoglycemia, particularly in the premature or newborn infant.

Hypoglycemia of Children

Persistent Hyperinsulinemic Hypoglycemia of Infancy

Hypoglycemia secondary to hyperinsulinemia, persistent hyperinsulinemic hypoglycemia of infancy (PHHI) most commonly appears during the first year of life. Early recognition and treatment of PHHI are of utmost importance to avoid or minimize permanent neurologic damage. A sigmoid relationship exits between the plasma glucose and insulin concentrations in normals. Only small amounts of insulin are secreted when the plasma glucose falls below 3.3 mM (60 mg·dL^{-1}). In children with PHHI, this relationship is disturbed or disrupted. Although insulin increases the transport and the metabolic clearance of glucose, the primary effect of insulin on glucose metabolism is to decrease hepatic glucose production.

The incidence of PHHI is ~1:50 000 in northern Europe. It is significantly higher in countries with a high prevalence of consanguinity. Four different gene defects on chromosome 11 have been identified: (a) sulfonyl urea receptor defects (SUR1); (b) defects on the inward rectifying potassium channel KIR6.2 gene; (c) regulatory mutations on the glutamate dehydrogenase gene; and (d) an activating glucokinase mutation. The SUR1 and KIR6.2 mutations result in absence of K_{ATP} activity in the β-cell, which leads to closure of the potassium channel, depolarization of the cell membrane, influx of calcium ions, and increased insulin release. Recently, a form of congenital hyperinsulinemia was described, characterized by hypoglycemia and hyperammonemia as a result of defects in the glutamate dehydrogenase gene impairing the control of the enzyme activity. Both a familial and a sporadic form have been described. In the sporadic cases, 4 different mutations were found, while the 2 familial cases shared the same mutation. Glucokinase controls glucose metabolism in the β-cell, which is responsible for glucose-mediated regulation of insulin secretion. A loss of function mutation (Val203Ala) of this gene is associated with maturity onset diabetes of the young (MODY). Recently, however, a mutation (Val455Met) was described in the glucokinase gene, which causes autosomal dominant familial hyperinsulinism. The Val455Met mutation results in lowering the K_m for glucose by 65%. The long-term effects of this mutation are not clear, but it is noteworthy that the oldest affected patient developed diabetes later in life. The Val203Ala and Val455Met gene defects occur in both autosomal recessive and dominant forms. The recessive form is more severe and difficult to treat, while the dominant is milder, presents later, and responds well to pharmacological treatment.[14–17]

Two types of histopathological abnormalities are associated with PHHI in infants, a focal and a diffuse form. The former is found in 30% to 50% of operated cases. In some patients with the focal form, a specific loss of maternal alleles in the p15 region of chromosome 11 (limited to the hyperplastic lesion) has been described. Further, in some of these patients, a mutant band in the

SUR1 gene inherited from the father was enhanced in the DNA derived from the hyperplastic lesion. Thus, in these cases, the loss of the maternal allele resulted in hemi- or homozygosity of the paternal defective allele of the SUR1 gene, causing a recessive endocrine disorder associated with focal β-cell hyperplasia and hyperinsulinemia.[14]

The primary aim of therapy in PHHI is to prevent neurologic symptoms and sequelae, including a permanent seizure disorder independent of plasma glucose, and mental retardation.[18] The therapeutic approaches to PHHI are directed at decreasing insulin secretion pharmacologically or surgically. It is of great importance to distinguish the focal and diffuse forms as early as possible because the focal forms respond very well to partial pancreatectomy.

Medical management of hyperinsulinemia includes diazoxide, which blocks the sulfonylurea receptors on the β-cells resulting in opening of the potassium channels and decreasing insulin release. In doses of 5 to 20 mg·kg^{-1}·d^{-1}, the side effects consist of hypertrichosis, advanced bone age, mild hyperuricemia, decreased IgG concentration and neutrophil counts, and sodium and water retention. Water retention can be reduced by hydrochlorothiazides, which, in addition, further reduces insulin secretion. If treatment with diazoxide is not successful, somatostatin analogues and Ca-channel blockers may be tried. However, long-term follow-up studies have not been carried out to assess the potential side effects of these drugs. In addition, infusion of glucagon may be useful during the initial stabilization period and prior to surgery. Finally, when hyperinsulinemia is proven and medical therapy fails to control hypoglycemia, surgical exploration is indicated in any child past the first weeks of life. Selective resection of focal lesions is often curative, while the diffuse form requires subtotal pancreatectomy, in which 95% to 99% of the pancreas is removed, while leaving the spleen intact. The variable results of surgery reflect the differences in the pathophysiology and the extent of pancreatectomy. Following subtotal pancreatectomy, exogenous insulin may be required for several months to control hyperglycemia. Conversely, the recurrence of hypoglycemia within days of surgery portends significant future problems with glucose homeostasis, requiring reinstitution of medical management and, in many cases, additional surgery.[14–18]

Careful follow-up of each patient is required to evaluate the long-term effects of subtotal pancreatectomy on endocrine and exocrine pancreatic function. When an islet cell adenoma is diagnosed, especially in the older child or adolescent, a search for other endocrine abnormalities (hyperparathyroidism, hypergastrinemia, and pituitary tumors) must be made in the patient and the patient's family to exclude multiple endocrine neoplasia syndrome type I. The plasma insulin response to fasting or insulin secretagogues does not clearly distinguish these various disorders. Because adenomas are generally less than 1 cm in size and are rare in infants and young children, celiac arteriography, MRI, and CT are of little diagnostic value. Percutaneous and intraoperative ultrasound has been used to identify some insulin-producing tumors of the pancreas.[17,19]

Hormone Deficiencies

Hypoglycemia is a frequent complication in children with growth hormone and cortisol insufficiency and has been reported in children with hypothyroidism. During hypoglycemia, patients with isolated ACTH and/or growth hormone deficiency are ketotic, have low plasma concentrations of insulin, alanine, and glutamine (the latter 2 are potential gluconeogenic substrates for hepatic and renal gluconeogenesis), and a blunted glycemic response to exogenous glucagon. However, several cases of panhypopituitarism and hyperinsulinemia have been reported in children. The pathophysiologic process of the hypoglycemia in these disorders is not completely understood. Appropriate hormone replacement is the treatment of choice.[13]

Enzyme Deficiency Conditions

Hereditary disorders associated with a deficiency of specific enzymes involved with substrate mobilization, interconversion, and utilization are individually rare disorders but frequently associated with hypoglycemia.[13] These enzymatic defects may involve carbohydrate, amino acid, or fat metabolism and are almost always inherited as autosomal recessive traits. Because of the interactions of fat, carbohydrate, and amino acid metabolism in the maintenance of normal fuel homeostasis, abnormalities in the metabolism of a single substrate can have primary and secondary effects on other metabolic pathways. A common expression of these derangements is the development of biochemical or symptomatic hypoglycemia.

Defective Carbohydrate Metabolism

Glycogen Storage Diseases

The glycogen storage diseases are inherited autosomal recessive defects characterized by a deficient or abnormally functioning enzyme involved in the formation or degradation of glycogen. Severe hypoglycemia is observed in newborns with glycogen synthetase deficiency. Patients with defects of debrancher enzyme or phosphorylase activation are commonly englycemic, because hepatic gluconeogenesis is intact and the defects in glycogenolysis are rarely complete. As a result, hypoglycemia is not usually a major clinical problem. When hypoglycemia does occur with these disorders, it can usually be managed with frequent feedings, supplemental raw cornstarch, or both. Lysosomal α-1,4-glucosidase deficiencies (glycogen storage diseases, type II) and amylo-1,4–1,6-transglucosidase (type III) and those due to specific muscle enzyme defects are not associated with hypoglycemia.[13,20]

Disorders in Hepatic Gluconeogenesis

Glucose-6-Phosphatase Deficiency (Glycogen Storage Disease, Type Ia)

Hydrolysis of glucose-6-phosphate is the final common enzymatic event in the hepatic release of glucose from the gluconeogenic and glycogenolytic pathways. Therefore, deficiency of glucose-6-phosphatase typically results in severe hypoglycemia and is associated with ketosis and lactic acidosis, particularly during early infancy. Some patients have only mild clinical and biochemical abnormalities with hypoglycemia after 15 to 20 hours of fasting and subnormal, but detectable, glycemic responses to glucagon, fructose, and galactose administration. Hepatomegaly, growth retardation, hyperlipidemia, and hyperuricemia are also common clinical features of this disorder. Other children with identical clinical and biochemical findings but normal hepatic activity of glucose-6-phosphatase have been described. These children have one of several transport defects. Glucose-6-phosphate translocase deficiency is known as glycogen storage disease, type Ib, and is associated with neutropenia and mucosa ulcerations. Type Ic is a defect in microsomal phosphate or pyrophosphate transport, and type Id is a microsome defect in glucose transport.[20]

The primary goal of therapy is to provide a constant source of exogenous glucose by frequent feeding or gastric infusion. Raw cornstarch provides a slow-release form of carbohydrate, thus avoiding gastric infusions of carbohydrate in older children and adults with this disease. Such dietary programs reduce the hyperlipidemia, hyperuricemia, lacticacidemia, and ketoacidemia and improve the low growth velocities observed. Allopurinol is frequently used to decrease further the abnormally high rates of uric acid production. Although the hepatomegaly remains or decreases only slightly, a striking and sustained increase in growth velocity has been observed in most children. Over time, a number of these individuals develop renal compromise and, in some cases, renal failure. The pathophysiology of this renal damage is not clear but most likely is related to glycogen storage in the kidney. Follow-up studies are needed to determine the long-term morbidity and mortality of this disease and the impact of current therapy.[13,20]

Fructose 1,6-Diphosphatase Deficiency

Hepatic fructose 1,6-diphosphatase deficiency results in a defect in gluconeo-genesis. The initial signs and symptoms can be similar to those of glycogen storage disease, type I (eg, failure to thrive, hepatomegaly, signs and symptoms referable to the lactic acidosis and hypoglycemia). However, excessive hepatic glycogen accumulation does not occur in this disease because the entire glycogenolytic pathway is intact. The mild to moderate hepatomegaly is caused by lipid storage, but results of hepatic function studies are generally normal or only mildly abnormal. Hypoglycemia, lactic acidosis, ketoacidosis, hyperlipidemia, and hyperuricemia are presumed to have the same patho-genesis as in glucose-6-phosphatase deficiency. Adherence to a relatively high-carbohydrate frequent feeding diet prevents hypoglycemia and hyperlac-tatemia and permits normal growth and development. However, in situations resulting in catabolic stress (eg, infection and burns), severe life-threatening lactic acidosis, ketoacidosis, and hypoglycemia can develop, necessitating hospitalization and parenteral glucose administration.[5,13,21]

Pyruvate Carboxylase and Phosphoenolpyruvate Carboxykinase Deficiencies

Pyruvate carboxylase converts pyruvate to oxaloacetate and is the first enzy-matic step of gluconeogenesis from 3-carbon precursors (eg, pyruvate, lactate, and alanine). Patients with pyruvate carboxylase deficiency are severely retard-ed, die early in infancy, and have neuropathologic evidence of subacute necro-tizing encephalopathy. Although hypoglycemia is an inconsistent finding in patients with proved hepatic pyruvate carboxylase deficiency, increased plasma concentrations of lactate, pyruvate, and alanine, metabolic acidosis, and ketonuria are consistently observed. The long-term prognosis remains bleak. A small number of cases of children with deficiency of hepatic phosphoenolpyru-vate carboxykinase have been reported. Although hypoglycemia is a common feature, in vivo biochemical studies have been limited or their findings are inconsistent with those observed in other patients with defects of hepatic glu-coneogenesis. A clear description of this enzymatic defect must await further in vitro and in vivo investigation.[5,13]

Galactose-1-Phosphate Uridyl Transferase Deficiency (Classic Galactosemia)

Infants with classic galactosemia are intolerant of products containing galac-tose. In addition to failure to thrive, sepsis, or both, these infants have hypoglycemia, diarrhea, and vomiting following meals containing galactose.

The accumulation of galactose-1-phosphate in tissues results in hepatic dysfunction (hepatosplenomegaly and elevation of plasma activities of hepatic enzymes and bilirubin), lenticular cataracts, mental retardation, and aminoaciduria. The occurrence of postprandial hypoglycemia seems to be due to inhibition of phosphoglucomutase by galactose-1-phosphate, thereby resulting in sudden inhibition of glycogenolysis. The diagnosis can be made by determining the activity of this enzyme in red blood cells, and most of these children today are identified on routine neonatal screen testing. Elimination of galactose from the diet prevents further manifestations of the disease, but mental deficiencies are present in most of these children, and a large number of women with this disorder experience ovarian failure.[13,22]

Fructose 1-Phosphate Aldolase, Isozyme B Deficiency (Hereditary Fructose Intolerance)

This disorder is dominated by symptoms of hypoglycemia and vomiting following ingestion of foods containing fructose. Fructosuria is present only after meals containing this simple sugar; patients frequently manifest hepatomegaly, jaundice, aminoaciduria, and failure to thrive. The hypoglycemia following fructose ingestion is presumed to be the result of accumulation of fructose 1-phosphate, which inhibits the activation of hepatic phosphorylase and gluconeogenesis at the level of fructose 1,6-diphosphatase. Elimination of dietary fructose will reverse and prevent or minimize nearly all of the manifestations of this disease but is difficult because of the ubiquitous use of sucrose in prepared foods.[13,21]

Defects in Amino Acid Metabolism

Maple Syrup Urine Disease (Branched-Chain α-Keto Acid Dehydrogenase Deficiency)

Hypoglycemia and profound hypoalaninemia are observed in patients with classic maple syrup urine disease at times when their branched-chain amino acids and α-keto acids are markedly elevated. With dietary therapy and correction of the plasma branched-chain amino acid abnormalities, fasting plasma alanine and glucose values increase toward normal. Other defects in the catabolism of the α-keto acids or the branched-chain amino acids can manifest by hypoglycemia and low plasma carnitine concentration and are discussed in the next section.[13]

Defects in Fatty Acid Metabolism

A group of rare but severe metabolic disorders have been described to be associated with abnormalities in fatty acid oxidation and ketone body formation and resulting in hypoglycemia and hypoketonemia. During periods of fasting or intercurrent illness, free fatty acids are mobilized from adipose tissue and are utilized directly by body tissue (eg, heart, skeletal muscle, gut, and skin) or undergo β-oxidation in the liver with the resultant production and release of ketone bodies. This process includes (a) activation of fatty acids by acyl-CoA synthetase, (b) transport into the mitochondrial matrix (in contrast to medium- and short-chain fatty acids, the long-chain fatty acids are dependent on carnitine for their transport across the mitochondrial membrane), and (c) mitochondrial β-oxidation of the fatty acids. Defects in the activities of these enzymes are depicted in Table 31.1. The most frequently occurring defect is the medium-chain acyl-CoA deficiency. Medium-chain acyl-CoA deficiency has been found in 1:10 000 births in a white population of Northern European origin. About 90% of the patients with medium-chain acyl-CoA deficiency are homozygous for a single point mutation (A985G) and can be diagnosed by

Table 31.1.
Disorders of Fatty Acid Oxidation

Transport across the mitochondrial membrane
Carnitine palmitoyltransferase (CPT I and II) deficiency
Carnitine/acylcarnitine translocase deficiency
β-oxidation in the mitochondrial matrix
Acyl dehydrogenase deficiencies
LCA-dehydrogenase (LCAD) deficiency
MCA-dehydrogenase (MCAD) deficiency
SCA-dehydrogenase (SCAD) deficiency
Tri-functional enzyme deficiency
LC-2-enoyl-CoA hydratase
LC-3-hydroxyacyl-CoA dehydrogenase (LCHAD)
LC-3-ketoacyl-CoA thiolase
SC-2-enoyl-CoA hydratase (Crotonase) deficiency
SC-3-hydroxyacyl-CoA dehydrogenase (SCHAD) deficiency
SC-3-ketoacyl-CoA thiolase deficiency
Deficiency of enzymes of unsaturated β-oxidation
LC Δ^3, Δ^2 – enoyl-CoA isomerase
SC Δ^3, Δ^2 – enoyl-CoA isomerase
2, 4-Dienoyl-CoA reductase

simple molecular techniques or electrospray ionization tandem mass spectrometry using newborn filter paper bloodspots. The latter technique has also been used to diagnose trifunctional protein deficiency.[23–26]

In patients with organic acidemias (methylmalonic, propionic, and isovaleric acidemia), carnitine deficiency occurs secondary to renal losses of carnitine as acylcarnitine derivatives. These disorders have been associated with hypoglycemia, the pathophysiology of which must be presumed to be the same as that of the defects in fatty acid oxidation.

Children with disorders of fatty acid oxidation can present with profound hypoglycemia (frequently <1 mM or <15 to 20 mg·dL^{-1}) and profound disturbance of consciousness that may not improve when the plasma glucose is normalized. In addition, they may have absolute or relative hypoketonemia, remarkably high plasma free fatty acid concentrations, hypotonia, hepatomegaly with microvesicular fat accumulation, elevated plasma activities of both liver and muscle enzymes, congestive heart failure, rhabdomyolysis, and, frequently, cerebral edema. The combination of these features has a striking resemblance to Reye syndrome. The pathophysiology of the hypoglycemia in these children is not known. Two mechanisms might be considered: (1) decreased hepatic glucose production, because gluconeogenesis and ketogenesis are intimately linked to the production and utilization of phosphopyridine nucleotides; or (2) accelerated rates of glucose utilization, because glucose might serve as the primary substrate for all tissues in the absence of ketone body availability and defective free fatty acid oxidation.

The physician should have a high index of suspicion for these disorders when a child presenting with severe hypoglycemia has decreased plasma concentrations of free and total carnitine and relatively low plasma ketone body concentrations but very high free fatty acid concentrations. At such times, parenteral glucose should be infused at a rate (5 to 10 mg·kg^{-1}·min^{-1}) sufficient to increase plasma insulin and, thus, maximally suppress lipolysis and proteolysis. Once the diagnosis has been established, fasting must be avoided and frequent high-carbohydrate feeds should be instituted during periods of catabolic stress. If oral carbohydrate is not tolerated, parenteral glucose must be provided. Depending on the defect, special diets and/or oral carnitine replacement must be considered. Such treatment of these children should not be presumed to be curative because, under catabolic conditions (illness, trauma), mobilization of endogenous substrate could once again evoke the potentially devastating metabolic abnormalities present at the time of initial presentation.

Drug-Induced Hypoglycemia
Hypoglycemia in Children With Diabetes Treated With Insulin (see also Chapter 30)

The most common cause of hypoglycemia in the pediatric age is iatrogenic insulin-induced hypoglycemia in children with type 1 diabetes or type 2 diabetes receiving parenteral insulin and/or sulfonylrea derivative drugs. It is now clearly established in patients with both type 1 and type 2 diabetes mellitus that the incidence of long-term microvascular complications of diabetes can be reduced by bringing the blood glucose into the near normal range.[27,28] As a result, we attempt to maintain tight metabolic control of children with diabetes. However, this occurs at a real cost of significantly more hypoglycemia. In the Diabetes Control and Complications Trial, the experimental group (tight metabolic control group) had an incidence of severe insulin reactions of 61.2 per 100 patient years, an increase of more than threefold when compared to the standard treatment group (18.7 per 100 patient years).[29]

Children with type 1 diabetes who genuinely try to control their diabetes may have 2 to 5 (or more) mild hypoglycemic episodes each week. A number of factors result in increased hypoglycemia in these children. Since their insulin is generally administered in subcutaneous boli, the mass of insulin delivered, as well as the carbohydrate consumed at a meal, becomes critical in maintaining metabolic control. Errors in insulin administration, whether using a syringe or a pump or failure to mix the NPH or ultralente, can result in both hyper- and hypoglycemia. Failure to consume the planned carbohydrates will leave the insulin unopposed and will result in hypoglycemia. But perhaps the most frequent cause of severe hypoglycemia is late-afternoon or evening exercise with hypoglycemic seizures occurring in the middle of the night. In addition, very young children with type 1 diabetes are also at increased risk for severe hypoglycemia. Several factors have been attributed to this increased risk in these young children: (1) dramatic fluctuations in exercise and food intake, (2) increased insulin sensitivity, and (3) our inability to make sufficiently small adjustments in their insulin doses. A critical factor in the management of these children is frequent measurement of the blood glucose using a variety of commercially available self-glucose monitoring devices. However, when objectively analyzed, we truly have inadequate tools with which to manage children (and adults) with diabetes.

With the onset of hypoglycemia in the patient without diabetes, the body decreases the release of insulin and secretes counter regulatory hormones (glucagon, cortisol, and growth hormone) to increase glucose production and the blood glucose concentration. In the patient with diabetes, the insulin entry cannot be acutely modulated from its subcutaneous depot of injected insulin, and glucagon does not increase for reasons that are unclear. Therefore, the primary mechanism for counter regulation is the secretion of epinephrine. With recurrent moderate or severe insulin reactions, the difference in threshold for the autonomic and the neuroglycopenic symptoms disappears and the patient's first signs and symptoms are those of a severe insulin reaction. This is hypoglycemic unawareness as discussed above. In the patient with diabetes, this can be very dangerous and can lead to very severe and prolonged episodes of hypoglycemia, which may cause permanent neurologic damage or even death.

Patient (friend and parent) recognition of hypoglycemic signs and symptoms is extremely important. When the early autonomic symptoms of hypoglycemia are recognized, the patient with diabetes must consume sufficient carbohydrate to raise blood glucose, but not enough to cause hyperglycemia. With the secretion of counter regulatory hormones, the patient becomes insulin resistant, which further contributes to post-hypoglycemic hyperglycemia. When the patient is unable to treat him- or herself, another individual must intervene to provide oral carbohydrate. If the patient becomes combative, comatose, or seizes, the blood glucose needs to be increased using either parenteral glucose or large doses of glucagon (which can cause nausea and vomiting) administered by a trained individual. During times of gastroenteritis or with oppositional behavior of a young child, the patient is unable or unwilling to retain or to consume oral carbohydrate. Under these circumstances, the individual will benefit from very small doses of subcutaneous glucagon.[30]

A variety of new devices to improve the delivery of insulin (pen injectors, pumps, glucose monitoring devices) and new pharmaceutical agents (short- and aqueous long-acting insulins) have improved our ability to accomplish this arduous task for the patient with diabetes. However, we continue to fall significantly short of dramatically improving the glycemic control of these children.

Sulfonylurea

With the wide use of sulfonylurea derivative drugs in type 2 diabetes mellitus, accidental ingestion of these compounds must be considered for any child with hypoglycemia, and appropriate historical and laboratory information must be sought. Use of these drugs to treat gestational diabetes has resulted in transplacental transfer of these compounds and profound hypoglycemia in the newborn during the first several days of life. For this reason, use of oral hypoglycemic agents in pregnant women with diabetes is contraindicated. With the broader use of metformin and the thiazoladiendione class drugs, the risk of this occurring will hopefully be less.

Hypoglycemia as a result of malicious administration of insulin or an oral hypoglycemic agent to infants and young children (as in Munchausen syndrome by proxy) is fortunately rare but must be considered if the parents or guardians have access to these drugs. Therefore, analysis of blood for insulin and C peptide and urine for oral hypoglycemic agents may aid in the diagnosis and treatment of these abused children.[13]

Ethyl Alcohol

Ingestion of ethyl alcohol, particularly by young children, can lead to profound hypoglycemia, seizures, and, in some cases, death. An unexpectedly large anion gap at the time of diagnosis of the hypoglycemia should alert the physician to the possibility of accidental ingestion of ethanol or a number of other compounds, the identification of which will facilitate appropriate treatment of the child.

Salicylate and Related Compounds

Salicylates, their ester derivatives, and acetaminophen have been associated with hypoglycemia and ketosis. The child with salicylism may have vomiting, mental confusion, delirium, hyperventilation, and, occasionally, hypoglycemia. Clinically, this entity may be confused with pneumonia, encephalitis, Reye syndrome, or diabetic ketoacidosis. Therefore, even in the absence of a history of salicylate exposure or inappropriate salicylate administration, the diagnosis must still be suspected and plasma salicylate levels determined.[13]

Cyanotic Congenital Heart Disease

Patients with a variety of congenital heart diseases and patients with congestive heart failure, regardless of age or cause, appear to be at greater risk for the development of hypoglycemia. Decreased hepatic perfusion could compromise the rate of glucose production.[13]

Abnormalities in Substrate Availability

Ketotic Hypoglycemia

The number of children with ketotic hypoglycemia has inexplicably decreased over the past 20 years. This disorder classically manifests itself between the ages of 18 months and 5 years and generally remits spontaneously before 8 to 9 years of age. Early studies failed to identify defects in hepatic gluconeogenesis or functional disturbances of insulin, glucagon, or cortisol. As the supply of endogenous substrates increases relative to glucose demand (ie, with age), spontaneous remission could be expected.[19] Because of the striking decrease in the number of children with this condition, the pathophysiologic factor(s) responsible for the hypoglycemia may never be fully understood.[13]

Hypoglycemia Associated With Surgery

A number of cases of severe hypoglycemia have been reported among young children, complicating the postoperative course. Whether the hypoglycemia was related to the antecedent period of fasting or some intraoperative stress or medication is not clear; however, minimizing the period of fasting and/or providing parenteral glucose preoperatively and appropriate monitoring of the plasma glucose level during the postoperative period in young children may prevent this unexpected complication. In contrast, neonates and premature infants frequently develop hyperglycemia with surgery. This may be a result of the stress associated with surgery in combination with continuous parenteral glucose both prior to and during the surgery.[13]

Diagnostic Evaluation

When the diagnosis of hypoglycemia is suspected and supported by a rapid indicator of the blood glucose concentration, sufficient blood should be obtained *before* therapeutic intervention to confirm the diagnosis by an established quantitative laboratory method, to determine the actual glucose concentration, and to permit additional biochemical determinations. Further analysis of this plasma for glucoregulatory hormones (eg, insulin, cortisol, and growth hormone), metabolic substrates (eg, NEFAs, ketone bodies, lactate, ammonia, alanine, and liver enzymes), and plasma-free and total carnitine and specific acyl carnitine concentrations (if available) will be invaluable in facilitating subsequent evaluation and management of the patient's condition.

A large number of diagnostic procedures are available to clarify the pathogenesis of the various hypoglycemic disorders, but a systematic approach is necessary. The results obtained from the history, physical examination, and initial plasma sample should guide further testing. For most children with a history of hypoglycemia, a diagnostic fast under carefully controlled conditions should be considered. Because of the potential risk of provoking an episode of severe encephalopathy in a child with a defect in fatty acid or carnitine metabolism, the plasma carnitine concentration should be proved normal before initiating an elective fast. For infants and very young children who are normally fed every 4 to 6 hours, the fast can be easily accomplished by omitting one or more feedings. For the older child who normally fasts overnight at home, a 24- to 30-hour fast beginning after the evening meal has been useful in the evaluation of hypoglycemia. Normal plasma values of glucose, counter regulatory hormones, and substrates are available for comparison. This fasting protocol places most of these children at risk for hypoglycemia between 10:00 am and 6:00 pm, a time when the patient should be awake and alert and when physician and laboratory staff availability is optimal. Plasma concentrations of glucose, ketone bodies, lactate, alanine, and insulin should be serially monitored throughout the fast. In addition, plasma growth hormone and cortisol concentrations should also be obtained at the time of hypoglycemia (although their interpretation is not always clear).

Hypoglycemia without (or with only minimal) hepatomegaly and the absence of substantial ketonuria or ketonemia should focus attention on abnormalities of insulin secretion, or disorders of ketogenesis or fatty acid oxidation. Hyperinsulinism is best documented by obtaining a number of plasma samples for simultaneous determination of the glucose and insulin levels at times of hypoglycemia. The plasma insulin concentration after 24 hours of fasting in normal children is rarely above 35 pmol/L (5 μU/mL), except in markedly obese children; levels less than 15 pmol/L (2 μU/mL) are generally noted. Plasma insulin concentrations greater than 35 pmol/L (5 μU/mL) with a concomitant plasma glucose value less than 2.8 mmol/L (50 mg/dL), regardless of the period of fasting, are distinctly abnormal and are an indication for further studies to document hyperinsulinism.

Administration of intravenous glucagon (0.03 mg/kg; glucagon challenge test) at the time of hypoglycemia may be of therapeutic and diagnostic value. A clear glycemic response (>20 to 30 mg/dL or 1 to 2 mM) during the first 10 to 20 minutes following glucagon administration would reflect inappropriate sequestration of hepatic glycogen and strongly suggests hyperinsulinemia or glucagon deficiency. Provocative testing of insulin secretion with tolbutamide and leucine may have some diagnostic values. In addition, some investigators are advocating portal vein catheterization and pancreatic venous blood sampling for insulin in an attempt to localize a focal lesion. Such procedures may provide significant new data to the diagnostic fast and glucagon. However, at the present time, these diagnostic tests must be considered experimental and unproven and should only be carried out in the context of a research protocol.

References

1. Cahill GF Jr, Herrera MG, Morgan AP, et al. Hormone-fuel interrelationships during fasting. *J Clin Invest.* 1966;45:1751–1769
2. Chaussain JL, Georges P, Calzada L, Job JC. Glycemic response to 24-hour fast in normal children, III. Influence of age. *J Pediatr.* 1977;91:711–714
3. Haymond MW, Karl IE, Clarke WL, Pagliara AS, Santiago JV. Differences in circulating gluconeogenic substrates during short-term fasting in men, women and children. *Metabolism.* 1982;31:33–42
4. Kalhan SC, D'Angelo LJ, Savin SM, Adam PA. Glucose production in pregnant women at term gestation. Sources of glucose for the human fetus. *J Clin Invest.* 1979;63:388–394
5. Darmaun D, Haymond MW, Bier DM. Metabolic aspects of fuel homeostasis in the fetus and neonate. In: DeGroot LJ, Besser M, Burger HG, et al, eds. *Endocrinology.* 3rd ed. Philadelphia, PA: WB Saunders Co; 1995:2258–2286
6. Sunehag A, Ewald U, Gustafsson J. Extremely preterm infants (<28 weeks) are capable of gluconeogenesis from glycerol on their first day of life. *Pediatr Res.* 1996;40:553–557
7. Cornblath M, Schwartz R. *Disorders of Carbohydrate Metabolism in Infancy.* 3rd ed. Boston, MA: Blackwell Scientific Publications; 1991
8. Haymond MW, Sunehag A. Controlling the sugar bowl: regulation of glucose homeostasis in children. *Endocrinol Metab Clin North Am.* 1999;28:663–694
9. Haymond MW, Howard C, Ben-Galim, DeVivo DC. Effects of ketosis on glucose flux in children and adults. *Am J Physiol.* 1983;245:E373–E378
10. Bier DM, Leake RD, Haymond MW, et al. Measurement of "true" glucose production rates in infancy and childhood with 6,6-dideuteroglucose. *Diabetes.* 1977;26:1016–1023
11. Amiel SA, Simonson DC, Sherwin RS, Lauritano AA, Tamborlane WV. Exaggerated epinephrine responses to hypoglycemia in normal and insulin-dependent diabetic children. *J Pediatr.* 1987;110:832–837
12. Cryer PE. Banting Lecture. Hypoglycemia: the limiting factor in the management of IDDM. *Diabetes.* 1994;43:1378–1389
13. Haymond MW. Hypoglycemia in infants and children. *Endocrinol Metab Clin North Am.* 1989;18:211–252
14. Schwitzgebel VM, Gitelman SE. Neonatal hyperinsulinism. *Clin Perinatol.* 1998;25:1015–1038
15. Stanley CA, Lieu YK, Hsu BY, et al. Hyperinsulinism and hyperammonemia in infants with regulatory mutations of the glutamate dehydrogenase gen. *N Engl J Med.* 1998;338:1352–1357
16. Grimberg A, Ferry RJ Jr, Kelly A, et al. Dysregulation of insulin secretion in children with congenital hyperinsulinism due to sulfonylurea receptor mutations. *Diabetes.* 2001;50:322–328

17. Menni F, de Lonlay P, Sevin C, et al. Neurologic outcomes of 90 neonates and infants with persistent hyperinsulinemic hypoglycemia. *Pediatrics*. 2001;107: 476–479

18. Glaser B, Chiu KC, Anker R, et al. Familial hyperinsulinism maps to chromosome 11p14–15.1, 30 cM centromeric to the insulin gene. *Nat Genet*. 1994;7:185–188

19. Thorton PS, Alter CA, Katz LE, Baker L, Stanley CA. Short- and long-term use of octreotide in the treatment of congenital hyperinsulinism. *J Pediatr*. 1993;123: 637–643

20. Chen YT, Burchall A. Glycogen storage diseases. In: Scriver CR, Beaudet AL, Sly WS, Valle D, eds. *The Metabolic and Molecular Bases of Inherited Disease*. Vol 1. 7th ed. New York, NY: McGraw-Hill, Inc; 1995:935–961

21. Gitzelmann R, Steinmann B, Van der Berghe G. Disorders of fructose metabolism. In: Scriver CR, Beaudet AL, Sly WS, Valle D, eds. *The Metabolic and Molecular Bases of Inherited Disease*. Vol 1. 7th ed. New York, NY: McGraw-Hill, Inc; 1995:905–934

22. Segal S, Berry GT. Disorders of galactose metabolism. In: Scriver CR, Beaudet AL, Sly WS, Valle D, eds. *The Metabolic and Molecular Bases of Inherited Disease*. Vol 1. 7th ed. New York, NY: McGraw-Hill, Inc; 1995:967–1000

23. Stanley CA, Hale DE. Genetic disorders of mitochondrial fatty acid oxidation. *Curr Opin Pediatr*. 1994;6:476–481

24. Kelly DP, Strauss AW. Inherited cardiomyopathies. *N Engl J Med*. 1994;330:913–919

25. Bougneres PF, Saudubray JM, Marsac C, Bernard O, Odievre M, Girard J. Fasting hypoglycemia resulting from hepatic carnitine palmitoyl transferase deficiency. *J Pediatr*. 1981;98:742–746

26. Bennett MJ, Rinaldo P, Strauss AW. Inborn errors of mitochondrial fatty acid oxidation. *Crit Rev Clin Lab Sci*. 2000;37:1–44

27. Diabetes Control and Complications Trial Research Group. The effect of intensive treatment of diabetes on the development and progression of long-term complications in insulin-dependent diabetes mellitus. *N Engl J Med*. 1993;329:977–986

28. UK Prospective Diabetes Study Group. Intensive blood glucose control with sulfonylureas or insulin compared with conventional treatment and risk of complications in patients with type 2 diabetes (UKPDS 33). *Lancet*. 1998;352:837–853

29. Diabetes Control and Complications Trial Study Group. Adverse events and their association with treatment regimens in the diabetes control and complications trial. *Diabetes Care*. 1995;18:1415–1427

30. Haymond MW, Schreiner B. Mini-dose glucagon rescue for hypoglycemia in children with type I diabetes. *Diabetes Care*. 2001;24:643–645

32

Hyperlipidemia

Coronary artery disease and blood cholesterol levels are statistically related. Although the incidence of coronary artery disease is now declining in the United States, it remains the leading cause of death in adults in the United States and most industrialized countries. The familial occurrence of coronary heart disease has been known since the 19th century; however, the familial risk factors have been delineated only in recent decades. The Framingham study[1] and subsequent studies have identified the following risk factors for coronary heart disease:

1. Family history
2. Male gender
3. Reduced level of high-density lipoprotein (HDL)
4. Elevated serum cholesterol level
5. Hypertension
6. Cigarette smoking
7. Impairment of carbohydrate tolerance
8. Lack of physical activity
9. Elevated serum triglyceride level

Not all investigators agree that an elevated level of plasma triglycerides is an independent risk factor for coronary heart disease. Although a direct correlation is evident in univariate analysis, this effect is lost when the influences of obesity, diabetes mellitus, cholesterol, and HDL are removed.[1]

In 1992, and again most recently in 1998, the Committee on Nutrition of the American Academy of Pediatrics (AAP), endorsed the findings and recommendations of the Expert Panel on Blood Cholesterol in Children and Adolescents of the National Cholesterol Education Program (NCEP).[2-4] The AAP Committee on Nutrition and the NCEP found that

1. Certain inborn or acquired diseases accompanied by hypercholesterolemia are associated with premature atherosclerosis.

2. Serum cholesterol levels are higher than usual in persons with coronary heart disease.
3. Persons with high serum cholesterol levels develop coronary heart disease more often than those with normal levels.
4. The mortality rate from coronary heart disease in different countries varies in relation to the average blood cholesterol values (and with dietary fat and animal protein intake).
5. Experimentally induced hypercholesterolemia in animals is associated with atherosclerotic deposits.
6. Atherosclerotic plaques contain lipids similar in composition to those in the blood.

Evidence that atherosclerosis begins in childhood includes the following:

1. In autopsies of black and white males and females between 15 and 19 years old, the coronary arteries showed fatty streaks in 71% to 83% and raised atherosclerotic lesions in 7% to 22%.[5]
2. When bodies of US soldiers killed at a mean age of 22 years were examined, 77% of those from the Korean Conflict[6] and 45% of those from the Vietnam War[7] showed evidence of coronary vessel atherosclerosis.
3. United States adolescents who died of non-atherosclerotic causes show atherosclerotic changes of a magnitude directly related to postmortem low-density lipoprotein (LDL)-cholesterol plus very low-density lipoprotein (VLDL)-cholesterol levels and inversely related to HDL-cholesterol levels.[8]

Lipoproteins

Lipoproteins are necessary to make fats soluble so they can be transported in the plasma. All lipoproteins contain an outer polar layer of phospholipid, unesterified cholesterol, and protein (called apoprotein). The inner, nonpolar core contains cholesterol ester and triglyceride in varying proportions. The types of lipoproteins are

1. Chylomicrons, which are formed from dietary fat and enter the plasma via the thoracic duct, are removed from the blood by the activity of lipoprotein lipase (LPL) with the fatty acids, stored in adipose tissue as triglyceride, or catabolized by the liver. They do not form other lipoproteins.
2. Very low-density lipoproteins (also called pre-β-lipoproteins) are formed from dietary glucose and nonesterified fatty acids in the liver and are then secreted into the plasma. The outer surface of VLDLs contains apoproteins

β-100 and E. The LPL on capillary endothelium of adipose tissue and cardiac and skeletal muscle partially metabolizes the VLDLs to nonesterified fatty acids for storage or for energy, with a remnant remaining. The apoprotein E allows the remnant to be taken up by the liver. Several types of hyperlipoproteinemia have been identified.[9]

3. If the remnant also contains apoprotein β-100, it can be used for synthesis of LDL in the liver.

4. Low-density lipoprotein is formed in the liver from VLDL remnants containing apoprotein β-100; LDL is an important source of cholesterol for peripheral tissues. An important step in the regulation of cholesterol metabolism is the attachment of LDL to receptor sites on cell surfaces.

5. High-density lipoprotein is secreted by the liver and small intestine and is important in helping to remove cholesterol from cells (high levels are protective; low levels are a strong risk factor for coronary heart disease).

Types of Hyperlipidemia

The hereditary types of hyperlipidemias are sometimes difficult to distinguish from the hyperlipidemias related to diabetes and other conditions, but an attempt should be made to do so by family studies and other tests.[9,10]

Type I

Type I hyperlipoproteinemia is found in children and is usually associated with pancreatitis and abdominal pain. The triglycerides in this disorder are primarily chylomicron triglycerides. The activity of LPL is diminished or absent. This enzyme is responsible for hydrolysis and removal of chylomicrons from the blood. Thus the pathophysiologic mechanism is decreased triglyceride catabolism. Type I hyperlipoproteinemia is relatively rare; it may occur secondarily in children with lupus erythematosus, pancreatitis, or immunologic disorders.

Type II-a

Type II-a hyperlipoproteinemia, which consists of elevation of the level of serum cholesterol and LDL, is probably the most common of the 5 lipoprotein disorders to manifest in childhood. The homozygous form can be seen during the first year of life, and the differential diagnosis can be made on the basis of the following:

1. Serum cholesterol higher than 12.95 mmol/L (500 mg/dL)
2. Concentrations of LDL about twice that of heterozygotes in the same kindred
3. Both parents with elevated serum cholesterol levels

4. Xanthomas appearing before the age of 10 years
5. Vascular disease before age 20 years
6. Exclusion of clinically similar secondary hyperlipidemias

In the heterozygous condition, usually no skin xanthomas are present, and the serum cholesterol level is lower than 12.95 mmol/L (500 mg/dL); yet these individuals have a definite predisposition to coronary heart disease during early adulthood. The basic metabolic defect is a lack of functional LDL receptors on the cell membrane, with 3 different classes of mutations.[11] As a result of the LDL not attaching to the cell membrane, cholesterol is not released to suppress the rate-limiting enzyme in cholesterol synthesis, hydroxymethylglutaryl-coenzyme A (CoA) reductase.

Type II-b

Type II-b hyperlipoproteinemia, which includes familial combined hyperlipidemia, consists of elevated triglyceride and cholesterol levels, with concomitant increased LDL and VLDL. This is the third most frequent of the types with the onset during childhood, but the situation frequently is confusing because the parents may have other types of hyperlipoproteinemia and because of the variations in the cholesterol and triglyceride levels caused by changes in diet and exercise.

Type III

Type III hyperlipoproteinemia, "floating beta" with the LDL having an abnormal density and consisting of an abnormal protein, is rare. The onset is usually after age 20 years. The basic defect is thought to be in the conversion of VLDL to LDL (abnormal remnant catabolism) because of an abnormal apoprotein E. Increased remnants, VLDL, chylomicrons, and apoprotein E are all present. Xanthomas may occur, and early coronary and peripheral vascular disease have been reported.

Type IV

Type IV hyperlipoproteinemia, "familial hypertriglyceridemia," is associated with elevated levels of serum triglycerides and is the second most common of the disorders found in children, although the elevation in level of serum triglycerides may not occur in some patients until a later age. This condition is a monogenic autosomally inherited disorder. It involves an increase in production and secretion of triglyceride-rich VLDL. Elevated triglyceride levels can occur in relation to other factors, such as infrequent exercise, stress, an inadequate period of fasting before obtaining blood samples, diabetes, and obesity. Establishing that the patient has the genetic disease and excluding another cause for the elevation is important. This is best done by studying parents and other family members as well as the patient.

Type V

Type V hyperlipoproteinemia is rare in childhood and is associated with increased triglyceride levels related to increased chylomicrons and increased VLDL. This condition may be primarily familial, or it may be secondary to diabetes, nephrotic syndrome, or hypothyroidism. The onset may be similar to that of type I, although it occurs in adulthood rather than childhood.

Prevention of Atherosclerosis and Prudent Lifestyle and Diet

In 1983, 1986, 1992, and 1998,[2,3,11,12] the AAP Committee on Nutrition made recommendations about the risks of atherosclerosis and, when possible, the avoidance of risks. Of these, avoidance of smoking, increased physical activity, and treatment of hypertension and diabetes are emphasized. After 1 year of age, it was recommended that a varied diet best assures nutritional adequacy. Decreased consumption of saturated fats, cholesterol, and sodium and increased intake of monounsaturated and polyunsaturated fats were recommended. No restriction of fat or cholesterol intake was recommended for infants younger than 2 years because this is a period of rapid growth and development with high energy requirements. Early recognition and treatment of obesity and hypertension, a regular exercise program, and counseling about the dangers of smoking were recommended for all children older than 2 years. The family history should include information about family members who had (before 55 years of age) heart attack, stroke, hypertension, obesity, diabetes mellitus, or hyperlipidemia, with screening by at least 2 serum cholesterol measurements for children older than 2 years with a positive family history. The optimal fat intake was suggested to be a total fat intake of approximately 30% of calories for children older than 2 years.

Intake of skim or partly skimmed milk is not recommended during the first 2 years because of the high-protein, high-electrolyte concentration. Furthermore, the low-calorie density of these milks increases the volume necessary to satisfy caloric requirements.

While some studies have shown safety in lowering fat intakes in infants,[13] the transition to a lower fat diet beginning at the age of 2 years requires special consideration. Approximately 50% of the calories in the diet of the exclusively breastfed infant comes from the fat content of the milk. As solids are introduced during the first and second years of life, the percentage of calories in the diet contributed by fat decreases. At 2 to 3 years, if only 30% of total calories are derived from fat, for some infants the protein content would have to provide 15% or more of calories for the diet to meet the recommended dietary allowances for minerals. Early childhood then should be considered a transition period during which the fat and cholesterol content of the diet should gradually decrease to the recommended amounts. Particular care should be taken to avoid excessive restriction of dietary fat. The consumption of lower fat dairy products and lean meats, critical sources of protein, iron, and calcium, as well as grains, cereals, fruits, and vegetables should be encouraged throughout childhood and adolescence.

The NCEP Expert Panel on Blood Cholesterol Levels in Children and Adolescents and the AAP offer the following specific recommendations for the population older than 2 years[3,4]:

1. Nutritional adequacy should be achieved by eating a wide variety of foods.
2. Energy (calories) should be adequate to support growth and to reach or maintain desirable body weight.
3. The following intake pattern is recommended: saturated fatty acids, less than 10% of total energy intake (serum cholesterol appears most responsive to dietary saturated fatty acids); total fat, averaged over several days, no less than 20% of total calories and no more than 30% of calories; and dietary cholesterol, less than 300 mg/d.

Carbohydrate content of the diet should be 55% to 60% of the calories, of which the majority should be complex carbohydrates. Fiber is an important dietary constituent that can affect blood cholesterol levels. Current recommendations for fiber intake in children range from 0.5 g/kg to approximately 12 g/1000 kcal. Protein should provide 10% to 15% of dietary calories.

This diet is similar to the American Heart Association Step I Diet recommended for moderate reduction of serum cholesterol levels. Similarly composed diets are useful in controlling obesity.

Screening for Hyperlipidemia

The AAP endorses an individualized approach to screening and treating children (over age 2 years) and adolescents whose risk of developing coronary vas-

> The AAP endorses an individualized approach to screening and treating children and adolescents whose risk of developing coronary vascular disease as adults can be identified through family history. If the family history cannot be ascertained and other risk factors are present, screening should be at the discretion of the physician.
>
> *Pediatrics.* 1998:101:141–147

cular disease as adults can be identified through family history. If the family history cannot be ascertained and other risk factors are present, screening should be at the discretion of the physician.

The poor predictive value of a total cholesterol level for an elevated LDL-cholesterol level[4] and the imperfect tracking of blood cholesterol values from childhood to adulthood[15,16] are among the factors that weigh against a recommendation for universal cholesterol testing. Universal screening by any method other than family history will continue to be inadvisable until tests become available that better predict later coronary vascular disease. An elevated blood cholesterol value in childhood is only a risk factor for an elevated blood cholesterol value as an adult, which in turn is a risk factor for coronary vascular disease. The possibility of unwarranted anxiety and unnecessary dietary restriction from false-positive results is significant.[17]

Children with elevated blood cholesterol values undoubtedly will be missed by selective screening.[18–20] Family history may be unavailable or unknown. However, a universal (population-based) approach to dietary modification of fat and cholesterol intake and the reversibility of coronary vascular lesions when diet and drug therapy are used during middle age suggests that selective screening of children is an appropriate recommendation. Children whose parents or grandparents had a documented myocardial infarction, positive results on a coronary angiogram, or cerebrovascular or peripheral vascular disease before the age of 55 years qualify for screening blood tests. For these children, the initial test should be determination of blood lipoprotein values, obtained after a 12-hour fast. Children (over age 2 years) whose parents have a serum cholesterol level greater than or equal to 6.2 mmol/L (240 mg/dL) should be screened for total serum cholesterol level. Figures 32.1 and 32.2 present algorithms for screening and initiating therapy.

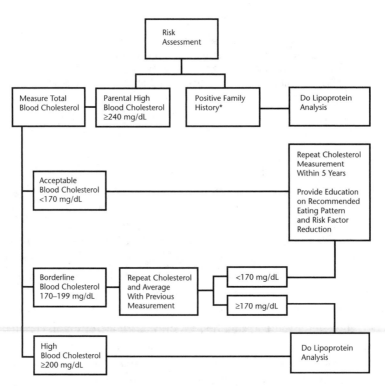

Figure 32.1. Risk assessment. *Positive family history is defined as a history of premature (before age 55 years) cardiovascular disease in a parent or grandparent (from National Cholesterol Education Program [NCEP][4]). To convert mg/dL to mmol/L, multiply by 0.02586.

For a youth at risk, blood determinations are recommended. For initial screening of those whose parents have high levels of serum cholesterol, total cholesterol should be determined. For children with a family history of cardiovascular disease, the child should fast for 12 hours. Blood is drawn with the patient in the sitting position. Levels of total cholesterol, HDL cholesterol, and triglycerides are determined; the LDL cholesterol level is estimated from these. Interpretations are given in Table 32.1 for children and adolescents.

Appropriate examinations or tests for secondary causes of hypercholesterolemia should be performed (Table 32.2) before treatment.

To accomplish the Step II diet, the meat serving size should be taken and the calories increased from the other food groups.

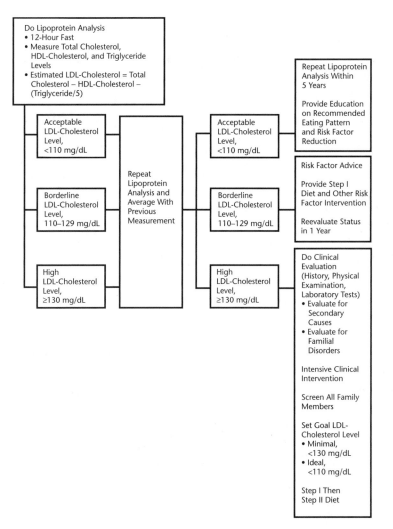

Figure 32.2. Classification, education, and follow-up based on low-density lipoprotein cholesterol (from National Cholesterol Education Program [NCEP][4]). HDL indicates high-density lipoprotein; LDL, low-density lipoprotein. To convert mg/dL to mmol/L, multiply by 0.02586.

Table 32.1.
Interpretation of Cholesterol Levels for Children and Adolescents*

Term	Total Cholesterol, mg/dL	LDL Cholesterol, mg/dL
Acceptable	<170	<110
Borderline	170–199	110–129
High	>200	>130

*From National Cholesterol Education Program (NCEP).[4] To convert mg/dL to mmol/L, multiply by 0.02586.

Table 32.2.
Causes of Secondary Hypercholesterolemia

Exogenous	**Storage Diseases**
Drugs	Glycogen storage diseases
Oral contraceptives, corticosteroids, isotretinoin (Accutane), thiazides, anticonvulsants, β-blockers, anabolic steroids	Sphingolipidoses
	Obstructive Liver Diseases
Alcohol	Biliary atresia
Obesity	Biliary cirrhosis
Endocrine and Metabolic	**Chronic Renal Diseases**
Hypothyroidism	Nephrotic syndrome
Diabetes mellitus	**Others**
Lipodystrophy	Anorexia nervosa
Pregnancy	Progeria
Idiopathic hypercalcemia	Collagen vascular disease
	Klinefelter syndrome

Bread, Cereal, Rice, and Pasta Group (Grains group)—whole grain and refined
- 1 slice bread
- About 1 c of ready-to-eat cereal
- 1 c of cooked cereal, rice, or pasta

Vegetable Group
- 1 c raw leafy vegetables
- 1/2 c of other vegetables—cooked or raw
- 1 c vegetable juice

Fruit Group
- 1 medium apple, banana, orange, pear
- 1 c chopped, cooked, or canned fruit
- 1 c fruit juice

Milk, Yogurt, and Cheese Group (Milk Group)
- 2 c fat free milk or yogurt
- 1 oz of natural cheese (such as Cheddar)
- 2 oz of processed cheese (such as American)

Meat, Poultry, Fish, Dry Beans, Eggs, and Nuts Group (Meat and Beans Group)
- 2–3 oz of cooked lean meat, poultry, or fish
- 1/2 c of cooked dry beans or 1/2 c of tofu counts as 1 oz of lean meat
- 2 oz of soy burger or 1 egg counts as 1 oz of lean meat
- 2 tbsp of peanut butter or 1/3 c of nuts counts as 1 oz of meat

Treatment

Therapy should be initiated after the diagnosis of hyperlipidemia is confirmed by 2 separate blood tests done at least 2 weeks apart. Dietary therapy is the first mode of treatment in almost all instances, whether or not elevations are due to a genetic cause. A 3-day diet record is extremely helpful for suggesting changes; this record should be as typical as possible of the child's usual intake. Consultation with a dietitian or nutritionist is helpful.

The step I diet (Table 32.3) suggests an average intake of saturated fatty acids less than 10% of total calories, total fat no more than 30% of calories, and cholesterol less than 300 mg/d. The polyunsaturated fatty acids constitute up to 10%; and the monounsaturated fatty acids, 10% to 15% of the total calories.

Avoidance of smoking, the value of exercise, attaining weight appropriate for age and body build, and correction or treatments of other risk factors are emphasized. If after 3 months desired lipid levels are not achieved, the step II diet is initiated. Saturated fatty acids are reduced to about 7% of the caloric

Table 32.3.
Step I and Step II Diets*

Nutrient	Recommended Intake	
	Step I Diet	Step II Diet
Total fat	Average of no more than 30% of total calories and no less than 20%	Same as step I diet
Saturated fatty acids	Less than 10% of total calories	Less than 7% of total calories
Polyunsaturated fatty acids	Up to 10% of total calories	Same as step I diet
Monounsaturated fatty acids	Remaining dietary fat calories	Same as step I diet
Cholesterol	Less than 300 mg/d	Less than 200 mg/d
Carbohydrates	About 55% of total calories	Same as step I diet
Protein	About 15% of total calories	Same as step I diet
Calories	To promote growth and development	Same as step I diet

*Adapted from National Cholesterol Education Program (NCEP) and AAP Committee on Nutrition.[3,4]

Table 32.4.
Number of Servings From Each of the Food Groups That Should Be Taken for the Step I Diet*

FOOD GROUPS	Children aged 2 to 6 years, women, some older adults (about 1600 calories)	Older children, teen girls, active women, most men active men (about 2200 calories)	Teen boys, active men (about 2800 calories)
Bread, Cereal, Rice, and Pasta Group (Grains group)—especially whole grain	6	9	11
Vegetable Group	3	4	5
Fruit Group	2 or 3	2 or 3	2 or 3
Meat, Poultry, Fish, Dry Beans, Eggs, and Nut Groups, (Meat and Beans Group—preferably lean or low fat)	2, for a total of 5 ounces	2, for a total of 6 ounces	3, for a total of 7 ounces

*Adapted from *Dietary Guidelines for Americans*; 2000.[21]

intake; cholesterol is reduced to less than 200mg/d. Dietary fat must be even further restricted in patients with type I hyperlipoproteinemia.

The NCEP Panel for Children and Adolescents recommends that after an adequate trial of diet therapy has been completed (6 months to 1 year), drug therapy should be considered in children 10 years or older under the following conditions:

1. If LDL cholesterol remains above 4.9 mmol/L (190 mg/dL); or
2. If LDL cholesterol remains above 4.1 mmol/L (160 mg/dL) *and* there is a positive family history of cardiovascular disease before age 55; *or* 2 or more other risk factors for cardiovascular disease are present.

The goal of drug therapy is to achieve an LDL-cholesterol level to approach 2.85 mmol/L (110 mg/dL). Drugs recommended for children and adolescents are the bile acid sequestrants, cholestyramine and cholestipol, because of their apparent safety. Drugs that cause profound metabolic effects, such as niacin, hydroxymethylglutaryl-CoA reductase inhibitors, probucol, gemfibrozil, thyroxine, and clofibrate, are not recommended for routine use in children and adolescents because no long-term clinical trials of these agents in children have been completed.

Since 1992, when these recommendations were made by National Cholesterol Education Program Expert Panel on Blood Cholesterol Levels in Children and Adolescents,[4] several short-term studies of the use of hydroxymethylglutaryl-CoA reductase inhibitors in adolescents have shown their efficacy, acceptability, and safety.[22] However, because the long-term effects of these drugs have not been tested, careful monitoring of liver function and the presence of skeletal myolysis should be regularly assessed throughout childhood and adolescence.

References

1. Kannel WB, Castelli WP, Gordon T. Cholesterol in the prediction of atherosclerotic disease. New perspectives based on the Framingham study. *Ann Intern Med.* 1979;90: 85–91
2. American Academy of Pediatrics, Committee on Nutrition. Statement on cholesterol. *Pediatrics.* 1992;90:469–473
3. American Academy of Pediatrics, Committee on Nutrition. Cholesterol in childhood. *Pediatrics.* 1998;101:141–147
4. National Cholesterol Education Program (NCEP): highlights of the report of the Expert Panel on Blood Cholesterol Levels in Children and Adolescents. *Pediatrics.* 1992;89:495–501
5. Strong JP, McGill HC Jr. The pediatric aspects of atherosclerosis. *J Atherosclerosis Res.* 1969;9:251–265
6. Enos WF Jr, Beyer JC, Holmes RH. Pathogenesis of coronary disease in American soldiers killed in Korea. *JAMA.* 1955;158:912–914
7. McNamara JJ, Molot MA, Stremple JF, Cutting RT. Coronary artery disease in combat casualties in Vietnam. *JAMA.* 1971;216:1185–1187

8. Strong JP, Malcom GT, McMahan CA, et al. Prevalence and extent of atherosclerosis in adolescents and young adults: implications for prevention from the Pathobiological Determinants of Atherosclerosis in Youth Study. *JAMA*. 1999;281: 727–735

9. Fredrickson DS, Goldstein JL, Brown MS. The familial hyperlipoproteinemias. In: Stanbury JB, Wyngaarden JB, Fredrickson DS, eds. *The Metabolic Basis of Inherited Disease*. 4th ed. New York, NY: McGraw-Hill Book Co; 1978:604–655

10. Havel RJ, Kane JP. Introduction: structure and metabolism of plasma lipoproteins. In: Scriver CR, Beaudet AL, Sly WS, Valle D, eds. *The Metabolic Basis of Inherited Disease*. Vol 1. 6th ed. New York, NY: McGraw-Hill Book Co; 1989:1129–1138

11. Goldstein JL, Brown MS. The LDL receptor defect in familial hypercholesterolemia. Implications for pathogenesis and therapy. *Med Clin North Am*. 1982; 66:335–362

12. American Academy of Pediatrics, Committee on Nutrition. Toward a prudent diet for children. *Pediatrics*. 1983;71:78–80

13. Simell O, Niinikoski H, Viikari J, Rask-Nissila L, Tammi A, Ronnemaa T. Cardiovascular disease risk factors in young children in the STRIP baby project. *Ann Med*. 1999;31(suppl):55–61

14. American Academy of Pediatrics, Committee on Nutrition. Prudent life-style for children: dietary fat and cholesterol. *Pediatrics*. 1986;78:521–525

15. Dennison BA, Kikuchi DA, Srinivasan SR, Webber LS, Berenson GS. Serum total cholesterol screening for the detection of elevated low-density lipoprotein in children and adolescents: the Bogalusa Heart Study. *Pediatrics*. 1990;85:472–479

16. Lauer RM, Clarke WR. Use of cholesterol measurements in childhood for the prediction of adult hypercholesterolemia. The Muscatine Study. *JAMA*. 1990;264: 3034–3038

17. Stuhldreher WL, Orchard TJ, Donahue RP, Kuller LH, Gloninger MF, Drash AL. Cholesterol screening in childhood: sixteen-year Beaver County Lipid Study experience. *J Pediatr*. 1991;119:551–556

18. Newman TB, Browner WS, Hulley SB. The case against childhood cholesterol screening. *JAMA*. 1990;264:3039–3043

19. Griffin TC, Christoffel KK, Binns HJ, McGuire PA. Family history evaluation as a predictive screen for childhood hypercholesteremia. Pediatric Practice Research Group. *Pediatrics*. 1989;84:365–373

20. Dennison BA, Kikuchi DA, Srinivasan SR, Webber LS, Berenson GS. Parental history of cardiovascular disease as an indication for screening for lipoprotein abnormalities in children. *J Pediatr*. 1989;115:186–194

21. US Department of Agriculture, US Department of Health and Human Services. *Nutrition and Your Health: Dietary Guidelines for Americans*. 5th ed. Washington, DC: US Government Printing Office; 2000

22. Stein EA, Illingworth DR, Kwiterovich PO Jr, et al. Efficacy and safety of lovastatin in adolescent males with heterozygous familial hypercholesterolemia: a randomized controlled trial. *JAMA*. 1999;281:137–144

33

Pediatric Obesity

Definition

Obesity or overweight may be defined functionally as a maladaptive increase in the mass of somatic fat stores. An ideal definition of obesity in children will reflect both the likelihood that the child will become an obese adult, as well as present and future risk of adiposity-related morbidity. In evaluating diagnostic criteria for obesity, the following should be considered:

1. The risk of persistence of pediatric obesity into adulthood increases with age, independent of the length of time that the child has been obese.[1]
2. The risk of adiposity-related morbidity is strongly influenced by family history of such morbidities, regardless of whether affected family members are obese.[1,2]
3. Growth patterns are familial. A mildly overweight teenager with a family history of excessive weight gain in adulthood may be at greater risk for subsequent obesity than a more severely overweight teenager without a family history of obesity in adulthood.[2]

Direct assessment of body fatness by hydrodensitometry (underwater weighing) or various radiologic methods are not feasible in the pediatrician's office. Plots of weight, height, and weight-for-height measures versus reference "standards" are the indices of body fatness generally used by clinicians to assess body fatness in children. However, these standards are neither sufficiently sensitive to identify all children at risk for adiposity-related morbidity, nor sufficiently specific to identify only children at such risk. Interpretation of these weight and height measures must be highly individualized for each child by assessing obesity and morbidity risk in the context of family history and other risk factors for disease.

Body mass index (BMI, weight [kg]/[height (m)]^2) is a surrogate measure of body fatness that correlates quite well with direct measures of body fatness within a population.[3,4] An American Medical Association Expert Panel on Obesity has recently suggested that adults with a BMI >25 kg/m^2 be defined as overweight or "at risk" for adiposity-related morbidity, while those with a BMI >30 kg/m[2] be defined as obese.[5] Because normative values for BMI are highly age dependent[6] (see Table 33.1), these adult definitions based on BMI cannot be used in children.

Table 33.1.
Mean Body Mass Index (kg/m[2]) of Children Enrolled in the National Health Examination Survey (NHES) II or III (1963–1970) or the National Health and Nutrition Examination Survey (NHANES) III (1988–1994)[6]

Age (years)	6	7	8	9	10	11	12	13	14	15	16	17
Males NHES II or III	15.6	15.9	16.3	16.9	17.1	17.9	18.4	19.4	20.2	20.9	21.3	22.1
NHANES III	16.3	16.5	17.3	18.0	18.4	19.4	20.1	20.5	22.3	22.3	22.3	23.4
Females NHES II or III	15.4	15.8	16.4	17.0	17.6	18.2	19.2	19.9	20.8	21.4	21.9	21.7
NHANES III	16.1	16.9	17.3	18.2	18.4	19.4	20.2	21.8	22.4	21.9	23.0	23.3

The International Life Sciences Institute and American Academy of Pediatrics Expert Panels have recently suggested a classification system for overweight in children similar to that described in adults.[6] Children with a BMI in the 85th percentile to 95th percentile of BMI for age and gender, based on National Health and Nutrition Examination Survey I (NHANES I, 1971–1974) data, are defined as "at risk" for overweight, while those with a BMI >95th percentile are defined as overweight[7] (see Table 33.2B). It should also be noted that individuals at the extremes of body composition (either extremely high or extremely low percentages of body fat) may be incorrectly labeled as non-overweight or as overweight, respectively, solely based on BMI. However, in most cases, the clinician should be able to visually distinguish the obese child from the extremely muscular child. If this distinction cannot readily be made (ie, if the clinician is uncertain whether a child with an elevated BMI has an elevated body weight predominantly due to an abnormally large adipose tissue or lean body mass), then further evaluation of body fat by triceps skinfold thicknesses (see Table 31.2A) may be indicated. Growth charts of age- and gender-specific BMI percentiles are now available (see Appendix J) and can be downloaded directly from the Centers for Disease Control and Prevention (www.cdc.gov/nchs/data/ad/ad314.pdf).

Table 33.2A.
85th Percentile/95th Percentile Body Mass Index (kg/m²) and Triceps Skinfold Thickness (mm) (Midpoint Between the Acromion and Olecranon on the Posterior Surface of the Arm) of Children Enrolled in National Health and Nutrition Examination Survey I (1971–1974)[7]

Age (years)	6	7	8	9	10	11	12	13	14	15	16	17
Body Mass Index (kg/m²)												
Males 85th percentile	16.5	17.3	18.1	18.9	19.7	22.3	21.3	22.1	23.0	23.8	24.6	25.4
95th percentile	17.8	19.0	20.2	21.5	20.5	23.9	25.0	20.5	26.1	27.0	28.7	29.5
Females 85th percentile	16.1	17.2	18.2	19.2	20.2	21.2	22.3	23.3	23.9	24.3	24.7	25.1
95th percentile	17.5	18.9	20.4	21.8	23.0	24.6	26.0	27.1	28.0	28.5	29.1	29.7
Triceps Skinfold Thickness (mm)												
Males 85th percentile	11.1	12.4	13.7	14.9	16.0	16.9	17.3	17.1	16.4	15.8	16.0	16.6
95th percentile	14.1	15.6	17.2	18.8	20.7	22.2	23.3	23.7	23.5	22.3	21.5	21.5
Females 85th percentile	13.4	14.9	16.4	17.9	19.0	20.1	21.3	22.3	23.3	24.3	25.1	25.8
95th percentile	15.6	17.9	20.2	22.5	24.4	26.2	28.0	29.5	30.9	32.2	33.2	34.8

Table 33.2B.
Prevalence of overweight and obesity among different children in different ethnic groups in the National Health and Nutrition Examination Survey III[8] based on 85th percentile and 95th percentile in the National Health Examination Survey II and III

	At-Risk for Overweight (BMI 85th to 95th percentile)				Overweight (BMI >95th percentile)			
	Age 6–11 years		Age 12–17 years		Age 6–11 years		Age 12–17 years	
	Boys	Girls	Boys	Girls	Boys	Girls	Boys	Girls
All	21.6±2.4	22.7±2.4	22.0±2.2	21.4±2.7	11.3±1.8	12.8±1.9	10.6±1.3	8.8±1.4
White	20.5±2.8	21.5±3.7	23.1±3.1	20.3±3.5	10.4±2.4	14.4±2.7	9.8±2.0	8.3±1.6
African American	26.5±2.7	31.4±4.0	21.1±3.7	29.9±4.5	13.4±2.3	9.3±2.4	16.9±2.8	14.4±3.1
Hispanic American	33.3±3.0	29.0±2.1	26.7±4.6	23.4±3.0	17.7±2.3	12.8±3.2	14.3±1.7	8.7±2.5

Epidemiology

Sociodemographic Data

In the United States, obesity is more prevalent among children raised in urban communities and in smaller families. The prevalence of obesity also varies among different ethnic groups (more prevalent among African Americans and Hispanic Americans) (see Table 33.2B), geographic regions (more prevalent in the northeast > midwest > south > west; urban > rural) and socioeconomic classes (more prevalent in poorer, less-educated families or single parent/older parent families, less prevalent in large families).[8–16] These strong demographic trends demonstrate that there is potent environmental interaction with whatever genetic predispositions toward obesity may exist.

Prenatal and Postnatal Influences on Adiposity

Prenatal undernutrition has been studied by examining the prevalence of obesity in children conceived during periods of natural or man-made famine such as the Nazi-imposed Dutch famine of 1944–1945 (the "Winter Hunger").[17] There was a small but statistically significant increase in the prevalence of obesity (defined as weight for height greater than 120% of World Health Organization standards for 1948) in 19-year-old male military recruits whose mothers were malnourished only during the first trimester of pregnancy (2.77% prevalence if mother was in famine area versus 1.45% if mother was outside of famine area during pregnancy), and a decrease in the prevalence of obesity among recruits whose mothers were malnourished during the child's immediate postnatal period (0.82% if mother was in famine area vs 1.32% if mother was outside of famine area during pregnancy). It has been hypothesized that early intrauterine malnutrition might affect hypothalamic ("appetite center") development while the anti-obesity effects of early postnatal malnutrition might be due to suppression of adipocyte formation. Despite the lower mean birthweight and adult BMI of recruits who had experienced prenatal malnutrition in the second or third trimester of pregnancy, these same adults had a higher incidence of type 2 diabetes mellitus than the cohort of subjects who were exposed to prenatal malnutrition early in pregnancy and who were slightly fatter.[18] In general, birth weight has been shown to be negatively correlated with the incidence of adiposity-related morbidities, including type 2 diabetes mellitus, hypertension, stroke, and cardiovascular disease in adulthood, even when corrected for adult adiposity.[19–23] This association implies an interaction between the prenatal environment and development/function of pancreatic beta cells or other organs (eg, hypothalamus, liver) that are involved in the regulation of adult-energy homeostasis and cardiovascular function. As hypothesized by Barker,[22,24,25] the metabolic, cardiovascular, and endocrine bases for adult adiposity-related morbidities may originate through adaptations that the fetus makes in response to undernourishment. Therefore, the small-for-gestational-age baby may be considered to be at increased risk for adult morbidities that are exacerbated by increased adiposity.[26] It should be noted, however, that the concept of "metabolic programming" of the human fetus or neonate for chronic illness later in adult life, based on retrospective observational data, remains controversial.

The infant of a diabetic mother (IDM) is a model for the influences of fetal overnutrition on postnatal adiposity. Exposure of the fetus to high ambient glucose concentrations stimulates fetal hyperinsulinemia, increased lipogenesis, and macrosomia. Since women with gestational diabetes are often obese, it is difficult to separate the metabolic effects of gestational diabetes on subsequent adiposity of the IDM from the possibility that the mother has transmitted a genetic tendency toward obesity to her offspring. In studies controlled for the effects of maternal adiposity, being an IDM is still associated with an increased risk of obesity, independent of the degree of maternal obesity.[27-29] The effects of early infant feeding practices on subsequent adiposity remain controversial. Many studies fail to control for possible effects of maternal socioeconomic status and adiposity on ability to breastfeed. Some studies that do control for these effects suggest that predominantly breastfeeding for at least 6 months is associated with an approximately 20% to 30% reduction in the prevalence of obesity (defined as BMI >95th percentile for age and gender) through early adolescence.[30,31] Other well-controlled studies do not show a reduction in adult adiposity in those who were breastfed as infants.[32,33]

Neither the age at which specific foods are introduced into the diet nor the proportions of fat, carbohydrate, or protein in the diet significantly influences subsequent adult adiposity.[34,35] However, the institution of a well-balanced diet in childhood may form the basis for long-term healthy dietary habits that will significantly lower cardiovascular disease risk even if the diet composition does not substantially affect body composition. Significant negative correlations have been reported between physical activity and body fatness in preschool children, while positive correlations have been noted between adiposity and the amount of time spent watching television in adolescence.[36-40] More than 60% of television commercials during children's programs are food related, and television watching promotes both inactivity and increased caloric intake.[41]

Demographic Trends in the Prevalence of Pediatric Obesity

The increasing fatness of the pediatric population is especially evident at the extremes of body fatness. In a study of US adolescents conducted between 1988 and 1991, the prevalence of obesity (defined as BMI >85th percentile based on data obtained in the NHES I survey, 1963–1970) rose from 15% to 22.5% in 6- to 11-year-olds and 15% to 21.5% in 12- to 17-year-olds.[8] Using the criteria of BMI described (defining obesity in children as BMI >95th percentile based on NHES I survey (see Table 33.2A), the prevalence of obesity among children aged 6 to 11 years has risen from 5% to 10.8%, and from 5% to 10.5% in 12- to 17-year-olds.[8,13,42] Thus, while the prevalence of overweight increased by an average of about 40% over this time period, the prevalence of obesity has more than doubled. Such skewing of weight increases is consistent with impact of relevant environmental changes on a genetically susceptible subgroup within the population. Changes in the mean BMI of children aged 6 to 17 from NHES II or III to NHANES III are illustrated in Table 33.1.

Although there are clearly genetic influences on susceptibility to obesity (described in this chapter), the current demographics of obesity and the large increases in the prevalence of obesity over a single decade must reflect major changes in nongenetic factors. The interaction of genetic factors favoring storage of calories as fat and an environment, which is permissive to the clinical expression of this genetic tendency, is thus evident in the increasing prevalence of pediatric (and adult) obesity. Such secular trends may also be taken as tacit evidence that some instances/aspects of obesity are responsive to, and, therefore, preventable by, environmental manipulation (eg, diet, physical activity). However, the resistance of obesity to current therapies (including a variety of environmental and behavioral manipulations) is reflected in an overall 75% to 95% reported recidivism rate to obesity among formerly obese adults and children.[43–48]

Pathophysiology

The first law of thermodynamics dictates that the accumulation of stored energy (fat) must be due to caloric intake in excess of energy expenditure. A small excess of energy intake relative to expenditure will, over time, lead to a substantial increase in body weight. For example, an individual increasing daily caloric intake by 150 kcal (8 oz of whole milk) above usual daily energy expenditure, would gain approximately 8 lbs before a new equilibrium between energy intake and expenditure (due to increased body mass) was reached. Despite the potentially large effects of small imbalances in energy intake versus expenditure, adults maintain a relatively constant body weight and most children tend to grow steadily along their respective weight percentile isobars for age, with little conscious effort to regulate energy intake or expenditure.

The high rate of recidivism to previous levels of fatness of reduced-obese children and adults[43–48] and the tendency for individuals to maintain a relatively stable body weight over long periods of time, despite variations in caloric intake,[49] provide empirical evidence that body weight is regulated, and that energy intake and expenditure are not independent processes, but rather are regulated by complex interlocking control mechanisms. Data generated from studies of energy homeostasis in adults must be applied cautiously to children. Unlike adults, children accrete both fat mass and fat-free mass as they grow and, unlike adults, the magnitude and composition of this weight gain is highly age- and gender-dependent.[3,50,51]

The energy expended in growth is a combination of the energy stored as protein, carbohydrate, or fat and the energy expended in the process of storing these calories. Though the amount of energy stored per gram of fat (~7 kcal/g) is about twice that of protein or carbohydrate (~4 kcal/g), the energy cost of synthesis and deposition of stored energy as protein (1.4 kcal/1 kcal energy stored or approximately 0.3 kcal/g protein stored) is much greater than the cost of fat synthesis and storage (0.17 kcal/kcal energy stored or approximately 0.2 kcal/g fat stored).[52,53] The number of calories to be deposited for energy storage is maximal, and the energy cost of caloric deposition is minimal, in the infant at 2 to 3 months of age, when approximately 40% of weight gain is fat and 10% is protein (the remaining weight gain is due mostly to water and, to a lesser degree, skeletal growth). The converse is true at age 1 year when the average composition of weight gain is 10% fat and 17% protein.[52] Therefore, in calculating infant energy expenditure, one must include not only weight-maintenance calories, but also the fraction of calories that will be stored as lean or adipose tissue as normal growth occurs.

Because of the slower growth rate in the toddler and preadolescent years, the energy cost of growth after infancy constitutes only about 1% of total energy expenditure. In adolescence, the average male increases muscle mass out of proportion to weight gain while the average female increases fat mass out of proportion to weight gain. The average adult male has approximately 150% of the lean body mass and twice as many muscle cells as the average adult female, while females have, on the average, approximately 25% greater fat mass despite their average smaller stature and lower body weight. The comparatively greater cost of protein synthesis in the adolescent male is offset by the increased number of calories stored as fat versus protein in the adolescent female. Because of the increased lean body mass, males have significantly greater rates of resting energy expenditure than females and, therefore, require more calories to maintain their body composition at the same weight than the average female. These differences in resting metabolic rate, body composition, and the energy cost of growth may account for some features of the greater appetite that characterizes the mid-pubertal male, even when compared to a female of the same weight.

Energy Intake

Feeding behavior consists of "decisions" about initiation, composition, and termination of meals; these decisions are influenced by many internal and external factors. Voluntary food intake is increased in rodents and humans following intentional undernutrition relative to the same animal or person prior to food restriction.[54] The observed hyperphagia, relative to usual food intake, following caloric restriction ceases once "usual" body weight or, in the case of rodents, body weight similar to nonfood-restricted littermates is reached. Reciprocal changes are seen following imposed weight gain by overfeeding. Once the overfeeding is terminated, relative hypophagia ensues until the individual has returned to usual weight.[55–60] These transient changes in spontaneous food intake support the view that systems regulating energy intake are directly responsive to changes in stored calories.

Energy Expenditure

Total energy expenditure (TEE) can be viewed as the sum of the energy expended at rest in cardiorespiratory work and the maintenance of transmembrane ion gradients (resting energy expenditure, ~50% to 60% of TEE), the work of digestion and absorption of nutrients (thermic effect of feeding, ~5% to 10% of TEE), and energy expended as physical activity (non-resting energy expenditure, ~20% to 40% of total), and, to a small extent in the growing child beyond infancy, energy expended in the process of storing fat and nonfat mass in growth.[61] As discussed previously, energy costs of growth reflect both rates of growth (highest in infancy and adolescence) and the percentage of calories being stored as high-caloric density (approximately 7 kcal/g) fat (higher in females, especially during adolescence) versus carbohydrate or protein (approximately 4 kcal/g). The differences in caloric density of carbohydrate versus fat are exacerbated by the hydration of carbohydrate (actual caloric density of wet carbohydrate is approximately 1 kcal/g) versus hydrophobic fat, which contains less than 5% water.[50,51]

A number of studies have found that, in adults, the maintenance of a reduced body weight and/or the process of weight loss are associated with significant declines in 24-hour energy expenditure (weight-maintenance caloric requirements) beyond those expected solely on the basis of diminished tissue mass[62–73] and that the maintenance of a reduced body weight is associated with a decline in weight maintenance caloric requirements that is significantly (~300 kcal/d) greater than would be predicted solely on the basis of weight lost or compared to body composition-matched control subjects. Fewer studies have reported that 24-hour energy expenditure does not remain suppressed during maintenance of a reduced body weight[74,75]; and that weight-maintenance caloric need, corrected for changes in body composition following weight loss, is unchanged. However, as the long reference list (listed previously) suggests, this is a very active area of research with differing results probably arising from methodological differences between studies. Results of studies evaluating the effects of weight loss on energy expenditure may be strongly affected by lack of weight stability (declines in energy expenditure may be accentuated by weight loss) and whether the investigators have controlled for changes in physical activity. While carefully controlled studies of the effects of weight loss on energy expenditure in children are not yet available, the high rate of recidivism to at least previous levels of fatness among reduced obese children and adolescents suggests that these same systems are operant.[2,44,76–78]

Systems Integrating Energy Intake and Energy Expenditure Physiology and Molecular Genetics

Overview: The relative long-term constancy of body weight in humans, their lack of success in sustaining therapeutic weight loss, and the hypometabolism and hyperphagia that accompany weight decrease provide strong evidence that weight (fat) is biologically regulated. The amount of energy stored in the body as fat exerts potent effects on growth, pubescence, fertility, autonomic nervous system activity, and thyroid function, suggesting that humoral "signals" reflecting adipose tissue mass interact directly or indirectly with many neuroendocrine systems.[54,79–83] Weight loss and maintenance of a reduced body weight are accompanied by changes in autonomic nervous system function (increased parasympathetic and decreased sympathetic nervous system tone), circulating concentrations of thyroid hormones (decreased triiodothyronine and thyroxine without a compensatory increase in thyroid stimulating hormone [TSH]), and circulating concentrations of glucocorticoids (increased cortisol)[79,84,85] that are consistent with a homeostatic resistance to altered body weight, acting, in part, through effectors that mediate energy expenditure. Such a neurohumoral system to protect body energy stores would convey clear evolutionary advantages. During periods of undernutrition, the perceived reduction in energy stores would result in hyperphagia, hypometabolism, and decreased fertility (protecting females from the increased metabolic demands of pregnancy and lactation and the delivery of progeny into inhospitable environments).

The anatomy of body weight regulation: Classically, investigators of central nervous system regulation of energy intake and expenditure have viewed the brain as having discrete hunger and satiety centers that are located in the ventromedial and lateral regions of the hypothalamus, respectively. The view of the hypothalamus as having distinct areas regulating hunger and satiety was largely based on studies of rodents with lesions of the so-called satiety center in the ventromedial hypothalamus. These lesioned rodents became hyperphagic and hypometabolic until they had eaten their way to a higher body weight. The human hypothalamus also regulates both energy intake and expenditure. Traumatic or infectious injury to the human ventromedial hypothalamus results in a syndrome characterized by hyperphagia, hyperinsulinism, and hyperactivity of the parasympathetic nervous system. In fact, the hypothalamus is only a part of a complex regulatory system for energy homeostasis through which signals about the nutritional state of the organism, as well as hedonic signals about the palatability of available food, are integrated by a number of neuronal tracts that include the hypothalamus, cerebral cortex, and brain stem.

Outflow tracts from the hypothalamus to the nucleus tractus solitarius in the brainstem serve to integrate signals about the nutritional state of the organism from the gastrointestinal tract, endocrine glands, adipose tissue, and the central and peripheral nervous system with systems regulating energy expenditure and food intake (see Figure 33.1).[86] The hypothalamic pro-opiomelanocortin (POMC)-melanocortin-4 receptor (MC4R) pathway, by virtue of its constituent arcuate neurons' ability to affect the autonomic nervous system, neuroendocrine axes, pancreatic-cell function, and cortical tracts subserving food intake, may provide a central nexus for the integrated effects on energy expenditure and intake that have been detected in weight perturbation experiments.[80,86,87] Human autosomal recessive mutations leading to defects in POMC production result in central hypoadrenalism (due to lack of adrenocorticotropic hormone production), red hair (due to lack of α-MSH production), hyperphagia due to lack of transduction of leptin-stimulated hypothalamic POMC/α-MSH (melanocyte stimulating hormone) production resulting in lack of MC4R-induced appetite suppression,[86] and obesity.[87] Inactivating mutations of MC4R have been implicated in human obesity. In some studies, up to 5% of individuals with a BMI >40 kg/m² are heterozygous for such mutations.[87] Arcuate nucleus POMC is processed post-translationally in the hypothalamus to yield multiple neuropeptides including –melanocyte-stimulating hormone (–MSH), 3-MSH, and –endorphin (–EP). –EP inhibits the release of corticotropin releasing factor (CRF).[88]

Major chemical mediators of ingestive behavior and energy expenditure include peptides, hormones, and neurotransmitters, and are schematized in Figure 33.1.

Leptin: Leptin is secreted from adipose tissue and provides a signal linking fat mass to food intake and energy expenditure. Mice homozygous for the Lep^{ob} mutation (leptin-deficient) are obese due to increased food intake and

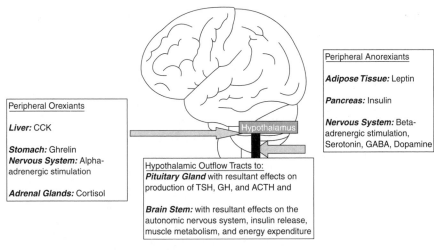

Figure 33.1. Major molecules affecting food intake by primary site of secretion. All of these molecules directly or indirectly input to the hypothalamus whose outflow tracts afftect energy expenditure. GHRH, Growth Hormone Releasing Hormone; NPY, Neuropeptide Y; AGRP, Agouti Related Peptide; SRIF, Somatostatin; MCH, Melanocyte Concentrating Hormone; MSH, Melanocyte Stimulating Hormone; CRF, Corticotropin Releasing Factor; CART, Cocaine-amphetamine-related transcript; GABA, Gamma-amino-butyric Acid; TSH, Thyroid Stimulating Hormone; GH, Growth Hormone; ACTH, Adrenocorticotropic Hormone. These molecules are described in detail in reference.[87]

reduced energy expenditure. Administration of leptin in the region of the hypothalamus or peripherally to Lep^{ob} mice decreases food intake and increases energy expenditure. In contrast to neuropeptide Y (NPY), which is associated with decreased thermogenesis, leptin administration to mice increases thermogenesis. Rare families have been identified in which hypoleptinemia (leptin gene mutation)[89,90] or leptin nonresponsiveness (leptin receptor mutation)[91] is inherited as an autosomal recessive disorder associated with obesity. As predicted from the leptin-deficient mouse, administration of physiological doses of leptin to a leptin-deficient child has been shown to promote weight loss. However, gross deficiency of leptin or its receptor do not appear to be frequent causes of human obesity. Administration of very high doses of leptin that produce circulating leptin concentrations per unit of fat mass 20 to 30 times above normal for fat mass are required to promote even modest weight loss in leptin-sufficient rodents or humans.[92,93]

The Molecular Genetics of Body Fatness

Heritability of Body Fatness: The ability to store calories as fat would presumably have conferred a survival advantage to our progenitors by enabling them to survive periods of prolonged caloric restriction, as well as increasing the fertility of women and enhancing their ability to breastfeed their offspring. Thus, it is likely that the human genome would be enriched with genes favoring the storage of calories as adipose tissue.[26,94]

There are rare instances of single gene/locus disorders, which result in human obesity (eg, Prader-Willi syndrome, Bardet-Biedl syndrome, Ahlstrom, Cohen), in association with other often dysmorphic phenotypes.[87,95] However, as indicated earlier, in most humans, body fatness is a continuous quantitative trait reflecting the interaction of development and environment with genotype. The calculation of heritability in twin studies is based on the assumption that each member of a monozygotic or dizygotic pair is reared in the same environment, and that the degree to which body fatness is more similar within mono- than dizygotic twin pairs is due to the greater genetic similarity of identical versus nonidentical twins. Studies comparing adopted children with their adoptive and their biological parents assume that each child shares little or none of the immediate environment with each biological parent, and that the degree to which body fatness is more similar between children and their biologic versus adoptive parents is due to the 50% of their genotype that each child shares with each biological parent. Twin and adoption studies indicate that the heritability of body fatness and of body fat distribution in adulthood is

65% to 80%, (approximately equal to the heritability of height and greater than the heritability of schizophrenia (68%) or breast cancer (45%).[96] Recent studies have also identified significant genetic influences (heritability greater than 30%) on resting metabolic rate, feeding behavior, food preferences, and changes in energy expenditure that occur in response to overfeeding.[87,97] Genetic influences on resting energy expenditure (REE) are evidenced by studies demonstrating that African American children tend to have lower REE than white children, even when adjusted for body composition, gender, age, and pubertal status.[98]

Single Gene Mutations Producing Obesity: The pivotal role of genetics in the control of body weight is confirmed by the existence of single gene mutations capable of producing profound increases in body fat content. The fact that mutations in different genes can produce obesity suggests that these genes may be part of a control system for the regulation of body weight (ie, that feeding behavior and energy expenditure are integrated in a system with complex control mechanisms that can be disrupted at many loci). In fact, as summarized in Figure 33.2 and Table 33.3, many of these mutations affect specific aspects of the signaling system described.

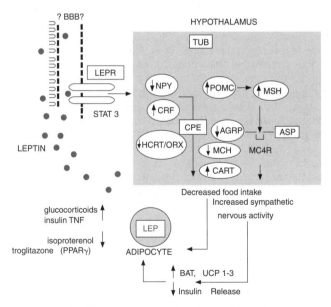

Figure 33.2. Legend follows on the next page

Figure 33.2. Possible functional relationships among products of the rodent obesity genes. The genes *Lepr, Cpe, tub,* and *agouti (asp)* in hypothalamus and *Lep*, which encodes leptin in adipocytes, are depicted in white boxes. Changes in adipocyte volume and fat mass affect leptin production as would be anticipated if leptin were part of a regulatory loop to control body fat by modulating food intake and energy expenditure. Cell size effects may be secondary to changes in substrate fluxes (fatty acids, glucosamine) and/or to associated endocrine changes (eg, insulin). Leptin production is also experimentally increased by glucocorticoids, TNF (tumor necrosis factor), or insulin, and reduced the isoproterenol (-adrenoreceptor agonist). Leptin may also play a role in peripheral sensitivity to insulin and in insulin synthesis in the islets. Leptin reaches its receptor (LEPR) in the hypothalamus via active transport into CSF (cerebrospinal fluid) (across the blood-brain barrier) and/or by acting upon hypothalamic nuclei that are functionally outside of the BBB (blood brain barrier). The major signal-transducing form of LEPR (Leptin receptor) in the hypothalamus is probably a dimer of the "long form" (1162aa) of the LEPR protein. Occupation of LEPR causes JAK (Janus kinase)-mediated activation of STAT3 (signal transducer and activator of transcription 3), resulting in decreased production of NPY (Neuropeptide Y—a stimulator of food intake) and increased release of CRF (corticotropin releasing hormone), which suppresses food intake. Carboxypeptidase (CPE), via its role in processing and intracellular transport of proneuropeptides for NPY, CRF (corticotropin releasing factor), galanin, and CCK (cholecystokinin) could affect food intake and energy expenditure (autonomic nervous system activity). However, there is no direct evidence at present to indicate that the *Cpe^fat* phenotype is conveyed by such effects on central neuropeptides. Agouti signalling protein (ASP), which is not normally expressed in the rodent brain, increased food intake in the *A^y* mouse, apparently through competitive inhibition of a normal ligand for melanocortin receptor MC4R (melonocortin receptor 4). The predicted *tub* gene product bears some sequence similarly to a cyclic nucleotide phosphodiesterase. A role in apoptosis of hypothalamic neurons has been suggested because the *tub* mutation results in the death of neurons in the retina and organ of Corti. Sympathetic nervous system efferent output is affected by the hypothalamic centers in which these peptides act. Intracerebral ventricular leptin administration, for example, increases energy expenditure in BAT (brown adipose tissue) and reduces insulin secretion by SNS-mediated mechanisms (sympathetic nervous system). Uncoupling protein (UCP3) is a mitochondrial uncoupling protein expressed in skeletal muscle and fat that may play a role in energy expenditure. By analogy to uncoupling protein 1 in BAT, the sympathetic nervous system would be expected to influence the activity of this pathway. These influences on energy intake and expenditure are shown converging on the amount of fat stored in the adipocyte. For reasons discussed elsewhere, it is most likely that the major role of the leptin axis is to prevent excessive depletion of fat stores rather than to prevent obesity. Additional abbreviations: MSH (melanocyte stimulating hormone); PPAR (peroxisome proliferator activated receptor); HCRT (hypocretin—also called orexin); ORX (orexin); CART (Cocaine- and amphetamine-regulated transcript peptide); MCH (melanocyte-concentrating hormone).
(Reprinted with permission from Leibel RL, Chua SC, Rosenbaum M. Obesity. In: Scriver CR, Beaudet AL, Sly WS, Valle D, eds. *The Metabolic and Molecular Bases of Inherited Disease.* New York, NY: McGraw-Hill; 2001:3977.)

Table 33.3A.
Human Single Gene Mutations Associated With Obesity[87]

Syndrome	Chromosome	Phenotype
Prader-Willi	15q11-q12 (Uniparental Maternal Disomy)	Short stature, small hands and feet, mental retardation, neonatal hypotonia, failure to thrive, cryptorchidism, almond-shaped eyes, and fish-mouth
Alström	2p14-p13 (Recessive)	Childhood blindness due to retinal degeneration, nerve deafness, acanthosis nigricans, chronic nephropathy, primary hypogonadism in males only, type 2 diabetes mellitus, or infantile obesity, which may diminish in adulthood
Bardet-Biedl	16q21 15q22-q23 (Recessive)	Retinitis pigmentosa, mental retardation, polydactyly, hypothalamic hypogonadism, rarely glucose intolerance, deafness, or renal disease[99]
Carpenter	Unknown (Recessive)	Mental retardation, acrocephaly, poly- or syndactyly, or hypogonadism (males only)
Cohen	8q22-q23 (Recessive)	Mental retardation, microcephaly, short stature, or dysmorphic facies
Prohormone Convertase	5q15-q21 (Recessive)	Abnormal glucose homeostasis, hypogonadotropic hypogonadism, Hypocortisolism, and elevated plasma proinsulin and POMC
Beckwith-Wiedemann	11p15.5 (Recessive)	Hyperinsulinemia, hypoglycemia, neonatal hemihypertrophy (Beckwith-Wiedemann syndrome), or intolerance of fasting
Neisidioblastosis	11p15.1 (Recessive or Dominant)	Hyperinsulinemia, hypoglycemia, or intolerance of fasting
Pseudohypoparathyroidism (type IA)	20q13.2 (Recessive)	Mental retardation, short stature, short metacarpals and metatarsals, short thick neck, round facies, subcutaneous calcifications, or increased frequency of other endocrinopathies (hypothyroidism, hypogonadism)
Leptin	7q31.3 (Recessive)	Hypometabolic rate, hyperphagia, pubertal delay, infertility, or impaired glucose tolerance due to leptin deficiency
Leptin Receptor	1p31-p32 (Recessive)	Hypometabolic rate, hyperphagia, or pubertal delay due to deranged leptin signal transduction
POMC	2p23.3 (Recessive)	Red hair, hyperphagia, adrenal insufficiency, or hyperpigmentation of skin due to impaired α-MSH production
MC4 receptor	18q22 (Dominant)	Obesity, early onset hyperphagia, increased bone density

Table 33.3B.
Rodent Single Gene Mutations Associated With Obesity[87,100]

Gene Name (rodent) Symbol	Mutation Name Rodent Chromosome	Phenotype	Human Chromosome
Agouti (mouse) *A*	*A^y* (yellow) 2	Adult-onset obesity, yellow coat color, hyperphagia, due to ectopic overexpression of agouti signaling protein (ASP) leading to MC4 receptor blockade.	20q11.2
Carboxypeptidase E (mouse); *Cpe*	*Cpe^fat* (fat) 8	Adult obesity, possibly due to impaired processing of prohormones.	4q32
Leptin (mouse) *Lep*	*Lep^ob* (obese) 6	Early-onset obesity, hyperphagia, hypometabolic rate, infertility, diabetes, increased partitioning of stored calories as fat due to leptin deficiency.	7q31.3
Leptin Receptor (mouse/rat); *Lepr*	*Lepr^db* (diabetes) *Lepr^fa* (fatty rat)	Early-onset obesity, hyperphagia, hypometabolic rate, infertility, diabetes, increased partitioning of stored calories as fat due to deranged leptin signal transduction.	1p31-p22
Tubby (mouse) *Tub*	*Tub* (tubby) 7	Impaired Gα-protein coupled receptor (possibly serotonin) signaling in the hypothalamus due to a mutation in this transcription factor may result in earlier cellular apoptosis.	11p15
OLETF (rat) *Cckar*	*Cckar^OLETF*	Adult obesity and hyperphagia due to CCK receptor deficiency	4p16.2-p15.1

Table 33.3. Single gene mutations associated with obesity in humans (Table 33.3A) and rodents (Table 33.3B). Human orthologs are known for all rodent genes that are associated with obesity and, in the case of Lep and Lepr, human mutations associated with obesity have been reported. The primary physiological sites of the derangements in all of the rodent mutations and in some of the human mutations can be seen in Figures 33.1 and 33.2.

Clinical and Laboratory Correlates of Obesity in Children

As summarized in Table 33.4, obesity adversely affects virtually every organ system. *Obesity in childhood may also constitute an independent risk factor for adult morbidity and mortality, even if the childhood obesity does not persist.* In 40- to 50-year follow-up studies of obese and lean adolescents (defined on the basis of body weight-for-height indices), adolescent fatness was a powerful predictor of mortality, cardiovascular disease, colorectal cancer, gout, and arthritis, irrespective of body fatness at the time that the morbidity was diagnosed.[101] Also, adiposity-related morbidities, such as hyperlipidemia, which are evident in childhood, track into adulthood.[102]

Table 33.4.
Potential Effects of Increased Adiposity on Organ Systems in Children[103],[104]

	Nonendocrine
Cardiovascular	Common identifiable cause of pediatric hypertension, ↑ [total cholesterol], ↑ [low density lipoproteins], ↓ [high density lipoproteins], syndrome X
Respiratory	Abnormal respiratory muscle function and central respiratory regulation, difficulty with ventilation during surgery, lower arterial oxygenation, sleep apnea, pickwickian syndrome, more frequent and severe upper respiratory infections, snoring, daytime somnolence
Orthopedic	Coxa vara, slipped-capital femoral epiphyses, Blount disease, Legg-Calve-Perthe disease, degenerative arthritis
Dermatologic	Intertrigo, furunculosis, acanthosis nigricans
Immunologic	Impaired cell-mediated immunity, polymorphonuclear leukocyte killing capacity, lymphocyte generation of migration inhibiting factor, and maturation rates of monocytes into macrophages
Gastro-intestinal	Gallstones, hepatic steatosis, steatohepatitis
	Endocrine
Somatotroph	↓ basal and stimulated growth hormone release, normal concentration of insulin-like growth factor-I, accelerated linear growth and bone age
Lactotroph	↑ basal serum prolactin but ↓ prolactin release in response to provocative stimuli
Gonadotroph	Early entrance into puberty with normal circulating gonadotropin concentrations
Thyroid	Normal serum T_4 and reverse T_3, normal or ↑ serum T_3, ↓ TSH-stimulated T_4 release
Adrenal	Normal serum cortisol but ↑ cortisol production and excretion, early adrenarche, ↑ adrenal androgens and dehydroepiandrosterone, normal serum catecholamines and 24-hour urinary catecholamine excretion
Gonad	↓ circulating gonadal androgens in males; ↑ androgens in females with ↓ sex-hormone binding globulin, dysmenorrhea, dysfunctional uterine bleeding, polycystic ovarian syndrome
Pancreas	↑ fasting plasma [insulin], ↑ insulin and glucagon release, ↑ resistance to insulin-mediated glucose transport

Some morbidities, such as slipped capital-femoral epiphyses, are physical consequences of excessive body weight. Other morbidities, cardiovascular disease in particular, are more closely correlated with the centrality of body fat distribution than absolute body fatness per se. In long-term (40 to 50 years) follow-up studies of adolescents, adiposity-related morbidities, such as hyperlipidemia, which are evident in childhood, track into adulthood. While certain endocrinopathies, such as hypothyroidism, may precipitate weight gain, the vast majority of endocrine disorders associated with obesity are secondary to excess body fat and will correct with weight loss. There are, however, a number of endocrine or genetic syndromes in which obesity is part of a distinct symptom complex that often includes poor statural growth (eg, hypercortisolism, hypothyroidism) (see Table 33.5) and/or very distinct heritable phenotypes (eg, Prader-Willi syndrome; Bardet-Biedl syndrome) (see Table 33.3). Assessment of skeletal maturation by bone age, and physical examination for the presence or absence of age-appropriate secondary sexual characteristics as well as syndrome-specific morphology or symptomatology (eg, hypotension, constipation in hypothyroidism, centripetal distribution of fat in hypercortisolism) can usually rule out these syndromes as causes of obesity.

Type 2 diabetes mellitus (type 2 DM) has emerged over the past decade in almost epidemic proportions among obese adolescents, and the clinician must now consider type 2 DM as a pediatric illness. Until recently, type 2 diabetes was considered an "adult" disease and constituted less than 2% of the new cases of diabetes in children as recently as a decade ago. Now, however, between 25% and 60% of new-onset childhood diabetics are type 2. Thus, over the last decade and along with the increasing prevalence of obesity among children,

Table 33.5.
Other Diseases and Injuries Associated With Obesity[87]

Disease	Structural/Biochemical Lesion	Clinical Features
Acquired hypothalamic lesions	Infectious (sarcoid, tuberculosis, arachnoiditis, encephalitis), vascular malformations, neoplasms, trauma	Adipocyte hypotrophy with little hyperplasia, headache and visual disturbance, hyperphagia, hypodipsia, hypersomnolence, convulsions, central hypogonadism-hypothyroidism-hypoadrenalism, diabetes insipidus, hyperprolactinemia, hyperinsulinism, type IV hyperlipidemia
Cushings	Hypercortisolism	Moon faces, central obesity, ↓ lean body mass, glucose intolerance, short stature
Growth Hormone Deficiency	Impaired production of GH (pituitary) or GHRH (hypothalamus)	Short stature, obesity, increased risk of elevated cholesterol (especially in GHRH deficiency), central distribution of body fat
Hypothyroidism	Hypothalamic, pituitary, or thyroidal	Hypometabolic state (constipation, anemia, hypotension, bradycardia, cold intolerance), cretinism (if congenital)

type 2 diabetes has become a "pediatric" disease, and children with type 2 diabetes experience the same morbidities as adults.[105]

Obesity is the major risk factor for type 2 DM in adolescents,[106,107] and adiposity accounts for approximately 55% of the variance in insulin sensitivity in children.[108] As in adults, 50% to 90% of children with type 2 DM have a BMI >85th percentile.[106,107] This is especially true in African American and Mexican American adolescents who have experienced the greatest increase in the prevalence of adolescent obesity over the past generation.[6,8,9,109,110] The prevalence of obesity in African Americans relative to other ethnic groups increases specifically during puberty.[8,111,112] Similarly, insulin sensitivity has been shown to be approximately 35% lower in African American than in white adolescents[113] and approximately 40% lower in pubertal children after controlling for adiposity and body fat distribution in most,[114–116] but not all[117] studies.

Body fat distribution, usually defined on the basis of waist circumference or the ratio of waist-to-hip circumference, is an independent predictor of adiposity-related insulin insensitivity in adolescents and adults.[107,118] There appear to be effects of ethnicity on the relative impact of body fat distribution on insulin sensitivity. In white children, visceral adiposity is the best correlate of hyperinsulinism and insulin secretion during oral glucose tolerance tests (OGTT) and of glucose disposal during glucose clamp studies.[107] In African American, but not white, prepubertal children, intra-abdominal adipose tissue volume measured by magnetic resonance imaging was significantly correlated with fasting insulin concentrations and with insulin sensitivity as measured by area under the curve (AUC) during oral glucose tolerance testing.[114,115,119] Other studies of prepubertal children have found that fasting insulin concentrations and insulin sensitivity are significantly correlated with subcutaneous, but not visceral, adipose tissue volume in African American prepubertal girls.[117] Because of the increasing frequency of type 2 DM among obese adolescents, and the worsening of diabetes-related morbidities that may result from delayed diagnosis, the clinician should be alert to the possible of type 2 DM in all obese adolescents, and especially those with a family history of early-onset (<40 years of age) type 2 diabetes.[120]

The psychological stress of social stigmatization imposed on obese children may be just as damaging to some children as the medical morbidities. These negative images of the obese are so strong that growth failure and pubertal delay have been reported in children due to self-imposed caloric restriction arising from fears of becoming obese.[121]

Identification of the Obese Child and Decisions Regarding Therapeutic Intervention

The rapid increase in prevalence of obesity in the US pediatric population during the last 25 years demonstrates the potent effects of environment on adiposity. The pediatrician should seek to identify the child at risk for adiposity-related morbidity, as well as the already obese child, with the goal of encouraging a lifestyle (environment), which will minimize obesity and its comorbidities. A detailed history and physical examination should be performed to assess each child for current obesity-related morbidities and for family history that suggests risk of such morbidities. Anthropometric data should be plotted on height and weight velocity charts, as well as standard curves of body mass index (see Appendix J), with the aim of detecting increased weight gain velocity before actual obesity occurs. Any child, regardless of body weight, with a history in first-degree relatives of obesity, type 2 diabetes mellitus, hypertension, hyperlipidemia, or premature myocardial infarction, and any child with a BMI above the 85th percentile (see Table 33.2B) should be considered to be at risk for adiposity-related morbidity.

Not every obese child requires or will benefit from treatment. The likelihood of persistence of pediatric obesity into adulthood increases with age. The obese 2-year-old is about twice as likely as a non-obese 2-year-old to become an obese adult. In contrast, that risk increases to sixfold or sevenfold by adolescence, independent of the duration of the obesity. In large epidemiologic studies, if neither of a child's parents is obese, the likelihood of childhood obesity persisting into adulthood may actually be less than the risk for a non-obese child with 1 or 2 obese parents.[1]

Because risk of persistence is lower and risk of treatment-associated impairment of statural or brain growth is higher, caloric restriction to reduce weight should not be used in infants less than age 2 years. Though hypothyroidism is an unusual cause of obesity in infants, the profound neurologic sequelae of untreated hypothyroidism in infancy justify heightened attention to this possibility. Similarly, children less than age 2 years who are severely obese, especially if they have concurrent adiposity-related morbidities, evidence of developmental delay, or other phenotypic features associated with the rare obesity syndromes (such as Prader-Willi) discussed previously (see Table 33.3A), should be referred to a physician who specializes in the treatment and evaluation of pediatric obesity.[122]

The decision as to whether to initiate therapy in the toddler (aged 2 to 9) should be strongly influenced by family history of obesity and adiposity-related morbidities. For the pre-adolescent or adolescent child with obesity-related morbidity (eg, hypertension), the child with central obesity and/or the child with a strong family history of adiposity-related morbidity (eg, hyperlipidemia, hypertension, diabetes mellitus), medical evaluation might also include screening for hyperlipidemia (fasting cardiovascular disease risk profile), an oral glucose tolerance test with concurrent serum insulin levels and serum transaminases.

Before beginning any type of therapy, it is essential to have the cooperation of the child and the child's family. Clinicians should not assume that the obese child is necessarily depressed, or that every obese child is significantly motivated to lose weight. Initiating weight-loss therapy in an overweight child and the child's family who are not motivated to do so is likely to be unsuccessful and may have negative influences on the child's self-esteem and likelihood of future successful weight loss. The clinician should begin assessment of family therapeutic readiness by asking the entire family how concerned they are about the patient's overweight. The clinician should make these inquiries in a supportive manner designed to elicit cooperation from the family and patient (ie, ask "Do you feel that weight is a problem?" or "What do you think that you could change to help you lose weight?" rather than, "Why can't you control your eating?") If they are not concerned, or feel that it cannot be changed, initiation of therapy should be delayed. Depending on the degree of obesity and adiposity-related morbidity, noncooperative families may benefit from further counseling to improve motivation.[122] Issues that should be addressed in such counseling include the following:

1. The risk of persistence of obesity into adulthood increases with age.
2. There are potential medical complications of obesity, some of which may already be evident in other family members.
3. The cooperation of the entire family (including all caregivers) in any therapeutic regimen is essential.
4. There are potential benefits to the entire family, regardless of whether any individual family member is obese, of adopting a healthier lifestyle.
5. The major goal is long-term maintenance of reduced body fatness, not just short-term weight reduction.
6. The increased likelihood that good health habits (diet and exercise) that are started early will persist into adulthood.

The importance of family based therapy and of the setting of realistic weight-loss goals is illustrated by the work Epstein et al,[123,124] which followed 55 obese children and their families over a 10-year study period. At the start of the study, children and their families received a total of 14 therapy sessions. Subjects were randomly assigned to receive either therapy targeted to both the parents and child with reinforcement directed toward parent and child weight loss and behavioral modification, treatment of the child alone with reinforcement directed only toward weight loss and behavior change in the child, and a control group where reinforcement was given for attendance at meetings. All 3 treatment groups received identical information on diet, exercise, and behavioral principles. During the initial treatment period, all children were placed on weight-reduction diets of 1200 to 1500 kcal/d and lost weight to within 5% to 25% of ideal body weight. Children in the parent and child targeted group were, on the average, 42% above ideal body weight upon entrance into the study and 34% above ideal body weight at the 10-year follow-up. In contrast, children in the child-alone targeted and control groups were approximately 44% and 46% above ideal body weight, respectively, at the start of the study and 48% and 60% above ideal body weight, respectively, at the 10-year follow up. Thus, while the family oriented therapeutic approach did not result in children maintaining their maximally reduced level of body fatness outside of the 6-month treatment period, it did result in a modest sustained level of weight loss well beyond the initial 6-month therapeutic trial and the maintenance of a significantly lower level of body fatness than subjects in other treatment groups.

Obesity is only one of many possible risk factors for cardiovascular disease. Since the adverse cardiovascular effects (such as hyperlipidemia, diabetes, and hypertension) are often cumulative, a combination of a cholesterol-lowering diet and program of regular exercise may be sufficient to reduce cardiovascular morbidity even if body weight is not significantly altered.[125-129] Children with a strong family history of any morbidity, which can be exacerbated by obesity, should be firmly and repeatedly counseled about good dietary and exercise habits, regardless of whether there is a family history of obesity per se.

Treatment of the Obese Child

Overview of Therapy (see Figures 33.3 and 33.4)
Initial evaluation should include a dietary history of the child and family's typical eating habits (including snacks beverages, who, if anyone, they eat with, and the frequency with which they eat foods prepared outside of the home). A physical activity history should also be obtained, including school physical education, after-school activities, activities of daily living (such as walking to

school), family activities, and sedentary activities (such as television watching). Treatment of the overweight child must, of necessity, be individualized and the clinician should remain sensitive to issues such as ability of the parents to prepare meals for the patient and neighborhood safety or availability of adult supervision, which may impact on the availability of physical activity after school. A complete physical examination should also be performed with special attention to the possibility of adiposity-related morbidities (hypertension, dyslipidemia, acanthosis nigricans [indicative of insulin resistance]; see Table 33.4). As discussed later in this chapter, the morbidly obese child requires more aggressive therapeutic intervention.

The major goal of obesity therapy should be to diminish morbidity and morbidity risk rather than to achieve a "cosmetically endorsed" body weight. Overweight in children (BMI >95th percentile for age and gender), the presence of concurrent morbidities in any child at risk for overweight (BMI >85th percentile for age and gender), and a high risk of future adiposity-related morbidity (based on family history) indicate that therapy is needed.[122]

In the otherwise healthy overweight child with no evidence of adiposity-related morbidity, clinicians and parents are generally concerned that the child will become an obese adult. Initial therapy in such instances should be directed toward decreasing or eliminating weight growth while allowing height growth to continue at age- and gender-appropriate velocity so that height eventually becomes appropriate for weight. Avoidance of calorically dense foods and substitution of fruit and vegetable snacks for sugared sodas, juices, and cookies, without restricting access to such snacks, will, in most cases, result in significant slowing of weight velocity.[130] The time required to significantly reduce adiposity can be estimated. One to 2 years of weight maintenance (1 year during normally rapid weight gain periods such as adolescence, and 2 years during periods of slower weight gain) compensates for 20% of excess weight for height.

If gradual statural growth into the child's weight is not possible because weight is already obese by **adult** standards (ie, body mass is so great that BMI will still be >85th percentile even if weight remains stable until adult stature is achieved), then a weight loss regimen should be considered. Therapeutic weight reduction is usually indicated for the child with evidence of current adiposity-related morbidity. The child with hypertension or diabetes should endeavor to reduce weight or alter body composition within 1 year to the point that the morbidity is no longer evident. Needless to say, if the morbidity is more severe (eg, pickwickian syndrome), then more rapid weight reduction, even in an inpatient setting, may be necessary. The obese child with a poor self-image, feelings of isolation from peers, and depression should also attempt weight reduction, perhaps with adjunctive psychotherapy. The initial therapeutic approach for children with predominantly psychiatric obesity-related morbidities should combine exercise and a closely supervised dietary plan, preferably with the involvement of a dietitian. Studies of compliance with weight-reduction plans have emphasized the importance of a family-oriented approach. Any therapeutic regimen should involve the entire family, as well as the child's school. Frequent physical examination of the child and monitoring of school performance should be included. Patients and their families should be made aware that the treatment period does not end once the prescribed reduction in body fatness has been achieved, and that caloric restriction must continue beyond the period of weight reduction.

Diet

Dietary restriction should never be presented in a punitive manner and, if possible, the obese child and the entire family should adhere to a similar diet to minimize feelings of isolation by the obese child. Parents, pediatricians, and patients (especially adolescents) will be frustrated by the need for prolonged attention to diet and exercise that is required to achieve and maintain a reduced level of body fatness. Encouragement can be provided by examining growth and growth velocity curves with patients and their families to illustrate progress. If appropriate, the significance of any evident reduction in morbidity (eg, lowering of blood pressure or cholesterol) can be reinforced. Reasonable goals in the form of a "target" body weight at the next visit should be set at each office visit so that the patient and parents are aware of what is expected. These goals should be modest and attainable even if patients are only moderately compliant with their diet and exercise regimens, since achievement of an interval "target weight" will also encourage the patient.

Dietary Intervention

The prescribed diet, especially in prepubertal children, should initially provide 300 to 400 kcal/d below weight-maintenance requirements as assessed by dietary history or as calculated based on formula relating anthropometry to energy expenditure (eg, the Harris-Benedict Equation[131]). (See also Chapter 15.) Self-reported caloric intake is generally very inaccurate. The child's *ad libitum* diet should be directly observed and recorded by the parents for a minimum of 5 consecutive days. A 300 to 400 kcal/d energy deficit should result in weight loss of approximately 300 to 400 g/week. Older children may, with supervision, further restrict their caloric intake to as much as 500 to 700 kcal/d below weight maintenance requirements, which will produce an approximately 0.5 kg weight loss per week.[132] Further caloric restriction in the form of very low calorie diets (VLCDs), usually the protein-sparing modified fast, have not been shown to be of any greater benefit in the long-term maintenance of a reduced body weight than the hypocaloric diet, and have been reported to promote cholelithiasis, hyperuricemia, orthostatic hypotension, diarrhea, halitosis, and significant declines in various serum proteins, including transferin and complement β1C.[132]

Weight loss per se may result in declines in energy expenditure beyond that predicted solely on the basis of changes in body composition.[72] This phenomenon, plus the ongoing loss of metabolic mass, necessitates periodic downward adjustments of energy intake needed to sustain ongoing weight loss. The family should be instructed in long-term monitoring of caloric intake within, and outside of, the home and cautioned not to become overly critical or punitive toward the child if weight loss is slow or compliance is suboptimal.

The composition of the diet should be in accordance with the American Heart Association "Heart Healthy" recommendations and contain at least the minimal recommend amounts of protein, essential fatty acids, vitamins, and minerals, and be low in saturated fats (less than 30% of calories as fat and less than 10% of calories as saturated fat). The American Academy of Pediatrics Statement on Cholesterol in Children describes a healthful, cardiovascular-disease, risk-lowering diet.[133] (See also Chapter 32.) Diets consisting of drastically altered proportions of nutrients may be dangerous and yield no better results than a limited intake of a nutritionally balanced diet. Nutritional counseling should encourage decreasing the use of calorically dense (high-fat or fried) foods, and adding more fruits and vegetables to the daily diet. The substitution of water for nonnutritious high-calorie sugar-containing drinks (juices, iced teas, and soda) may be very helpful.[130] (See also Chapter 7.) In some cases, reductions in calorically dense foods and sugar-containing drinks through substitution and/or elimination alone can decrease calories and weight without changing the general pattern of food consumption in the family. When families eat at restaurants and fast-food vendors, they have less control over food choices than they do at home. Thus, reduction in the number of meals prepared outside the home may also be an effective weight-loss strategy. Parents and adult caregivers should understand the important role they play in the development of proper eating habits in their young children. The parents' food preferences, the quantities and variety of foods in the home, the parents' eating behavior, and physical activity patterns all determine how supportive the home environment is to the obese child.

Therapeutic Exercise

Regular exercise will promote increased muscle mass, thereby raising total metabolic rate and the putative effects of exercise to reduce visceral adipose tissue mass independently lower the risk of hyperlipidemia and diabetes mellitus.[134–136] However, the energy cost of even vigorous exercise is low when compared to the caloric content of many fast foods or other snacks, and exercise should not be viewed as a license to eat. For example, walking at 3 miles per hour for 1 hour consumes about 200 kcal, about the same number of calories contained in a 1-oz bag of potato chips. Obviously, treats, such as ice cream and potato chips, should not be used as incentives to exercise.

While no specific aspect of the sedentary lifestyle has been shown to directly cause obesity, behaviors such as television viewing, reading, working at a computer, driving a car, or commuting do exert effects on health. Television viewing appears to be directly associated with the incidence of obesity, and inversely associated with the remission of obesity. The impact of television viewing on obesity seems to be due to both displacing more vigorous activities and its effect on diet. Not only is television viewing a sedentary behavior, but also food has constituted the most heavily advertised product on children's television in the United States. In Mexican American children, adiposity was significantly correlated with time spent watching television but not with time spent watching videos,[137] suggesting that the bulk of the positive association of television watching and adiposity is due to the approximately 60% of advertising that is devoted to food.[41] Children and adolescents should be encouraged to view as little television as possible. Limitation of television, video games, and Internet surfing will encourage greater participation in physical activity. Clinicians should encourage children to participate in organized or individual sports (participate, not watch from the bench) and advocate for better community- and school-based activity programs.

If the patient is unable to lose weight and/or co-morbid conditions persist, consideration should be given to referral of the child to a physician specializing in the treatment of pediatric obesity. Weight-loss programs and weight-reduction camps are often not covered by medical insurance and should be considered for the morbidly obese child with some caution. Enrollment in a highly supervised environment may demonstrate to an overweight child that weight loss is possible and encourage the child to continue. However, rapid weight loss may precipitate cholelithiasis[138] or eating disorders. A child may become overly preoccupied with his or her weight and, even if a moderate degree of weight loss is achieved, lose self-esteem. Obsession with weight on the part of the child or the family may lead to serious deterioration of intra-family relationships.

Surgical Intervention

In obese adults, surgery is usually recommended only for subjects with severe obesity (BMI >40 kg/m^2) obesity, or those with BMI values between 35 and 40 kg/m^2 who have significant co-morbid conditions. Gastroplasty with gastro-duodenal bypass can lead initially to a great deal of weight loss, and approximately 80% of patients remain at least 10% below their preoperative body weight for 10 years postsurgery. There is evidence that insulin sensitivity may be improved in patients with hyperinsulinemia and type 2 diabetes following gastroplasty, even before significant weight loss has occurred,[139] suggesting that bariatric surgery may, perhaps via effects on the secretion of other gastrointestinal peptide hormones (incretins), improve insulin sensitivity in some patients. Patients who have such procedures must be carefully followed since it is possible to overeat liquid or semi-solid diets or to develop intestinal obstruction and electrolyte disturbances. While there is no documented role at present for surgical therapy in pediatric obesity, in some extremely obese children with life-threatening morbidity (eg, with pickwickian syndrome) in whom all other interventions have failed, it may be appropriate to consider such treatments. While some adolescents have been included in various reports on gastroplasty-induced weight loss, there are few studies specifically examining safety and efficacy of this procedure or other obesity surgeries in children.[140,141] There are few studies of this procedure in adolescents.[132] However, such studies are needed to evaluate surgery in adolescence as a response to the rapidly increasing prevalence of adolescent obesity, as well as type 2 diabetes mellitus and other adiposity-related morbidities such as hypertension.

Pharmacotherapy

Drug therapy in children is not recommended, and there are currently no Food and Drug Administration (FDA)-approved medications for use in children less than 16 years of age. However, in some extremely obese adolescent patients with life-threatening morbidities, this approach may be necessary with the warning that, though clinical studies are ongoing, studies of the effectiveness of these drugs in children have not yet been reported.

Pharmacotherapies can be subdivided into those that are designed primarily to (1) increase energy expenditure, (2) decrease caloric intake, or (3) decrease nutrient absorption. Catecholaminergic agonists, such as the Schedule IV (low abuse potential) drug phentermine (Adipex-P, Ionomin) have been shown to decrease food intake and to increase energy expenditure in short-term studies. However, this drug has been withdrawn from the market in the United States because of significant side effects, including life-threatening arrhythmias, insomnia, nervousness, dry mouth, and increased heart rate and blood pressure.[142,143] Sibutramine (Meridia) has been available in this country since November 1997, and acts by inhibiting the neuronal reuptake of both norepinephrine and serotonin. Like phentermine, sibutramine suppresses appetite and increases energy expenditure. Side effects include elevation in blood pressure, increase in heart rate, insomnia, constipation, increased sweating, headache, and dry mouth.[144,145] A long-acting pancreatic lipase inhibitor, Orlistat (Xenical) was approved in 1999 for use in adults. Decreased lipase activity results in decreased hydrolysis of dietary fat and thus allows about 30% of the fat ingested to pass through the gut undigested. The most frequent side effects are loose stools, flatulence, and oily discharge leading to soiling of underwear. Inhibition of pancreatic lipase also causes loss of fat-soluble vitamins (A, D, E, and K) in the stool, and vitamin supplementation is recommended.[146,147] The use of lipase inhibitors has not been well studied in adolescents. Because of the possible effects of impaired vitamin D absorption on the extensive bone mineralization that occurs in adolescence, the use of any therapy that inhibits such absorption should be thoroughly investigated before it is prescribed for teens. Combinations of caffeine and ephedrine (derived from ephedra in the commonly available herb ma huang) are available as thermogenic agents but have not been approved for the treatment of obesity. The combination of ephedrine and caffeine may participate serious cardiac arrhythmias.[142]

Summary of Therapeutic Options

Before prescribing any type of treatment for obesity, health personnel should assess the risk-benefit ratio in the particular patient. In the older and otherwise healthy overweight child without family history of adiposity-related morbidity, the fact that adolescent obesity may constitute an independent risk factor for adult mortality and morbidity must be weighed against the possible morbidities (poor statural growth, precipitation of eating disorders) associated with therapeutic weight reduction. Long-term studies of children and adults who experienced weight reduction have shown that 80% to 90% return to their previous weight percentiles. Obese children and their families must recognize that maintenance of a reduced degree of body fatness will probably require a lifetime of attention to energy intake and expenditure. The cautions emphasized in deciding who should undergo a therapeutic weight reduction and the relatively slow rate at which weight reduction of slowing down of weight gain should be prescribed reflect the significant morbidities associated with these processes. Diets extremely low in caloric content or with unusual distribution of calories as fat, protein, and carbohydrate may precipitate cardiac arrhythmias, severe electrolyte disturbances, or other morbidities. As many as 80% of children using unsupervised diets obtained from popular magazines have been found to experience weakness, headaches, fatigue, nausea, constipation, nervousness, dizziness, poor concentration, dysmenorrhea, and/or fainting. Children on a supervised diet must also be closely monitored for treatment-associated psychological morbidities (stigmatization of the child, precipitation of anorexia nervosa or bulimia).

Therapeutic intervention should emphasize the need for participation of the entire family and lifelong attention to, and benefits of, a healthy lifestyle, as well as positive reinforcement for even small degrees of compliance. Preparation of the family and child for therapeutic intervention is as important as the intervention itself. Among the most important recommendations that the primary care physician can offer include the following (see also Figures 33.3 and 33.4):

1. Limit television to 1 to 2 hours per day.
2. Do not eat in front of the television.
3. Do not use the remote while watching television.
4. Do exercise during television commercials instead of surfing the channels.
5. Do not have TV, VCR, or video games in the child's room.
6. Decrease calories being consumed from beverages (eg, soda, juice drinks).
7. Do not use food as a reward.
8. Have parents act as role models in terms of eating and exercise.
9. Encourage the family to eat meals and exercise together.
10. Encourage multiple types of physical activity so that the child does not get bored and take into account different times of day and weather conditions.
11. Encourage daily physical activity.

Summary/Conclusions

The American Academy of Pediatrics recommends:

1. Prevalence of overweight and its significant comorbidities in pediatric populations has rapidly increased and reached epidemic proportions.
2. Prevention of overweight is critical, because long-term outcome data for successful treatment approaches are limited.
3. Genetic, environmental, or combinations of risk factors predisposing children to obesity can and should be identified.
4. Early recognition of excessive weight gain relative to linear growth should become routine in pediatric ambulatory care settings. BMI (kg/m2 [see http://www.cdc.gov/growthcharts]) should be calculated and plotted periodically.
5. Families should be educated and empowered through anticipatory guidance to recognize the impact they have on their children's development of lifelong habits of physical activity and nutritious eating.
6. Dietary practices should be fostered that encourage moderation rather than overconsumption, emphasizing healthful choices rather than restrictive eating patterns.
7. Regular physical activity should be consciously promoted, prioritized, and protected within families, schools, and communities.
8. Optimal approaches to prevention need to combine dietary and physical activity interventions.
9. Advocacy is needed in the areas of physical activity and food policy for children; research into pathophysiology, risk factors, and early recognition and management of overweight and obesity; and improved insurance coverage and third-party reimbursement for obesity care.

Recommendations

1. Health supervision
   a. Identify and track patients at risk by virtue of family history, birth weight, or socioeconomic, ethnic, cultural, or environmental factors.
   b. Calculate and plot BMI once a year in all children and adolescents.
   c. Use change in BMI to identify rate of excessive weight gain relative to linear growth.
   d. Encourage, support, and protect breastfeeding.
   e. Encourage parents and caregivers to promote healthy eating patterns by offering nutritious snacks, such as vegetables and fruits, low-fat dairy foods, and whole grains; encouraging children's autonomy in self-regulation of food intake and setting appropriate limits on choices; and modeling healthy food choices.
   f. Routinely promote physical activity, including unstructured play at home, in school, in child care settings, and throughout the community.
   g. Recommend limitation of television and video time to a maximum of 2 hours per day.
   h. Recognize and monitor changes in obesity-associated risk factors for adult chronic disease, such as hypertension, dyslipidemia, hyperinsulinemia, impaired glucose tolerance, and symptoms of obstructive sleep apnea syndrome.

2. Advocacy
   a. Help parents, teachers, coaches, and others who influence youth to discuss health habits, not body habitus, as part of their efforts to control overweight and obesity.
   b. Enlist policy makers from local, state, and national organizations and schools to support a healthful lifestyle for all children, including proper diet and adequate opportunity for regular physical activity.
   c. Encourage organizations that are responsible for health care and health care financing to provide coverage for effective obesity prevention and treatment strategies.
   d. Encourage public and private sources to direct funding toward research into effective strategies to prevent overweight and obesity and to maximize limited family and community resources to achieve healthful outcomes for youth.
   e. Support and advocate for social marketing intended to promote healthful food choices and increased physical activity.

American Academy of Pediatrics. Prevention of pediatric overweight and obesity. *Pediatrics.* 2003;112:424–430

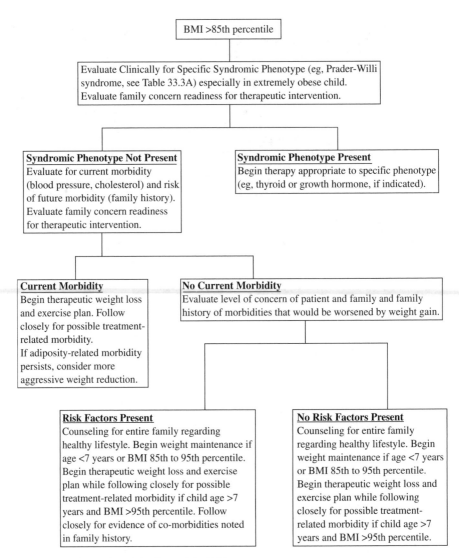

Figure 33.3. Evaluation of the Overweight Child

Physician	Parent
1. Identify child at risk for adiposity-related morbidity and initiate therapy early.	1. Encourage your child and give positive reinforcement for healthy lifestyle changes. Be consistent.
2. Educate families about the complications of obesity and benefits of therapy.	2. Never use food as a reward or punishment.
3. Assess factors in the child's environment that increase the risk of adiposity-related morbidity and can be modified.	3. Adopt similar lifestyle changes to those that the child is being asked to make. Ask for nonfood rewards from children for good parental behavior.
4. Recommend gradual lifestyle changes that are not disruptive.	4. Establish a regular schedule of meals, snacks, and exercise.
5. Involve the entire family in the treatment plan, including non-parent caregivers.	5. Remove calorically dense foods from the home for everyone.
6. Educate parents to monitor child's eating behavior and activity.	6. Offer only healthy meals.
7. Set reasonable and achievable weight goals from visit to visit.	7. Limit television watching to a maximum of 1 to 2 hours per day.
8. Emphasize need for long-term lifestyle changes rather than just loss of body fatness.	8. Encourage physical activity.
9. Be supportive, not critical of child and family.	9. Be a role model to the child.
10. Be alert to therapy-associated morbidities.	10. Stay in close contact with the physician, even if compliance with the recommended lifestyle changes is poor.

Child
1. Realize that being overweight is not the same as being lazy and greedy.
2. Realize that losing weight takes time and that someone who is overweight is not less of a person.
3. Realize that small changes in diet and exercise over time will produce big changes in fatness.
4. Remind the entire family that everyone benefits from a healthier lifestyle.
5. Do not hesitate to discuss fears, frustrations, and any other feelings about weight, diet, and exercise with your family and your doctor.
6. Be patient.
7. Be honest.
8. Do your best.
9. Respect your best.
10. Respect yourself.

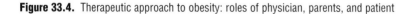

Figure 33.4. Therapeutic approach to obesity: roles of physician, parents, and patient

References

1. Whitaker RC, Wright JA, Pepe MS, Seidel KD, Dietz WH. Predicting obesity in young adulthood from childhood and parental obesity. *N Engl J Med.* 1997;337:869–873

2. Rosenbaum M, Leibel RL. The physiology of body weight regulation: relevance to the etiology of obesity in children. *Pediatrics.* 1998;101:525–539

3. Pietrobelli A, Faith MS, Allison DB, Gallagher D, Chiumello G, Heymsfield SB. Body mass index as a measure of adiposity among children and adolescents: a validation study. *J Pediatr.* 1998;132:204–210

4. Reilly JJ, Dorosty AR, Emmet PM, et al. Identification of the obese child: adequacy of the body mass index for clinical practice and epidemiology. *Int J Obes Relat Metab Disord.* 2000;24:1623–1627

5. Expert Panel on the Identification, Evaluation, and Treatment of Overweight in Adults. Clinical guidelines on the identification, evaluation, and treatment of overweight and obesity in adults: executive summary. *Am J Clin Nutr.* 1998;68:899–917

6. Troiano RP, Flegal KM. Overweight children and adolescents: description, epidemiology, and demographics. *Pediatrics.* 1998;101:497–504

7. Must A, Dallal GE, Dietz WM. Reference data for obesity: 85th and 95th percentiles of body mass index (wt/ht^2) and triceps skinfold thickness. *Am J Clin Nutr.* 1991;53:839–846

8. Troiano RP, Flegal KM, Kuczmarski RJ, Campbell SM, Johnson CL. Overweight prevalence and trends for children and adolescents. *Arch Pediatr Adolesc Med.* 1995;149:1085–1091

9. Flegal KM, Troiano RP. Changes in the distribution of body mass index of adults and children in the US population. *Int J Obes Relat Metab Disord.* 2000;24:807–818

10. Kuczmarski RJ, Flegal KM, Campbell SM, Johnson CL. Increasing prevalence of overweight among US adults. *JAMA.* 1994;272:205–211

11. Overpeck MD, Hedger ML, Ruan WJ, et al. Stature, weight, and body mass among US children born at term with appropriate birth weights. *J Pediatr.* 2000;137:205–213

12. Rosner B, Prineas R, Loggie J, Daniels SR. Percentiles for body mass index in US children 5 to 17 years of age. *J Pediatr.* 1998;132:211–222

13. Kuczmarski RJ. Trends in body composition for infants and children in the US. *Crit Rev Food Sci Nutr.* 1993;33:375–387

14. Dietz WM Jr. Childhood obesity: susceptibility, cause, and management. *J Pediatr.* 1983;103:676–686

15. Dietz WH Jr, Gortmaker SL. Factors within the physical environment associated with childhood obesity. *Am J Clin Nutr.* 1984;39:619–624

16. Ravelli GP, Belmont L. Obesity in nineteen-year-old men: family size and birth order associations. *Am J Epidemiol.* 1979;109:66–70

17. Ravelli GP, Stein ZA, Susser MW. Obesity in young men after famine exposure in utero and early infancy. *N Engl J Med.* 1976;295:349–353

18. Ravelli AC, van der Meulen JH, Michels RP, et al. Glucose tolerance in adults after prenatal exposure to famine. *Lancet.* 1998;351:173–177

19. Moore VM, Cockington RA, Ryan P, Robinson JS. The relationship between birth weight and blood pressure amplifies from childhood to adulthood. *J Hypertens.* 1999;17:883–888

20. Hattersley AT, Tooke JE. The fetal insulin hypothesis: an alternative explanation of the association of low birthweight with diabetes and vascular disease. *Lancet.* 1999;353:1789–1792

21. Yarborough DE, Barrett-Connor E, Kritz-Silverstein D, Wingard DL. Birth weight, adult weight, and girth as predictors of the metabolic syndrome in post-menopausal women: the Rancho Bernardo Study. *Diabetes Care.* 1998;21:1652–1658

22. Barker DJ. Maternal nutrition, fetal nutrition, and diseases later in life. *Nutrition.* 1997;3:807–813

23. Godfrey KM, Barker DJ. Fetal nutrition and adult disease. *Am J Clin Nutr.* 2000;71(suppl 5):1344S–1352S

24. Barker DJ, Clark PM. Fetal undernutrition and disease in later life. *Rev Reprod.* 1997;2: 105–112

25. Barker DJ. Fetal origins of cardiovascular disease. *Ann Med.* 1999;31(suppl):3–6

26. Stern MP, Bartley M, Duggirala R, Bradshaw B. Birth weight and the metabolic syndrome: thrifty phenotype or thrifty genotype? *Diabetes Metab Res Rev.* 2000;16: 88–93

27. Pettitt DJ, Baird HR, Aleck KA, Bennett PH, Knowler WC. Excessive obesity in offspring of Pima Indian women with diabetes during pregnancy. *N Engl J Med.* 1983;308:242–245

28. Pettitt DJ, Knowler WC, Bennett PH, Aleck KA, Baird HR. Obesity in offspring of diabetic Pima Indian women despite normal birth weight. *Diabetes Care.* 1987;10: 76–80

29. Pettitt DJ, Aleck KA, Baird HR, Carraher MJ, Bennett PH, Knowler WC. Congential susceptibility to NIDDM. Role of intrauterine environment. *Diabetes.* 1988;37:622–628

30. Gillman MW, Rifas-Shiman SL, Camargo CA Jr, et al. Risk of overweight among adolescents who were breastfed as infants. *JAMA.* 2001;285:2461–2467

31. Kries R, Koletzko B, Sauerwald T, et al. Breast feeding and obesity: cross sectional study. *BMJ.* 1999;319:147–150

32. Hediger ML, Overpeck MD, Kuczmarski RJ, Ruan WJ. Association between infant breastfeeding and overweight in young children. *JAMA.* 2001;285:2453–2460

33. Ravelli AC, van der Meulen JH, Osmond C, Barker DJ, Bleker OP. Infant feeding and adult glucose tolerance, lipid profile, blood pressure, and obesity. *Arch Dis Child.* 2000;82: 248–252

34. Agras WS, Kraemer HL, Berkowitz RI, Hammer LD. Influence of early feeding style on adiposity at 6 years of age. *J Pediatr.* 1990;116:805–809

35. Wolman PG. Feeding practices in infancy and prevalence of obesity in preschool children. *J Am Diet Assoc.* 1984;84:436–438

36. Dietz WH Jr, Gortmaker SL. Do we fatten our children at the television set? Obesity and television viewing in children and adolescents. *Pediatrics.* 1985;75:807–812

37. Salbe AD, Nicolson M, Ravussin E. Total energy expenditure and the level of physical activity correlate with plasma leptin concentrations in five-year-old children. *J Clin Invest.* 1997;99:592–595

38. Ku LC, Shapiro LR, Crayford PB, Huenemann RL. Body composition and physical activity in 8 year old children. *Am J Clin Nutr.* 1981;34:2770–2775

39. Davies PS, Gregory J, White A. Physical activity and body fatness in pre-school children. *Int J Obes Relat Metab Disord.* 1995;19:6–10

40. Crespo CJ, Smit E, Troiano RP, Bartlett SJ, Macera CA, Andersen RE. Television watching, energy intake, and obesity in US children: results from the third National Health and Nutrition Examination Survey, 1988–1994. *Arch Pediatr Adolesc Med.* 2001;155:360–365

41. Borzekowski DL, Robinson TN. The 30-second effect: an experiment revealing the impact of television commercials on food preferences of preschoolers. *J Am Diet Assoc.* 2001;101:42–46

42. Flegal KM, Ogden CL, Wei R, Kuczmarski RL, Johnson CL. Prevalence of overweight in US children: comparison of US growth charts from the Centers for Disease Control and Prevention with other reference values for body mass index. *Am J Clin Nutr.* 2001;73:1086–1093

43. Wadden TA. Treatment of obesity by moderate and severe caloric restriction. Results of clinical research trials. *Ann Intern Med.* 1993;119:688–693

44. Knip M, Nuutinen O. Long-term weight control in obese children: persistence of treatment outcome and metabolic changes. *Int J Obes Relat Metab Disord.* 1992;16:279–287

45. McGuire MT, Wing RR, Hill JO. The prevalence of weight loss maintenance among American adults. *Int J Obes Relat Metab Disord.* 1999;23:1314–1319

46. Klem ML, Wing RR, Lang W, McGuire MT, Hill JO. Does weight loss maintenance become easier over time? *Obes Res.* 2000;8:438–444

47. Klem ML, Wing RR, McGuire MT, Seagle HM, Hill JO. A descriptive study of individuals successful at long term maintenance of substantial weight loss. *Am J Clin Nutr.* 1997;66:239–246

48. Wing RR, Hill JO. Successful weight loss maintenance. *Annu Rev Nutr.* 2001;21:323–341

49. Belanger AJ, Cupples LA, D'Agostino RB. *The Framingham Study: The Epidemiological Investigation of Cardiovascular Disease, Section 36. Means at Each Examination and Interexamination Consistency of Specified Characteristics.* Bethesda, MD: National Heart, Lung, and Blood Institute; 1988

50. Johnston FE. Sex differences in fat patterning in children and youth. In: Bouchard C, Johnston FE, eds. *Fat Distribution During Growth and Later Health Outcomes.* New York, NY: Alan R. Liss, Inc; 1988:85–102

51. Horlick M, Thornton JC, Wang J, Fedun B, Levine LS, Pierson RN. The relationship of central adiposity to total body fatness in children and adolescents varies with sex, puberty, and black/white ethnicity [abstract]. *Pediatr Res.* 2000;47:132A

52. Jequier E. Energy cost of growth in infants. *Bibl Nutr Dieta.* 1996;53:129–134

53. Butte NF, Hopkinson JM, Wong WW, Smith EO, Ellis KJ. Body composition during the first 2 years of life: an updated reference. *Pediatr Res.* 2000;47:578–585

54. Rosenbaum M, Leibel RL, Hirsch J. Obesity. *N Engl J Med.* 1997; 337:396–407

55. Bouchard C, Bray GA, eds. *Regulation of Body Weight: Biological and Behavioral Mechanisms.* Chichester, England: John Wiley & Sons Ltd; 1996

56. Sims EA, Goldman RF, Gluck CM, Horton ES, Kelleher PC, Rowe DW. Experimental obesity in man. *Trans Assoc Am Physicians.* 1968;81:153–170

57. Bouchard C, Tremblay A, Despres JP, et al. The response to long-term overfeeding in identical twins. *N Engl J Med.* 1990;322:1477–1482

58. Sims EA. Experimental obesity, dietary-induced thermogenesis, and their clinical implications. *Clin Endocrinol Metab.* 1976;5:377–395

59. Sims EA, Danforth E Jr, Horton ES, Bray GA, Glennon JA, Salans LB. Endocrine and metabolic effects of experimental obesity in man. *Rec Prog Horm Res.* 1973;29:457–496

60. Tremblay A, Despres JP, Theriault G, Fournier G, Bouchard C. Overfeeding and energy expenditure in humans. *Am J Clin Nutr.* 1992;56:857–862

61. Ravussin E, Lillioja S, Anderson TE, Christin L, Bogardus C. Determinants of 24-hour energy expenditure in man. Methods and results using a respiratory chamber. *J Clin Invest.* 1986;78:1568–1578

62. Wadden TA, Foster GD, Letizia KA, Mullen JL. Long-term effects of dieting on resting metabolic rate in obese outpatients. *JAMA.* 1990;264:707–711

63. Elliot DL, Goldberg L, Kuehl KS, Bennett WM. Sustained depression of the resting metabolic rate after massive weight loss. *Am J Clin Nutr.* 1989;49:93–96

64. Dulloo AG, Girardier L. 24 hour energy expenditure several months after weight loss in the underfed rat: evidence for a chronic decrease in whole-body metabolic efficiency. *Int J Obes. Relat Metab Disord.* 1993;17:115–123

65. Schoeller DA. Balancing energy expenditure and body weight. *Am J Clin Nutr.* 1998;68:956S–961S

66. Raben A, Mygind E, Astrup A. Lower activity of oxidative key enzymes and smaller fiber areas in skeletal muscle of postobese women. *Am J Physiol.* 1998;275: E487–E494

67. Weigle DS, Brunzell JD. Assessment of energy expenditure in ambulatory reduced-obese subjects by techniques of weight stabilization and exogenous weight replacement. *Int J Obes.* 1990(suppl);14:69–81

68. Froidevaux F, Schutz Y, Christin L, Jequier E. Energy expenditure in obese women before and during weight loss, after refeeding, and in the weight-relapse period. *Am J Clin Nutr*. 1993;57:35–42

69. van Gemert WG, Westerterp KR, van Acker BA, et al. Energy, substrate and protein metabolism in morbid obesity before, during and after massive weight loss. *Int J Obes Relat Metab Disord*. 2000;24:711–718

70. deBoer JO, van Es AJ, van Raaij JM, Hautvast JG. Energy requirements and energy expenditure of lean and overweight women, measured by indirect calorimetry. *Am J Clin Nutr*. 1987;46:13–21

71. de Boer JO, van Es AJ, Roovers LC, van Raaij JM, Hautvast JG. Adaptation of energy metabolism of overweight women to low-energy intake, studied with whole-body calorimeters. *Am J Clin Nutr*. 1986;44:585–595

72. Leibel RL, Rosenbaum M, Hirsch J. Changes in energy expenditure resulting from altered body weight. *N Engl J Med*. 1995;332:621–628

73. Rosenbaum M, Ravussin E, Matthews DE, et al. A comparative study of different means of assessing long-term energy expenditure in humans. *Am J Physiol*. 1996; 270:R496–R504

74. Welle S, Forbes GB, Statt M, Bernard RR, Amatruda JM. Energy expenditure under free-living conditions in normal-weight and overweight women. *Am J Clin Nutr*. 1992;55:14–21

75. Weinsier RL, Hunter GR, Zuckerman PA, et al. Energy expenditure and free-living physical activity in black and white women: comparison and after weight loss. *Am J Clin Nutr*. 2000;71:1138–1146

76. Mossberg HO. 40-year follow-up of overweight children. *Lancet*. 1989;2:491–493

77. Maffeis C, Schutz Y, Pinnelli L. Effects of weight loss on resting energy expenditure in obese prepubertal children. *Int J Obes Relat Metab Disord*. 1992;16:41–47

78. Kiortsis D, Duraced I, Turpin G. Effects of a low-calorie diet on resting metabolic rate and serum tri-iodothyronine levels in obese children. *Eur J Pediatr*. 1999; 158:446–450

79. Rosenbaum M, Hirsch J, Murphy E, Leibel RL. The effects of changes in body weight on carbohydrate metabolism, catecholamine excretion, and thyroid function. *Am J Clin Nutr*. 2000;71:1421–1432

80. Wardlaw SL. Clinical review 127: obesity as a neuroendocrine disease: lessons to be learned from proopiomelanocortin and melanocortin receptor mutations in mice and men. *J Clin Endocrinol Metab*. 2001;86:1442–1446

81. Rosenbaum M, Leibel RL. Leptin: a molecule integrating somatic energy stores, energy expenditure, and fertility. *Trends Endocrinol Metab*. 1998;9:117–124

82. Ahima RS, Prabakaran D, Mantzoros C, et al. Role of leptin in the neuroendocrine response to fasting. *Nature*. 1996;382:250–252

83. Ahima RS, Kelly J, Elmquist JK, Flier JS. Distinct physiologic and neuronal responses to decreased leptin and mild hyperleptinemia. *Endocrinol*. 1999;140:4923–4931

84. Aronne LJ, Mackintosh R, Rosenbaum M, Leibel RL, Hirsch J. Autonomic nervous system activity in weight gain and weight loss. *Am J Physiol*. 1995;38:R222–R225

85. Rosenbaum M, Nicolson M, Hirsch J, Murphy E, Chu F, Leibel RL. Effects of weight change on plasma leptin concentrations and energy expenditure. *J Clin Endocrinol Metab*. 1997;82:3647–3654

86. Schwartz MW, Woods SL, Porte D Jr, Seeley RJ, Baskin DG. Central nervous system control of food intake. *Nature*. 2000;404:661–671

87. Leibel RL, Chua SC, Rosenbaum M. Obesity. In: *The Metabolic and Molecular Bases of Inherited Disease*. Vol 1. 8th ed. New York, NY: McGraw-Hill; 2001:3965–4028

88. Vale W, Rivier C, Brown MR, et al. Chemical and biological characterization of corticotropin releasing factor. *Recent Prog Horm Res*. 1983;39:245–270

89. Farooqi IS, Jebb SA, Langmack G, et al. Effects of recombinant leptin therapy in a child with congenital leptin deficiency. *N Engl J Med*. 1999;341:879–884

90. Montague CT, Farooqi IS, Whitehead JP, et al. Congenital leptin deficiency is associated with severe early-onset obesity in humans. *Nature*. 1997;387:903–908

91. Clement K, Vaisse C, Lahlou N, et al. A mutation in the human leptin receptor gene causes obesity and pituitary dysfunction. *Nature*. 1998;392:398–401

92. Heymsfield SB, Greenberg AS, Fujioka K, et al. Recombinant leptin for weight loss in obese and lean adults: a randomized, controlled, dose-escalation trial. *JAMA*. 1999;292:1568–1575

93. Rosenbaum M, Leibel RL. The role of leptin in human physiology. *N Engl J Med*. 1999;341:913–915

94. Garrow JS, Webster J. Are pre-obese people energy thrifty? *Lancet*. 1985;1:670–671

95. Leibel RL, Bahary N, Friedman JM. Genetic variation and nutrition in obesity. In: Simopoulos AP, Childs B, eds. *Genetic Variation and Nutrition*. Basel, Switzerland: Karger; 1990:90–101

96. Stunkard AJ, Foch TT, Hrubec Z. A twin study of human obesity. *JAMA*. 1986;256: 51–54

97. Rosenbaum M, Leibel RL. Pathophysiology of childhood obesity. *Adv Pediatr*. 1998; 35:73–137

98. Sun M, Gower BA, Bartolucci AA, Hunter GR, Figueroa-Colon R, Goran MI. A longitudinal study of resting energy expenditure relative to body composition during puberty in African American and white children. *Am J Clin Nutr*. 2001;73:308–315

99. Beales PL, Katsanis N, Lewis RA, et al. Genetic and mutational analyses of a large multiethnic Bardet-Biedl cohort reveal a minor involvement of BBS6 and delineate the critical intervals of other loci. *Am J Hum Genet*. 2001;68:606–616

100. Santagata S, Boggon TJ, Baird CL, et al. G-protein signaling through tubby proteins. *Science*. 2001;292:2041–2050

101. Must A, Jacques PF, Dallai GE, Bajema CJ, Dietz WH. Long-term morbidity and mortality of overweight adolescents. A follow-up of the Harvard Growth Study of 1922 to 1935. *N Engl J Med*. 1992;327:1350–1355

102. Webber LS, Srinivasan SR, Wattigney WA, Berenson GS. Tracking of serum lipids and lipoproteins from childhood to adulthood. The Bogalusa Heart Study. *Am J Epidemiol.* 1991;133:884–899

103. Daniels SR. Obesity in the pediatric patient: cardiovascular complications. *Prog Pediatr Cardiol.* 2001;12:161–167

104. Sothern MS, Loftin M, Blecker U, Udall JN Jr. Impact of significant weight loss on maximal oxygen uptake in obese children and adolescents. *J Investig Med.* 2000;48: 411–416

105. Rosenbloom AL, Joe JR, Young RS, Winter WE. Emerging epidemic of type 2 diabetes in youth. *Diabetes Care.* 1999;22:345–354

106. Young TK, Dean HJ, Flett B, Wood-Steinman P. Childhood obesity in a population at high risk for type 2 diabetes. *J Pediatr.* 2000;136:365–369

107. Caprio S, Tamborlane WV. Metabolic impact of obesity in childhood. *Endocrinol Metab Clin North Am.* 1999;28:731–747

108. Arslanian S, Suprasongsin C. Insulin sensitivity, lipids, and body composition in children: is "syndrome X" present? *J Clin Endocrinol Metab.* 1996;81:1058–1062

109. Harris MI, Flegal KM, Cowie CL, et al. Prevalence of diabetes, impaired fasting glucose, and impaired glucose tolerance in US adults. The Third National Health and Nutrition Examination Survey, 1988–1994. *Diabetes Care.* 1998;21:518–524

110. Dabelea D, Pettitt DJ, Jones KL, Arslanian SA. Type 2 diabetes mellitus in minority children and adolescents. An emerging problem. *Endocrinol Metab Clin North Am.* 1999;28:709–729

111. Campaigne B, Morrison JA, Schumann BC, et al. Indexes of obesity and comparisons with previous national survey data in 9- and 10-year-old black and white girls: the National Heart, Lung, and Blood Institute Growth and Health Study. *J Pediatr.* 1994;124:675–680

112. Morrison JA, Barton B, Biro FM, Sprecher DL, Falkner F, Obarzanek E. Sexual maturation and obesity in 9- and 10-year-old black and white girls: the National Heart, Lung, and Blood Institute Growth and Health Study. *J Pediatr.* 1994;124:889–895

113. Arslanian S, Suprasongsin C. Differences in the in vivo insulin sensitivity in healthy black vs white adolescents. *J Pediatr.* 1996;129:440–443

114. Gower BA, Nagy TR, Trowbridge CA, Dezenberg C, Goran MI. Fat distribution and insulin response in prepubertal African American and white children. *Am J Clin Nutr.* 1998;67:821–827

115. Gower BA, Nagy TR, Goran MI. Visceral fat, insulin sensitivity, and lipids in prepubertal children. *Diabetes.* 1999;48:1515–1521

116. Svec F, Nastasi K, Hilton C, Bao W, Srinivasan SR, Berenson GS. Black-white contrasts in insulin levels during pubertal development. The Bogalusa Heart Study. *Diabetes.* 1992;41:313–317

117. Yanovski JA, Yanovski SZ, Filmer KM, et al. Differences in body composition of black and white girls. *Am J Clin Nutr.* 1996;64:833–839

118. Freedman DS, Srinivasan SR, Burke GL, et al. Relationship of body fat distribution to hyperinsulinemia in children and adolescents: the Bogalusa Heart Study. *Am J Clin Nutr*. 1987;46:403–410

119. Osei K, Schuster DP. Effects of race and ethnicity on insulin sensitivity, blood pressure, and heart rate in three ethnic populations: comparative studies in African-Americans, African immigrants (Ghanaians), and white Americans using ambulatory blood pressure monitoring. *Am J Hypertens*. 1996;9:1157–1164

120. Mitchell BD, Kammerer CM, Reinhart LJ, Stern MP. NIDDM in Mexican-American families. Heterogeneity by age of onset. *Diabetes Care*. 1994;17:567–573

121. Pugliese MT, Lifshitz F, Grad G, Fort P, Marks-Katz M. Fear of obesity. A cause of short stature and delayed puberty. *N Engl J Med*. 1983;309:513–518

122. Barlow SE, Dietz WH. Obesity evaluation and treatment: expert committee recommendations. The Maternal and Child Health Bureau, Health Resources and Services Administration and the Department of Health and Human Services. *Pediatrics*. 1998;102:E29

123. Epstein LH. Family-based behavioural intervention for obese children. *Int J Obes Relat Metab Disord*. 1996;20(suppl):S14–S21

124. Epstein LH, Valoski A, Wing RR, McCurley J. Ten-year follow-up of behavioral, family-based treatment of obese children. *JAMA*. 1990;264:2519–2523

125. Blair SN. Evidence for success of exercise in weight loss and control. *Ann Intern Med*. 1993;119:702–706

126. Gordon NF, Scott CB, Wilkinson WJ, Duncan JJ, Blair SN. Exercise and mild essential hypertension. Recommendations for adults. *Sports Med*. 1990;10:390–404

127. Kriska AM, Blair SN, Pereira MA. The potential role of physical activity in the prevention of non-insulin-dependent diabetes mellitus: the epidemiological evidence. *Exerc Sport Sci Rev*. 1994;22:121–143

128. Wei M, Macera CA, Hornung CA, Blair SN. Changes in lipids associated with change in regular exercise in free-living men. *J Clin Epidemiol*. 1997;50:1137–1142

129. Wei M, Schwertner HA, Blair SN. The association between physical activity, physical fitness, and type 2 diabetes mellitus. *Compr Ther*. 2000;26:176–182

130. Epstein LH, Gordy CC, Raynor HA, Beddome M, Kilanowski CK, Paluch R. Increasing fruit and vegetable intake and decreasing fat and sugar intake in families at risk for childhood obesity. *Obes Res*. 2001;9:171–178

131. Roza AM, Shizgal HM. The Harris Benedict equation reevaluated: resting energy requirements and the body cell mass. *Am J Clin Nutr*. 1984;40:168–182

132. Yanovski JA. Intensive therapies for pediatric obesity. *Pediatr Clin North Am*. 2001; 48:1041–1053

133. American Academy of Pediatrics, Committee on Nutrition. Cholesterol in childhood. *Pediatrics*. 1998;101:141–147

134. Albright A, Franz M, Hornsby G, et al. American College of Sports Medicine position stand. Exercise and type 2 diabetes. *Med Sci Sports Exerc*. 2000;32:1345–1360

135. Epstein LH, Wing RR, Penner BC, Kress MJ. Effect of diet and controlled exercise on weight loss in obese children. *J Pediatr*. 1985;107:358–361

136. Kelley DE, Goodpaster BH. Effects of exercise on glucose homeostasis in type 2 diabetes mellitus. *Med Sci Sports Exerc.* 2001;33(suppl 6):S495–S501

137. Hernandez B, Gortmaker SL, Colditz GA, Peterson KE, Laird NM, Parra-Cabrera S. Association of obesity with physical activity, television programs and other forms of video viewing among children in Mexico city. *Int J Obes Relat Metab Disord.* 1999;23:845–854

138. Schweizer P, Lenz MP, Kirschner HJ. Pathogenesis and symptomatology of cholelithiasis in childhood. A prospective study. *Dig Surg.* 2000;17:459–467

139. Yashkov YI, Vinnitsky LI, Poroykova MV, Vorobyova NT. Some hormonal changes before and after vertical banded gastroplasty for severe obesity. *Obes Surg.* 2000; 10:48–53

140. van de Weijgert EJ, Ruseler CH, Elte JW. Long-term follow-up after gastric surgery for morbid obesity: preoperative weight loss improves the long-term control of morbid obesity after vertical banded gastroplasty. *Obes Surg.* 1999;9:426–432

141. Soper RT, Mason EE, Printen KJ, Zellwegger H. Gastric bypass for morbid obesity in children and adolescents. *J Pediatr Surg.* 1975;10:51–58

142. Bray GA. A concise view of the therapeutics of obesity. *Nutrition.* 2000;16:953–960

143. Bray GA, Tartaglia LA. Medicinal strategies in the treatment of obesity. *Nature.* 2000;404:672–677

144. Lean ME. Sibutramine—a review of clinical efficacy. *Int J Obes Relat Metab Disord.* 1997;21(suppl):S30–S39

145. Stock MJ. Sibutramine: a review of the pharmacology of a novel anti-obesity agent. *Int J Obes Relat Metab Disord.* 1997;21(suppl):S25–S29

146. Finer N, James WP, Kopelman PG, Lean ME, Williams G. One-year treatment of obesity: a randomized, double-blind, placebo-controlled, multicentre study of orlistat, a gastrointestinal lipase inhibitor. *Int J Obes Relat Metab Disord.* 2000;24:306–313

147. Hill JO, Hauptman J, Anderson JW, et al. Orlistat, a lipase inhibitor, for weight maintenance after conventional dieting: a 1-y study. *Am J Clin Nutr.* 1999;69:1108–1116

34

Food Sensitivity

Adverse reactions to foods have been implicated as the causes of many clinical problems ranging from life-threatening anaphylaxis to the tension-fatigue syndrome.[1-4] This topic is controversial and complex. The literature is replete with documented and anecdotal accounts of symptoms attributed to food ingestion. Unfortunately, although some adverse responses such as anaphylactic (immunoglobulin [Ig]E-mediated) reactions have been systematically studied, the precise pathogenesis of other responses, such as tension-fatigue syndrome, behavioral and learning problems, and others are unproved and unresolved. Nevertheless, studies indicate that about 2% to 8% of infants and children less than 3 years experience food hypersensitivity reactions.[5] Overall, approximately 2.5% of infants will experience allergic reactions to cow milk in the first 3 years of life, 1.5% to eggs, and 0.6% to peanuts.[2] Fortunately, about 85% of infants who are allergic to milk and eggs will "outgrow" [develop tolerance to] their food allergy within the first 5 years of life, and about 20% of infants who are allergic to peanuts will "outgrow" their peanut allergy.[6] However, food allergies are the leading single cause of anaphylactic reactions treated in emergency departments in the United States and Europe,[7,8] and account for about 30 000 emergency room visits in the United States and about 100 to 125 deaths per year.[9] Peanut allergy is the leading cause of fatal and near-fatal food allergic reactions in the United States. Delayed introduction of peanut products into the diet of infants identified as being at high risk for developing allergy by a strong (biparental; parent and sibling) family history of allergy and a complete allergy evaluation of any child suspected of peanut allergy is recommended.[10]

Definitions

Food allergy is the term that has been used generically by physicians and patients to refer to many different types of clinical reactions and has resulted in confusion in terminology. To standardize nomenclature, the American Academy of Allergy and Immunology Committee on Adverse Reactions to Foods[11] suggested that the following definitions be used for food-induced reactions:

- *Adverse reaction to a food:* clinically abnormal response believed to be caused by an ingested food or food additive.
- *Food hypersensitivity (allergy):* immunologic reaction resulting from the ingestion of a food or food additive.
- *Food anaphylaxis:* classic allergic hypersensitivity reaction to food or food additives involving IgE antibody and release of chemical mediators.
- *Food intolerance:* general term describing an abnormal physiologic response to an ingested food or food additive; can include idiosyncratic, metabolic, pharmacologic, or toxic response. Note: In European literature, this term is used to mean an adverse reaction to food.
- *Food idiosyncrasy:* quantitatively abnormal response to a food or food additive; response differs from its physiologic or pharmacologic effect and resembles a hypersensitivity reaction but does not involve an immune mechanism.
- *Food toxicity (poisoning):* an adverse effect caused by direct action of a food or food additive on the host recipient without the involvement of immune mechanisms; nonimmune release of chemical mediators may occur; toxins may be from the food itself or from microorganisms.
- *Anaphylactoid reaction to a food:* anaphylaxis-like reaction to a food or food additive as a result of non–IgE-mediated release of chemical mediators.
- *Pharmacologic food reaction:* adverse reactions to a food or food additive as a result of a naturally derived or added chemical that produces a drug-like or pharmacologic effect in the host.
- *Metabolic food reaction:* adverse reactions to a food or food additive as the result of the effect of the substance on the metabolism of the host recipient.

Manifestations commonly ascribed to hypersensitivity to food, but not exclusively caused by food are as follows:

1. *Systemic:* anaphylaxis, failure to thrive[3,12]
2. *Gastrointestinal:* vomiting, abdominal pain, diarrhea, malabsorption, enteropathies[3,13,14]
3. *Respiratory:* rhinitis, cough, wheezing, pulmonary infiltration[3,15]
4. *Cutaneous:* rash, urticaria, atopic dermatitis[1,3]

Hypersensitivity reactions to food may be categorized according to the interval between ingestion and the appearance of symptoms: *immediate* (minutes to 2 hours) or *delayed* (more than 2 hours, usually within 48 hours).

These intervals may be associated with corresponding immunologic mechanisms involving IgE antibodies (immediate) and possibly immune complexes
containing IgG and IgM or sensitized lymphocytes (delayed). Any of the manifestations may occur at any period during infancy or childhood. As depicted in
Table 34.1, a number of food-allergic disorders have been identified.

Diagnosis of Hypersensitivity to Food

Symptoms associated with the ingestion of foods may stem from microbial,
parasitic, or chemical contaminants, deficiencies of digestive enzymes, psychological aversion, hypersensitivity, and other causes.[3,16] Before making the
diagnosis of food hypersensitivity, other possibilities to account for adverse
food reactions should be considered.

A diagnosis of hypersensitivity to food requires (1) verification that the
food in question causes an adverse reaction, (2) exclusion of other causes of
adverse reactions, and (3) identification of immunologic sensitization.[17]

Complete delineation of the immunologic basis may be an elaborate
undertaking that is not essential to practical management but is necessary
for full comprehension. Certain signs of an immunologic pathogenesis are
discussed later.

Table 34.1.
Food-Allergic Disorders

IgE-mediated -▶		Non–IgE-mediated
Cutaneous Urticaria Angioedema Erythematous macular rash	Atopic dermatitis	Contact dermatitis
Gastrointestinal Oral allergy syndrome Gastrointestinal anaphylaxis	Allergic eosinophilic esophagitis Allergic eosinophilic gastritis Allergic eosinophilic gastroenteritis	Food-induced enterocolitis Food-induced proctocolitis Food-induced enteropathy
Respiratory Rhinoconjunctivitis Laryngeal edema Acute bronchospasm	Asthma	Food-induced pulmonary hemosiderosis [Heiner syndrome]

Confirmation of Food as the Cause of Symptoms

Various symptoms are commonly ascribed to some foods recently eaten. A feeble suspicion readily becomes a strong conviction, especially when no objective test is applied. Unwarranted enthusiasm can lead to overzealous incrimination of foods as the basis of many complaints.

The role of food as the cause of symptoms must be confirmed by some process that excludes the bias of the subject and observers. A double-blind placebo-controlled food challenge may be necessary if errors in the diagnosis of adverse reactions to food and needless dietary restrictions are to be avoided. In some instances, the simpler challenge-withdrawal test provides the same information.

Food Challenge

Recommended detailed procedures for performing food challenge have been published.[16] With infants and children up to 6 years, the suspected food may be successfully camouflaged by mixing it with some other food.* For older children, the suspected food or a placebo may also be camouflaged in a liquid or another food, or administered in opaque capsules. These should be prepared by someone other than the subject or observer and designated by a code number. When capsules are not used, the suspected food can be camouflaged in milk shakes or other liquids that mask taste (eg, Vivonex, Elecare, and Neocate One +). The most common offending foods can be obtained in the dry state (eg, milk, eggs, peanuts, and wheat). Wet foods can be freeze-dried and powdered.

Before the challenge, the suspected foods are excluded from the diet for 2 weeks or longer (until symptoms subside). If the foods that may be causing symptoms are unknown, a diet of foods unlikely to cause hypersensitivity may be given. Diets with decreasing levels of food restriction have been helpful in formulating elimination diets for diagnostic and therapeutic reasons (Tables 34.2 through 34.4). The restricted diet is used in place of regular meals during the limited period of observation. Overly restrictive diets used for a prolonged period of time may result in nutritional deficiencies.

During the challenge procedure, the suspected foods are swallowed under close supervision. The test dose in the capsules or test substance is chosen according to the impressiveness of the history and ranges from 20 to 2000 mg

---

* Warning: Testing a food strongly implicated in the induction of an anaphylactic reaction is unnecessary and unsafe.

Table 34.2.
Allergy Diet No. 1*

Foods and Beverages Allowed†	Items To Be Avoided
Lamb	Milk
	Tea
	Coffee
	Cola
	Soft drinks
Poi	
Rice	
Rice wafers	
Rice cereals	Chewing gum
Pineapples	All medications except those prescribed
Loganberries	by a physician
Pears	
Blueberries	
	All foods not listed under Foods and
	Beverages Allowed
Lettuce†	
Artichokes	
Beets	
Spinach	
Celery	
Parsnips	
Salt	
Sugar (cane or beet)	
Water	
Any vegetable oil, such as olive oil	
or Crisco, except oleomargarine‡	

* Modified from Golbert TM. Food allergy and immunologic diseases of the gastrointestinal tract. In: Patterson R, ed. *Allergic Disease, Diagnosis and Management.* 2nd ed. Philadelphia, PA: JB Lippincott Co; 1980:418.
† All fruits and vegetables, except lettuce, must be cooked.
‡ Kosher pareve oleomargarines contain no milk and may be allowed.

as an initial dose. With immediate-type hypersensitivity, symptoms will occur within 2 to 4 hours. If no reaction occurs, the amount in the test material may be increased twofold to 10-fold in subsequent challenges. If 8 to 10 g of a dried food or 60 to 100 g of a wet food provoke no symptoms, usual portions of the food can be added openly to the diet without expectation of an immediate-type reaction. A single unequivocal reaction in a double-blind challenge may be considered as definitive evidence of an adverse reaction to the food, but it is

Table 34.3.
Allergy Diet No. 2: Cereal-, Milk-, and Egg-Free Diet*

Foods and Beverages Allowed†		Items To Be Avoided
Lamb	Arrowroot	Tea
Chicken, turkey	Potatoes, potato chips	Coffee
Beef, all-beef wieners	Rice	Cola
Ham (boiled), bacon	Yams, sweet potatoes	Soft drinks
	Tapioca (whole or pearl, not minute)	
Lettuce		Chewing gum
Artichokes		
Beets		
Spinach		
Celery		
Carrots		
	Lentils	All medications except those
	Navy beans	prescribed by physician
	Kidney beans	
	Asparagus	
		All foods not listed under Foods and Beverages Allowed
Soybeans	Water	
Soy milk	Ginger ale	
Soybean sprouts	White soda	
Pineapples	Poi	
Apricots	Olive oil	
Cherries	White vinegar	
Blueberries	Vanilla extract	
Plums, prunes		
Any vegetable shortening or oleomargarine that contains no milk solids‡		
Salt		
Sugar (cane or beet)		
Maple syrup or maple-flavored cane syrup		

*Modified From Rowe's Cereal-Free 1–2–3 Diet. Adapted from Golbert TM. Food allergy and immunologic diseases of the gastrointestinal tract. In: Patterson R, ed. *Allergic Diseases, Diagnosis and Management*. Philadelphia, PA: JB Lippincott Co; 1972:363.
† All fruits and vegetables, except lettuce, must be cooked.
‡ Kosher pareve oleomargarines, Mazola margarine, and Crisco contain no milk.

Table 34.4.
Allergy Diet No. 3*

Only Foods Allowed		
Rice	White potatoes	Water
Lamb	Sweet potatoes, yams	Ginger ale (dry)
Beef	Squash	
Chicken, turkey	Carrots	Sugar (cane or beet)
Bacon	Soybeans	Salt
Apples	String beans	Maple or maple-flavored
Peaches	Peas	syrup
Apricots	Spinach	White vinegar
Pears	Chard	Vanilla extract
Pineapples	Beets	Crisco
Cranberries	Artichokes	Safflower oil margarine
	Asparagus	Pearl tapioca
	Lettuce	

Possible milk substitutes: I-Soyalac (corn-free), ProSobee, Isomil, Coffee Rich

Suggested Menu		
Breakfast	**Dinner**	**Supper**
Rice cereal	Lamb or beef patty	Chicken or turkey
Milk substitute	Baked potato	Mashed potatoes
Bacon	Lettuce and carrot salad	Peas
Tapioca and peaches	Baked pears	Lettuce and pineapple
Apple juice	Ginger ale	Salad
Water	Water	Frozen peaches
		Water

*Adapted from Rowe AH. Elimination diets in the control of food allergy. In: Rowe AH Sr, Rowe AH Jr, eds. *Food Allergy, Its Manifestations and Control in the Elimination Diets.* Springfield, IL: Charles C Thomas Publisher; 1972:41–75.

not necessarily due to an immunologic process. Other mechanisms of adverse reactions, such as deficiency of digestive enzymes, may produce similar symptoms in some cases.

With the use of blind food challenges in confirmation of delayed-type reactions, the elimination diet should be continued as long as an adverse reaction is thought to have occurred after ingestion of the suspected food. Double-blind, placebo-controlled food challenge is particularly needed for confirmation of delayed adverse reactions to food because the long interval between ingestion and the supposed reaction makes the association prone to error. The elimination diet, although not suitable for long-term use, can be used during the food challenge period without concern.

The testing of suspected foods by double-blind challenges may seem elaborate, yet it can be highly rewarding. In many instances, adverse reactions to foods elicited by history will not be confirmed, and incriminated foods can be restored to the diet. Neurotic and subjective complaints are especially susceptible to erroneous association with foods eaten; this can be verified through blind challenges.

Eat and drink only the foods listed. Avoid coffee, tea, cola, and other soft drinks, and chewing gum.

Differential Diagnosis

When an adverse reaction to a food has been confirmed by blind challenge, customary procedures differentiate hypersensitivity disorders from various causes of disturbances of the gastrointestinal, respiratory, or cutaneous systems (ie, mucosal digestive enzyme deficiencies, cystic fibrosis, infections, and immunologic deficiencies). The diagnosis of hypersensitivity must be supported by detection of immunologic sensitization.[3,16]

Identification of an Immunologic Basis for an Adverse Reaction to Food

At present, a convenient technique for identification of a definitive component of the immunologic basis for a hypersensitivity reaction to food is available only for food-induced anaphylaxis. The immunologic mechanisms responsible for delayed-type hypersensitivity reactions have not been elucidated sufficiently to permit selection of a definitive laboratory test for identification.[3,16]

Symptoms of food anaphylaxis are caused by release of mediators (histamine) when food antigen combines with specific IgE antibody attached to basophils and mast cells. In children older than 1 year, the presence of IgE antibody to food may be identified by serologic tests (see following text) or by a specific wheal and flare reaction in the skin induced by prick skin testing. Certain precautions are necessary to make skin tests with food extracts reliable. Commercially prepared extracts must be subjected to verification.[18] The concentration and technique used must not cause reactions in the skin of persons not hypersensitive, but produce wheal and flare responses in hypersensitive individuals.

Food antigens used for skin testing should, in general, be obtained from reputable manufacturers as 1:20 weight-volume glycerinated extracts. After prick skin testing with these materials, a wheal reaction 3 mm in diameter greater than or equal to the negative control [usually 0] in diameter 15 minutes after application is considered a positive reaction. Since some food extracts (eg, fruits and vegetables) may lack appropriate antigens because of enzymatic degradation during preparation, direct prick testing with the suspected food may also be performed; in these instances, a control individual should be simultaneously tested to exclude the possibility that a positive response is due to a local irritant effect.[19] The use of intradermal skin tests is generally not warranted since they frequently evoke "nonspecific" irritant responses or wheal and flare reactions that indicate low level sensitivity that is not associated with symptoms following ingestion of the food in a double-blind challenge. In addition, intradermal skin tests are more often associated with systemic reactions, including fatal anaphylaxis.

Immediate skin test responses can be helpful to include or exclude possible culprit foods in equivocal cases.[3,16] Not all positive skin tests reflect clinical sensitivity to that food (ie, false-positive responses are seen frequently).[2] Standard radioallergosorbent tests (RASTs) are no more diagnostic. Thus, it is potentially harmful to exclude foods from the diet based on skin test results alone; careful comparisons between skin test results and clinical symptoms are necessary.

Despite frequent false-positive skin test results, the incidence of false-negative results is very low (<5%). Thus, a negative skin test response to a suspected food indicates a very low probability that a double-blind food challenge will result in an immediate or early onset hypersensitivity. Recently, it has been demonstrated that quantification of food-specific IgE antibodies are highly predictive of clinical reactivity, and can be used to preclude the use of food challenges in some cases.[20]

Diagnostic Approach

When a history suggestive of an adverse reaction to a specific food is obtained, the following is recommended:

1. For children (older than 1 year), serologic tests or skin prick skin tests with 1:20 food extract should be done if an "immediate-type" reaction is suspected. If the wheal response in the skin prick test is less than 3 mm in diameter or the serologic test is negative, significant clinical sensitivity to the food does not exist. If the wheal response on the skin test is more than 3 mm, a double-blind food challenge should be performed to ascertain that the reaction is clinically significant. For serologic evaluation of egg, milk, peanut, and fish hypersensitivity, food-specific IgE concentrations may be obtained [eg, CAP-System FEIA®]. If the level exceeds the 95% predictive value [egg – 7 kU_A/L (2 kU_A/L for children ≤2 years); milk – 15 kU_A/L

(5 kU$_A$/L for children ≤2 years); peanut – 14 kU$_A$/L; and fish – 20 kU$_A$/L] food challenges are not generally required to confirm the diagnosis of food hypersensitivity.[20]

2. For infants (younger than 1 year), a double-blind food challenge should be performed if a response occurs to an open challenge. If positive, skin or serologic tests to determine that the reaction is based on immediate-type immunologic sensitization may be performed. Double-blind challenges are not always necessary, particularly if no response occurs with open challenge.

Radioallergosorbent Test

The radioallergosorbent test (RAST) was developed for the estimation of antigen-specific IgE in serum. The level of specific IgE reflects the degree of sensitization. As with the skin test, RAST reveals that only the higher degrees of hypersensitivity are correlated with clinical symptoms on exposure to the antigen. Except when the skin is unsuitable, as in patients with widespread atopic dermatitis, the standard RAST has no practical advantage over skin tests.[21] The same verification suggested for skin tests is required for RAST.

CAP-System FEIA

The CAP-System FEIA (Fluorescein Enzyme Immunoassay) uses a cellulose matrix system that allows quantification of allergen-specific IgE antibodies. Studies comparing the outcome of double-blind placebo-controlled food challenges and the level of food-specific IgE antibodies have demonstrated a correlation between clinical reactions and the quantity of food-specific IgE.[20,22]

Food Hypersensitivity Not Involving IgE Antibody

In addition to immediate or anaphylactic food reactions that involve IgE antibody and mast cell or basophil mediator release, food antigens may induce a state of hypersensitivity through the formation of other classes of immunoglobulins (ie, IgG, IgM, or IgA) or sensitized lymphocytes. No clinically reliable test exists to confirm an immune-mediated basis for non–IgE-mediated

Food	>95% PPV*
Egg	7 kU$_A$/L
Milk	15 kU$_A$/L
Peanut	14 kU$_A$/L
Fish	20 kU$_A$/L

*Where ">95% positive predictive value (PPV)" = greater than 95% probability of clinical reaction for children ≥2 years of age.

food hypersensitivity. Tests to determine serum levels of IgG antibodies to food antigens are not clinically useful. With gastrointestinal manifestations, histopathologic examination of tissue may help determine the presence of immunoglobulins, complement, eosinophils, or lymphocytes. Although these findings suggest an immunologic pathogenesis, they do not necessarily confirm a cause and effect relationship. However, until more precise diagnostic tools are available, these types of analyses have provided insight into potential immune mechanisms responsible for perplexing clinical symptomatology.

Milk Allergy

Cow milk hypersensitivity develops in 2.2% to 2.8% of infants, but 85% of these children outgrow the reactivity (ie, develop tolerance) by 4 years of age.[2] Prick skin tests at 1 year of age are valuable for predicting the outcome of the milk sensitivity and the likelihood of developing other food sensitivities.[23] Soy protein-based formulas are no less allergenic than cow milk protein-based formulas.[24] Symptoms include diarrhea, vomiting, and failure to thrive.[12,25] Colitis with gastrointestinal bleeding and colic may occur, as well as skin and respiratory symptoms.[2,3]

A rare syndrome (Heiner syndrome) alleviated by the elimination of milk was described by Lee et al[26] as recurrent otitis, bronchitis, sinusitis, and eosinophilia. Pulmonary hemosiderosis with anemia and hemosiderin-laden cells in the saliva may be found.[26]

There is evidence that milk-induced enterocolitis, proctocolitis, eosinophilic esophagitis and gastroenterocolitis, and enteropathies (including celiac disease) induced by other foods are caused by immunologic mechanisms and fit the definition of food allergy. Nevertheless, the diet of many infants who vomit, spit up, or have colicky symptoms is often altered without fulfilling the criteria as outlined.

If neither soy nor cow milk can be consumed, consideration should be given to increase consumption of other foods with calcium (Appendix N, Table N-2) or a calcium supplement to meet the recommended dietary allowance.

Treatment

Rational treatment must be based on a correct diagnosis. Clinically significant hypersensitivity to food may be far less common than generally supposed.[2] A relatively small number of foods are responsible for most confirmable hypersensitivity reactions to foods. The long-term elimination of staple items such as milk, eggs, and wheat should be done only when clearly justified by proper diagnostic procedures. Infants with milk or soy hypersensitivity should be fed a substitute hypoallergenic formula until they are 1 year of age or older. A rechallenge with milk or soy should be undertaken in a controlled setting in which intravenous fluids, epinephrine, oxygen and personnel familiar with resuscitation are available. For children, elimination diets should be designed with appropriate dietetic counseling.

Exclusion of a food for 2 to 4 weeks should serve to evaluate any contribution it may make to symptoms. Small amounts of a food may be tolerated, but larger quantities of it may cause symptoms. Since many antigens (eg, soy protein) can be present in multiple foods, dietetic consultation should be

---

In summary, the American Academy of Pediatrics recommends:

1. Breast milk is an optimal source of nutrition for infants through the first year of life or longer. Those breastfeeding infants who develop symptoms of food allergy may benefit from:
   a. maternal restriction of cow's milk, egg, fish, peanuts and tree nuts and if this is unsuccessful,
   b. use of a hypoallergenic (extensively hydrolyzed or if allergic symptoms persist, a free amino acid-based formula) as an alternative to breastfeeding. Those infants with IgE-associated symptoms of allergy may benefit from a soy formula, either as the initial treatment or instituted after 6 months of age after the use of a hypoallergenic formula. The prevalence of concomitant reactions is not as great between soy and cow milk in these infants compared with those with non–IgE-associated syndromes such as enterocolitis, proctocolitis, malabsorption syndrome, or esophagitis. Benefits should be seen within 2 to 4 weeks and the formula continued until the infant is 1 year of age or older.
2. Formula-fed infants with confirmed cow's milk allergy may benefit from the use of a hypoallergenic or soy formula as described for the breastfed infant.
3. Infants at high risk for developing allergy, identified by a strong (biparental; parent and sibling) family history of allergy may benefit from exclusive breastfeeding or a hypoallergenic formula or possibly a partial hydrolysate formula. Conclusive studies are not yet available to permit definitive recommendations. However, the following recommendations seem reasonable at this time:
   a. Breastfeeding mothers should continue breastfeeding for the first year of life or longer. During this time, for infants at risk, hypoallergenic formulas can be used to supplement breastfeeding. Mothers should eliminate peanuts and tree nuts (eg, almonds, walnuts, etc) and consider eliminating eggs, cow's milk, fish, and perhaps other foods from their diets while nursing. Solid foods should not be introduced into the diet of high-risk infants until 6 months of age, with dairy products delayed until 1 year, eggs until 2 years, and peanuts, nuts, and fish until 3 years of age.
   b. No maternal dietary restrictions during pregnancy are necessary with the possible exception of excluding peanuts.
4. Breastfeeding mothers on a restricted diet should consider the use of supplemental minerals (calcium) and vitamins.

American Academy of Pediatrics. Hypoallergenic infant formulas. *Pediatrics*. 2000;106:346–349.

---

obtained to avoid equivocal results and the establishment of a diet nutritionally adequate for various age groups. Drug therapy (eg, cromolyn sodium) has not been proven to be consistently helpful, although the efficacy of anti-IgE therapy is currently under investigation for the treatment of patients at risk for food-induced anaphylaxis. Those who have had an anaphylactic reaction to food in the past should carry a readily injectable form of epinephrine that they are trained to use in case of inadvertent exposure to the offending food.

Prognosis

For IgE-mediated reactions, 44% of children younger than 3 years will likely outgrow the clinical response in 1 to 7 years. Of infants with milk allergy, 70% to 85% will tolerate milk by 4 years.[2] Recent evidence indicates that ~20% of infants who experience allergic reactions to peanuts will "outgrow" their sensitivity.[6] Children in whom food sensitivities develop after age 3 are less likely outgrow the problem. Although many children outgrow the clinical sensitivity, the immediate skin test response to the food allergen may remain positive for an extended period of time.

Prevention

Several studies have demonstrated that elimination of food allergens (eg, peanuts, milk, and eggs) from the diet of infants at high risk for atopic disease and their lactating mothers can delay or prevent some food allergy and atopic dermatitis,[27,28] although during pregnancy, maternal dietary restrictions, with the possible exception of peanuts, do not decrease the risk of most allergic diseases later in childhood. Based on these studies, recommending the following guidelines for high-risk infants seems reasonable: (1) maternal dietary avoidance of peanuts and nuts during pregnancy; (2) exclusive breastfeeding for the first 4 to 6 months of life or use of a hypoallergenic formula if breastfeeding is not possible or supplementation is required (mothers should eliminate all peanut and tree nuts from their diet, and, if highly motivated, consider eliminating eggs and milk; dietary counseling to achieve the recommended allowances of minerals and other nutrients is important with these highly restricted diets); (3) delay introduction of solid foods until after 6 months of age; and (4) delay introduction of cow milk until 1 year of age; eggs until 2 years; and peanuts, nuts, fish, and shellfish until 3 years of age.

References

1. Bock SA, Atkins FM. Patterns of food hypersensitivity during sixteen years of double-blind, placebo-controlled food challenges. *J Pediatr.* 1990;117:561–567

2. Sampson HA. Food allergy. Part 1: immunopathogenesis and clinical disorders. *J Allergy Clin Immunol.* 1999;103:717–728

3. Sampson HA. Food allergy. Part 2: diagnosis and management. *J Allergy Clin Immunol.* 1999;103:981–989

4. Sampson HA, Mendelson L, Rosen JP. Fatal and near-fatal anaphylactic reactions to food in children and adolescents. *N Engl J Med.* 1992;327:380–384

5. Bock SA. Prospective appraisal of complaints of adverse reactions to foods in children during the first 3 years of life. *Pediatrics.* 1987;79:683–688

6. Skolnick HS, Koerner CB, Connover-Walker MK, Sampson HA, Burks W, Wood RA. The natural history of peanut allergy. *J Allergy Clin Immunol.* 2001;107: 367–374

7. Yocum MW, Butterfield JH, Klein JS, Volcheck GW, Schroeder DR, Silverstein MD. Epidemiology of anaphylaxis in Olmsted County: a population-based study. *J Allergy Clin Immunol.* 1999;104:452–456

8. Novembre E, Cianferoni A, Bernardini R, et al. Anaphylaxis in children: clinical and allergologic features. *Pediatrics.* 1998;101:E8

9. Bock SA, Munoz-Furlong A, Sampson HA. Fatalities due to anaphylactic reactions to foods. *J Allergy Clin Immunol.* 2001;107:191–193

10. Sampson HA. Peanut allergy. *N Engl J Med.* 2002;346:1294–1299

11. Anderson JA. The establishment of common language concerning adverse reactions to foods and food additives. *J Allergy Clin Immunol.* 1986;78:140–144

12. Bock SA, Sampson HA. Food allergy in infancy. *Pediatr Clin North Am.* 1994;41: 1047–1067

13. Wang LF, Lin JY, Hsieh K, Lin RH. Epicutaneous exposure of protein antigen induces a predominant Th2-like response with high IgE production in mice. *J Immunol.* 1996;156:4077–4082

14. Trier JS. Celiac sprue. In: Sleisenger MH, Fordtran JS, eds. *Gastrointestinal Disease: Pathophysiology/Diagnosis/Management.* Vol 2. 5th ed. Philadelphia, PA: W.B. Saunders Company; 1993:1078–1096

15. James JM, Eigenmann PA, Eggleston PA, Sampson HA. Airway reactivity changes in asthmatic patients undergoing blinded food challenges. *Am J Respir Crit Care Med.* 1996;153:597–603

16. Sampson HA. Differential diagnosis in adverse reactions to foods. *J Allergy Clin Immunol.* 1986;78:212–219

17. Bock SA, Sampson HA, Atkins FM, et al. Double-blind, placebo-controlled food challenge (DBPCFC) as an office procedure: a manual. *J Allergy Clin Immunol.* 1988;82:986–997

18. Bock SA. In vitro diagnosis: skin testing and oral challenge procedures. In: Metcalfe DD, Sampson HA, Simon RA, eds. *Food Allergy: Adverse Reactions to Foods and Food Additives.* 2nd ed. Cambridge, MA: Blackwell Science; 1997:151–168

19. Rosen JP, Selcow JE, Mendelson LM, Grodofsky MP, Factor JM, Sampson HA. Skin testing with natural foods in patients suspected of having food allergies: is it a necessity? *J Allergy Clin Immunol.* 1994;93:1068–1070

20. Sampson HA, Ho DG. Relationship between food-specific IgE concentrations and the risk of positive food challenges in children and adolescents. *J Allergy Clin Immunol.* 1997;100:444–451

21. Sampson HA, Albergo R. Comparison of results of skin tests, RAST, and double-blind, placebo-controlled food challenges in children with atopic dermatitis. *J Allergy Clin Immunol.* 1984;74:26–33

22. Sampson HA. Utility of food-specific IgE concentrations in predicting symptomatic food allergy. *J Allergy Clin Immunol.* 2001;107:891–896

23. Host A. Cow's milk protein allergy and intolerance in infancy. Some clinical, epidemiological and immunological aspects. *Pediatr Allergy Immunol.* 1994;5(suppl 5):1–36

24. Zeiger RS. Development and prevention of allergic disease in childhood. In: Middleton E, Reed C, Ellis E, Adkinson N, Yunginger J, Busse W, eds. *Allergy: Principles and Practice.* Vol 2. 4th ed. St Louis, MO: Mosby; 1993:1137–1171

25. Baehler P, Chad Z, Gurbindo C, Bonin AP, Bouthillier L, Seidman EG. Distinct patterns of cow's milk allergy in infancy defined by prolonged, two-stage double-blind, placebo-controlled food challenges. *Clin Exp Allergy.* 1996;26:254–261

26. Lee SK, Kniker WT, Cook CD, Heiner DC. Cow's milk-induced pulmonary disease in children. *Adv Pediatr.* 1978;25:39–57

27. Zeiger RS, Heller S, Mellon MH, Halsey JF, Hamburger RN, Sampson HA. Genetic and environmental factors affecting the development of atopy through age 4 in children of atopic parents: a prospective randomized study of food allergen avoidance. *Pediatr Allergy Immunol.* 1992;3:110–127

28. Hide DW, Matthews S, Matthews L, et al. Effect of allergen avoidance in infancy on allergic manifestations at age two years. *J Allergy Clin Immunol.* 1994;93:842–846

35

Nutrition and Immunity

Introduction

Nutrients play integral roles in the development and function of the immune system. The keystones of an effective immune response are rapid cellular proliferation and early synthesis of regulatory and/or protective proteins, all of which require a ready supply of nutrients as substrates, cofactors, and structural components. Therefore, insufficiency of one or more essential nutrients is potentially rate limiting in the development and maintenance of immune responses. Similarly, inflammation and other immune responses alter a person's nutritional status through sequestration of minerals (eg, iron and zinc), impaired absorption, increased nutrient loss, or altered nutrient utilization. Although the effects of the immune system on nutritional status are important during inflammation and other acute disease states, this discussion focuses on the role of nutrition in immune system development and the impact of primary nutrient deficiencies on immune responses.

Nutrient-immune interactions are of special concern in infants and children because of the increased vulnerability of the developing immune system. Early in life, systemic humoral immunity is strongly dependent on maternal IgG acquired transplacentally and specific mucosal immunity relies to a great extent on secretory IgA supplied via breastfeeding. This reliance on maternal factors is due to the paucity of production of those immunoglobulin isotypes during early infancy, the decreased repertoire of antibody binding specificities during that period, and the slow development of antibody responses to polysaccharide antigens during the first 2 to 3 years of age.[1] Adult concentrations of serum IgM and IgG do not develop until 4 to 6 years of age.[2] The thymus and other immune tissues continue to grow and develop through puberty. Thus, definitions of "normal" immune status and responses depend on a child's age and stage of development. Factors such as prematurity or low birth weight will further delay the development of the immune system.

To appreciate the importance to the child of nutrient-immune interactions, the ontogeny of the immune system must be considered in the context of the child's overall growth and development. Periods of rapid growth velocity increase the demands of muscle, organ, and other tissues on the available nutrient pool. If there is an insufficient supply of any nutrient, growth retardation and/or other functional deficits will occur. In some cases (eg, "catch-up" growth), nutrient repletion will promote nearly full recovery from a prior insult. In other cases (eg, cognitive development), moderate to severe nutritional insults early in life may overcome the system's plasticity and recovery may not be possible.

In the case of the immune system, the degree and reversibility of an immune defect depends on the timing, duration, severity, and type of nutritional insufficiency. Early and/or severe nutrient deficiencies appear to cause long-lasting effects on the immune system. Thymic involution and reduced immune responsiveness occur during moderate to severe general undernutrition and various single nutrient deficiencies. Even after nutritional supplementation, immune responsiveness may not recover fully in previously malnourished children. Animal studies indicate that severe nutrient deficiencies during early development, especially in utero and in the pre-weaning period, may result in lifelong and even perhaps transgenerational immune deficiencies.[3] For example, in the prenatal zinc deficiency mouse model, immune deficits appears to carry over to the second and third generation.[4] Thus, in the growing child with nutrient deficiencies, the combination of increased nutrient demands and a rapidly developing immune system provide great potential for permanent adverse outcomes.

Nutritional status influences the immune system at different levels. Subclinical or frank deficiencies of some micronutrients (see Micronutrients and Immunity section in this chapter) reduce the circulating levels and functional capacities of key immune cells and proteins. Other micronutrient deficiencies, including essential fatty acids, folate, zinc, and vitamin A, cause mucosal lesions or reduce mucosal integrity, thus increasing susceptibility to infections. The most severe outcomes occur among children in the developing world where severe, combined nutrient deficiencies adversely affect many parts of the immune system. This review focuses on nutrient-immune interactions likely to be encountered among children in the United States or other developed countries.

Early Nutritional-Immunologic System Interactions

Current research amply documents the influence of early nutrition on (a) immunologic responses, (b) the immediate risks to infectious diseases, and

(c) possibly, the risks to immune-related conditions expressed in later life stages. These influences have played major roles in the formulation of recommendations for the nutritional management of infants. Recognition of these influences comes principally from studies of infants fed human milk or synthetic formulas.[5,6]

Beyond the well-recognized nutritional roles of the major organic macronutrients (proteins, carbohydrates, and lipids), the macronutrients in human milk also play functional roles related to the infant's immune competence and ontogenic stage of development. These immunologic roles are expressed either actively (ie, by modulating the infant's ability to respond to an immunologic challenge) or passively (ie, attenuating or preventing infection without altering the infant's immunologic development or ability to respond to a specific challenge).[7]

Several proteins in human milk have the potential to modulate specific and/or nonspecific immune responses before their degradation to amino acids and the subsequent fulfillment of the classical metabolic roles associated with dietary proteins. Among the 2 most frequently studied examples of proteins with this characteristic are secretory IgA and lactoferrin. Although breastfeeding's general protective roles against infection are well documented, the only specific human milk component clinically proven to be protective is secretory IgA. Its efficacy against *Vibrio cholerae* O antigen and enterotoxin, *Campylobacter*, and enterotoxin-producing *Escherichia coli* has been documented by various investigators.[8] Secretory IgA provides passive protection presumably by neutralizing pathogens and their toxins and interfering with their adherence to the infant's gastrointestinal and upper respiratory tracts.

Human milk secretory IgA, however, also may provide a mechanism for active protection. The identification of anti-idiotypic antibodies in milk suggests that human milk may aid the infant's production of the corresponding idiotypic antibody.[8] Secretion of anti-idiotypic antibodies and excretion in milk of potential pathogens such as cytomegalovirus concomitantly with the secretion of corresponding neutralizing antibodies may serve as important natural immunization strategies in early infancy.[9]

Other human milk proteins such as cytokines may influence the infant's immune system through alternative mechanisms. The identification in human milk of substantial amounts of immunomodulating cytokines, including those that are ordinarily pro-inflammatory (eg, tumor necrosis factor α, interleukin 1β (IL-1β), IL-6),[10–13] anti-inflammatory (eg, transforming growth factor β and

IL-10),[14,15] colony stimulating (eg, granulocyte-colony stimulating factor and macrophage colony stimulating factor),[16,17] chemotactic (IL-8),[18] and others[19] raises the possibility of roles for human milk cytokines in leukocyte development, mobilization, and activation; the regulation of cytokine production; the expression of class I and class II histocompatibility antigens; the up-regulation of secretory component production by epithelial cells; and the production of IgA dimers required for the assembly of secretory IgA in the recipient infant.

The earlier demonstrations of urinary excretion of intact and large fragments of lactoferrin by premature infants fed human milk[20,21] and their maternal origin[22] raise the possibility of the postnatal uptake of other intact or biologically active fragments of immunoregulatory molecules of maternal origin by the infant at this and other developmental stages. The roles that these and other immunoregulatory components and antigenic exposure play in determining disparate antibody responses to immunization and to differences in "baseline" serum immunoglobulin levels between breastfed and bottle-fed infants remain unclear.[23]

Lactoferrin's strong iron-binding capacity is a well-described example of a "nonspecific" immune modulating activity of a major human milk protein. This capacity presumably limits the availability to potentially pathogenic enteric flora of an essential mineral in the infant's gastrointestinal lumen by competing effectively with bacterial enterochelins for iron.[24] This competition limits the growth of iron-dependent pathogens in the infant's gastrointestinal lumen. Lactoferrin also appears to modulate inflammatory responses by influencing macrophage responses. Lactoferrin also is able to kill certain bacterial and fungal pathogens by the membrane damaging effect of a peptide C (lactoferrin-H) located near the terminus of the lactoferrin molecule.

Anti-inflammatory capacity is not unique to lactoferrin. It is shared by several of the antimicrobial agents and other factors in human milk.[25] Beyond its actions as a single agent, lactoferrin also acts with secretory IgA to mutually enhance each other's antibacterial efficacy.[23]

Although infants rely on carbohydrates as a key energy source, human milk carbohydrates also serve immune-related roles. Oligosaccharides and more complex glycoproteins and glycolipids serve as receptor analogs that interfere with the adherence of pathogens such as pneumococci and *Haemophilus influenzae* and of enterotoxins such as those of *V cholerae* and *E coli* to epithelial cells.[26] These molecules may account partially for human milk's protection against gastroenteritis, possibly otitis media, and respiratory infections.[8]

Similarly, lipids provide essential fatty acids for structuring membranes, serving as an important energy source, and contributing to the infant's immunologic responses. The precursor role of essential fatty acids in the synthesis of functional components such as prostaglandins and the antiviral and antibacterial properties of the shorter-chain fatty acids such as lauric acid are examples of the immunologically related functions of dietary lipids. Certain products from the hydrolysis of human lipids lyse enveloped viruses.[27] The human fat globule membrane and its mucin component's ability to bind s-fimbriated *E coli* suggest another potential protective property of the milk's lipid fraction.[28]

Human milk also plays another important role. The normal development of the gastrointestinal tract is subdivided into 4 phases.[29] In the first phase, the infants' intestinal microflora resemble maternal flora and those of the surroundings encountered by infants during birth and the immediate postnatal period. The second phase is affected significantly by whether infants are breastfed or formula-fed. Although there is some inconsistency among published studies, due presumably to methodological differences, generally, initial similarities between the floras of breastfed and bottle-fed infants on day 7 of postnatal life diminish substantially by day 30. Bottle-fed infants have more *enterococci* and *clostridia* in their flora than do breastfed infants, and the latter have more *staphylococci*, more so at younger ages.[30] Generally, breastfed infants have fewer *Klebsiella, Enterobacter*, and *Citrobacter* in their flora and the strains of *E coli* found in the flora differ between feeding groups. For example, P-fimbriated *E coli* are less common and type 1-fimbriated *E coli* are more common in the flora of breastfed infants than in the flora of bottle-fed infants. P-fimbriae is the virulence factor most often associated with urinary tract infections.[30] Previous reports of highly marked differences between breastfed and bottle-fed infants in the bifidobacteria content of their flora have not been confirmed for unexplained reasons by more recent investigations.[30] The third phase relates to the period following the initial introduction of solid foods. During this period, enterococci, bacteriodes, clostridia, anaerobic streptococci, and other bacteria increase in the breastfed infants' flora. Less marked changes occur in the flora of bottle-fed infants.[29] In the fourth phase (the time following the introduction of an adult diet), although the intestinal flora of infants remains distinct from that of adults, the flora increasingly resemble adult patterns.

The short-term benefits of these nutritional-immunologic interactions are clear.[5,31] The frequency in breastfed infants of gastrointestinal infections is lower in industrialized and industrially developing populations. Also, even when rates of infections are similar among breastfed and non-breastfed infants, the duration and severity of infection often are less for breastfed infants. Attenuation of clinical responses has been reported for both gastrointestinal (eg, rotavirus infection) and respiratory infections (eg, respiratory syncytial virus infections). Such positive outcomes become progressively more significant as the frequency and severity of microbial challenges rise.

The possibility that the antimicrobial, anti-inflammatory, and immunoregulatory components in human milk have longer lasting effects on the infant's immune system and the effects of breastfeeding on the development of allergic diseases remain controversial. If breastfeeding prevents certain allergic disorders, it is unclear whether those positive outcomes are due to delays in the introduction of potentially allergenic foods, immunoregulatory components in the milk, or the balance among specific nutrients. For example, Wright and Bolton[32] reported a significantly greater proportion of linoleic acid and a smaller proportion of dihomogamma-linolenic acid in the human milk lipid fraction of mothers of infants with atopic eczema compared with controls.

In addition, there is evidence that some breastfed infants become sensitized to certain maternally ingested foods by the passage of those food antigens into human milk.[33] The topic is, however, controversial because some of these same dietary proteins may be detected in human milk from mothers whose infants are asymptomatic and one of the major suspected dietary allergens, bovine β-lactoglobulin, immunologically cross-reacts with a fragment of human β casein.[34] Therefore, the diagnosis of allergic reactions in the breastfed infant due to food allergens passed via breastfeeding depends upon tedious dietary elimination-oral provocation procedures in the lactating woman. The management of such problems requires either a cessation of breastfeeding or a long-term elimination of the food allergen from the maternal diet and severely atopic infants may require support by a pediatric allergist. Recent studies suggest that prophylactic dietary elimination of suspected food allergens from the maternal diet, with the possible exception of peanuts (and subsequent development of peanut allergy), does not decrease the risk of the development of most atopic diseases in later childhood in breastfed infants.[35] (See also Chapter 34.)

Publications linking the length of breastfeeding to the risk of type 1 diabetes mellitus, childhood lymphoma, acute lymphocytic leukemia, and Crohn's disease suggest that maturational changes may be effected in early life by the provision of immunoactive components found in milk.[36–39] These provocative, retrospective studies require the investigation of more specific mechanisms of action relating nutritional management in early life to immune system function in later development.

Prematurity and Low-Birth-Weight Infants

Interactions between nutritional status and immune system function in infants of low birth weight, because of prematurity and/or intrauterine growth retardation, have not been studied systematically. Therefore, these interactions are difficult to describe beyond the qualitative assessment of immune function deficiencies that are imposed by premature birth[40] (eg, decreased placental transfer of maternal IgG to the fetus, developmental delays in many components of the immune system and/or intrauterine growth retardation) and are also linked inextricably to inadequate micronutrient status in low-birth-weight infants. Premature separation from the mother prevents the normal transfer of nutrients with key immunologic roles, since the transfer of nutrients, such as iron and zinc, mostly occurs in the third trimester. The vitamin status of such infants also is impaired (eg, vitamin A). The inadequate nutrient transfer to the fetus that often accompanies growth retardation may be due to maternal nutrient deficiency states and/or secondary to impaired placental perfusion. In either case, the postnatal unavailability of adequate nutrient stores likely interferes with functions described in the nutrient-specific sections of this discussion. Schlesinger and Uauy[41] have reviewed potential nutrient-immune interactions in low-birth-weight infants.

Micronutrients and Immunity

Primary nutrient deficiencies are seen rarely in children in the United States, with the exception of iron deficiency. On the other hand, aberrant diets lacking key nutrients (eg, ascorbic acid[42]), certain medical conditions (eg, fat malabsorption, acrodermatitis enteropathica) and lifestyle choices (eg, vegan or macrobiotic) can induce moderate or severe nutrient deficiencies that may influence immune competence. Even in mild cases of nutrient deficiency, concern has been raised that immunological effects of nutrient deficiency may precede the appearance of classic nutritional deficiency sequelae. Unfortunately, the bulk of scientific literature on nutritional deficiency and immune competence is based largely on data from severely malnourished individuals, cell culture experiments, animal models, and clinical trials with adult or elderly subjects. The greatest caution must be taken in extrapolating suggestive data from animals or adults into recommendations for children.

Conversely, a number of vitamins, minerals, and other dietary ingredients are marketed and sold in the United States for their putative immune system-enhancing properties. Given the high rates of common infectious diseases (eg, cold, flu) among young children, parents may chose to use such supplements. A recent population survey found that half of all mothers gave vitamin supplements to their preteen children.[43] Thus, pediatricians often are challenged by the need to be familiar with the scientific evidence about individual nutrients and other dietary supplement ingredients.

Iron

Iron deficiency is the most prevalent micronutrient deficiency among children in the United States, ranging from 2% to 3% of 3- to 11-year-old children up to 9% to 11% of girls aged 12 to 19 years,[44] with higher prevalence among certain at-risk groups like Mexican Americans.[45] Studies in France[46] and the United States[47] showed that iron supplementation of children of low socioeconomic status (SES) who are iron deficient can normalize blood T-cell counts, delayed-type hypersensitivity skin responses, or in vitro IL-2 production, but the clinical consequences are unknown. A small placebo-controlled trial among 6- to 36-month-old children in Togo, West Africa (n = 163), found no change in infectious disease incidence after 6 months of iron supplementation.[48] Iron supplementation of iron-replete children is not known to improve immune function further, and increased availability of elemental iron in the gut has the potential to promote the growth and survival of pathogenic organisms.[49] Also, high-dose supplementation with iron alone can interfere with zinc absorption and, therefore, exacerbate zinc deficiency.[50]

Zinc

Moderate or severe zinc deficiency can impair immune system function in humans,[51] but this degree of zinc deficiency is encountered rarely in the United States. In developing countries, zinc supplementation reduces infectious disease morbidity, especially respiratory and diarrheal diseases, among infants and preschool children.[52-54] Zinc supplements have been used to modify the immune status of institutionalized elderly,[55] or as high-dose oral lozenges to treat the common cold in adults,[56] but there is no direct evidence that zinc supplementation may benefit zinc-replete children. Furthermore, there is a risk of zinc supplements impairing copper absorption at daily intakes above 7 mg for children under 3 years, 12 mg for children 4 to 8 years old, or 23 mg for children 9 to 13 years old.[57]

Vitamin A

In developing countries, vitamin A supplementation of deficient children reduces overall mortality[58,59] and morbidity from diarrhea,[60] measles,[61] and possibly other diseases.[62] There is no direct evidence that vitamin A supplementation benefits the immune system of vitamin A-replete children. Daily intakes of retinol above 600 µg for children under 3 years old, 900 µg for children 4 to 8 years old, or 1700 µg for children 9 to 13 years old[57] should be avoided to reduce the risk of vitamin A toxicity. This form of toxicity is not seen when vitamin A is supplied by pro-vitamin A carotenoids (eg, β-carotene, α-carotene).

Vitamin E

Although high-dose vitamin E supplements can improve immune function in healthy elderly subjects,[63] it is unclear whether that occurs in children. Vitamin E supplements did not affect tetanus antibody titers in 2-month-old infants[64] or neutrophil function in preterm infants.[65] On the other hand, smaller increases in vitamin E intake may serve the child's overall nutritional adequacy since few children in the United States consume the recommended amounts of vitamin E.[66]

Vitamin C

Vitamin C is commonly believed to benefit the immune system largely because Nobel laureate Linus Pauling advocated high-dose vitamin C to prevent the common cold.[67] A recent, comprehensive meta-analysis indicates that high-dose vitamin C (1 g or more daily) does not reduce the incidence of the common cold, but it may slightly reduce the duration of the infection.[68] Five of the 11 studies evaluated in this meta-analysis were conducted in children, and the results in this subset were consistent with the overall finding. Few studies have addressed the role of vitamin C more generally in the immune system although neutrophils are known to maintain high concentrations of the vitamin in vivo[69] and vitamin C may inactivate histamine chemically.[70] Overall, it is unclear whether high-dose vitamin C supplements have any general immunological benefit for pediatric populations.

B Vitamins

Moderate to severe deficiencies of vitamin B_6,[71,72] vitamin B_{12},[73,74] pantothenic acid,[75,76] folate,[77] or biotin[78,79] suppress immune responses in adult humans and/or animal models. Biotin and pantothenic acid are nearly ubiquitous in the US diet[80] and deficiency only occurs in unusual circumstances. Vitamin B_{12} deficiency may occur in breastfed infants of vegan (a person who consumes no animal products) mothers[81] or, theoretically, in vegan children who do not consume a supplemental source of vitamin B_{12}. Much less information is available on the effects of B-vitamin supplements on immune responses, although a few preliminary studies indicate that pharmacological intakes of riboflavin[82] or vitamin B_6[83–85] can affect immunological parameters. B-vitamin deficiency or supplementation studies have not been conducted in children, and the clinical relevance of these findings for the pediatric population is unknown.

Nucleotides

Nucleotides (components of RNA and DNA) are found normally in human milk at concentrations ranging from 189 ± 70 µmol/L.[86] Currently, nucleotides are added to several infant formula brands in the United States. The mechanism by which dietary nucleotides may modify immune function is unknown,[87] although recent mouse-model studies indicate they may augment Th1-biased immune responses.[88,89] Studies in human infants have reported that adding nucleotides to infant formula increases NK cell activity, IL-2 production by monocytes, serum IgM and IgA concentrations, and serum antibody titers to food antigens.[90–92] The clinical relevance of these changes is unknown. Two studies have reported more clinically specific endpoints. One study showed higher antibody titers to Hib (*H influenzae* type b) vaccine in treated infants[93] and another study reported a reduced duration and frequency of diarrheal disease in a group of children of low SES.[94] Such data are promising, but additional studies are needed to understand the mechanism of action, confirm clinical endpoints, and monitor the long-term effects of adding nucleotides to infant formula.

Long-Chain Polyunsaturated Fatty Acids

Human milk fat contains 0.10% to 0.35% docosahexaenoic acid (DHA) and 0.30% to 0.65% arachidonic acid (AA), depending on the mother's polyunsaturated fatty acid intake.[95] Some term infant formulas now also contain DHA and AA.[96] Both DHA and AA may contribute to visual acuity and cognitive development,[97,98] but their impact on infant immune function is not understood well. Arachidonic acid is the precursor for prostaglandins and leukotrienes that regulate normal inflammatory processes.[99,100] In vivo, DHA feeding can inhibit both inflammation responses and T-cell signaling in animal models and adult humans.[101,102] Infant data related to these responses are limited and difficult to interpret. Observational studies indicate that mothers of atopic infants have lower concentrations of DHA and AA in their milk compared to mothers of non-atopic infants.[103,104] On the other hand, Field et al[105] found that preterm infants fed formula with DHA and AA had more mature CD4+ T-cells with higher ex vivo IL-10 production (indicating a potential bias toward antibody and atopic responses) than infants fed formula without DHA and AA. Additional studies are needed to determine if DHA and AA can have clinically significant effects on in vivo inflammation, immune responses, mucosal immune system development, or long-term immunocompetence.

Probiotics

Yogurt, certain other milk-based products, and some dietary supplements contain live, nonpathogenic bacteria of the *Lactobacillus* or *Bifidobacterium* spp., collectively termed probiotics. Certain human milk carbohydrates naturally enhance the growth of probiotic bacteria in the infant's gut[106] that may benefit the child by competitively reducing colonization of the gastrointestinal tract with pathogenic organisms. A number of studies have used probiotic-containing foods or infant formula to successfully prevent or treat chronic,[107,108] acute[109-113] or antibiotic-induced diarrhea[114] in children, although not all studies showed an effect.[115] Some infants with atopic dermatitis have benefited from probiotic supplements[116] and pre- and postnatal probiotic consumption by mothers with at least one first-degree atopic relative may reduce the frequency of atopic dermatitis in their infants.[117] A wide range of other health effects have been ascribed to probiotic organisms, but considerably less data are available to substantiate other claims.[118]

Herbal Products

An emergent issue in children's nutrition is the use of dietary supplements or fortified foods for purposes other than achieving nutritional adequacy. A subcategory of dietary supplements, herbal products, often are promoted and claimed to be safe based on history of use in folk remedies or among aboriginal cultures. Health care providers should be aware that there are currently no premarket federal standards of quality, safety, or efficacy testing for herbal treatments. The Food and Drug Administration (FDA) can exercise enforcement power only if the manufacturer (1) claims the herb works like a drug, (2) the herb contains illegal substances or substances not declared on the label, or (3) if the herb causes unambiguous, serious harm to people who have purchased and used the supplement. With these cautions in mind, the health care professional must discern judiciously between benign actions that may have special significance for the family (religion, tradition, self-empowerment) and potentially hazardous misuse of potent bioactive compounds. Additional information on common dietary supplements is available from the American Dietetic Association's *The Health Professional's Guide to Popular Dietary Supplements*[119] and the *Physician's Desk Reference (PDR) for Herbal Medicines*.[120]

Summary

Adequate nutrition is necessary for proper development and function of a child's immune system. Both human milk and synthetic formula can provide adequate nutrition, but human milk is clearly best for infants because it provides unique components proven to protect and stimulate the developing immune system and contributes positively to growth and development in other ways. In older children, immune function appears to be preserved except in the most severe micronutrient deficiencies. The use of high-dose nutrient supplements and other dietary components to stimulate immune function in otherwise well-nourished children is controversial. Overall, considerably more research is needed to better understand how the maturation and function of the immune system interacts with the changing nutrient requirements of growth.

References

1. Adderson EE, Johnston JM, Shackerford PG, Carroll WL. Development of the human antibody repertoire. *Pediatr Res.* 1992;32:257–263
2. Burgio GR, Ugazio AG, Notarangelo LD. Immunology of the neonate. *Curr Opin Immunol.* 1989-1990;2:770–777
3. Gershwin ME, Beach RS, Hurley LS. Nutritional factors and immune ontogeny. In: *Nutrition and Immunity.* Orlando, FL: Academic Press, Inc; 1985:99–127
4. Beach RS, Gershwin ME, Hurley LS. Gestational zinc deprivation in mice: persistence of immunodeficiency for three generations. *Science.* 1982; 218:469–471
5. Institute of Medicine. *Nutrition During Lactation.* Washington, DC: National Academy Press; 1991
6. Stevens S. Maturation of the immune system in breast-fed and bottle-fed infants. In: Cunningham-Rundles S, ed. *Nutrient Modulation of the Immune Response.* New York, NY: Marcel-Dekker, Inc; 1993:301–318
7. Garza C, Schanler RJ, Butte NF, Motil KJ. Special properties of human milk. *Clin Perinatol.* 1987;14:11–32

8. Hanson LA, Adlerberth I, Carlsson BUM, et al. Human milk antibodies and their importance for the infant. In: Cunningham-Ruddles S, ed. *Nutrient Modulation of the Immune Response*. New York, NY: Marcel Dekker, Inc; 1993:525–532

9. Peckham CS, Johnson C, Ades A, Pearl K, Chin KS. Early acquisition of cytomegalovirus infection. *Arch Dis Child*. 1987;62:780–785

10. Rudloff HE, Schmalstieg FC Jr, Mushtaha AA, Palkowetz KH, Liu SK, Goldman AS. Tumor necrosis factor-alpha in human milk. *Pediatr Res*. 1992;31:29–33

11. Munoz C, Endres S, van der Meer J, Schlesinger L, Arevalo M, Dinarello C. Interleukin-1β in human colostrum. *Res Immunol*. 1990;141:505–513

12. Saito S, Maruyama M, Kato Y, Moriyama I, Ichijo M. Detection of IL-6 in human milk and its involvement in IgA production. *J Reprod Immunol*. 1991;20:267–276

13. Rudloff HE, Schmalstieg FC, Palkowetz KH, Paszkiewicz EJ, Goldman AS. Interleukin-6 in human milk. *J Reprod Immunol*. 1993;23:13–20

14. Okada M, Ohmura E, Kamiya Y, et al. Transforming growth factor (TGF)-alpha in human milk. *Life Sci*. 1991;48:1151–1156

15. Garofalo R, Chheda S, Mei F, et al. Interleukin-10 in human milk. *Pediatr Res*. 1995;37:444–449

16. Gilmore WS, McKelvey-Martin VJ, Rutherford S, et al. Human milk contains granulocyte colony stimulating factor. *Eur J Clin Nutr*. 1994;48:222–224

17. Hara T, Irie K, Saito S, et al. Identification of macrophage colony-stimulating factor in human milk and mammary gland epithelial cells. *Pediatr Res*. 1995;37:437–443

18. Palkowetz KH, Royer CL, Garofalo R, Rudloff HE, Schmalstieg FC Jr, Goldman AS. Production of interleukin-6 and interleukin-8 by human mammary gland epithelial cells. *J Reprod Immunol*. 1994;26:57–64

19. Garofalo RP, Goldman AS. Cytokines, chemokines, and colony-stimulating factors in human milk: the 1997 update. *Biol Neonate*. 1998;74:134–142

20. Goldblum RM, Schanler RJ, Garza C, Goldman AS. Human milk feeding enhances the urinary excretion of immunologic factors in low birth weight infants. *Pediatr Res*. 1989;25:184–188

21. Goldman AS, Garza C, Schanler RJ, Goldblum RM. Molecular forms of lactoferrin in stool and urine from infants fed human milk. *Pediatr Res*. 1990;27:252–255

22. Hutchens TW, Henry JF, Yip TT, et al. Origin of intact lactoferrin and its DNA-binding fragments found in the urine of human milk-fed preterm infants. Evaluation by stable isotopic enrichment. *Pediatr Res*. 1991;29:243–250

23. Stephens S, Dolby JM, Montreuil J, Spik G. Differences in inhibition of the growth of commensal and enteropathogenic strains of *Escherichia coli* by lactotransferrin and secretory immunoglobulin A isolated from human milk. *Immunology*. 1980;41:597–603

24. Griffths E, Humphreys J. Bacteriostatic effect of human milk and bovine colostrum on Escherichia coli: importance of bicarbonate. *Infect Immun.* 1977;15:396–401

25. Goldman AS, Thorpe LW, Goldblum RM, Hanson LA. Anti-inflammatory properties of human milk. *Acta Paediatr Scand.* 1986;75:689–695

26. Newburg DS. Oligosaccharides and glycoconjugates in human milk: their role in host defense. *J Mammary Gland Biol Neoplasia.* 1996;1:271–283

27. Isaacs CE, Thormar H. The role of milk-derived antimicrobial lipids as antiviral and antibacterial agents. *Adv Exp Med Biol.* 1991;310:159–165

28. Schroten H, Hanisch FG, Plogmann R, et al. Inhibition of adhesion of S-fimbriated Escherichia coli to buccal epithelial cells by human milk fat globule membrane components: a novel aspect of the protective function of mucins in the nonimmunoglobulin fraction. *Infect Immun.* 1992;60:2893–2899

29. Orrhage K, Nord CE. Factors controlling the bacterial colonization of the intestine in breastfed infants. *Acta Paediatr Suppl.* 1999;430:47–57

30. Wold AE, Adlerberth I. Breast feeding and the intestinal microflora of the infant – implications for protection against infectious diseases. *Adv Exp Med Biol.* 2000;478:77–93

31. Kramer MS, Chalmers B, Hodnett ED, et al. Promotion of Breastfeeding Intervention Trial (PROBIT): a randomized trial in the Republic of Belarus. *JAMA.* 2001;285:413–420

32. Wright S, Bolton C. Breast milk fatty acids in mothers of children with atopic eczema. *Br J Nutr.* 1989;62:693–697

33. Goldman AS. Association of atopic diseases with breast-feeding: food allergens, fatty acids, and evolution. *J Pediatr.* 1999;134:5–7

34. Conti A, Giuffrida MG, Napolitano L, et al. Identification of the human beta-casein C-terminal fragments that specifically bind to purified antibodies to bovine beta-lactoglobulin. *J Nutr Biochem.* 2000;11:332–337

35. Herrmann ME, Dannemann A, Gruters A, et al. Prospective study of the atopy preventive effect of maternal avoidance of milk and eggs during pregnancy and lactation. *Eur J Pediatr.* 1996;155:770–774

36. Davis MK, Savitz DA, Graubard BI. Infant feeding and childhood cancer. *Lancet.* 1988;2:365–368

37. Koletzko S, Sherman P, Corey M, Griffiths A, Smith C. Role of infant feeding practices in development of Crohn's disease in childhood. *BMJ.* 1989;298:1617–1618

38. Mayer EJ, Hamman RF, Gay EC, Lezotte DC, Savitz DA, Klingensmith GJ. Reduced risk of IDDM among breast fed children. The Colorado IDDM Registry. *Diabetes.* 1988;37:1625–1632

39. Shu XO, Linet MS, Steinbuch M, et al. Breast-feeding and risk of childhood acute leukemia. *J Natl Cancer Inst.* 1999;91:1765–1772

40. Goldman AS. Back to basics: host responses to infection. *Pediatr Rev.* 2000;21:342–349

41. Schlesinger L, Uauy R. Nutrition and neonatal immune function. *Semin Perinatol.* 1991;15:469–477

42. Tamura Y, Welch DC, Zic JA, Cooper WO, Stein SM, Hummell DS. Scurvy presenting as painful gait with bruising in a young boy. *Arch Pediatr Adolesc Med.* 2000; 154:732–735

43. Roche Vitamins. *Vitamin Consumption in the US.* Parsippany, NJ: Roche Vitamins Inc; 2000

44. Centers for Disease Control and Prevention. Recommendations to prevent and control iron deficiency in the United States. *MMWR Recomm Rep.* 1998;47(RR-3):1–29

45. Frith-Terhune AL, Cogswell ME, Khan LK, Will JC, Ramakrishnan U. Iron deficiency anemia: higher prevalence in Mexican American than in non-Hispanic white females in the third National Health and Nutrition Examination Survey, 1988–1994. *Am J Clin Nutr.* 2000;72:963–968

46. Thibault H, Galan P, Selz F, et al. The immune response in iron-deficient young children: effect of iron supplementation on cell-mediated immunity. *Eur J Pediatr.* 1993;152:120–124

47. Krantman HJ, Young SR, Ank BJ, O'Donnell CM, Rachelefsky GS, Stiehm ER. Immune function in pure iron deficiency. *Am J Dis Child.* 1982;136:840–844

48. Berger J, Dyck JL, Galan P, et al. Effect of daily iron supplementation on iron status, cell-mediated immunity, and incidence of infections in 6–36 month old Togolese children. *Eur J Clin Nutr.* 2000;54:29–35

49. Kent S, Weinberg ED, Stuart-Macadam P. The etiology of the anemia of chronic disease and infection. *J Clin Epidemiol.* 1994;47:23–33

50. Couzy F, Keen C, Gershwin ME, Mareschi JP. Nutritional implications of the interactions between minerals. *Prog Food Nutr Sci.* 1993;17:65–87

51. Shankar AH, Prasad AS. Zinc and immune function: the biological basis of altered resistance to infection. *Am J Clin Nutr.* 1998;68(suppl 2):447S–463S

52. Sazawal S, Black RE, Bhan MK, Bhandari N, Sinha A, Jalla S. Zinc supplementation in young children with acute diarrhea in India. *N Engl J Med.* 1995;333:839–844

53. Rosado JL, Lopez P, Munoz E, Martinez H, Allen LH. Zinc supplementation reduced morbidity, but neither zinc nor iron supplementation affected growth or body composition of Mexican preschoolers. *Am J Clin Nutr.* 1997;65:13–19

54. Sazawal S, Black RE, Jalla S, Mazumdar S, Sinha A, Bhan MK. Zinc supplementation reduces the incidence of acute lower respiratory infections in infants and preschool children: a double-blind, controlled trial. *Pediatrics.* 1998;102:1–5

55. Girodon F, Galan P, Monget AL, et al. Impact of trace elements and vitamin supplementation on immunity and infections in institutionalized elderly patients: a randomized controlled trial. MIN. VIT. AOX. geriatric network. *Arch Intern Med.* 1999;159:748–754

56. Mossad SB, Macknin ML, Medendorp SV, Mason P. Zinc gluconate lozenges for treating the common cold. A randomized, double-blind, placebo-controlled study. *Ann Intern Med.* 1996;125:81–88

57. Institute of Medicine. *Dietary Reference Intakes for Vitamin A, Vitamin K, Arsenic, Boron, Chromium, Copper, Iodine, Iron, Manganese, Molybdenum, Nickel, Silicon, Vanadium, and Zinc.* Washington, DC: National Academy Press; 2001

58. West KP Jr, Pokhrel RP, Katz J, et al. Efficacy of vitamin A in reducing preschool child mortality in Nepal. *Lancet.* 1991;338:67–71

59. Rahmathullah L, Underwood BA, Thulasiraj RD, et al. Reduced mortality among children in southern India receiving a small weekly dose of vitamin A. *N Engl J Med.* 1990;323:929–935

60. Glasziou PP, Mackerras DE. Vitamin A supplementation in infectious diseases: a meta-analysis. *BMJ.* 1993;306:366–370

61. Hussey GD, Klein M. A randomized, controlled trial of vitamin A in children with severe measles. *N Engl J Med.* 1990;323:160–164

62. Shankar AH, Genton B, Semba RD, et al. Effect of vitamin A supplementation on morbidity due to *Plasmodium falciparum* in young children in Papua New Guinea: a randomised trial. *Lancet.* 1999;354:203–209

63. Meydani SN, Meydani M, Blumberg JB, et al. Vitamin E supplementation and in vivo immune response in healthy elderly subjects. A randomized controlled trial. *JAMA.* 1997;277:1380–1386

64. Kutukculer N, Akil T, Egemen A, et al. Adequate immune response to tetanus toxoid and failure of vitamin A and E supplementation to enhance antibody response in healthy children. *Vaccine.* 2000;18:2979–2984

65. Mino M. Clinical uses and abuses of vitamin E in children. *Proc Soc Exp Biol Med.* 1992;200:266–270

66. US Department of Agriculture-Agricultural Research Service. *Food and Nutrient Intakes by Children 1994–96, 1998.* Table Set 17. Available at: http://www.barc.usda.gov/bhnrc/foodsurvey/Products9496.html. Accessed April, 8, 2003

67. Pauling L. The significance of the evidence about ascorbic acid and the common cold. *Proc Natl Acad Sci U S A.* 1971;68:2678–2681

68. Douglas RM, Chalker EB, Treacy B. Vitamin C for preventing and treating the common cold. *Cochrane Database Syst Rev.* Oxford: Update Software; 2000

69. Muggli R. Vitamin C and phagocytes. In: Cunningham-Rundles S, ed. *Nutrient Modulation of the Immune Response.* New York, NY: Marcel-Dekker; 1993:75–90

70. Johnston CS. The antihistamine action of ascorbic acid. *Subcell Biochem.* 1996; 25:189–213

71. Frydas S, Reale M, Vacalis D, et al. IgG, IgG1 and IgM response in *Trichinella spiralis*-infected mice treated with 4-deoxypirydoxine or fed a Vitamin B6-deficient diet. *Mol Cell Biochem.* 1999;194:47–52

72. Rall LC, Meydani SN. Vitamin B6 and immune competence. *Nutr Rev.* 1993; 51:217–225

73. Tamura J, Kubota K, Murakami H, et al. Immunomodulation by vitamin B12: augmentation of CD8+ T lymphocytes and natural killer (NK) cell activity in vitamin

B12-deficient patients by methyl-B12 treatment. *Clin Exp Immunol.* 1999;116: 28–32

74. Fata FT, Herzlich BC, Schiffman G, Ast AL. Impaired antibody responses to pneumococcal polysaccharide in elderly patients with low serum vitamin B12 levels. *Ann Intern Med.* 1996;124:299–304

75. Hodges RE, Bean WB, Ohlson MA, Bleiler RE. Factors affecting human antibody response. IV. pyridoxine deficiency. *Am J Clin Nutr.* 1962;11:180–186

76. Hodges RE, Bean WB, Ohlson MA, Bleiler RE. Factors affecting human antibody response. V. combined deficiencies of pantothenic acid and pyridoxine. *Am J Clin Nutr.* 1962;11:187–199

77. Dhur A, Galan P, Hercberg S. Folate status and the immune system. *Prog Food Nutr Sci.* 1991;15:43–60

78. Baez-Saldana A, Diaz G, Espinoza B, Ortega E. Biotin deficiency induces changes in subpopulations of spleen lymphocytes in mice. *Am J Clin Nutr.* 1998;67: 431–437

79. Rabin BS. Inhibition of experimentally induced autoimmunity in rats by biotin deficiency. *J Nutrition.* 1983;113:2316–2322

80. Institute of Medicine. *Dietary Reference Intakes for Thiamin, Riboflavin, Niacin, Vitamin B6, Folate, Vitamin B12, Pantothenic Acid, Biotin, and Choline.* Washington, DC: National Academy Press; 1998

81. Specker BL, Black A, Allen L, Morrow F. Vitamin B12: low milk concentrations are related to low serum concentrations in vegetarian women and to methylmalonic aciduria in their infants. *Am J Clin Nutr.* 1990;52:1073–1076

82. Araki S, Suzuki M, Fujimoto M, Kimura M. Enhancement of resistance to bacterial infection in mice by vitamin B2. *J Vet Med Sci.* 1995;57:599–602

83. Gebhard KJ, Gridley DS, Stickney DR, Shulz TD. Enhancement of immune status by high levels of dietary vitamin B6 without growth inhibition of human malignant melanoma in athymic nude mice. *Nutr Cancer.* 1990; 14:15–26

84. Talbott MC, Miller LT, Kerkvliet NI. Pyridoxine supplementation: effect on lymphocyte responses in elderly persons. *Am J Clin Nutr.* 1987;46:659–664

85. Debes SA, Kirksey A. Influence of dietary pyridoxine on selected immune capacities of rat dams and pups. *J Nutr.* 1979;109:744–759

86. Motil KJ. Infant feeding: a critical look at infant formulas. *Curr Opin Pediatr.* 2000;12:469–476

87. Grimble GK, Westwood OM. Nucleotides as immunomodulators in clinical nutrition. *Curr Opin Clin Nutr Metab Care.* 2001;4:57–64

88. Jyonouchi H, Sun S, Abiru T, Winship T, Kuchan MJ. Dietary nucleotides modulate antigen-specific type 1 and type 2 T-cell responses in young C57Bl/6 mice. *Nutrition.* 2000;16:442–446

89. Nagafuchi S, Hachimura S, Totsuka M, et al. Dietary nucleotides can up-regulate antigen-specific Th1 immune responses and suppress antigen-specific IgE responses in mice. *Int Arch Allergy Immunol.* 2000;122:33–41

90. Carver JD, Pimentel B, Cox WI, Barness LA. Dietary nucleotide effects upon immune function in infants. *Pediatrics.* 1991;88:359–363

91. Martinez-Augustin O, Boza JJ, Del Pino JI, Lucena J, Martinez-Valverde A, Gil A. Dietary nucleotides might influence the humoral immune response against cow's milk proteins in preterm neonates. *Biol Neonate.* 1997;71:215–223

92. Navarro J, Maldonado J, Narbona E, et al. Influence of dietary nucleotides on plasma immunoglobulin levels and lymphocyte subsets of preterm infants. *Biofactors.* 1999;10:67–76

93. Pickering LK, Granoff DM, Erickson JR, et al. Modulation of the immune system by human milk and infant formula containing nucleotides. *Pediatrics.* 1998; 101:242–249

94. Brunser O, Espinoza J, Araya M, Cruchet S, Gil A. Effect of dietary nucleotide supplementation on diarrhoeal disease in infants. *Acta Paediatr.* 1994;83:188–191

95. Jensen RG, Bitman J, Carlson SE, Couch SC, Hamosh M, Newburg DS. Milk lipids: human milk lipids. In: Jensen RG, ed. *Handbook of Milk Composition.* San Diego, CA: Academic Press; 1995:495–576

96. Rulis AM, Lewis CJ. FDA agency response letter to Martek Biosciences Corp. regarding GRAS notice GRN 000041. FDA Office of Premarket Approval. Available at: http://www.cfsan.fda.gov/~rdb/opa-g041.html. Accessed April 8, 2003

97. SanGiovanni JP, Berkey CS, Dwyer JT, Colditz GA. Dietary essential fatty acids, long-chain polyunsaturated fatty acids, and visual resolution acuity in healthy full-term infants: a systematic review. *Early Hum Dev.* 2000;57:165–188

98. Gibson RA, Makrides M. The role of long chain polyunsaturated fatty acids (LCP-UFA) in neonatal nutrition. *Acta Paediatr.* 1998;87:1017–1022

99. Griffiths RJ. Prostaglandins and inflammation. In: Gallin JI, Snyderman R, eds. *Inflammation: Basic Principles and Clinical Correlates.* 3rd ed. Philadelphia, PA: Lippincott Williams and Wilkins; 1999:349–360

100. Penrose JF, Austen F, Lam BK. Leukotrienes: biosynthetic pathways, release, and receptor-mediated actions with relevance to disease states. In: Gallin JI, Snyderman R, eds. *Inflammation: Basic Principles and Clinical Correlates.* 3rd ed. Philadelphia, PA: Lippincott Williams and Wilkins; 1999:361–372

101. Calder PC. N-3 polyunsaturated fatty acids, inflammation and immunity: pouring oil on troubled waters or another fishy tale? *Nutr Res.* 2001;21:309–341

102. McMurray DN, Jolly CA, Chapkin RS. Effects of dietary n-3 fatty acids on T cell activation and T cell receptor-mediated signaling in a murine model. *J Infect Dis.* 2000;182(suppl):S103–S107

103. Duchen K, Casas R, Fageras-Bottcher M, Yu G, Björkstén B. Human milk polyunsaturated long-chain fatty acids and secretory immunoglobulin A antibodies and early childhood allergy. *Pediatr Allergy Immunol.* 2000;11:29–39

104. Businco L, Ioppi M, Morse NL, Nisini R, Wright S. Breast milk from mothers of children with newly developed atopic eczema has low levels of long chain polyunsaturated fatty acids. *J Allergy Clin Immunol.* 1993;91:1134–1139

105. Field CJ, Thomson CA, Van Aerde JE, et al. Lower proportion of CD45RO+ cells and deficient interleukin-10 production by formula-fed infants, compared with human-fed, is corrected with supplementation of long-chain polyunsaturated fatty acids. *J Pediatr Gastroenterol Nutr.* 2000;31:291–299

106. Kunz C, Rudloff S, Baier W, Klein N, Strobel S. Oligosaccharides in human milk: structural, functional, and metabolic aspects. *Annu Rev Nutr.* 2000;20:699–722

107. Boudraa G, Touhami M, Pochart P, Soltana R, Mary JY, Desjeux JF. Effect of feeding yogurt versus milk in children with persistent diarrhea. *J Pediatr Gastroenterol Nutr.* 1990;11:509–512

108. Touhami M, Boudraa G, Mary JY, Soltana R, Desjeux JF. Clinical consequences of replacing milk with yogurt in persistent infantile diarrhea [French]. *Ann Pediatr (Paris).* 1992;39:79–86

109. Oberhelman RA, Gilman RH, Sheen P, et al. A placebo-controlled trial of Lactobacillus GG to prevent diarrhea in undernourished Peruvian children. *J Pediatr.* 1999;134:15–20

110. Pant AR, Graham SM, Allen SJ, et al. Lactobacillus GG and acute diarrhoea in young children in the tropics. *J Trop Pediatr.* 1996;42:162–165

111. Raza S, Graham SM, Allen SJ, Sultana S, Cuevas L, Hart CA. Lactobacillus GG promotes recovery from acute nonbloody diarrhea in Pakistan. *Pediatr Infect Dis J.* 1995;14:107–111

112. Majamaa H, Isolauri E, Saxelin M, Vesikari T. Lactic acid bacteria in the treatment of acute rotavirus gastroenteritis. *J Pediatr Gastroenterol Nutr.* 1995;20:333–338

113. Saavedra JM, Bauman NA, Oung I, Perman JA, Yolken RH. Feeding of Bifidobacterium bifidum and Streptococcus thermophilus to infants in hospital for prevention of diarrhoea and shedding of rotavirus. *Lancet.* 1994;344:1046–1049

114. Contardi I. Oral bacterial therapy in prevention of antibiotic-induced diarrhea in childhood [Italian]. *Clin Ter.* 1991;136:409–413

115. Millar MR, Bacon C, Smith SL, Walker V, Hall MA. Enteral feeding of premature infants with Lactobacillus GG. *Arch Dis Child.* 1993;69:483–487

116. Isolauri E, Arvola T, Sutas Y, Moilanen E, Salminen S. Probiotics in the management of atopic eczema. *Clin Exp Allergy.* 2000;30:1604–1610

117. Kalliomaki M, Salminen S, Arvilommi H, Kero P, Koskinen P, Isolauri E. Probiotics in primary prevention of atopic disease: a randomized placebo-controlled trial. *Lancet.* 2001;357:1076–1079

118. Naidu AS, Bidlack WR, Clemens RA. Probiotic spectra of lactic acid bacteria (LAB). *Crit Rev Food Sci Nutr.* 1999;39:13–126

119. Sarubin A. *The Health Professional's Guide to Popular Dietary Supplements.* Chicago, IL: American Dietetic Association; 2000

120. Medical Economics Co. *PDR for Herbal Medicines.* 2nd ed. Montvale, NJ: Medical Economics Co; 2000

36

Nutritional Support for Children Who Are Neurologically Impaired

Introduction

Feeding difficulties and poor growth are well-recognized problems among the neurologically impaired population. Mothers often report feeding difficulties such as poor suck, vomiting, and choking as the first indications that something is wrong with the child.[1] In fact, in 60% of patients, severe feeding problems preceded the diagnosis of cerebral palsy.[2] As a consequence, children with developmental disabilities are at very high risk for malnutrition and are often in a poor nutritional state, exhibiting marked linear growth failure, poor weight gain, decreased lean body mass, and fat stores.[3–5] The true prevalence of malnutrition in this population is not known but a significant proportion are shorter and lighter than the reference standard and this worsens as the child grows older.[6] A small proportion is overweight. Nutrient requirements and expected growth pattern of children with severe disabilities are difficult to determine. Krick et al have developed a growth reference standard for patients with quadriplegic cerebral palsy,[6] but this reference may be seen as a reflection of the current situation and not a standard.

Despite the well-documented poor linear growth in this population, the exact cause remains unclear. The role of neurologic disease, genetic and endocrine factors, immobility, and lack of weight bearing might be added to nutritional factors. In patients with cerebral palsy, height and weight Z-scores (standard deviation scores) are highly correlated, indicating that nutritional factors indeed play a role in linear growth failure. However, height Z-score declines with advancing age independently of weight Z-score and was significantly lower in children with seizures, those who were non-ambulatory, and those with spastic quadriplegia, suggesting that non-nutritional factors also contribute to linear growth failure.[7] Linear growth of children with diplegia or hemiplegia is less affected than those with spastic quadriplegia, but 30% exhibit signs of malnutrition with decreased weight and triceps skinfold thickness and 23% are stunted.[4]

Monitoring of nutritional status and provision of adequate nutrition are essential in the care of the neurologically impaired patient. Promotion of growth and well-being must be an integral part of medical management. Because of the numerous factors that need to be considered, nutritional intervention is best accomplished by a multidisciplinary team involving dieticians, speech and occupational therapists, physicians, and nurses.

Causes of Malnutrition

Nutritional factors such as inadequate intake, excess losses, and altered energy requirements clearly contribute to the poor nutritional status of patients with neurological disability.

Inadequate Intake

Inadequate intake seems to be a major factor contributing to malnutrition since aggressive nutritional supplementation improves growth.[8–11] An increase in weight for length Z-score from −2.71 to −1.18 was seen 23 months after gastrostomy.[11] Some noted an increase of 10% to 46% in body weight over 5 weeks with a 50% increase of intake by means of nasogastric tube.[8]

Children with cerebral palsy spontaneously consume less calories than age-matched control children.[1] Reasons for inadequate intake are numerous. Oral-motor dysfunction is found in more than 90% of children with cerebral palsy.[2] Sucking and swallowing problems, inadequate lip closure, drooling, and persistent extrusion reflex make oral feedings difficult. It is a major factor in the pathogenesis of malnutrition in patients with cerebral palsy since weight, height, and weight-for-height Z-scores are significantly lower in patients with oral-motor dysfunction than in patients without.[12] Because of their poor oral and fine motor skills, these children depend on a caretaker for feedings. Since they are often unable to communicate hunger and satiety, the caretaker regulates their intake. Oftentimes, the task of feeding such a child is difficult and time consuming, and inadequate intake may ensue. It has been shown that the caretaker often overestimates caloric intake[13] and time spent feeding the child.[2] Gastroesophageal reflux (GER) may also lead to food refusal especially if reflux esophagitis is present.

Increased Losses

In addition to decreased intake, excessive losses may occur from spillage and frequent emesis.

Energy Requirements

Defining energy needs is very important because of the patient's inability to communicate hunger and satiety and because of abnormal physical activity, body composition, and food intake. Unfortunately, energy needs are poorly defined in this heterogeneous population. Energy intake in normally growing patients with spastic quadriplegic cerebral palsy (SQCP) fed exclusively by gastrostomy was estimated at 60 ± 15% of recommended daily allowance (RDA) for gender and age, and 103 ± 32 % of RDA for weight.[14] Resting energy expenditure (REE) by indirect calorimetry in well-nourished, non-ambulatory, bedridden patients was significantly less than healthy age-matched controls or from those calculated from World Health Organization (WHO) equations based on weight, age, and gender.[15] In addition, REE per unit of body cell mass was significantly reduced, suggesting a role of central nervous system in energy regulation. Therefore calculation of total energy needs based on WHO standards for healthy children (1.5 to 1.6 × calculated REE) would overestimate energy requirements in children with SQCP (1.1 × measured REE).[15]

Muscle tone (hypotonicity, spasticity and athetosis) and activity level (bedridden, moderately active, ambulatory) will influence energy needs. Additional calories must be given to achieve normal growth and catch-up growth. Also, energy needs may be increased in periods of infection such as aspiration pneumonia.

Assessment

Medical History
Assessment of health status must include knowledge of the underlying disease to better understand its natural history (ie, static vs degenerative vs temporary neurological impairment). The type of intervention will differ whether it is a terminal disease, a short-term reversible condition, or a chronic condition. In addition, the duration and the severity of the neurological disability correlate with greater risk of malnutrition. Other medical problems such as chronic respiratory symptoms, recurrent pneumonia, symptoms of GER, constipation, and the use of medication must be sought.

Nutritional History
Nutritional history is of the utmost importance and must encompass all aspects of the feeding process. A good evaluation of oral motor skills must be done since oromotor impairment is a major factor leading to malnutrition.[16] Swallowing function, including adequacy of lip closure, drooling, spilling, extrusion reflex, incoordination, gagging, delayed swallowing, and symptoms suggestive of aspiration, such as choking and coughing, should be evaluated. The amount of time spent feeding the child should be estimated. Feeding efficiency in patients with severe cerebral palsy is far below normal, as it may take

them 12 to 15 times longer to chew and swallow than normal controls of the same weight. Even longer mealtime does not compensate for the child's feeding impairment and, as a consequence, caloric intake is often insufficient.[17] Appetite and ability to self feed, as well as feeding schedule, must be taken into account. Sixty percent of patients with cerebral palsy are totally dependent on a caretaker for their intake.[2] For the caretaker, often the parent, too much time spent around meals may impair the parent-child relationship and take time away from other activities. It is also important to assess parental perception of mealtime, as it is often perceived as a stressful and not enjoyable experience.

A review of a typical day's food intake or a full 3-day food record will help assess caloric intake but also adequacy of fiber, vitamin, and mineral intake. Food refusal or a recent change in feeding pattern may be indicative of an underlying problem.

A careful review of previous growth pattern is very important and growth charts for height and weight as well as weight gain or weight loss must be recorded. Infants with cerebral palsy who had low birth weight are at greater nutritional risk.

Social/Familial History

Social situations, including school schedule, family situation, siblings, parents' working schedule, and availability of the caretaker must be taken into account. If the child's condition involves a considerable amount of care, integration of that care and its impact on work, social life, family life, and the patient's siblings are important to evaluate. Interventions should be as efficient as possible and disrupt the family's routine as little as possible.

The height of the biological parents should be recorded to estimate the patient's genetic potential for linear growth.

Physical Examination

Physical examination includes weight, height or length, and head circumference (see next section) and signs of malnutrition or specific nutrient deficiency. In addition, muscle tone, activity level, and skeletal deformities such as scoliosis and contractures should be assessed.

Anthropometrics

Weight and length or height must be obtained at every visit and should be as accurate as possible, always using the same technique and equipment. Weight should be measured on the same scale every time with the child wearing little or no clothing. Length should be obtained supine in children under age 2 years or in older children unable to stand. Linear growth assessment is important to detect chronic malnutrition but may be difficult to obtain in children with severe contractures or scoliosis. For these patients, length measurements are inappropriate and alternative techniques such as upper arm length (UAL) or lower leg length (LLL) using an anthropometer may be used as a proxy for body length.[18] Both measurements are significantly lower than normal in quadriplegic cerebral palsy but should be normal in hemiplegic or diplegic patients.[18] Upper arm length is usually less compromised than LLL in patients with cerebral palsy.[5] The right side is measured unless the patient is hemiplegic, in which case the less-affected side is used. In children aged less than 2 years, the UAL is obtained by measuring the distance between the top of the shoulder and the bottom of the elbow with joints at a right angle, and the LLL is obtained by measuring the distance between the top of the knee to the sole of the heel, again with both joints at a right angle. In children over age 2 years, the UAL is obtained using an anthropometer to measure the distance between the acromion and the head of the radius, and the LLL is obtained by measuring the distance between the superomedial border of the tibia and the inferior border of the medial malleolus with the child sitting, one leg crossed horizontally across the other. The LLL can be measured with a tape, but the UAL requires an anthropometer. Lower leg length is affected by race (longer in black patients) while UAL is less affected by race.[18] Head circumference must also be obtained under the age of 3 but may be of limited use in children with brain damage.

Mid-arm circumference combined with triceps skinfold thickness are useful to estimate upper arm muscle and fat area. They should preferably be obtained by the same observer every time to guarantee a reproducible and reliable measurement. Subscapular skinfold measurement is also useful in SQCP. Fat stores are usually reduced in all areas, but triceps skinfold thickness is more affected than subscapular skinfold (60% vs 85% of healthy controls).[3] This pattern of retention of truncal fat is seen in malnourished patients. Normal values for mid-arm circumference and triceps skinfold thickness are available in Appendix L.

Laboratory Evaluation

Basic laboratory evaluation includes a complete blood count and iron studies, as iron-deficiency anemia occurs frequently. Serum albumin and prealbumin will reflect nutritional adequacy in the previous month and week respectively. Serum electrolyte and blood urea nitrogen may help assessing hydration status.

In addition, for patients taking anticonvulsants, vitamin D levels, serum calcium, and phosphorus, as well as alkaline phosphatase, are often warranted since anticonvulsants interfere with vitamin D metabolism by increasing its conversion to inactive metabolites. The literature on osteopenia in patients with cerebral palsy is conflicting. Some have found that approximately 25% of neurologically impaired children who receive anticonvulsants develop osteomalacia with hypocalcemia, hypophosphatemia, and elevated alkaline phosphatase levels regardless of ambulatory status.[19] Others report that ambulatory status is more important than anticonvulsant use in determining serum calcium levels.[20] There is, however, general agreement that calcium and vitamin D intake are insufficient in patients with cerebral palsy[14,20] and deficiency leading to osteopenia can be the cause of very debilitating pathological fractures. Parathyroid hormone and bone densitometry may be done if necessary.

Specific Investigation

In addition, specific investigation is often warranted, according to the medical history and physical findings. Videofluoroscopy evaluates swallowing function using liquids and different food textures and will help determine the efficiency of the entire swallowing process as well as the risk of aspiration. An upper gastrointestinal series is useful to see if complications of gastroesophageal reflux, such as peptic stenosis or hiatal hernia, are present. Superior mesenteric artery syndrome may be found in patients with severe undernutrition. In addition, the anatomy and position of the stomach (which is often abnormally located in the thorax in patients with severe scoliosis) can be determined. This will be useful if a percutaneous gastrostomy is considered.

Esophageal pH monitoring is the gold standard in evaluating reflux and may be warranted in patients with food refusal or significant emesis, especially if a gastrostomy is considered. Gastric emptying scans can help determine the presence of delayed gastric emptying, GER, and possible aspiration from reflux.

Nutritional Intervention

Improvement of nutritional status is likely to improve well-being, behavior, and peripheral circulation. It can lead to better resistance to infections and promote healing of decubitus ulcers.[8] A decrease in spasticity may also be seen.[8] Improvement of lower esophageal sphincter tone has been shown to be associated with nutritional repletion.[21]

Early intervention in patients with neurological disability is important since the best response to nutritional repletion is seen in children with the shortest duration between the neurological insult and institution of nutritional therapy. When nutritional therapy (nasogastric or gastrostomy) was initiated within a year of the insult, length and weight for length improved, and weight increased by 3.3 g/kg/d. Between 1 and 8 years, nutritional therapy improved both linear growth and weight for length, but led to a lesser weight gain (2.8 g/kg/d). When nutritional intervention was delayed after 8 years of the neurological insult, weight gain was only 1.5 g/kg/d and linear growth did not improve.[10] After careful evaluation of nutritional status, feeding abilities, and medical status, the decision whether to intervene may be taken. A multidisciplinary approach is preferred. It involves issues as simple as providing an appropriate chair and finding adequate positioning at mealtime. Improvement of oral motor skills can be accomplished with speech and occupational therapy. Medical treatment of GER with prokinetics and/or H-2 blockers and treatment of constipation often make a remarkable difference.

Nutrient Requirements

Recommended dietary allowance for age often overestimates the caloric needs of children with developmental disabilities. Caloric needs should be individualized, taking into account Basal Metabolic Rate (BMR), muscle tone, activity level, and desired growth. A formula to calculate energy needs in children with severe cerebral palsy has been developed by Krick et al.[22] It uses BMR and accounts for muscle tone, activity level, and growth factors (normal growth-for-height age and catch-up growth):

Culley et al also estimated caloric needs of 14.7 cal/cm in children without motor dysfunction, 13.9 cal/cm in ambulatory patients with motor dysfunction, and 11.1 cal/cm in non-ambulatory patients with motor dysfunction.[23] The

---

Calories (kcal/d) = (BMR × muscle tone factor × activity factor) + growth factor.
Where:
BMR (kcal/d) = Body surface area (m^2) × standard metabolic rate (kcal/m^2/h) × 24 h

muscle tone factor	0.9 decreased muscle tone
	1.0 normal muscle tone
	1.1 increased muscle tone
activity factor	1.15 bedridden
	1.2 dependant (wheel chair)
	1.25 crawling
	1.3 ambulatory
growth factor	5 kcal/g of desired weight gain

best way to evaluate adequacy of nutritional therapy is to monitor the response in terms of weight gain. Caloric intake should be readjusted accordingly.[24]

Goal of Nutritional Intervention

Ideal body weight for children whose activity level is normal should be on the 50th percentile on the weight-for-height or BMI chart. If the patient is wheelchair bound but able to do independent transfer, weight for height should be around the 25th percentile, and, for patients who are bedridden, the 10th percentile is sufficient for adequate nutrition but low enough to facilitate the care and mobilization of the child. Overfeeding carries the risks of overfatness, which can also compromise respiratory function and care. An exception should be made for patients under 3 years (chronological or height age), where weight for height should be between the 25th and the 50th percentile independent of activity level.[22]

Source of Nutrients

The choice of formula depends on the age of the patient, specific nutrient deficiency, medical problems, and caloric requirements. In children younger than 1 year, the liquid feeding of choice is breast milk or infant formula. Formula may be concentrated or modular nutrients may be added to increase caloric content and reduce the volume in patients with high caloric needs (Appendix E, Table E-4).

Nutrient modules such as carbohydrates, fat, and intact protein are combined to add nutrients or to change the composition of the diet. Carbohydrates may be added in the form of glucose polymers; they are bland in taste and add little osmolality. Lipid can be supplied as long-chain or medium-chain triglycerides (MCT); they are calorie dense and have little influence on osmolality.

Table 36.1.
Modular Nutrients (see also Appendix O)

Carbohydrate		
Polycose powder	glucose polymer	23 kcal/tbsp
Moducal	maltodextrin	30 kcal/tbsp
Duocal	dried glucose syrup and refined vegetable oils	
Fat		
Microlipid	safflower oil emulsion	4.5 kcal/mL
MCT oil	coconut oil	7.7 kcal/mL

Medium-chain triglyceride oil is absorbed without the need for chylomicron formation but does not contain essential fatty acids.

Precautions should be taken to avoid preparation errors. By concentrating the formula, the renal solute load (RSL) increases and the amount of free water decreases. Renal solute load should not exceed 250 mOsm/L and can be estimated as follows: RSL (mOsm) = [protein (g) − 4] + [Na (mEq) + K (mEq) + Cl (mEq)].

When nutrient modules are used to modify the caloric content, the final composition of the diet must be determined to ensure that the final diet provides 35% to 65% of the calories as carbohydrates, 7% to 16% as protein, and 30% to 55% as fat. If more than 55% of calories are fat, ketosis may develop, excess carbohydrate may overwhelm absorption capacity and cause diarrhea, and protein intakes exceeding 5 g/kg/d may cause azotemia.

After 1 year of age, a 1 cal/mL formula is preferred. A fiber-containing formula will help with constipation. Since caloric needs are lower than the normal population, the use of an adult solution with lower vitamin and mineral content may be inadequate. A pediatric solution with a higher vitamin and mineral content should be used to avoid deficiencies (especially vitamin D, phosphorus, and calcium).[14] The use of a 1.5 or 2 cal/mL formula may be required but, if used, hydration status and micronutrient intake must be carefully evaluated. Specific nutritional deficiencies (iron, vitamin D) must be corrected.

Route of Enteral Feedings

The best way to administer feeds should be decided after evaluation of caloric needs. Enteral nutrition is preferred when the gastrointestinal tract is intact.

If oral intake is safe (no risk of aspiration) but insufficient, attempts to maximize caloric intake orally can be made. Caloric density of food can be increased. Adequate positioning and improvement of oral feeding technique may help. Food consistency should be adjusted according to swallowing study results. Liquids and purees can be thickened with thickening agents.

Nasogastric feedings are usually a good option and should be attempted initially in patients with mild or no gastroesophageal reflux. They can be administered at home and are minimally invasive. A trial of nasogastric feeds is helpful to determine the patient's tolerance to gastric feeds before a more permanent solution is decided upon. Nasojejunal feeds are preferred in patients with reflux or those who do not tolerate nasogastric feeds.

If long-term enteral nutrition is required (>3 months), a more convenient, more permanent, and more esthetically acceptable route, such as gastrostomy, is preferred. The gastrostomy will either be placed surgically or percutaneously. Whether a prior evaluation for reflux is warranted and whether patients with preexisting reflux should undergo an antireflux procedure (ARP) with surgical gastrostomy tube placement is debated. The decision must be carefully evaluated since ARP failures, postoperative complications, and need for reintervention are more common in neurologically impaired than non-neurologically impaired patients. The failure rate of ARP in neurologically impaired children is between 19% and 28%, and the incidence of major complications is between 10% and 33%.[25–27] Also, Nissen procedures may induce myoelectrical disturbances and inappropriate activation of the emetic reflex, inducing very debilitating postoperative retching in neurologically impaired patients.[28]

For patients without reflux, the role of protective ARP is debated. In neurologically impaired patients without reflux undergoing a surgical gastrostomy, between 14% and 44% developed reflux and 14% to 33% subsequently required an ARP.[29,30] Sixty-six percent of patients with normal pH probe studies prior to surgical gastrostomy had a positive study after the procedure, making ARP in conjunction with the surgical gastrostomy warranted according to some.[31]

The development of new techniques such as percutaneous endoscopic gastrostomy (PEG) offers more alternatives for neurologically impaired patients. It is a simple technique that requires a short anesthesia, involves minimal discomfort, and can be used within hours of placement. The rate of major complications following PEG placement is 2% to 17.5% in the pediatric population.[32–34] In neurologically impaired patients without prior clinical reflux, there was a lower incidence of symptomatic gastroesophageal reflux requiring an ARP after PEG, compared to surgical gastrostomy (10% versus 39%), and fewer major complications (0% versus 9%).[35] In patients (mostly neurologically impaired) undergoing PEG placement, 5% of those with a normal pre PEG pH probe study eventually required ARP versus 29% if the study was abnormal.[32] In neurologically impaired patients without prior clinical symptoms, post-PEG gastroesophageal reflux occurred in 25% to 27%, and 16.6% to 17% of patients required ARP,[36,37] while 20% of those with preexisting clinical reflux subsequently required an ARP or a gastrojejunal tube.[37] In summary, a PEG would be a good option in patients with no or mild reflux. If reflux develops, optimal medical treatment should be attempted before considering ARP.

A percutaneous endoscopic or radiological gastrojejunostomy may also be an option in some patients if the risk of a prolonged anesthesia and a surgical procedure is unacceptable. Even if preexisting reflux is a problem, a percutaneous gastrojejunal tube is an option that has fewer complications in neurologically impaired patients than a Nissen procedure with a surgical gastrostomy (11.8% vs 33.3%).[38] In patients with severe scoliosis in whom the stomach may be abnormally positioned in the rib cage and not accessible percutaneously, an upper gastrointestinal study is useful before the procedure is performed. A severely malnourished child should always be repleted nutritionally before a surgical intervention is performed.

Method of Administration
Initially, continuous nasogastric or gastric infusion of formula is preferred, given the poor nutritional status and the high caloric requirements of the patient. Subsequently, a gradual charge to daytime bolus infusions may be attempted as they are often more convenient, especially in ambulatory patients. A combination of both can be used. When the child requires transpyloric feeds, a continuous infusion is necessary.

Outcome
Children with cerebral palsy demonstrate improvement of nutritional status with a weight gain of 33% or 1.5 to 3.3 g/kg/d with a caloric intake of 40 to 150 cal/kg/d.[8,10] They may also show a 20% increase in weight for age as well as weight for height, and a 4% increase in height for age. Eighty-five percent of the gain is body fat and 15% is lean body mass.[9] Early nutritional intervention is associated with a more favorable outcome.[9,10]

Conclusion
Children with neurological disabilities cannot be nutritionally evaluated against conventional standards because of growth retardation, abnormal energy requirements, and abnormal body composition, but they should not be expected to be malnourished. One of the most basic components of care is provision of adequate nutrition. Therefore, medical management of these patients must include careful monitoring of their nutritional status, and early, multidisciplinary nutritional intervention is essential to promote growth and well-being.

References
1. Reilly S, Skuse D. Characteristics and management of feeding problems of young children with cerebral palsy. *Dev Med Child Neurol.* 1992;34:379–388
2. Reilly S, Skuse D, Poblete X. Prevalence of feeding problems and oral motor dysfunction in children with cerebral palsy: a community survey. *J Pediatr.* 1996;129:877–882

3. Stallings VA, Charney EB, Davies JC, Cronk CE. Nutrition-related growth failure of children with quadriplegic cerebral palsy. *Dev Med Child Neurol.* 1993;35:126–138

4. Stallings VA, Charney EB, Davies JC, Cronk CE. Nutritional status and growth of children with diplegic or hemiplegic cerebral palsy. *Dev Med Child Neurol.* 1993;35:997–1006

5. Stallings VA, Cronk CE, Zemel BS, Charney EB. Body composition in children with spastic quadriplegic cerebral palsy. *J Pediatr.* 1995;126:833–839

6. Krick J, Murphy-Miller P, Zeger S, Wright E. Pattern of growth in children with cerebral palsy. *J Am Diet Assoc.* 1996;96:680–685

7. Stevenson RD, Hayes RP, Cater LV, Blackman JA. Clinical correlates of linear growth in children with cerebral palsy. *Dev Med Child Neurol.* 1994;36:135–142

8. Patrick J, Boland M, Stoski D, Murry GE. Rapid correction of wasting in children with cerebral palsy. *Dev Med Child Neurol.* 1986;28:734–739

9. Rempel GR, Colwell SO, Nelson RP. Growth in children with cerebral palsy fed via gastrostomy. *Pediatrics.* 1988;82:857–862

10. Sanders KD, Cox K, Cannon R, et al. Growth response to enteral feeding by children with cerebral palsy. *JPEN J Parenter Enteral Nutr.* 1990;14:23–26

11. Shapiro BK, Green P, Krick J, Allen D, Capate AJ. Growth of severely impaired children: neurological versus nutritional factors. *Dev Med Child Neurol.* 1986;28:729–733

12. Krick J, Van Duyn MA. The relationship between oral-motor involvement and growth: a pilot study in a pediatric population with cerebral palsy. *J Am Diet Assoc.* 1984;84:555–559

13. Stallings VA, Zemel BS, Davies JC, Cronk CE, Charney EB. Energy expenditure of children and adolescents with severe disabilities: a cerebral palsy model. *Am J Clin Nutr.* 1996;64:627–634

14. Fried MD, Pencharz PB. Energy and nutrient intakes of children with spastic quadriplegia. *J Pediatr.* 1991;119:947–949

15. Azcue MP, Zello GA, Levy LD, Pencharz PB. Energy expenditure and body composition in children with spastic quadriplegic cerebral palsy. *J Pediatr.* 1996;129:870–876

16. Thommessen M, Heiberg A, Kase BF, Larsen S, Riis G. Feeding problems, height and weight in different groups of disabled children. *Acta Paediatr Scand.* 1991;80:527–533

17. Gisel EG, Patrick J. Identification of children with cerebral palsy unable to maintain a normal nutritional state. *Lancet.* 1988;1:283–286

18. Spender QW, Cronk CE, Charney EB, Stallings VA. Assessment of linear growth of children with cerebral palsy: use of alternative measures to height or length. *Dev Med Child Neurol.* 1989;31:206–214

19. Tolman KG, Jubiz W, Sannella JJ, et al. Osteomalacia associated with anticonvulsant drug therapy in mentally retarded children. *Pediatrics.* 1975;56:45–50

20. Baer MT, Kozlowski BW, Blyler EM, Trahms CM, Taylor ML, Hogan MP. Vitamin D, calcium, and bone status in children with developmental delay in relation to anticonvulsant use and ambulatory status. *Am J Clin Nutr.* 1997;65:1042–1051

21. Lewis D, Khoshoo V, Pencharz PB, Golladay ES. Impact of nutritional rehabilitation on gastroesophageal reflux in neurologically impaired children. *J Pediatr Surg.* 1994;29:167–170

22. Krick J, Murphy PE, Markham JF, Shapiro BK. A proposed formula for calculating energy needs of children with cerebral palsy. *Dev Med Child Neurol.* 1992;34:481–487

23. Culley WJ, Middleton TO. Caloric requirements of mentally retarded children with and without motor dysfunction. *J Pediatr.* 1969;75:380–384

24. Motil KJ. Enteral nutrition in the neurologically impaired child. In: Baker SB, Baker RD, Davis A, eds. *Pediatric Enteral Nutrition.* New York, NY: Chapman & Hall; 1994:217–237

25. Pearl RH, Robie DK, Ein SH, et al. Complications of gastroesophageal antireflux surgery in neurologically impaired versus neurologically normal children. *J Pediatr Surg.* 1990;25:1169–1173

26. Smith CD, Othersen HB Jr, Gogan NJ, Walker JD. Nissen fundoplication in children with profound neurologic disability. High risks and unmet goals. *Ann Surg.* 1992;215:654–659

27. Spitz L, Roth K, Kiely EM, Brereton RJ, Drake DP, Milla PJ. Operation for gastro-oesophageal reflux associated with severe mental retardation. *Arch Dis Child.* 1993;68:347–351

28. Richards CA, Andrews PL, Spitz L, Milla PJ. Nissen fundoplication may induce gastric myoelectrical disturbance in children. *J Pediatr Surg.* 1998;33:1801–1805

29. Langer JC, Wesson DE, Ein SH, et al. Feeding gastrostomy in neurologically impaired children: is an antireflux procedure necessary? *J Pediatr Gastroenterol Nutr.* 1988;7:837–841

30. Wheatley MJ, Wesley JR, Tkach DM, Coran AG. Long-term follow-up of brain-damaged children requiring feeding gastrostomy: should an antireflux procedure always be performed? *J Pediatr Surg.* 1991;26:301–305

31. Jolley SG, Smith EI, Tunell WP. Protective antireflux operation with feeding gastrostomy. Experience with children. *Ann Surg.* 1985;201:736–740

32. Sulaeman E, Udall JN Jr, Brown RF, et al. Gastroesophageal reflux and Nissen fundoplication following percutaneous endoscopic gastrostomy in children. *J Pediatr Gastroenterol Nutr.* 1998;26:269–273

33. Khattak IU, Kimber C, Kiely EM, Spitz L. Percutaneous endoscopic gastrostomy in paediatric practice: complications and outcome. *J Pediatr Surg.* 1998;33:67–72

34. Behrens R, Lang T, Muschweck H, Richter T, Hofbeck M. Percutaneous endoscopic gastrostomy in children and adolescents. *J Pediatr Gastroenterol Nutr.* 1997;25:487–491

35. Cameron BH, Blair GK, Murphy JJ III, Fraser GC. Morbidity in neurologically impaired children after percutaneous endoscopic versus Stamm gastrostomy. *Gastrointest Endosc.* 1995;42:41–44

36. Heine RG, Reddihough DS, Catto-Smith AG. Gastro-oesophageal reflux and feeding problems after gastrostomy in children with severe neurological impairment. *Dev Med Child Neurol*. 1995;37:320–329
37. Isch JA, Rescorla FJ, Scherer LR 3rd, West KW, Grosfeld JL. The development of gastroesophageal reflux after percutaneous endoscopic gastrostomy. *J Pediatr Surg*. 1997;32:321–322
38. Albanese CT, Towbin RB, Ulman I, Lewis J, Smith SD. Percutaneous gastrojejunostomy versus Nissen fundoplication for enteral feeding of the neurologically impaired child with gastroesophageal reflux. *J Pediatr*. 1993;123:371–375

37

Nutrition of Children Who Are Critically Ill

Critical illness is often accompanied by a constellation of metabolic aberrations that tend to be profound and predictable. More than 60 years ago, Sir David Cuthbertson described the fundamental aspects of this metabolic response in adults.[1] The metabolic sequelae of illness and operation seen in neonates and children qualitatively resemble those of adults though marked quantitative differences exist. To design optimal nutritional therapy for the critically ill child, an understanding of these metabolic changes and their effect upon nutrient requirements is necessary.

Metabolic Reserves and Baseline Requirements

The most striking difference in body composition between the healthy adult and child is the quantity of protein available in times of injury. As a percentage of body weight, the protein stores of adults are twice those of neonates (Table 37.1). Lipid stores are also decreased in children as compared to adults, while carbohydrate reserves are constant across age groups. Not only do neonates and children have reduced stores, they have much higher baseline requirements. The resting energy expenditure for low-birth-weight neonates is 3 times that for adults. Protein requirements for the premature neonate to maintain growth rates approximating those in utero are 3.5 times the requirement for protein balance in the adult.[2] Thus, critically ill children are potentially much more susceptible to the deleterious effects of protracted catabolic stress.

Table 37.1.
The Body Composition of Neonates, Children, and Non-obese Adults as a Percent of Total Body Weight*

Age	Percent Protein	Percent Fat	Percent Carbohydrates
Neonates	11	14	0.4
Children (age 10 yr)	15	17	0.4
Adults	18	19	0.4

*Based on the data of Forbes,[3] Foman,[4] Munro.[5]

Protein Metabolism

Amino acids are the key building blocks required for growth and tissue repair. The majority of amino acids reside in proteins, with the remainder being in the free amino acid pool. Proteins themselves are not static, as they are continually degraded and synthesized in a process termed protein turnover. The reutilization of amino acids released from protein breakdown is extensive as evidenced by protein turnover contributing more than 2 times the amino acids derived from protein intake. In critically ill children, such as those with severe burn injury or respiratory failure requiring extracorporeal membrane oxygenation (ECMO), protein turnover is doubled when compared to normal subjects.[6] Generally, in critical illness, amino acids are redistributed away from skeletal muscle to injured tissues, cells involved in the inflammatory response, and the liver. Acutely needed enzymes, serum proteins, and glucose (by way of gluconeogenesis) are thus synthesized. There is also a marked rise in the circulation of hepatically derived acute-phase proteins (ie, C-reactive protein, fibrinogen, haptoglobin, α-1 antitrypsin, and α-1-acid glycoprotein) and a concomitant decrease in hepatically derived nutrient transport proteins such as albumin and retinol binding protein. A salient advantage of high protein turnover is that it allows for the immediate synthesis of proteins needed for the inflammatory response and tissue repair. The process does require energy, hence either an increase in resting energy expenditure or a redistribution of energy normally used for growth is required. Although critically ill children demonstrate both an increase in whole-body protein degradation and whole body synthesis, it is the former that predominates. Thus, these patients manifest net negative protein balance, which clinically may be noted by weight loss, negative nitrogen balance and skeletal muscle wasting.

The catabolism of skeletal muscle to generate glucose is necessary as glucose is the preferred substrate for the brain, red blood cells, and renal medulla, and provides an energy source for injured tissues. Illness enhances gluconeogenesis in adults, children, and neonates. On a per kg body weight basis, gluconeogenesis seems to be particularly elevated in the ill, low-birth-weight neonates (presumably because of their relatively large brain-body weight ratio).[7] Interestingly, the provision of dietary glucose is relatively ineffective in quelling endogenous glucose production in stressed states.[8]

The catabolism of skeletal muscle to generate glucose is an excellent short-term adaptation in the ill child; however, it is limited in duration due to the reduced stores available. Without elimination of the inciting stress for catabolism, the progressive loss of diaphragmatic and intercostal muscle, as well as cardiac muscle, can precipitate cardiopulmonary failure. Fortunately amino acid nutritional supplementation does improve protein balance, and the mechanism for this change in ill neonates appears to be an increase in protein synthesis, while protein degradation rates remain relatively unaffected.[9]

The amount of protein required to optimally enhance protein accretion is higher in sick children than in healthy children. Infants demonstrate 25% higher protein degradation after surgery, 100% increase in urinary nitrogen excretion with bacterial sepsis, and 100% increase in protein breakdown if they are ill enough to require ECMO.[6] Children treated for cancer also show increased net protein breakdown.[10] The provision of dietary protein sufficient to optimize protein synthesis and facilitate wound healing and the inflammatory response, as well as to preserve skeletal muscle protein mass, is the single most important nutritional intervention in ill children. The quantity of protein (or amino acid solution) administered in critical illness should be 3 to 4 g/kg/d for low-birth-weight infants, 2 to 3 g/kg/d for full-term neonates, and 1.5 g/kg/d for older children. Certain severely stressed states may require additional protein supplementation, hence, growth rates should be carefully monitored in chronically ill patients. Excessive protein administration should be avoided because toxicity is possible, particularly in patients with marginal renal function. Low-birth-weight neonates fed protein allotments of 6 g/kg/d have demonstrated azotemia, pyrexia, a higher incidence of strabismus, and somewhat lower IQ.[11,12]

Two important issues relating to the protein metabolism of critically ill children remain to be elucidated. At present, there is no specific recommendation on a specific or special amino acid composition that may be of specific benefit to critically ill children. The use of glutamine supplementation remains investigational. Similarly, quelling the extreme protein catabolism found in sick children using hormonal modulation also remains experimental.

Energy Metabolism

A careful appraisal of energy requirements in critically ill children is required as both underestimates and overestimates are associated with potentially deleterious consequences. Inadequate caloric allotment will result in poor protein retention, particularly if protein administration is marginal. The provision of excess glucose calories in neonates on ECMO results in increased CO_2 production rates (hence, exacerbating ventilatory failure) and an apparent paradoxical increase in net protein degradation.[13]

The energy needs of critically ill patients are governed by the severity and persistence of the illness. The resting energy expenditure in the flow phase of injury is increased by 50% in children with severe burns and returns to normal during convalescence.[14] Preterm neonates with bronchopulmonary dysplasia similarly have a 25% increase in energy needs over basal requirements.[15] Conversely, stable extubated neonates have resting energy expenditures that resemble normal infants.[16] Newborns undergoing major operations have only a transient 20% increase in energy expenditure that returns to baseline levels within 12 hours, unless complications develop.[17] Very-low-birth-weight neonates undergoing patent ductus arteriosus ligation do not manifest any discernible increase in resting energy expenditure the first day postoperatively.[18]

Total energy requirements encompass resting energy expenditure, energy needed for physical activity, and diet-induced thermogenesis. Resting energy expenditure itself includes the caloric requirement for growth. Although critically ill children have increased energy requirements due to increased protein turnover, their growth is often halted during extreme physiologic stress. Due to intrinsic illness and sedation, the levels of physical activity are low in critical illness. Using a stable isotopic technique, the mean energy expenditures of critically ill neonates on ECMO and an age- and diet-matched non-stressed control were found to be nearly identical.[19] The critically ill cohort did, however, have a greater variability in energy expenditure. Further, as previously noted, a surfeit of calories in critically ill neonates does not necessarily result in improved protein accretion. Thus, for practical purposes, the recommended dietary caloric intake for healthy children is a reasonable starting point in critically ill patients. Postoperative parenterally fed neonates, when given an adequate amino acid intake, require a total of 85 to 90 kcal/k/d of energy to achieve adequate protein accretion rates during the first 3 days postoperatively.[9] Ventilated extremely low-birth-weight neonates receiving 3.0 g/k/d of protein and 105 kcal/k/d remain in positive protein balance before and after patent ductus arteriosus ligation.[18] Enterally fed critically ill children as a rule require a further 10% increment in calories due to obligate malabsorption.

Once protein needs have been met, both carbohydrate and lipid energy sources have similar beneficial effects on net protein synthesis in ill patients.[20] A rational partitioning of these energy-yielding substrates is predicated on the knowledge of carbohydrate and lipid utilization in illness.

Carbohydrate Metabolism

Glucose production and availability is a priority in ill children. Injured and septic adults have a threefold increase in glucose turnover and oxidation, and an elevation in gluconeogenesis.[21,22] An important feature of the metabolic stress response is that the provision of dietary glucose does not halt gluconeogenesis; consequently, the catabolism of muscle proteins continues.[8] It is clear, however, that a combination of glucose and amino acids effectively improves protein balance in illness, even in premature neonates with respiratory distress during the first week of life, primarily by augmenting protein synthesis.[23] In early nutritional support regimens for surgical patients, glucose and amino acid formulations with minimal lipids (only to obviate fatty acid deficiency) were often used. A further tendency existed to provide energy allotments well over requirements. As may be predicted, the excess glucose was synthesized to fat resulting in a net generation of carbon dioxide. The synthesis of fat from glucose has a respiratory quotient (RQ), defined as the ratio of CO_2 produced to O_2 consumed, of about 8.7. In clinical situations, this high RQ is not attained, as glucose is never purely used for fatty acid synthesis. Nonetheless, the provision of excess glucose results in an elevated RQ and, thus, increases the ventilatory burden placed on the child. The mean RQ in postsurgical neonates fed a high glucose diet is approximately 1.0 while comparable neonates fed with less glucose, and lipids at 4.0 g/kg/d, have an RQ of 0.83.[20] In contrast to glucose metabolism, excess lipids are merely stored as triglycerides and do not result in an augmentation of CO_2 production. Using high glucose total parenteral nutrition, hypermetabolic adult patients fed excess caloric allotments have a 30% increase in O_2 consumption, a 57% rise in CO_2 production, and 71% elevation in minute ventilation.[24] Thus, avoidance of overfeeding and the use of a mixed fuel system of nutrition employing both glucose and lipids to yield energy is theoretically and practically of utility in stressed patients, many of whom are also have respiratory failure. Such an approach also often obviates problems with hyperglycemia in the relatively insulin-resistant ill child.

Lipid Metabolism

Lipid metabolism, analogous to protein and carbohydrate metabolism, is generally accelerated by illness and trauma.[25] Initially, during the brief ebb phase following trauma or in early septic shock, lipid use is compromised, and triglyceride levels rise with an attendant decrease in the metabolism of intravenously administered lipids. In the predominant flow phase of injury, however, adult patients demonstrate lipid turnover rates twofold to fourfold higher than in comparable controls and they are proportionate to the degree of injury.[26,27] Conceptually similar to the increased protein turnover noted in illness, this process involves the recycling of free fatty acids and glycerol into, and hydrolysis from, triglycerides. Both metabolic processes result in a continual stream of substrates through the plasma pool, though at an energy cost, which is reflected by an elevation in the resting metabolic rate. Approximately 30% to 40% of the released fatty acids are oxidized for energy and the RQ values post injury are in the vicinity of 0.8. Thus, this suggests that free fatty acids are, in fact, the prime source of energy in stressed patients. When subjected to uncomplicated abdominal surgery, infants and children have a reduction in RQ and a decline in plasma triglycerides, implying an increased oxidation of free fatty acids.[28] The glycerol, released along with free fatty acids from triglycerides, may be converted to pyruvate that then, in turn, is used as a gluconeogenic precursor. As with other catabolic processes in illness and trauma, the provision of dietary glucose does not decrease glycerol clearance nor diminish lipid recycling.

Normal ketone body metabolism is markedly altered by severe illness. The product of incomplete fatty acid and pyruvate oxidation is acetyl-CoA, which, through a condensation reaction within the hepatocyte, forms the ketone bodies acetoacetate and β-hydroxybutyrate. In starved healthy subjects, a major adaptation to help preserve skeletal muscle mass is the use of ketone bodies generated by the liver as an energy source for the brain (which cannot directly oxidize free fatty acids). However, in the 3-day period following trauma, there is a negligible elevation in serum ketone body levels when compared with healthy fasting subjects.[29] This observation may be understood in light of serum insulin levels as ketogenesis is inhibited by even low concentrations of the hormone, a phenomenon evident to physicians by the absence of ketotic problems in type 2 diabetes. Hence, the high insulin concentrations seen in severe injury and after major operations ablate the ketotic adaptation of starvation.

The energy needs of the injured patient are met largely by the mobilization and oxidation of free fatty acids. In conjunction with these increased demands, ill neonates have limited lipid stores. Thus, they may suffer biochemical essential fatty acid deficiency within 1 week if administered a fat-free diet.[30,31] In infants, linoleic and linolenic acid are considered essential with arachidonic acid and docosahexaenoic acid is deemed as conditionally essential. When there is a lack of dietary linoleic acid, the formation of arachidonic acid (a tetraene) by desaturation and chain elongation cannot occur, and the same pathway entrains available oleic acid to form 5,8,11-eicosatrienoic acid (a triene). Empirically, a triene-tetraene ratio of greater than 0.4 is characteristic of essential fatty acid deficiency. The clinical syndrome consists of dermatitis, alopecia, thrombocytopenia, susceptibility to bacterial infection, and failure to thrive.[30,31] To obviate essential fatty acid deficiency in injured infants, the prompt administration of linoleic acid and linolenic acid is recommended.

The provision of commercially available lipid solutions to parenterally fed critically ill neonates obviates the risk of essential fatty acid deficiency, results in improved protein use, and does not significantly increase CO_2 production or metabolic rate.[32] These advantages, however, are balanced by some potential risks of excess administration—hypertriglyceridemia, increased infections, and decreased alveolar oxygen diffusion capacity.[33–35] Although the evidence is far from conclusive, the possible adverse effects of lipid administration have resulted in most centers starting lipid supplementation in ill neonates and children at 0.5 g/kg/d, and advancing over a period of days to 2 to 4 g/kg/d, while closely monitoring triglyceride levels. Lipid administration is usually restricted to a maximum of 30% to 40% of total calories, although this practice has not been validated by clinical trials.

Vitamin and Trace Mineral Metabolism

Vitamin and trace mineral metabolism in ill and postoperative pediatric patients has not been well studied. For the neonate and child, the fat-soluble vitamins A, D, E, and K, as well as the water-soluble vitamins, ascorbic acid, thiamine, riboflavin, pyridoxine, niacin, pantothenate, biotin, folate, and vitamin B_{12}, are all required and are routinely administered. Since vitamins are not stoichiometrically consumed in biochemical reactions, but rather act as catalysts, the administration of large supplements of vitamins in stressed states is not logical from a nutritional standpoint. The trace minerals that are required for normal development are zinc, iron, copper, selenium, manganese, iodide, molybdenum, and chromium. Trace minerals are usually used in the synthesis of the active sites of an ubiquitous and extraordinarily important class of enzymes called metalloenzymes. As with vitamins, the role of metalloenzymes is to act as catalysts. Hence, unless there are excessive losses, such as enhanced zinc loss with severe diarrhea, large nutritional requirements would not be anticipated in illness. The vitamin and trace mineral needs of healthy children and neonates are outlined in Appendix C. These levels have been used in critically ill patients and little evidence exists that they are nutritionally inadequate. In children with severe hepatic failure, copper and manganese accumulation occurs and, thus, parenteral trace mineral supplementation should be limited to once per week.

The pharmacologic use of vitamins and trace minerals in pediatric illness is controversial. Reviews of both vitamin and trace mineral toxicity demonstrate that excessive dosage is clearly a health risk.[36,37]

Routes of Nutrient Provision

In the critically ill child, the enteral route of nutrient provision is preferable to parenteral nutrition whenever the gastrointestinal tract is functional. Enteral nutrition is physiologic, safer, and more cost effective. The use of nasojejunal feeding tubes placed at bedside or by interventional radiology is a very useful adjunct to the nutritional management of the critically ill child. Continuous feedings using standard formulas can adequately nourish the majority of patients. At the time of extubation, feeds are held for a period of 6 to 12 hours. If parenteral nutrition is necessary, central venous access is sought. Peripheral percutaneously placed intravenous lines that are threaded centrally and central lines are the preferred routes of administration. Central access may be garnered at bedside in most patients in the intensive care unit. Groin lines are not a favored access route for nutritional therapy because of their propensity for infection.

Conclusion

Neonates and children are particularly susceptible to the loss of lean body mass and its attendant increased morbidity and mortality. Critical illness results in increased protein, carbohydrate, and lipid use, and net negative protein balance. The judicious administration of carbohydrates, lipids, vitamins, trace minerals, and particularly protein can optimize wound healing and reduce or even eliminate the consequences of this catabolic response.

References

1. Cuthbertson DP. Further observations on the disturbance of metabolism caused by injury, with particular reference to the dietary requirements of fracture cases. *Br J Surg*. 1936;23:505–520
2. Kashyap S, Schulze KF, Forsyth M, et al. Growth, nutrient retention, and metabolic response in low birth weight infants fed varying intakes of protein and energy. *J Pediatr*. 1988;113:713–721

3. Forbes GB, Bruining GJ. Urinary creatinine excretion and lean body mass. *Am J Clin Nutr.* 1976;29:1359–1366

4. Foman SJ, Haschke F, Zeigler EE, Nelson SE. Body composition of reference children from birth to age 10 years. *Am J Clin Nutr.* 1982;35(suppl 5):1169–1175

5. Munro HN. Nutrition and muscle protein metabolism: introduction. *Fed Proc.* 1978;37:2281–2282

6. Keshen TH, Miller RG, Jahoor F, Jaksic T. Stable isotopic quantitation of protein metabolism and energy expenditure in neonates on and post extracorporeal life support. *J Pediatr Surg.* 1997;32:958–963

7. Keshen T, Miller R, Jahoor R, Jaksic T, Reeds PJ. Glucose production and gluconeogenesis are negatively related to body weight in mechanically ventilated, very low birth weight neonates. *Pediatr Res.* 1997;41:132–138

8. Long CL, Kinney JM, Geiger JW. Nonsuppressibility of gluconeogenesis by glucose in septic patients. *Metabolism.* 1976;25:193–201

9. Duffy B, Pencharz P. The effects of surgery on the nitrogen metabolism of parenterally fed human neonates. *Pediatr Res.* 1986;20:32–35

10. Daley SE, Pearson AD, Craft AW, et al. Whole body protein metabolism in children with cancer. *Arch Dis Child.* 1996;75:273–281

11. Goldman HI, Freudenthal R, Holland B, Karelite S. Clinical effects of two different levels of protein intake on low birth weight infants. *J Pediatr.* 1969;74:881–889

12. Goldman HI, Liebman OB, Freudentahal R, Reuben R. Effects of early dietary protein intake on low-birth weight infants: evaluation at 3 years of age. *J Pediatr.* 1971;78:126–129

13. Shew SB, Keshen TH, Jahoor F, Jaksic T. The determinants of protein catabolism in neonates on extracorporeal membrane oxygenation. *J Pediatr Surg.* 1999;34:1086–1090

14. Jahoor F, Desai M, Herndon DN, Wolfe RR. Dynamics of the protein metabolic response to burn injury. *Metabolism.* 1988;37:330–337

15. Weinstein MR, Oh W. Oxygen consumption in infants with bronchopulmonary dysplasia. *J Pediatr.* 1981;99:958–961

16. Shew SB, Beckett PR, Keshen TH, Jahoor F, Jaksic T. Validation of a [^{13}C]bicarbonate tracer technique to measure neonatal energy expenditure. *Pediatr Res.* 2000;47:787–791

17. Jones MO, Pierro A, Hammond P, Lloyd DA. The metabolic response to operative stress in infants. *J Pediatr Surg.* 1993;28:1258–1263

18. Shew SB, Keshan TH, Glass NL, Jahoor F, Jaksic T. Ligation of a patent ductus arteriosus under fentanyl anesthesia improves protein metabolism in premature neonates. *J Pediatr Surg.* 2000;35:1277–1281

19. Jaksic T, Shew SB, Keshen TH, Dzakovic A, Jahoor F. Do critically ill surgical neonates have increased energy expenditure? *J Pediatr Surg.* 2001;36:63–67

20. Jones MO, Pierro A, Garlick PJ, McNurlan MA, Donnell SC, Lloyd DA. Protein metabolism kinetics in neonates: effect of intravenous carbohydrate and fat. *J Pediatr Surg.* 1995;30:458–462

21. Long CL, Spencer JL, Kinney JM, Geiger JW. Carbohydrate metabolism in normal man and effect of glucose infusion. *J Appl Physiol.* 1971;31:102–109

22. Long CL, Spencer JL, Kinney JM, Geiger JW. Carbohydrate metabolism in normal man: effect of elective operations and major injury. *J Appl Physiol.* 1971;31: 110–116

23. Rivera A Jr, Bell EF, Bier DM. Effect of intravenous amino acids on protein metabolism of preterm infants during the first three days of life. *Pediatr Res.* 1993;33: 106–111

24. Askanazi J, Rosenbaum SH, Hyman AI, Silverberg PA, Milic-Emili J, Kinney JM. Respiratory changes induced by the large glucose loads of total parenteral nutrition. *JAMA.* 1980;243:1444–1447

25. Jeevanandam M, Young DH, Schiller WR. Nutritional impact on energy cost of fat fuel mobilization in polytrauma victims. *J Trauma.* 1990;30:147–154

26. Wiener M, Rothkop MM, Rothkop G, Askanazi J. Fat metabolism in injury and stress. *Crit Care Clin.* 1987;3:25–56

27. Nordenstrom J, Carpentier YA, Askanazi J, et al. Metabolic utilization of intravenous fat emulsion during total parenteral nutrition. *Ann Surg.* 1982;196:221–231

28. Powis MR, Smith K, Rennie M, Halliday D, Pierro A. Effect of major abdominal operations on energy and protein metabolism in infants and children. *J Pediatr Surg.* 1998;33:49–53

29. Birkhahn RH, Long CL, Fitkin DL, Basnardo AC, Geiger JW, Blakemore WS. A comparison of the effects of skeletal trauma and surgery on the ketosis of starvation in man. *J Trauma.* 1981;21:519

30. Paulsrud JR, Pensler L, Whitten CF, Stewart S, Holman RT. Essential fatty acid deficiency in infants induced by fat-free intravenous feeding. *Am J Clin Nutr.* 1972;25:897–904

31. Friedman Z, Danon A, Stahlman MT, Oates JA. Rapid onset of essential fatty acid deficiency in the newborn. *Pediatrics.* 1976;58:640–649

32. Van Aerde JE, Sauer PJ, Pencharz PB, Smith JM, Heim T, Swyer PR. Metabolic consequences of increasing energy intake by adding lipid to parenteral nutrition in full-term infants. *Am J Clin Nutr.* 1994;59:659–662

33. Cleary TG, Pickering LK. Mechanisms of intralipid effect on polymorphonuclear leukocytes. *J Clin Lab Immunol.* 1983;11:21–26

34. Periera GR, Fox WW, Stanley CA, Baker L, Schwartz JG. Decreased oxygenation and hyperlipidemia during intravenous fat infusions in premature infants. *Pediatrics.* 1980;66:26–30

35. Freeman J, Goldmann DA, Smith NE, Sidebottom DG, Epstein MF, Platt R. Association of intravenous lipid emulsion and coagulase-negative staphylococcal bacteremia in, neonatal intensive care units. *N Engl J Med.* 1990;323:301–308

36. Marks J. The safety of vitamins: an overview. *Int J Vitam Nutr Res Suppl.* 1989;30: 12–20

37. Flodin NW. Micronutrient supplements: toxicity and drug interactions. *Prog Food Nutr Sci.* 1990;14:277–331

38

Anorexia Nervosa and Bulimia Nervosa

Anorexia nervosa and bulimia nervosa are associated with significant health problems due to nutritional and weight control practices used by patients either to lose weight or to minimize weight gain.[1] Therefore, medical and nutritional consultation is of particular importance in the management of this condition, which is generally classified as a disorder of mental health. Affected individuals are typically intellectually bright and strong willed, making them simultaneously receptive to professional input and challenging. Clinicians working with young people with an eating disorder require (1) general knowledge about the disorder and specific understanding of the individual (and the individual's family) affected by the disorder and (2) practical information about the management of common problems related to health, food, nutrition, and weight control. This section will focus on these elements as they relate to pediatric practice and nutrition consultation.[2]

Clinical Features

Weight and Food-Related Characteristics

Common features of eating disorders include *dysfunctional eating habits* (frequently related to underlying psychosocial issues related to developing autonomy and identity, low self-esteem, family dynamics, or environmental problems), *body image disturbance* (generally focused on the abdomen, hips, and thighs) and *change in weight* (ranging from extreme loss of weight in anorexia nervosa to fluctuation around a normal to moderately high weight in bulimia nervosa). The *Diagnostic and Statistical Manual of Mental Disorders-Primary Care* (*DSM-PC*) (Tables 38.1 and 38.2) classification describes a continuum of severity from variations (minor deviations from normal that might still be of concern), to *problems* (more serious manifestations representing subthreshold eating disorders), to full *eating disorders* (meeting full *Diagnostic and Statistical Manual of Mental Disorders, Fourth Edition* [*DSM-IV*] criteria).

Anorexia nervosa is an eating disorder characterized by an insufficient and voluntarily restricted caloric intake resulting in weight loss (or failure to gain

Table 38.1.
Combined *Diagnostic and Statistical Manual of Mental Disorders, Primary Care (DSM-PC)/Diagnostic and Statistical Manual of Mental Disorders, Fourth Edition (DSM-IV)* **Criteria for Eating Disorders: Dieting-Anorexia Nervosa Spectrum**

V65.49 Dieting/Body Image Variation
• A significantly overweight child changes eating habits in a realistic, healthy way.
• The child does not completely eliminate any food group, but generally decreases intake of food, especially of sweets and fats or is eating an appropriate diet.
• The child favors a thin appearance but has a realistic image.
• The individual can stop dieting voluntarily.
V69.1 Dieting/Body Image Problem
• Dieting and voluntary food restrictions are more restrictive and result in weight loss or failure to gain weight as expected during growth but these behaviors are not sufficiently intense to qualify for the diagnosis of anorexia nervosa or eating disorder, NOS.
• The individual begins to become obsessed with the pursuit of thinness and develops systematic fears of gaining weight.
• The individual also begins to develop a consistent disturbance in body perception and starts to deny that weight loss or dieting is a problem.
307.1 Anorexia Nervosa (from DSM-IV)
• Refusal to maintain body weight at or above a minimally normal weight for age and height (eg, weight loss leading to maintenance of body weight less than 85% of that expected; or failure to make expected weight gain during period of growth, leading to body weight less than 85% of that expected).
• Body mass index (BMI) is <17.5 kg/m² for older adolescents.
• Intense fear of gaining weight or becoming fat, even though underweight.
• Disturbance in the way in which one's body weight, shape or size is experienced, undue influence of body weight or shape on self-evaluation, or denial of the seriousness of the current low body weight.
• In postmenarchal females, amenorrhea (ie, the absence of at least 3 consecutive menstrual cycles). (A female is considered to have amenorrhea if her periods occur only following hormone [eg, estrogen] administration.)

From: Wolraich ML, Felice ME, Drotar D, eds. *The Classification of Child and Adolescent Mental Diagnoses in Primary Care, Diagnostic and Statistical Manual for Primary Care (DSM-PC)*, Child and Adolescent Version. Elk Grove Village, IL: American Academy of Pediatrics; 1996. And from: American Psychiatric Association. *Diagnostic and Statistical Manual of Mental Disorders, Fourth Edition*. Washington, DC: American Psychiatric Association; 1994.

weight during puberty) that is accompanied by an obsession to be thinner and a delusion of being fat. Weight loss can be extreme, but there is no specific amount of weight loss required in diagnostic criteria. The *DSM-IV* suggests, as an example, 85% of ideal body weight. However, patients with less severe eating patterns in the categories of *DSM-PC variations* or *problems* (Table 38.1),

Table 38.2.

Combined *Diagnostic and Statistical Manual of Mental Disorders, Primary Care (DSM-PC)/Diagnostic and Statistic Manual of Mental Disorders, Fourth Edition (DSM-IV)* **Criteria for Eating Disorders: Purging/Binge Eating-Bulimia Nervosa Spectrum**

V65.49 Purging/Binge-Eating Variation
• Occasional overeating or perception of overeating, either objective or subjective binges occurs.
• Intermittent concern about body image or getting fat is present in specific situations during which too much food was eaten. Concerns are not pervasive or cross-situational and do not change eating behaviors.
• Normal weight gain is typically present.
V69.19 Purging/Binge-Eating Problem
• Experimentation with vomiting, laxatives, fasting, or exercises to prevent weight gain.
• Isolated episodes are far apart in time.
• Individual has increased episodes of uncontrolled eating, and perceptions of body shape or size become more systematically distorted. Negative self-evaluation is often influenced by weight and body shape.
• The behaviors are not sufficiently intense to qualify for a diagnosis of bulimia nervosa or eating disorder, NOS.
307.51 Bulimia Nervosa (from DSM-IV)
• Recurrent episodes of binge eating, characterized by both of the following:
– Eating, in a discrete period of time (eg, within any 2-hour period), an amount of food that is definitely larger than most people would eat during a similar period of time and under similar circumstances.
– A sense of lack of control over eating during the episode (eg, a feeling that one cannot stop eating or control what or how much one is eating).
• Recurrent inappropriate compensatory behavior in order to prevent weight gain, such as self-induced vomiting; misuse of laxatives, diuretics, enemas, or other medications; fasting; or excessive exercise.
• The binge eating and inappropriate compensatory behaviors both occur, on average, at least twice a week for 3 months.
• Body shape and weight unduly influence self-evaluation.
• The disturbance does not occur exclusively during episodes of Anorexia Nervosa.

From: Wolraich ML, Felice ME, Drotar D, eds. *The Classification of Child and Adolescent Mental Diagnoses in Primary Care, Diagnostic and Statistical Manual for Primary Care (DSM-PC)*, Child and Adolescent Version. Elk Grove Village, IL: American Academy of Pediatrics; 1996. And from: American Psychiatric Association. *Diagnostic and Statistical Manual of Mental Disorders, Fourth Edition*. Washington, DC: American Psychiatric Association; 1994.

may not experience this degree of emaciation for various reasons, but still deserve medical and nutritional attention. More than 75% of persons with anorexia nervosa exercise compulsively to accelerate weight loss. Less than 10%

may attempt to rid themselves of calories by vomiting or taking laxatives; such purging is more commonly associated with bulimia nervosa.

The key feature of bulimia nervosa is repeated episodes of consuming large amounts of food in a brief period (binge eating). Binges are followed by some type of compensatory behavior intended to rid the body of the effects of food: fasting; "purging" through vomiting, laxatives, or diuretics; or exercise. Depending on the balance between intake and output, patients range from moderately thin to moderately overweight, and an individual's weight can fluctuate depending on the pattern of weight control over time. Episodic binges make binge eating disorder similar to bulimia nervosa, but binge eating disorder does not include any compensatory behavior to rid the body of the effects of excessive calories. In fact, for patients with binge eating disorder, self-deprecating thoughts following a binge may best be relieved by another binge. Thus, individuals with binge eating disorder may become massively overweight.

Typically, patients with bulimia nervosa have strong feelings of guilt and shame about both the binge eating and the compensatory behaviors, such as vomiting. However, the relief of anxiety that patients with bulimia nervosa experience after getting rid of the food is strong enough to temporarily help them feel better. This relief is short-lived, as the cycle of behaviors tends to repeat itself in an addictive fashion. A personal and/or family history of depression and/or addictions is commonly found in patients with bulimia nervosa.

Meals

Meals are typically restricted to eating small amounts of a monotonously narrow range of low-calorie, low-fat foods and drinking low-calorie beverages.[3] Breakfast is generally avoided. If not entirely vegetarian, the intake of meat is typically severely restricted, eaten primarily at dinner—under duress from parents and confined to small amounts of skinless poultry or broiled fish. Snacks and desserts are assiduously avoided in anorexia nervosa. When they occur, binges typically consist of "forbidden foods" considered to be fattening and occur in the late afternoon or evening. Immediately after a binge, patients may go to the bathroom to vomit or take laxatives, or exercise.

Clinical Approach

Comerci[4] has noted 4 main elements of successful treatment of eating disorders: (1) early recognition and restoration of physiologic stability, (2) establishment of a trusting, therapeutic partnership with the patient, (3) involvement of the family in treatment, and (4) a team approach. Levenkron[5] has emphasized the "nurturant-authoritative" approach, in contrast to an unsupportive, authoritarian one. With respect to medical and nutritional management, eating disorders are a final common pathway allowing affected individuals to cope with unresolved adolescent developmental conflicts. Parents often search for a specific cause, emotional flaw, set of family traits, or precipitating event, but this is rarely helpful in the short-term. Mental health services may focus on these issues, but these are needed over a period of months to years. At one level, the conflict is metaphorical and has nothing to do with food, eating, or weight—the struggle for control over these concrete and measurable realities is symbolic of the intangible, confusing, and often illusory internal struggles that accompany adolescent development. However, this conflict also can result in serious health consequences that perpetuate dysfunctional patterns. It is essential that both levels be addressed in treatment. Nutritional, medical, and psychological interventions should occur simultaneously.

Epidemiology/Prevalence

Eating disorders most commonly affect white, adolescent females. There is an increasing awareness of these conditions, especially bulimia nervosa, among females in minority groups and among males, however. Prevalence is estimated at between 0.5% and 5% of adolescent females.[6] Certain groups, such as athletes or dancers, may have a substantially higher risk for developing anorexia nervosa. However, the prevalence of unrecognized, atypical or subclinical anorexia nervosa is undoubtedly several times greater, and these individuals may be at greater risk of health consequences since they are less likely to come to clinical attention and more likely to persist in unhealthy nutritional and weight control habits.

Assessment

General Issues

The initial assessment of the adolescent with an eating disorder should focus on weight loss and health, per se, and not to attempt to determine underlying psychologic or emotional factors.[7] The denial that patients so frequently project when threatened with direct confrontation about their eating disorder is less likely to be exhibited when they are questioned about their nutritional habits, physical symptoms, and health. The first step in the assessment is to determine if weight loss is intentional and/or desired and ensure that the symptoms are not related to a medical disease, such as inflammatory bowel disease, endocrinopathy, cancer, or an occult infection. However, some patients recover from a medical condition, such as infectious mononucleosis, only to continue to lose weight because they then diet intentionally. This occurs because of positive reinforcement received for the weight loss that accompanied the initial illness. Pubertal adolescents, on the other hand, may fail to increase caloric intake during their growth spurt, or may increase their caloric expenditure playing sports, and lose weight unintentionally. Finally, many healthy adolescents lose weight while attempting to get in shape or look better.

The second step in the assessment of a person with a suspected eating disorder is to determine if weight control habits are excessive or unhealthy. Young people with eating disorder *variations* or *problems* in the *DSM-PC* classification may have significant health problems associated with weight control. Questionnaires assessing symptoms related to malnutrition, such as those in Table 38.3, can be used to identify individuals who may be experiencing health problems associated with weight control.

The third step in conducting the nutritional assessment is to determine the degree to which the pursuit of thinness is an overriding concern and a driving force in the individual's daily activities. Typically the adolescent with anorexia nervosa restricts intake to <1000 cal/d, is unwilling to accept a body weight >85% of average weight for height, and has a self-concept that is directly linked to his or her weight or how he or she feels about his or her weight. It is useful to have the patient identify a desired goal weight, especially if the patient is still within a normal weight range. Adolescents with anorexia nervosa either have an unrealistically low goal weight, or cannot identify a specific weight with which they would be satisfied. Although a distorted body image is included in diagnostic criteria for anorexia nervosa, many adolescent females without eating disorders are also dissatisfied with their bodies, especially their hips, buttocks, and thighs, limiting the specificity of this finding. Instruments such as the Eating Disorder Inventory (EDI) can also be used to measure features, including body dissatisfaction or drive for thinness.

If the evidence indicates that the adolescent has anorexia nervosa, the fourth step is to determine an immediate plan of action. The biopsychosocial approach recognizes that patients require attention to their biological, psychological, and social needs. For patients who have lost a significant amount of weight and are exhibiting signs of starvation and hypometabolism, or who have intractable vomiting and electrolyte imbalance, hospitalization should be

Table 38.3.
Questionnaire for Adolescents With Weight Loss

1. SYMPTOMS: Do you have any of the following symptoms?	NO	YES
Cold or blue hands or feet	☐	☐
Constipation	☐	☐
Dizziness or fainting	☐	☐
Headaches	☐	☐
Tired or weak	☐	☐
Loss of appetite	☐	☐
Difficulty concentrating or making decisions	☐	☐
Feeling irritable	☐	☐
Being sad or bored	☐	☐
Not wanting to be around friends or family	☐	☐
Thinking about food	☐	☐
Worrying about gaining weight	☐	☐
Loss or irregularity of menstrual periods (females)	☐	☐

2. WEIGHT AND ACTIVITY HISTORY

What is the *most* you have ever weighed? .... _____

What is the *least* you have weighed in the last year? .... _____

What do you weigh *now*? .... _____

What would you *like* to weigh? .... _____

Are you trying to lose weight? .... ☐ No   ☐ Yes

Do you exercise at least once a week? .... ☐ No   ☐ Yes

    If yes, check all that apply:

	No	Yes	Hours/Week
Running/jogging	☐	☐	_____
Aerobics/calisthenics	☐	☐	_____
Dancing/ballet	☐	☐	_____
Gymnastics	☐	☐	_____
Swimming	☐	☐	_____
Team sport(s)	☐	☐	_____
Other: _____			_____

Do you exercise to lose weight? .... ☐ No   ☐ Yes

3. Check all the methods that you have used to try to control your weight in the past 2 months.

Dieting	☐	Vomiting	☐
Exercising	☐	Laxatives	☐
Diet Pills	☐		

4. EATING HISTORY

Rate on a scale of 0 to 5 how much you eat at each of the following times during a typical day. (Nothing=0; Snack=1; Small meal=2; Meal=3; Large Meal=4; Binge=5)

At	Between	After
Breakfast _____	Breakfast and lunch _____	Going to bed _____
Lunch _____	Lunch and dinner _____	Something upsetting _____
Dinner _____	Dinner and bedtime _____	

Table 38.3.
Questionnaire for Adolescents With Weight Loss *(continued)*

5. Please describe your typical breakfast, lunch, and dinner.	
Food/Beverage	Amount
Breakfast _____	_____
_____	_____
_____	_____
Lunch _____	_____
_____	_____
_____	_____
Dinner _____	_____
_____	_____
_____	_____
_____	

considered. However, with early recognition, hospitalization can usually be avoided, as long as appropriate outpatient treatment is available.

Physical Health Issues

No organ system is spared the effects of the malnutrition that occurs in anorexia nervosa. Keys and colleagues studied young adult males who were "voluntarily" starved to determine the effects of starvation and the best means of refeeding extremely malnourished individuals.[8] These subjects exhibited findings remarkably similar to those found in anorexia nervosa; much of the clinical syndrome can be traced to the physiologic adaptation to low caloric intake. Among patients with eating disorders, the most concerning health problems are amenorrhea, hypothermia, bradycardia, and orthostatic cardiovascular instability; low weight, amenorrhea, and poor nutrition predispose females to osteoporosis. Hypothermia can be extremely uncomfortable and profound, so temperature measurement is essential. Cardiovascular instability can lead to weakness, fatigue, dizziness, loss of energy, fainting, and death. Orthostatic pulse change of more than 20 beats per minute indicates significant compromise.

Cardiovascular instability can also occur in bulimia nervosa, but it is generally due to volume depletion and electrolyte imbalance (hypokalemic, hypochloremic metabolic alkalosis). Erosion of the dental enamel (due to stomach acid), abrasion of the knuckles of metacarpophalangeal joints (rubbing against the maxillary central incisors), and enlargement of the salivary glands indicate significant binge eating and vomiting.

Anthropometry

The most important anthropometric measurements in the assessment of an adolescent with an eating disorder are height and weight. The latter should be determined with the patient in a gown, immediately after voiding. The body mass index (BMI) is a calculated anthropometric variable that standardizes weight for height, but which increases throughout childhood (see Appendix J).

Skinfold thickness, either as triceps or multiple-site determination, can be used to assess subcutaneous fat, but the standards apply only for older adolescents and skilled personnel using research-quality instruments must obtain the measurements. Thus, plastic calipers are unreliable and should not be used. The 4-site (triceps, biceps, subscapular, iliac) method of body fat determination is probably the most accurate. Also, the measurement may not be accurate in states of dehydration and there have been few studies in which skinfold thickness in adolescents with anorexia nervosa has been compared to reference methods of body composition determination. The primary use of this tool is in following the progress of a patient during treatment, rather than to define a level of body fat at any one time.

Early in recovery, over two thirds of the weight gained is lean.[9,10] As the body approaches a more normal distribution of lean and fat, an increasing amount of tissue laid down is fat. The composition does not appear to be influenced by dietary composition, but can be influenced by activity. That is, if patients increase their energy intake in a well-balanced diet and also engage in a combination of aerobic exercise and resistance training, the majority of tissue that is added will be lean. This point deserves emphasis, since most patients believe that all of their weight gain is or will be as fat. In addition, it is worthwhile to emphasize to patients that lean body mass has a higher metabolic rate than fat, which is relatively inert. Therefore, an increase in temperature can be interpreted as due to an increase in lean body tissue, not fat. Likewise, cold, acrocyanotic hands and feet with poor peripheral circulation and slow capillary refill can be interpreted to mean a low lean body (muscle) mass, while warm hands and feet with good circulation and rapid capillary refill indicate an improved metabolic rate and lean, not fat, body mass.

Laboratory Studies

The laboratory evaluation of patients with anorexia nervosa is primarily directed at detecting unsuspected underlying medical conditions. Nutrition-related tests include levels of hepatic secretory proteins, measures of immune function, and measurement of vitamin or mineral levels.[11] Serum albumin and pre-albumin (transthyretin) with half-lives of 20 and 2 days respectively, can be used to assess energy balance and protein synthesis in the liver. Levels of these proteins are typically normal, due to adequate protein intake in the context of extreme restriction of carbohydrates and fat, or to dehydration. Transferrin, with a half-life of 8 days, tends to be nonspecifically increased in anorexia nervosa. Visceral protein levels can be assessed with the calculation of creatinine height index (CHI) and then compared to reference standards.[12] A 20% to 40% reduction of CHI is evidence of moderate visceral protein depletion, while severe depletion is indicated by a reduction of more than 40%. Measurement of immune function by various methods have not produced consistent results in the literature, but can sometimes be useful in assessing the physiologic response to nutritional status. Vitamin and mineral levels in circulating compartments, such as the serum, may not be related to actual deficiencies at the tissue level. In vitro assay of dependent enzymes with and without the vitamin cofactor may be a more useful measure, but is not routinely available.

Routine laboratory tests obtained during medical evaluation usually include a complete blood count and erythrocyte sedimentation rate, a chemistry panel, and urinalysis. These are usually normal, a reflection of the remarkable ability of the body to maintain homeostatic balance. An electrocardiogram may be indicated if there is significant bradycardia or rhythm disturbance. Thyroid screening is often obtained, but rarely useful, since the clinical picture in anorexia nervosa combines symptoms of hyperthyroidism and hypothyroidism. An unusual finding is elevated serum cholesterol, with both elevated and normal low-density lipoprotein fractions being reported, despite an extremely low fat and low cholesterol intake.

Diet and Activity Records

Recording food and drink intake by an adolescent is helpful both in assessment and in treatment. It helps the clinician identify dietary patterns, deficiencies, excesses, and strengths; and helps the patient become more aware of his or her nutritional habits.[13] Seven-day food diaries are superior to 24-hour recall. However, since adolescents with anorexia nervosa overestimate their serving size (often by as much as 50%), it is important to verify their reports. In this respect, food models are helpful tools that simultaneously inform the professional about the patient's intake and teach the patient how to estimate serving size. The weekly journals used to evaluate nutrition can also be used to determine dysfunctional habits (such as eating a rice cake for breakfast), associated mood disturbances (such as not eating dinner because of an argument with mother), as well as episodes where the patient makes a breakthrough toward recovery (such as eating a "forbidden food" like peanut butter).

To understand the balance between energy intake and output, it is also important to record the type, intensity, frequency, and duration of exercise. In addition, one should determine if there are other ways in which energy is expended without qualifying as exercise. For example, walking to and from school while carrying a heavy book bag, bounding repeatedly up and down stairs at home to "get some things," or "stretching" twice a day all add to the daily expenditure of calories, but generally go unmeasured.

Energy Intake and Needs

The measurement of metabolic rate by indirect calorimetry can be very helpful in determining the metabolic needs of the patient. This also allows the expected increase in resting energy expenditure (REE) that occurs with refeeding to be monitored over time. Measurement of REE is not widely available, so an estimate of energy needs is usually required, generally between 2000 and 3000 kcal/d, sometimes more.[14] When patients ask how many calories they need to eat, it may be helpful to remind them that a calorie is a unit of energy required to raise the temperature of $1cm^3$ of water by $1°C$. By emphasizing to patients that food provides their body with energy and heat, it may become easier to increase their energy intake. Patients who have a high level of anxiety, or who engage in "fidgeting" (formally known as *nonexercise activity thermogenesis*) appear to need a much higher energy intake than calculated by REE or mathematical formula. Thus, the answer to the question of "How many calories are needed to gain weight?" is "Enough to cover the amount that is expended each day, plus an additional amount for new tissue."

Vitamins and Minerals

Elevated plasma levels of retinol (the primary form of vitamin A in plasma) and retinyl esters (a transient form of vitamin A associated with chylomicrons) have been reported by some investigators. These changes are not typical of protein-energy malnutrition and may be due to altered metabolism (closely related to low T_3 levels) or delayed clearance of chylomicrons. It is not clear why adolescents with anorexia nervosa have a tendency to become hypercarotenemic. The intake of β-carotene can be quite high in patients whose diet consists largely of yellow vegetables. However, Rock and Curran-Celentano[12] pointed out that elevated plasma carotenoids in anorexia nervosa may also indicate a diminished ability to clear or metabolize these compounds. There is little evidence for these increased levels posing a risk of hypervitaminosis A, however.

Investigators have reported increased, decreased, and normal plasma concentrations of tocopherol. Because vitamin E is known to be associated with lipoproteins, levels may reflect the effects of binding to blood lipids rather than tissue concentrations. Vitamin E deficiency has been related to cognitive and neuropsychological problems, even though there is no consistent pattern of deficiency yet recognized. Further investigation is required to elucidate the circumstances in which alteration of vitamin E status might be expected. Thiamin, riboflavin, and vitamin B_6 may also contribute to cognitive problems and physiological features associated with semi-starvation in many patients with anorexia nervosa. The dietary requirements for these vitamins are determined by substrate utilization, the severity of malnutrition, the refeeding process, and the stage of recovery. Measurements of blood levels are of little clinical use unless the history and physical examination suggest the presence of a specific deficiency.

The primary minerals that are of concern in anorexia nervosa are calcium and zinc.[11] Although calcium intake is typically much less than the recommended dietary allowance, serum levels are usually normal and urinary excretion is often increased. This may be due to the resorption of bone that commonly occurs in association with the low estrogen and high cortisol levels typically found in anorexia nervosa. There is little evidence that variation in calcium intake has measurable effects on bone density.

Zinc is known to be lost in catabolic states such as occurs in anorexia nervosa, but serum levels do not always reflect body stores. There is also theoretical evidence to consider zinc deficiency as possibly related to some of the symptoms of anorexia nervosa, but little evidence to suggest that it is clinically relevant. A double-blind, placebo-controlled clinical trial of zinc supplementation demonstrated improvement in some psychological functioning, but no effect on weight gain.

Treatment

Daily Structure

The daily structure should include eating 3 meals a day. Eating an adequate breakfast (not merely a rice cake) maximizes the likelihood of adequate daily caloric intake and deserves repeated emphasis. If about half of the daily energy requirement is not consumed by the end of lunch, patients tend to put off eating until late in the day, and find themselves unable to take in adequate nutrition without binge eating. The consequence of eating an insufficient amount of food at meals will be failure to gain weight, which will elicit responses by the treatment team. Thus, parents should be encouraged to ensure that healthy food is available and that mealtimes are planned into the day, but not to assume responsibility for eating. If parents feel it is their duty to make their child eat, eating becomes a battle that cannot be won. If the adolescent acquiesces and eats merely to please parents, there is the possibility that purging will develop as a means of avoiding weight gain after being forced to eat.

Nutrition Prescription

The initial caloric prescription is generally between 1000 and 1400 kcal/d, although the use of 130% of REE as determined by indirect calorimetry or adjusted Harris-Benedict equation are more precise methods of determining actual resting energy requirements. These values need to be adjusted for estimated energy expenditure in daily activity especially for adolescents involved in sports or vigorous physical exercise. The nutrition prescription should work toward gradually increasing weight at the rate of about 1/2 to 1 lb per week, by increasing energy intake at 100 to 200 kcal increments every few days. In addition, the gradual inclusion of forbidden foods should be part of the nutrition prescription once the adolescent has shown evidence of being able to eat adequately to gain weight. A standard nutritional balance of 15% to 20% protein, 55% to 60% carbohydrate, and 20% to 25% fat is appropriate. However, the fat content may need to be lowered to 15% to 20% early in treatment because of continued fat phobia.

Rock and Curran-Celentano note that if refeeding is accomplished with an increasing energy containing diet consisting of a variety of regular foods, sufficient amounts of vitamins and minerals will be provided so that correction of deficiencies without supplementation is anticipated.[12] Treating the nutritional problems with nutrient-dense foods will also help to correct the multitude of metabolic and physiological abnormalities associated with semi-starvation, in addition to reversing specific micronutrient deficiencies. Low-dose multiple vitamins with minerals at recommended dietary allowance levels may be appropriate for chronically ill adolescents who are unable to maintain adequate nutrition. On the other hand, the use of high-dose supplements can have unfavorable effects either through excessive levels of the micronutrient itself or through adverse interactions with other elements (such as occurs between zinc and copper).

Nutrition-specific Issues

It is useful to return to the physical evidence that nutrition is inadequate when discussing meal planning with an adolescent with an eating disorder. Emphasizing food as fuel for the body, the source of energy in our daily lives grounds the goal of increasing a patient's energy level, endurance, and strength in the need for food. It is also important to recognize cognitive distortions of adolescents with anorexia nervosa. Examples include dichotomous, all-or-none thinking; overgeneralization; jumping to conclusions; catastrophizing; emotional reasoning; personalization; and the use of "should" statements. These generate behaviors such as breaking foods down into good or bad categories, having a day ruined because of one unexpected event, or choosing foods based on rigid restrictions rather than personal desires or wishes. In combination with the perfectionism that characterizes adolescents with anorexia nervosa, cognitive patterns can lead to extreme levels of fat restriction (<5 g/d) or strict vegetarianism.

Finally, delayed gastric emptying occurs with malnutrition, leading to early satiety and fullness with small meals. Although this generally abates with a few weeks of healthy eating, it can preclude adequate nutrition, especially if low-calorie foods and drinks continue to be ingested. Therefore, frequent, small meals that are high in carbohydrates, starting early in the day can be helpful. Some patients find liquid nutritional supplements helpful, since they occupy a small volume and have more rapid transit time than solid food. Prokinetic agents, such as metoclopramide, can be used if these symptoms are debilitating, but may be associated with limiting side effects.

Hospitalization

Some clinicians include falling below a predetermined minimum weight as an indication for hospitalization for an adolescent with moderate anorexia nervosa. Low weight is only one index of malnutrition. Weight should not be used as the sole criterion for admission to the hospital. Most adolescents with moderate anorexia nervosa realize the wisdom in the adage "a pint is a pound the world around." They may drink fluids, or hide heavy objects in their underwear prior to weigh-in if weight, alone, determines hospital admission. This may result in acute hyponatremia or dangerous degrees of unrecognized weight loss. A focus on health that includes a physical examination and consideration of body temperature, pulse, blood pressure, and orthostatic cardiovascular changes generally is more physiologically defensible than an arbitrary minimum. However, some patients need to know a concrete minimum threshold to avoid hospitalization.

Energy Needs and Dietary Prescription for Hospitalized Patients

Most adolescents with severe anorexia nervosa who are hospitalized require at least 1500 cal/d to maintain weight. Their reduced basal metabolic rate (BMR) may be as low as 800 to 1000 cal/d, and maintenance requirements are 130% to 150% of BMR. Approximately 1 g of weight is gained for every 5 cal of intake in excess of output; to accrue an additional 100 g of weight requires an excess of 500 cal. At low weight, few calories are expended in exercise than at higher weights; even with 1 hour of vigorous exercise, the patient expends ≤400 cal. If an adolescent appears to eat >3000 cal daily and still does not gain weight, it is likely that food is being vomited or discarded or that unrecognized exercise is occurring. Younger patients require slightly more energy to gain weight than older patients, since some of their intake is allocated to growth.

In prescribing an initial caloric intake, the clinician must recognize that gaining weight is frightening and that patients who demonstrate decreased metabolic rate (hypothermia, bradycardia, hypotension, and lethargy) may gain weight more readily than physiologically stable individuals. Initial weight gain can be rapid for 3 reasons. First, many malnourished adolescents are hypovolemic and gain weight in the form of extracellular fluid. Second, their basal metabolic rate can be half of normal. This reduction in energy expenditure enables calories ingested to exceed calories expended even at low levels of intake, resulting in weight gain in the form of body tissues. Third, these newly formed tissues are two thirds lean, not entirely fat as presumed by most patients, regardless of the protein content of the diet. It requires much less energy to produce protein-rich lean tissues than it does to produce fat-rich storage tissues (that are formed in quantity only after restoration of the lean body mass). Thus, more weight is gained initially for each excess calorie over expenditure than will be gained later as the patient approaches normal weight and body composition.

Therefore, although the daily requirement may eventually exceed 2500 calories, one should not attempt to prescribe an increase of more than 50% over present average daily intake of energy. Not only is the patient unlikely to respond favorably to a normal diet, but it is also unnecessary and can be physically and psychologically dangerous if the patient gains weight too quickly. Parents, especially, need to recognize that "more" is not necessarily "better" with respect to eating and weight gain. By focusing on a gradual, monitored increased intake, the dietitian can often lessen the adolescent's resistance to changing eating habits.

The minimal daily caloric intake can begin at about 1000 to 1200 calories, but may need to be lower if the patient was ingesting only a few hundred calories per day prior to admission. Intake is increased, as necessary, at 250- to 500-calorie increments every 2 days. In severely malnourished patients fluid retention, congestive heart failure,[15] hypophosphatemia,[16] and other manifestations of the refeeding syndrome can occur with too-rapid replacement. Careful monitoring of serum mineral values, including sodium, potassium, calcium, magnesium, and phosphorus is very important. It is rarely advisable to decrease the daily caloric minimum once it is established at a higher level. Lowering energy intake should be considered only if the patient has demonstrated consistent weight gain not attributable to fluid.

Food Choices

An adolescent with anorexia nervosa typically agonizes obsessively over decisions relating to choosing and consuming food—eating means he or she will disappoint himself or herself by giving in, but not eating means he or she will disappoint those whom he or she would like to please. Therefore, he or she should be allowed ≤10 minutes to make menu selections and ≤30 minutes to complete a meal. If the patient is unable to choose sufficient food within the 10-minute allotment, additional foods are chosen by the dietitian. If the patient does not clear a food tray within the 30-minute allotment, the tray can be removed, and the uneaten portions can be returned at the next meal time or replaced with fresh food. Alternatively, the balance of energy needs for the meal can be taken as a liquid supplement. In extremely resistant cases, in which the medical stability of the patient is tenuous, that nutrition may need to be supplied via nasogastric tube or by parenteral nutrition.[17] Attempts to increase appetite with medications, such as selective serotonin reuptake inhibitors, have not been found to be effective[18] and pharmacotherapy is not recommended unless also combined with adequate nutrition.[19]

References

1. Becker AE, Grinspoon SK, Klibanski A, Herzog DB. Eating disorders. *N Engl J Med.* 1999;340:1092–1098
2. American Dietetic Association. Position of the American Dietetic Association: nutrition intervention in the treatment of anorexia nervosa, bulimia nervosa, and eating disorders not otherwise specified (EDNOS). *J Am Diet Assoc.* 2001;101:810–819
3. van der Ster Wallin G, Norring C, Lennemas MA, Holmgren S. Food selection in anorectics and bulimics: food items, nutrient content and nutrient density. *J Am Coll Nutr.* 1995;14:271–277

4. Comerci GD. Eating disorders in adolescents. *Pediatr Rev.* 1988;10:37–47

5. Levenkron S. *Anatomy of Anorexia.* New York, NY: W. W. Norton; 2001

6. Fisher M, Golden NH, Katzman DK, et al. Eating disorders in adolescents: a background paper. *J Adolesc Health.* 1995;16:420–437

7. Kreipe RE, Dukarm CP. Eating disorders in adolescents and older children. *Pediatr Rev.* 1999;20:410–421

8. Keys A, Brozek J, Henschel A, Mickelsen O, Taylor HL. *The Biology of Human Starvation.* Minneapolis, MN: University of Minnesota Press; 1950

9. Forbes GB, Kreipe RE, Lipinski BA, Hodgman CH. Body composition changes during recovery from anorexia nervosa: comparison of two dietary regimes. *Am J Clin Nutr.* 1984;40:1137–1145

10. Scalfi L, Marra M, Caldara A, Silvestri E, Contaldo F. Changes in bioimpedance analysis after stable refeeding of undernourished anorexic patients. *Int J Obes Relat Metab Disord.* 1999;23:133–137

11. Hadigan CM, Anderson EJ, Miller KK, et al. Assessment of macronutrient and micronutrient intake in women with anorexia nervosa. *Int J Eat Disord.* 2000;28:284–292

12. Rock CL, Curran-Celentano J. Nutritional management of eating disorders. *Psychiatr Clin North Am.* 1996;19:701–713

13. Melchior JC. From malnutrition to refeeding during anorexia nervosa. *Curr Opin Clin Nutr Metab Care.* 1998;1:481–485

14. Marcason W. Nutrition therapy and eating disorders: what is the correct calorie level for clients with anorexia? *J Am Diet Assoc.* 2002;102:644

15. Kohn MR, Golden NH, Shenker IR. Cardiac arrest and delirium: presentations of the refeeding syndrome in severely malnourished adolescents with anorexia nervosa. *J Adolesc Health.* 1998;22:239–243

16. Fisher M, Simpser E, Schneider M. Hypophosphatemia secondary to oral refeeding in anorexia nervosa. *Int J Eat Disord.* 2000;28:181–187

17. Mehler PS, Weiner KA. Treatment of anorexia nervosa with total parenteral nutrition. *Nutr Clin Pract.* 1995;10:183–187

18. Ferguson CP, La Via MC, Crossan PJ, Kaye WH. Are serotonin selective reuptake inhibitors effective in underweight anorexia nervosa? *Int J Eat Disord.* 1999;25:11–17

19. Casper RC. How useful are pharmacological treatments in eating disorders? *Psychopharmacol Bull.* 2002;36:88–104

39

Nutrition of Children With HIV-1 Infection

Infection with the human immunodeficiency type-1 virus (HIV-1) is a worldwide problem of increasing magnitude. The World Health Organization estimates that 25.8 to 41.8 million adults and children are infected with HIV, the majority of whom are in developing countries.[1] In 1999, the cause of death worldwide in up to 670 000 children aged 0 through 14 years was attributed to HIV/acquired immunodeficiency syndrome (AIDS).[1] With the advent of highly active antiretroviral therapy (HAART) and improved prophylactic regimens, HIV-1 has become a chronic illness in developed nations. With the increasing number of children surviving with HIV/AIDS, the need for appropriate supportive care is paramount. Clinicians who care for children with HIV/AIDS should be aware of potential nutritional problems and their consequences. Knowledge and implementation of effective nutritional therapies is important to improve medical outcomes and quality of life. With appropriate combination of antiviral therapy and nutrition support, many of these patients are now able to lead relatively normal lives.

The Wasting Syndrome

During the early 1980s, AIDS was first recognized in Africa as an epidemic and was initially termed *slim disease* because people in Uganda were dying of severe malnutrition for otherwise unknown reasons.[2] Eventually, the virus causing AIDS was found. Wasting is included as one of the principal criteria for the diagnosis of severely symptomatic AIDS (category C, Table 39.1).[3]

The Centers for Disease Control and Prevention (CDC)[3] defines wasting in children younger than 13 years as (1) persistent weight loss of more than 10% of baseline, (2) downward crossing of at least 2 percentile lines on the weight-for-age chart in a child 1 year or older, or (c) less than the 5th percentile on weight-for-height chart on 2 consecutive measurements at least 30 days apart plus chronic diarrhea or documented fever for at least 30 days, whether intermittent or constant.

The relationship between protein-energy malnutrition (PEM) and adverse effects on the immune system resulting in immune deficiency states has been

Table 39.1.
Pediatric Criteria for Diagnosis of AIDS*

Immunologic Category, by Evidence of Suppression	Clinical Category, by Symptom Severity			
	N, None	A, Mild	B, Moderate	C, Severe
1, None	N1	A1	B1	C1
2, Moderate	N2	A2	B2	C2
3, Severe	N3	A3	B3	C3

* Centers for Disease Control and Prevention classification system of HIV infection in children younger than 13 years (revised, 1994). Children born to women infected with HIV and whose status is not confirmed are classified by using the above grid with a letter E (for perinatally exposed) placed before the appropriate classification code (eg, EN2). From Centers for Disease Control and Prevention.[3]

recognized for many years.[4] Table 39.2 lists the differences and similarities between the effects of PEM and HIV-1 on the immune system. Thus on a basic level, PEM may exacerbate the immunologic effects of HIV-1. Epidemiologic studies of both adult and pediatric HIV-1 infection suggest that nutritional status can impact independently on quality of life and survival, likely due to the effect of malnutrition on immune function. Wasting is related to length of survival.[5,6] Weight loss has been associated with increased infectious complications in patients with AIDS. Conversely, HIV-1 and its complications have been associated with nutritional disorders. Higher HIV-1 viral load has been associated with a greater risk of growth failure.[7,8] In addition, other factors such as lower CD4 T lymphocyte counts, infectious complications such as pneumonia, maternal drug use during pregnancy, lower infant CD4+ T-cell count, and exposure to antiretroviral therapy (non-protease inhibitor) have been associated with growth problems.[9] (Unpublished data.)

A variety of disturbed growth patterns have been described for children infected with HIV-1,[9–13] ranging from symmetric delays in weight and height to severe wasting with normal height. The differences in growth patterns are likely due to the variable manifestations of the disease in children infected with HIV-1, associated with factors such as viral load and infections as mentioned previously. In developed countries, children infected with HIV-1 show decline in both weight and length as early as the first 1 to 3 months of life. Sequential follow-up shows that growth in children infected with HIV-1 remains below growth in age- and gender-matched uninfected children.

Table 39.2.

Comparison of Body Composition, Energy Expenditure, and Immunologic Function in Protein-Energy Malnutrition (PEM), Sepsis, and HIV Infection

Condition	Body Composition	Energy Expenditure	Immune Function
PEM (starvation)	Decreased fat leading to decreased lean body mass	Decreased	Decreased white blood cell count, cell-mediated immunity, and T-cell function; Decreased immuno-globulin (Ig) A and E; Increased or decreased IgG
Sepsis	Decreased lean body mass leading to decreased fat	Increased	Activated (?effective)
HIV	Decreased lean body mass leading to decreased fat	Unchanged to increased according to severity of infection	Increased IgG; Decreased CD4 count and lymphocyte function

Many pediatric studies have shown progressive declines in lean body mass over time in children with HIV/AIDS, while measures of fat stores remain constant, yet low.[10,11] Currently, there is conflicting literature on whether there is more of a pattern of cachexia (preferential wasting of muscle over fat) or normal weight loss with initial loss of fat over lean body mass[14,15] in adults with HIV/AIDS. Cytokines may be responsible for some of the growth, metabolic, and immunologic effects associated with HIV-1 infection.[16] Elevated serum triglyceride levels are seen in patients with HIV/AIDS and correlate with de novo hepatic lipogenesis.[17]

Causes of Malnutrition in AIDS

Nutritional problems in children with HIV/AIDS may be due to several mechanisms working independently or synergistically. These causes are summarized in Table 39.3. Insufficient consumption of nutrients is one factor that may lead to poor nutritional status. A variety of potential factors may lead to abnormal intake as outlined in Table 39.3. For example, inflammation and ulcers of the upper gastrointestinal tract can lead to anorexia owing to odynophagia, dysphagia, or abdominal pain that is associated with eating. In one series, 70% of upper gastrointestinal endoscopies in children infected with HIV-1 revealed abnormal histology.[18] These lesions may be due to acid-related injury or infectious agents such as *Candida albicans*, cytomegalovirus, or herpes simplex virus, all of which may cause inflammation and pain with swallowing or after

Table 39.3.

Causes of Nutritional Deficiencies and Wasting in Human Immunodeficiency Virus (HIV)/Acquired Immunodeficiency Syndrome (AIDS)

1. Decreased nutrient intake
Primary anorexia
Peptic disease
Opportunistic infections of upper GI tract (Candida, CMV, HSV)
Idiopathic aphthous ulcers
Dysgeusia (zinc deficiency)
Pancreatic/hepatobiliary disease
Encephalopathy

2. Gastrointestinal malabsorption
Mucosal disease
    Infectious
    Inflammatory
    Disaccharidase deficiency
    Protein-losing enteropathy
    Fat malabsorption
Hepatobiliary
    Sclerosing cholangitis
    Chronic pancreatitis
    Co-infection with HBV/HCV

3. Increased nutritional requirements or tissue catabolism
Protein wasting
Hypermetabolism/related to degree of immune suppression
Futile metabolic cycling
    Secondary to:
Fever, infections, sepsis
Neoplasms (Kaposi's sarcoma, lymphoma)
Medications
Release of catabolic factors (cytokines, tumor necrosis factor)

4. Psychosocial factors
Poverty
Illness in biological family members
Limited access to health care
Substance abuse

eating. As well, oral ulcers that are due to viral agents or idiopathic oral ulcers[19] are common and may cause pain with eating and reduce oral intake.

Pancreatic and biliary tract disease can also cause vomiting and abdominal pain in children infected with HIV-1 leading to poor oral intake. Pancreatic disease has been linked to medications (eg, pentamidine, 2′, 3′ dideoxyinosine

[ddI], sulfa medications, and some protease inhibitors [Table 39.4]) and opportunistic infections (eg, cytomegalovirus, *Cryptosporidium*, and myco-bacterial disease).[20,21] Biliary tract disease with sclerosing cholangitis and papillary stenosis has been linked to *Cryptosporidium*, cytomegalovirus, and *Microsporidia*.[22,23] Primary anorexia, described in patients with cancer and other chronic disorders, may also contribute to inadequate oral intake. It is postulated that increased cytokine production (eg, tumor nerosis factor, interferon-gamma, and interleukins 1 and 6) may be associated with anorexia. In animal models, administration of exogenous tumor necrosis factor (TNF) has produced anorexia and cachexia.[24] Tumor necrosis factor also causes delayed gastric emptying, which can increase anorexia as well.[25] Currently, the scientific data that implicate these cytokines as mediators of anorexia are controversial.[26]

Human immunodeficiency virus encephalopathy, which can be present in up to 16% of children with HIV-1 infection,[27] may result in the physical inabil-ity to consume enough calories to sustain growth. Oral administration of feed-ings under this condition may also be dangerous, owing to the high risk of aspiration in children who are neurologically compromised. Finally, many medications that children infected with HIV are required to take may result in gastric irritation, vomiting, nausea, and diarrhea. These medications are listed in Table 39.4.

A few small studies have shown differences in energy intake between chil-dren with HIV-1 and noninfected children, suggesting substandard intakes may relate to growth differences.[8,28,29] However, a large prospective study has shown that stable children with HIV-1 in an ambulatory setting whose growth was below a control group, received well over the recommended dietary allowance (RDA) in total calories and protein, similar to the noninfected control children.[28] However, in this study, higher intake was associated with improve-ment in weight and fat mass.

Malabsorption may also contribute to malnutrition. The etiology of malab-sorption is multifactorial but includes gastrointestinal mucosal abnormalities leading to macro- and micronutrient malabsorption. These mucosal changes can be due to local HIV-1 infection of the gut or secondary enteric infections. There is evidence that certain gastrointestinal epithelial cells bind and selec-tively transfer HIV-1 from the cells' apical to basolateral surface, where viral translocation across the epithelium encounters lamina propria macrophages and T cells.[30] As a result of either local HIV-1 infection or of the damage caused by a secondary infection, mucosal function is compromised with result-

Table 39.4.
Medications and Common Gastrointestinal Side Effects

Medication	Action	Side Effects
Abacavir	nucleoside analogue-reverse transcriptase inhibitor (NRTI) antiviral	nausea, vomiting, abdominal pain, pancreatitis, abnormal liver function tests
Acyclovir	antiviral	nausea, abdominal pain, diarrhea, abnormal liver function tests
Amprenavir	protease inhibitor (PI)	abdominal pain, diarrhea
Azithromycin	antibacterial	nausea, vomiting, melena, jaundice
Ciprofloxacin	antibacterial	ileus, jaundice, bleeding, diarrhea, anorexia, oralulcers, hepatitis, pancreatitis, vomiting, abdominal pain
Clarithromycin	antibacterial	nausea, diarrhea, abdominal pain, abnormal taste
Dideoxycytidine (ddC)	NRTI	nausea, vomiting, abdominal pain
Dideoxyinosine (ddl)	NRTI	nausea, vomiting, abdominal pain, pancreatitis, abnormal liver function tests
Efavirenz	NRTI	nausea, vomiting, abnormal liver function tests
Erythromycin	antibacterial	nausea, vomiting, abdominal pain
Ganciclovir	antiviral	nausea, vomiting, diarrhea, anorexia, abnormal liver function tests
Indinavir	protease inhibitor	nausea, vomiting, abdominal pain, diarrhea, changes in taste, jaundice, abnormal liver function tests
Ketoconazole	antifungal	hepatotoxicity
Lamivudine (3TC)	NRTI	nausea, diarrhea, vomiting, abdominal pain, pancreatitis, abnormal liver function tests
Nelfinavir	protease inhibitor	nausea, diarrhea, vomiting, abdominal pain, pancreatitis, abnormal liver function tests
Nevirapine	NRTI	stomatitis, nausea, abdominal pain, elevated gamma glutamyl transpeptidase
Pentamidine	antiparasitic	abdominal pain, bleeding, hepatitis, pancreatitis, nausea, vomiting

Table 39.4.
Medications and Common Gastrointestinal Side Effects *(continued)*

Medication	Action	Side Effects
Rifampin	antibacterial	abdominal pain, nausea, vomiting, diarrhea, jaundice
Ritonavir	protease inhibitor	nausea, vomiting, diarrhea, abdominal pain, pancreatitis, abnormal liver function tests
Saquinavir	protease inhibitor	mouth ulcers, nausea, abdominal pain, diarrhea, pancreatitis, abnormal liver function tests
Stavudine (d4T)	NRTI	nausea, vomiting, abdominal pain, diarrhea, pancreatitis, abnormal liver function tests
Sulfonamides	antibacterial	hepatitis, pancreatitis, stomatitis, nausea, vomiting, abdominal pain
Zidovuding (ZDV)	NRTI	nausea, vomiting, abdominal pain, abnormal liver function tests

ing malabsorption. Because of the difficulty in treating many of these infections, the diarrhea may be unremitting and predispose to the severe malnutrition that may lead to eventual mortality, especially in developing nations.

The evaluation of diarrhea in patients with AIDS yields a specific cause in 50% to 85% of patients, with most being effectively treated.[31] The nonspecific AIDS enteropathy[32] may be due in part to undiagnosed infections or to HIV-1 itself. Several investigators have reported impaired carbohydrate, fat, and protein absorption in children with HIV/AIDS[33,34]; the extent of malabsorption is not always correlated with the degree of malnutrition.[33]

In addition to nutrient losses as a result of diarrhea, gastrointestinal bleeding due to mucosal ulcerations leads to loss of nutrients with the loss of blood. Opportunistic infections affect the hepatobiliary system and pancreas in addition to the gastrointestinal tract and may lead to malabsorption. The site and severity of infection vary according to the infecting organism (Table 39.5).

Other nutrient deficiencies often seen in patients with AIDS-related gastrointestinal disease include vitamin B_{12}, folic acid, thiamine, zinc, selenium, calcium, and magnesium. Fat-soluble vitamins, particularly vitamins A and D, may be malabsorbed, and deficiencies of these vitamins have been described.

Table 39.5.

Infectious Gastrointestinal Manifestations of Human Immunodeficiency Virus (HIV)/Acquired Immunodeficiency Syndrome (AIDS)*

Site	Manifestations or Infecting Organisms
Oral	Candidiasis HSV Human papillomavirus Oral hairy leukoplakia Kaposi's sarcoma Lymphoma
Esophagus	Candidiasis CMV HSV Cryptosporidiosis Kaposi's sarcoma Lymphoma
Stomach	CMV Cryptosporidiosis Kaposi's sarcoma *Helicobacter pylori*
Small intestine	Giardiasis Cryptosporidiosis CMV *Salmonella* species Enteroaggregative *E Coli* *Blastocystis hominis* *Isospora belli* Rotavirus, calcivirus, astrovirus, coronavirus, picobirnavirus Adenovirus *Shigella* species *Mycobacterium* species Lymphoma
Colon	CMV *Salmonella* species *Shigella* species *Campylobacter* species *Entamoeba* species Lymphoma *C Difficile* Adenovirus
Anus/rectum	Kaposi's sarcoma Lymphoma Squamous cell carcinoma Papovavirus

Table 39.5.
Infectious Gastrointestinal Manifestations of Human Immunodeficiency Virus (HIV)/Acquired Immunodeficiency Syndrome (AIDS)* *(continued)*

Site	Manifestations or Infecting Organisms
Hepatobiliary	*Mycobacterium* species CMV *Cryptococcus, histoplasmosis* Hepatitis B, C, or D Cryptosporidiosis Kaposi's sarcoma Microsporida
Pancreas	CMV *Mycobacterium* species Cryptosporidiosis

* HSV indicates herpes simplex virus; CMV, cytomegalovirus.

Fat malabsorption and protein-losing enteropathy are likely a result of severe enteritis usually caused by secondary infections. Small-bowel bacterial overgrowth, a result of gastrointestinal dysmotility or hypochlorhydria, may also predispose the individual to malabsorption. Pancreatic insufficiency is rarer, although it has been described in some patients infected with HIV-1.[35] Diarrhea may also be caused by antiretroviral therapy (Table 39.4), other medications (especially antibiotics), malignancies, and, rarely, inflammatory bowel disease.

Asymptomatic chronic viral infections may have some effect on energy utilization, and can predispose children to secondary infections, which can alter energy utilization patterns. These infections can increase or shunt effective use of energy substrates from normal, healthy growth patterns to abnormal ones, as in many children with chronic illness, including cystic fibrosis, inflammatory bowel disease, congenital heart disease, and childhood cancer.[34–36] The chronic viral activity of HIV-1 is likely no different. In small studies of energy expen-diture, there are, in general no differences in resting energy expenditure (REE)[8,29,36] or total energy expenditure (TEE)[8,37] between children with HIV-1 with growth failure and those with normal rates of growth. However, adults with HIV-1 infection show increasing REE with increasing severity of illness,[38] especially with secondary infection and more advanced HIV-1 disease.[39,40]

Psychosocial factors are also important contributors to suboptimal growth of children infected with HIV-1. An unstable home environment and inadequate emotional and social support may obviously affect growth in both children infected with HIV-1[41] and noninfected children.[42,43] Children with HIV-1 infection are at risk for living with parents who are ill, who have limited access to social services and support, and who may have ongoing problems with drug and substance abuse.[44] Investigators have found maternal crack and cocaine use during pregnancy to be a predictor of growth and nutritional problems for the child.[9] This finding is not unique for HIV-1, as it has been reported in other non-HIV-1 cohorts.[45] Children born to women who use drugs are often small, suggesting that drugs have a prenatal effect, but the post-natal home environment is likely to influence growth as well. Current studies have also found that home care providers can both positively or negatively influence functional status of children infected with HIV-1.[41]

The Nutritional Effects of Highly Active Antiretroviral Therapy (HAART)

Protease inhibitors are highly potent antiretroviral agents that act by selectively blocking HIV-1 protease, an enzyme necessary for HIV-1 replication in the later stages of virus production.[46] Studies in children suggest that protease inhibitor therapy is associated with a reduction in viral load and an increase in CD4 cell count,[47,48] although longitudinal studies are essential to determine the duration of this immune response. Current pediatric treatment guidelines include a protease inhibitor in the recommended combination therapy regimen for any child infected with HIV-1 with the following: clinical symptoms (CDC Class A, B, C); immune suppression (CDC Class 2,3) (Table 39.1); or any child diagnosed under the age of 1 year, due to the high viral load during this period.[49] Thus, the majority of children with HIV-1 in developed countries are given these medications.

Over the past several years, coincident with the introduction of HAART, a clinical syndrome of body fat redistribution and metabolic changes have been described predominantly in adults.[50] Adults infected with HIV-1 receiving protease inhibitor therapy or HAART regimens have developed a syndrome of peripheral insulin resistance, hyperlipidemia, and lipodystrophy (truncal obesity, dorso-cervical fat pad, and extremity and facial wasting).[50] Clinical and biochemical abnormalities associated with the lipodystrophy syndrome are shown in Table 39.6. Risk factors associated with the development of the fat redistribution syndrome in adults include female gender, increasing age, and higher pre-therapy body weight.[51] Complications associated with the development of the fat redistribution syndrome include higher rates of diabetes mellitus and

Table 39.6.
Clinical and Biochemical Abnormalities Associated With the Lipodystrophy Syndrome

Clinical Features	Laboratory Features

Increased abdominal (visceral) fat
  Increased waist-to-hip ratio (more
  reliable in adults)
Buffalo hump
Fat atrophy
  Wasting of extremities
  Wasting of buttocks
  Loss or thinning of facial fat,
  prominence of nasolabial fold
No change to increased weight
Fatigue and weakness
	Hyperlipidemia
	  Increased triglycerides
	  Increased total cholesterol
	  Increased LDL
	  Decreased HDL
	Insulin resistance
	  Normal to increased serum glucose
	  Increased insulin
	  Increased C peptide
	  Decreased glucose tolerance/insulin resistance

premature cardiovascular disease. Medical compliance with drug therapy may be poorer owing to the cosmetic side effects of therapy. This entity has not been as well defined in children, although many centers are reporting anecdotal experience.[52]

One recently published study showed that protease inhibitor therapy affects weight, weight-for-height, and mid-arm muscle circumference (AMC) of children infected with HIV-1, independent of the concurrent decrease in HIV-1 viral load and improved CD4 T-lymphocyte counts.[53] The immediate treatment effects were most apparent with an improvement in weight and AMC and there was a trend toward increased height and lean body mass. Therapeutic strategies to diminish the clinical and biochemical features of the fat redistribution syndrome include oral hypoglycemic agents such as metformin[54] and troglitazone (although liver toxicity limits its use).[55] Results of similar studies in children are not yet available.

Recommendations for Nutritional Support

Wasting contributes significantly to the morbidity and mortality of patients infected with HIV-1. With the advent of HAART and its attendant nutritional consequences, potential metabolic complications are likely to ensue over the years as children age with HIV-1 infection. The most effective role the pediatrician can play in the nutritional care of the child infected with HIV-1 is close surveillance of nutritional and metabolic complications over time and with evolving medical therapy. The efficacy of nutritional support in children with

HIV/AIDS is emerging as an important ancillary treatment. A gross assessment of nutritional status can be achieved by vigilant monitoring of weight status (ie, weight-for-age and weight-for-height). The very early detection of failure to gain weight allows the opportunity for prevention of malnutrition, clearly a more effective intervention approach than repletion once malnutrition or failure to thrive has occurred. In addition, changes in body composition become a very important sign of disease progression and can be determined through serial measurements of midarm circumference, triceps skinfolds, and bioelectric impedance analysis.

Enteral tube feeding can be administered in the hospital and at home to children with HIV-1 infection. Children supported in this way show an increase in weight-for-age, weight-for-height, and adipose store but no improvement in height-for-age or lean body mass over the short term.[6,56] There is evidence that nutritional status independently predicts morbidity and mortality; children whose weight improved with gastrostomy tube feedings survived longer than those whose weight did not improve.[6] Nutrition also improves functional status.[41] The influence of socioeconomic factors on the development of wasting syndrome, HIV-1 infection itself, and nutritional status needs to be considered and targeted because populations of lower socioeconomic status who are at higher risk for nutritional and other health problems predominate among patients with HIV/AIDS. The influence of the socioeconomic environment on the provision of adequate nutrition may be particularly critical. Limiting factors that may be present include poor health of the caregiver because of HIV-1 infection or AIDS, inadequate cooking facilities, poverty and limited food availability, emotional deprivation, and inexperienced parenting.

Complete data on which to base nutrition interventions for children infected with HIV-1 are lacking. Optimal treatment to decrease viral load is important, as high viral loads are directly linked with poorer nutritional state. The following are guidelines to provide optimal nutritional care of children infected with HIV-1.

1. *Nutrition assessment* should be performed on all patients regardless of symptoms. This assessment should include a review of the medical and dietary history, a dietary diary with calorie count, anthropometric measurements (ie, weight, height, head circumference, muscle circumferences, skinfolds [4-site], and measurement of baseline laboratory values [eg,

complete blood count, albumin, prealbumin, iron, zinc, lipid profile, and absorptive tests as indicated]). When inadequate weight gain or weight loss is identified, aggressive diagnostic evaluation should be pursued to detect opportunistic infections or other inflammatory lesions of the gastrointestinal tract. With clinical symptoms, an evaluation of gastrointestinal absorption is indicated. Treatment of underlying infections will likely improve the response to nutritional and medical management. Determining the degree and extent of gastrointestinal malabsorption will help guide dietary recommendations. Indirect calorimetry may be useful to guide nutrition support by determining basal energy expenditure. With clinically evident fat redistribution syndrome, an oral glucose tolerance test and C-peptide levels should be ascertained. If these studies are abnormal, dietary and exercise advice and an oral hypoglycemic agent should be considered.

2. *Nutritional counseling* should provide guidance for patients to maintain a diet that provides the RDAs or dietary reference intakes (DRIs) of nutrients. The intake and dietary composition should be adjusted according to the degree of gastrointestinal dysfunction and insulin resistance and may include a low-fat, lactose-free, low-fiber, caffeine-free diet. Infants may benefit from increased caloric density of a formula that is achieved by adding cereal or modular nutrient supplements (eg, glucose polymers, protein powders, medium-chain triglycerides if needed [this is an expensive supplement] and vegetable oils) or by concentrating the caloric density of the formula. Patients with diarrhea may benefit from an elemental formula. Fad diets, including megavitamins and amino acid supplementation, should be discouraged. Frequent nutritional assessment is necessary to determine the response to the nutritional intervention. Further recommendations should be made if the child fails to respond to a specific intervention.

3. *Specialized nutrition support* is indicated before the onset of malnutrition, because undernutrition will complicate the disease course for patients with HIV/AIDS. Oral nutrition supplementation is preferable. However, enteral tube feedings (eg, nasogastric or gastrostomy) may be necessary to provide supplemental or total nutritional support for patients with inadequate oral intake. Appropriate diagnostic studies to treat an underlying gastrointestinal disorder that results in inadequate intake should be performed prior to initiating supplemental enteral feedings. If inadequate intake is due to delayed feeding skills, support by a team including a

speech or occupational therapist, a behavioral therapist, and a registered dietitian may be effective. Parenteral nutrition is reserved for children in whom the enteral route is not feasible and includes those with severe malabsorption, gastrointestinal dysfunction due to infection or dysmotility, and pancreatitis. Parenteral nutrition should not be instituted with an ongoing disseminated infection.

4. *Vitamin and mineral supplementation* should be provided so the dietary intake of vitamins and minerals is 1 to 5 times the RDA. Megadoses (10 times the RDA) are discouraged. Routine monitoring and supplementation of selected micronutrients (vitamin A, E, folate, B12, iron, zinc) are recommended.

5. *Nutritional appetite stimulants and growth hormone* may be useful in selected patients. Megesterol acetate should not be used in children who have documented insulin resistance as this therapy may exacerbate it. Growth hormone may be useful in the preadolescent whose growth is significantly stunted, although it is unclear whether overall adult height will be ultimately improved.

6. *Drug-nutrient interactions* should be considered. In addition, many of the antiretroviral drugs and medications used to treat illness or symptoms related to HIV-1 infection may cause nausea, anorexia, abdominal pain, diarrhea, dry mouth, and alterations in taste. The adverse effects of medications and their administration schedules on intake should be considered.

7. *A nutrition support team* should be involved to ensure optimal nutrition monitoring and care. A core team of physician, nutritionist, and social worker collaborating with other health care providers offers the best opportunity to achieve optimal nutritional health for individual patients.

Conclusion

The cause of nutritional problems in children with HIV-1 infection is complex and likely multifactorial. While the incidence of malnutrition in developed countries has decreased with HAART, a significant number of children continue to have problems with malnutrition, gastrointestinal dysfunction, and some with emerging insulin resistance. Optimal nutritional support includes complete nutritional assessment and follow-up of every child and adolescent with HIV/AIDS. Enteral nutrition support with improved body weight appears to be associated with survival.

References

1. Joint United Nations Programme on HIV/AIDS. Report on the global HIV/AIDS epidemic, June 2000. Geneva, Switzerland: World Health Organization; 2000. Available at: http://www.unaids.org/epidemic_update/report_june00/index.htm. Accessed March 7, 2003

2. Serwadda D, Mugerwa RD, Sewankambo NK, et al. Slim disease: a new disease in Uganda and its association with HTLV-III infection. *Lancet*. 1985;2:849–852

3. Centers for Disease Control and Prevention. 1994 revised classification system for human immunodeficiency virus infection in children less than 13 years of age. *MMWR Morb Mortal Wkly Rep*. 1994;43(RR-12):1–10

4. Chandra RK, Kumari S. Nutrition and immunity: an overview. *J Nutr*. 1994; 124(suppl 8):1433S–1435S

5. Carey VJ, Yong FH, Frenkel LM, McKinney RE Jr. Pediatric AIDS prognosis using somatic growth velocity. *AIDS*. 1998;12:1361–1369

6. Miller TL, Awnetwant EL, Evans S, Morris VM, Vazquez IM, McIntosh K. Gastrostomy tube supplementation for HIV-infected children. *Pediatrics*. 1995;96:696–702

7. Johann-Liang R, O'Neill L, Cervia J, et al. Energy balance, viral burden, insulin-like growth factor-1, interleukin-6 and growth impairment in children infected with human immunodeficiency virus. *AIDS*. 2000;14:683–690

8. Arpadi SM, Cuff PA, Kotler DP, et al. Growth velocity, fat-free mass and energy intake are inversely related to viral load in HIV-infected children. *J Nutr*. 2000; 130:2498–2502

9. Moye J Jr, Rich KC, Kalish LA, et al. Natural history of somatic growth in infants born to women infected by human immunodeficiency virus. *J Pediatr*. 1996;128:58–69

10. Miller TL, Evans SJ, Orav EJ, Morris V, McIntosh K, Winter HS. Growth and body composition in children infected with the human immunodeficiency virus-1. *Am J Clin Nutr*. 1993;57:588–592

11. Arpadi SM, Horlick MN, Wang J, Cuff P, Bamji M, Kotler DP. Body composition in prepubertal children with human immunodeficiency virus type 1 infection. *Arch Pediatr Adolesc Med*. 1998;152:688–693

12. Saavedra JM, Henderson RA, Perman JA, Hutton N, Livingston RA, Yolken RH. Longitudinal assessment of growth in children born to mothers with human immunodeficiency virus infection. *Arch Pediatr Adolesc Med*. 1995;149:497–502

13. McKinney RE Jr, Robertson RW. Effect of human immunodeficiency virus infection on the growth of young children. *J Pediatr*. 1993;123:579–582

14. Kotler DP, Wang J, Pierson RN. Body composition studies in patients with acquired immunodeficiency syndrome. *Am J Clin Nutr*. 1985;42:1255–1265

15. Mulligan K, Tai VW, Schambelan M. Cross-sectional and longitudinal evaluation of body composition in men with HIV infection. *J Acquir Immune Defic Syndr Hum Retroviral*. 1997;15:43–48

16. de Martino M, Galli L, Chiarelli F, et al. Interleukin-6 release by cultured peripheral blood mononuclear cells inversely correlates with height velocity, bone age, insulin-like growth factor-I, and insulin-like growth factor binding protein-3 serum levels in children with perinatal HIV-1 infection. *Clin Immunol.* 2000; 94:212–218

17. Hellerstein MK, Grunfeld C, Wu K, et al. Increased de novo hepatic lipogenesis in human immunodeficiency virus infection. *J Clin Endocrinol Metab.* 1993;76: 559–565

18. Miller TL, McQuinn L, Orav EJ. Endoscopy of the upper gastrointestinal tract as a diagnostic tool for children with human immunodeficiency virus infection. *J Pediatr.* 1997;130:766–773

19. Kotler DP, Reka S, Orenstein JM, Fox CH. Chronic idiopathic esophageal ulceration in the acquired immunodeficiency syndrome. Characterization and treatment with corticosteroids. *J Clin Gastroenterol.* 1992;15:284–290

20. Miller TL, Winter HS, Luginbuhl LM, Orav EJ, McIntosh KS. Pancreatitis in pediatric human immunodeficiency virus infection. *J Pediatr.* 1992;120:223–227

21. Butler KM, Venzon D, Henry N, et al. Pancreatitis in human immunodeficiency virus-infected children receiving dideoxyinosine. *Pediatrics.* 1993;91:747–751

22. Bouche H, Housset JL, Carnot F, et al. AIDS-related cholangitis: diagnostic features and course in 15 patients. *Hepatol* 1993;17:34–39

23. Pol S, Romana CA, Rich S, et al. Microsporidia infection in patients with human immunodeficiency virus and unexplained cholangitis. *N Engl J Med.* 1993;328: 95–99

24. Beutler B, Milsark IW, Cerami AC. Passive immunization against cachectin/tumor necrosis factor protects mice from lethal effect of endotoxin. *Science.* 1985;229: 869–871

25. Langhans W. Bacterial products and the control of ingestive behavior: clinical implications. *Nutrition.* 1996;12:303–315

26. Rimaniol AC, Zylberberg H, Zavala F, Viard JP. Inflammatory cytokines and inhibitors in HIV infection: correlation between interleukin-1 receptor antagonist and weight loss. *AIDS.* 1996;10:1349–1356

27. Tardieu M, Le Chenadec J, Persoz A, Meyer L, Blanche S, Mayaux MJ. HIV-1-related encephalopathy in infants compared with children and adults. French Pediatric HIV Infection Study and the SEROCO Group. *Neurology.* 2000;54:1089–1095

28. Henderson RA, Talusan K, Hutton N, Yolken RH, Caballero B. Resting energy expenditure and body composition in children with HIV infection. *J Acquir Immune Defic Syndr Hum Retroviral.* 1998;19:150–157

29. Miller TL, Evans S, Vasquez I, Orav EJ. Dietary intake is an important predictor of nutritional status in HIV-infected children [abstract]. *Pediatr Res.* 1997;41:85A

30. Meng G, Sellers MT, Mosteller-Barnum M, Rogers TS, Shaw GM, Smith PD. Lamina propria lymphocytes, not macrophages, express CCR5 and CXCR and are the likely target cell for human immunodeficiency virus type 1 in the intestinal mucosa. *J Infect Dis.* 2000;182:785–791

31. Weber R, Ledergerber B, Zbinden R, et al. Enteric infections and diarrhea in human immunodeficiency virus-infected persons: prospective community-based cohort study. *Arch Int Med.* 1999;159:1473–1480

32. Ullrich R, Zeitz M, Heise W, Líage M, Hoffken G, Riecken EO. Small intestinal structure and function in patients infected with human immunodeficiency virus (HIV): evidence for HIV-induced enteropathy. *Ann Intern Med.* 1989;111:15–21

33. Miller TL, Orav EJ, Martin SR, Cooper ER, McIntosh K, Winter HS. Malnutrition and carbohydrate malabsorption in children with vertically transmitted human immunodeficiency virus 1 infection. *Gastroenterology.* 1991;100:1296–1302

34. Yolken RH, Hart W, Oung I, Shiff C, Greenson J, Perman JA. Gastrointestinal dysfunction and disaccharide intolerance in children infected with human immunodeficiency virus. *J Pediatr.* 1991;118:359–363

35. Carroccio A, Fontana M, Spagnuolo MI, et al. Pancreatic dysfunction and its association with fat malabsorption in HIV infected children. *Gut.* 1998;43:558–563

36. Alfaro MP, Siegel RM, Baker RC, Heubi JE. Resting energy expenditure and body composition in pediatric HIV infection. *Pediatr AIDS HIV Infect.* 1995;6:276–280

37. Johann-Liang R, O'Neill L, Cervia J, et al. Energy balance, viral burden, insulin-like growth factor-1, interleukin-6 and growth impairment in children infected with human immunodeficiency virus. *AIDS.* 2000;14:683–690

38. Melchior JC, Raguin G, Boulier A, et al. Resting energy expenditure in human immunodeficiency virus-infected patients: comparison between patients with and without secondary infections. *Am J Clin Nutr.* 1993;57:614–619

39. Grunfeld C, Pang M, Shimizu L, Shigenaga JK, Jensen P, Feingold KR. Resting energy expenditure, caloric intake, and short-term weight change in human immunodeficiency virus infection and the acquired immunodeficiency syndrome. *Am J Clin Nutr.* 1992;55:455–460

40. Hommes MJ, Romijn JA, Godfried MH, et al. Increased resting energy expenditure in human immunodeficiency virus-infected men. *Metabolism.* 1990;39:1186–1190

41. Missmer SA, Speigelman D, Gorbach SL, Miller TL. Predictors of change in the functional status of children with human immunodeficiency virus infection. *Pediatrics.* 2000;106:E24

42. Money J. The syndrome of abuse dwarfism (psychosocial dwarfism or reversible hyposomatotropism). *Am J Dis Child.* 1977;131:508–513

43. Boulton TJ, Smith R, Single T. Psychosocial growth failure: a positive response to growth hormone and placebo. *Acta Paediatr.* 1992;81:322–325

44. Children whose mothers are infected with HIV. *Commun Dis Rep CDR Wkly.* 1995;5:111

45. Lifschitz MH, Wilson GS, Smith EO, Desmond MM. Fetal and postnatal growth of children born to narcotic-dependent women. *J Pediatr.* 1983;102:686–691

46. Kakuda TN, Struble KA, Piscitelli SC. Protease inhibitors for the treatment of human immunodeficiency virus infection. *Am J Health Syst Pharm.* 1998;55: 233–254

47. Mueller BU, Sleaseman J, Nelson RP Jr, et al. A phase I/II study of the protease inhibitor indinavir in children with HIV infection. *Pediatrics*. 1998;102:101–109

48. Rutstein RM, Feingold A, Meislich D, Word B, Rudy B. Protease inhibitor therapy in children with perinatally acquired HIV infection. *AIDS*. 1997;11:F107–F111

49. Working Group on Antiretroviral Therapy and Medical Management of HIV-Infected Children. *Guidelines for the Use of Antiretroviral Agents in Pediatric HIV Infection*. December 14, 2001. Available at: http://aidsinfo.nih.gov/guidelines/default_db2.asp?id-51. Accessed March 7, 2003

50. Carr A, Samaras K, Chisholm DJ, Cooper DA. Pathogenesis of HIV-1 protease inhibitor-associated peripheral lipodystrophy, hyperlipidemia, and insulin resistance. *Lancet*. 1998;351:1881–1883

51. Bartnof HS. New anti-HIV drug interactions, toxicities, and dosing options. *BETA*. 1999;12:60–63, 66

52. Arpadi SM, Cuff PA, Horlick M, Kotler DP. Visceral obesity, hypertriglyceridemia and hypercortisolism in a boy with perinatally acquired HIV infection receiving protease inhibitor-containing antiviral treatment. *AIDS*. 1999;13:2312–2313

53. Miller TL, Mawn B, Orav EJ, et al. The effect of protease inhibitor therapy on growth and body composition in human immunodeficiency virus type 1-infected children. *Pediatrics*. 2001;107:E77

54. Hadigan C, Corcoran C, Basgoz N, Davis B, Sax P, Grinspoon S. Metformin in the treatment of HIV lipodystrophy syndrome: a randomized controlled trial. *JAMA*. 2000;284:472–477

55. Walli R, Michl GM, Muhlbayer D, Brinkmann L, Geobel FD. Effects of troglitazone on insulin sensitivity in HIV-infected patients with protease inhibitor-associated diabetes mellitus. *Res Exp Med (Berl)*. 2000;199:253–262

56. Henderson RA, Saavedra JM, Perman JA, Hutton N, Livingston RA, Yolken RH. Effect of enteral tube feeding on growth of children with symptomatic human immunodeficiency virus infection. *J Pediatr Gastroenterol Nutr*. 1994;18:429–434

40

Nutrition for Children With Sickle Cell Disease

Introduction

Sickle cell disease is a general term for the genetic disorder related to the production of hemoglobin S, anemia, and a collection of acute and chronic clinical events caused by the blockage of blood flow by the abnormal sickle-shaped red blood cells. The hallmark is a chronic hemolytic anemia with acute and chronic tissue injury.

Sickle cell anemia, the homozygous hemoglobin S state, is the most common variant type of sickle cell disease and affects more than 50 000 African Americans. An estimated prevalence of hemoglobin SS in African American newborn infants is about 1 in 375. There are 2 less common types of sickle cell disease in the United States. Hemoglobin SC disease occurs about 1 in 835 African American live births, and sickle β-thalassemia occurs in about 1 in 1700 African American live births. Thus, sickle cell disease, with an autosomal recessive inheritance pattern, is the most common, medically significant genetic condition in African American children, but also occurs in Americans with Mediterranean, East Indian, Middle Eastern, Caribbean, and South and Central American ancestry. The discussion that follows uses hemoglobin SS disease (SCD) as the example as it is the most common and presents the greatest challenges for nutrition support.

Nutritional Consequences

Hemoglobin SS disease is frequently associated with growth failure, delayed pubertal development, and poor nutritional status.[1–6] The exact etiology of this pattern of poor growth and abnormal body composition has not been completely established, yet it is generally recognized that nutritional factors are implicated, and likely a major cause. Various nutritional factors have been identified, including increased energy requirements as the result of increased resting energy expenditure, poor dietary intake, and increased calorie and micronutrient requirements as a result of the chronic hemolysis and increased erythropoiesis and increased protein turnover.[7–14]

Several studies have documented increased resting energy expenditure in children and adults with SCD in the United States and other countries. Generally the increase is in the 10% to 20% range above predicted or above the measured energy expenditure of healthy control children.[1] Studies have indicated that children with SCD do not necessarily show the desired, adaptive increase in dietary intake, although dietary intake is always difficult to accurately document in free living children.[1] A recent study of children with SCD showed about a 15% increase in resting energy expenditure compared to control children. These same children with SCD did not increase their dietary intake and showed a trend toward decreasing energy used for normal childhood physical activity. The common SCD acute illness event does not appear to increase the resting energy expenditure above baseline values.[15] Some of the new treatments, such as hydroxyurea therapy, may decrease the elevated resting energy expenditure, but extensive data and clinical experience are not yet available.[16]

When comparing children and adolescents with SCD to healthy control children and to national reference data, those with SCD have many indications of growth faltering and abnormal body composition.[17] This is shown by a variety of anthropometric measures, including lower body weight, height, arm circumference, and arm fat stores. In addition, bone age is often delayed, indicating delayed sexual maturation. More direct measures of body composition by several research methods showed lower total body fat stores and total body fat-free mass.[17] This is a pattern of impaired growth, delayed puberty, and poor nutritional status with reduced energy stores and muscle wasting, in a group of children with a common chronic disease.

In addition, there is evidence that children with SCD are at risk for deficiencies of folate, vitamin B_6, and zinc.[18–20] The low folate status was documented in a group of patients who were prescribed a daily folate supplement (1 mg/d). This study was conducted before the recent changes in food folate fortification in the United States. Folate supplementation is a common but not universal practice in SCD care centers in the United States. Iron status is unclear, although a recent study suggested that iron depletion and deficiency are uncommon in children and adolescents with SCD.[21] Preliminary data suggest that vitamin D and antioxidant (vitamin A, vitamin E, and selenium) levels are low in children and adolescents with SCD.

Nutrition Support

Given these general findings in children with SCD, careful nutrition and growth assessment should be a routine component of care. However, there are neither nutrition intervention trials nor nutrition consensus statements to suggest a standard of care. In usual practice, there is rarely a pediatric nutritionist/dietitian in the hematology outpatient care area on a routine basis. Therefore, the nutrition assessment and support care are based on good practice patterns for infants, children, and adolescents with chronic disease. For a full review of these issues, please refer to Chapters 24 and 37.

The nutritional concern that is routinely addressed and stressed by most clinical care teams is the importance of maintaining adequate hydration and encouraging fluid intake, particularly during warm weather.[22] Children with SCD have increased fluid needs due to hyposthenuria.[22] Dehydration can precipitate an acute pain event. Some care must be taken to avoid use of fluids that contain only water and carbohydrates and few other nutrients. This may lead to inadequate dietary nutrient density due to excess fluids from "empty calories." Anorexia and/or nausea secondary to fever, pain, analgesics, or other medications may contribute to poor overall calorie intake. The suboptimal intake during periods of illness at home and when hospitalized may contribute to the pattern of poor growth.[15]

The major concern for nutritional support is to ensure that children with SCD routinely consume adequate calories to maintain a normal pattern of growth and development. Protein needs are somewhat increased, but, for most patients living in the United States, this is not a significant problem, as the usual diet contains 1.5 to 2 times the recommended protein intake. Routine longitudinal growth and nutritional status assessment is essential to care. These data should be the basis of diagnosis of growth failure or malnutrition, and the basis for planning the nutrition intervention strategy. Given the common occurrence of linear growth failure, the biological parental heights should be obtained, recorded on the patient's growth chart and used to assess the pattern of linear growth. Short stature is not a part of the genetic expression of this hemoglobinopathy. With optimal nutritional intake, most children will be able to grow to their genetic potential for height. The care team should take this into account and not accept poor height growth as an unavoidable part of SCD. An accurate longitudinal growth (length, height, weight, head circumference) and body composition (fat stores measurements) record is essential to monitoring nutritional status and evaluating the results of nutrition intervention efforts. At least every 6 months, the progression through pubertal development should be documented in the physical examination and in the nutrition assessment sections of the medical record for children aged 10 years and older.

Specific recommendations are not available for vitamin or mineral supplementation above the age- and gender-based Dietary Reference Intakes (DRIs). Current commercially available vitamin and mineral compounds for children routinely contain iron and, due to concerns over iron overload syndrome, are generally not recommended. There are no data to demonstrate safety or efficacy of vitamin and mineral intakes above the DRIs.

Many African American children have a low intake of dairy products, due to lactose intolerance or family dietary or cultural practices that limit dairy intake. This information should be noted, and an effort made to promote adequate calcium and vitamin D intake. Families and patients should also be asked about other important nutrition information, such as the use of a vegetarian diet or other restrictive food practices.

Summary

In summary, the nutritional goal for infants, children, and adolescents with SCD is to support normal growth and development and not be limited by the nutritional effects of SCD. Energy requirements can be met most often by nutrition and behavior education (patient and family) for a calorie and nutrient-dense diet. When necessary, specific calorie supplements and feeding tubes are important components of care. Less is known about increased micronutrient requirements, and appropriate monitoring (usually blood levels) should be obtained before and after implementation of nutrient supplementation in any individual patient.

References

1. Barden EM, Zemel BS, Kawchak DA, Goran MI, Ohene-Frempong K, Stallings VA. Total and resting energy expenditure in children with sickle cell disease. *J Pediatr.* 2000;136:73–79

2. Platt OS, Rosenstock W, Espeland MA. Influence of sickle hemoglobinopathies on growth and development. *N Engl J Med.* 1984;311:7–12

3. Phebus CK, Gloninger MF, Maciak BJ. Growth patterns by age and sex in children with sickle cell disease. *J Pediatr.* 1984;105:28–33

4. Heyman MB, Vinchinsky E, Katz R, et al. Growth retardation in sickle cell disease treated by nutritional support. *Lancet.* 1985;1:903–906
5. Stevens MC, Maude GH, Cupidore L, Jackson H, Hayes RJ, Serjeant GR. Prepubertal growth and skeletal maturation in children with sickle cell disease. *Pediatrics.* 1986; 78:124–132
6. Finan AC, Elmer MA, Sasanow SR, McKinney S, Russel MO, Gill FM. Nutritional factors and growth in children with sickle cell disease. *Am J Dis Child.* 1988; 142:237–240
7. Borel MJ, Buchowski MS, Turner EA, Peeler BB, Goldstein RE, Flakoll PJ. Alterations in basal nutrient metabolism increase resting energy expenditure in sickle cell disease. *Am J Physiol.* 1998;274:E347–E364
8. Modebe O, Ifenu SA. Growth retardation in homozygous sickle cell disease: role of calorie intake and possible gender-related differences. *Am J Hematol.* 1993;44: 149–154
9. Gray NT, Barlett JM, Kolasa KM, Marcuard SP, Holbrook CT, Horner RD. Nutritional status and dietary intake of children with sickle cell anemia. *Am J Pediatr Hematol Oncol.* 1992;14:57–61
10. Badaloo A, Jackson AA, Jahoor F. Whole body protein turnover and resting metabolic rate in homozygous sickle cell disease. *Clin Sci (Lond).* 1989;77:93–97
11. Salman EK, Haymond MW, Bayne E, et al. Protein and energy metabolism in prepubertal children with sickle cell anemia. *Pediatr Res.* 1996;40:34–40
12. Singhal A, Davies P, Sahota A, Thomas PW, Serjeant GR. Resting metabolic rate in homozygous sickle cell disease. *Am J Clin Nutr.* 1993;57:32–34
13. Singhal A, Thomas P, Cook R, Wierenga K, Serjeant G. Delayed adolescent growth in homozygous sickle cell disease. *Arch Dis Child.* 1994;71:404–408
14. Singhal A, Davies P, Wierenga KJ, Thomas P, Serjeant G. Is there an energy deficiency in homozygous sickle cell disease? *Am J Clin Nutr.* 1997;66:386–390
15. Fung EB, Malinauskis BM, Kawchak DA, et al. Energy expenditure and intake in children with sickle cell disease during acute illness. *Clin Nutr.* 2001;20:131–138
16. Fung EB, Barden EM, Kawchak DA, Zemel BS, Ohene-Frempong K, Stallings VA. Effect of hydroxyurea therapy on resting energy expenditure in children with sickle cell disease. *J Pediatr Hematol Oncol.* 2001;23:604–608
17. Barden EM, Kawchak DA, Ohene-Frempong K, Stallings VA, Zemel BS. Body composition in children with sickle cell disease. *Am J Clin Nutr.* 2002;76:218–225
18. Kennedy TS, Fung EB, Kawchak DA, Zemel BS, Ohene-Frempong K, Stallings VA. Red blood cell folate and serum vitamin B_{12} status in children with sickle cell disease. *J Pediatr Hematol Oncol.* 2001;23:165–169
19. Leonard MB, Zemel BS, Kawchak DA, Ohene-Frempong K, Stallings VA. Plasma zinc status, growth and maturation in children with sickle cell disease. *J Pediatr.* 1998;132:467–471

20. Nelson MC, Zemel BS, Kawchak DA, et al. Vitamin B_6 status of children with sickle cell disease. *J Pediatr Hematol Oncol.* 2002;24:463–469
21. Stettler N, Zemel BS, Kawchak DA, Ohene-Frempong K, Stallings VA. Iron status of children with sickle cell disease. *JPEN J Parenter Enteral Nutr.* 2001;25:36–38
22. Smith JA, Wethers DL. Health care maintenance. In: Embury SH, Hebbel RP, Mohandas N, Steinberg MH, eds. *Sickle Cell Disease: Basic Principles and Clinical Practice.* New York, NY: Raven Press; 1994:739–744

41

Nutritional Management of Children With Renal Disease

Introduction

There are a number of unique considerations in the nutritional management of children with renal disease. In particular, if renal function is significantly compromised, it is frequently necessary to restrict the intake of selected nutrients (see Table 41.1) while at the same time providing adequate amounts of nutrients to maintain homeostasis and support growth. Whenever possible, evidence-based recommendations for nutritional support of children with specific renal disorders will be given. Since many of these disorders are rare, recommendations based on randomized controlled trials are often not available.

General Philosophy of Medical Nutrition Therapy in Children With Renal Disease

Children whose diets are restricted frequently respond by consuming insufficient nutrients for age-appropriate growth and development. Traditionally, many physicians have been taught to restrict certain nutrients to very low limits, when, in fact, less restriction may achieve the desired result and increase the potential for long-term compliance. For example, minimum sodium intake recommendations range from 120 to 500 mg/d, according to age and weight. Achievement of these sodium intakes past 6 months of age in the outpatient setting is unrealistic, given current food purchasing, consumption patterns, and psychosocial situations. A diet history may reveal specific foods of food groups that can be limited to achieve decreased sodium intakes, such as chips, fast foods, or microwave convenience foods.

Urinary Tract Infections, Vesicoureteral Reflux, and Urinary Incontinence

Urinary tract infections are among the more common renal conditions in children. They are often associated with vesicoureteral reflux. There are no data that demonstrate a clear role for special nutritional management of children

Table 41.1.
Food Sources of Selected Nutrients

General overview	Evaluating patient and family lifestyle eating patterns may reveal areas that can be improved without limiting all sources of the nutrient in question. Ongoing nutritional follow-up is important to monitor nutrient intake and assess adequacy.
Sodium	Fast food, microwavable products, and snack foods, such as chips, contribute significant sodium to the diet. Appealing to parents to make lifestyle changes for the entire family may be effective and necessary. Foods that should be limited when sodium restriction is recommended include the following: • Convenience products (frozen, packaged, or canned), including pizza, macaroni and cheese, meat stew, spaghetti, and burritos. **Use** frozen entrees with the lowest sodium content. • Cured, salted, canned, or smoked meats, including ham, corned beef, jerky, salt pork, luncheon meats, bacon, sausage, hot dogs/frankfurters, sausage, canned tuna or salmon, and sardines. **Use** fresh meats or those frozen without added sauces. • Processed cheese, cheese spreads, or buttermilk. **Use** low-sodium cheese, ricotta/mozzarella cheese, and cream cheese. • Regular canned or frozen soups and bouillon cubes, and instant soup or dried noodle cups. **Use** low-sodium soups or homemade soups without salt or bouillon cubes, and fresh-cooked pasta and grains. • Salted crackers and snack foods, such as potato chips. **Use** unsalted chips, pretzels, and unsalted popcorn or crackers. • Regular canned vegetables, vegetable juices, or those frozen with salt. **Use** fresh or frozen vegetables without added salt; if canned, use "no salt added" vegetables, and sauces.
Potassium	Juices, fruits, vegetables, and nuts contribute the most significant sources of potassium to the diet. If restricted, a multivitamin supplement may be necessary to provide micronutrient needs. Herbal products may provide significant potassium and should be avoided in children. Examples of high-potassium foods: orange juice, carrot juice; avocados, bananas, cantaloupes, dried fruits (raisins, apricots, banana, etc), oranges; potatoes, sweet potatoes, tomatoes; chocolate; lentils, dried beans (cooked); nuts. Examples of **low**-potassium foods: cranberry juice and apple juice; apples, grapes, peaches, pears, pineapple, strawberries, watermelon; green beans, lettuce, zucchini; bread; dried pasta (cooked); and tortillas.
Phosphorus	Milk and milk products, plus meat, chicken, fish, eggs, and nuts provide the most significant sources of phosphorus in the diet. Ironically, dairy products generally are the most popular protein source for children. Limiting dairy products and utilizing phosphate binders with meals is the treatment goal. Calcium supplementation may be required, since limiting phosphorus in the diet automatically limits calcium as well.

Table 41.1.
Food Sources of Selected Nutrients *(continued)*

Phosphorus *(continued)*	*800-mg Phosphorus Diet* Goal: Limit milk, milk-rich foods (cheese, cottage cheese, yogurt), beans, nuts. Plan: Drink 8 oz milk **or** select *one* of the foods below instead of milk. 2 oz cheese 1 c cottage cheese (8 oz) 1 c hot chocolate (8 oz) 1/4 c nuts (over age 3 y) 4 tbsp peanut butter (over age 3 y) 1/2 c dried cooked beans (4 oz) 1/2 c macaroni and cheese (4 oz) 6 pieces nachos 1 large slice pizza Items from other food groups should be included in age-appropriate quantities.
Hypertension	Hypertension either is *secondary*, arising from a specific pathophysiologic state, or *essential*, meaning there is no identifiable etiology. Secondary hypertension in children is most often related to renal parenchymal or renal vascular diseases. Nutritional considerations for the hypertension resulting from renal parenchymal diseases will be discussed in the sections of this chapter specific for the renal condition. Renovascular hypertension may be amenable to definitive treatment and, once treatment is achieved, will require no specific dietary modification. When this form of hypertension is not curable, or until it can be definitively treated, a reduced sodium diet is advised. Renovascular hypertension is often treated with angiotensin enzyme inhibitors or angiotensin II receptor antagonists. The efficacy of these drugs can be enhanced by sodium restrictions. See Table 41.2 for recommendations on minimum sodium requirements at different ages.

with recurrent urinary tract infections, whether or not there is associated reflux. However, recurrent urinary tract infections (UTIs) have been associated with constipation, which certainly may respond to dietary manipulation. There are some preliminary data suggesting that cranberry juice may be helpful in minimizing the risk of infection, but no compelling data are available from studies in children.[1,2] There are also no nutritional issues associated with urinary incontinence, although there is anecdotal evidence that elimination diets have been of benefit for children with nocturnal enuresis.

Essential hypertension in children is often associated with a family history of early-onset hypertension and/or obesity in the affected child. Dietary modification aimed at weight stabilization (or slow weight loss in the older adolescent) to normalize body mass index (BMI) (see also Chapter 33) is appropriate. Sodium restriction is also often recommended, although, in real-

Table 41.2.
Diet Restrictions in Pediatric Renal Patients

GENERAL GUIDELINES
• Obtain a detailed diet history to determine current food and beverage intake. All diet changes are based on evaluation of this current intake.
• Resist the temptation to restrict nutrients until there is a need demonstrated.
• Focus on decreasing the amount of frequently consumed high sources of nutrients that need to be decreased.
• Selective micronutrient restrictions may result in the patient refusing to consume adequate amounts of macronutrients (calories, protein, fat). Follow-up is important to ensure adequacy of intake to meet growth needs.
• A phosphorous restriction will automatically restrict protein and potassium intake.
• A sodium restriction will automatically decrease fat intake in most children.

Starting Points		
Sodium	Outpatient:	<20 kg: Begin with 2 to 3 g/d >20 kg: Begin with 3 to 4 g/d Note: It is difficult to achieve compliance with <2 g/d as an outpatient
	Inpatient:	<20 kg with severe edema or HTN: begin with 1 g/d; otherwise begin with 2 g/d >20 kg: Begin with 3 to 4 g/d
Potassium	If serum potassium level is >5.0 mEq/L with normal CO_2, limit high sources of potassium the patient is currently eating or drinking.	
Phosphorous	When serum phosphorus is >5.5, limit intake to 800 mg/d and consider phosphate binders. Note: Infants require higher serum phosphorous levels for adequate bone mineralization.	
Protein	Limit only if intake consistently exceeds recommended dietary allowance (RDA) for chronological age and gender. If so, use the RDA as the maximum and minimal target level of intake.	

ity, the safety and efficacy of long-term sodium restriction in children and adolescents has not been established.[3–6] However, high-sodium foods in general are calorie dense and should, therefore, be limited in the diet of the obese hypertensive child. Depending on the child's usual salt intake, restriction to 3 to 4 g/d of sodium is a reasonable starting point. Epidemiological and some clinical data are accumulating that suggest that increased dietary calcium and potassium may be effective in helping to lower blood pressures.[7–12] The Dietary Approaches to Stop Hypertension (DASH) diet is an example of such a diet.[13,14] There are scant data to substantiate a salutary effect of potassium or calcium supplementation in children with hypertension. Manipulations of dietary magnesium or fiber may prove to be beneficial, but data in children are also lacking.[15,16]

Renal Stone Disorders

Although there are a variety of diseases that predispose children to renal stones, there are certain common therapeutic interventions. In all cases, increased fluid intake is critical. Children should be encouraged to drink at least $1\frac{1}{2}$ times their calculated maintenance fluid requirements. The fluids the child chooses to drink may have an impact on the total caloric intake of the child, and the family needs to be instructed in providing a varied fluid intake, with at least 50% from water. Water alone is sufficient, but the monotony of high water intake may make it difficult to enforce in some children.

A second consistent nutritional consideration in children with recurrent renal stones is sodium restriction. Expansion of total body water and sodium spaces leads to enhanced sodium excretion in the urine. This is often accompanied by increased excretion of the components of renal stones, particularly calcium and cystine (the latter important for the recurrent stone disease associated with cystinuria).[17,18] An initial limitation to 3 to 4 g/d of salt is recommended; smaller children will take in less due to decreased portion sizes.

There is a considerable body of literature concerning the role of dietary calcium in children with hypercalciuria, a condition that predisposes these children to recurrent calcium stones.[19–21] Attempts to differentiate hypercalciuria into absorptive and renal-leak subgroups have not been successful. While it was originally thought that children with absorptive hypercalciuria might benefit from calcium restriction, it has become clear that these children benefit from sodium restriction. In fact, epidemiological data in adults suggest that high-calcium diets may be effective in decreasing the risk of recurrent calcium stones.[19–22]

Many renal stones in children are composed of calcium and oxalate. The role of oxalate restriction in decreasing urinary oxalate excretion is not clearly established. In children with hereditary hyperoxaluria, which is a metabolic defect, dietary oxalate restriction has little impact on urinary oxalate. For children with hypercalciuria and mild hyperoxaluria, avoidance of high oxalate foods (see Table 41.3) may be prudent.[23,24] Vitamin C should be limited to 100 mg/d or less, due to ascorbate breakdown to oxalate under alkaline conditions.

A small percentage of children with recurrent renal stones pass stones composed predominantly of uric acid. There has been no demonstration that

Table 41.3.
Foods With High Oxalate Content*

Spinach
Rhubarb
Beets
Nuts
Chocolate
Tea
Wheat bran
Strawberries

*Massey L, Sutton R. Modification of dietary oxalate and calcium reduces urinary oxalate in hyperoxaluric patients with kidney stones. *J Am Diet Assoc.* 1993;93:1305.

restriction of foods high in purines decrease recurrent stones in these patients.[25,26] The goal is to achieve, but not exceed, the RDA for protein.

Renal Tubular Defects

There are a number of rare disorders characterized by abnormal renal tubular function. These include the proximal tubular disorders that present with Fanconi syndrome and some of the distal tubular disorders, such as Bartter syndrome. Each of these results in the wasting of important electrolytes, which, in turn, necessitates supplementation. In the proximal tubular Fanconi syndrome, there is usually wasting of bicarbonate, resulting in a form of renal tubular acidosis. Replacement with large doses of alkali is required to achieve a normal serum bicarbonate level. Doses exceeding 10 m/Eq/kg/d of alkali may be needed. In addition, phosphate wasting is also a feature of proximal tubular disorders (and is a key feature of X-linked hypophosphatemic rickets). Phosphorus supplementation is necessary to assist in achieving a more normal growth velocity. Doses of 30 to 90 mg/kg/d in 3 to 4 divided doses may be necessary. Phosphate supplements may cause diarrhea. A low once-daily dose may be used to start, with slow increases as needed and tolerated. In many of these conditions, renal activation of vitamin D is impaired and children may need supplemental 1α-hydroxylated forms of this vitamin. Table 41.4 lists currently available forms and doses.

Children with distal tubular defects may have distal renal tubular acidosis (dRTA); a condition characterized by an inability to excrete an acid urine, or may have tubular wasting disorders, most commonly potassium or magnesium wasting. Children with dRTA require alkali, but usually in doses far

Table 41.4.
Vitamin D Preparations

Comparison Factor	Vitamin D₂	Dihydrotachysterol	1,25-Dihydroxy-vitamin D₃
Name	Calciferol,™ Drisdol®	DHT™, Hytakerol®	Rocaltrol®
Pharmacologic dose (μg/d)	25–125 (1000–5000 units) for nutritional rickets with normal absorption 75–125 (3000–5000 units); maximum dose: 1500 for vitamin D-dependent rickets	500 as a single dose or 13–50 daily until healed for nutritional rickets	0.01–0.05 three times weekly IV or 0.25–2 (oral) for hypocalcemia in chronic kidney failure; <1 year: 0.04–0.08 1 to 5 years: 0.25–0.75 >6 years: 0.5–2.0 for hypoparathyroidism
Dosage forms	Capsule (Drisdol®): 50 000 units [1.25 mg] Injection (Calciferol™): 500 000 units/mL [1.25 mg/mL] Liquid (Calciferol™), Drisdol®): 8000 units/mL [200 μg/mL] Tablet (Calciferol™): 50 000 units [1.25 mg]	Capsule (Hytakerol®): 0.125 mg Solution: oral concentrate (DHT™): 0.2 mg/mL oral, in oil (Hytakerol®): 0.25 mg/mL Tablet (DHT™): 0.125 mg, 0.2 mg, 0.4 mg	Capsule: 0.25 μg, 0.5 μg Injection: 1 μg /mL; 2 μg /mL Solution, oral: 1 μg/mL

*Modified from Alpers DH, Stenson WF, Bier DM. *Manual of Nutritional Therapeutics.* 3rd ed: 1995, and Kumar R, Riggs BL. Vitamin D in the Therapy of Disorders of Calcium and Phosphorus Metabolism. *Mayo Clin Proc.* 1981;56:327.

lower than in children with the proximal variety. In dRTA, children are also at risk of developing nephrocalcinosis, as a result of excess calcium in the urine, which occurs predictably in children with low serum bicarbonate levels. In the other tubular wasting disorders, titrated replacement of potassium and/or magnesium is indicated.

Nephrotic Syndrome

Nephrotic syndrome is defined clinically by the presence of proteinuria, hypoproteinemia, edema, and hypercholesterolemia. In young children, nephrotic syndrome is usually due to minimal change nephrotic syndrome, a condition that responds to steroid therapy. In all forms of nephrotic syndrome, there is a tendency for renal sodium and water retention (the prime cause of the edema) during a relapse. The mainstay of dietary therapy for children with nephrotic syndrome is sodium restriction. While there are no studies that define the optimal level to which sodium should be restricted in these children, a reasonable starting point is 2 to 3 g/d. The sodium restriction can be liberalized when the child achieves remission.

At times, children are found to be at the extremes of renal compensation, with severe edema and evidence of salt and water overload. These children often have nephrotic syndrome or oliguric acute renal failure. They require aggressive, short-term, inpatient treatment. Under these circumstances, in which total intake can be reasonably controlled, much more restricted intake can be delivered reliably, especially sodium. The guidelines for such aggressive sodium restriction are found in Table 41.5. It must be emphasized that restriction to this degree cannot be successfully employed for extended periods, and cannot be expected to be followed outside the hospital.

In light of the hypercholesterolemia that typifies the nephrotic syndrome, and the negative impact on plasma lipids of the corticosteroids that are used as treatment, attention to the lipid content of the diet is prudent. Data demonstrating the efficacy of this approach to diet in the nephrotic syndrome are scant,[27,28] particularly in pediatric patients. Limiting sodium in the diet virtually limits the consumption of high-fat foods popular with children (hot dogs, pizza, cheese). In addition, in the acute phase, the presence of edema frequently results in poor appetite (despite the use of steroids) and, potentially, malabsorption. Therefore, one should approach sodium and other nutrient restrictions with caution and insure adequate, consistent nutrient intake with dietary counseling from a registered dietitian.

Table 41.5.
Diet Restrictions in Pediatric Renal Patients

Age	Weight (kg)	Sodium (mg)
0–5 mo	4.5	120
6–11 mo	8.9	200
1 y	11.0	225
2–5 y	16.0	300
6–9 y	25.0	400
10–18 y	50.0	500

Some children will not respond to corticosteroid treatment for the nephrotic syndrome, and their heavy proteinuria will persist, as will the hypoproteinemia. Often, a medication regimen can be selected that minimizes the edema, but the efficacy of this regimen is enhanced by ongoing sodium restriction. Hypercholesterolemia will persist as long as there is proteinuria, and attention should be given to achieving or maintaining appropriate BMI and regular physical activity, in addition to limiting sodium in the diet.

Glomerulonephritis

From a histologic perspective, there are many etiologies for the glomerulonephritic syndrome, which is characterized by hematuria and proteinuria, and often associated with hypervolemia and consequent hypertension. Renal function may also be reduced. Hyperlipidemia is an occasional finding. The nutritional management of these patients depends on how well renal function is maintained. In the setting of hypervolemia and hypertension, the prime nutritional intervention is sodium restriction to 2 to 4 g/d. If the clinical circumstances indicate, fluid restriction may be necessary. This restriction may be as severe as a limitation to insensible fluid losses only (40% of calculated daily maintenance fluids) or range up to full maintenance fluids. If proteinuria is significant, hyperlipidemia may ensue, and further dietary modifications may be indicated (see discussion under Nephrotic syndrome in this chapter). Close attention must be paid, however, to the achievement of adequate calories and protein for growth.

Acute Renal Failure (ARF)

Acute renal failure is defined as an abrupt decline in the glomerular filtration rate and is most often caused by either underperfusion of the kidneys (eg, during hypovolemic shock) or intrinsic renal disease. The intrinsic renal diseases are usually forms of acute glomerulonephritis or the hemolytic-uremic syndrome. Acute renal failure is associated with either oliguria or a non-oliguric state. In non-oliguric ARF, the patient's volume status is usually easy to maintain, with little need for fluid or sodium restriction. However, given the diminished glomerular filtration rate, children can be expected to have difficulty excreting potassium and phosphorus. Recommendations for potassium and phosphorus restrictions are detailed in Table 41.1. Since protein restriction may limit the rate of urea production, as well as the generation of other uremic toxins, protein intake should, therefore, be restricted early in ARF, and provision of adequate nonprotein calories to minimize use of protein for energy and catabolism ensured. Enteral or parenteral nutrition may be necessary to achieve this, depending on the patient's medical condition.

Children with the oliguric forms of ARF will benefit from fluid and sodium restriction, as well as from potassium, phosphorus, and protein restriction. As stated previously, provision of adequate calories within the above restrictions is essential, and may require enteral feedings if the child is unable to cooperate with oral feeds.

Chronic Renal Failure

Chronic renal failure (CRF) is generally defined by the presence of a glomerular filtration rate less than 25 mL/min/1.73m². There are many etiologies of CRF in children, but, as with ARF, they tend to fall into 2 categories—oliguric and non-oliguric. Dietary protein restriction is commonly recommended for both forms of CRF. Nitrogenous waste products that are derived from dietary protein sources may accumulate and lead to progressive azotemia. In addition, there are experimental data in animals that suggest that standard protein intake in the setting of renal failure enhances the progression of the renal failure and the development of uremia.[29] In clinical trials conducted in humans, dietary protein restriction has not clearly delayed the progression of renal disease.[30,31]

When allowed an unrestricted diet, children with renal insufficiency eat an average 120% of the RDA for dietary protein for age.[32,33] It would, therefore, seem reasonable to prescribe a diet that limits protein intake to the reference standards for age and ensures the consumption of adequate nonprotein calories.[34,35] Protein restriction, on the other hand, may be deleterious.[31] Dietary protein restriction should be initiated only after a detailed dietary history of intake has determined that protein intake exceeds the RDA for age and gender. Commonly, these patients do not consume significantly excess protein, but, instead, restrict nonprotein-derived calories needed for protein sparing. Analogous to the setting of acute renal failure, children with chronic renal failure should restrict potassium and phosphorus intake as the glomerular filtration rate declines.

Children with oliguric chronic renal failure usually have had an acute glomerular injury, such as rapidly progressive glomerulonephritis or the hemolytic-uremic syndrome, or have experienced acute cortical necrosis. They have a limited ability to excrete salt and water and, as a result, are often hypertensive. Thus, sodium and fluid restrictions are critical. A reasonable sodium intake would be 3 to 4 g/d initially. Fluid intake is usually a fraction of the calculated daily maintenance volume, adjusted for the degree of oliguria. Children with oliguric chronic renal failure also develop an elevated serum phosphorus level, with the resulting hypocalcemia and hyperparathyroidism, and require limitation of dietary phosphorus and often require the initiation of phosphate binders.

One subset of children with CRF requires special mention—infants and toddlers with non-oliguric CRF, usually as a result of congenital renal dysplasia. These children often waste sodium despite advanced degrees of renal failure, and they will, therefore, require supplementation of dietary sodium. Signs of sodium depletion are often subtle, and include listlessness, failure to gain weight despite adequate caloric intake, and hypercalcemia. It is reasonable to initiate supplementation with 1 to 2 mEq/kg/d of sodium, either as sodium chloride or a sodium-based alkali. Substantially greater amounts of sodium may be necessary to ensure optimal growth.

Children on Dialysis

The National Kidney Foundation's Kidney Disease Outcomes and Quality Initiative (KDOQI) recently addressed dietary and nutritional issues related to children on dialysis.[36] The following summarizes the recommendations of that work group. There are 2 common forms of maintenance dialysis for children with end-stage renal disease—peritoneal dialysis (PD) and hemodialysis (HD). The KDOQI workgroup separated its recommendations for these 2 forms when there were data to justify that separation.

Protein and energy requirements were based on the RDA for the child's age and gender as a starting point for a diet prescription. Incremental protein to account for protein and amino acid losses during the dialysis process was suggested (Table 41.6). Supplemental vitamins were not routinely recommended for those children whose diet achieved the DRIs, for the individual vitamins. Supplemental nutritional support (oral and/or enteral) is suggested for those children who cannot consistently consume the RDAs for protein and energy, or who are not growing despite good biochemical control and seemingly adequate intake.[36]

Renal Transplantation

Current immunosuppressive regimens for children after a renal transplant include steroids and calcineurin inhibitors in the large majority of children. In part as a result of this therapy, a high percentage of children are hypertensive post-transplant, and are in need of a sodium-controlled diet. In the initial 2

Table 41.6.
Recommended Nutrient Intakes for Dialysis Patients[36]

	Age (y)	Protein Intake* for HD	Protein Intake* for PD
Infants	0-0.5	2.6	2.9-3.0
	0.6-1.0	2.0	2.3-2.4
Children	1-3	1.6	1.9-2.0
	4-6	1.6	1.9-2.0
	7-10	1.4	1.7-1.8
Males	11-14	1.4	1.7-1.8
	15-18	1.3	1.4-1.5†
	19-21	1.2	1.3†
Females	11-14	1.4	1.7-1.8
	15-18	1.2	1.4-1.5†
	19-21	1.2	1.3†

*Values are expressed in grams of protein per kilogram per day. HD: Hemodialysis; PD: Peritoneal dialysis.
†Based on growth potential.

months post-transplant, the focus of medical nutrition therapy should be on limitation of sodium (3 to 4 g/d), and weight control. Long-term goals include achieving or maintaining age- and gender-appropriate BMI, regular physical activity, and eating a variety of foods, including fruits and vegetables, with moderate consumption of high-fat and high-sodium foods. Children should have their lipid levels monitored post-transplant.[37,38]

References

1. Henig YS, Leahy MM. Cranberry juice and urinary-tract health: science supports folklore. *Nutrition.* 2000;16:684–687
2. Jepson RG, Mihaljevic L, Craig J. Cranberries for preventing urinary tract infections. *Cochrane Database Syst Rev.* 2000;3:CD001321
3. Mo R, Omvik P, Lund-Johansen P, Myking OL. The Bergen blood pressure study: sodium intake and ambulatory blood pressure in offspring of hypertensive and normotensive families. *Blood Press.* 1993;2:278–283
4. Geleijnse JM, Grobbee DE, Hofman A. Sodium and potassium intake and blood pressure change in childhood. *BMJ.* 1990;300:899–902
5. Falkner B, Michel S. Blood pressure response to sodium in children and adolescents. *Am J Clin Nutr.* 1997;65(suppl 2):618S–621S
6. Staessen JA, Lijnen P, Thijs L, Fagard R. Salt and blood pressure in community-based intervention trials. *Am J Clin Nutr.* 1997;65(suppl 2):661S–670S
7. Resnick LM. The role of dietary calcium in hypertension: a hierarchical overview. *Am J Hypertens.* 1999;12:99–112

8. Allender PS, Cutler JA, Follmann D, Cappuccio FP, Pryer J, Elliott P. Dietary calcium and blood pressure: a meta-analysis of randomized clinical trials. *Ann Intern Med.* 1996;124:825–831

9. Karanja N, Morris CD, Rufolo P, Snyder G, Illingworth DR, McCarron DA. Impact of increasing calcium in the diet on nutrient consumption, plasma lipids, and lipoproteins in humans. *Am J Clin Nutr.* 1994;59:900–907

10. Kristal-Boneh E, Green MS. Dietary calcium and blood pressure—a critical review of the literature. *Public Health Rev.* 1990;18:267–300

11. Falkner B, Sherif K, Michel S, Kushner H. Dietary nutrients and blood pressure in urban minority adolescents at risk for hypertension. *Arch Pediatr Adolesc Med.* 2000; 154:918–922

12. Sorof JM, Forman A, Cole N, Jemerin JM, Morris RC. Potassium intake and cardiovascular reactivity in children with risk factors for essential hypertension. *J Pediatr.* 1997;31:87–94

13. Harsha DW, Lin PH, Obarzanek E, Karanja NM, Moore TJ, Caballero B. Dietary Approaches to Stop Hypertension: a summary of study results. *J Am Diet Assoc.* 1999;99(suppl 8):S35–S39

14. Appel LJ, Moore TJ, Obarzanek E, et al. A clinical trial of the effects of dietary patterns on blood pressure. *N Engl J Med.* 1997;336:1117–1124

15. Mizushima S, Cappuccio FP, Nichols R, Elliott P. Dietary magnesium intake and blood pressure: a qualitative overview of the observational studies. *J Hum Hypertens.* 1998;12:447–453

16. He J, Whelton PK. Effect of dietary fiber and protein intake on blood pressure: a review of epidemiologic evidence. *Clin Exp Hypertens.* 1999;21:785–796

17. Rodriguez LM, Santos F, Malaga S, Martinez V. Effect of a low sodium diet on urinary elimination of cystine in cystinuric children. *Nephron.* 1995;71:416–418

18. Norman RW, Manette WA. Dietary restriction of sodium as a means of reducing urinary cystine. *J Urol.* 1990;143:1193–1195

19. Burtis WJ, Gay L, Insogna KL, Ellison A, Broadus AE. Dietary hypercalciuria in patients with calcium oxalate kidney stones. *Am J Clin Nutr.* 1994;60:424–429

20. Osorio AV, Alon US. The relationship between urinary calcium, sodium, and potassium excretion and the role of potassium in treating idiopathic hypercalciuria. *Pediatrics.* 1997;100:675–681

21. Cirillo M, Ciacci C, Laurenzi M, Mellone M, Mazzacca G, De Santo NG. Salt intake, urinary sodium, and hypercalciuria. *Miner Electrolyte Metab.* 1997;23:265–268

22. Hess B, Jost C, Zipperle L, Takkinen R, Jaeger P. High-calcium intake abolishes hyperoxaluria and reduces urinary crystallization during a 20-fold normal oxalate load in humans. *Nephrol Dial Transplant.* 1998;13:2241–2247

23. Laminski NA, Meyers AM, Kruger M, Sonnekus MI, Margolius LP. Hyperoxaluria in patients with recurrent calcium oxalate calculi: dietary and other risk factors. *Br J Urol.* 1991;68:454–458

24. Massey LK, Sutton RA. Modification of dietary oxalate and calcium reduces urinary oxalate in hyperoxaluric patients with kidney stones. *J Am Diet Assoc.* 1993;93: 1305–1307

25. Cattini Perrone H, Bruder Stapleton F, Toporovski J, Schor N. Hematuria due to hyperuricosuria in children: 36-month follow-up. *Clin Nephrol.* 1997;48:288–291

26. La Manna A, Polito C, Marte A, Iovene A, Di Toro R. Hyperuricosuria in children: clinical presentation and natural history. *Pediatrics.* 2001;107:86–90

27. Coleman JE, Watson AR. Hyperlipidaemia, diet and simvastatin therapy in steroid-resistant nephrotic syndrome of childhood. *Pediatr Nephrol.* 1996;10:171–174

28. D'Amico G, Gentile MG, Manna G, et al. Effect of vegetarian soy diet on hyperlipidaemia in nephrotic syndrome. *Lancet.* 1992;339:1131–1134

29. Motomura K, Okuda S, Sanai T, Ando T, Onomaya K, Fujishima M. Importance of early initiation of dietary protein restriction for the prevention of experimental progressive renal disease. *Nephron.* 1988;49:144–149

30. Wingen AM, Fabian-Bach C, Mehls O. Multicentre randomized study on the effect of a low-protein diet on the progression of renal failure in childhood: one-year results. *Miner Electrolyte Metab.* 1992;18:303–308

31. Uauy RD, Hogg RJ, Brewer ED, Reisch JS, Cunninham C, Holliday MA. Dietary protein and growth in infants with chronic renal insufficiency: a report from the Southwest Pediatric Nephrology Study Group and the University of California, San Francisco. *Pediatr Nephrol.* 1994;8:45–50

32. Ratsch IM, Catassi C, Verrina E, et al. Energy and nutrient intake of patients with mild-to-moderate chronic renal failure compared with healthy children: an Italian multicentre study. *Eur J Pediatr.* 1992;151:701–705

33. Wingen AM, Fabian-Bach C, Mehls O. Evaluation of protein intake by dietary diaries and urea-N excretion in children with chronic renal failure. *Clin Nephrol.* 1993;40:208–215

34. Hellerstein S, Holliday MA, Grupe WE, et al. Nutritional management of children with chronic renal failure. Summary of the Task Force on Nutritional Management of Children with Chronic Renal Failure. *Pediatr Nephrol.* 1987;1:195–211

35. Sedman A, Friedman A, Boineau F, Strife CF, Fine R. Nutritional management of the child with mild to moderate chronic renal failure. *J Pediatr.* 1996;129:S13–S18

36. K/DOQI, National Kidney Foundation. Clinical practice guidelines for nutrition in chronic renal failure. II. Pediatric guidelines. Kidney Foundation. *Am J Kidney Dis.* 2000;35(suppl 2):S105–S136

37. Locsey L, Asztalos L, Kincses Z, Berczi C, Paragh G. The importance of obesity and hyperlipidaemia in patients with renal transplants. *Int Urol Nephrol.* 1998; 30:767–775

38. Broyer M, Tete MJ, Laudat MH, Goldstein S. Plasma lipids in kidney transplanted children and adolescents: influence of pubertal development, dietary intake and steroid therapy. *Eur J Clin Invest.* 1981;11:397–402

42

Nutritional Management of Children With Cancer

Malnutrition, often related to advanced disease or consequences of therapy, is not uncommon in children with cancer.[1-4] Malnutrition is associated with poor growth and development, decreased immune function (including anergy to intradermal antigens), decreased tolerance for chemotherapy, and increased rates of infection.[5-8] Studies suggest that children with cancer and malnutrition have a higher risk for chemotherapy toxicity, have a higher incidence of infectious complications, and tolerate chemotherapy poorly when compared with children with normal nutritional status.[1,5,7,9-15]

Whether malnutrition leads to less favorable outcomes in children with cancer is currently not clear.[16-18] Nevertheless, the effects of poor nutrition on a child's physical and emotional well-being and overall quality of life are well established.[15,18] The goals for nutrition support in children with cancer are to promote normal growth and development, minimize morbidity and mortality, and maximize quality of life. The pathogenesis of malnutrition in children with cancer is multifactorial and includes the individual and overlapping effects of the tumor, the host-response to the malignancy, the effects of therapy, and psychological effects.

Tumor-Related Effects on Nutritional Status

Malnutrition in pediatric oncology patients is related to therapy and its complications and, to a lesser degree, to specific tumor characteristics.[6] Childhood cancer often presents with an acute onset (eg, acute leukemia) with a relatively low incidence of malnutrition at the time of diagnosis. Children with solid tumors, especially those causing intestinal obstruction or demonstrating widespread metastatic disease, may have a higher incidence of malnutrition.[9] The incidence of malnutrition has been reported to range from 6% in children with newly diagnosed leukemia to as high as 50% in patients with stage IV neuroblastoma.[9,19]

Host-Related Effects on Nutritional Status

Cancer can affect host metabolism of protein, fat, and carbohydrate. This has been demonstrated both in animal models and humans.[20] These changes include an increase in protein turnover and a loss of normal compensatory mechanisms seen in starvation, which contributes to skeletal muscle depletion.[20–22] Additionally, accelerated lipolysis results in depletion of fat stores and increased free fatty acid turnover with the net effect of wasting of body fat and hyperlipidemia.[19,20] Changes in carbohydrate metabolism result in an energy-losing cycle. Studies of adult patients with large tumor burdens have shown that tumors consume glucose by anaerobic glycolysis, producing lactic acid. Lactic acidosis, during infusions of glucose, has also been reported in children with cancer.[6,19] In general, the data on changes in a patient's metabolic rate due to a malignancy tend to be inconsistent, although an increased resting energy expenditure occurs fairly consistently in children with a very high tumor burden.[22]

The most common characteristic of cancer-associated malnutrition is anorexia. Anorexia occurs as a result of both malignancy and cancer therapy.[23] Side effects of chemotherapy such as nausea, vomiting, diarrhea, mucositis, food aversion, and an altered sense of taste and smell are major causes of anorexia in children undergoing cancer treatment. In addition, infection, chemotherapy-induced ulcers, delayed gastric emptying, pain, and psychological factors can play a significant role in the development of anorexia. There is a clear relationship between treatments for cancer and anorexia, malnutrition, and growth retardation.[9,24–26]

Therapy-Related Effects on Nutritional Status

Multimodal treatments (chemotherapy, radiation, and surgery) may contribute either directly or indirectly to altered nutritional status in children with cancer. Most chemotherapeutic agents adversely affect dietary intake. In a study of 100 newly diagnosed pediatric oncology patients, 44 were found to be consuming less than 80% of their estimated caloric requirements compared to none of the controls.[27] Oral-mucositis is one of the frequent side effects of intensive cancer treatment.[28] Many chemotherapy agents cause nausea and vomiting, altered food intake, impaired digestion and absorption and increased nutrient losses.[10] Antineoplastic drugs can be a cause of diarrhea, constipation, ileus, and morphological changes in the intestine, resulting in alteration of digestive enzymes.[29] Factors such as constipation, related to use of vincristine or narcotics, and lactose malabsorption with diarrhea can result in significant abdominal discomfort and loss of appetite.

The majority of children diagnosed with cancer in the United States are treated by one of the institutions affiliated with the Children's Oncology Group. Toxicity of chemotherapy treatment depends on the type of agent, the dose, and combination of chemotherapeutic medications. The child receiving chemotherapy may experience significant pain, dysphagia, and an alteration in nutritional status associated with these complications. While new approaches in supportive care have decreased the nausea, vomiting, and mucositis associated with some of the treatment protocols, these side effects are often difficult to control in *intensive* treatment protocols.[30]

Radiation therapy alone or in combination with chemotherapy can severely impact nutritional status. The effect is influenced by dose, fractionation, location, and the field size.[9,10,31] Radiotherapy to the head and neck can result in anorexia, altered taste sensation, and mucositis. Radiation to the chest can cause dysphagia or swallowing difficulties. Therapy to the abdomen or pelvis can result in gastrointestinal side effects (nausea, vomiting with poor food intake) or late effects on intestinal mucosa leading to radiation enteritis.[9,10]

Infection is a common occurrence in children with cancer. Among the factors that contribute to an increased risk of infection are myelosuppression and changes in humoral and cellular immunity that may, in part, be a result of poor nutrition.[32] An infected child with myelosuppression may experience a poor appetite and exhibit suboptimal nutritional intake during the course of the infection. Antibiotics as well as antifungal agents can cause gastrointestinal and urinary losses of nutrients, malabsorption, and anorexia with associated weight loss.

Psychological Factors

Loss of appetite secondary to learned food aversions can also play a significant role in a child's nutritional status during cancer therapy. Children may develop aversions to foods in their usual diet when these foods are consumed prior to "gastrointestinal-toxic" chemotherapy treatments.[6,33,34] Learned food aversions and anticipatory vomiting may be seen in adolescents confronting an unfamiliar environment, an altered body image, the disruption of normal life, and frequent medical procedures.[6,35] Knowledge of treatment protocols and expected side effects of therapy will permit early intervention to prevent significant nutrition deterioration.

Nutritional Screening

The nutritional status of all children diagnosed with cancer should be evaluated at the time of diagnosis and throughout therapy. The purpose of a nutrition evaluation is to identify the child at risk for malnutrition and to establish baseline nutrition information for future follow-up examinations.

The following criteria are used to identify children at risk[9,19,36]:

- Total weight loss of >5% of the pre-illness body weight over the past month
- Weight less than fifth percentile for age
- Height less than fifth percentile for age
- Weight for height less than fifth percentile
- Weight <90% of ideal body weight for height
- Triceps skinfold less than tenth percentile for age and gender
- Arm circumference less than fifth percentile for age and gender
- BMI less than fifth percentile for age and gender
- Serum albumin <3.2 g/dL
- Oral intake <80% of estimated needs

Children receiving high-dose chemotherapy or combination therapy for aggressive cancers are at high risk for developing malnutrition and may need early nutrition intervention based on their oral intake and the treatment protocol.

Nutritional Assessment

The goals for nutrition assessment are to identify and define nutrition problems, to establish individual nutrition needs and care plans, and to assess the appropriate route of nutrition. Follow-up is essential in monitoring the effectiveness of nutrition support therapy. The nutritional assessment of a child diagnosed with cancer should include the following:

- Medical and surgical history, including history of gastrointestinal symptoms, such as diarrhea, vomiting, and constipation
- Medication history, to include review of chemotherapy, antibiotics, and antifungal agents and their potential impact on nutritional status
- Diet history
  - Type and amount of foods or formula consumed
  - Feeding and eating patterns
  - Feeding problems and skills
  - Food aversions or intolerance
  - Food preferences

- Food intake in relation to treatment schedule
- Supplements, herbs and/or complementary therapies
- Anthropometric Assessment
  The National Center for Health Statistics (NCHS) growth charts are widely used to assess the nutritional status of children. Measurements of height (length) for age, weight for age, weight for length (height), and head circumference for age (<3 years old) at diagnosis and throughout therapy should be a routine aspect of nutritional evaluation of the child with cancer.[9,36] Calculation of weight for height percentile, percent of weight loss from usual body weight, and percent of ideal body weight for height are used regularly to determine nutritional status.[9,36] Longitudinal data on each child's growth pattern is most helpful for detecting deviations from a child's normal growth pattern. Flattening of the weight/growth curve may be an early indicator of decreased energy and protein intake.[37,38] Skinfold measurements and body mass index (BMI=weight/height^2) are more sensitive measures of lean body mass and fat stores.[16]
- Biochemical Assessment
  Biochemical determinations in combination with anthropometric data are helpful in the evaluation of the nutritional status. Serum albumin and pre-albumin levels are obtained to determine visceral protein status. These values are altered by poor protein intake, impaired absorption, inadequate synthesis, chronic losses, hydration status, and abnormal liver and renal function.[37,38] Their specificity is limited because they are also acute phase-reactant proteins. An abnormal serum albumin level may more often reflect the acute metabolic response to fever and infection or chronic catabolic stress from infection rather than the depletion of lean body mass.

  Transthyretin (pre-albumin), with its shorter half-life of 2 to 3 days versus 21 days for serum albumin, is often used to determine the effectiveness of nutrition interventions. Other serum biochemical indices, such as sodium, potassium, chloride, bicarbonate, glucose, creatine, urea nitrogen, calcium, phosphorous, magnesium, triglycerides, and transaminases, should be monitored closely since dietary intake as well as chemotherapy and antibiotic medications can alter their values.
- Clinical Evaluation
  The clinical evaluation of the child with cancer should include monitoring for signs of muscle or fat depletion, wasting, edema, or mouth sores and must be a routine part of the comprehensive nutritional assessment.

● Estimating nutrient requirements

Actual nutrient requirements of children with cancer may vary with individual needs, disease activity, and treatment modalities. It is necessary to establish intake goals for calories, protein, vitamins, minerals, and fluids, especially for children receiving parenteral and enteral nutrition support. The Dietary Reference Intakes (DRIs) for age and gender are often used to estimate the nutrient requirements for infants and children.[36] The Recommended Daily Allowance for calories may not be the most appropriate method for estimating the calorie requirements of children with cancer.[31,39] Children receiving intensive therapy are generally less active and require less energy than their healthy counterparts. However, they may need additional calories during infections or other stresses. Protein requirements for children with cancer are not known. Children with significant metabolic stress (eg, major surgery, infection) or increased losses may have a higher protein requirement. During stress-related illness, the usual estimate of the protein requirement in children is 1.5 to 2.5 g/kg/d, which is approximately 50% higher than normal.[31]

There is little information about vitamin and mineral requirements of children with cancer. Recommendations for vitamins and minerals are based on the DRI for age and gender. If the oral intake is suboptimal, a multivitamin-mineral supplement with 100% of the DRI is recommended.[39] Additional iron supplementation is not recommended for children receiving frequent blood products.[39] Children receiving methotrexate should not receive additional folic acid as a supplement.

Mineral wasting and deficiencies associated with the side effects of chemotherapy are commonly seen in children. The nutrients most frequently affected include magnesium, calcium, phosphorus, potassium, and zinc.[31] Intravenous or oral electrolyte supplementation is often needed. In these cases, monitoring of the serum electrolyte levels is essential. The provision of adequate fluid is important throughout therapy. Fluid requirements are highly individualized; however, the following guidelines may be used as estimates of maintenance fluid requirements[35,36,39]:

<10 kg:	100 mL/kg/24 hr
11 kg to 20 kg:	1000 mL plus 50 mL/kg for each kg >10 kg/24 hr
21 kg to 40 kg:	1500 mL plus 20 mL/kg for each kg >20 kg/24 hr
>40 kg:	1500 mL/m^2/24 hr

Nutrition Therapy

Nutrition therapy involves oral feeding, enteral tube feeding, and parenteral nutrition. Although the oral route is the preferred method of providing nutrition, the challenges for children on intensive treatment protocols are their inability to eat an adequate amount of food in the face of nausea, vomiting, aversion to smells and tastes, mucositis, and stomatitis. Children should be encouraged to try calorie-dense foods; however, they should not be threatened or punished for not being able to eat enough food.

Initial nutritional counseling on the impact of cancer and its treatment on nutrition is an important part of the comprehensive care of children with cancer. Information on appropriate food choices to meet daily nutrient requirements with or without supplements may be adequate for some children on low-risk protocols. Guidelines for management of nutritional complications from oncology treatments should be provided during initial or ongoing counseling. Food safety and appropriate food handling should be a part of overall nutrition education for the caregiver.

Tube Feeding

When oral intake remains inadequate, tube feedings may provide an effective and safe method for nutrition support. Although nasogastric tube feeding has been accepted for nutrition support of children with other illnesses,[40] it not the preferred method for children with cancer. This is due to the discomfort of nasogastric tube placement, the psychological impact of alterations in body image, and poor compliance. An additional concern with nasogastric tube feeding is possible trauma to the fragile mucosal surfaces of a patient with a low platelet and white blood cell count resulting in bacterial translocation into the bloodstream. However, pilot data have demonstrated the safety and feasibility of nasogastric tube feedings for the nutritional support of children with cancer when other routes of feeding are inappropriate.[41]

Gastrostomy feedings have been used for nutritional support in pediatric oncology patients with some concern for site infections, leakage of gastric contents on to the skin, and poor healing at the site.[42,43] In general, enteral tube feedings have a number of distinct advantages over parenteral nutrition.[43-46] These advantages include the following:

- Decreased risk of infection
- Maintenance of structural and functional gastrointestinal integrity
- Decreased potential for bacterial translocation

- Greater ease and safety of administration
- Decreased hepatobiliary complications
- Lower cost

Tube feeding should be the first choice for nutritional support of children with an inadequate oral intake. The following criteria should be considered when tube feeding is recommended:

- The patient and family consent
- A functional gastrointestinal tract
- The inability of the child to maintain normal nutrition by the oral route
- The patient's status regarding nausea, vomiting, and diarrhea
- An adequate platelet count (>20 000)
- A normal mucosal surface in the upper gastrointestinal tract

A team approach with support from a dietician, a child life specialist, social workers, a psychiatrist, oncologists, and nursing staff will help facilitate the successful initiation and continuation of nasogastric tube feedings of children with cancer.[41]

The optimal access route for enteral nutrition is based on anticipated duration of the tube feeding, the neurological status of patient, and risk of aspiration. In general, nasoenteric tubes are considered for short-term use (less than 6 weeks), although successful long-term use of nasogastric feeding has been reported.[41] Other routes of enteral tube feeding include naso-duodenal, naso-jejunal, gastrostomy, and jejunostomy tubes. The use of a silicone or polyurethane tube with the smallest diameter (6F to 8F) is recommended for nasoenteric tubes.

Enteral formulas are selected based on age and gastrointestinal function. Infant formulas with 20 to 30 kcal/oz are appropriate choices for oral or enteral tube feedings of infants. Lactose-free infant formulas may be required due to chemotherapy-induced lactose intolerance. The need for nutrient-dense formulas (>20 cal/oz) is based on the fluid tolerance. Increasing the formula concentration may increase renal solute load or cause gastrointestinal intolerance with abdominal distention, vomiting, or diarrhea. Thus, the concentration of a formula should be increased slowly with close monitoring of potential side effects. A concentrated formula may be achieved by adding "modular" supplements to standard infant formulas. Age-appropriate standard formulas may be used for patients with normal gut function. Unflavored formulas with lower osmolality are better tolerated than flavored ones and are recommended for tube feedings. Children with abnormal gastrointestinal function may benefit from protein hydrolysate or elemental formulas (see Appendix O).

Tube feeding may be administered by continuous drip using a feeding pump for a reliable, constant infusion rate. Continuous feeding may be better tolerated with delayed gastric emptying. Tube feedings may also be delivered by intermittent bolus feeding, which is more physiologic and mimics normal feeding. Nocturnal continuous feedings with daytime oral and/or bolus feedings work well to meet nutritional goals. Small-bowel feedings should be considered for children who are neurologically impaired with higher risk for aspiration and those with frequent vomiting. Continuous tube feedings may be initiated with full-strength isotonic formula at 1 to 2 cc/kg body weight/h/d. They may be advanced by 1 to 2 cc/kg/h/d as tolerated until the volume goal is achieved.[9,31,36]

Parenteral Nutrition

Parenteral nutrition is indicated when the child's nutrition status cannot be maintained by enteral route. This may occur with tumors producing gastrointestinal obstruction, severe mucositis, uncontrolled nausea and vomiting, or inability to absorb nutrients. The parenteral route may also be required to supplement enteral tube feedings. The use and risk of parenteral nutrition in children with cancer has been extensively reviewed.[19,36,47,48] The risk of catheter-related infections and gastrointestinal and metabolic complications should be considered when parenteral nutrition is selected for nutrition support of a child with normal gastrointestinal function. An aggressive approach with enteral tube feedings has greatly reduced the need for total parenteral nutrition, thereby reducing potential side effects and cost.[41]

References

1. Fernandez CV, Stutzer CA, MacWilliam L, Fryer C. Alternative and complementary therapy in pediatric oncology patients in British Columbia: prevalence and reasons for use and nonuse. *J Clin Oncol*. 1998;16:1279–1286
2. Zlotkin SH, Stallings VA, Pencharz PB. Total parenteral nutrition in children. *Pediatr Clin North Am*. 1985;32:381–400
3. Pencharz P. Identifying the patient at nutritional risk. *J Can Diet Assoc*. 1988; 49:108–112
4. Wilson DC, Pencharz PB. Nutritional care of the chronically ill. In: Tsang RC, Zlotkin SH, Nichols BL, Hansen JW, eds. *Nutrition During Infancy: Principles and Practice*. 2nd ed. Cincinnati, OH: Digital Educational Publishing; 1997:37–56

5. Elhasid R, Laor A, Lischinsky S, Postovsky S, Weyl Ben Arush M. Nutritional status of children with solid tumors. *Cancer.* 1999;86:119–125

6. Mauer AM, Burgess JB, Donoldson SS, et al. Special nutritional needs of children with malignancies: a review. *JPEN J Parenter Enteral Nutr.* 1990;14:315–324

7. Pietsch JB, Meakins J, MacLean LD. The delayed hypersensitivity response: application in clinical surgery. *Surgery.* 1977;82:349–355

8. Spanier AH, Pietsch, JB, Meakins JL, Maclean LD, Shizgal HM. The relationship between immune competence and nutrition. *Surg Forum.* 1976;27:332–336

9. Barale KV, Charuhas PM. Oncology and marrow transplantation. In: Samour PQ, Helm KK, Lang CE, eds. *Handbook of Pediatric Nutrition.* 2nd ed. Gaithersburg, MD: Aspen Publishers, Inc; 1999:465–491

10. Donoldson SS, Lenon RA. Alterations of nutritional status impact of chemotherapy and radiation therapy. *Cancer.* 1979;43(suppl 5):2036–2052

11. Andrassy RJ, Chwals WJ. Nutritional support of the pediatric oncology patient. *Nutrition.* 1998;14:124–129

12. Gomez-Almaguer D, Ruiz-Arguelles GJ, Ponce-de-Leon S. Nutritional status and socio-economic conditions as prognostic factors in the outcome of therapy in childhood acute lymphoblastic leukemia. *Int J Cancer Suppl.* 1998;11:52–55

13. Murry DJ, Riva L, Poplack DG. Impact of nutrition on pharmacokinetics of antineoplastic agents. *Int J Cancer Suppl.* 1998;11:48–51

14. Viana MB, Murao M, Ramos G, et al. Malnutrition as a prognostic factor in lymphoblastic leukemia: a multivariate analysis. *Arch Dis Child.* 1994;71:304–310

15. Taj MM, Pearson AD, Mumford DB, Price L. Effect of nutritional status on the incidence of infection in childhood cancer. *Pediatr Hematol Oncol.* 1993;10:283–287

16. Barr RD, Gibson BE. Nutritional status and cancer in childhood. *J Pediatr Hematol Oncol.* 2000;22:491–494

17. Pedrosa F, Bonilla M, Liu A, et al. Effect of malnutrition at the time of diagnosis on the survival of children treated for cancer in El Salvador and northern Brazil. *J Pediatr Hematol Oncol.* 2000;22:502–505

18. Van Eys J. Benefits of nutritional intervention on nutritional status, quality of life and survival. *Int J Cancer Suppl.* 1998;11:66–68

19. Alexander HR, Rickard KA, Godshall B. Nutritional supportive care. In: Pizzo PA, Poplack DG, eds. *Principles and Practices of Pediatric Oncology.* 3rd ed. Philadelphia, PA: Lippincott-Raven Publishers; 1997:1167–1182

20. Picton SV. Aspects of altered metabolism in children with cancer. *Int J Cancer.* 1998;11:62–64

21. Kurzer M, Meguid, MM. Cancer and protein metabolism. *Surg Clin North Am.* 1986;66:969–1001

22. Pencharz PB. Aggressive oral, enteral or parenteral nutrition: prescriptive decisions in children with cancer. *Int J Cancer Suppl.* 1998;11:73–75

23. Kern KA, Norton, JA. Cancer cachexia. *JPEN J Parenter Enteral Nutr.* 1988;12:286–298

24. Katz JA, Chambers B, Everhart C, Marks JF, Buchanan GR. Linear growth in children with acute lymphoblastic leukemia treated without cranial irradiation. *J Pediatr.* 1991;118:575–578

25. Katz JA, Pollock BH, Jacaruso D, Morad A. Final attained height in patients successfully treated for childhood acute lymphoblastic leukemia. *J Pediatr.* 1993;123:546–552

26. Sempoux P, Moell C, Cornu G, Malvaux P, Maes M. Subnormal growth during puberty in children treated for acute lymphoblastic leukemia. *Pediatr Hematol Oncol.* 1992;9:217–222

27. Smith DE, Stevens MC, Booth IW. Malnutrition at diagnosis of malignancy in childhood: common but mostly missed. *Eur J Pediatr.* 1991;150:318–322

28. Kennedy L, Diamond J. Assessment and management of chemotherapy-induced mucositis in children. *J Pediatr Oncol Nurs.* 1997;14:164–177

29. Pettelo-Mantovani M, Guandaline S, diMartino L, et al. Prospective study of lactose absorption during cancer chemotherapy: feasibility of a yogurt-supplemented diet in lactose malabsorbers. *J Pediatr Gastroenterol Nutr.* 1995;20:189–195

30. Betcher DL, Ablin AR. Chemotherapy-induced nausea and vomiting. In: Ablin AR, ed. *Supportive Care of Children with Cancer.* Baltimore, MD: The Johns Hopkins University Press; 1993:59–66

31. Sheard NF, Clark NG. Nutritional management of pediatric oncology patients. In: Baker SB, Baker RD, Davis A, eds. *Pediatric Enteral Nutrition.* New York, NY: Chapman & Hall; 1994:387–398

32. Altman AJ, Barnard DR, Iacuone JJ, Wiener ES, Wolff LJ, Ablin AR. The prevention of infection. In: Ablin AR, ed. *Supportive Care of Children with Cancer.* Baltimore, MD: The Johns Hopkins University Press; 1993:1–11

33. Nielsen SS, Theologides A, Vickers ZM. Influence of food odors on food aversions and preferences in patients with cancer. *Am J Clin Nutr.* 1980;33:2253–2261

34. Bernstein IL, Webster MM, Bernstein ID. Food aversions in children receiving chemotherapy for cancer. *Cancer.* 1982;50:2961–2963

35. Chan AK, Sacks N. Enteral nutrition in pediatric oncology. *Oncology Nutrition Connection;* 8:1–11. Available at: http://www.oncologynutrition.org/public/newsletter/index.php. Accessed July 22, 2003

36. Singher L, Lukens JN, Ablin AR. Nutrition support. In: Ablin AR, ed. *Supportive Care of Children with Cancer.* Baltimore, MD: The Johns Hopkins University Press; 1993:107–112

37. Neumann CG, Jelliffe DB, Zerfas AJ, Jelliffe EF. Nutritional assessment of the child with cancer. *Cancer Res.* 1982;42(suppl 2):699s–712s

38. Holcomb GW III, Ziegler MM Jr. Nutrition and cancer in children. *Surg Annu.* 1990;22:129–142

39. Nutrition management of cancer. In: Williams CP, ed. *Pediatric Manual of Clinical Dietetics.* Chicago, IL: American Dietetic Association; 1998:151–160

40. Heland DK, Cook DJ, Guyatt GH. Enteral nutrition in the critically ill patient: a critical review of the evidence. *Intensive Care Med.* 1993;19:435–442

41. DeSwarte-Wallace J, Firouzbakhsh S, Finklestein JZ. Using research to change practice: enteral feedings for pediatric oncology patients. *J Pediatr Oncol Nurs*. 2001; 18:217–223

42. Mathew P, Bowman L, Williams R, et al. Complications and effectiveness of gastrostomy feedings in pediatric cancer patients. *J Pediatr Hematol Oncol*. 1996;18:81–85

43. Szeluga DJ, Stuart RK, Brookmeyer R, Utermohlen V, Santos GW. Nutritional support of bone marrow transplant recipients: a prospective, randomized clinical trial comparing total parenteral nutrition to an enteral feeding program. *Cancer Res*. 1987;47:3309–3316

44. Ford C, Whitlock JA, Pietsch JB. Glutamine-supplemented tube feedings versus total parenteral nutrition in children receiving intensive chemotherapy. *J Pediatr Oncol Nurs*. 1997;14:68–72

45. Deitch EA, Winterton J, Li M, Berg R. The gut as a portal of entry for bacteremia. *Ann Surg*. 1987;205:681–692

46. Pietsch JB, Ford C, Whitlock JA. Nasogastric tube feedings in children with high-risk cancer: a pilot study. *J Pediatr Hematol Oncol*. 1999;21:111–114

47. Charuhas PM, Gautier ST. Parenteral nutrition in pediatric oncology. In: Baker SB, Baker RD, Davis A, eds. *Pediatric Parenteral Nutrition*. New York, NY: Chapman & Hall; 1997:331–353

48. American Society for Parenteral and Enteral Nutrition. Guidelines for the use of parenteral and enteral nutrition in adult and pediatric patients. *JPEN J Parenter Enteral Nutr*. 1993;17(suppl 4):1SA–52SA

43

Diet in the Prevention of Cancer and Hypertension

The preponderance of evidence to date indicates that diet contributes to the development of chronic diseases. Observational studies over the past several decades have shown an association between diet in adult years and cancer and hypertension, and are responsible in part for federal diet and health policies in place since 1980 when the first Dietary Guidelines for Americans was published.[1] Causal relationships between diet and cancer and hypertension largely remain to be established. There are no consistent prospective studies available to establish a relationship between diet during childhood and the development of cancer and hypertension during adulthood.

Diet and Cancer

Many aspects of the relationship between diet and cancer, including both excessive or suboptimal levels of dietary components, remain under investigation. A recent review related dietary factors to breast and colorectal cancer.[2] Many breast cancer risk factors, such as age, family history of breast cancer, reproductive history, mammographic densities, previous breast disease, and race and ethnicity, are not subject to intervention. Being overweight, however, is an established breast cancer risk for postmenopausal women.[3] Risk factors for colorectal cancer may include age, personal and family history of polyps or colorectal cancer, inflammatory bowel disease, inherited syndromes, physical inactivity, obesity, alcohol use, and a diet high in fat and low in fruits and vegetables.[4] Research that relates diet to cancer is provided by animal experiments and epidemiological observational and prospective cohort studies. Very few intervention studies have investigated the relation between diet and cancer. The Women's Health Initiative, a prospective, randomized clinical trial, may help clarify the relationship between total fat and the risk of cancer. This multicenter trial investigates several risk factors for chronic disease in US women. One of the dietary interventions reduces fat intake to 25% of dietary calories to determine whether a low-fat diet has any effect on breast cancer risk.[5] At this time, there are no conclusive data about a causal relationship between cancer and fat intake, or cancer and any particular dietary factor.[2–4] Current dietary guidelines acknowledge the complex relationship that exists between the environment, including dietary patterns, and genotypes. Observational data suggest that a healthful dietary pattern to reduce the risk of cancer is one that emphasizes a variety of grains, especially whole grains, fruits, and vegetables, a moderate intake of total fat, and is low in saturated fat and cholesterol.[6]

Diet and Hypertension

A current goal of public health policy is to prevent the development of hypertension, which affects 1 in 4 US adults, more African Americans than whites, and more older than younger Americans.[7] In formulating a strategy to achieve this goal, it must be recognized that a significant portion of cardiovascular disease occurs in people whose blood pressure is above the optimal level (120/80 mm Hg) but not so high as to be diagnosed or treated with antihypertenisve medications. An effective intervention to prevent the rise in blood pressure with age and to reduce the mean blood pressure of the US population could substantially lower cardiovascular morbidity and mortality as much or more than a focus on treatment of individuals with diagnosed hypertension.

Lifestyle modifications have been promoted among adults to prevent or treat hypertension. These include (1) lose weight if overweight, (2) limit alcohol intake to no more than 2 drinks for men and one drink for women, (3) increase aerobic physical activity to 60 minutes most days of the week, (4) reduce sodium intake to not more than 100 mmol/d (2.4 g sodium or 6 g sodium chloride), (5) achieve daily recommended intakes of other nutrients that may affect blood pressure (ie, potassium, magnesium, and calcium) (see Appendix C), and (6) reduce intake of dietary saturated fat and cholesterol. The successful application of these 6 diet and lifestyle factors may also reduce other cardiovascular risk factors.[7]

In the past, researchers tried to find clues about what in the diet affects blood pressure by testing various nutrients, such as calcium and magnesium, individually. These studies were done mostly with dietary supplements of these nutrients, and their findings were not conclusive. In contrast, the Dietary Approaches to Stop Hypertension (DASH) study compared 3 eating plans for their effect on blood pressure: (1) a plan similar in nutrients to what many Americans consume, (2) a plan similar to what Americans consume but higher in fruits and vegetables, (3) the DASH diet.[8] All 3 plans used about 3000 mg of sodium daily. The DASH eating plan is low in saturated fat, cholesterol, and total fat, and emphasizes fruits, vegetables, and low-fat dairy foods. This eating plan includes whole grain products, fish, poultry, and nuts. It is reduced in red meat, sweets, and sugar-containing beverages. It is rich in magnesium, potassium, and calcium, as well as protein and fiber.[9]

The DASH study involved 459 adults with systolic blood pressures of less than 160 mm Hg and diastolic pressures of 80 to 95 mm Hg.[10] About 27% of the participants had hypertension. About 50% were women and 60% were African Americans.[11] Results showed that both the fruits and vegetables plan and the DASH diet reduced blood pressure. The DASH diet, however, had the greatest effect, especially for those with high blood pressure.[10] The blood pressure reduction averaged 11/6 mm Hg among those with hypertension and 4/2 mm Hg among those without hypertension, with the greatest reduction in African American hypertensive persons.[11] Further, the blood pressure reductions were seen within 2 weeks of starting the plan. The DASH trial showed that, in addition to calorie balance and intake of sodium chloride and alcohol, multiple nutrients influence blood pressure in adults.

An extension of the Dash study (Dash-Sodium) examined the effect on blood pressure of a reduced dietary sodium intake as participants followed either the DASH diet or an eating plan typical of what many Americans consume.[12] Participants were randomly assigned to one of the 2 successful eating plans described in the DASH study and then followed for a month at each of 3 sodium levels—about 3300 mg/d (the level consumed by many Americans) about 2400 mg/d (the daily value [DV] indicated on the Nutrition Facts food label) and about 1500 mg/d.

Reducing dietary sodium lowered blood pressure for subjects consuming both eating plans. At the 2 lower sodium intake levels, blood pressure was lower on the DASH diet than on the other eating plan. The biggest blood pressure reductions were for the DASH diet at the sodium intake of 1500 mg/d. Compared with the control diet, the DASH diet with the 1500 mg sodium resulted in a mean systolic blood pressure which was 7.1 mm Hg lower. Those with hypertension saw the biggest reductions, but those without it also had large decreases.[12] Thus, a dietary pattern with a lower sodium intake reduces blood pressure more than the DASH diet alone.

These 2 randomized controlled trials established both that blood pressure levels are lowered with a particular dietary pattern—the DASH diet—and that establishing a ceiling for sodium intake, such as the DV level of 2400 mg/d or an even lower target of 1500 mg/d, lowers blood pressure further. In summary, the total data from a myriad of studies conducted in US adults now establish that blood pressure can be lowered with dietary change and that lower blood pressure predicts lower rates of coronary heart disease and greater longevity.

Children and adolescents with the upper distribution of blood pressure are at risk of developing hypertension as adults.[13] In addition, children with a family history of high blood pressure have 2 mm Hg (2%) higher systolic blood pressure and 1 mm Hg (1.5%) higher diastolic blood pressure than children without a family history of hypertension.[14] A review of 25 observational and 12 intervention studies[15] that examined the relationship between nutrient intake and blood pressure in children found that sodium intake is positively related to higher blood pressure in children and adolescents. In comparison, the review found no clear relationship in children and adolescents between blood pressure and the intake of potassium or magnesium or calcium—other nutrients often associated with blood pressure levels in adults. Among adolescents, a relationship between sodium intake and blood pressure is linked with being overweight and having a family history of hypertension or African American ancestry.[16] While these studies relate sodium intake to blood pressure levels, there is no conclusive evidence that relates sodium intake or other dietary factors in infancy and childhood and the development of chronic hypertension.

References

1. Ballard-Barbash R. Designing surveillance systems to address emerging issues in diet and health. *J Nutr.* 2001;131:437S–439S
2. US Department of Health and Human Services, Office of Disease Prevention and Health Promotion. Healthy People 2010: Objectives for Improving Health. Washington, DC: US Government Printing Office; 2001
3. Henderson BE, Pike MC, Bernstein L, Ross RK. Breast cancer. In: Schottenfeld D, Fraumeni JF Jr, eds. *Cancer Epidemiology and Prevention.* 2nd ed. New York, NY: Oxford University Press; 1996:1022–1039
4. Scottenfeld D, Winawer SJ. Cancers of the large intestine. In: Schottenfeld D, Fraumeni JF Jr, eds. *Cancer Epidemiology and Prevention.* 2nd ed. New York, NY: Oxford University Press; 1996:813–840
5. Whittemore AS, Henderson BE. Dietary fat and breast cancer: where are we? *J Natl Cancer Inst.* 1993;85:764–765
6. US Department of Agriculture and US Department of Health and Human Services. *Nutrition and Your Health: Dietary Guidelines for Americans.* 5th ed. Washington, DC: US Government Printing Office; 2000

7. Joint National Committee on Detection, Evaluation, and Treatment of High Blood Pressure. The sixth report of the Joint National Committee on the Detection, Evaluation and Treatment of High Blood Pressure. *Arch Intern Med.* 1997;157: 2413–2446

8. Sacks FM, Obarzanek E, Windhauser MM, et al. Rationale and design of the Dietary Approaches to Stop Hypertension trial (DASH). A multicenter controlled-feeding study of dietary patterns to lower blood pressure. *Ann Epidemiol.* 1995;5:108–118

9. Karanja NM, Obarzanek E, Lin PH, et al. Descriptive characteristics of the dietary patterns used in the Dietary Approaches to Stop Hypertension Trial. *J Am Diet Assoc.* 1999;99(suppl 8):S19–S27

10. Appel LJ, Moore TJ, Obarzanek E, et al. A clinical trial of the effects of dietary patterns on blood pressure. *N Engl J Med.* 1997;336:117–1124

11. Svetkey LP, Simons-Morton D, Vollmer WM, et al. Effects of dietary patterns on blood pressure: subgroup analysis of the Dietary Approaches to Stop Hypertension (DASH) randomized clinical trial. *Arch Intern Med.* 1999;159:285–293

12. Sacks FM, Svetkey LP, Vollmer WM, et al. Effects on blood pressure of reduced dietary sodium and the Dietary Approaches to Stop Hypertension (DASH) diet. DASH-Sodium Collaborative Research Group. *N Engl J Med.* 2001;344:3–10

13. Shear CL, Burke GL, Freedman DS, Berenson GS. Value of childhood blood pressure measurements and family history in predicting future blood pressure status: results from 8 years of follow-up in the Bogalusa Heart Study. *Pediatrics.* 1986;77: 862–869

14. Lauer RM, Burns TL, Clarke WR, Mahoney LT. Childhood predictors of future blood pressure. *Hypertension.* 1991;18(suppl 3):I74–I81

15. Simons-Morton DG, Obarzanek E. Diet and blood pressure in children and adolescents. *Pediatr Nephrol.* 1997;11:244–249

16. Falkner B, Michel S. Blood pressure response to sodium in children and adolescents. *Am J Clin Nutr.* 1997;65(suppl 2):618S–621S

44

Gastrointestinal Disease

This chapter discusses some general principles of nutritional treatment for disorders of the gastrointestinal tract. Some of the diseases for which there is specific nutritional therapy are discussed in detail elsewhere in this text, but the principles presented here should be an integral part of therapy for these diseases.

Diseases of the Gastrointestinal Tract

The Esophagus

Gastroesophageal Reflux

The reflux of gastric contents into the esophagus is common early in life. Thickened formulas have been used for infants with gastroesophageal reflux (GER), but their benefit remains unproven. Solids may retard gastric emptying, and the role of delayed gastric emptying in the pathogenesis of GER in infants continues to be evaluated.

Studies of gastric emptying in infants have shown it to be altered by the composition, osmolarity, and calorie density of feedings, and several investigators have suggested that delayed gastric emptying may contribute to GER. In one study of children with spastic quadriplegia, gastric emptying, evaluated by scintigraphy, was shown to be accelerated with whey-based formulas when compared to a casein-based formula.[1] When fed whey-based formulas, patients had significantly fewer episodes of emesis than when fed a casein-based formula.

In another study of GER, chronic gastrointestinal symptoms and histologic changes of the esophagus unresponsive to standard treatments for GER were improved by the use of an elemental formula.[2] There is now some support for the concept that cow milk protein allergy may contribute to GER in some patients.

Dysmotility

Esophageal motility and gastroesophageal sphincter function is a complex, highly coordinated process that may be influenced by ingested nutrients. One report described an infant with delayed development and peripheral myopathy who was nourished using a soy-based liquid diet deficient in carnitine.[3] The investigators proposed that dysmotility of the upper gastrointestinal tract in infants may occur in carnitine deficiency. However, this observation needs to be further examined.

The Stomach

Dumping Syndrome

Dumping syndrome, thought to result from the rapid gastric emptying of carbohydrates with consequent hyperglycemia followed by reactive symptomatic hypoglycemia, is relatively rare in children. When encountered in children, dumping syndrome is usually a complication of a Nissen fundoplication. The syndrome has been treated with continuous nasogastric or gastrostomy feedings and by the frequent administration of small amounts of thickened feeds to which are added complex carbohydrates such as fiber and/or uncooked cornstarch.

Bezoars

Bezoars of the gastrointestinal tract have been the subject of medical curiosity and historical interest for decades. Lactobezoars ("milk curd bezoars") tend to occur during the first 3 weeks of life in infants with birth weights of less than 1500 g and gestational ages of less than 33 weeks. Operative intervention may be necessary, but early diagnosis and treatment, including cessation of oral intake for 24 hours, gentle gastric lavage with saline, and a change in formula, should resolve this problem relatively promptly. Most cases develop in the first 2 weeks of life in infants fed formulas of high-caloric density (24 calories per ounce). Some authors have suggested that when infants with this condition are recognized early, a predigested elemental formula devoid of intact casein should be used to help clear the obstruction.

Pernicious Anemia

Individuals with pernicious anemia require intramuscular supplements of vitamin B_{12} every month or 2. However, recently, it has been noted that 300- to 1000-μg daily doses of oral cyanocobalamin have led to acceptable serum levels of vitamin B_{12} in patients with pernicious anemia. In Sweden, oral cobalamin "has proved to be a completely safe alternative to B_{12} injections."[4] Others have suggested that intranasal cobalamin is more effective than the oral administration of cobalamin.[5]

Peptic Ulcer Disease

There are no conclusive studies implicating constituents of the diet as causative factors in the establishment of *Helicobacter pylori* infection, and the use of diet in the treatment of this infection does not appear to be efficacious. However, recent studies suggest that smoking may impair the eradication of *H pylori*, and children who eat several servings of fruits and vegetables a day and drink 2 or more cups of milk a day are less likely to acquire the infection. Most reports of *H pylori* infection in developing countries support the role of food prepared under unhygienic conditions as the probable mechanism of transmission of the organism and suggest that the cause of childhood acquisition of *H pylori* infection is limited to unhygienic practices.

The Intestine

Celiac Disease

Celiac disease is a gluten-sensitive disorder characterized by malabsorption and a typical histologic lesion of the small intestine. Treatment with a strict gluten-free diet results in complete clinical and histologic recovery. The conventional gluten-free diet prohibits the use of wheat, barley, and rye. Whether oat should be eliminated from the diet remains controversial, with the weight of evidence in favor of permitting moderate oat intake. Studies evaluating the increased risk of intestinal malignancy in celiac disease have shown that the risk is not increased compared with that of the general population if celiac patients adhere to a gluten-free diet for 5 years or more.

Lactose Intolerance

Lactase deficiency and lactose malabsorption can cause abdominal pain and distention, flatulence, and the passage of loose, watery stools. Lack of awareness and misunderstanding of lactose intolerance are quite prevalent in the public. It has been reported that the consumption of 1 cup (8 oz) of milk produces negligible symptoms in lactase-deficient individuals, and some have concluded that lactase-deficient patients may tolerate 2 cups of milk per day without appreciable symptoms.[6]

Patients with inflammatory bowel disease (IBD) tend to avoid dairy products more than is necessary, partly because of incorrect patient perceptions and partly because of arbitrary advice from physicians and popular diet books. Adequate scientific and clinical information is now available to permit recommendations about the intake of dairy products for each patient with IBD.[7]

Food Allergy

Allergic disorders have been linked to a variety of factors, including genetic predisposition, environment, smoke exposure, and infection. Some authors suggest that cow milk protein intolerance (CMPI) symptoms regress within 3 to 4 years in most children. As mentioned earlier, CMPI may be associated with gastroesophageal reflux. The protein may also induce gastric dysrhythmia in infants with cow milk allergy that, in turn, may contribute to reflux and vomiting.[8] (See also Chapter 34.)

Short-Bowel Syndrome

Before the introduction of parenteral nutrition (PN), the prognosis for newborn infants undergoing extensive small-bowel resection was poor, survival being determined by both the length of the residual intestine and the presence or absence of the ileocecal valve. The availability of PN has transformed the outcome for these children, allowing them to grow normally during the long period required for adaptation of the remaining small intestine after surgery.

After significant intestinal resection, amino acids and peptides should be used because they are better tolerated than intact protein. Fat is poorly tolerated in many of these children, especially if the ileum has been resected. This results in a diminished bile acid pool size and steatorrhea. Medium-chain triglycerides (MCTs) are usually a better source of dietary lipid under these circumstances because they are partially water soluble and do not require bile acids for absorption; however, some long-chain fat must be provided for essential fatty acid needs.

Inflammatory Bowel Disease

Nutritional therapy may be important in the treatment of inflammatory bowel disease, at least for Crohn's disease. Some authors suggest that increased enteral nutrition should be a first-line treatment for Crohn's disease. The value of good nutrition in ulcerative colitis is not clearly established, but some recent studies suggest that dietary fish oil may reduce colonic inflammation in this disease.

Two recent randomized, double-blind, placebo-controlled crossover studies examined the role of fish oil supplementation in patients with ulcerative colitis. Although fish-oil supplementation provides only modest benefits to patients with ulcerative colitis, this research may establish a precedent for further work on modulating inflammatory processes by using dietary manipulation of long-chain fatty acids.

Intestinal Atrophy

The intestine is known to atrophy extensively when children and adults are fed exclusively by parenteral nutrition. Recent studies have shown glutamine

to be a primary respiratory fuel source for enterocytes as well as for lymphocytes and macrophages. When stimulated, these cell types appear to metabolize large quantities of glutamine through partial oxidation. Under normal
conditions, sufficient glutamine is synthesized in the body to meet physiologic
requirements, but, during severe illness or stress, this requirement may not be
met, and a deficiency state may develop. Addition of sufficient glutamine to
PN solution has been shown in animals to attenuate gut atrophy and seemed
to reduce intestinal immune dysfunction observed with standard PN.[9] This
has not been studied extensively in children.

Pseudo-obstruction

Studies of children with pseudo-obstruction have suggested that enteral feedings using standard and elemental formulas should be tried, but that many
individuals will eventually require PN. Early nutritional intervention for these
patients is critical for sustaining growth and many improve their gut and
bladder function with early nutritional intervention.

Abetalipoproteinemia/Hypobetalipoproteinemia

In abetalipoproteinemia, there is inefficient or defective chylomicron formation, resulting from a generalized defect in cell membranes. The disease is
characterized by malformed erythrocytes (acanthocytes), retinitis pigmentosa,
and a form of Friedreich's ataxia. Vitamin E deficiency may explain part of the
symptoms. Treatment consists of dietary restriction of triglycerides. Medium-
chain triglycerides should initially be substituted for long-chain triglycerides,
and substantial fat-soluble vitamin supplements plus essential fatty acids
should be provided.

Intestinal Lymphangiectasia

Intestinal lymphangiectasia is characterized by dilated mucosal, submucosal,
or subserosal lymphatics and by protein-losing enteropathy leading to hypoalbuminemia, peripheral edema, and lymphopenia. The disease may be severe
or mild, chronic or transitory, and, on occasion, none of the classic signs or
symptoms may be manifest.

Treatment consists of a high-protein, very low long-chain-fat diet with added
MCT. While this diet has no effect on the underlying pathology, it reduces enteric lymph flow, and, in theory, enteric protein loss. It seems reasonable to
assume that the absence of fat in the diet reduces engorgement of the intestinal
lymphatics; MCT being absorbed directly into the portal system provides an
energy source but avoids lacteal engorgement.

Nonspecific Diarrhea

Prolonged nonspecific idiopathic diarrhea is common is young children. Symptoms begin usually between 6 and 30 months of age, with 3 to 6 loose stools per day. With the cause and pathophysiology remaining ill-defined, the cornerstone of therapy has been reassurance. Experience indicates that because the problem eventually resolves spontaneously, some patients may benefit from restoration of normal amounts of fat in their diet, which may be fat deficient. Malabsorption of carbohydrates (particularly in hyperosmolar beverages like juices and sodas), sorbitol found in juices, and excessive fluid intake may contribute to loose stools in some children.

Irritable Bowel Syndrome

Irritable bowel syndrome (IBS) is a motor disorder of the gut associated with altered bowel habits, abdominal pain, and the absence of any detectable organic pathologic process. Its diagnosis requires the exclusion of organic disease because it is without precise motility or structural correlates. The identity may begin in childhood as recurrent abdominal pain.

Increased dietary fiber has been a suggested treatment for IBS. Children in the United States, like adults, probably consume inadequate amounts of dietary fiber for optimal health.[10] The recommendation now is that dietary fiber should be increased in children 3 years of age and older, as well as in adults. This is best accomplished by increasing the intake of a variety of fiber-rich fruits, vegetables, and cereals and other grain products. A reasonable goal for minimal intake of dietary fiber for ages 3 through 20 years is suggested to be the equivalent of the age of an individual plus 5. Accordingly, fiber intake will range from 8 g/d for a 3-year-old child to 25 g/d at age 20 years, and remain constant thereafter.[10] Certainly, in children with recurrent abdominal pain, IBS, or other functional gastrointestinal problems, fiber intake should be assessed, and fiber should be recommended if the diet is deficient. Gastrointestinal distress, as occurs in IBS, may be provoked by malabsorption of small amounts of fructose, sorbitol, and fructose-sorbitol mixtures in patients with functional bowel disease. Nevertheless, these patients invariably have interrelated multifactorial and complex problems.

Disease of the Liver

Intestinal absorption and metabolism of key nutrients may play critical roles in the development of hepatic encephalopathy (HE). It is generally agreed that nutrition and diet are important factors in the pathophysiology and management of HE. Most available data on nutrition and the use of diet in the treatment of HE come from studies of adult patients.

Hepatocellular Failure

The provision of adequate nutrition to patients with severe liver disease is a major concern since limited protein intake may be advisable when hepatic function is compromised. It has been suggested that increased dietary protein in hepatocellular failure is a factor in the precipitation of hepatic encephalopathy.

Branch-chain amino acid (BCAA)-enriched formulas, both parenteral and enteral, have been used in the treatment of acute and chronic liver failure. They are expensive, and the clinical application and usefulness of these formulas in the nutritional support of patients, especially those in the pediatric age group with hepatic dysfunction, needs to be more clearly defined.

Poorly absorbed dissacharides as well as soluble fiber in the diet may have profound effects on nitrogen metabolism in the colon and significant therapeutic benefits in patients with hepatocellular failure. Lactulose, which consists of galactose and fructose, is neither broken down nor absorbed in the small intestine. When lactulose reaches the colon, it is metabolized by intraluminal bacteria with the production of organic acids. The dual effects of lactulose on colonic microflora to acidify the fecal stream and increase utilization of nitrogen, thereby reducing ammonia production, are the likely mechanisms, whereby lactulose reduces the amount of ammonia absorbed into the portal system. Through these mechanisms, lactulose might also alter the production or absorption of a number of potential cerebral toxins in addition to ammonia.

Dietary Treatment Guidelines (see Table 44.1)

Subclinical Hepatic Encephalopathy

This subclinical form of HE, which can adversely affect quality of life, is rare in children. If suspected, this condition does warrant some dietary precautions. Reduction of dietary protein, the use of lactulose (or lacititol therapy), vegetable protein diets, zinc supplementation, and BCAA-enriched enteral supplements have been reported to reduce the severity of psychometric test performance deficits in this form of encephalopathy.

Overt Hepatic Encephalopathy

Initially, a zero-protein diet with parenteral dextrose should be used for patients in deep coma. Failure of patients to improve in 48 to 72 hours is often due to unidentified precipitating factors rather than end-stage liver failure. The

Table 44.1.
Dietary Treatment of Hepatic Encephalopathy

Protein
Limited to adequate intake
Vegetable source preferred
Branched-chain amino acids
Carbohydrate
High intake
Soluble fiber
Fat
Adequate to high intake
Minerals
Adequate intake
Zinc supplementation

physician faced with a patient who has unresolved HE after standard therapy must determine if precipitating factors are present and whether enteral or parenteral nutrition is to be used. Lactulose delivery via a nasogastric tube should be commenced except in patients with bowel obstruction. Stool pH should be monitored and kept below 6. Lacitol (B-galactosidosorbitol) is as effective as lactulose in controlling HE, and patient compliance may be better.[11] In cases of severe upper gastrointestinal bleeding, enemas should also be used.

Gallbladder Disease

Cholelithiasis occurs in children, and consequently the interaction of diet and cholelithiasis has been studied only in adults. Clinical experience has documented that very low-calorie diets used in treating obesity are associated with an increased risk of developing cholelithiasis. If substantial or rapid weight loss increases the risk of developing gallstones, a more gradual weight loss may lessen the risk. However, additional studies are necessary to further elucidate the relationship of cholelithiasis and diet.

Diseases of the Pancreas

Cystic Fibrosis

Although an entire chapter is devoted to cystic fibrosis (Chapter 46), several points should be underscored. Inadequate weight gain is hypothesized to be the direct result of an energy imbalance caused by malabsorption of nutrients, chronic respiratory infections, and increased metabolic rate or inadequate intake. However, there appear to be behavioral differences in eating and parents' perceptions of cystic fibrosis children's eating habits, which may contribute to the failure to achieve dietary recommendations in these children.[12,13] There is a need for individualized assessment of the energy needs of children with cystic fibrosis and comprehensive programs to teach parents behavioral strategies to motivate their children to meet the high energy needs required for these patients to grow.

Acute Pancreatitis

During the past 2 decades, nutritional support has come to be a significant component of the general supportive therapy for acute pancreatitis. The recommendation for the nutritional support of children with acute pancreatitis is based on studies of adults. Generally, most patients with mild, uncomplicated pancreatitis do not benefit from nutritional support; however, nutritional support should begin early in patients with moderate to severe disease. In moderate to severe acute pancreatitis, initial nutritional support should be through the parenteral route and include fat emulsions in amounts sufficient to prevent essential fatty acid deficiency. It has been suggested that patients requiring an operation for the diagnosis of complications of the disease should have a feeding jejunostomy placed at the time of the operation for subsequent enteral nutrition using a low-fat formula. When oral feedings are instituted, they should be low in fat content and should be reinstituted using traditional clinical criteria, including the symptoms of the patient, physical examination, and appearance of the pancreas on computed tomography (CT). These guidelines must be individualized to incorporate what is perhaps the most important clinical variable—the premorbid nutritional state of the patient. Most importantly, it must be remembered that these recommendations are based on data from studies of adults and not children.

Chronic Pancreatitis

A high-energy diet adequately supplemented with fat is recommended to achieve usual growth. However, voluntary intake of nutrients by a child or teenager with chronic pancreatitis may be inadequate for normal or catch-up growth. Therefore, enteral feedings (nasogastric or gastrostomy tube) or total parenteral nutrition may be required.

Pancreatic insufficiency due to chronic pancreatitis may lead to symptomatic malabsorption of both starch and fat. The use of pancreatic enzymes in patients with pancreatic insufficiency due to chronic pancreatitis very often reduces abdominal pain and discomfort because of improved absorption of complex carbohydrates. Because of malabsorption, additional fat-soluble vitamins are usually required to compensate for increased losses.

Conclusion

Diet and nutritional intervention is useful in the treatment of many gastrointestinal diseases, but additional research and more clinical trials are needed to better define the importance of dietary therapy in gastrointestinal disease.

References

1. Fried MD, Khoshoo V, Secker DJ, Gilday DL, Ash JM, Pencharz PB. Decrease in gastric emptying time and episodes of regurgitation in children with spastic quadriplegia fed a whey-based formula. *J Pediatr.* 1992;120:569–572

2. Kelly KJ, Lazenby AJ, Rowe PC, Yardley JH, Perman JA, Sampson HA. Eosinophilic esophagitis attributed to gastroesophageal reflux: improvement with an amino acid-based formula. *Gastroenterology.* 1995;109:1503–1512

3. Weaver LT, Rosenthal SR, Gladstone W, Winter HS. Carnitine deficiency: a possible cause of gastrointestinal dysmotility. *Acta Paediatr.* 1992;81:79–81

4. Lederle FA. Oral cobalamin for pernicious anemia. Medicine's best keep secret? *JAMA.* 1991;265:94–95

5. Romeo VD, Sileno A, Wenig DN. Intranasal cyanocobalamin. *JAMA.* 1992;268: 1268–1269

6. Suarez FL, Savaiano D, Arbisi P, Levitt MD. Tolerance to the daily ingestion of two cups of milk by individuals claiming lactose intolerance. *Am J Clin Nutr.* 1997;65: 1502–1506

7. Mishkin S. Dairy sensitivity, lactose malabsorption and elimination diets in inflammatory bowel disease. *Am J Clin Nutr.* 1997;65:564–567

8. Ravelli AM, Tobanelli P, Volpi S, Ugazio AG. Vomiting and gastric motility in infants with cow's milk allergy. *J Pediatr Gastroenterol Nutr.* 2001;32:59–64

9. Glutamine in parenteral solutions enhances intestinal mucosal immune function in rats. *Nutr Rev.* 1993;51:152–155

10. American Academy of Pediatrics. A summary of conference recommendations on dietary fiber in childhood. Conference on Dietary Fiber in Childhood, New York, May 24, 1994. *Pediatrics.* 1995;96:1023–1028

11. Morgan MY, Hawley KE. Lactitol vs lactulose in the treatment of acute hepatic encephalopathy in cirrhotic patients: a double-blind, randomized trial. *Hepatology.* 1987;7:1278–1284

12. Stark LJ, Mulvihill MM, Jelalian E, et al. Descriptive analysis of eating behavior in school-age children with cystic fibrosis and healthy control children. *Pediatrics.* 1997;99:665–671

13. Stark LJ, Jelalian E, Mulvihill MM, et al. Eating in preschool children with cystic fibrosis and healthy peers: behavioral analysis. *Pediatrics.* 1995;95:210–215

45

Cardiac Disease

Growth retardation is prevalent in children with congenital heart disease (CHD). Growth failure in heart disease has a multifactorial etiology and follows a pattern identical to acute and chronic protein-calorie undernutrition with wasting and stunting, once termed cardiac cachexia. Cyanosis, congestive heart failure (CHF), and pulmonary hypertension (pulmonary-systemic pressure ratio >0.4) are all consequences of lesions producing circulatory shunts of varying direction and magnitude. These physiologic alterations are the sentinel features of CHD implicated in growth failure. The growth failure often begins before birth. Infants with most forms of cardiac malformations (transposition of the great arteries [TGA] being a notable exception) have a lower than normal birth weight.[1] Approximately 6% of infants with symptomatic heart disease may present with intrauterine growth retardation.[2] In addition, extracardiac malformations or recognizable syndromes (eg, trisomy 21, trisomy 18, Turner, VACTERL, CHARGE) with noncardiac reasons for impaired growth are also more common in children with heart disease.[3]

Acute undernutrition, defined as reduced weight relative to the weight predicted by length (wasting) and chronic undernutrition, based on reduced length relative to that predicted for age (stunting), are more prevalent among hospitalized patients with CHD. Acute undernutrition, or wasting, may affect up to one third of patients and chronic undernutrition, or stunting, may be found in about two thirds of patients. As many as 60% of patients with left-to-right shunts and up to 70% of patients with either cyanosis or CHF meet criteria for undernutrition.[4] The most severe undernutrition may occur in severe CHF associated with ventricular septal defect (VSD), patent ductus arteriosus (PDA), TGA, or coarctation of the aorta. Infants with these defects may present as appropriate for gestational age at birth but incur early weight deficits or wasting, followed by linear growth deficits or stunting. In cyanotic lesions such as tetralogy of Fallot or TGA, symmetric failure to thrive is observed with weight and length gain depressed concurrently. In acyanotic lesions such as atrial septal defect (ASD), VSD, or PDA, slow weight gain or wasting predominates over linear growth retardation or stunting, especially with CHF and/or large left-to-right shunts. The incidence of growth failure is highest in patients with VSD, perhaps because of the greater prevalence of pulmonary hypertension and CHF in children with large left-to-right shunts.[5] A recent retrospective study of 123 children with CHD showed the worst growth retardation in patients with a large VSD (CHF) and tetralogy of Fallot (cyanotic heart disease). Delay in skeletal maturation as assessed by bone age is related to severity of hypoxemia in cyanotic heart disease but also is seen in CHF.[5] Conversely, asymptomatic acyanotic lesions (aortic stenosis, coarctation, pulmonary stenosis) without CHF or pulmonary hypertension may not be associated with undernutrition. Surgical repair or correction allows normalization of most height deficits.[6]

The following text describes the components of undernutrition in CHD, the nutritional impact of the hemodynamic features of CHD, and the effects of nutrients on cardiac function, providing a basis for optimal nutritional management and monitoring.

Undernutrition in Congenital Heart Disease
Undernutrition occurs when metabolic demands for protein or energy (expenditure) combined with nutrient losses (regurgitation or malabsorption) exceed energy and protein nutrient intake. Investigators have attempted to study each of these components of nutrient balance.

Energy Expenditure
A number of studies have confirmed that total daily energy expenditure (TDEE), including components of physical activity such as cardiorespiratory work associated with movement, and dietary thermogenesis, is increased significantly in children with CHD, with relatively insignificant increases in resting energy expenditure (REE) relative to lean body mass. Total daily energy expenditure is composed of REE, physical activity, and dietary-induced thermogenesis. Metabolizable, or absorbed, energy intake must exceed TDEE to permit normal growth. Although REE in children with CHD seems to be similar to age-matched reference children, infants from 3 to 5 months of age with CHD have approximately 40% increased TDEE (94.2 + 6.9 kcal/kg/d vs 67.1 + 7.3 kcal/kg for healthy infants).[7–11] Surgery does not seem to alter REE.[5]

Nutrient Losses
Some patients with CHD have abnormalities of gastrointestinal function or renal losses that may affect nutrition. Urinary losses of energy as glucosuria and

proteinuria may be significant in certain patients with renal disease or glucose intolerance. Approximately 8% of infants with CHD have associated major gastrointestinal malformations, such as tracheoesophageal fistula and esophageal atresia, malrotation, or diaphragmatic hernia, that generally will limit intake and cause losses of nutrients.[12] Fecal losses of energy in subclinical steatorrhea or of protein in protein-losing enteropathy may be more significant and prevalent than expected, affecting up to 50% of patients with a variety of congenital heart lesions. In one study, protein-losing enteropathy was found in 8 of 21 infants with severe CHD[13] and is a major complication common to patients who undergo the Fontan procedure or have severe right-sided CHF. Steatorrhea, indicative of disturbed digestion or absorption, was found in 5 of 21 infants with CHD (1 of 8 patients with CHF and 4 of 12 cyanotic patients).[13] In these patients, mucosal small-bowel biopsies were normal. Mean resting oxygen consumption was higher in infants with CHF than in those with cyanotic heart disease.[13]

No significant malabsorption of energy or fat in stools was observed in the study of children receiving diuretics by Vaisman et al.[14] Total body water and extracellular water excess were measured and correlated directly with fat losses and inversely with energy intake, suggesting a relationship to the degree of CHF and diuretic efficacy. Therefore, infants with increased total body water (ie, not effectively diuresed) had more malabsorption than euvolemic diuresed patients.[14]

Yahav et al studied malabsorption relative to energy requirements in 14 infants with CHD aged 2 to 36 months (mean 10.4 months).[15] Ten infants with CHF and 4 with cyanosis were studied in 3 periods of 3 to 7 days each, comparing baseline oral intake, supplemented oral intake, and nasogastric feedings of a high-caloric density formula. Nasogastric feedings of a high-caloric density formula 1.5 kcal/mL or 45 kcal/oz were administered to 11 patients. Consistent weight gain averaging 13 g/d was observed only in patients receiving >170 kcal/kg/d, with only 50% of the children gaining weight on 149 kcal/kg/d. Increased cardiac and respiratory rates were observed in patients after feeding and were attributed to dietary thermogenesis but did not appear to be clinically significant. Minor intestinal losses of fat were observed in 3 patients and protein-losing enteropathy in no patients, and were not considered significant limiting factors.[15]

Nutrient Intake

Several studies have examined energy/nutrient intake requirements of infants and young children with CHD (Table 45.1). Approximately 140 to 150 kcal/kg/d is required to effect linear growth and increase subcutaneous fat and muscle in infants with CHD and CHF. In one study of 19 infants randomly assigned to 3 groups, only the group receiving continuous 24-hour NG feedings over a 5-month study period were able to achieve intake >140 kcal/d (mean 147).[16] Only this group of patients was able to demonstrate improved nutritional status manifested as increased weight, length, and anthropometric measures of fat and muscle stores. The groups who received either 12-hour supplemental nocturnal infusions or oral feedings failed to achieve such intakes and growth responses, perhaps due to increased REE. The 12-hour oral plus infusion group received only 122 kcal/kg, well below the threshold for growth. Fatigue during oral feedings was considered a limiting factor in both of these groups. In addition, in the 12-hour infusion group, daytime oral intake (52 kcal/kg) actually dropped to approximately 50% of the pre-study mean caloric intake (98 kcal/kg). The investigators concluded that only 24-hour continuous enteral feeding by nasogastric tube of a 1 kcal/mL formula was able to provide >140 kcal/kg/d and affect improved nutritional status.[16]

Two studies have concluded that children with CHD who are not growing appear to consume insufficient calories since they respond to supplementation, supporting the fact that failure to gain weight can be simply a matter of inadequate intake, not intrinsic genetic or cardiac factors. The type of cardiac defect does not necessarily predict or limit the response to dietary counseling and oral supplementation.[17,18]

Delayed gastric emptying[19] and gastroesophageal reflux[20] in children with CHD as well as oral aversion may be significant features that reduce voluntary intake and compromise nutrition. There may be early satiety induced by gastroparesis and gut hypomotility related to edema or hypoxia as well as by distention from hepatomegaly associated with CHF.

Congestive Heart Failure

Growth failure in CHF in children is common. The pathogenesis of this growth failure in CHF is not always clear and is likely to be multifactorial. Congestive heart failure may impair growth disturbance as a consequence of increased energy requirements due to increased myocardial and respiratory work and increased catecholamines, as well as intestinal malabsorption and anorexia or fatigability during feedings. In adults with CHF, total energy expenditure appears to be lower than that of controls. High protein-calorie feeds do not reverse the growth impairment, suggesting that the wasting has a metabolic basis rather than resulting from negative protein and energy balance.[21] In addition, malnutrition in adults with CHF is associated with increased right atrial pressure and tricuspid regurgitation.[22] Elevated right atrial pressures could thus cause intestinal protein losses and fat malabsorption and/or anorexia because of splanchnic and mesenteric venous congestion. In adults, REE is increased and may be caused by the increased work of breathing or elevated sympathetic innervation.[23] Cytokines such as tumor necrosis factor are elevated in adults with heart failure and may contribute to the cachexia seen in this condition.[24]

Both oxygen consumption and basal metabolic rate are increased in infants with CHF when compared with normal children or children with cyanotic CHD.[13,25,26] Traditionally, growth failure has been most common in infants with CHF due to pulmonary overcirculation from large left-to-right shunts such as a VSD or atrioventricular septal defect. This has been most evident in children with a VSD and large left-to-right shunt and pulmonary hypertension.[18] Fortunately, the increasing success of complete repairs of such defects in infancy has greatly lessened this problem.

There are many possible reasons for growth failure in children with CHF. There may be insufficient caloric intake due to inability to consume adequate calories for growth, intestinal malabsorption due to passive congestion and/or low cardiac output, or increased metabolic demands, mainly due to increased work of breathing. Insufficient caloric intake could be caused by a variety of factors, including excessive fatigue with oral feeding, excessive vomiting, or iatrogenic fluid restriction and diuresis because of the severity of heart failure.[16,27] Decreased gastric capacity caused by pressure on the stomach from an enlarged, congested liver, or from ascites may also interfere with the amount of nutrients a patient can ingest.[28] Children with CHF also may have abnormal intestinal function. They can demonstrate excessive intestinal protein losses, possibly secondary to elevated venous and lymphatic pressure.[13] Because of the obvious negative consequences of chronic fluid (and thus caloric) restriction in children, fluid restriction is now only temporarily used in patients who are either awaiting some type of intervention (eg, surgery or heart transplantation) or recovering from some type of acute process (eg, surgery, acute decompensation, pleural effusions).

Cyanotic Heart Disease

The role of hypoxia as a primary cause of growth retardation in children is unclear. Cyanotic CHD (eg, tetralogy of Fallot, tricuspid atresia) with chronic hypoxemia is frequently associated with undernutrition and linear growth retardation, especially if prolonged and if complicated by CHF (TGA or single ventricle). Isolated hypoxemia or desaturation does not necessarily result in tissue hypoxia since tissue aerobic metabolism may not be impaired until arterial pO$_2$ falls below 30 mm Hg, a threshold also affected by such factors as oxygen carrying capacity determined by erythroid mass or hemoglobin and tissue perfusion. Therefore, the added complication of CHF probably contributes to chronic tissue hypoxia limiting growth.

Some studies have demonstrated significant differences in growth between cyanotic and acyanotic children, whereas others have failed to do so.[5] Children without pulmonary hypertension who are cyanotic can demonstrate a normal nutritional state with stunting of growth being more common than poor weight gain.[29] Children with cyanotic CHD have also been shown to have excessive stool protein loss.[13] Cyanotic patients with pulmonary hypertension had the worst growth, with hypoxemia or cyanosis (right-to-left shunting) and pulmonary hypertension having additive effects.[29] However, after surgical repair of cyanotic CHD, resting and total energy expenditures in these children are no different than controls.[30]

Circulatory Shunts

Cardiac lesions with nutritional implications may also be categorized by shunt direction and magnitude: left-to-right shunts associated with CHF and right-to-left shunts associated with hypoxemia or cyanosis. As previously described, cyanotic patients with pulmonary hypertension appear to have the worst growth, with hypoxemia or cyanosis (right-to-left shunting) and pulmonary hypertension having additive effects.[18,29] Infants with a clinically significant VSD have significantly higher total energy expenditure than healthy control infants suggesting that they are unable to meet additional energy demands from activity of dietary thermogenesis, resulting in growth retardation.[31]

Pulmonary Hypertension

Increased resting oxygen consumption in CHD has been demonstrated, especially in patients with CHF or pulmonary hypertension, and attributed to the oxygen demands of increased catecholamine secretion and other factors. Pulmonary hypertension is a complication frequently implicated in growth failure, correlated with stunting in VSD, an acyanotic lesion.[32] Children with both cyanotic heart disease and pulmonary hypertension demonstrated both moderate to severe wasting and linear growth retardation.[29]

Significant protein-calorie undernutrititon may delay surgical correction and impair post-operative recovery and growth. Recently, growth failure has been added to the heart transplant criteria for the United Network for Organ Sharing, such that children with growth failure complicating CHD are listed at a higher status than children without growth failure.[33] Children demonstrate improvement in growth following corrective or palliative repair of a congenital heart lesion, and available data support the use of early surgical correction of major cardiac malformations to optimize growth.[9,30]

Within 1 week of surgery in infants with heart disease, energy expenditures fall sharply to reach levels significantly below preoperative levels. By approximately 2.5 years following surgery, weight, body composition, REE, TDEE, or energy expended during physical activity are similar to other healthy children without CHD.[30] Studies have demonstrated a reversal of decreased growth velocity in infants who have undergone repair of VSD, tetralogy of Fallot, and TGA in the first year of life.[34] There are conflicting data about somatic growth in patients who have undergone the Fontan procedure. Some studies have demonstrated improvement in growth parameters,[35] whereas others have shown persistent growth failure.[36] These differences may relate to many factors, including different malformations and timing for surgery. Catch-up linear growth is more likely with corrective than palliative surgery and with early repair. Residual, although reduced, CHF or shunt may still prevent normal nutritional recovery.[34,37]

Nutritional Assessment

A complete nutritional history includes feeding pattern and schedule, including frequency, duration, and volume of feedings. The volume of each feeding may actually be inversely related to the duration of feeding as the child fatigues. Diaphoresis with feedings reflects autonomic stimulation effects. Gastrointestinal function should be assessed to identify reflux and vomiting losses, irritability due to esophagitis or cramping, diarrhea, or constipation, and early satiety, which may respond to acid control and motility medications or be signs of associated anomalies. The physical examination must include accurate nude weight, length or height, and head circumference plotted on a growth curve. Consider changes in rate of growth or growth velocity as well as the relation of actual body weight to the ideal body weight predicted by height or length age. Use appropriate charts for preterm, Down syndrome, Turner syndrome, or Trisomy 18. Assessment of subcutaneous fat and muscle mass may be helpful, if measured by a skilled dietitian with calipers, although dehydration or edema may affect validity. Signs of CHF, pulmonary hypertension, clubbing, cyanosis, and hepatomegaly connote increased risk for nutritional failure.

Laboratory evaluation initially should include hemoglobin, oxygen saturation, albumin, and prealbumin. Protein-losing enteropathy as a cause of hypoalbuminemia can be confirmed by fecal α-1-antitrypsin assay and is encountered in conditions of systemic venous hypertension which occur with right-sided CHF, constrictive pericardial disease, restrictive cardiac disease, or post-Fontan operation. A low alkaline phosphatase or cholesterol may signify zinc deficiency that may affect taste and linear growth.

Nutritional Support

The goals of nutritional intervention are as follows:

1. Achieve nutritional balance by providing sufficient energy to stop catabolism of lean body mass and sufficient protein to match nitrogen losses.
2. Provide additional nutrients to restore deficits and allow growth, thus normalizing weight for height and promoting linear growth.
3. Provide enteral feedings to replace parenteral nutrition as tolerated by the gastrointestinal system.
4. Develop and maintain oral feeding competence to enable voluntary independent feeding.

Nutrient Prescription

The optimal nutritional support should provide sufficient energy and protein to not only prevent breakdown or catabolism of protein and maintain body composition and weight but also to restore deficits and permit growth toward genetic potential. Electrolyte losses with diuretics and deficiencies in micronutrients, such as the trace minerals iron and zinc or vitamins, may be limiting factors. As a general principle, for any given level of nitrogen (or protein) provided in the diet, increasing the energy (calories) will improve nitrogen balance and protein synthesis or accretion. Similarly, for a given level of energy intake, increasing the protein intake will improve the nitrogen balance or protein accretion. If energy provided by carbohydrate and fat in the diet is below the patient's requirements, protein will be catabolized as an energy source and not used in synthesis of lean body mass. Even if sufficient calories are provided to stop gluconeogenesis and restore body glycogen and fat stores, enough protein must be provided as a nitrogen source to allow accretion of lean body protein mass and effective growth. A marginal or negative electrolyte balance, such as low net sodium or potassium intake in the setting of fluid restriction and diuretic use, required for some patients in CHF, may impair growth independent of energy and protein sufficiency. Iron and zinc deficiencies have been implicated in cases of failure to thrive, with improved growth demonstrated after supplementation.

Energy Requirement

Additional energy above the recommended dietary allowance for age is required to permit normal growth rates, with even greater amounts required to restore nutritional deficits in "catch-up" or accelerated growth. A portion of this incremental energy requirement may be explained by simply calculating needs based on the patient's ideal or median body weight predicted from body length or even head circumference. This calculation assumes that metabolic needs for energy and protein are determined by the relatively preserved brain, visceral, and lean body mass with a minimal contribution from the adipose or fat mass that is depleted with undernutrition. In this reasoning, a lean but longer infant's energy requirement would exceed that of a robust infant of the same weight, whose lean mass is less and reflected in a shorter length. In undernutrition, the ratio of metabolically active lean body mass to total weight is increased. For example, children with CHD who are leaner than normal and at a weight-for-height age of 82% of ideal weight, 150 kcal/kg of actual body weight corresponds to 123 kcal/kg for a healthy robust infant of the same length but at ideal body weight.

Increased cardiac and respiratory work in the child with CHF, shunt, or cyanosis undoubtedly adds to the energy requirement. Increased catecholamines in CHF will increase energy expenditure as will the demands of increased respiratory rate and hematopoiesis in cyanotic heart disease. The myocardium itself is a significant consumer of energy with demands increased with pulmonary hypertension, hypertrophy, shunting, and CHF. Barton et al estimated the energy requirement of an infant with CHD—Energy cost of normal tissue deposition is 21 kJ/g (5 kcal/g).[38] This is 30% less than the 31 kJ/g (7.4 kcal/g) estimated in infants with CHD on high energy feeds.[39] This suggests a greater fat content (more energy per weight) of the tissue replenished in infants with CHD, supported by measuring increased skinfold thickness during high energy feeding. Assuming 75% of energy cost of growth is stored in this new tissue and the remainder used in synthesis (part of TDEE),

Table 45.1.
Energy Requirements for Normal Growth in Infants With CHD*

Study (ref.)	Age range	Mode	% IBW	kcal/kg/d	kcal/kg IBW
Bougle 1986[40]	2 week to 6 months	NG	–	137	–
Vanderhoof 1982[41]	1 week to 9 months	NG	–	120–150	–
Schwarz 1990[16]	1 to 10 months	NG	82	147	120
Yahav 1985[15]	2 to 36 months	NG/PO	76	149–169	113–128
Barton 1994[7]	0 to 3 months	NG/PO	80	143	114
Summary:	**0 to 36 months**	**NG**	**80**	**145**	**115**

* IBW=Ideal body weight or wt/ht; NG=nasogastric; PO=oral.

they calculated an intake of 600 kJ/kg/d (143 kcal/kg/d) to allow average weight gain during the first 3 months of life. Table 45.1 summarizes a number of studies of energy required to achieve growth in patients with CHD, comparing requirements calculated for actual body weight and ideal body weight-for-height age. Parenteral requirements for energy will be approximately 70% to 80% of these enteral estimates.

One must also consider the metabolic load imposed by feeding. Cardiac output is determined by tissue metabolic demand. As additional nutrients are provided, cardiac output must increase to oxygenate these tissues, and ventilatory demands on the lungs increase to eliminate the CO_2 generated by metabolic activity. This phenomenon of increased energy demands of nutrition support known as dietary thermogenesis, the thermic effect of food or specific dynamic action, varies for different nutrients, being minimal for fat metabolism and quite significant, up to 5% of calories, for carbohydrate. Carbohydrates are used for fat synthesis when carbohydrates or equivalent glucose amounts are administered at a rate exceeding 8 mg/kg/min. This endothermic process requires energy and oxygen and liberates CO_2 which must be expired. For this reason, the energy provided should be distributed between fat and carbohydrate, with fat providing at least 30% of the total caloric intake. At least 6% of the fat should be long-chain triglycerides (linoleic acid as in corn, soy, safflower oils) and some linolenic acid to provide essential fatty acids. The value and safety of additional α 3 fatty acids beyond essential fatty acid requirements are the subject of research.

Overfeeding or too-rapid increments in nutrition support can precipitate or worsen CHF. A refeeding syndrome has been described in which overzealous nutritional support has caused complications, not only with cardiac failure, but also with conduction disturbances and dysrhythmias related to electrolyte and mineral shifts with anabolism. Provision of glucose leads to an insulin-mediated influx of potassium and intermediary metabolism demands for phosphorus lead to an intracellular shift, causing profound hypokalemia, hypophosphatemia, hypomagnesemia, and hypocalcemia. Prolongation of QT_c interval may be observed. Sudden death suspected to be related to lethal arrhythmias such as torsade de pointes has been attributed to the refeeding of patients accommodated to the undernourished state.

In premature and full-term neonates with CHD, there is a higher incidence of necrotizing enterocolitis. This fact dictates gradual advancement of feeding in the newborn period and monitoring tolerance in terms of abdominal distention, accumulating gastric residual, and hematochezia. For those on parenteral nutrition, trophic feedings of approximately 10 cc/kg of formula, preferably expressed breast milk, for enteral and enterohepatic stimulation is beneficial.

Protein Intake

There is little discussion in the literature about nitrogen balance or protein intake in children with CHD. In general, if sufficient nonprotein energy is provided to prevent gluconeogenesis from catabolism of dietary amino acids, provision of more protein (up to specific limits) leads to greater incorporation of protein and its nitrogen in lean body mass. Protein generally constitutes 5% to 12% of total calories, reflected in the composition of breast milk and infant formulas modeling breast milk. Fomon and Ziegler suggested a formula caloric composition of 9% protein, 60% carbohydrate, and 31% fat provided in a density of 1 kcal/mL for infants with CHD.[42] The ratio of energy to protein in infant formulas is 30 to 50 kcal/g protein (corresponding to nonprotein calorie-nitrogen ratios of 287:140). Thus, a child receiving 140 kcal/kg/d of energy would receive 2.9 to 4.25 g/kg of protein, if derived from standard or concentrated formula, with protein constituting 8% to 12% of total calories. To avoid excessive hepatic protein metabolic and renal solute load, assuming a limit of 3.5 g/kg/d of protein, the additional energy required above 120 kcal/kg based on ideal body weight for length should be provided by either glucose polymers (polycose or starch) or by fat (microlipid or oils) added to the formula, unless using a standard infant formula or breast milk (see Table 45.2). These formulas are low enough in protein content that their high calorie-protein ratio allows concentration of the formula to achieve a higher calorie intake

Table 45.2.
Protein Load in Relation to Energy Provided in Selected Formulas

Formula	gm/dL (% kcal) protein	kcal/mL	kcal/g protein	kcal/kg @ 3.5 g/kg protein	Protein g/kg @:	
					140 kcal/kg/d	150 kcal/kg/d
Human Milk	0.9	.69	77	268	1.83	1.96
Enfamil/Similac	1.4	.67	48	167	2.9	3.1
Pediasure	3	1	33	116	4.25	4.5
Portagen	2.4	.67	28	98	5	5.36
Nutramigen	1.9	.67	35	123	4	4.25
Pregestimil	1.9	.67	35	123	4	4.25
Neocate-1+	2	.69	35	121	4	4.3
Vivonex Ped.	2.4	.8	33	117	4.2	4.3

without exceeding the threshold for protein tolerance. Once the child is older than 1 year, a protein-based 1 kcal/mL formula (Pediasure, Kindercal), a protein-hydrolysate (Peptamen Jr.), or an amino acid-based (Neocate – 1 +, Elecare, Vivonex Pediatric) formula should be substituted for infant formula.

Protein-losing enteropathy is diagnosed by hypoalbuminemia, lack of proteinuria, and positive fecal I-1-antitrypsin assay. Typically, protein-losing enteropathy is encountered in patients with Fontan anatomy or constrictive pericarditis. Additional protein is probably necessary and the fat provided may be limited to predominantly medium-chain triglycerides (MCT), transported via portal circulation, to reduce mesenteric lymphatic flow and pressures contributing to the protein loss. A similar rationale leads to the use of MCT in patients with chylothorax or chylous ascites. Formulas with predominant MCT as fat source are Portagen, a lactose-free protein hydrolysate formula with 85% of its fat as MCT oil, Vivonex Pediatric (68% MCT), Peptamen Jr. (60% MCT), Pregestimil (55% MCT), and Alimentum (50% MCT). The older child may be given Liposorb (85% MCT), similar in content to Portagen. Breast milk will be unable to supply these protein needs without supplementation and is very high in long-chain triglycerides assimilated via the lymphatic system.

Electrolytes, Minerals, and Micronutrients

Disturbances in electrolyte and mineral homeostasis accompany diuretic therapy or refeeding. Hypokalemia or hypocalcemia may cause changes in myocardial conduction and contractility. Diuretic therapy is irrational if sodium intake is not controlled. Potassium and chloride depletion commonly occur and may require supplementation. Calcium, magnesium, and zinc may also be depleted. Calciuria may be diminished by using chlorothiazide instead of furosemide. Calcium absorption from the gut is limited in magnesium deficiency (magnesium-dependent ATPase). Potassium may be spared by addition of spironolactone in selected cases.

Zinc depletion may manifest as a low alkaline phosphatase activity and cholesterol level (zinc-dependent enzymatic products). Iron needs are increased in cyanotic heart disease to maintain the increased erythroid mass demanded by hypoxemia. Anemia contributes to tissue hypoxia in patients with ventricular pressure overload, volume overload, CHF, or hypoxemia/cyanosis. In aortic valve stenosis, anemia may contribute to subendocardial ischemia causing angina or arrhythmia. In patients with a large VSD, anemia causes decreased blood viscosity and pulmonary vascular resistance that allows increased left-to-right shunting and increased CHF and pulmonary blood flow.[43] Selenium and carnitine deficiency may occur in unsupplemented parenteral nutrition and may manifest as cardiomyopathy.

Thiamine (vitamin B_1) deficiency may present as the syndrome of wet beriberi with varying severity of CHF due to impaired myocardial function and impaired autonomic regulation of circulation. Clinical manifestations include edema, fatigue, dyspnea, and tachycardia with signs of CHF. Shoshin is a severe form of beriberi that may affect infants with pulmonary edema and CHF. Thiamine depletion may occur in settings of high carbohydrate intake without thiamine as in a nursing mother on an inadequate diet or alcohol, and settings of prolonged parenteral nutrition or glucose administration without a multivitamin supplement. Thiamine requirements are increased with the stress of surgery and critical illness, and losses of thiamine increase with loop diuretics such as furosemide, putting patients with CHD at risk for deficiency. Shamir et al identified thiamine deficiency in 4 of 22 children with CHD before surgery, 3 of whom had adequate thiamine intakes, and 6 of 22 after surgery. However, no relationship to the level of undernutrition, thiamine intake, or furosemide use could be proved.[44] Vitamin K-containing foods, such as green leafy vegetables, may interfere with coumadin effectiveness.

Fluids

Many patients, especially those with CHF, are restricted in fluid intake with or without diuretic treatment. Providing adequate calories in the setting of fluid restriction is challenging and requires a concentrated formula, often requiring continuous administration via nasogastric or transpyloric tube.

Feeding Strategies

Oral or enteral feedings are preferred. Restriction in volume of formula in infants with CHF or cyanosis is not needed if they feed voluntarily. Many patients with CHD have limited oral voluntary intake insufficient to supply nutrient requirements to maintain growth. The increased cardiopulmonary demands of eating or associated problems such as gastrointestinal dysmotility, prematurity, and airway or pulmonary disease may prevent adequate intake. Volume may also be restricted, especially in patients with lesions associated with CHF or pulmonary hypertension, requiring diuretic therapy, fluid, and sodium restriction. Reparative or palliative surgery may be safer if performed after achieving a target weight. Formula concentration is frequently increased to provide more energy and protein in a restricted volume. If volume is the limiting factor, a more concentrated formula will be necessary to provide up to 3.5 g/kg/d of protein, above which additional calories may be added with carbohydrates (polycose powder or liquid) or fats (microlipid). Medium-chain triglycerides are not miscible in formula and may contribute to diarrhea and cramping, but are valuable as the principal fat source in patients with chylothorax. Concentrating a formula leads to increased protein and solute load, osmolarity or tonicity, and decreased free water.

Supplemental enteral nutrition is frequently instituted to achieve nutritional goals via nasogastric tube or gastrostomy. Some studies have concluded that only 24-hour continuous enteral feeding by nasogastric tube of a concentrated or augmented formula is able to provide the minimum of 140 kcal/kg/d necessary to improve nutritional status.[16] Consequences of coercive oral feeding efforts or nasopharyngeal tube placement and feeding include a high incidence of oral aversion, which may prove quite refractory long after the cardiac issues have improved. Patients who are considered likely to require chronic nasogastric tube feedings for greater than 6 months should be considered early for gastrostomy placement. Given the possibility that gastrostomy may alter motility and increase gastroesophageal reflux, evidence of airway penetration, impaired airway protective reflexes such as absent gag or cough, or lower respiratory tract disease may mandate protective anti-reflux surgery (Nissen fundoplication or variants). If airway protective reflexes are intact (eg, no vocal cord recurrent laryngeal nerve palsy), and there is no evidence of respiratory compromise, such as reactive airway disease, laryngospasm/stridor, or aspiration pneumonia, then percutaneous gastrostomy without anti-reflux surgery may be considered. The anatomy of the upper gastrointestinal tract should be evaluated by contrast studies to exclude associated anomalies of tracheoesophageal fistula, vascular ring, gross airway penetration directly or with reflux, and intestinal rotational anomalies. For patients with aspiration risks who are not considered safe candidates for anti-reflux fundoplication surgery, transpyloric feeding with a nasojejunal or percutaneous gastrojejunal tube is an alternative. Although transpyloric duodenal or jejunal feeding may prevent formula entry into the stomach, gastroduodenal motility may be inhibited and duodenogastric reflux of bile or gastroesophageal reflux of acid and/or bile may still occur.

The breastfed infant may require manual or pump expression of the milk if there is fatigue or problems suckling either due to inability to latch on, excessive respiratory effort and/or tachypnea competing with sucking and swallowing. Tube feeding either fortified breast milk or a high-caloric density formula continuously to augment a marginal nursing intake will be required for sufficient calories.

Parenteral nutrition is reserved for patients who cannot be fed effectively or safely fed by the enteral routes described above. Examples would be patients with associated gastrointestinal disease such as necrotizing enterocolitis or at risk for aspiration due to tachypnea and gastroesophageal reflux. Since cardiac output is determined by the demands of peripheral tissue metabolism, advancement of feedings, whether parenteral or enteral, in the patient accommodated to chronic malnutrition should be gradual and monitored for refeeding complications. Peripheral capillary vasodilation in response to tissue anabolism can lead to high output cardiac failure; excessive volume administration can provoke CHF and anasarca. Glucose uptake and metabolism will cause intracellular influx of potassium, magnesium, calcium and, most dramatically, phosphate. Dysrhythmias, particularly atrial arrhythmias related to changes in venous return, and ventricular arrhythmias, related to conduction disturbances associated with electrolyte fluxes (hypokalemia, hypocalcemia, hypophosphatemia), can manifest in changes in the corrected QT interval on electrocardiogram. Other cardiac complications of nutritional support include volume overload, increased viscosity, and pulmonary artery pressures with high lipid infusions (exceeding 0.15 g/kg/h or 3.5 g/kg/d), increased tissue metabolic demand for cardiac output, arrhythmias, and endocarditis/sepsis related to the central venous catheter.

Monitoring Outcome

Precise weights and lengths (or standing heights for patients greater than 3 years of age) should be obtained at each encounter and plotted on the appropriate growth curve (eg, Down syndrome specific curve, infant 0 to 36 months (lengths), or child 2 to 18 years (heights). The same dietitian should obtain measurements of mid-arm circumference and triceps skinfolds to help assess muscle and fat stores, understanding that fluid status and edema may affect the measures. Review of the diet is important. The current formula and methods for mixing and adding supplements should be reviewed to eliminate errors in formulation. The family should be instructed to bring a 3- or 5-day diet record to the clinic visit for evaluation by the dietitian for nutrient analysis. Attention should be paid to total caloric intake, proportion of fat and carbohydrate intake, protein intake, and adequacy of micronutrients, including iron, zinc, and vitamins. Fluid volume intake, urinary frequency, and hydration status in the context of diuretic therapy should be assessed. More sophisticated measures of body composition, including bone mineral status, may be obtained in certain groups or research settings if the technology such as dual energy x-ray absorptiometry or bioelectrical impedance analysis is available. Indirect calorimetry can assess REE and respiratory quotient to assess energy requirements and avoid overfeeding in patients in the intensive care unit. In the absence of direct measures of lean body mass or energy requirements, the surrogate parameter of weight expected for length age or ideal body weight for length, can be helpful in estimating energy and protein requirements for the very lean or obese child (see table 45.1). However, serial measurement of changes in weight, length, and anthropometry are the best indicators of nutrient adequacy.

References

1. Levy RJ, Rosenthal A, Castaneda AR, Nadas AS. Growth after surgical repair of simple D-transposition of the great arteries. *Ann Thorac Surg.* 1978;25:225–230
2. Levy RJ, Rosenthal A, Fyler DC, Nadas AS. Birthweight of infants with congenital heart disease. *Am J Dis Child.* 1978;132:249–254
3. Rosenthal GL, Wilson PD, Permutt T, Boughman JA, Ferencz C. Birth weight and cardiovascular malformations: a population-based study. The Baltimore-Washington Infant Study. *Am J Epidemiol.* 1991;133:1273–1281
4. Cameron JW, Rosenthal A, Olson AD. Malnutrition in hospitalized children with congenital heart disease. *Arch Pediatr Adolesc Med.* 1995;149:1098–1102
5. Leitch CA. Growth, nutrition and energy expenditure in pediatric heart failure. *Prog Pediatr Cardiol.* 2000;11:195–202

6. Schuurmans FM, Pulles-Heintzberger CF, Gerver WJ, Kester AD, Forget PP. Long-term growth of children with congenital heart disease: a retrospective study. *Acta Paediatr.* 1998;87:1250–1255

7. Barton JS, Hindmarsh PC, Scrimgeour CM, Rennie MJ, Preece MA. Energy expenditure in congenital heart disease. *Arch Dis Child.* 1994;70:5–9

8. Leitch CA, Karn CA, Peppard RJ, et al. Increased energy expenditure in infants with cyanotic congenital heart disease. *J Pediatr.* 1998;133:755–760

9. Mitchell IM, Davies PS, Day JM, Pollock JC, Jamieson MP. Energy expenditure in children with congenital heart disease, before and after cardiac surgery. *J Thorac Cardiovasc Surg.* 1994;107:374–380

10. Huse DM, Feldt RH, Nelson RA, Novak LP. Infants with congenital heart disease. Food intake, body weight, and energy metabolism. *Am J Dis Child.* 1975;129:65–69

11. Menon G, Poskitt EM. Why does congenital heart disease cause failure to thrive? *Arch Dis Child.* 1985;60:1134–1139

12. Rosenthal A. Congenital cardiac anomalies and gastrointestinal malformations. In: Pierpont MEM, Moller JH, eds. *Genetics of Cardiovascular Disease.* Boston, MA: Martinus Nijhoff, 1987:113–126

13. Sondheimer JM, Hamilton JR. Intestinal function in infants with severe congenital heart disease. *J Pediatr.* 1978;92:572–578

14. Vaisman N, Leigh T, Voet H, Westerterp K, Abraham M, Duchan R. Malabsorption in infants with congenital heart disease under diuretic treatment. *Pediatr Res.* 1994;36:545–549

15. Yahav J, Avigad S, Frand M, et al. Assessment of intestinal and cardiorespiratory function in children with congenital heart disease on high-caloric formulas. *J Pediatr Gastroenterol Nutr.* 1985;4:778–785

16. Schwarz SM, Gewitz MH, See CC, et al. Enteral nutrition in infants with congenital heart disease and growth failure. *Pediatrics.* 1990;86:368–373

17. Unger R, DeKleermaeker M, Gidding SS, Christoffel KK. Calories count. Improved weight gain with dietary intervention in congenital heart disease. *Am J Dis Child.* 1992;146:1078–1084

18. Salzer HR, Haschke F, Wimmer M, Heil M, Schilling R. Growth and nutritional intake of infants with congenital heart disease. *Pediatr Cardiol.* 1989;10:17–23

19. Cavell B. Gastric emptying in infants with congenital heart disease. *Acta Paediatr Scand.* 1981;70:517–520

20. Forchielli ML, McColl R, Walker WA, Lo C. Children with congenital heart disease: a nutrition challenge. *Nutr Rev.* 1994;52:348–353

21. Sole MJ, Jeejeebhoy KN. Conditioned nutritional requirements and the pathogenesis and treatment of myocardial failure. *Curr Opin Clin Nutr Metab Care.* 2000; 3:417–424

22. Carr JG, Stevenson LW, Walden JA, Heber D. Prevalence and hemodynamic correlates of malnutrition in severe congestive heart failure secondary to ischemic or idiopathic dilated cardiomyopathy. *Am J Cardiol.* 1989;63:709–713

23. Freeman LM, Roubenoff R. The nutrition implications of cardiac cachexia. *Nutr Rev.* 1994;52:340–347

24. Feldman AM, Combes A, Wagner D, et al. The role of tumor necrosis factor in the pathophysiology of heart failure. *J Am Coll Cardiol.* 2000;35:537–544

25. Krauss AN, Auld PA. Metabolic rate of neonates with congenital heart disease. *Arch Dis Child.* 1975;50:539–541

26. Stocker FP, Wilkoff W, Miettinen OS, Nadas AS. Oxygen consumption in infants with heart disease. Relationship to severity of congestive failure, relative weight, and caloric intake. *J Pediatr.* 1972;80:43–51

27. Weintraub RG, Menahem S. Growth and congenital heart disease. *J Paediatr Child Health.* 1993;29:95–98

28. Gervasio MR, Buchanan CN. Malnutrition in the pediatric cardiology patient. *CCQ.* 1985;8:49–56

29. Varan B, Tokel K, Yilmaz G. Malnutrition and growth failure in cyanotic and acyanotic congenital heart disease with and without pulmonary hypertension. *Arch Dis Child.* 1999;81:49–52

30. Leitch CA, Karn CA, Ensing GJ, Denne SC. Energy expenditure after surgical repair in children with cyanotic congenital heart disease. *J Pediatr.* 2000;137:381–385

31. Ackerman IL, Karn CA, Denne SC, Ensing GJ, Leitch CA. Total but not resting energy expenditure is increased in infants with ventricular septal defects. *Pediatrics.* 1998;102:1172–1177

32. Levy RJ, Rosenthal A, Miettinen OS, Nadas AS. Determinants of growth in patients with ventricular septal defect. *Circulation.* 1978;57:793–797

33. Renlund DG, Taylor DO, Kfoury AG, Shaddy RS. New UNOS rules: historical background and implications for transplantation management. United Network for Organ Sharing. *J Heart Lung Transplant.* 1999;18:1065–1070

34. Sholler GF, Celermajer JM. Cardiac surgery in the first year of life: the effect on weight gains of infants with congenital heart disease. *Aust Paediatr J.* 1986;22:305–308

35. Stenbog EV, Hjortdal VE, Ravn HB, Skjaerbaek C, Sorensen KE, Hansen OK. Improvement in growth, and levels of insulin-like growth factor-I in the serum, after cavopulmonary connections. *Cardiol Young.* 2000;10:440–446

36. Cohen MI, Bush DM, Ferry RJ Jr, et al. Somatic growth failure after the Fontan operation. *Cardiol Young.* 2000;10:447–457

37. Baum D, Beck RQ, Haskell WL. Growth and tissue abnormalities in young people with cyanotic congenital heart disease receiving systemic-pulmonary artery shunts. *Am J Cardiol.* 1983;52:349–352

38. Payne PR, Waterlow JC. Relative energy requirements for maintenance, growth, and physical activity. *Lancet.* 1971;2:210–211

39. Jackson M, Poskitt EM. The effects of high-energy feeding on energy balance and growth in infants with congenital heart disease and failure to thrive. *Br J Nutr.* 1991;65:131–143

40. Bougle D, Iselin M, Kahyat A, Duhamel JF. Nutritional treatment of congenital heart disease. *Arch Dis Child.* 1986;61:799–801

41. Vanderhoof JA, Hofschire PJ, Baluff MA, et al. Continuous enteral feedings. An important adjunct to the management of complex congenital heart disease. *Am J Dis Child.* 1982;136:825–827

42. Fomon SJ, Ziegler EE. Nutritional management of infants with congenital heart disease. *Am Heart J.* 1972;83:581–588

43. Lister G, Hellenbrand WE, Kleinman CS, Talner NS. Physiologic effects of increasing hemoglobin concentration in left-to-right shunting in infants with ventricular septal defects. *N Engl J Med.* 1982;306:502–506

44. Shamir R, Dagan O, Abramovitch D, Abramovitch T, Vidne BA, Dinari G. Thiamine deficiency in children with congenital heart disease before and after corrective surgery. *JPEN J Parenter Enteral Nutr.* 2000;24:154–158

46
Nutrition in Cystic Fibrosis

Cystic fibrosis (CF) is an autosomal recessive disease affecting multiple organ systems, including the airways, exocrine pancreas, intestine, hepatobiliary system, and the genital tract of males. There is considerable heterogeneity of disease phenotype. It is caused by mutations in the cystic fibrosis conductance regulator gene (CFTR), which encodes a cyclic adenosine monophosphate (cAMP)-activated chloride channel localized on the apical surface of epithelial cells. Since the CF gene was cloned in 1989, more than 900 different CFTR gene mutations have been identified. At least some of the variability of the CF phenotype can be explained by genotype. The strongest relation between the genotype and the phenotype is observed in the exocrine pancreas.[1,2] The majority of conventionally diagnosed patients with CF (85% to 90%) have evidence of pancreatic failure or pancreatic insufficiency (PI). Most patients with the PI phenotype present with signs and symptoms of maldigestion and/or failure to thrive at an early age. A smaller subset of patients have evidence of pancreatic dysfunction, but retain sufficient residual pancreatic function to permit normal digestion without the need for exogenous pancreatic enzyme supplements with meals.[3] The term pancreatic sufficiency (PS) is used to describe patients with this phenotype who tend to have a milder form of CF disease. Analysis of large patient cohorts have revealed that different mutations in the CFTR gene confer either the PI or the PS phenotypes.[2] Specifically, the PI phenotype is associated with 2 mutations that are classified as "severe," whereas a single "mild" mutation, which appears to be dominant over the "severe" allele, confers the PS phenotype. From a nutritional perspective, patients with the PI phenotype are at greatest risk of developing malnutrition and/or growth failure.

Diagnosis
In certain countries throughout the world and in specific states within the United States, the diagnosis of CF is established by newborn screening using measurement of the immunoreactive trypsinogen concentration in dried blood spots. Many of these patients are asymptomatic at diagnosis and may remain pancreatic sufficient for a period of time.[4] However, a surprisingly large number

of patients with PI have evidence of malnutrition at approximately 7 weeks of age when the diagnosis of screened patients is usually confirmed.[5] If newborn screening is not performed, the diagnosis of CF is established by characteristic signs and symptoms or, in some cases, based on knowledge of an affected first-degree relative. Common presenting signs and symptoms of CF, which can occur alone or in combination, include the following:

- Meconium ileus at birth (can be diagnosed in utero)
- Failure to thrive
- Severe malnutrition with anemia, hypoalbuminemia, and edema
- Greasy, foul-smelling, and bulky stools
- Pulmonary disease (recurrent pneumonia, persistent cough, or wheezing)
- Excessive appetite with increased energy intake
- Poor appetite with decreased energy intake
- Hyponatremia due to excessive salt loss from sweating (especially hot climates)
- Salty taste (parents often describe a salty taste when kissing their infants)

In the majority of cases, the diagnosis of CF is confirmed by characteristic clinical features of the disease plus an elevated sweat chloride concentration (>60 mmol/L), which should be performed on 2 occasions in a medical center with significant experience in the diagnosis of CF. Other clinical evaluations of the patient are helpful in establishing the diagnosis and/or to perform a baseline assessment. These include the following:

- Analysis of CF genotypes
- Chest x-ray
- Pulmonary function tests and sputum analysis (if older than 5 to 7 years of age)
- Liver function tests
- Serum albumin and protein
- Complete blood count
- Serum vitamins A, E, and 25-hydroxy D
- Seventy-two-hour fecal fat balance study
- Alternative tests of pancreatic function (fecal chymotrypsin, fecal elastase-1, or serum trypsinogen)
- Height, weight, weight as a percentage of ideal body weight for height (IBW), skinfold measurements

Assessment of Pancreatic Function Status

Exocrine pancreatic function should be assessed in the following situations:

- All newly diagnosed patients (before enzyme therapy is initiated)—to provide objective evaluation of pancreatic status and to determine the severity of nutrient maldigestion
- To monitor patients with PS for evidence of developing fat maldigestion due to PI, particularly when frequent bulky bowel movements or unexplained weight loss occur
- Before and after changes in enzyme therapy and/or initiation of adjunctive treatment to provide objective evidence of a response to treatment

At diagnosis, a 72-hour fecal fat balance study provides the most information.[6] It can be completed at home or in hospital. If collections are to be done at home, the family should be given a dietary scale, and equipment for collecting the bowel movements, including a stool collection can. Details of the test should be carefully explained to the patient and/or family and clear, written instructions should be provided. Food should be weighed and recorded so that fat intake can be accurately calculated. If food or the formula contains medium-chain triglycerides (MCTs), the stool must be analyzed by a specialized method.[7] For infants less than 6 months, fat losses exceeding 15% of fat intake are indicative of PI. In patients older than 6 months, fat losses exceeding 7% of intake are considered to be abnormal.

Seventy-two-hour fecal fat studies cannot be performed accurately in the infant who is being breastfed, because the nutrient content of breast milk cannot be determined accurately. The fat content of breast milk, in particular, varies considerably. In these circumstances, the caregivers should encourage the mother to breastfeed and rely on other clinical and laboratory evidence of PI before initiating enzyme therapy. The vast majority of patients who present with meconium ileus will have PI. In addition, young infants with severe failure to thrive, with or without hypoalbuminemia and edema, are likely to have PI. The presence of hypovitaminosis A and/or E,[8,9] microscopic evidence of fat droplets in stool, and low fecal elastase-1 concentrations[10] are strongly suggestive of PI. In these circumstances, a 72-hour fecal fat balance study is still recommended, but should be deferred until breastfeeding has been discontinued.

Nutritional Care

Goals

The goal of nutritional care in patients with CF is to achieve normal growth and nutritional status and, for those with PI, to provide enzyme therapy, which optimizes micronutrient and macronutrient absorption (see Enzyme Therapy in this chapter).[11] A high-energy, nutritionally balanced diet is encouraged with liberal use of fat to provide additional calories. In patients with insulin-dependent diabetes, careful control of blood sugars with appropriate insulin therapy must be balanced with the need to maintain energy balance through regular meals and snacks.[12,13]

Assessment and Monitoring

A complete nutritional assessment includes a diet history and relevant laboratory and clinical data. Height and weight measurements, appropriate mid-arm parameters, as well as assessment of pubertal development in the adolescent are used to assist in the determination of nutritional status.

Nutritional monitoring is considered to be a routine part of every clinic visit, which, in most CF centers, occurs every 3 to 4 months. Routine assessment should include measurement of height and weight and mid-arm parameters. Written dietary records may be obtained along with documentation of enzyme intake if growth or weight gain is a concern. Attention should be given to determine compliance with enzyme therapy.

Seventy-two-hour fecal fat collections should be arranged if indicated, particularly if there is poor weight gain and/or signs and symptoms of maldigestion. If the patient exhibits evidence of severe steatorrhea, adjustments should be made to enzymes and/or adjuvants may be used (see Enzyme Therapy in this chapter). Laboratory indices of nutritional status should be obtained at least once each year or more frequently if there is a concern. This should include vitamins A, E, 25-hydroxy D, albumin, liver function tests, and a complete blood count.

Nutritional Requirements

For most patients with CF, energy requirements only moderately exceed the recommended dietary allowance (RDA).[14] If a patient is healthy and has minimal pulmonary disease, energy requirements hardly ever exceed 5% to 10% of RDA. However, in patients with significant lung disease (ie, FEV_1 <40%), or in those who have severe maldigestion/malabsorption, energy requirements may be greatly increased, ranging from 20% to 50% or more of RDA.[15] Some patients, particularly those with advanced lung disease, may reduce energy expenditure by decreasing physical activity. To calculate energy needs, the following formulas are used (modified from CF consensus report).[16]

1. Less than 1 year of age:

$$\frac{RDA \times 1.25^* \times IBW\ (kg)}{Actual\ weight\ (kg)} = kcal/kg/d$$

   *After diagnosis, infants may require 125% RDA to achieve catch-up weight gain.

2. More than 1 year of age

   BMR [using actual wt] × (1.5–1.7 [activity factor]) × $\underline{0.93}$ =kcal/d

   0.85 (represents absorption of fat)

- Add 200 to 400 kcal/d to achieve weight gain if <90% to 95% IBW.
- Use actual fraction of absorption if available from 72-hour fat balance studies (ie, replace 0.85 with known value).

RDA=Recommended Dietary Allowance
IBW=Ideal Body Weight for height, age, and gender
BMR= Basal Metabolic Rate

Vitamins

Supplemental fat-soluble vitamins (A, D, E, and K) are usually required to counter malabsorption of these micronutrients in patients with PI.[8] Daily requirements for vitamins A and D are approximately 1 to 2 times the Dietary Reference Intakes (DRIs), and for E are estimated to be approximately 5 to 20 times the DRIs.[17] The precise requirement for vitamin K has not been established.[18] In patients with clinically significant liver disease with evidence of multilobular cirrhosis, additional fat-soluble vitamins may be required. In particular, supplemental vitamin K (5 mg/d) is recommended, particularly in a patient with laboratory evidence of vitamin K deficiency. (See also Chapter 21.)

Salt

Patients with CF, particularly young infants, are at risk of developing hyponatremia if sweat losses are excessive. The risk is greatest in patients exposed to hot environments. To prevent hyponatremia, a liquid mineral mix (1 mL = 1.6 mmol Na^+, 1.6 mmol K^+, 2 mmol Cl^-, 0.84 mmol PO_4^{2-}) can be offered to infants receiving only formula. The mineral mix solution can be added to the patient's food or formula (1 mL/100 mL formula [based on 150 mL formula/kg body weight] or 1.5 mL/kg/d for breastfed infant—divided into 6 to 8 doses/d).

The dose may require adjustment depending on individual salt losses. Salt tablets are usually unnecessary for older the children. However, sports drinks that contain significant quantities of electrolytes are recommended for older individuals who are undertaking strenuous exercise or individuals who are living in or visiting hot climates.

Patient and Parent Education

Education of patients and their caregivers is a vital and routine component of the multidisciplinary care of patients with CF. A solid grounding in the special nutritional needs of a patient with CF should be established at diagnosis. This should include an explanation of the role of the pancreas and how enzyme replacement therapy helps to correct maldigestion. Parents should be given specific instructions on how to provide an appetizing, high-energy, nutritionally balanced diet, particularly with a liberal use of fat to provide extra calories. It is important to communicate the expectation that most children with CF are able to grow and gain weight normally. Patients and their parents require education about the importance of fat-soluble vitamins. Details on when to administer enzymes and vitamins must be reviewed in several occasions. In older children, concerns about compliance should be emphasized at diagnosis and assessed at each follow-up visit.

Specific Guidelines

Infants

Breastfeeding is encouraged, though some patients may require fortification with formula or a concentrated formula as a supplement. Milk-based formulas are recommended as an alternative to breastfeeding. There is no evidence that partially digested or MCT-containing formulas offer any nutritional advantage to the patient with CF.[19] If a young infant with CF is not thriving or is failing to exhibit catch-up growth, strategies should include increasing the strength of formula to at least 3300 kJ/L (24 kcal/oz) to ensure adequate energy intake.

When solids are introduced into the diet, extra energy can be provided by adding 2.5 to 5 mL (1/2 to 1 tsp) of butter or margarine to each 128-mL (4-oz) jar of meat or vegetables. Commercially prepared infant foods contain very little salt and additional salt (0.6 mL of mineral mix or 1/8 of a tsp of table salt) should be added twice daily to solids to ensure adequate salt intake.

Children Older Than 1 year

A high-energy diet is encouraged. In addition to 3 regular meals, 3 daily snacks are recommended. Adding butter or margarine to food will increase total energy intake. Milkshake supplements may be offered if required. Homemade milkshakes are less expensive than commercially prepared ones. Commercial dietary supplements are not proven to be of benefit to the nutritional status of patients with CF.[20] Nevertheless, these expensive sources of energy are often used in CF centers, despite lack of evidence to support their use. Nutritional supplements may actually substitute for normal dietary energy intake rather than as a supplement to increase total energy intake. Strategies to improve nutritional intake through enriching the energy content of regular meals and snacks should be entertained before costly supplements are introduced.

Aggressive Nutritional Support

Provided lung function is not severe, most patients will grow normally in childhood and remain well nourished during adulthood. Pulmonary exacerbations may cause acute weight loss but, following appropriate therapy, healthy patients will regain weight quite rapidly. Unfortunately, a subset of individuals, especially those with advanced lung disease, will be unable to maintain energy balance.[21] In such cases, more aggressive approaches to nutritional therapy may be indicated, because patients are incapable of increasing energy intake voluntarily.

Supplemental nutritional support via gastrostomy or jejunostomy tube are indicated in patients who exhibit poor weight gain over a period of 6 months to 1 year or show persistent malnutrition (weight as a percentage of ideal body weight for height of <85%).[22] Patients with end-stage lung disease who are listed for lung transplantation frequently experience reduced energy intake and decline in weight. In these circumstances, early and careful use of supplemental tube feedings may help to maintain energy balance.

Feeds are usually run overnight by continuous pump infusion. The energy needs and rate of infusion are determined on an individual basis. Patients are encouraged to eat normal meals during the day. However, voluntary intake, particularly at breakfast time, may be decreased. The choice of feed depends on individual tolerance and cost. Most patients can tolerate a complete formula (1.0 to 2.0 kcal/mL)[23] provided adequate enzyme therapy is prescribed (1000 to 2000 U lipase/g fat) and adjusted according to individual needs. Enzymes should be taken at intervals—at the beginning of the infusion, when they go to bed and at the end of the tube feeding. In patients who experience cramping or diarrhea, lowering the concentration of the formula may help to alleviate symptoms. Predigested feeds are more expensive than regular complete formulas, but those with a low fat content can be given without the use of supplemental enzymes and may be better tolerated by some patients. Low carbohydrate-containing formulas may be chosen for individuals with insulin-dependent diabetes mellitus. Occasionally, initiation of tube feedings will expose manifestations of diabetes mellitus, especially in older patients with PI. To anticipate this problem, an oral glucose tolerance test should be considered prior to placing the gastrostomy tube. To determine supplemental energy requirements from tube feeding, total energy requirements, normal dietary intake, nutritional status, and the degree of malabsorption must be considered. Higher supplemental energy requirements may be required to begin with to achieve catch-up growth and/or nutritional rehabilitation. Once patients achieve catch-up-growth, maintenance needs may be considerably lower. In most patients, delivery of approximately one third of total energy needs by tube feeding will achieve improvement of nutritional status. However, the amounts will vary considerably according to various factors, including individual energy needs, severity of malnutrition, degree of malabsorption, and the patient's ability to ingest calories voluntarily.

Total parenteral nutrition (TPN) is rarely indicated in patients with CF and may be important to nourish neonates immediately following surgery from meconium ileus. In addition, short-term TPN may be required if oral intake is inadequate due to vomiting or severe respiratory distress, especially if symptoms are accompanied by acute weight loss.

Commonly Encountered Nutritional Problems

Feeding Difficulties or Poor Growth in Infancy

When the diagnosis of CF is established in infancy, the patient may be severely malnourished. In these circumstances, it may take more than a year to achieve full catch-up in growth. Young infants have high energy requirements and frequently have severe malabsorption, which may require several adjustments to enzyme therapy in the first year after diagnosis. If poor weight gain is observed or the patient is failing to exhibit catch-up growth, careful assessment of energy intake and/or malabsorption may be needed. Breastfed infants may require formula supplements, while those receiving a formula should receive additional energy by increasing the concentration of the formula. Gastroesophageal reflux is quite common in the infant with CF, particularly in individuals with respiratory disease. Drugs to suppress gastric acid may be indicated if reflux is severe. A predigested formula should be only considered in individuals who have had significant bowel resection following complicated meconium ileus.[19]

Malabsorption

A large number of patients with CF experience some degree of maldigestion despite adequate dosing with potent pancreatic enzymes.[24,25] Subjective symptoms, such as abdominal bloating or cramps, or bulky stools, cannot reliably assess the severity of maldigestion. Instead, objective assessment is advocated by a 72-hour fat collection (while eating a regular diet) and the prescribed dose of enzymes. If severe fat maldigestion is identified (fecal fat losses exceeding 20% of intake or more) and is clearly contributing to abdominal symptoms or malnutrition, the dose of enzymes could be increased up to the maximum recommended amount. Alternatively, inhibition of gastric acid secretion with a histamine antagonist or a proton pump inhibitor may raise intestinal pH and improve the efficacy of enzyme therapy (see Enzyme Therapy in this chapter). Several weeks after the adjustment to therapy has been made, the individual patient should be reassessed by a repeat 72-hour fecal fat collection.

Distal Intestinal Obstruction Syndrome and Constipation

Distal intestinal obstruction syndrome (DIOS) is unique to CF and is characterized by cramping abdominal pain, which may be periumbilical or in the right, lower quadrant. A mass is usually palpable in the ileocecal area. Unlike simple constipation, the frequency and consistency of bowel motions are normal. It should be emphasized that simple constipation is a common problem in individuals with CF. Consequently, a careful history, abdominal examination, and abdominal x-ray is indicated when abdominal pain due to DIOS is suspected to distinguish it from constipation and other CF-associated complications such as intussusception and appendiceal abscess. Distal intestinal obstruction syndrome is treated by several different approaches. In our experience, if the DIOS is severe, a balanced electrolyte solution (used for cleansing the bowel prior to colonoscopy) is very effective in relieving the subacute obstruction. In children over age 2 years, mineral oil, n-acetylcysteine, and, in severe cases, large-volume enemas with hyperosmolar contrast agents are used.

Insulin-Dependent Diabetes

Adolescents and adults with CF and pancreatic insufficiency are at increased risk of developing CF-associated diabetes mellitus.[12,13] In many instances, patients exhibit no clear-cut signs and symptoms of diabetes. Furthermore, hemoglobin A1C values are not reliable tests of CF-associated diabetes. The diagnosis should be considered in any patient who is exhibiting weight loss or poor weight gain. Some CF centers are recommending annual screening for diabetes by a modified oral glucose tolerance test after the age of 18 years. In the patient who has CF-associated diabetes, high-energy meals and snacks are encouraged but energy needs and insulin requirements must be carefully balanced. Foods high in simple sugars may be limited according to insulin needs. Multidisciplinary care and the support of an endocrinologist is essential.

Enzyme Therapy

Patients with CF and PI are treated with pancreatic enzyme extracts of porcine origin. A large variety of enzyme products are available, including enteric-coated microspheres, enteric-coated tablets, and conventional powder enzymes.[24,25] All products contain the various enzymes synthesized by the pancreas comprising amylase, proteases, and lipase. The actual activities of these enzymes and the ratio to one another varies considerably according to specific batches and the commercial manufacturer. Enzyme potency is usually based on the content of lipase in each capsule. This is because lipase is required to treat fat maldigestion, which is the nutrient most vulnerable to maldigestion in CF. Commercial products vary in lipase activity from 4000 to 25 000 U lipase/capsule. The stated activity in each product is the minimum amount of activity during its shelf life, as dictated by national regulatory agencies. The actual activity may be considerably higher than stated (sometimes by as much as 200%).[26]

The enteric coated forms vary considerably in their biochemical coating, biophysical dissolution properties, and size of microspheres or microtablets.[24,27] There are few carefully performed clinical studies comparing the different formulations and little in vivo data are available that demonstrate the superiority of a single product. In fact, all currently available enzyme products fail to completely correct nutrient maldigestion in all patients with CF.[24] The reasons are likely multiple and variable from patient to patient. The enteric coating of enzyme microsphere or microtablets require a pH >5.2–6.0 for dissolution to occur in the proximal intestine, which may be acidic in the CF patient. Unprotected conventional enzymes are subject to destruction by the harsh acid-peptic gastric environment.[28] Patients with CF and PI have gastric acid hypersecretion and a relative deficiency of bicarbonate secretion from the pancreaticobiliary tree. This results in a more acidic proximal intestinal environment, which may be below the ideal optimal pH for maximal pancreatic enzyme activity and may hasten the inactivation of enzymes, especially lipase within the small intestine. Nevertheless, enzymes do improve nutrient digestion and absorption in CF patients, but the caregiver must be aware of the less than ideal efficacy of these products in individual patients.

Enzyme Administration

Dosing guidelines have been established by the US CF Foundation and the Food and Drug Administration.[29] These guidelines were established when it was recognized that many CF centers were giving excessive doses of enzymes. Overdosage was, in turn, strongly associated with a newly recognized and severe intestinal complication termed fibrosing colonopathy.[30] The response to treatment by individual patients will vary considerably, as will their required dosing schedule. Though dosing is best calculated using U lipase/g fat ingested, it is perhaps more practical to use a dosing schedule with age-adjusted guidelines. These take into account the fact that fat intake varies at different ages, with infants taking much larger amounts per body weight than an adult. Age-adjusted guidelines, with a limit of 4000 U lipase/g fat beyond 1 year of age, would avoid overdosing (see Table 46.1).

There are no convincing data concerning timing of enzyme dosing with meals, but, for practical reasons, we recommend that enzymes be taken in

Table 46.1.
Dosing Guidelines

	Conventional Products	Enteric-Coated Products*
Infants	8000–16 000 lipase units per 120 mL (4 oz) formula 8000 lipase units per 60 mL (4 tbsp) solids 8000–16 000 lipase units per breastfeed	8000 lipase units per 240 mL (8 oz) formula 8000 lipase units per 120 mL (8 tbsp) solids 4000–8000 lipase units per breastfeed
1–4 yr	...	16 000–24 000 lipase units per meal† 8000–16 000 lipase unit per snack‡
5–12 yr	...	24 000–40 000 lipase units per meal† 8000–24 000 lipase units per snack‡
>12 yr	...	40 000–64 000 lipase units per meal† 16 000–24 000 lipase units per snack‡

* The majority of patients with CF require approximately 1800 to 2000 lipase units/g fat/d (range 500 to 4000).
† Infants and Children <4 yr: 1000 lipase units/kg/meal; Children and Adults >4yr: 500 lipase units/kg/meal to a maximum of 2500 lipase units/kg/meal.
‡ The dose should vary according to the size of each snack. This should be assessed for each patient individually.

divided doses before and during meals.[31] Theoretically, this would provide
a more evenly distributed dose, though this has not been clinically proven.
Enzymes are not required with simple carbohydrates (eg, hard candy, popsi-
cles, pop, jello) but are needed for starch-containing foods (eg, rice, potatoes).
Specific guidelines for administration of enzymes in infants and older children
are outlined as follows.

Infants

Conventional enzymes or enteric-coated products can be offered to infants.
Furthermore, there are no published studies of the efficacy of enteric coated
products in infants with CF. In our experience, enteric-coated products offer no
advantage over conventional powder enzymes. In fact, in some infants, parents
report seeing the beads intact in the stools. In either case, offer enzymes right
before feeding. Enzymes can be mixed with 2 to 3 mL (1/2 tsp) applesauce and
given by spoon. Conventional enzymes should be offered in applesauce immediately after mixing because the acidity of the applesauce will destroy the enzymes.
Other strained fruit can be tried if applesauce is not taken, but parents should
try to use only one type of food to avoid problems with overall food refusal if
many different types of food are used as the vehicle for enzyme delivery.

Mouth care is important for infants prior to administration of enzymes.
Petroleum jelly (Vaseline) should be applied around the outside of the mouth
for skin protection. After administration, the inside of the mouth should be
cleaned with a Toothette (sponge) or Q-tip soaked in water, to avoid irritation
of the mouth by residual enzymes. Once an infant is taking solids, mouth
cleaning is not necessary as the action of saliva and food mixing in the mouth
cleans the mouth. A zinc-based cream is recommended for buttocks care at the
start of enzyme therapy and for a few weeks or months afterward. We recommend a cream that contains 33% Nystatin, 60% zincoderm (40% zinc cream),
and 1% hydrocortisone, which should be applied generously to buttocks with
each diaper change.

Over 1 Year

By age 1 year, children can be offered enteric-coated products, mixed with one
food. Patients should be discouraged from chewing the capsules, as this will
destroy the protective coating. Swallowing of capsules is encouraged as soon
as parents consider the child to be ready. This varies considerably for patient to
patient but occurs usually around 4 to 5 years of age. Some older patients continue to experience difficulties swallowing capsules. In this case, they should

open the capsule and sprinkle the beads in the mouth, which can be ingested by drinking a liquid.

Adjunctive Therapy

Histamine (H_2) antagonists (Ranitidine) and proton pump inhibitors (Omeprazole) inhibit gastric acid *and* can be used to assist enzyme activity (by decreasing gastric acidity) resulting in (1) less destruction of unprotected conventional powder enzymes in the stomach or (2) increasing pH in the upper intestine allowing for more rapid dissolution of the enteric coating dissolution and optimal conditions for enzyme to catalyze nutrients. In the case of Ranitidine, a higher dose is recommended (10 mg/kg/d divided into 2 to 3 doses/d). There are no safety data on the long-term use of Omeprazole.

For patients who continue to have symptoms of maldigestion and malabsorption with maximum prescribed enzyme dose for age, a combination of enteric coated and conventional enzyme should be tried. We recommend substituting about 25% of the enteric-coated product with conventional products. For example, if a patient is receiving six 8000-unit enteric-coated products per meal, then offer 4 enteric products and 2 conventional enzymes of the same strength.

Vitamin Therapy

The fat-soluble vitamins (A, D, E, & K) are absorbed with dietary fat and, therefore, need to be supplemented in the CF diet. The multivitamin ADEKs (Axcan Scandipharm Inc.) has been formulated for CF patients, but other commercial and multivitamin preparations are available. ADEKs, which contains other vitamins (including B vitamins and Vitamin C) and minerals, is available in a liquid form for infants, and in a capsule form for older children. Compliance with vitamin therapy is important. Deficiency of the fat-soluble vitamins (especially vitamins A, E, and D) are not uncommon.[8] Therefore, yearly monitoring of vitamin levels is recommended. Side effects of severe deficiencies have been reported, including severe xerophthalmia (vitamin A), hematologic and neurologic complications (vitamin E), clotting abnormalities (vitamin K), and loss of bone density (vitamin D).[32]

Since overdosing of fat-soluble vitamins (especially vitamins A and D) can be harmful, it is important to instruct patients to take only the amount prescribed and to ensure that they are not taking other over-the-counter vitamin products in addition to the prescribed vitamins. Again, yearly monitoring of serum levels is recommended.

Table 46.2.
Vitamin Therapy

Vitamins*	<2 years		2–8 years		8 years-adult
A	1500 IU		5000 IU		5000–10 000 IU
D	400 IU		400 IU		400–800 IU
	0–6 years	6–12 years	1–4 years	4–10 years	>10 years
E	25 IU	50 IU	100 IU	100–200 IU	200–400 IU
K	Unknown: see text				

*Vitamins should be taken with meals since enzymes will help assimilation.

References

1. Kerem E, Corey M, Kerem BS, et al. The relation between genotype and phenotype in cystic fibrosis—analysis of the most common mutation (ΔF508). *N Engl J Med.* 1990;323:1517–1522

2. Kristidis P, Bozon D, Corey M, et al. Genetic determination of exocrine pancreatic function in cystic fibrosis. *Am J Hum Genet.* 1992;50:1178–1184

3. Gaskin K, Gurwitz D, Durie P, Corey M, Levison H, Forstner G. Improved respiratory prognosis in patients with cystic fibrosis with normal fat absorption. *J Pediatr.* 1982;100:857–862

4. Waters DL, Dorney SF, Gaskin KJ, Gruca MA, O'Halloran M, Wilcken B. Pancreatic function in infants identified as having cystic fibrosis in a neonatal screening program. *N Engl J Med.* 1990;322:303–308

5. Reardon MC, Hammond KB, Accurso FJ, et al. Nutritional deficits exist before 2 months of age in some infants with cystic fibrosis identified by screening test. *J Pediatr.* 1984;105:271–274

6. van de Kamer JH, Huinink H, Weyers HA. Rapid method for determining fat in feces. *J Biol Chem.* 1949;177:347–355

7. Jeejeebhoy KN, Ahmed S, Kozak G. Determination of fecal fats containing both medium and long chain triglycerides and fatty acids. *Clin Biochem.* 1970;3:157–163

8. Feranchak AP, Sontag MK, Wagener JS, Hammond KB, Accurso FJ, Sokol RJ. Prospective, long-term study of fat-soluble vitamin status in children with cystic fibrosis identified by newborn screening. *J Pediatr.* 1999;135:601–610

9. Kalnins D, Corey M, Durie P, Ellis L. Do serum vitamin E levels correlate with 72-hour fecal fat at time of CF diagnosis? [abstract]. *Pediatr Pulmonol Suppl.* 1995; 12:266

10. Loser C, Mollgaard A, Folsch UR. Faecal elastase1: a novel, highly sensitive, and specific tubeless pancreatic function test. *Gut.* 1996;39:580–586

11. Durie PR, Pencharz PB. Nutritional management of cystic fibrosis. *Ann Rev Nutr.* 1993;13:111–136

12. Lanng S, Thorsteinsson B, Lund-Andersen C, Nerup J, Schiotz PO, Koch C. Diabetes mellitus in Danish cystic fibrosis patients: prevalence and late diabetic complications. *Acta Paediatr.* 1994;83:72–77

13. Consensus conference on CF-related diabetes mellitus. I (IV): 1990 (CF Foundation)

14. National Research Council. *Recommended Dietary Allowances.* 10th ed. Washington, DC: National Academy Press; 1989

15. Fried MD, Durie PR, Tsui LC, Corey M, Levison H, Pencharz PB. The cystic fibrosis gene and resting energy expenditure. *J Pediatr.* 1991;119:913–916

16. Ramsey BW, Farrell PM, Pencharz P. Nutritional assessment and management in cystic fibrosis: a consensus report. *Am J Clin Nutr.* 1992;55:108–116

17. Institute of Medicine. *Dietary Reference Intakes: Proposed Definition of Dietary Fiber.* Washington, DC: National Academy of Sciences; 2001

18. Rashid M, Durie P, Andrew M, et al. Prevalence of vitamin K deficiency in cystic fibrosis. *Am J Clin Nutr.* 1999;70:378–382

19. Ellis L, Kalnins D, Corey M, Brennan J, Pencharz P, Durie P. Do infants with cystic fibrosis need a protein hydrolysate formula? A prospective, randomized, comparative study. *J Pediatr.* 1998;132:270–276

20. Kalnins D, Durie PR, Corey, et al. Are oral dietary supplements effective in the nutritional management of adolescents and adults with CF? [abstract]. *Pediatr Pulmonol.* 1997;13(suppl):314

21. Pencharz PB, Durie PR. Pathogenesis of malnutrition in cystic fibrosis, and its treatment. *Clin Nutr.* 2000;19:387–394

22. Levy LD, Durie PR, Pencharz PB, Corey ML. Effects of long-term nutritional rehabilitation on body composition and clinical status in malnourished children and adolescents with cystic fibrosis. *J Pediatr.* 1985;107:225–230

23. Erskine JM, Lingard CD, Sontag MK, Accurso FJ. Enteral nutrition for patients with cystic fibrosis: comparison of a semi-elemental and nonelemental formula. *J Pediatr.* 1998;132:265–269

24. Durie P, Kalnins D, Ellis L. Uses and abuses of enzyme therapy in cystic fibrosis. *J R Soc Med.* 1998;91(suppl 34):2–13

25. Lebenthal E, Rolston DD, Holsclaw DS Jr. Enzyme therapy for pancreatic insufficiency: present status and future needs. *Pancreas.* 1994;9:1–12

26. Kraisinger M, Hochhaus G, Stecenko A, Bowser E, Hendeles L. Clinical pharmacology of pancreatic enzymes in patients with cystic fibrosis and in vitro performance of microencapsulated formulations. *J Clin Pharmacol.* 1994;34:158–166

27. Carroccio A, Pardo F, Montalto G, et al. Effectiveness of enteric-coated preparations on nutritional parameters in cystic fibrosis. A long-term study. *Digestion.* 1988;41: 201–206

28. Barraclough M, Taylor CJ. Twenty-four hour ambulatory gastric and duodenal pH profiles in cystic fibrosis: effect of duodenal hyperacidity on pancreatic enzyme function and fat absorption. *J Pediatr Gastroenterol Nutr.* 1996;23:45–50

29. Borowitz DS, Grand RJ, Durie PR. Use of pancreatic enzyme supplements for patients with cystic fibrosis in the context of fibrosing colonopathy. *J Pediatr.* 1995;127:681–684

30. FitzSimmons SC, Burkhart GA, Borowitz D, et al. High-dose pancreatic-enzyme supplements and fibrosing colonopathy in children with cystic fibrosis. *N Engl J Med.* 1997;336:1283–1289

31. Brady MS, Rickard K, Yu PL, Eigen H. Effectiveness of enteric coated pancreatic enzymes given before meals in reducing steatorrhea in children with cystic fibrosis. *J Am Diet Assoc.* 1992;92:813–817

32. Bhudhikanok GS, Wang MC, Marcus R, Harkins A, Moss RB, Bachrach LK. Bone acquisition and loss in children and adults with cystic fibrosis: a longitudinal study. *J Pediatr.* 1998;133:18–27

47

The Ketogenic Diet

The ketogenic diet is a high-fat, low-carbohydrate, and low-protein diet designed to increase the body's reliance on fatty acids rather than glucose for energy. Thus, it is intended to mimic the fasting state, which can be useful in treating disorders affecting the brain, such as intractable epilepsy or some metabolic defects involving glucose metabolism. Variations on the ketogenic diet have been proposed over the years, including the medium-chain triglyceride (MCT) oil diet. The classical ketogenic diet, now the preferred form of the ketogenic diet, will be discussed in this chapter. This chapter briefly reviews the history, physiology, efficacy, indications, contraindications, and mechanism of action of the ketogenic diet. The emphasis will be on implementing and maintaining the diet, while preventing and managing its complications.

History

The benefits of fasting on seizures have been known for ages.[1-4] Although the first scientific report did not appear until 1911, fasting was used to treat seizures by Hippocrates and was also recommended in the Bible (Mark 9:14–29). Since fasting is not a practical long-term treatment, Wilder proposed using a high-fat, low-carbohydrate diet to mimic fasting in 1921.[5] Several studies reported improved seizure control on the ketogenic diet by the end of the 1920s. Interest in the diet then waned as new anticonvulsants became available, though it has experienced a resurgence of interest during the last decade.

Physiological Basis of the Ketogenic Diet

The basis of the ketogenic diet is the brain's ability to obtain 30% to 60% or more of its energy during fasting from serum ketones derived from β-oxidation of fatty acids.[6-13] Some of the most relevant aspects are briefly reviewed in Figure 47.1.

Fasting lowers serum glucose, resulting in a lower insulin-glucagon ratio. The fall in this ratio and the effect of changes in other hormones, such as epinephrine, stimulate lipolysis in adipocytes. The free fatty acids released in the blood undergo β-oxidation in liver, cardiac muscle, and skeletal muscle. β-oxidation of

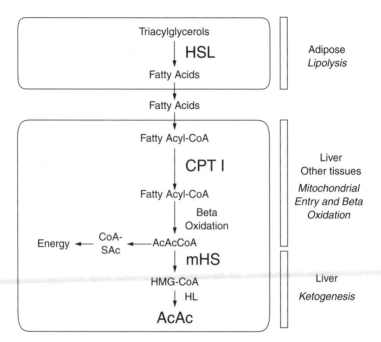

Figure 47.1. Summary of ketogenesis. HSL = hormone sensitive lipase, CPT I = carnitine palmitoyltransferase I, AcAcCoA = acetoacetyl CoA, CoA = coenzyme A, mHS = mitochondrial HMG-CoA synthease, HMG = 3-hydroxy-3-methyl glutaric acid, HL = HMG-CoA lyase, AcAc = acetoacetate. Adapted from Reference 13.

free fatty acids in the mitochondria of these tissues results in the formation of acetyl coenzyme A (CoA). Acetyl CoA condenses with oxaloacetate to enter the Krebs cycle. However, liver oxaloacetate levels are low during fasting because it is used to synthesize glucose. Instead, the liver converts acetyl CoA to acetoacetate, a ketone, during fasting. Reduction of acetoacetate forms another ketone, β-hydroxybutyrate. After these ketones are transported across the blood brain barrier, they can be converted to acetyl CoA and enter the Krebs cycle (Figure 47.2). The mitochondrial electron transport chain then oxidizes the resulting reduced nicotinamide adenine dinucleotide (NADH) and reduced flavin adenine dinucleotide ($FADH_2$) to yield adenosine triphosphate (ATP). Although cardiac and skeletal muscle can use both free fatty acids and ketones, the conversion of free fatty acids to ketones is necessary because free fatty acids do not cross the blood brain barrier.

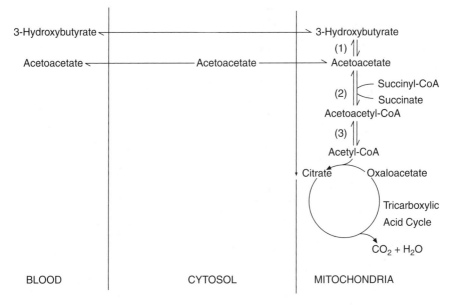

3-Hydroxybutyrate

Acetoacetate

Acetoacetate

3-Hydroxybutyrate

(1)

Acetoacetate

Succinyl-CoA

(2)

Succinate

Acetoacetyl-CoA

(3)

Acetyl-CoA

Citrate — Oxaloacetate

Tricarboxylic
Acid Cycle

$CO_2 + H_2O$

BLOOD   CYTOSOL   MITOCHONDRIA

Figure 47.2. Pathways of ketone utilization. 1 = hydroxybutyrate dehydrogenase, 2 = 3-oxoacid-coenzyme A (CoA) transferase, 3 = acetoacetyl-CoA thiolase. Adapted from reference 9.

β-oxidation occurs in the mitochondrial matrix and, therefore, free fatty acids must cross the inner mitochondrial membrane. Long-chain fatty acids have 14 to 20 carbons and are activated to fatty acyl CoA thioesters on the outer mitochondrial membrane. The carnitine cycle transports the long-chain fatty acyl CoA thioesters across the inner mitochondrial membrane (Figure 47.3). Short- and medium-chain fatty acids, which have <6 and 8 to 14 carbons respectively, cross the inner mitochondrial membrane directly without the help of the carnitine cycle.

Effectiveness of the Ketogenic Diet

Treatment of Seizures

Since the early 1920s, multiple case series and open-label studies have been published describing the effectiveness of the ketogenic diet.[2–4] Most of these studies have reported a reduction in seizure frequency, and a few have described its use in treating inborn errors of metabolism[12] and even rheumatoid arthritis.[14] As a result of these studies, the diet is primarily used to treat children with either intractable epilepsy or specific inborn errors of metabolism, such as pyruvate dehydrogenase deficiency.

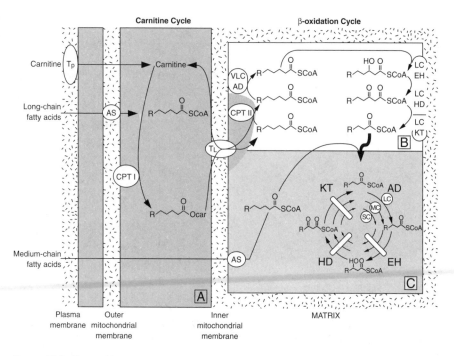

Figure 47.3. Fatty acid oxidation. A, carnitine cycle. B, inner mitochondrial membrane system. C, mitochondrial matrix system. The carnitine cycle includes the plasma membrane transporter, CPT I = carnitine palmitoyltransferase I, T_L = carnitine-acylcarnitine translocase, and CPT II = carnitine palmitoyltransferase II. The inner mitochondrial system includes the VCL AD = very-long-chain acyl-coenzyme A (CoA) dehydrogenase, and the trifunctional protein with 3 catalytically active sites. Long-chain acylcarnitines enter the mitochondrial matrix by the action of the CPT II to yield long-chain acyl-CoAs. These thioesters undergo 1 or more cycles of chain shortening catalyzed by the membrane-bound system. Chain-shortened acyl-CoAs are degraded further by the matrix β-oxidation system. T_p = carnitine transporter, EH = 2-enoyl-CoA hydratase, HD = 3-hydroxyacyl-CoA dehydrogenase, KT = 3-ketoacyl-CoA thiolase, MC = medium chain, SC = short chain, AS = acyl-CoA synthase. Adapted from Reference 11.

Two recent open-label studies evaluated the effectiveness of the ketogenic diet in children with medically intractable seizures.[15,16] The children ranged from age 4 months to 16 years. Their seizure types included absence, myoclonic, atonic, generalized tonic, clonic, tonic clonic, complex partial, simple partial, and partial seizures with secondary generalization. Several children included in these open-label studies had multiple seizure types and electroencephalographic (EEG) features consistent with Lennox-Gastaut syndrome. About 70% and 50% of those who initiated the diet remained on the diet at 6 and 12 months, respectively. At both 6 and 12 months, about 20% to 30% of children starting the diet had greater than 90% reduction in seizure frequency, and about 5% of children were seizure free. About 20% of those starting the diet had a 50% to 90% reduction in seizure frequency at both time points. No statistically significant differences in outcome were found with respect to age, sex, seizure type, or EEG findings, though some studies report greatest efficacy against myoclonic, astatic, and atypical absence seizures.[2,15] Remarkably, these findings are similar to the multiple reports published over the last 80 years.[2–4] Preliminary results from the first randomized, blinded, placebo-controlled study of the ketogenic diet, which is currently in progress, are promising.[17]

The other benefits to children include a reduction in the number of medications, increased alertness, and improved behavior even if seizure control is not improved.[15,16,18–20] The ketogenic diet has been associated with reduced seizure frequency among adults with either partial or generalized epilepsy.[21–23]

Treatment of Inborn Errors of Metabolism

Since ketones are essentially transportable units of acetyl CoA, which can enter the Krebs cycle, they provide a means for generating ATP that bypasses glycolysis and the pyruvate dehydrogenase complex.[10] The pyruvate dehydrogenase complex links glycolysis to the Krebs cycle by decarboxylating pyruvate to form acetyl CoA. Thus, the ketogenic diet should benefit those who cannot metabolize glucose or pyruvate because of pyruvate dehydrogenase complex deficiency or the glucose transporter protein syndrome. Pyruvate dehydrogenase complex deficiency is clinically heterogeneous but includes lactic acidosis, neuroanatomic lesions, developmental delay, and early death.[24] The ketogenic diet has produced clinical and biochemical improvement in children with mutations in pyruvate dehydrogenase, one of the enzymes in the pyruvate dehydrogenase complex.[25,26] Clinically, the glucose transporter protein syndrome is characterized by hypoglycorrhachia (low CSF glucose), infantile seizures, ataxia, hypotonia, acquired microcephaly, and developmental delay.[27] Glucose transporter protein syndrome is caused by a defect in GLUT1, which transports glucose across the blood brain barrier. The ketogenic diet provides clinical benefit probably by providing the brain with ketones as an alternative energy source.[27] Infantile phosphofructokinase deficiency may also respond to the ketogenic diet since phosphofructokinase is the rate limiting enzyme of glycolysis.[28]

Mechanism of Action

When the ketogenic diet is used to provide an alternative energy source because of an inborn error of metabolism, the mechanism of action is intuitive.

However, the mechanism by which it acts as an anticonvulsant remains a mystery.[29] The diet has been hypothesized to alter acid-base balance, water and electrolyte balance, lipid composition, energy balance, hormonal balance, neurotransmitter levels, neuropeptide function, and the blood brain barrier to change glial function or neuronal membrane properties.[3,4,30,31] Alternatively, ketones could interact directly with ion channels.

Indications

Although the ketogenic diet has efficacy in treating multiple seizure types, the difficulty implementing and maintaining the ketogenic diet and the poorly characterized long-term effects of the ketogenic diet make it at best a second-line therapy for treating epilepsy. Unlike anti-epileptic drugs (AEDs) that are monitored with post-marketing surveillance systems allowing for estimates of the risk of rare, but potentially fatal, idiosyncratic adverse events, it is not possible to determine whether the ketogenic diet has less or more risk for serious rare adverse events than AEDs. The ketogenic diet is indicated for selected patients with seizures that fail to respond to standard AEDs without side effects.

The 2 inborn errors of metabolism for which the ketogenic diet are indicated are the glucose transporter protein syndrome and pyruvate dehydrogenase complex deficiency as discussed previously. Although the diet should be considered soon after diagnosis, the decision to use it should be made in consultation with a pediatric neurologist familiar with the ketogenic diet. The diet may be a treatment option for other inborn errors such as phosphofructokinase deficiency in which providing fatty acids or ketones as an energy source may be beneficial. Using the diet for these diseases requires careful consideration of the enzyme or protein involved and the metabolic pathways in which it participates.

Contraindications

The contraindications to the ketogenic diet are apparent from its physiological actions. The ketogenic diet is contraindicated in primary and secondary carnitine deficiency, carnitine cycle defects, known mitochondrial disorders, including those involving β-oxidation defects and electron transport chain deficiencies, ketogenic defects, ketolytic defects, pyruvate carboxylate deficiency, and pyruvate dehydrogenase phosphatase deficiency.[12,13,26,32,33] Although high-fat diets can exacerbate ketotic hypoglycemia, the ketogenic diet is not absolutely contraindicated in this condition, but requires expert management.[34] Acetozolamide should be discontinued before beginning the ketogenic diet.[35]

The use of zonisamide, topiramate, or valproate with the ketogenic diet, although not absolutely contraindicated, require careful monitoring by epilepsy specialists. Zonisamide and topiramate, although helpful for young children with multiple seizure types, are known to increase the risk of nephrolithiasis. Some authors have reported an increase in adverse events associated with the ketogenic diet among children co-treated with valproate.[36] There are very limited data on the use of the ketogenic diet among children above the age of 10 years. Most normal children, adolescents, and adults who are able to obtain their own food are not compliant with the ketogenic diet.

Micronutrient Deficiencies of the Diet

The ketogenic diet requires supplementation of several micronutrients, and it may also be deficient in carnitine. It is deficient in water-soluble vitamins B and C, calcium, magnesium, and iron.[4,37] In addition, it is deficient in vitamin D despite the high fat content, because the diet is low in fluid milk. Through a variety of mechanisms, the diet or concurrently used seizure medications such as valproic acid may cause a secondary carnitine deficiency.[11,12] A recent consensus conference on carnitine supplementation recommended supplementing carnitine if carnitine levels decrease while on the diet, if low levels reduce the efficacy of the diet and accentuate hypoglycemia, and if carnitine supplementation produces a clinical response.[11]

Adverse Effects

Growth and Nutrition

The nature of the ketogenic diet raises concerns about growth, although it is calculated to provide adequate nutrients to maintain growth, with a calorie intake at 75% of the recommended dietary allowance (RDA) for age and gender. The deficiencies in the diet are addressed by supplementation with vitamins and minerals. However, few studies have specifically addressed this issue. One study reporting quantitative data showed that linear growth and weight gain were maintained in children on the diet for 6 months.[38] These findings were confirmed in some but not all studies that have monitored growth, with children under 2 years being particularly vulnerable to poor growth.[22,39,40]

Nephrolithiasis

The effects of the ketogenic diet on urine composition and the fluid restriction increase the risk of nephrolithiasis. Renal calculi occur in about 5% of children treated with the diet.[15,19,39,41,42] The presenting symptoms and signs include gross and microscopic hematuria, abdominal or flank pain, and/or sand-like sediment in the urine. The calculi may be composed of uric acid, calcium oxalate, or calcium phosphate. Their formation may be promoted by a combination of hypercalciuria, hypocitruria, hyperuricosuria, acidic urine, and fluid restriction.[15,41,43] Treatment may require hydration and lithotripsy. Additional episodes may be prevented by liberalization of fluids and alkalinization of urine with bicitrate. Chlorthiazide may be considered for hypercalciuria.

Cardiovascular Effects

The ketogenic diet may have untoward effects on the cardiovascular system through 2 different mechanisms. The high fat content of the diet raises obvious concerns about the development of atherosclerosis and its complications. Although serum cholesterol and triglycerides are often elevated among children on the ketogenic diet,[44,42] not all studies report such increases.[45] The long-term consequences of these alterations in the lipid profile are unknown. The ketogenic diet has also been associated with a prolonged corrected QT (QT_c) interval and cardiomyopathy among children on the ketogenic diet who have no other risk factors.[46] Longer QT_c intervals correlate with higher serum β-hydroxybutyrate and lower serum bicarbonate levels; these effects can be reversed by stopping the ketogenic diet.

Immunosuppression

The ketogenic diet may lead to an immunosuppressed state. A study examining neutrophils from children on the diet found impaired phagocytosis and bacteriocidal function, which appeared to be secondary to serum metabolites.[47] While a few studies have reported that 2% to 4% of children have more frequent infections while on the diet,[16,19] most studies have not reported such a finding. Thus, the immunosuppression does not appear to be clinically significant.[14]

Initiation of the Ketogenic Diet

Traditionally, the ketogenic diet is initiated by an inpatient fast, followed by initiation of the ketogenic diet when the patient is documented to be ketotic, as evidenced by large ketones on urine dipstick tests for ketones. All major studies of the ketogenic diet have included fasting; studies have not been published that determine whether fasting at the time of initiation of the diet improves outcome compared to initiation of the diet without fasting. Fasting of young children requires careful in-hospital monitoring for acute adverse events such as symptomatic hypoglycemia, dehydration, and fluid-electrolyte imbalances. Initiation of the ketogenic diet outside the hospital in young children has been associated with reports of serious adverse events, including isolated reports of sudden death.

Prior to scheduling the admission, parents should be given information about the ketogenic diet and make a commitment to maintain the diet under close supervision for at least 2 months—usually the minimum amount of time required to determine if the diet will be effective. Monographs describing the ketogenic diet, written for parents are available.[48] Well-informed and motivated families are the best predictor of reduction of seizure frequency among children on the ketogenic diet.

The child generally is asked to fast after dinner the night prior to the admission to initiate the diet. Fasting continues in the hospital, with monitoring of blood glucose (Dextrostix) every 4 hours until the child is in ketosis and eating the ketogenic diet. Once eating the diet and in ketosis, the child is monitored clinically and the Dextrostix is monitored only if there are clinical concerns about possible symptomatic hypoglycemia. Unless the child is symptomatic, blood glucose levels as low as 25 mg/dL are not treated.

The traditional approach has been to begin the diet at a 4:1 ratio of ketogenic to anti-ketogenic foods (4 g of fat for every 1 g of protein and carbohydrate). With the traditional approach, it is usually necessary to begin the child on one third of the total calories of the diet the first day and increase to the full diet over 3 days. Beginning children on a 3:1 ratio of the ketogenic diet usually allows them to start on the full diet in the hospital almost immediately. Children tend to tolerate the 3:1 ratio diet better, and are, therefore, discharged faster. The fat can then be increased to a maximum ration of 4.5 g fat for every gram of protein, based on seizure control and presence or absence of adverse events. Typically, the diet allows 1 g of protein per kg of body weight daily, although protein intake can be increased if linear growth slows unacceptably. Fluid intake is usually maintained at about 60 to 70 mL/kg/d; more fluid often makes maintaining ketosis difficult, while less fluid risks dehydration and increases the risk of nephrolithiasis.

Calculation of the Ketogenic Diet

The calculations required for the ketogenic diet should be performed with consultation from a registered pediatric dietician with experience in the ketogenic diet. These calculations are assisted with the recent availability of software designed for the ketogenic diet (eg, KetoPerfect for Windows, 1999; KetoCalculator, Scientific Hospital Supplies). Families can begin with 4 simple meal plans, and then gradually become more sophisticated—often using the ketogenic diet software themselves under the supervision of the dietician.

The steps typically taken in the calculation of the ketogenic diet are outlined in Table 47.1. In general, the patient's calorie level should meet approximately 75% of the RDA. The content of the fat is the critical part of the diet calculation. One can calculate the heavy cream (30% to 36% fat) for each meal first, which is consumed in a wide variety of creative ways, including as liquids, whipped as toppings, or flavored ice cream-like substances. The amount of carbohydrate used in the heavy cream must be taken into account during the first calculation. Consistent use of the same brand of heavy cream, and careful calculations using nutritional tables[48] or standard software are mandatory. Once the fat and carbohydrate are calculated, the remaining protein (meat/fish/poultry, cheese, egg) required is then calculated by subtracting the protein in the cream and vegetable from the total protein allowance. A 4:1(fat-protein) powdered formula is now also available (Ketocal, Scientific Hospital Supplies) and can be used as a meal substitute. For those children who are tube fed, Ketocal or a carbohydrate-free powdered formula (RCF) can be used with added carbohydrate and lipid (Microlipid).

Table 47.1.
Ketogenic Diet Calculations

1. Calculate calories needed per day
   (Example: 15 kg child × 68 cal/kg/d = 1000 cal/d).
2. Calculate number of dietary units needed per day*
   (For example, on a 4:1 diet, each dietary unit (4 g fat + 1 g protein or carbohydrate) = 40 calories. (1000 calories/d)/(40 calories/unit) = 25 units/d).
3. Calculate the number of grams of fat required per day
   (Fat: 25 units/d × 4 g/unit = 100 g/d).
4. Calculate the remainder of units/calories, allotted to protein and carbohydrate
   (Protein and carbohydrate: 25 units/d × 1 g/unit = 25 g/d).
5. Maintain at least the minimum protein requirement (1 g/kg/d)
   (Protein: 1 g/kg/d × 15 kg = 15 g/d of protein).
6. Calculate remainder, allotted to carbohydrate
   (Carbohydrate: 25 g/d − 15 g/d protein = 10 g/d carbohydrate).
7. Divide the allotments into 3 meals per day.

*The calories per dietary unit vary with the ratio of the ketogenic diet as follows: for a 2:1 diet, 22 calories per dietary unit; for a 3:1 diet, 31 calories per dietary unit; for a 4:1 diet, 40 calories per dietary unit; and for a 5:1 diet, 49 calories per dietary unit.

Supplementation of the Ketogenic Diet

The ketogenic diet is deficient in several vitamins (including vitamin D and B vitamins) and minerals (including magnesium, potassium, and calcium). Children on the ketogenic diet must receive supplements of these vitamins and minerals. Parents must understand that these supplements are not elective. Prior to understanding these vitamin requirements in the 1920s and 1930s, serious complications of vitamin and mineral deficiencies, such as blindness, were reported among patients on the ketogenic diet. A typical patient (toddler-school age) receives the following supplements consistent with American Dietetic Association (ADA) recommendations—*Bugs Bunny Complete Sugar-Free* multivitamins (1 per day), or an equivalent multivitamin without sugar; calcium tribasic, 1 tsp per day; ergocalciferol (vitamin D) 8000 IU (0.2 mg) per mL, 1 mL per week. Whether this additional vitamin D is required in addition to what is present in the multivitamin is debatable and is based on early recommendations.[48] Selected patients receive carnitine supplementation based on previous published recommendations.[11] A registered dietitian should develop the supplementation plan, in concert with the pediatrician/neurologist and nursing staff.

Maintenance of the Ketogenic Diet

Children on the ketogenic diet require close supervision by the treating pediatric neurologist/epilepsy specialist, the pediatric dietitian, and the pediatrician. Menus, records of seizure frequency, and records of urine dipsticks for ketones should be provided from the child's caregivers to the neurologist and the dietician. Routine laboratory studies are performed at clinic visits on months 1, 2, 6, 9, and 12, including urinalysis, electrolytes, transaminases, bilirubin, glucose, serum calcium, lipid profile, and prealbumin. Weight and length/height should be monitored regularly and alterations in the diet made if growth slows unacceptably.

Intercurrent Illnesses

Minor viral illnesses and more serious infections typically make it difficult to maintain ketosis. During intercurrent illnesses, breakthrough seizures can be managed with benzodiazepines instead of adding another maintenance AED.

Use of Over-the-Counter and Prescription Medications

The parents should know that virtually all chewable tablets and almost all syrups contain carbohydrates (including lactose, starch, and other sugars), and must, if possible, be avoided. Pediatricians who care for children on the ketogenic diet should consult with references[48] and a dietician about medication choice. Crushing tablets and eating them with meals is often an alternative. All medications must be reviewed and any added carbohydrates must be included in the diet calculations.

Adjusting the Diet for Optimal Seizure Control

The experienced pediatric neurologist will learn to adjust the ketogenic diet like an AED. The time of day of breakthrough seizures in combination with the degree of ketosis at different times of day are used to modify the diet. For example, breakthrough seizures upon waking in the early morning, if ketones are not "large" upon waking, may be addressed with a small high-fat snack at bedtime (eg, olives).

Discontinuation of the Ketogenic Diet

Like most children who are seizure-free on an AED for more than 2 years, the ketogenic diet may be discontinued in children who have been seizure free for 2 years or longer. The weaning process is usually accomplished by reducing the ratio gradually over several months until the child is eating a normal diet. If seizures occur during the weaning process, the diet can be immediately restarted at a 4:1 ratio without fasting and prompt reevaluation of the child.

Most children who try the diet without significant improvement stop the diet within months. Occasionally, children experience significant reductions in seizure frequency on the ketogenic diet, have no other good therapeutic options, and stay on the ketogenic diet for many years. These atypical patients who are on the ketogenic diet for many years should be managed at a major pediatric epilepsy center, where all seizure treatment alternatives can be considered and close monitoring of potential complications of these therapies can be accomplished.

Conclusion

When managed in a meticulous manner, with careful monitoring of the child, the ketogenic diet can be helpful for many children with intractable epilepsy. However, without an expert team managing the ketogenic diet, the risk of adverse events appears to be significant. Parents should be discouraged from attempting the ketogenic diet on their own without careful supervision at an epilepsy center.

References

1. Wheless JW. The ketogenic diet: Fa(c)t or fiction. *J Child Neurol.* 1995;10:419–423
2. Prasad AN, Stafstrom CF, Holmes GL. Alternative epilepsy therapies: the ketogenic diet, immunoglobulins, and steroids. *Epilepsia.* 1996;37(suppl 1):S81–S95
3. Swink TD, Vining EP, Freeman JM. The ketogenic diet: 1997. *Adv Pediatr.* 1997; 44:297–329
4. Tallian KB, Nahata MC, Tsao CY. Role of the ketogenic diet in children with intractable seizures. *Ann Pharmacother.* 1998;32:349–361
5. Wilder RM. The effect of ketonemia on the course of epilepsy. *Mayo Clinic Bull.* 1921;2:307
6. Owen OE, Morgan AP, Kemp HG, Sullivan JM, Herrera MG, Cahill GF Jr. Brain metabolism during fasting. *J Clin Invest.* 1967;46:1589–1595
7. Kraus H, Schlenker S, Schwedesky D. Developmental changes of cerebral ketone body utilization in human infants. *Hoppe-Seylers Z Physiol Chem.* 1974;355:164–170
8. Edmond J, Auestad N, Robbins RA, Bergstrom JD. Ketone body metabolism in the neonate: development and the effect of diet. *Fed Proc.* 1985;44:2359–2364
9. Williamson DH. Ketone body metabolism during development. *Fed Proc.* 1985;44: 2342–2346
10. Stryer L. *Biochemistry.* 4th ed. New York, NY: W. H. Freeman; 1995
11. De Vivo DC, Bohan TP, Coulter DL, et al. L-carnitine supplementation in childhood epilepsy: current perspectives. *Epilepsia.* 1998;39:1216–1225
12. Sankar R, Sotero de Menezes M. Metabolic and endocrine aspects of the ketogenic diet. *Epilepsy Res.* 1999;37:191–201
13. Mitchell GA, Fukao T. Inborn errors of ketone body metabolism. In: Scriver CR, Beaudet AL, Sly WS, Valle D, eds. *The Metabolic and Molecular Bases of Inherited Disease.* Vol 2. 8th ed. New York, NY: McGraw-Hill; 2001:2327–2356
14. Fraser DA, Thoen J, Bondhus S, et al. Reduction in serum leptin and IGF-1 but preserved T-lymphocyte numbers and activation after a ketogenic diet in rheumatoid arthritis patients. *Clin Exp Rheumatol.* 2000;18:209–214
15. Freeman JM, Vining EP, Pillas DJ, Pyzik PL, Casey JC, Kelly LM. The efficacy of the ketogenic diet-1998: a prospective evaluation of intervention in 150 children. *Pediatrics.* 1998;102:1358–1363
16. Vining EP, Freeman JM, Ballaban-Gil K, et al. A multicenter study of the efficacy of the ketogenic diet. *Arch Neurol.* 1998;55:1433–1437
17. Freeman JM, Vining EP. Seizures decrease rapidly after fasting: preliminary studies of the ketogenic diet. *Arch Pediatr Adolesc Med.* 1999;153:946–949
18. Huttenlocher PR, Wilbourn AJ, Signore JM. Medium-chain triglycerides as a therapy for intractable childhood epilepsy. *Neurology.* 1971;21:1097–1103
19. Kinsman SL, Vining EP, Quaskey SA, Mellits D, Freeman JM. Efficacy of the ketogenic diet for intractable seizure disorders: review of 58 cases. *Epilepsia.* 1992;33: 1132–1136

20. Katyal NG, Koehler AN, McGhee B, Foley CM, Crumrine PK. The ketogenic diet in refractory epilepsy: the experience of Children's Hospital of Pittsburgh. *Clin Pediatr (Phila).* 2000;39:153–159

21. Barborka CJ. Epilepsy in adults: results of treatment by ketogenic diet in 100 cases. *Arch Neurol Psych.* 1930;23:904–914

22. Schwartz RH, Eaton J, Bower BD, Aynsley-Green A. Ketogenic diets in the treatment of epilepsy: short-term clinical effects. *Dev Med Child Neurol.* 1989;31:145–151

23. Sirven J, Whedon B, Caplan D, et al. The ketogenic diet for intractable epilepsy in adults: preliminary results. *Epilepsia.* 1999;40:1721–1726

24. Lyon G, Adams RD, Kolodny EH. *Neurology of Hereditary Metabolic Diseases of Children.* 2nd ed. New York, NY: McGraw-Hill; 1996

25. Wijburg FA, Barth PG, Bindoff LA, et al. Leigh syndrome associated with a deficiency of the pyruvate dehydrogenase complex: results of treatment with a ketogenic diet. *Neuropediatrics.* 1992;23:147–152

26. Wexler ID, Hemalatha SG, McConnell J, et al. Outcome of pyruvate dehydrogenase deficiency treated with ketogenic diets. Studies in patients with identical mutations. *Neurology.* 1997;49:1655–1661

27. De Vivo DC, Trifiletti RR, Jacobson RI, Ronen GM, Behmand RA, Harik SI. Defective glucose transport across the blood-brain barrier as a cause of persistent hypoglycorrhachia, seizures, and developmental delay. *N Engl J Med.* 1991;325: 703–709

28. Swoboda KJ, Specht L, Jones HR, Shapiro F, DiMauro S, Korson M. Infantile phosphofructokinase deficiency with arthrogryposis: clinical benefit of a ketogenic diet. *J Pediatr.* 1997;131:932–934

29. Thio LL, Wong M, Yamada KA. Ketone bodies do not directly alter excitatory or inhibitory hippocampal synaptic transmission. *Neurology.* 2000;54:325–331

30. Nordli DR Jr, De Vivo DC. The ketogenic diet revisited: back to the future. *Epilepsia.* 1997;38:743–749

31. Schwartzkroin PA. Mechanisms underlying the anti-epileptic efficacy of the ketogenic diet. *Epilepsy Res.* 1999;37:171–180

32. Robinson BH, Sherwood WG. Pyruvate dehydrogenase phosphatase deficiency: a cause of congenital chronic lactic acidosis in infancy. *Pediatr Res.* 1975;9:935–939

33. De Vivo DC, Haymond MW, Leckie MP, Bussman YL, McDougal DB Jr, Pagliara AS. The clinical and biochemical implications of pyruvate carboxylase deficiency. *J Clin Endocrinol Metab.* 1977;45:1281–1296

34. DeVivo DC, Pagliara AS, Prensky AL. Ketotic hypoglycemia and the ketogenic diet. *Neurology.* 1973;23:640–649

35. Vining EPG. Ketogenic diet. In: Engel J Jr, Pedley TA, eds. *Epilepsy: A Comprehensive Textbook.* Philadelphia. PA: Lippincott-Raven; 1998:1339–1344

36. Ballaban-Gil K, Callahan C, O'Dell C, Pappo M, Moshe S, Shinnar S. Complications of the ketogenic diet. *Epilepsia.* 1998;39:744–748

37. Dodson WE, Prensky AL, DeVivo DC, Goldring S, Dodge PR. Management of seizure disorders: selected aspects. Part II. *J Pediatr*. 1976;89:695–703

38. Couch SC, Schwarzman F, Carroll J, et al. Growth and nutritional outcomes of children treated with the ketogenic diet. *J Am Diet Assoc*. 1999;99:1573–1575

39. Hopkins IJ, Lynch BC. Use of ketogenic diet in epilepsy in childhood. *Aust Paediatr J*. 1970;6:25–29

40. Vining EP. Clinical efficacy of the ketogenic diet. *Epilepsy Res*. 1999;37:181–190

41. Herzberg GZ, Fivush BA, Kinsman SL, Gearhart JP. Urolithiasis associated with the ketogenic diet. *J Pediatr*. 1990;117:743–745

42. Chesney D, Brouhard BH, Wyllie E, Powaski K. Biochemical abnormalities of the ketogenic diet in children. *Clin Pediatr (Phila)*. 1999;38:107–109

43. Kielb S, Koo HP, Bloom DA, Faerber GJ. Nephrolithiasis associated with the ketogenic diet. *J Urol*. 2000;164:464–466

44. Huttenlocher PR. Ketonemia and seizures: metabolic and anticonvulsant effects of two ketogenic diets in childhood epilepsy. *Pediatr Res*. 1976;10:536–540

45. Schwartz RM, Boyes S, Aynsley-Green A. Metabolic effects of three ketogenic diets in the treatment of severe epilepsy. *Dev Med Child Neurol*. 1989;31:152–160

46. Best TH, Franz DN, Gilbert DL, Nelson DP, Epstein MR. Cardiac complications in pediatric patients on the ketogenic diet. *Neurology*. 2000;54:2328–2330

47. Woody RC, Steele RW, Knapple WL, Pilkington NS Jr. Impaired neutrophil function in children with seizures treated with the ketogenic diet. *J Pediatr*. 1989;115:427–430

48. Freeman JM, Freeman JB, Kelly MT. *The Ketogenic Diet: A Treatment for Epilepsy*. 3rd ed. New York, NY: Demos Medical Publishing; 2000

48
Nutrition and Oral Health

Introduction

The oral health of children living in industrialized countries has improved over the last 2 decades in a remarkable way, but there are many children who continue to experience the effects of dental decay.[1] The prevalence of early childhood caries (ECC) is approximately 6% in children under the age of 3 years.[2] Segments of our population continue to experience a disproportionate amount of dental decay and have a more difficult time obtaining care. Children who experience ECC tend to remain at high risk for dental decay in the primary as well as the permanent dentition.

The prevalence of caries in the 3- to 5-year-old US Head Start program has been reported as high as 90% in some groups.[3] Untreated dental decay leads to pain, poor eating, infection, speech problems, crowding of the permanent teeth, and self-esteem issues. In a study by Acs,[4] 8.7% of children with ECC weighed less than 80% of their ideal weight compared with only 7% of the control group. In addition, 19.1% of children with ECC were in the tenth percentile or less for weight compared with only 7% of the control group. Early childhood caries has also been implicated in contributing to other health problems such as otitis media.

Many times, treatment for ECC has to be completed in the operating room under general anesthesia due to the amount of treatment and the young age of the child. The average costs for dental treatment in a hospital setting can be very expensive. Not only can treatment of ECC be expensive to society, but the child's overall health and well-being also can be compromised.

Oral Bacteria

It has been well established that the group of cariogenic bacteria thought to have the highest association with caries is *Streptococcus mutans*. These bacteria are not detectable in children's mouths until the teeth have begun eruption. The predominant source for this infection seems to be associated with the mother's saliva. Studies have shown that mothers with high levels of salivary

S mutans tended to have children with high levels. This places the child at a high risk for developing caries. Dental caries is an infectious disease. These findings give support for the need to address oral issues and preventive measures in mothers during their pregnancy in hopes of reducing the mother's overall *S mutans* levels. In a recent study, a group of pregnant women were given an oral examination and a comprehensive preventive dental program.[4] This included monitoring of oral bacteria levels and referral for dental treatment as needed. When their infants were born, they were given additional instruction on caring for their infants' teeth, including examinations. Compared with a control group who received no prenatal or postnatal dental care, the children in the intervention group showed significant benefits in various measures of oral health. The mothers also reported significant improvement in their oral health.

As the carbohydrate intake increases, *S mutans* colonizes in plaque and metabolizes the carbohydrates into acid. This, in turn, provides the appropriate environment for a drop in the plaque pH, and subsequent demineralization of the enamel. Saliva serves an important role as a buffering agent and by providing calcium and phosphorous to remineralize the demineralized enamel. In addition, the presence of fluoride facilitates the transformation of calcium phosphates to hydroxyapatite during remineralization, and aids in the formation of fluoridated hydroxyapatite and fluorapatite. Both of these are less soluble than hydroxyapatite when placed in an acidic environment. If demineralization exceeds remineralization over time, cavitation of the enamel surface will occur leading to decay. As the decayed area continues to grow in size, eventually the pulp/nerve of the tooth will become involved, leading to pain, infection, early tooth loss, and potential crowding problems.

Dietary Influences

In many cases, early childhood caries is thought to be the result of the inappropriate use of a bottle or sippy cup while sleeping, or of its unsupervised use during the day with a liquid other than water. Dipping the child's pacifier in a sweetened substance also increases the risk of ECC. Early childhood caries usually affects the maxillary anterior teeth first followed by the primary molars. The lower anterior teeth are usually not involved due to protection by the tongue. Perhaps 20% of bottle-fed infants and children are put to bed with a bottle with contents other than water.[5] Many children continue to drink a bottle between the ages of 2 and 5 years. Like many foods, some infant formulas are acidogenic and promote the development of caries when prolonged contact

with teeth occurs.[6] Because of the decrease in salivary flow during sleep, there
is a decrease in the clearance of sugars from the mouth by saliva. This, in
turn, will allow any sugar substrate present in the mouth to have an increased
cariogenic effect.

Sucrose, glucose, and fructose found in fruit juices, foods, and candy are
probably the main sugars associated with ECC. Fructose and glucose are as cariogenic as sucrose in their ability to cause a drop in the oral pH.[7] In addition,
starchy foods such as breads or biscuits have been shown to cause a variable pH
drop. As the levels of starch increase, the acid production found in plaque also
increases. This is probably the result of the increased stickiness of starchy foods.[8]

The frequency of eating and drinking also plays a role in the decay process
of teeth during childhood. Children who are constantly snacking and drinking
sugar-containing substances are at higher risk for caries than children who
eat 3 meals and a few snacks per day. The more frequent the food intake, the
greater the risk for caries. A high frequency of eating encourages the growth
of the S mutans, that, in turn, leads to increased acidity in the oral cavity.

It is well known that acids found in fruit juices and soft drinks may cause
an increase in the overall acidity of the mouth if high quantities are consumed.
Parents must be reminded that their child should not walk around the house
throughout the day with a bottle or sippy cup containing sweetened drinks.
Consumption of these drinks should be limited, and, in any event, consumed
at mealtimes and snack times only.

The teeth are most susceptible to decay the first few years after eruption due
to their immaturity. In addition, the teeth may have actual structural defects or
hypoplastic areas. This could be the result of hereditary diseases, birth trauma,
birth prematurity, and low birth weight, infections, malnutrition, metabolic
disorders, and chemical toxicity.[9] Enamel defects can be common in newborns,
with a prevalence ranging from 12.8% in infants weighing >2500 g at birth, to
more than 62% in those born preterm with very low birth weight (<1500 g).[10]
In one study, defects were noted to have occurred in 85% of 40 intubated
preterm infants, compared with approximately 22% of non-intubated
children.[11] Chronically ill children are also at high isk for ECC. These children
can have increased enamel hypoplastic areas as well. In addition, many of these
children may be comforted with bottles containing sweetened liquids or by frequently ingesting medications that have a high sugar content. This allows the
teeth to be surrounded by a constant source of sugar, leading to rapid demineralization of the enamel.

The role on demand breastfeeding plays in contributing to ECC has been controversial. There have been a few studies that have implicated at-will breastfeeding with caries. Breastfeeding alone, however, has not been shown to cause any significant drop in the pH of plaque, or to be cariogenic. Human breast milk was demonstrated to be a poor buffering agent when acid from other carbohydrate sources was added.[2,6] With the addition of sucrose to human milk, the rate of in vitro caries formation is faster than for sucrose alone. Thus, breast milk alone is not cariogenic. However, if an infant is given a sugar-rich food in combination with on-demand breastfeeding, the combination is highly cariogenic.

Malnutrition

The teeth may reflect nutritional disturbances that occur during their formation. Tooth development begins during the second month of embryonic life, and, by age 8 years, the crowns of all permanent teeth except the third molars are formed. Enamel and dentin cannot regenerate, and any defect in their structure is permanent. A longitudinal study of Peruvian children confirmed previous studies in animals and indirect epidemiological evidence in humans that suggested a cause-effect relationship between early malnutrition and increased dental caries.[12] The study also reported the eruption of primary teeth was significantly delayed.

Vitamin A deficiency during tooth formation is reported to interfere with tooth calcification and result in hypoplasia of the enamel. The effect of vitamin C deficiency in humans occurs chiefly in the gingival and periodontal tissues. The gingiva is bright red with a swollen, smooth, shiny surface that may become boggy, ulcerate, and bleed.

When vitamin D deficiency occurs during childhood, eruption of the deciduous and permanent teeth is delayed, and the sequence of eruption is disturbed. Histologically, widening of the predentin layer, the presence of interglobular dentin, and interference with enamel formation have been reported. Some authors report hypoplasia of the enamel with a symmetrical distribution of thinning and pitting enamel defects. With riboflavin deficiency, glossitis begins with soreness of the tip and lateral margins of the tongue. The tongue surface appears reddened and coarsely granular. The lips are pale, and cheilosis develops at the oral commissures. Niacin deficiency leads to pellagra. In the acute stages, the oral mucosa becomes fiery red and painful, accompanied by profuse salivation. As pellagra progresses, the epithelium of the tongue sloughs.[13]

Fluoride

Since the introduction of fluoride through water fluoridation and topical fluorides, cavities in the primary teeth of children have decreased by as much as 60%. Fluoride reduces dental decay by (1) reducing the solubility of enamel, (2) reducing the ability of bacteria to produce acid, and (3) promoting remineralization. At one time, fluoride was thought to exert a pre-eruptive effect on teeth, but now it is generally accepted that its main benefit is topical. Systemic fluoride exerts its topical effects following secretion from the salivary glands. Drinking fluoridated water protects more than 360 million people worldwide in approximately 60 countries. Slightly less than two thirds of the municipalities in the United States optimally fluoridate water. The cost of water fluoridation is $0.50 per person per year. Based on extensive research by the United States Public Health Service, the optimum concentration of fluoride in the drinking water ranges from 0.7 to 1.2 ppm. This range effectively reduces dental decay while minimizing the risk for dental fluorosis.[14] The effectiveness of prenatal fluoride exposure is still in question today but, generally, is not thought to be beneficial.

Fluoride Supplements

Fluoride supplements may be of some benefit to children living in fluoride-deficient areas (Table 48.1).[15]

The decision to recommend a supplement should be based on the total amount of fluoride from all sources available to a child daily.

For example, a child may be living in a non-fluoridated community but attend school in an area where fluoride is at optimal levels. If the fluoride content of a child's water source is unknown, then it is important to have the water

Table 48.1.
Fluoride Supplementation Schedule*

Age	Fluoride Concentration in Local Water Supply, ppm		
	<0.3	0.3–0.6	>0.6
6 mo to 3 y	0.25ᵁ	0.00	0.00
3–6 y	0.50	0.25	0.00
6 y to at least 16 y	1.00	0.50	0.00

*Must know fluoride values of drinking water prior to making a prescription.
All values are milligrams of fluoride supplement per day.
From the American Academy of Pediatrics, American Dental Association, and the American Academy of Pediatric Dentistry.

tested for the fluoride content prior to prescribing a fluoride supplement. Foods and beverages that are produced in communities with optimally fluoridated water are consumed not only in the area where they are made, but also can be shipped to an area that is non-fluoridated. This is termed the "halo or diffusion" effect and can benefit people in non-fluoridated communities. A child's overall risk for decay should also be considered.

Because of the widespread availability of fluoride, the difference in the tooth decay rate in communities with fluoridated water compared with those that are not fluoridated has lessened. The question has been raised as to the need for fluoride supplements in the United States, given the fact that fluoride can be found in so many varied sources such as drinking water, toothpaste, gels, rinses, professionally applied fluorides, and processed foods and beverages. The evidence for the benefit of fluoride supplements when used from birth or soon after is weak, and supplements are a risk factor for fluorosis.[16] It is essential, as we look towards ways to reduce dental decay, that we maximize protection from caries while minimizing the risk for fluorosis.

However, dietary supplements alone are unlikely to be the cause of the reported increase in fluorosis because compliance with recommendations to use supplemental fluoride continues to be extremely poor[17] (as it is with prescription medications).[18,19] In addition, few children use supplements for more than 1½ years.[17] In contrast, many children are still at high risk for dental caries, and may not have access to fluoridated drinking water or professionally administered fluoride regimens. Some studies have shown the greatest benefit for the primary and permanent teeth when fluoride supplements are given before the age of 2,[20] although it is unclear how fluoride affects the permanent teeth at this young age if its main benefit is topical.

Another factor that may need to be considered in assessing a child's total fluoride exposure is the increasing popularity of bottled water and home water filtration systems. The majority of bottled water sold on the market today does not contain adequate amounts of fluoride (0.7–1.2 ppm). In a 1991 study of 39 different bottled-water brands, 34 of them had fluoride levels less than 0.3 ppm.[21] Home water treatment systems also have the ability to reduce fluoride levels. Reverse osmosis and distillation units remove significant amounts of fluoride. Therefore, it is conceivable that a preschool child could live in an optimally fluoridated area, but not receive adequate amounts of fluoride. However, the most common type of home water filtration is a carbon or charcoal filter systems and generally, this does not remove significant levels of fluoride. Studies have also shown that water softeners cause no significant changes in fluoride levels.[22]

Prescriptions for supplemental fluoride should be specific about when and how the supplement is to be given. Fluoride ingested on an empty stomach is 100% bioavailable, while fluoride administered with milk or a meal will not be completely absorbed. The best time to administer the supplement is at bedtime or at least 1 hour prior to eating.[23] The American Academy of Pediatrics endorses and accepts as its policy the Recommendations for Using Fluoride to Prevent and Control Dental Caries in the United States. (See www.cdc.gov/mmwr/pdf/rr/rr5014.pdf.)

Fluorosis

How much fluoride a child should receive on a daily basis varies with both age and body weight (Table 48.2 and Appendix W). The adequate intake of fluoride from all sources on a daily basis is 0.05 mg/kg/d. This is the amount of fluoride needed for optimal health without incurring the risks of fluorosis. The tolerable upper intake level has been set at 0.10 mg/kg/d for infants, toddlers, and children up to age 8 years. For those that are older, the upper limit has been set at 10 mg/d.[14]

Over the past several years, an increase in enamel fluorosis has been noted in both optimally fluoridated and non-fluoridated areas. Fluorosis is the result of too much fluoride and affects approximately 22% of children. Ninety-four

Table 48.2.
DRI: Fluoride*

Age Group	Adequate Intake (mg/d)	Tolerable Upper Intake (mg/d)
Infants 0–6 months	0.01	0.7
Infants 7–12 months	0.5	0.9
Children 1–3 years	0.7	1.3
Children 4–8 years	1.0	2.2
Children 9–13 years	2.0	10
Boys 14–18 years	3.0	10
Girls 14–18 years	3.0	10
Males 19 years and older	4.0	10
Females 19 years and older	3.0	10

*Institute of Medicine, Food and Nutrition Board. *Dietary Reference Intakes for Calcium, Phosphorus, Magnesium, Vitamin D, and Fluoride.* Washington, DC: National Academy Press; 1997. (See also Appendix C.)

percent of children have only mild to moderate fluorosis.[14] This condition results in a change in the appearance of the teeth when higher than optimal levels of fluoride are ingested before the age of 7 years, during the calcification stage of tooth development. Dental fluorosis is a cosmetic effect with little consequence to health. The risk of fluorosis can be greatly reduced by proper supervision of children around fluoride products. Clinically, fluorosis ranges from minor white lines running across the teeth to a very chalky appearance. In severe cases, the teeth may demonstrate pitting and brown staining.

One factor that has contributed to the overall increase in fluorosis has been the inappropriate prescribing of fluoride supplements for children already receiving adequate intakes of fluoride. Inappropriate supplementation may account for 25% of the cases of fluorosis in children living in an optimally fluoridated area.[24] Studies have found that those drinking non-fluoridated water and taking a fluoride supplement had a marked increase in dental fluorosis.[25,26] In Europe and Canada, the fluoride supplement schedules are used as guidelines only for those children aged 3 years and older considered to be at high risk for caries.[16]

Because the use of fluoridated toothpaste in early childhood significantly increases the risk of fluorosis,[25,27] it is recommended that children should not use a fluoridated toothpaste until after reaching the age of 2 years, and then only a small pea-size amount up to the age of 6 years. Over the past several years, many companies have marketed toothpaste with special colors and flavors to increase use by children. There is concern this type of marketing may encourage children to use more toothpaste and potentially ingest significant amounts of fluoride, thereby contributing to dental fluorosis. Preschool children use significantly more children's toothpaste than the adult brands and brush their teeth for a longer period of time, and only about 50% of the children expectorate and half as many rinse following brushing.[28] Parents should be reminded of the need to supervise their preschool children during toothbrushing to ensure that the proper amount of toothpaste is used regardless of whether their water is optimally fluoridated or not. Parents should encourage their children to expectorate and rinse with water after brushing to lessen the amount swallowed. All fluoride products should be kept out of reach of young children. The fact that nearly all children use fluoride toothpaste and relatively few take fluoride supplements means that fluoride toothpaste undoubtedly has had a greater overall impact on fluorosis in the United States than have fluoride supplements.[18]

Having considered the risks and benefits of fluoride, the idea of assessing the child's overall risk for developing decay becomes important. One can look at the child's previous dental history, family history, medical complications, diet, hygiene, fluoride status, and use of chronic medications in determining a child's risk for developing caries and the need for a fluoride supplement.

Fluoride Toxicity

Although fluoride has been shown to be beneficial, it can be toxic to children if more than 5 mg/kg is ingested. Since the majority of toothpaste in the United States contains fluoride, it is theoretically possible for a child to ingest enough toothpaste to cause toxic effects. The probable toxic dose for a 1-year-old (10 kg) is contained in 50 mL of a 1000-ppm fluoride toothpaste. For a 5-year-old (19 kg), it is found in 95 mL. For these reasons, parents are to be reminded that close supervision of the use of all fluoride products for their children is essential. Children should be encouraged not to swallow or eat toothpaste or other fluoride products, and these products should be stored out of reach. Nausea and vomiting are common side effects of too much fluoride. The certain lethal dose for fluoride has been shown to be 16 to 32 mg/kg. Symptoms include nausea, vomiting, electrolyte imbalance, arrhythmia's, central nervous system excitation, and coma, followed by death within a few hours.[29]

Access to Dental Care

Tooth decay is the most common chronic disease of childhood. Despite the clear importance of health insurance, an estimated 1.3 million children with special health care needs were uninsured during 1994–1995. These children were disproportionately represented among low-income families. In addition, there are problems with access to health care for some children with special health care needs despite having insurance.[30] Children with dental problems lose more than 51 million school hours annually.[31] Substantial numbers of children with untreated caries are seen in emergency departments around the United States, and for those that are 3.5 years and younger, 52% have never seen a dentist before.[32] Only 1 in 5 children covered by Medicaid receive preventive oral care for which they are eligible.[33]

The infectious nature of dental caries, its early onset, and the potential benefit of early interventions require an emphasis on preventive oral care in the primary pediatric setting.[33] Most caries in children today occur in only 25% of the childhood-age population. These children could greatly benefit from early referral by their primary health care professional for appropriate dental care.

The major risk factors for caries in infants include a low socioeconomic status, mothers of a low educational level and/or immigrant background, consumption of sugary beverages and foods, or high salivary S mutans levels.[34] Children who exhibited all of these risk factors are 32 times more likely to have decay by the age of 3.5 years than children who have no risk factors. The presence of plaque on the upper front teeth of infants is predictive of future caries.[35] This is why it is essential for parents and pediatricians to learn to lift children's lips and look for developing decay before it becomes more serious. Dental decay usually presents itself as obvious dental lesions with minor, chronic pain and is often missed. Undetected caries can present dramatically if left untreated. When the decay spreads to the nerve of the tooth, infection can result, leading to a cellulitis.

Role of the Pediatrician

Because all children are susceptible to oral conditions including caries, pediatricians play a pivotal role in guidance, screening, and coordination of needed care.[36] The American Academy of Pediatric Dentistry recommends that the first oral evaluation be completed within 6 months of the eruption of the first primary tooth and no later than 12 months of age.[37] The American Academy of Pediatrics Section on Pediatric Dentistry recommends that every child should begin to receive oral health risk assessments by 6 months of age by a qualified pediatric health care provider. Between 6 and 12 months of age infants identified as having a significant risk of caries should be entered into an aggressive anticipatory guidance and intervention program, provided by a dentist.[38]

Regardless of the time of the first visit to the dentist, parents need to be reminded that any teeth that have erupted should be cleaned daily with a washcloth. A toothbrush can be introduced once the back molars begin to erupt, but the child should not be allowed to walk around the house with the toothbrush to avoid the possibility of injury. Parents should brush their child's teeth at least 2 times per day, and their child should be encouraged to brush as well. A good rule of thumb is once a child can easily tie their shoes, the child should have the hand skills to brush well. Parents should always supervise the brushing of their children's teeth to ensure that the proper amount of toothpaste is used, and flossing should be started once the teeth begin to contact each other.

References

1. Nowak AJ. Rationale for the timing of the first oral evaluation. *Pediatr Dent.* 1997;19:8–11
2. Erickson PR, Mazhari E. Investigation of the role of human breast milk in caries development. *Pediatr Dent.* 1999;21:86–90
3. Tinanoff N, O'Sullivan DM. Early childhood caries: overview and recent findings. *Pediatr Dent.* 1997;19:12–16
4. Acs G, Lodolini G, Kaminsky S, Cisneros GJ. Effect of nursing caries on body weight in a pediatric population. *Pediatr Dent.* 1992;14:302–305
5. Kaste LM, Gift HC. Inappropriate infant bottle feeding. Status of the Healthy People 2000 objective. *Arch Pediatr Adolesc Med.* 1995;149:786–791
6. Sheikh C, Erickson PR. Evaluation of plaque pH changes following oral rinse with eight infant formulas. *Pediatr Dent.* 1996;18:200–204
7. Neff D. Acid production from different carbohydrate sources in human plaque in situ. *Caries Res.* 1967;1:78–87
8. Mormann JE, Muhlemann HR. Oral starch degradation and its influence on acid production in human dental plaque. *Caries Res.* 1981;15:166–175
9. Seow WK. Enamel hypoplasia in the primary dentition: a review. *ASDC J Dent Child.* 1991;58:441–452
10. Seow WK, Humphrys C, Tudehope DI. Increased prevalence of developmental dental defects in low birthweight, prematurely born children: a controlled study. *Pediatr Dent.* 1987;9:221–225
11. Seow WK, Brown JP, Tudehope DI, O'Callaghan M. Developmental defects in the primary dentition of low birth-weight infants: adverse effects of laryngoscopy and prolonged endotracheal intubation. *Pediatr Dent.* 1984;6:28–31
12. Alvarez JO, Caceda J, Woolley TW, et al. A longitudinal study of dental caries in the primary teeth of children who suffered from infant malnutrition. *J Dent Res.* 1993; 72:1573–1576
13. Oral aspects of metabolic disease. In: Shafer WG, Hine MK, Levy BM, Tomich CE, eds. *A Textbook of Oral Pathology.* 4th ed. Philadelphia, PA: WB Saunders Co; 1983:616–672
14. American Dental Association. Fluoridation Facts. Available at: http://www.ada.org/public/topics/fluoride/facts-toc.html. Accessed March 7, 2003
15. American Academy of Pediatric Dentistry. Fluoride. *Pediatr Dent.* 1999;21:40
16. Burt BA. The case for eliminating the use of dietary fluoride supplements for young children. *J Public Health Dent.* 1999;59:269–274
17. Moss SJ. The case for retaining the current supplementation schedule. *J Public Health Dent.* 1999;59:259–262
18. Horowitz HS. The role of dietary fluoride supplements in caries prevention. *J Public Health Dent.* 1999;59:205–210
19. Adair SM. Overview of the history and current status of fluoride supplementation schedules. *J Public Health Dent.* 1999;59:252–258

20. Mellberg JR, Ripa LW, Leske GS. Dietary fluoride supplementation. In: *Fluoride in Preventive Dentistry: Theory and Clinical Applications.* Chicago, IL: Quintessence; 1983:123–149

21. Tate WH, Chan JT. Fluoride concentrations in bottled and filtered water. *Gen Dent.* 1994;42:362–366

22. Robinson SN, Davies EH, Williams B. Domestic water treatment appliances and the fluoride ion. *Br Dent J.* 1991;171:91–93

23. Shulman ER, Vallejo M. Effect of gastric contents on the bioavailability of fluoride in humans. *Pediatr Dent.* 1990;12:237–240

24. Pendrys DG. Risk of fluorosis in a fluoridated population. Implications for the dentist and hygienist. *J Am Dent Assoc.* 1995;126:1617–1624

25. Lalumandier JA, Rozier RG. The prevalence and risk factors of fluorosis among patients in a pediatric dental practice. *Pediatr Dent.* 1995;17:19–25

26. Pendrys DG. Risk of enamel fluorosis in nonfluoridated and optimally fluoridated populations: considerations for the dental professional. *J Am Dent Assoc.* 2000; 131:746–755

27. Osuji OO, Leake JL, Chipman ML, Nikiforuk G, Locker D, Levine N. Risk factors for dental fluorosis in a fluoridated community. *J Dent Res.* 1988;67:1488–1492

28. Adair SM, Piscitelli WP, McKnight-Hanes C. Comparison of the use of a child and an adult dentifrice by a sample of preschool children. *Pediatr Dent.* 1997;19:99–103

29. Whitford GM. Fluoride in dental products: safety considerations. *J Dent Res.* 1987; 66:1056–1060

30. Newacheck PW, McManus M, Fox HB, Hung YY, Halfon N. Access to health care for children with special health care needs. *Pediatrics.* 2000;105:760–766

31. Gift HC, Reisine ST, Larach DC. The social impact of dental problems and visits. *Am J Public Health.* 1992;82:1663–1668

32. Sheller B, Williams BJ, Lombardi SM. Diagnosis and treatment of dental caries-related emergencies in a children's hospital. *Pediatr Dent.* 1997;19:470–475

33. Mouradian WE, Wehr E, Crall JJ. Disparities in children's oral health and access to dental care. *JAMA.* 2000;284:2625–2631

34. Grindefjord M, Dahllof G, Nilsson B, Modeer T. Prediction of dental caries development in 1-year-old children. *Caries Res.* 1995;29:343–348

35. Alaluusua S, Malmivirta R. Early plaque accumulation—a sign for caries risk in young children. *Community Dent Oral Epidemiol.* 1994;22:273–276

36. Edelstein BL. Public and clinical policy considerations in maximizing children's oral health. *Pediatr Clin North Am.* 2000;47:1177–1189

37. American Academy of Pediatric Dentistry. Infant oral health care. *Pediatr Dent.* 1999;21:77

38. American Academy of Pediatrics Section on Pediatric Dentistry. Oral health risk assessment timing and establishment of the dental home. *Pediatrics.* 2003;111:1113–1116

49

Community Nutrition Services

Promoting the nutritional health of children and their families is a common goal of the nutrition services offered by a wide variety of public and private agencies, organizations, and individuals in communities across the nation. These include state health and education departments; local health agencies such as city and county health departments, community health centers, health maintenance and preferred provider organizations; hospital and ambulatory outpatient clinics; nutritionists and dietitians in public and private practice; voluntary health agencies such as the diabetes and heart associations; social service agencies; elementary and secondary schools; colleges and universities; and business and industry.

Nutrition Services Provided Through Federal, State, and Local Health Agencies

Each year Congress appropriates funds for a variety of health programs, many of which are targeted to mothers and children. Such programs are administered at the national level by the US Department of Agriculture (USDA) and the US Department of Health and Human Services (DHHS). These include USDA Child Nutrition Programs (National School Lunch Program, School Breakfast Program, Summer Food Service Program, and Child and Adult Care Food Program), Special Supplemental Nutrition Program for Women, Infants, and Children (WIC), Food Stamp Program, and the Commodity Supplemental Food Program (CSFP); and DHHS maternal and child health services block grant programs, preventive health services block grant programs, Early Periodic Screening, Diagnostic, and Treatment Program under Medicaid, Indian Health Services, and programs such as community health centers and migrant health projects that serve at-risk populations.[1] In addition to federal support, considerable state and local funds also support child health programs. An example of a local resource is community-based food programs that are nonprofit, nongovernmental, grass-roots, self-help community developmental programs. One such program is the Self-Help and Resource Exchange Program that has international, national, and local programs based on food distribution and community building through service (WORLD SHARE; see Table 49.1). Physicians and other primary care providers must be aware of the local food and nutrition programs so families become informed consumers and appropriate referrals can be made to emergency food and nutrition programs. An informed clinician can also serve as an advocate to strengthen policy and budget decisions that guide the provision of quality cost-effective nutrition programs focused on improving the health of the nation.

Although nutrition services were introduced into public health programs as early as the late 1920s, Title V of the Social Security Act of 1935 initiated the federal-state partnership for maternal and child health that served as the major impetus for the development of nutrition services for mothers and children.[2] A census of public health nutrition personnel in 1991 showed that approximately 4500 public health nutritionists are employed in federal, state, and local public health agencies.[3] Public health nutritionists provide a wide range of services based on the core public health functions, which include assessment, assurance, and policy development. These include provision of direct clinical services (eg, screening, assessment, monitoring); population-based research; development and implementation of nutrition services and policies that focus on disease prevention and health promotion; provision of technical assistance to a range of providers and consumers; collection and analysis of health-related data, including nutrition surveillance and monitoring; investigation and control of disease, injuries, and responses to natural disasters; protection of the environment, housing, food, water, and workplace; public information, education, and community mobilization; quality assurance; training and education; leadership, planning, policy development, and administration; targeted outreach and linkage to personal services; and other direct clinical services.[4]

Many community nutrition services include screening, education, counseling, and treatment of the nutritional status of an individual or a population. These services are designed to meet the preventive, therapeutic, and rehabilitative health care needs of all segments of the population. The focus of nutrition services in an agency is based on several factors, including the mission of the agency, funding, analysis of data from a community needs assessment, resources, and politics.[5] Nutrition services are provided in a variety of inpatient and outpatient settings. Public agencies provide nutrition services for individuals throughout the life cycle. The broadest range of nutrition services may be most evident in community-based nutrition programs in which services are

Table 49.1.
Professional and Federal Resources for Nutrition Services

Professional Nutrition Organizations
American Dietetic Association 216 West Jackson Blvd, Suite 800 Chicago, IL 60606–6995 Consumer Hotline Numbers: 312/899–0040; 800/877–1600; fax: 312/899–1758 www.eatright.org
American School Food Service Association 1600 Duke St, 7th floor Alexandria, VA 22314 800/877–8822; fax: 703/739–3915 www.asfsa.org
Association of Public Health State and Territorial Nutrition Directors 1015 15th St, NW, Suite 403 Washington, DC 20005 202/408–1330
National Association of WIC Directors PO Box 53405 Washington, DC 20009–3405 202/232–5492; fax: 202/387–5281
WORLD SHARE 6950 Friars Rd San Diego, CA 92108 619/686–5818
Federal Resources
Food and Drug Administration Office of Consumer Affairs 5600 Fishers Ln Rockville, MD 20857 301/827–4420
The National Center for Education in Maternal and Child Health 2000 15th St N, Suite 701 Arlington, VA 22201–2617 703/524–7802; fax: 703/524–9335
US Department of Agriculture Food and Nutrition Service 3101 Park Center Dr Alexandria, VA 22302 703/305–2062 Fact sheets on USDA programs are available from the USDA Web site: www.fns.usda.gov/fns

based on the core public health functions. The physician and other primary care providers must know where services are provided in their community. Resources to help identify federal and state nutrition services are listed in Table 49.1. A resource directory describing national organizations that provide technical assistance related to maternal and child health is a useful resource for pediatricians and other primary care providers.[6]

Qualified providers of nutrition services include physicians, registered and/or licensed dietitians (RDs), nurses, and others. The American Dietetic Association (ADA), the largest organization of professional dietitians and nutritionists, has identified qualified providers as the RD and other qualified professionals who meet licensing and other standards prescribed at the state level.[7]

Health Agencies: A Nutrition Resource to Provide Service and Identify Qualified Providers

Federal, state, and local health agencies, particularly those employing public health nutritionists, can be helpful resources for physicians and other primary care providers. Nutritionists provide extensive technical assistance to clients, their families, and the physician, especially for children with special health care needs. One example is services to persons with an inborn error of metabolism. The diet prescription includes special medical formulas and foods that are modified to meet medical and socioeconomic needs. The formulas and foods are expensive, and the costs are generally not reimbursed by insurance companies. Many states have provisions for coverage for special formulas and foods.[8] Physicians should contact the special needs program of their state health department for information about patient eligibility for coverage for these formulas and foods and procedures for obtaining them. Another example in which a nutritionist and nutrition services are instrumental in supporting feeding and growth is an early intervention program. In an early intervention program, nutritionists work with the child's family, other team members, and the child's primary care provider to optimize development from birth to 3 years.[9]

Other types of nutrition services provided in many state and local health agencies include nutrition counseling, classes on specific aspects of nutrition (eg, infant feeding, breastfeeding, diet and heart disease, and weight management), radio and cable TV programs on nutrition topics, publications and educational materials on a wide range of topics for the lay public, and nutrition seminars and workshops. Another local nutrition resource is available from the

USDA-funded Cooperative Extension Service. This service provides up-to-date information about the science of nutrition and its practical application in planning low-cost nutritious meals. Many nutrition publications provided by the extension service and other public health agencies are available in various foreign languages and for clients with low literacy skills.[5,10] The director of the nutrition department at the state health department is another excellent resource for identifying specific state, regional, or national resources and services. Similar information can be obtained from the Association of State and Territorial Public Health Nutrition Directors (Table 49.1). The state affiliate of the ADA or the ADA Consultant Directory can help identify an RD with specific clinical expertise (Table 49.1). Consumers may also call the ADA consumer hotline number and speak directly to an RD who can assist them with answers to general questions ranging from food labeling to food sanitation and other topics.

In addition to federal, state, and local health agencies, agencies such as visiting nurse associations, the American Diabetes Association, the American Heart Association, health maintenance organizations, and hospital inpatient and outpatient departments frequently employ personnel with nutrition expertise. They usually provide technical consultation in nutrition to physicians and nurses and nutrition counseling to patients and other agencies in the community. An increasing number of RDs have also established private or independent practices.

Food Assistance Programs

National policy has long provided for publicly supported food assistance programs to safeguard the health of individuals whose nutrition status is compromised because of poverty or complex physiologic, social, or other type of stress. The National School Lunch Act of 1946 provided for a major federal role in food service for school children. Two major types of food assistance programs are operated nationally by the USDA—the Food Stamp Program and the special nutrition programs that include the child nutrition programs and the supplemental nutrition programs for women, infants and children. The USDA Food and Nutrition Service provides updated fact sheets on each of its food programs (Table 49.1).

Food Stamp Program

Authorized as a permanent program in 1964, the Food Stamp Program is the primary source of nutrition assistance for low-income Americans. As an entitlement program, it is available to all persons who meet its eligibility standards. Reliable data indicate that only 3 in 5 of those eligible actually participate in the program. The program provides monthly benefits to help low-income households purchase foods for an adequate diet. More than half of the recipients are children. The average monthly household benefit level is $170.

To participate, most able-bodied applicants must meet certain work requirements; households may have no more than $2000 worth of countable resources ($3000 for households with at least one member aged 60 years or older); gross monthly incomes must be 130% or less of the federal poverty line; and net income after deductions must be 100% or less of the poverty line (households with an elderly or disabled member are subject only to the net income test). Income limits vary by household size and are adjusted each October to reflect changes in the cost of living.[11]

School Nutrition Programs

The National School Lunch Program, the School Breakfast Program, and the Special Milk Program are administered in most states by the state education agency, which enters into agreements with officials of local schools or school districts to operate nonprofit food services. Most public and private schools in the United States participate in the National School Lunch Program. Participating schools receive cash subsidies and donated USDA commodities. Any public or nonprofit private school of high school grade or less is eligible. Public and licensed, nonprofit, private residential child care institutions, such as orphanages, community homes for children who are disabled, juvenile detention centers, and temporary shelters for runaway children, are also eligible.

Schools participating in the federal meals programs agree to serve meals at a reduced price or free to children who are unable to pay the locally established full price. Children who can pay the full price are expected to do so. Local school officials determine the individual eligibility of each child for reduced-priced or free meals on the basis of family size and income. Each year the US Secretary of Agriculture issues uniform national standards for free and reduced-price eligibility based on national poverty guidelines. Although federal subsidies continue to be provided for meals served to children from all income levels, recent legislation has directed more of the program benefits to needy children. Free and reduced price meals served to children determined to be income eligible, are subsidized at a higher rate, although some federal subsidy is provided for meals served to children from all income levels.

To ensure that the nutrition goals of the school meal programs are met, federal nutrition requirements are specified in program regulations. The standard for lunch, averaged over a week's menu cycle, is one third of the RDAs of protein, vitamin A, vitamin C, iron, calcium, and calories for various age/grade groupings.

Through the 1994 Healthy Meals for Healthy Children's Act, the USDA, in 1995, undertook the first major reform in the nutritional quality of school meals since the program began with the School Meals Initiative for Healthy Children. In addition to the RDA for key nutrients, starting in 1996, school meals must also comply with the Dietary Guidelines for Americans, which call for less fat, saturated fat, cholesterol, and sodium and more fruits, vegetables, and grains.

To help schools implement the updated nutritional standards, the USDA launched the Team Nutrition initiative in June 1995. In addition to expanding training and technical assistance resources for schools, Team Nutrition brings together public and private networks to promote food choices for a healthy diet through 6 channels—the classroom, food service, the media, the entire school, families, and the community. Team Nutrition funds a limited number of competitive grants to states each year for Team Nutrition initiatives at the state and local levels. The Nutrition Education and Training (NET) Program was authorized in 1978 as the nutrition education component of the USDA food assistance programs for children. The NET Program provided the state and local infrastructure for the delivery of the Team Nutrition materials and resources to the local schools but, although NET is still authorized under current legislation, no funding for NET has occurred since 1998. More information on Team Nutrition can be found at http://www.fns.usda.gov/tn/.

The Special Milk Program reduces the cost of each half-pint of milk served to children by providing for cash reimbursement at an annually adjusted rate. A school district can choose to provide milk free to children who meet the eligibility guidelines. This program is available only to schools, child care institutions, and summer camps that do not participate in other federal meal service programs.

Child and Adult Care Food Program

The Child and Adult Care Food Program provides cash reimbursement, commodities, or both for the provision of meals and snacks to facilities providing nonresidential child care for children. Institutions eligible to participate include nonprofit child care centers, Head Start centers, and family or group child care homes. Some proprietary child care centers serving low-income children may also be eligible to participate in the program.

Although federal subsidies continue to be provided for meals served to children from all income levels, recent legislation has directed more program benefits to needy children. Children aged 12 and younger are eligible to receive up to 2 meals and one snack each day at a day care home or center. Children who reside in homeless shelters may receive up to 3 meals each day. Migrant children aged 15 and younger and persons with disabilities, regardless of their age, are eligible to receive reimbursable meals. After-school care snacks are available to children through age 18.

Summer Food Service Program

The Summer Food Service Program provides nutritious meals for children, aged 18 and younger, during school vacations at centrally located sites, such as schools or community centers in low-income neighborhoods, or in summer camps. Meals are served free to all eligible children and must meet the nutritional standards established by the USDA. Sponsors of the program must be public or private nonprofit schools, public agencies, or private nonprofit organizations.

Supplemental Food Programs

Special Supplemental Nutrition Program for Women, Infants, and Children

Since its initiation in 1972, funding for the WIC program has grown to about $4 billion yearly. The program serves low-income infants and pregnant, breastfeeding, and postpartum women, and children up to the age of 5 years who are nutritionally or medically at risk.

The WIC program differs from all other federal nutrition programs in its close association with health care services. These services include referral for ongoing routine pediatric and obstetric care, such as infant and child care and prenatal and postpartum referral for treatment. The WIC program provides specific food items and nutrition education to eligible participants. The program is operated as an adjunct to health care provided by state and local public and private nonprofit health or human service agencies, as well as the private sector.

The WIC program provides annual grants to state health departments or comparable agencies and to Indian Tribunal Organizations. Program funds are allocated to state agencies according to a formula that considers food and administrative costs.

Different food packages are provided for different categories of participants and are designed to provide nutrients frequently lacking in the diets of the target population. Participants generally receive food vouchers that can be redeemed at certain retail stores for specified foods. In some instances, participants receive food through home delivery or a warehouse distribution system. For infants, foods provided include iron-fortified infant formula, iron-fortified infant cereal, and vitamin C-rich fruit juice; for children and pregnant or lactating women, foods include milk, cheese, eggs, vitamin C-rich fruit or vegetable juice, iron-fortified cereal, and dry beans or peas, or peanut butter. Nonlactating postpartum women receive a similar package, except some quantities are reduced and legumes and peanut butter are not provided. Women who exclusively breastfeed can receive a special package that includes increased quantities of certain WIC foods, as well as tuna and carrots. The average monthly food package cost for FY 1999 was $32.52.

Nutrition education is an important benefit of the program and includes information about the participant's nutritional needs, breastfeeding, and referrals to health services, such as immunization, drug and alcohol abuse counseling, prenatal care, well-baby care, and smoking cessation. Efforts are made to adapt the educational activities to the individual participant's nutritional needs, cultural preferences, and education levels.[12–14]

The WIC Farmers' Market Nutrition Program provides additional coupons to WIC recipients that they can use to buy fresh fruits and vegetables from authorized farmers or farmers' markets.

The American Academy of Pediatrics recent Policy Statement: The WIC Program highlights the important collaboration between pediatricians and local WIC programs to ensure that infants and children receive high-quality, cost-effective health care and nutrition services.

Pediatrics. 2001;108:1216–1217

Commodity Assistance Programs
These programs include the Commodity Supplemental Food Program (CSFP), the Emergency Food Assistance Program (TEFAP), and the Soup Kitchens/ Food Banks Program (SK/FB).

Commodity Supplemental Food Program
The Commodity Supplemental Food Program operates in 25 states, including the District of Columbia, and on 2 Indian reservations. The program provides food packages to low-income pregnant, lactating, and postpartum women up

to 1 year, to infants and children up to 6 years, and to elderly people at least 60 years of age.

Like the WIC program, the CSFP provides food packages to supplement the diets of participants. The foods offered include infant formula and cereal, non-fat dry and evaporated milk, juice, farina, oats, ready-to-eat cereal, rice, pasta, egg mix, dehydrated potatoes, peanut butter, dried beans or peas, canned meat or poultry or tuna, and canned fruits or vegetables.

Unlike the WIC program, the CSFP distributes food rather than vouchers for redemption at grocery stores. Eligible people cannot participate concurrently in both programs. In fiscal year 2000, an average of more than 388 000 people each month participated in the CSFP.

State agencies set eligibility standards, store the food, and select local public and nonprofit private agencies to whom they distribute the food. Local agencies determine the eligibility of applicants, distribute the foods, and may provide nutrition education and referrals for health care and social services. In addition to donated food, the USDA provides funds to cover some of the administrative costs of outreach, warehousing, and client transportation.

Emergency Food Assistance Program

The Emergency Food Assistance Program provides surplus and purchased commodities for soup kitchens food banks and grants to help states with storage and distribution costs. States determine who is eligible to participate.

Food Distribution Program on Indian Reservations

The Food Distribution Program on Indian Reservations (FDPIR) provides commodity foods to low-income households, including the elderly, living on Indian reservations and to Native American families in designated areas near reservations. Many Native Americans participate in the FDPIR as an alternative to the Food Stamp Program, usually because they do not have easy access to food stores. The FDPIR participants receive a monthly food package consisting of meats, vegetables, fruits, dairy products, grains, and cereals.

Where to Seek Food Assistance for Clients

Food assistance programs are usually administered at the local level by the following agencies:

1. Local school food authority: School Lunch Program, School Breakfast Program, and Special Milk Program.
2. State and local health, social services, education, or agriculture agencies, public or private nonprofit health agencies, and Indian Tribal

Organizations or groups recognized by the US Department of the Interior: WIC, FDPIR, Summer Food Service Program, Child and Adult Care Food Program, TEFAP, SCFP.
3. Local social services, human services, or welfare department: Food Stamp Program.

Conclusion

As the key provider of child health care, the physician has a major role in ensuring that nutrition services for children include assessment of their nutritional status, provision of a safe food supply adequate in quality and quantity, nutrition counseling, and nutrition education for children and parents. As the primary expert on health in the community and as a concerned citizen, the physician, in coordination with members of the health care team, including the nutritionist or dietitian and nurse, can provide meaningful leadership in the formulation of sound nutrition policy and the education of legislators, administrators, and others who influence the response of the community to the nutritional needs of its children.

References

1. Eagan MC, Oglesby AC. Nutrition services in the maternal and child health program: a historical perspective. In: *Call to Action: Better Nutrition for Mothers, Children, and Families.* Washington, DC: National Center for Education in Maternal and Child Health; 1990:73–92
2. *Healthy People 2000: National Health Promotion and Disease Prevention Objectives.* Washington, DC: US Dept of Health and Human Services, Public Health Service; 1990
3. 1992 Public Health Nutrition Personnel Census. Data from the Association of State and Territorial Public Health Nutrition Directors.
4. Institute of Medicine. *The Future of Public Health.* Washington, DC: National Academy Press; 1988
5. Kaufman M. *Nutrition in Public Health: A Handbook for Developing Programs and Services.* Rockville, MD: Aspen Publishers Inc; 1990
6. Pickett OK, Clark EM, Kavanagh LD, eds. *Reaching Out: A Directory of National Organizations Related to Maternal and Child Health.* Arlington, VA: National Center for Education in Maternal Child Health; 1994
7. American Dietetic Association. Position of the American Dietetic Association: cost-effectiveness of medical nutrition therapy. *J Am Diet Assoc.* 1995;95:88–91
8. Bayerl CT, ed. *Report on H 5622: An Act Further Regulating Insurance Coverage for Certain Inherited Diseases.* Boston, MA: Office of Nutrition, Massachusetts Department of Public Health

9. Bayerl CT, Ries J, Bettencourt MF, Fisher P. Nutritional issues of children in early intervention programs: primary care team approach. *Semin Pediatr Gastrointest Nutr.* 1993;4:11–15

10. Owens AL, Frankle RT. *Nutrition in the Community: The Art of Delivering Services.* 3rd ed. St Louis, Mo: Mosby; 1993

11. Food and Nutrition Service. *Facts About the Food Stamp Program.* Washington, DC: US Department of Agriculture; 1992

12. US General Accounting Office. *Early Intervention: Federal Investments Like WIC Can Produce Savings: Report to Congressional Requesters.* Washington, DC: US General Accounting Office; 1992. Publication GAO/HRD-92-18

13. Mathematical Policy Research Inc. *The Savings in Medicaid Costs for Newborns and Their Mothers Resulting From Prenatal Participation in the WIC Program.* Alexandria, VA: US Department of Agriculture; 1991

14. Food Research and Action Center. *WIC: A Success Story.* 3rd ed. Washington, DC: Food Research and Action Center; 1991

50

Food Labeling

In 1990, Congress passed the Nutrition Labeling and Education Act (NLEA), mandating numerous changes in food labeling. Before the act, nutrition labeling on food products was voluntary, except for those that contained added nutrients or carried nutrition claims. As Americans became more interested in nutrition, however, food label regulations were revised to provide nutrition information that would help consumers make food choices to meet national dietary recommendations.

The NLEA took effect in 1994, when the labels of most packaged foods were required to feature the new "Nutrition Facts" panel.[1] Labeling is voluntary for fresh fruits and vegetables and raw meat, poultry, and seafood. For these raw foods, nutrition information may be printed on the package or on pamphlets or posters displayed near the food in the supermarket. Food labeling of meat and poultry products is regulated by the US Department of Agriculture (USDA), and the remainder of foods by the US Food and Drug Administration (FDA).

Ingredient Labeling

Ingredient labeling is an important source of information for consumers about the composition of packaged foods. Both FDA and USDA regulations require that food products with 2 or more ingredients list ingredients in descending order of their prominence by their common, specific names.[2-4] The source of some ingredients must be stated by name to help people with specific food needs because of religious or health reasons. These include protein hydrolysates and caseinate as a milk derivative in foods that claim to be nondairy. Certified color additives must also be listed by name (eg, FD&C Blue No. 1 or FD&C Yellow No. 5).

For families with food allergies, it is essential to read the ingredient listings on food labels to determine the presence of the 8 major allergens (milk, egg, wheat, soy, peanuts, tree nuts, fish, and crustacea). Since food and beverage manufacturers are continually making ingredient changes, people with food allergies and their caregivers should read the ingredient declaration on the food label of every product purchased, each time it is purchased.

The Nutrition Facts Panel

The updated food label carries a variety of nutrition information (Figure 50.1).
It is primarily presented within the Nutrition Facts panel that indicates the

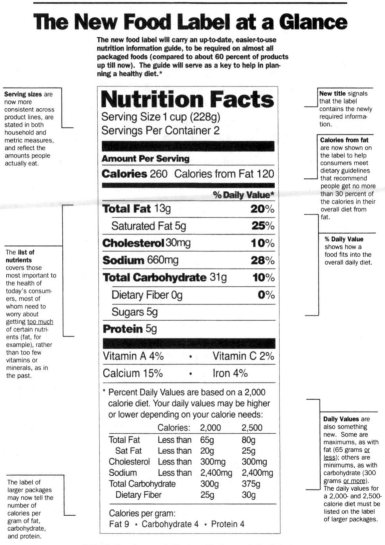

Figure 50.1. Sample Nutrition Facts label. Reproduced with permission from Gerber Products
Company, Fremont, Mich; 1994.

amount of target macronutrients and micronutrients. Simplified or shortened formats may be used for products that contain insignificant amounts (less than 1 g) of certain mandatory label nutrients. Package size constraints may also dictate different formats.

The following provides more details about the various features of the Nutrition Facts panel:

1. Serving size: Serving sizes are standardized for different food categories based on the average amount of food eaten at one time, using data from national food consumption surveys. Sizes do not always match serving sizes specified in the Food Guide Pyramid. Two measurements are provided— common household and metric measures.

2. Calories: Total calories in one serving are identified. In addition, calories from fat per serving are included. To calculate the total percentage of calories from fat in a diet, however, the fat grams in all food choices must be added. Dietary guidelines emphasize eating 30% or less of calories from fat over a few days, not in one food or one meal.

3. Nutrients: Information about the content of nutrients most related to today's health concerns must be listed. These nutrients include fat, saturated fat, cholesterol, sodium, total carbohydrate, fiber, sugars, protein, vitamins A and C, calcium, and iron. Other nutrients are listed voluntarily, and if foods contain insignificant amounts of a required nutrient, that nutrient may be omitted from the label. Information about other nutrients is required in 2 cases: (1) if a claim is made about the nutrients on the label, or (2) if the nutrients are added to the food, as in the case of fortified foods. Nutrient amounts are listed in one of 2 ways—in the metric amount or as a percentage of the daily value (DV).

4. Daily values: The "% Daily Value" suggests the nutritional value of a food and how it fits in a moderate, varied, and balanced diet. The term *daily value* is an umbrella term for 2 sets of reference values—daily reference values (DRVs) and daily reference intakes (DRIs). The DRVs are set for total fat, saturated fat, cholesterol, total carbohydrate, dietary fiber, sodium, potassium, and protein. They are established for adults and children 4 years or older, based on current nutrition recommendations. The DRVs for cholesterol, sodium, and potassium are set at a constant level for all calorie levels. The DRVs for total fat, saturated fat, total carbohydrate, dietary fiber, and protein are based on a 2000-calorie reference diet (Table 50.1). Current DRIs are listed in Appendix C.

Table 50.1.
Daily Values Used to Calculate % Daily Value for Nutrition Panel*

Food Component	Daily Value for Adults and Children Older Than 4 Years
Daily Reference Values	
Total fat	65 g[†]
Saturated fat	20 g[†]
Cholesterol	300 mg
Sodium	2400 mg
Potassium	3500 mg
Total carbohydrate	300 g[†]
Dietary fiber	25 g[‡]
Protein	50 g[†]

*Based on a 2000-calorie diet for adults and children older than 4 years.
[†]Daily value based on a 2000-calorie reference diet.
[‡]Daily value based on 11.5 g/1000 cal.

5. Label footnotes: A reference chart for a 2000- and a 2500-calorie diet also appears on the bottom of some Nutrition Facts panels. It suggests the upper limits for total fat, saturated fat, cholesterol, and sodium intake and the target intakes for total carbohydrate and dietary fiber. Some labels also show the number of calories supplied by 1 g of fat, carbohydrate, and protein.

Food Labels for Infants and Children Younger Than 4 Years

Food labels on products designed for infants and children younger than 4 years are different from food labels on adult products. Specifically, infant food labels differ in the listing of calories from fat, saturated fat, and cholesterol, DVs, and serving sizes. Fat information is not detailed because of the concern that adults may mistakenly apply this information to controlling the calories provided by fat for their infants.

The DVs for fat, cholesterol, sodium, potassium, carbohydrates, and fiber are not listed because the reference values have not been established for infants and children younger than 4 years. Protein is listed in grams per serving and as a percentage of the DV on foods for infants and children younger than 4 years. The DV used to calculate the nutrient percentages are calculated based on the DRI for each population.

Serving sizes of foods for infants and children younger than 4 years are based on government reference amounts and are smaller than the typical adult servings.

Nutrition Claims

Claims about nutrient contents describe the amount of a nutrient in a food, using terms such as free, low, high, reduced, and less. Using these terms in connection with a specific nutrient is strictly defined (Table 50.2).

Infant food labels may carry claims for vitamins and minerals. Claims about protein, fat, and sodium or the content of certain nutritional ingredients (ie, salt and sugar) are not allowed on products intended for infants younger than 2 years.

Claims about non-nutrient ingredients (eg, preservatives), the identification of ingredients (eg, made with apples), and taste (eg, unsweetened) are allowed.

Health Claims

In addition to the nutrient content claims, a food label may bear claims about the nutrient content and claims about the health benefits of the food or a component of the food. Products must meet strict nutrition requirements before they can carry these claims. Health claims are not allowed on the food labels of products intended for infants younger than 2 years.

To date, the FDA, based on scientific evidence, has approved 12 health claims.[5] Although the wording on packages may differ, the following summarizes the claims that link:

1. Calcium and osteoporosis: Physical activity and a calcium-rich diet may reduce the risk of osteoporosis, a condition in which the bones become soft or brittle.
2. Fat and cancer: A diet low in total fat may reduce the risk of some cancers.
3. Saturated fat and cholesterol and heart disease: A diet low in saturated fat and cholesterol may reduce the risk of heart disease.
4. Fiber-containing grain products, fruits, and vegetables, and cancer: A low-fat diet rich in fiber-containing grain products, fruits, and vegetables may reduce the risk of some cancers.
5. Fruits, vegetables, and grain products that contain fiber and heart disease: A diet low in saturated fat and cholesterol, and rich in fruits, vegetables, and grain products that contain some types of dietary fiber may reduce the risk of heart disease.

Table 50.2.
Nutrition Claims

	Definition, per Serving
Calories	
Calorie free	<5 cal
Low calorie	≤40 cal
Reduced or fewer calories	At least 25% fewer calories*
Light or lite	One third fewer calories or 50% less fat*
Sugar	
Sugar free	<0.5 g
Reduced sugar or less sugar	At least 25% less sugars
No added sugar; Without added sugar; No sugar added	No sugars added during processing or packaging, including ingredients that contain sugars, such as juice or dry fruit
Fat	
Fat free	<0.5 g
Low fat	<3 g
Reduced or less fat	At least 25% less fat*
Light or lite	One third fewer calories or 50% less fat*

Saturated fat
    Saturated fat free
    Low saturated fat
 	
    Reduced or less saturated fat
	
	<0.5 g
	≤1 g saturated fat and no more than 15% of calories from saturated fat
	At least 25% less saturated fat*

Cholesterol	
Cholesterol free	<2 mg cholesterol and <2 g fat
Low cholesterol	≤20 mg cholesterol and <2 g saturated fat
Reduced or less cholesterol	At least 25% less cholesterol* and 2 g saturated fat
Sodium	
Sodium free	<5 mg
Very low sodium	≤35 mg
Low sodium	≤140 mg
Reduced or less sodium	At least 25% less sodium*
Light in sodium	50% less sodium*
Fiber	
High fiber	≥5 g[†]
Good source of fiber	2.5 to 4.9 g
More or added fiber	At least 2.5 g more or added*

Table 50.2.
Nutrition Claims (continued)

	Definition, per Serving
Other Claims	
High, rich in, excellent source of [name of nutrient]	≥20% of daily value*
Good source, contains, provides…	10% to 19% of daily value*
More, enriched, fortified, added	≥10% or more of daily value*
Lean‡	<10 g fat, (4.5 g saturated fat, and <95 mg cholesterol
Extra lean‡	<5 g fat, 2 g saturated fat, and <95 mg cholesterol
Healthy	Meets standards for "low" fat and saturated fat; contains ≤480 mg sodium; ≤60 mg cholesterol; and at least 10% DRV for vitamin A, vitamin C, calcium, iron, protein, or fiber

*Compared with a standard serving size of the traditional food.
†Must also meet the definition for low fat, or the level of fat must appear next to the high-fiber claim.
‡On meat, poultry, seafood, and game meats.

6. Sodium and high blood pressure: A low-sodium diet may reduce the risk of high blood pressure, which is a risk factor for heart attacks and strokes.

7. Fruits and vegetables and some cancers: A low-fat diet rich in fruits and vegetables (foods that are low in fat and may contain dietary fiber, vitamin A, or vitamin C) may reduce the risk of some cancers.

8. Folic acid and neural tube birth defects: Women who consume 0.4 mg of folic acid daily may reduce their risk of giving birth to a child affected with a neural tube defect.

9. Dietary sugar alcohols and dental caries: Frequent eating of foods high in sugars and starches as between-meal snacks can promote tooth decay. The sugar alcohol used to sweeten this food may reduce the risk of dental caries.

10. Soluble fiber from certain foods and risk of coronary heart disease: Soluble fiber from foods such as oat bran, rolled oats, and whole oat flour, as part of a diet low in saturated fat and cholesterol, may reduce the risk of heart disease.

11. Soy protein and risk of coronary heart disease: Diets low in saturated fat and cholesterol that include 25 g of soy protein a day may reduce the risk of heart disease. One serving of [name of food] provides [x] grams of soy protein.

12. Plant sterol or stanol esters and risk of coronary heart disease: Diets low in saturated fat and cholesterol that include 2 servings of foods that provide a daily total of at least 1.3 g of vegetable oil sterol esters in 2 meals may reduce the risk of heart disease. A serving of [name of the food] supplies [x] grams of vegetable oil sterol esters. Diets low in saturated fat and cholesterol that include 2 servings of foods that provide a daily total of at least 3.4 g of vegetable oil stanol esters in 2 meals may reduce the risk of heart disease. A serving of [name of the food] supplies [x] grams of vegetable oil stanol esters.

In addition to these health claims, the FDA Modernization Act of 1997 (FDAMA) instituted an additional route to establish claims. The FDAMA procedures allow a health claim to be made if it is based on a published authoritative statement, which is currently in effect, about the relationship between a nutrient and a disease or health-related condition to which the claim refers, issued by a scientific body of the US Government with official responsibility for public health protection or research directly relating to human nutrition (eg, National Institutes of Health, National Academy of Sciences).

In July 1999, the first such health claim was established related to whole grain foods and risk of heart disease and cancer. The health claim states: "Diets rich in whole grain foods and other plant foods and low in total fat, saturated fat, and cholesterol, may help reduce the risk of heart disease and certain cancers. To qualify for the claim, a food must contain 51% or more whole grain ingredients per serving, be low in fat, and meet other general criteria for health claims."

In October 2000, the FDA announced a second FDAMA-authorized health claim, related to potassium-containing foods and high blood pressure and stroke. The health claim states: "Diets containing foods that are good sources of potassium and low in sodium may reduce the risk of high blood pressure and stroke. To qualify for the claim, a food must be a good source of potassium, and low in sodium, total fat, saturated fat, and cholesterol." (See nutrition claim.)

Juice Labeling

Since 1994, the percentage of juice must be specified on the food label if a beverage claims to contain fruit or vegetable juice.[6] Label statements must be declared using the language, "Contains [x] percent [name of fruit or vegetable] juice," "[x] percent juice," or similar phrase (eg, Contains 50% apple juice."). If a beverage contains minor amounts of juice for flavoring, the product may use the term "flavor," "flavored," or "flavoring" with a fruit or vegetable name, as long as the product does not bear the term "juice" (other than in the ingredient declaration) and does not visually depict the fruit or vegetable from which the flavor is derived. If the beverage contains no juice, but appears to contain juice, the label must state, "Contains no [name of fruit or vegetable] juice," or similar statements. These percentage juice statements appear near the top of the information panel of the beverage label.

Package Dating

Package dating provides a measure of a product's freshness. *Open dates* are stated alphanumerically (eg, Oct 15) or numerically (eg, 10–15 or 1015). An open date might be featured as:

1. Pull or "sell by" date: This is the last day that the manufacturer recommends sale of the product. Usually the date allows for additional storage and use time at home.
2. Freshness or quality assurance date: This date suggests how long the manufacturer believes the food will remain at peak quality. The label might read, "Best if used by October 1995." However, the product may be used after this date. A "freshness date" has a different meaning than the word "fresh" printed on the label, which often suggests that a food is raw or unprocessed.
3. Pack date: The date when the food was packaged or processed.
4. Expiration date: The last day the product should be eaten. State governments regulate these dates for perishable foods, such as milk and eggs. The FDA requires the expiration dates on infant formula.

In addition, the FDA regulates all package dating rules from states in the sense that they must first provide the consumer with labeling that is truthful and non-misleading.

Conclusion

Recent changes in food labeling help consumers make food choices to meet dietary recommendations by providing specific information about the content of certain nutrients in the product. This information may be used to compare foods, to choose foods that help provide a balance of recommended nutrients, and to plan meals and a total diet that is moderate, varied, and balanced. In addition, ingredient declarations are useful for consumers to make food choices based on religious, cultural, health, or food-allergy concerns.

References

1. Food and Drug Administration. *Focus on Food Labeling: An FDA Consumer Special Report.* Washington, DC: Government Printing Office; May 1993. Publication FDA 93-2262
2. Food; designation of ingredients, 21 CFR §101.4
3. Labels: definition; required features, 9 CFR §317.2
4. Ingredients statement, 9 CFR §381.118
5. 21 CFR §101.72–101.83
6. Percentage juice declaration for foods purporting to be beverages that contain fruit or vegetable juice, 21 CFR §101.30

51

Food Safety: Infectious Diseases

Introduction

In the United States, an estimated 76 million cases of food-borne illness occur every year, resulting in approximately 5000 deaths and 325 000 hospitalizations.[1] Because more than 200 infectious and noninfectious agents have been associated with food-borne and water-borne illness, there is a wide range of clinical manifestations.[2–5] Infants, children, pregnant women, the elderly, and immunocompromised persons are particularly vulnerable to more severe forms of disease. Education about food-borne illness and reporting of all cases to public health authorities will help minimize the impact of food-borne diseases. A primer on food-borne diseases developed by the American Medical Association, the Centers for Disease Control and Prevention (CDC), the Food and Drug Administration (FDA), and the Department of Agriculture contains information about the causes, clinical considerations, patient scenarios, patient handout material, and resources.[6] Since 1996, various preventive measures have resulted in a decrease in food-borne illness due to the 9 most common pathogens in the CDC's FoodNet program.[7,8] Achieving the public health goals for 2010 of reducing the national incidence of infections with *Salmonella, Escherichia coli* 0157:H7, *Campylobacter,* and *Listeria* to 50% of their 1997 incidence will require a great deal of effort including use of new technology.[9,10] Since physicians may be the initial contacts of persons with food-borne illness, an understanding of the issues involved in this area is critical. This chapter will focus on food-borne syndromes; outbreak detection, control, and prevention; and available resource material.

Food-Borne Diseases

There are numerous bacterial, viral, parasitic, and noninfectious causes of food-borne illness. These agents can be acquired from a variety of foods, with some agents being linked more frequently with specific foods. Table 51.1 shows recent food-borne outbreaks reported in 2000 and 2001 in the United States by location, vehicle, and cause,[11–20] indicating the diversity in vehicles and causes.

Table 51.1.
Ten Food-Borne Outbreaks by Location, Vehicle, and Cause Reported in the Literature in 2000 and 2001

Date Reported	Location	Vehicle	Cause
1995[11]	New Hampshire	Milk	*Yersinia enterocolitica*
1997[12]	Illinois	Home-pickled eggs	*Clostridium botulinum*
1998[13]	Ohio	Green onions	Hepatitis A virus
1998[14]	Texas	Raw oysters	*Vibrio parahaemolyticus*
1998–1999[15]	North Carolina	Tuna burgers	Histamine (scombrotoxin)
1999[16]	Missouri	Basil	*Cyclospora*
1999[17]	California	Fresh cilantro	*Salmonella*
1999[18]	US	Delicatessen meal	Norwalk-like virus
2000[19]	North Carolina	Mexican-style fresh soft cheese (raw milk)	*Listeria monocytogenes*
2000[20]	District of Columbia	Deli sandwich	Rotavirus

Etiology and Epidemiology

Food-borne disease can be associated with bacteria, viruses, and parasites and their toxins; marine organisms and their toxins; and chemical contaminants including heavy metals. Table 51.2 shows specific clinical syndromes, incubation periods, causative agents (microorganisms, marine organisms, toxins, and chemical contaminants) and commonly associated food vehicles reported to cause food-borne disease. Of the 2751 food-borne outbreaks reported to the CDC from 1993 through 1997, 878 (32%) had a known etiology of which bacteria accounted for 75%, chemical agents 17%, viruses 6%, and parasites 2%.[3] In most outbreaks (68%), the etiology was not determined, indicating the need for enhanced epidemiologic and laboratory investigations. *Salmonella* caused 55% of the 755 bacterial food-borne disease outbreaks with a known etiology from 1993 through 1997.[3] Reports to the passive surveillance system may be somewhat misleading since most people with food-borne illness do not have stool or blood specimens tested and specimens are not tested uniformly for all agents, especially viral enteropathogens.[21] Since more than 50% of outbreaks reported to the CDC had incubation periods of more than 15 hours, viral enteropathogens (especially caliciviruses) are probably a more important cause of food-borne disease then currently recognized. Foods implicated in Norwalk-like virus outbreaks are shellfish (oysters and clams), which concentrate these organisms in their tissues, and food contaminated by infectious

Table 51.2.
Clinical Manifestations, Incubation Periods, and Major Causes of Food-Borne Disease

Clinical Manifestations	Incubation Periods (Hours)	Main Causative Agents
Gastrointestinal tract		
● Vomiting	<1	Chemical
● Vomiting and diarrhea	1–6	*Bacillus cereus* and *Staphylococcus aureus* preformed toxins
● Watery diarrhea, abdominal cramps	8–72	Many organisms
● Bloody diarrhea	≥15	Many organisms
Neurologic	0–6	Fish, shellfish and monosodium glutamate
	0–24	Mushrooms
	18–24	*Clostridium botulinum*
Systemic	Varied	*Listeria monocytogenes* Brucella species Trichinella species *Toxoplasma gondii* *Vibrio vulnificus* Hepatitis A

food handlers.[21] In the FoodNet surveillance in the United States, bacterial agents, including *Campylobacter, Salmonella*, and *Shigella* species, are the most frequently identified causes of diarrheal illness.[8]

From 1993 through 1997, the most commonly reported food preparation practices that contributed to food-borne disease were improper holding temperatures of food and poor personal hygiene of preparers of food (Figure 51.1).

Clinical Manifestations

The majority of food-borne illness results in gastrointestinal tract signs and symptoms (vomiting, diarrhea, and abdominal cramps), although nonspecific extraintestinal manifestations including neurologic signs and symptoms may be the presenting manifestation. Important clues to determining the etiology of a food-borne disease and to identifying an outbreak of food-borne illness include obtaining information about the incubation period, duration of illness, clinical signs and symptoms, and the population and potential foods involved. If a food-borne outbreak is suspected, appropriate specimens should

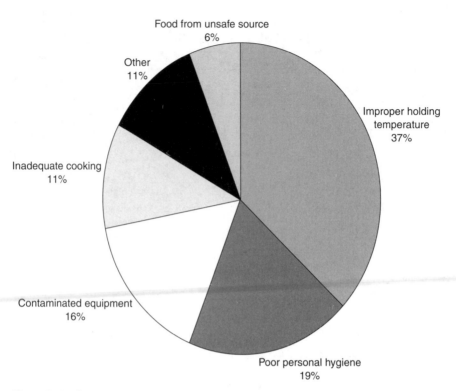

Figure 51.1. Food-borne disease outbreaks in the United States from 1993 through 1997 by reported contributing factor.[2]

be submitted for laboratory testing and the local health authorities should be notified for advice about outbreak evaluation, laboratory testing and disease containment. Table 51.2 shows various clinical syndromes of food-borne disease characterized by clinical manifestations (gastrointestinal tract, neurologic, and systemic), incubation periods, and main associated causative agents. In the gastroenteritis category, primary symptoms may include vomiting as occurs in short incubation period illness (chemical poisoning and *Bacillus cereus* and *Staphylococcus aureus* preformed toxin disease); watery (noninflammatory) diarrhea and bloody (inflammatory) diarrhea, both of which have many causes; or both vomiting and diarrhea as occurs with rotavirus infection in an infant and calicivirus infection in an older child or adult. Neurologic manifestations include paresthesias (fish, shellfish, and monosodium glutamate), hypotonia and descending muscle weakness (*Clostridium botulinum*), and a variety of other signs and symptoms (fish, shellfish, mushrooms). Systemic manifestations are varied and are associated with a variety of causes. In outbreaks reported to the CDC from 1993 through 1997 in which the incubation period was known, 3% had incubation periods reported less than 1 hour, 30% 1 to 7 hours, 20% 8 to 14 hours, and 46% greater or equal to 15 hours.[3]

Diagnosis and Treatment

Because so many infectious and noninfectious causes must be considered in people suspected of having food-borne illness, establishing a diagnosis may be difficult. This is compounded by the problem of not having specimens available for laboratory testing at the time an outbreak is evaluated. The extent of diagnostic evaluation depends on the clinical manifestations, epidemiologic factors, and the host. In general, laboratory testing should be considered for the following conditions: (1) patient populations, including infants, children, the elderly, pregnant women, and immunocompromised hosts; (2) in the presence of specific signs and symptoms, including bloody diarrhea, severe abdominal pain, fever, sudden onset of nausea, vomiting or diarrhea, dehydration associated with diarrhea, and neurologic involvement, including paresthesias, motor weakness, and cranial nerve palsies; (3) presence of gastrointestinal tract disease, including inflammatory bowel disease, malignancy, gastrointestinal tract surgery or radiation, certain medications, malabsorption syndromes, and other structural or functional conditions; and (4) association of illness with other factors such as travel, hospitalization, occupation, other ill persons, and child care or nursing home attendance. The occurrence of neurologic signs and symptoms as part of food-borne illness are particularly worrisome because of the potential for life-threatening complications. Food-related causes in this category include recent ingestion of contaminated seafood, mushroom poisoning, and chemical poisoning.

Collaboration and communication with clinical microbiology laboratory personnel and local public health officials will help optimize laboratory testing. Laboratory testing that may need to be performed include stool cultures and examination of stool for parasites by microscopy, direct antigen detection tests, use of molecular biology techniques, and blood cultures. More detailed information on laboratory procedures for detection of food-borne pathogens can be obtained from other sources,[2–6] from clinical specialists, and from microbiology and local or state public health personnel.

Enteric infections generally are self-limited conditions that require fluid and electrolyte therapy. (See also Chapter 28.) In some instances, specific antimicrobial therapy may eradicate fecal shedding of the causative organism, prevent transmission of the enteropathogen, abbreviate clinical symptoms, or prevent future complications. Guidelines and primers have been published to assist in managing patients with infectious diarrhea.[4,22]

Outbreak Detection and Control

Because of the extensive food distribution system in the United States, a contaminated food product may be distributed to people in many locations. Physicians are often the initial contact for people infected with a food-borne pathogen. Because of this initial exposure, an understanding of the clinical manifestations, incubation periods, involved food, epidemiologic factors, surveillance systems, and reporting mechanisms is critical.

Notifiable Diseases

National reporting requirements for food-borne diseases and conditions in the United States are determined collaboratively by the Council of State and Territorial Epidemiologists and the CDC. Table 51.3 lists food-borne diseases and conditions designated as nationally notifiable in the United States. Additional information about specific state requirements can be found at www.cste.org.

Table 51.3.
Nationally Notifiable Food-Borne Diseases and Conditions in the United States in the Year 2000

Category	Disease or Condition	Organism
Bacteria	Botulism	*Clostridium botulinum*
	Brucellosis	*Brucella species*
	Cholera	*Vibrio cholerae*
	Hemolytic uremic syndrome, post diarrhea	*Escherichia coli 0157:H7*
	Salmonellosis	*Salmonella species*
	Shigellosis	*Shigella species*
	Typhoid fever	*Salmonella typhi*
Viral	Hepatitis A	Hepatitis A virus
Parasitic	Cryptosporidiosis	*Cryptosporidium parvum*
	Cyclosporiasis	*Cyclospora cayetanensis*
	Trichinosis	*Trichinella spiralis*

Surveillance

In the United States, there are both active and passive surveillance systems established for detecting and reporting of food-borne and water-borne diseases. The present system of surveillance for food-borne and water-borne diseases began in 1966 when reports of enteric disease outbreaks attributed to microbial or chemical contamination of food or water were incorporated into an annual summary. Since 1966, more active participation by state and federal epidemiologists in outbreak investigations has improved the quality of investigative reports. Since 1978, outbreaks of food-borne and water-borne diseases have been reported in separate annual summaries.[2,3] Surveillance provides information about disease prevention and control; disease causation; guidance regarding trends over time; the prevalence of outbreaks caused by specific agents; food vehicles; and errors in food handling practices.

A food-borne disease outbreak is defined as the occurrence of 2 or more cases of a similar illness resulting from the ingestion of a common food. Sources of data for the food-borne disease outbreak surveillance system are a standard CDC form that was revised in 1999.[2] Most reports are submitted by state, local, and territorial health departments. The appropriate procedure for a physician to follow in reporting food-borne illnesses is to contact the local or state health department whenever a specific notifiable disease is identified. Prior to diagnostic testing, physicians also should report potential food-borne illnesses when 2 or more people present with a similar illness that may have resulted from ingestion of a common food. Local health departments then report the illnesses to the state health department and determine if further investigation is warranted. Each state health department then reports food-borne illnesses to the CDC, which compiles data nationally and disseminates information through annual summary reports.[2,3]

In 1996, the CDC established the Emerging Infections Program Food-Borne Diseases Active Surveillance Network (FoodNet) to collect data on laboratory-confirmed cases of 7 food-borne diseases. FoodNet now includes monitoring of 9 food-borne diseases in 8 US sites with a surveillance population of 29.5 million persons (11% of the 1999 US population).[8] Further expansion of sites will occur in 2001. In all 5 years of FoodNet data collection, *Campylobacter* was the most frequently diagnosed pathogen, followed by *Salmonella, Shigella*, and *E coli* 0157:H7 (Table 51.4).

Also in 1996, the CDC developed a national network of 10 laboratories that perform molecular fingerprinting of bacteria by pulsed field gel electrophoresis

Table 51.4.
Number and Incidence per 100 000 Population of Diagnosed Infections by Pathogens for the
Year 2000—Food-borne Diseases Active Surveillance Network, United States.[8]

Organism	Number	Incidence
Campylobacter	4640	15.7
Salmonella	4237	14.4
Shigella	2324	7.9
Escherichia coli 0157:H7	631	2.1
Cryptosporidium	484	1.5
Yersinia	131	0.4
Listeria	101	0.3
Vibrio	61	0.2
Cyclospora	22	0.1

to support epidemiologic investigations.[23] Initially only E coli 0157:H7 organisms were typed. Since then, PulseNet has expanded to include 46 states and
2 local public health laboratories and the Food Safety laboratories of the US
FDA and the Department of Agriculture. Four food-borne pathogens (E coli
0157:H7, nontyphoidal Salmonella, Listeria monocytogenes, and Shigella sonnei)
are being subtyped with Clostridium perfringens, Campylobacter jejuni, V parahaemolyticus, and V cholerae to be added in 2001. PulseNet has been useful in
the investigation of food-borne disease outbreaks.[23]

Prevention

Both general and specific measures or programs have been established to
prevent food-borne disease. Although these measures are important for all
people, they are especially relevant for specific high-risk segments of the population including infants, children, and the elderly, immunocompromised,
and pregnant women.[24,25]

General Measures

General measures that can be used to prevent food-borne illness include safe
food handling practices that encompass education of consumers in preparation, cooking, and storage of food; and use of technology including irradiation
and food processing methodologies.[10,26,27] For example, since 40% of persons
who die from Salmonella food-borne disease are residents of nursing homes,
hospitals and commercial kitchens should only use pasteurized egg products
for all recipes that require cooked or lightly cooked eggs.[28]

Anyone who prepares food should be familiar with food safety practices.[29] Major areas of concern with regard to food safety include caution when buying food, hand washing and surface cleaning, prevention of cross contamination, cooking of food at proper temperatures, and prompt and appropriate refrigeration of food before and after cooking or preparation.

Personal hygiene and cleaning of surfaces are critical in the prevention of food-borne disease. Microorganisms can be transmitted in the kitchen via hands, cutting boards, utensils, and countertops. Hands should be washed before and after handling food and after using the bathroom, changing diapers, or handling pets. Potential vehicles for transmission of organisms such as cutting board dishes, utensils, and countertops should be washed after preparing each food item.

Cross-contamination is a major problem when handling raw meat, poultry, seafood, and eggs. These food products and their juices should not come in contact with each other or other foods from the time of purchase until appropriately cooked. Hands, cutting boards, dishes, and utensils should be washed after each contact with raw meat, poultry, seafood, and eggs or their juices. In addition, separate plates should be used for raw and cooked foods.

Preparing food at appropriate temperatures will kill most pathogens that cause food-borne illness. Eggs should be cooked until they are firm, and raw eggs or foods that contain raw or partially cooked eggs should not be eaten. Poultry should be cooked until it has an internal temperature of 180°F, until the meat is white in the middle and until juices are clear. Fish should be cooked until it is opaque and flakes easily with a fork. Meat, especially hamburger meat, should be cooked to 160°F, until it is brown inside, and until the juices are clear.

Because bacteria grow at room temperature, hot foods should be maintained at 140°F or higher and cold foods at 40°F or lower. Perishables, prepared foods, and leftovers should be refrigerated or frozen within 2 hours of preparation. Foods should be defrosted in the refrigerator, under cold running water or in a microwave. Foods should be marinated in the refrigerator. Figure 51.1 shows food-borne disease outbreaks by contributing factor.

Specific Measures

Several measures have been enacted that are specific for defined food products and that have changed the incidence of food-borne infections.[30] These measure have included FDA prevention programs for seafood, increased attention to good agriculture practices aimed at fresh fruit and vegetables, new rules on egg and juice safety, increased regulation of imported foods, food safety education, radiation of meat, and introduction of the Hazard Analysis Critical Control Point (HACCP) regulations for meat and poultry in processing plants. Information about these and other measures enacted to reduce food-borne disease can be found at various Web sites shown in the directory of resources (Table 51.5).

Young children, pregnant women, older adults, and people with compromised immune systems are at higher risk for food-borne illness and more severe illness if disease occurs. People may have compromised immune systems due to medical treatments (corticosteroids, chemotherapy, radiation) or by conditions such as AIDS, malignancy, diabetes mellitus, or liver disease. People in these categories are advised to follow the general measures to prevent food-borne illness[29] and also should not eat the following foods:

- Raw fish or shellfish, including oysters, clams, mussels, and scallops
- Raw or unpasteurized milk or cheeses

Table 51.5.
Directory of Resources

Organizations	Telephone Hotlines	Web Sites
American Medical Association		www.ama-assn.org
Centers for Disease Control and Prevention		
● FoodNet World Wide Web		www.cdc.gov/foodnet
● Hand washing		www.cdc.gov/ncidod/hip/abc/practic6.htm
● Food safety information		www.cdc.gov/foodsafety
● Traveler's Health information		www.cdc.gov/travel/index.htm
Center for Food Safety and Applied Nutrition of the US Food and Drug Administration	888/723–3366	www.fda.gov
Food Safety and Inspection Service of the US Department of Agriculture	800/535–4555	www.usda.gov/fsis
● Foodborne illness education information center		www.nal.usda.gov/foodborne
US Government Safety information		www.foodsafety.gov
Partnership for Food Safety Education		www.fightbac.org/main.cfm

All of the above Web sites accessed on April 11, 2003.

- Soft cheeses, such as feta, Brie, Camembert, blue-veined, and Mexican-style cheese (Hard cheeses, processed cheeses, cream cheese, cottage cheese, and yogurt need not be avoided.)
- Raw or undercooked eggs or foods containing raw or lightly cooked eggs, including certain salad dressings, cookie and cake batters, sauces, and beverages such as unpasteurized egg nog (Foods made from commercially pasteurized eggs are safe to eat.)
- Raw or undercooked meat or poultry
- Raw vegetable sprouts (Alfalfa, clover, bean, and radish.)
- Unpasteurized fruit or vegetable juices (Unpasteurized juices will carry a warning.)
- Raw fruits with a rough texture (eg, raspberries)
- Undercooked or raw tofu
- Raw or unpasteurized honey (Infants less than 2 years of age should avoid all sources of honey.)
- Deli meats, hot dogs, and processed meats (Avoid unless further cooked.)
- All moldy and outdated food products

Travel

Travel to developing countries can result in significant risks for exposure to enteric pathogens in contaminated food and water. The CDC publishes biennially *Health Information for International Travelers*,[31] which contains basic advice to travelers on water treatment, food consumption, and how to avoid traveler's diarrhea. Parents of infants and children, the elderly, pregnant women, and immunocompromised hosts should consult their physician or a travel clinic before traveling to a developing country.

References

1. Mead PS, Slutsker L, Dietz V, et al. Food-related illness and death in the United States. *Emerg Infect Dis*. 1999;5:607–625
2. Centers for Disease Control and Prevention. Surveillance for foodborne-disease outbreaks—United States, 1993–1997. *MMWR CDC Surveill Summ*. 2000;49:1–62
3. Centers for Disease Control and Prevention. Surveillance for waterborne-disease outbreaks—United States, 1997–1998. *MMWR CDC Surveill Summ*. 2000;49:1–21
4. Guerrant RL, VanGilder T, Steiner TS, et al. Practice guidelines for the management of infectious diarrhea. *Clin Infect Dis*. 2001;32:331–351
5. Pickering LK. Approach to diagnosis and management of gastrointestinal tract infections. In: Long SS, Pickering LK, Prober CG, eds. *Principles and Practice of Pediatric Infectious Diseases*. 2nd ed. New York, NY: Churchill-Livingstone; 2003:362–368

6. Centers for Disease Control and Prevention. Diagnosis and management of food-borne illnesses: a primer for physicians. *MMWR Recomm Rep.* 2001; 50(RR-2):1–69

7. Centers for Disease Control and Prevention. Incidence of foodborne illnesses—FoodNet, 1997. *MMWR Morb Mortal Wkly Rep.* 1998;47:782–786

8. Centers for Disease Control and Prevention. Preliminary FoodNet data on the incidence of food-borne illnesses—selected sites, United States, 2000. *MMWR Morb Mortal Wkly Rep.* 2001;50:241–246

9. Office of Public Health and Science. *Healthy People 2010 Objectives.* Washington, DC: US Department of Health and Human Services; 2000. Available at: http://www.healthypeople.gov/Publications. Accessed April 8, 2003

10. Tauxe RV. Food safety and irradiation: protecting the public from food-borne infections. *Emerg Infect Dis.* 2001;7(suppl 3):516–521

11. Ackers ML, Schoenfeld S, Markman J, et al. An outbreak of *Yersina enterocolitica* O:8 infections associated with pasteurized milk. *J Infect Dis.* 2000;181:1834–1837

12. Centers for Disease Control and Prevention. Food-borne botulism from eating home-pickled eggs-Illinois, 1997. *MMWR Morb Mortal Wkly Rep.* 2000;49:778–780

13. Dentinger CM, Bower WA, Nainan OV, et al. An outbreak of hepatitis A associated with green onions. *J Infect Dis.* 2001;183:1273–1276

14. Daniels NA, Ray B, Easton A, et al. Emergence of a new *Vibrio parahaemolyticus* serotype in raw oysters: a prevention quandry. *JAMA.* 2000;284:1541–1545

15. Becker K, Southwick K, Reardon J, Berg R, MacCormack JN. Histamine poisoning associated with eating tuna burgers. *JAMA.* 2001;285:1327–1330

16. Lopez AS, Dodson DR, Arrowood MJ, et al. Outbreak of cyclosporiasis associated with basil in Missouri in 1999. *Clin Infect Dis.* 2001;32:1010–1017

17. Campbell JV, Mohle-Boetani J, Reporter R, et al. An outbreak of Salmonella serotype Thompson associated with fresh cilantro. *J Infect Dis.* 2001;183:984–987

18. Daniels NA, Bergmire-Sweat DA, Schwab KJ, et al. A food-borne outbreak of gastroenteritis associated with Norwalk-like viruses: first molecular traceback to deli sandwiches contaminated during preparation. *J Infect Dis.* 2000;181:1467–1470

19. Centers for Disease Control and Prevention. Outbreak of listeriosis associated with homemade Mexican-style cheese—North Carolina, October 2000-January 2001. *MMWR Morb Mortal Wkly Rep.* 2001;50;560–562

20. Centers for Disease Control and Prevention. Food-borne outbreak of group A rotavirus gastroenteritis among college students—District of Columbia, March-April 2000. *MMWR Morb Mortal Wkly Rep.* 2000;49:1131–1133

21. Centers for Disease Control and Prevention. "Norwalk-like viruses": public health consequences and outbreak management. *MMWR Recomm. Rep.* 2001; 50(RR-9):1–18

22. Pickering LK, Cleary TG. Therapy for diarrheal illness in children. In: Blaser MJ, Smith PD, Ravdin JI, Grenberg HB, Guerrant RL, eds. *Infections of the Gastrointestinal Tract.* 2nd ed. Philadelphia, PA: Lippincott Williams and Wilkins; 2002:1223–1240

23. Swaminathan B, Barrett TJ, Hunter SB, Tauxe RV. PulseNet: the molecular subtyping network for food-borne bacterial disease surveillance, United States. *Emerg Infect Dis.* 2001;7:382–389

24. Centers for Disease Control and Prevention. 1999 USPHS/IDSA guidelines for the prevention of opportunistic infections in persons infected with human immunodeficiency virus. *MMWR Recomm Rep.* 1999;48(RR-10):1–59, 61–66

25. Centers for Disease Control and Prevention. Guidelines for preventing opportunistic infections among hematopoietic stem cell transplant recipients. *MMWR Recomm Rep.* 2000;49(RR-10):1–125, CE1–7

26. Stephenson J. New approaches for detecting and curtailing food-borne microbial infections. *JAMA.* 1997;277:1337, 1339–1340

27. American Academy of Pediatrics Committee on Environmental Health. Technical report: irradiation of food. *Pediatrics.* 2000;106:1505–1510

28. Levine WC, Smart JF, Archer DL, Bean NH, Tauxe RV. Foodborne disease outbreaks in nursing homes, 1975 through 1987. *JAMA.* 1991;266:2105–2109

29. National Center for Infectious Diseases. *Handle and Prepare Food Safely.* Atlanta, GA: US Department of Health and Human Services, Centers for Disease Control and Prevention; 2000. Available at: http://www.cdc.gov.ncidod/op/food.htm. Accessed March 7, 2003

30. Centers for Disease Control and Prevention. Safer and healthier foods. *MMWR Morb Mortal Wkly Rep.* 1999;48:905–913

31. National Center for Infectious Diseases. *The Yellow Book: Health Information for International Travel 2001–2002.* Atlanta, GA: US Department of Health and Human Services, Centers for Disease Control and Prevention; 2001. Available at: http://www.cdc.gov/travel/yb/index.htm. Accessed March 7, 2003

52

Food Safety: Pesticides, Industrial Chemicals, Toxins, Antimicrobial Preservatives/ Irradiation, and Indirect Food Additives

Introduction

Foods available in the United States are among the safest found in the world.[1] However, there are a wide variety of nonnutritive chemical substances found in the food supply that are potentially harmful to children.

In contrast to the usually defined illnesses associated with microbial contamination of foods, the safety issues related to nonmicrobial substances in foods are less understood and more difficult to document. As a result, they are less-often recognized and less-easily diagnosed. Acute toxicity does occur, especially with the organophosphate insecticides, but it is not common and usually not recognized. The chronic effects of these substances are generally more significant for the fetus and young child because of potential neurotoxic and developmental effects, but these effects are even less recognized clinically than their acute effects. For the chronic effects, prevention of exposure is more significant than most treatments.

Three federal agencies are primarily involved in the regulation of many of the potentially toxic substances found in foods. The Environmental Protection Agency (EPA) establishes the level of pesticides, for example, allowed in foods; monitoring of many foods is done by the Food and Drug Administration (FDA), which carries out a market basket survey, the Total Diet Study; monitoring of meat, poultry, and eggs is done by the Food Safety and Inspection Service (FSIS) of the Department of Agriculture (USDA) and, with participating states, the USDA's Agriculture Marketing Service carries out its own residue testing survey. Other agencies also play a supporting role[1] (see Table 52.1).

A major problem had been that the allowable levels of nonnutritive substances in food were initially established primarily for adults. Concerns for the special vulnerability of infants and children led to the National Academy of Sciences' report, Pesticides in the Diets of Infants and Children in 1993.[2] The

Table 52.1.
Regulatory Agencies and Their Activities

Agency and Authority	Targets	Activities	Substances
FDA Federal Food Drug and Cosmetic Act-FFDCA-1958	All physical, chemical and microbial contaminants, and food and color additives	Enforces all laws governing domestic and imported foods and institutes recalls Review safety before marketing	All foods, including shell eggs, except meat, poultry, and egg products
	Irradiation	Radiological, toxicological and microbiological safety and nutritional adequacy	All foods and packaging subjected to irradiation
	Genetic modification	Reviews safety before marketing	Fruits, vegetables and grains
	Antibiotics and other antimicrobials	Reviews drugs for safety to animals and to humans who consume them	All animals
USDA Food Safety and Inspection Service–FSIS	All physical, chemical, and microbial contaminants	Enforces all laws governing domestic and imported foods and institutes recalls	Meat, poultry and egg products
Agricultural Marketing Service–AMS	Irradiation Genetic modification Antimicrobials	Reviews safety before marketing Reviews safety before marketing Reviews safety for animals	Meat, poultry and egg products All animals
CDC	All food contaminants	Monitors all acute and chronic toxic effects	All foods
	Antibiotics	Reviews safety for humans	All foods

http://vm.cfsan.fda.gov/~dms/opa-tg1.html

recommendations from that report led to the Food Quality and Protection Act (FQPA), which was passed in 1996.

Food Quality and Protection Act of 1966

Actions generated by the FQPA, modifying the Federal Insecticide Fungicide, and Rodenticide Act (FIFRA) and the Federal Food, Drug, and Cosmetic Act (FFDCA):

- Established a single health-based standards for all pesticides in food.
- Benefits, in general, cannot override the health-based standard.
- Prenatal and postnatal effects are to be considered.

- In the absence of data confirming the safety to infants and children, because of their special sensitivities and exposures, an additional uncertainty factor of up to 10X can be added to the safety values.
- Aggregate risk, the sum of all exposures to the chemical, must be considered in establishing safe levels.
- Cumulative risk, the sum of all exposures to chemicals with similar mechanisms of action, must be considered in establishing safe levels.
- Endocrine disrupters are to be included in the evaluation of safety.
- All existing pesticide registrations are to be reviewed by 2006.
- Expedited review is possible for safer pesticides.
- Risks are to be determined for both one year and lifetime exposure.

A major impact of this act has been the regulatory recognition that infants and children are potentially more sensitive than adults to environmental chemicals for a number of reasons. Increased susceptibility may result from the greater intake of foods per unit of body weight. This is especially true for foods that infants and young children already consume in large amounts such as milk, fruit juices, cereals, and fruits in general. The immaturity of developing organ systems is another potential hazard, especially for the nervous, immune, and endocrine systems, and particularly during sensitive periods of development when relatively brief insults may result in later long-term effects.[3] Altered pharmacokinetics are also of concern because of the immaturity of organs such as the liver and kidney and the changes in the amounts of body fat and extracellular water. Since children live longer than adults, the likelihood of long-term effects such as cancer is increased.[4]

Chemical substances that are potentially toxic may occur in foods as a result of environmental contaminants that enter the food chain during plant or animal growth (Polychlorinated biphenyls [PCBs] and metals), deliberate application during agricultural practices (pesticides), inadvertent contamination in processing (metals, phthalates), naturally occurring toxicants (patulin), substances added during processing (antimicrobials), substances created during processing (PAH–polycyclic aromatic hydrocarbons), and contaminants from the home environment. For additional information beyond what is in this chapter, see the *Handbook of Pediatric Environmental Health*, published by the American Academy of Pediatrics in 2003.[5]

Pesticides

Of the approximately 600 pesticides registered with the EPA, about 200 are routinely examined in food products in the United States.[6] They are used pri-

marily on fruits, vegetables, and grains. The chemicals included in the group
of pesticide substances are classified as insecticides, herbicides, fungicides,
rodenticides, and fumigants. While these products can increase both yield
and quality of produce, they may be toxic, especially to handlers, but also as
residues in the foods we eat. The residues an individual ingests from various
foods are determined by the amount of pesticide applied to the crop, the time
between application and harvesting, processing or storage, the type of processing, the treatment of the food in the home, and the amount of the food
ingested. When the EPA establishes the regulations for the application of pesticides to various crops, each of these factors is considered and residues present at various stages of movement from the field to the mouth are monitored
and can be enforced. The regulations governing these actions are contained in
the FIFRA and the FFDCA, as amended by the FQPA. As a result of regulations and voluntary withdrawals stemming from the FQPA, several high-use
pesticides have been, or are likely to be, significantly reduced in their usage.
These include chlorpyrifos and related compounds.

A significant problem in regulation arises because the sampling process can
never account for more than some fraction of the food supply. Additionally,
because of variations that occur in the application process, foods consumed
as single items, such as melons, bananas, and potatoes, may contain greater
residues than the crop as a whole.[7] For detailed information on pesticides
in foods, see Groth et al.[8]

Although the same rules about pesticide use apply to use in home gardens,
there is no monitoring or enforcement to assure proper use. Excessive applications or too short a time between application and harvesting can result in
greater residue levels than are tolerated in commercially produced foods.[9]

While pesticides in the food chain are not the major source for acute pesticide exposure in infants and children, such events do occur. It also seems clear
that chronic toxicity is related to the total exposure to the pesticides, including
exposures that occur in the home and outdoor environments as well as in
foods. Thus, exposure from consuming foods containing pesticide residues
is only one of the significant sources of exposure in infants and children.[2]

Most pesticides in common use and found in or on foods may be classified
as insecticides, herbicides, such as atrazine, 2,4-D, and glyphosphate, or fungicides that include a large number of compounds. In general, the insecticides
are most likely to result in acute illness. While pyrethroids are increasing in
use because of their lower toxicity, the commonly used insecticides belong to
1 of 2 major groups of compounds—organophosphates and carbamates, both

of which are acetylcholinesterase inhibitors. Their acute effects are the direct result of that inhibition. Acute symptoms and signs arise from muscarinic and nicotinic stimuli and usually occur within hours of exposure. These include nausea, vomiting, salivation, lacrimation, blurred vision, miosis, abnormal cardiac rhythm, fasciculations, convulsions, and, rarely, death. Treatment, when needed, is atropine initially, and this suffices for most acute situations. In severe cases of organophosphate poisoning, pralidoxime may be required.[10] Residues of pesticides above the allowable levels in domestic foods are generally found in less than 1% of foods tested. In foods imported from other countries, violative levels vary from year to year but have been found in up to 3% of the foods tested.[11] Because the organophosphates are increasingly recognized as potentially toxic to infants and small children, their use, beginning with chlorpyriphos, is being increasingly restricted by the EPA.

The effects of long-term exposures by various routes have been demonstrated in experimental animals, but chronic effects from food sources in human subjects have not been established. Effects that have been postulated on the basis of various epidemiological studies and animal experiments are shown in Table 52.2.[12] Undoubtedly any chronic effects that might occur from exposure through foods would depend on the age of the infant or child at the time exposure begins, the degree of exposure, and the duration. In general, one can assume that exposure in utero and early in infancy would be more harmful to the developing nervous system than exposure later in childhood. Because infants and children are exposed to many compounds that could have similar effects, and exposures may come from a variety of routes, it will likely

Table 52.2.
Examples of Effects of Long-Term Pesticide Exposure in Animals*[12]

Brain	Brain cell loss Impaired development of neurotransmitter receptors Decreased brain size
Behaviour	Generalized developmental delay Hyperactivity Altered exploratory behavior
Endocrine	Reproductive failure Delayed pubertal development Lactation inhibition
Carcinogenesis	Various sites and tumor types

*These vary based on compound tested, dose administered, route of exposure, animal species, timing, and duration of exposure.

be a long time before definitive effects of chronic exposure to pesticides in foods can be substantiated.

Reducing Pesticide Exposure From Foods

Although pesticide exposures from use in the home, gardens, lawns, day care centers, and schools may be a greater hazard to children than exposure from foods, reducing exposure from foods can certainly benefit the child. Measures that can be recommended to parents include the following:

- The thorough washing of fruits and vegetables with cold or warm tap water and scrubbing with a brush before consumption.
- Peeling of those fruits and vegetables when that is possible.
- Discarding the outer leaves of leafy vegetables such as lettuce and cabbage.
- Trimming the fat from meats and the skin and fat from poultry and fish.
- Avoiding pesticide use on home-grown fruits and vegetables.
- Avoiding fruits and vegetables from nonregulated sources such as other home gardens, country vegetable stands, and local produce markets.
- Limiting produce from other countries to those that can be peeled.
  The use of organic foods is controversial (see Chapter 13).

Industrial Chemicals

Another source of contaminants in the food supply are products from industrial processes that get into food supplies through precipitation from the atmosphere, direct contamination of underground or surface waters, which may, in turn, affect the water supply for irrigation or consumption, or unintentional contamination during food processing.

The most ubiquitous group of compounds resulting from industrial production are the polychlorinated biphenyls, dibenzofurans, and dibenzodioxins (PCBs, PCDFs, PCDDs, and TCDD, a particularly potent dioxin). These groups are often included in the larger group of compounds termed persistent organic pollutants (POPs), which also includes the pesticides DDT and its breakdown products, as well as aldrin, dieldrin, chlordane, endrin, heptachlor, hexachlorobenzene, mirex, and toxaphene.[13] Although the continued use of these products has been extensively curtailed, they persist in the environment and have accumulated in produce grown in contaminated soils and especially in the fat tissue of many animal species but primarily in fish—both salt and fresh water varieties. A major hazard is that the chronic ingestion of small amounts tends to accumulate in human fat. They can be transferred to the fetus from maternal stores and appear in human milk since they are fat soluble and are not significantly metabolized.

No acute exposures from food sources, other than some widely publicized accidental exposures, have been reported, but chronic effects are a potential problem.[14-18] Most chronic exposures that have been reported reflect effects on the developing fetus. These include a variety of central nervous system findings, including mental retardation and developmental delay. Endocrine function disruption and immune system disorders have been demonstrated in animals and possible similar effects on children are under study. The carcinogenic potential of the dioxins has also been recognized by the EPA, and TCDD has been upgraded from "probable carcinogen" to a "human carcinogen."[8]

No specific treatments are known and the prevention of excessive intakes are the only therapeutic approach. Since fish are the most common source of these compounds in human diets, levels in fish are regularly measured. States in which contaminated fish may be found routinely publish fish advisories about where such fish may exist, and their avoidance by pregnant women, lactating mothers, and young children need to be followed. Residues from the POPs and their breakdown products are still present in the soil and water. Through these routes they have become incorporated in a variety of foods.

The next most hazardous chemicals arising from industrial processes are the heavy metals, especially lead and mercury. Lead exposure rarely originates from food sources. One type of food exposure known to occur in some situations is lead-containing ceramic ware, in which acidic fluids, such as orange juice, may leach lead from the container.

Mercury, on the other hand, is ingested as methyl mercury, which arises from elemental mercury combining with organic molecules in the environment. It has been estimated that as much as 160 tons of mercury are released annually into the environment.[19] Methyl mercury, which is a neurotoxicant, is found in fish, just as the POP group of compounds, and the 2 often coexist. Most of the chronic effects of excessive methyl mercury ingestion have been found in the infants of mothers who had high levels of mercury ingestion during pregnancy, and neurodevelopmental delays have been the most recognized finding.[20-22] High intakes, by infants and toddlers, of fish with high levels of mercury could also result in neurodevelopmental problems.[23]

Most of the states in the United States have fish advisories that list fish with high levels of mercury and generally also report PCB levels. The majority of fish advisories on fresh water fish are in the area surrounding the Great Lakes.

Fresh water fish that are most likely to have high levels of methyl mercury and/or PCBs are pike and walleye. Fresh water fish with elevated levels of mercury, as with PCBs, need to be avoided by pregnant women, lactating women, and young children. Women of child-bearing age are also cautioned to limit their intake of such fish.[24]

The most common marine fish with high levels of methyl mercury are shark, swordfish, king mackerel, tilefish, and large tuna. The FDA now recommends that pregnant women, nursing mothers, women who may become pregnant, and young children should not consume shark, swordfish, king mackerel, or tilefish.[25]

Other metals that may have toxic effects on infants include manganese, aluminum, and cadmium. Manganese is an essential trace element in human metabolism. However, elevated levels have been tentatively associated with neurological problems in children, such as hyperactivity and learning disabilities.[26] Soy products are enriched in aluminum and manganese. For example, soy-based formulas contain 200 to 300 μg of Mn/L compared with other formulas that contain 77 to 100 μg/L.[27] (See also Chapter 4.) Cadmium is another metal found to have potential neurotoxicity and is found in foods such as leafy vegetables, grains, and shellfish. Although these metals raise some level of concern about the feeding of infants and small children, no specific guidelines have been promulgated regarding their ingestion.

Toxins

There are a wide variety of toxins found in various foods. Seafood may be toxic because of the accumulation of chemicals from the water (PCBs and mercury) or because the fish itself is toxic (tetrodotoxin from puffer fish), or from the ingestion by fish of toxin-producing algae. The most significant algae are the dinoflagellates, including Gymnodinium breve, which produces a severe neurotoxin and is the cause of the red tide. Gambierdiscus, which produces the most common fish toxin, ciguatera, and a large number of others that produce toxins affecting shellfish[28,29] (see Table 52.3).

Naturally occurring toxins found in other foods include the mushroom toxins, which are classified in 4 groups—protoplasmic poisons, neurotoxins, gastrointestinal irritants, and disulfram toxins. They are found in a wide variety of mushrooms that are not easily distinguished from nontoxic varieties. They are not inactivated by cooking. Of interest, the disulfram group is active only in the presence of alcohol ingestion. Pyrrolizide alkaloids are usually associated

Table 52.3.
Toxins in Seafoods[28,29]

Organism-Producing Toxin	Toxin	Seafood Affected	Health Effects
Gambierdiscus	Ciguatera	Barracudas, groupers, snappers, jacks, mackerel, triggerfish	Acute symptoms of the gastrointestinal, central nervous system, and cardiovascular systems; self-limited; usually subsides in several days
Many dinoflagellates	Saxitoxin derivatives	Mussels, clams, cockles, scallops	Paralytic Shellfish Poisoning (PSP)
	Polyethers	Mussels, oysters, scallops	Diarrheic Shellfish Poisoning (DSP)
	Brevetoxins	Shellfish from the Florida coast	Neurotoxic Shellfish Poisoning (NSP)
	Domoic acid	Mussels	Amnesic Shellfish Poisoning (ASP)
Various bacteria	Histamine, also called Scombrotoxin	Tuna, mahi mahi, bluefish, sardines, mackerel, amberjack, abalone Note: may also be in Swiss cheese	Burning mouth, upper-body rash, hypotension, headache, pruritis, vomiting and diarrhea

with home remedies that are derived from plants, especially legumes. Phytohaemagglutinins are found primarily in red kidney beans that are raw or only partially cooked as in slow cookers and in salads. Grayanotoxin is found in honey that comes from rhododendrons. Like most others in this group, the symptoms are usually acute. Aflatoxins are fungal in origin and may affect corn, nuts, and milk. They may have long-term carcinogenic effects.[28,29] The frequency of illness reported as resulting from these toxins is relatively rare but no specific data are available. Some of the rarity of cases may be related to lack of specific diagnoses.[28]

There are 2 other fungal toxins that are more widespread and are now under regulation by the EPA. These are patulin and fumonisin. Patulin is found in apple juice and apple juice products. It occurs in these products because of the use of rotten, or partially rotted, apples in the making of juice. The maximum recommended level for patulin in juice is 50 μg/kg and it is possible for infants and small children to exceed the limit of 0.43 μg/kg of body weight. The effects of patulin ingestion are considered to be chronic in nature and depend on long-term consumption. Toxicologic studies in animals indicate premature death, fetal and embryotoxic effects, and possible immunologic effects.[30] Studies in humans have not been done. Fumonisin is a mycotoxin and more than 10 types have been found worldwide.[31] They are present in corn and corn products that are used for animal feed and for human consumption. They may occur in products such as corn flour, corn meal, and grits. They have been found to be at very low levels in ready-to-eat breakfast cereals. They are not found in corn syrup. Low levels are found in corn chips and tortillas as well as in popcorn. The toxicity of the fumonisins in animals includes leukoencephalomalacia in horses, pulmonary edema in pigs, as well as liver, kidney, cardiac, and atherogenic effects in experimental animals. Rats and mice have been shown to develop liver cancers in chronic feeding experiments.[31] Possible carcinogenic effects in humans are somewhat inconclusive. However, because of the extensive nature of effects in animals, fumonisin action levels in corn products are now being established.

At this time there is little material available on how to protect children from these toxins. The EPA is increasing its evaluation of these substances and regulations are gradually being put into place about the most prevalent and serious of these materials. In the interim, there are several things families can do. In relation to seafood, the following suggestions are made:

- Do not use any seafood (fish or shellfish) that looks, smells, or tastes odd.
- Buy seafood from reputable sources.
- Buy only fresh seafood that is refrigerated or properly iced.
- Do not buy cooked seafood if displayed in the same case as raw fish.
- Do not buy frozen seafood with torn, open, or crushed package edges.
- Keep seafood refrigerated immediately after buying.
- For personal fishing, follow state advisories carefully.
  - As an example, the Michigan Fish Advisory (pages 6–9) states:
    - Choose smaller fish. Generally, panfish and fish just over the legal size will have fewer chemicals.
    - Choose lean fish. Panfish, brook trout, and brown trout that live in streams and rivers tend to be low in fat.
    - Choose fish that do not eat other fish. Large predator fish, especially large walleye, northern pike, muskie, bass, and lake trout tend to have more chemicals.

- Women of childbearing age and children under age 15 should eat no more than 1 meal per month of rock bass, perch, or crappie over 9 inches in length; and any size largemouth bass, smallmouth bass, walleye, northern pike, or muskie.
- Women who may become pregnant, pregnant women, lactating mothers, and young children should avoid fish that may have high levels of mercury and/or PCBs: shark, swordfish, king mackerel, and tilefish.

In addition, consumption of apple juice should be limited to 4 to 6 oz/d for children 1 to 6 years old and 8 to 12 oz/d for older children. (See also Chapter 7.)

Antimicrobial Preservatives

Among the approaches employed in achieving food preservation by inhibiting growth of undesirable microorganisms, is the use of chemical agents exhibiting antimicrobial activity. These chemicals may be either synthetic compounds intentionally added to foods or naturally occurring, biologically derived substances (ie, naturally occurring antimicrobials).[32] The vast majority of these substances are classified as GRAS (Generally Regarded as Safe). They include the traditional substances such as salt, sugar, or smoke. Other materials may be found naturally in some foods, or may be naturally occurring substances that are found in the food as it exists or are added to other foods. The most common of these compounds are the organic acids or their salts or derivatives— sorbic acid and benzoic acid are the most common but others include propionic, citric, acetic, lactic, and over 1/2 dozen others. Additionally, lipid materials such as monoaceylglcerols (from partially hydrolyzed fat), phenols, lytic enzymes such as egg white lysozyme, peroxidases and oxidases such as glucose oxidase, bacteriocins such as nisin, and hydrogen peroxide may be added to foods for their preservative function. No specific toxicity to any of these substances is known.

Food Irradiation

Food irradiation is a process by which food is exposed to a controlled source of ionizing radiation to prolong shelf life and reduce food losses, to improve microbiologic safety, and/or to reduce the use of chemical fumigants and additives. The dose of the ionizing radiation determines the effects of the process on foods. Food is generally irradiated at levels from 50 Gy to 10 kGy

(1 kGy = 1000 Gy), depending on the goals of the process. Low-dose irradiation (up to 1 kGy) is used primarily to delay ripening of produce, or kill or render sterile insects and other higher organisms that may infest fresh food. Medium-dose irradiation (1 to 10 kGy) reduces the number of pathogens and other microbes on food and prolongs shelf life. High-dose irradiation (>10 kGy) sterilizes food.

Food irradiation is regulated by the FDA as a food additive. The USDA also has regulatory responsibilities for some types of foods irradiated for defined purposes. All petitioners for FDA approval of food irradiation must complete a process that ensures that food irradiated for a specific purpose under precise conditions will remain radiologically, toxicologically, and microbiologically safe, and nutritionally adequate.[33]

All irradiated food sold in the United States must be labeled with the international sign of irradiation, the radura (Figure 52.1). Current labeling rules do not require that the dose of the irradiation or the purpose of the irradiation be specified. Thus, it is not possible for consumers to know if food has been treated to reduce pathogen loads or merely to prolong shelf life. Furthermore, current rules do not require food services to identify irradiated foods they serve.

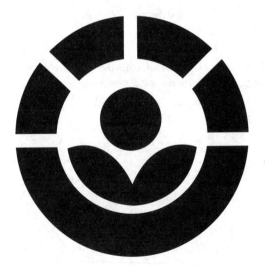

Figure 52.1. International Sign of Irradiation (Radura)

Radiological Safety
Neither the food nor the packaging materials become radioactive as a result of food irradiation.[34-36] The sources of radiation approved for use in food irradiation are limited to those producing energy too low to induce subatomic particles.

Toxicological Safety
Radiation absorbed by food causes a host of chemical reactions proportional to the dose of radiation applied. The desired reactions involve disrupting the DNA of spoilage and disease-causing microbes and pests. Undesired reactions could involve creation of toxic compounds. A number of approaches involving hundreds of studies have been employed over decades to determine whether such toxic compounds are created during irradiation and, if created, whether they are unique to the irradiation process (versus canning, freezing, drying) or created in amounts large enough to cause harm. Feeding studies and analytical chemical modeling studies have failed to identify any unusual toxicity associated with irradiation.[35,37,38] In fact, irradiated food often contains fewer changed molecules (also called radiolytic products) than food processed in conventional ways. For example, heat processed foods can contain 50 to 500 times more changed products than irradiated foods.[39] No compounds have been found in irradiated food that are not also found in foods processed in other ways (Personal Communication, Donald Thayer, USDA).

Microbiological Safety
Irradiation kills microbes primarily by fragmenting DNA. The sensitivity of organisms increases with the complexity of the organism. Thus, viruses are most resistant to destruction by irradiation, and insects and parasites are most sensitive. Spores, cysts, toxins, and prions are quite resistant to the effects of irradiation, because they are in highly stable resting states or are not living organisms. The conditions under which irradiation takes place (ie, temperature, humidity, and atmospheric content) can affect the dose required to achieve the food processing goal. Regardless, the quality of the food to be irradiated must be high, without heavy microbial contamination, for irradiation to achieve food-processing goals at any level.

When irradiation is used at non-sterilizing doses, the possibility of persistent pathogens is always present. While it is true that pathogen loads can be substantially reduced using this technique, it is always possible for foods to become recontaminated. Irradiation does not obviate the need for strict application of safe food-handling techniques, including adequate storage, hygienic preparation, and complete cooking, particularly of high-risk foods such as foods of animal origin, precooked processed foods, or imported foods.[40]

Nutritional Value

As with any food processing technique, irradiation can have a negative impact on some nutrients. It does not significantly damage carbohydrates or proteins, nor does it change the bioavailability or quantity of minerals or trace elements in foods. Slight loss of essential polyunsaturated fatty acids does occur with irradiation, but fats and oils that are major dietary sources of these nutrients tend to become rancid when irradiated and are not good candidates for this kind of treatment.[35]

Vitamin loss is the largest nutritional concern when foods are irradiated. Vitamin losses are most dramatic when studied in pure solutions. Whole foods exert a protective effect on vitamins since most of the radiation dose is absorbed by macromolecues (proteins, carbohydrates, and fats). Losses can be minimized by irradiating at low temperatures, at low doses, and by excluding oxygen and light.[41] When studied in pure solution, the water-soluble vitamins most sensitive to irradiation are thiamin (B_1), pyridoxine (B_6) and riboflavin (B_2). Vitamin C is converted by irradiation to dehydroascorbic acid (DHAA), which behaves like ascorbic acid in humans preserving nearly normal vitamin C activity after irradiation. Vitamins B_{12}, niacin, and pantothenic and folic acids are resistant to irradiation. Of the fat-soluble vitamins, vitamins E and A are sensitive. Plant carotenes are relatively resistant and vitamins D and K are quite resistant to irradiation.[39]

Thiamine loss can be 50% or more under some conditions in some foods. Loss is enhanced with increased irradiation doses, increased storage time after irradiation, and cooking after irradiation. Thiamin is found in meats, milk, whole grains, and legumes.[42] If all sources of thiamin come from irradiated products, a deficiency condition could develop, but this is unlikely in the United States. Irradiation losses of pyridoxine (found in meat, whole grains, corn, and soybeans) are not as severe as with thiamin and deficiency states are less likely to develop. The biological availability of riboflavin (found in meat, milk, eggs, green vegetables, whole grains, and legumes) can be paradoxically increased after irradiation by shortening required cooking time. For example, dried legumes irradiated at high doses require less than a quarter of the cooking time of untreated legumes and measured riboflavin is higher in irradiated versus nonirradiated cooked samples.[39]

Vitamin E loss can be significant. A study of effects of radiation plus heat shows that nonirradiated rolled oats lost 17% of their vitamin E after 10 minutes of cooking and 40% after 30 minutes, whereas rolled oats treated with 1 kGy lost 17% of their vitamin E after irradiation, 27.5% after cooking for 10 minutes, and 57% after cooking for 30 minutes.[39] Many of the sources of vitamin E, cereal grains, seed oils, peanuts, soybeans, milk fat, and turnip greens are unlikely to be treated with radiation and should provide for adequate alternative sources in a balanced and varied diet. Preformed vitamin A is found primarily in milk fat (Vitamin A-fortified milk) and eggs. Thus far, only eggs are approved for irradiation. Furthermore, plant carotenes found in dark green and yellow vegetables are converted by the body into vitamin A and are relatively resistant to irradiation.

While a few vitamins are significantly affected by irradiation, irradiated food is quite nutritious, in general. As long as a diet is balanced and food choices are varied, deficiency states are unlikely to develop.

Palatability

Taste, texture, color, and smell are all components of palatable foods. Some foods, particularly foods with high fat content, suffer unacceptable changes in these qualities when irradiated. Modified conditions, such as excluding oxygen from the atmosphere, lowering the temperature, excluding light, reducing water content, or lowering the radiation dose, can minimize or eliminate these changes. A welcome consequence of modifying irradiation conditions to preserve palatability is that the same modifications can also minimize vitamin loss.

Conclusion

Irradiation is increasingly suggested as an important adjunct to improving food safety and availability. Current rules by the FDA for food irradiation are listed in Table 52.4. Irradiated food is safe and nutritious and produces no toxicity as long as best management practices are followed. It can be safely used as part of a balanced and varied diet. It is important to remember, however, that irradiation of food does not substitute for careful food handling from farm to fork. Widespread use of food irradiation would necessitate construction of irradiation facilities in the United States and other countries. The benefits of expanding this technology and the risks involved must be thoroughly debated. Pediatricians should participate in the dialogue. As with any technology, unforeseen consequences are possible; therefore, careful monitoring and continuous evaluation of this and all food processing techniques are prudent precautions.

Table 52.4.
Rules From the United States Food and Drug Administration for Food Irradiation

Food	Purpose of Irradiation	Dose Permitted, kGy	Date of Rule
Spices, dry vegetable seasoning	Decontamination/ disinfest insects	30 (maximum)	7/15/63
Wheat, wheat powder	Disinfest insects	0.2–0.5	8/21/63
White potatoes	Extend shelf life	0.05–0.15	11/1/65
Dry or dehydrated enzyme preparations	Control insects and microorganisms	10 (maximum)	6/10/85
Pork carcasses or fresh noncut processed cuts	Control *Trichinella spiralis*	0.3 (minimum)– 1.0 (maximum	7/22/85
Fresh fruit	Delay maturation	1	4/18/86
Dry or dehydrated aromatic vegetable substances	Decontamination	30	4/18/86
Poultry	Control pathogens	3	5/2/90
Red meat	Control pathogens and prolong shelf life	4.5 (fresh)–7 (frozen)	12/3/97
Fresh shell eggs	Control *Salmonella* species	3.0	7/12/00

Indirect Food Additives

Indirect food additives are substances used in food-contact materials, including adhesives, dyes, coatings, paper, paperboard, and polymers (plastics), that may come into contact with food as part of packaging or processing equipment, but are not intended to be added directly to food.[43] They confer no nutritional value to food. While direct food additives undergo toxicological testing prior to approval based on structure-activity relationships as well as anticipated human exposure levels,[44] testing of indirect food additives is based primarily on anticipated exposure levels (Table 52.5). Exposures considered "virtually nil" (<0.05 ppm [parts per million]) or "insignificant" (0.05 to 1.0 ppm) receive subchronic testing (90 days or approximately 12% of post-weaning lifetime of test animals) unless "indicated by available data or information."[45] Petitioners for new indirect additive approvals may apply for an exemption from regulation if they can satisfy the agency that exposures will not exceed the regulatory threshold of 0.5 ppb (parts per billion) or are at or less than 1% of the acceptable dietary intake.[46] This regulatory approach is based on the concept that "the dose makes the poison," and adverse human health effects are unlikely for most substances when exposure levels are very small. The exposure level is calculated from labo-

Table 52.5.
Testing of Indirect Food Additives

Exposure Level	Required	Conditionally Required	Suggested
<0.05 ppm	Acute oral study—rodent	None	none
>0.05 ppm	Subchronic feeding study (90-day)—rodent Subchronic feeding study (90-day)—non-rodent	Acute oral study—rodent Multigenerational reproduction feeding study (minimum of 2 generations) with teratology phase—rodent Teratology study	Short-term tests for carcinogenic potential
>~1 ppm	Lifetime feeding study (2-year)—rodent with in-utero exposure for carcinogenesis and chronic toxicity Lifetime feeding study (2-year)—rodent for carcinogenesis Short-term feeding study (at least 1 year)—non-rodent Multigenerational reproduction feeding study (minimum of 2 generations) with teratology phase—rodent	Acute oral study—rodent Subchronic feeding study (90-day)—rodent Teratology study	Short-term tests for carcinogenic potential Metabolism studies

ratory generated migration data of the chemical into food simulants, and estimates of the percentage of total daily food intake that would contain the substance for an adult.[47]

EDI = 3000 g food/person/d × <M> × CF*
EDI: Estimated Daily Intake
<M> is the sum of the laboratory generated migration factors for each food fraction in contact with the material multiplied by the proportion of food from each fraction (aqueous and acidic, alcohol, fatty)

Additional calculations to estimate daily intake of indirect food additives of infants, children, or adolescents are not routinely performed as part of the approval process.

Many common packaging materials were approved for use prior to the 1958 Food Additives Amendment to the Federal Food, Drug, and Cosmetic Act

*CF is the Consumption Factor and represents the ratio of the weight of all food contacting a specific material to the total weight of the food packaged.

(1938), and thus "grandfathered in" for continued use as "prior-approved" substances.[39] Some of these substances have since been found to be hormonally active in laboratory animals, raising specific concerns about potential adverse impacts on the fetus and infants, children, and adolescents. Examples are plasticizers like the phthalate esters (used in polyvinyl chloride [PVC] plastics, inks, dyes, and adhesives in food packaging), nonyl phenol (used in PVC, juice boxes, and lid gaskets), and bisphenol A (found in some baby bottles, water bottles, and can-liner enamels). Considerable scientific uncertainty remains about the significance of the endocrine disrupting capacity of these chemicals to humans, the exposure levels at which toxicity might occur, and the extent of real world human exposures.[48] A recent analysis of infant formulas, baby food, and canned vegetables in the Washington, DC, area found levels of these chemicals in foods measuring in the low parts per billion.[49] This analysis reinforced earlier reports showing declining trends of contamination of infant food with phthalates over the past decade.[50-52] These declines correlate with the food industry's move to eliminate many uses of these chemicals in packaging of foods intended for small children.

Nonetheless, chemicals can and will migrate from processing equipment, packaging materials, and storage containers into foods. It is not feasible to subject all possible chemical contaminants to exhaustive toxicology testing. A reasonable approach, therefore, is to develop food preparation and storage practices that will minimize exposures. The following suggestions should help to minimize unnecessary exposure to indirect food contaminants:

- Avoid routine use of single-serving packaging. Such packaging maximizes contact between food and the packaging materials.
- When possible, buy fresh food to minimize contact with packaging materials.
- Use heat-safe glass or crockery when cooking or reheating food in the microwave. Heat increases migration of many contaminants into food, particularly foods containing fats.
- Make sure a generous air space separates the surface of stored food from cling wraps used to seal containers. Avoid using cling wraps when microwaving foods.

Finally, pediatricians are in an ideal position to provide important input and continued encouragement to regulatory agencies to ensure that the special exposures and vulnerabilities of children to toxic exposures remain under consideration as food-related materials and processes are developed, reviewed, and revised.

References

1. US Food and Drug Administration, FDA Backgrounder. *Food Safety: A Team Approach.* Available at: http://www.cfsan.fda.gov/~lrd/foodteam.html. Accessed May 16, 2003

2. National Research Council. *Pesticides in the Diets of Infants and Children.* Washington, DC: National Academy Press; 1993

3. Rice D, Barone S Jr. Critical periods of vulnerability for the developing nervous system: evidence from human and animal models. *Environ Health Perspect.* 2000;108(suppl 3):511–533

4. Bearer CF. How are children different from adults? *Environ Health Perspect.* 1995;103(suppl 6):7–12

5. American Academy of Pediatrics Commitee on Environmental Health. *Handbook of Pediatric Environmental Health.* Etzel RA, ed. Elk Grove Village, IL: American Academy of Pediatrics; 1999

6. Groth E III, Benbrook CM, Lutz K. *Do You Know What You're Eating? An Analysis Of U.S. Government Data on Pesticide Residues in Food.* Yonkers, NY: Consumers Union of the United States; 1999

7. Physicians for Social Responsibility. *Pesticides and Children: What the Pediatric Practitioner Should Know.* Washington, DC: Physicians for Social Responsibility; 1995:1–8

8. Groth E III, Benbrook CM, Lutz K. *Update: Pesticides in Children's Foods: An Analysis of 1998 USDA BDP Data on Pesticide Residues.* Yonkers, NY: Consumers Union of the United States; 2000

9. Grossman J. What's hiding under the sink: dangers of household pesticides. *Environ Health Perspect.* 1995;103:550–554

10. Reigart JR, Roberts JR. *Recognition and Management of Pesticide Poisonings.* 5th ed. Washington, DC: US Environmental Protection Agency; 1999

11. Food and Drug Administration Pesticide Program. *Residue Monitoring, 1999.* Washington, DC: US Food and Drug Administration; 2000

12. US Environmental Protection Agency. *Pesticides and National Strategies for Health Care Providers: Draft Implementation Plan.* Washington, DC: US Environmental Protection Agency; 2000

13. Shafer KS, Kegley SE, Patton S. *Nowhere to Hide: Persistent Toxic Chemicals in the U.S. Food Supply.* San Francisco, CA: Pesticides Action Network; 2001

14. Peterson RE, Theobald HM, Kimmel GL. Developmental and reproductive toxicity of dioxins and related compounds: cross species comparisons. *Crit Rev Toxicol.* 1993;23:283–335

15. Longnecker MP, Klebanoff MA, Zhou H, Brock JW. Association between maternal serum concentrations of the DDT metabolite DDE and preterm and small-for-gestational-age babies at birth. *Lancet.* 2001;358:110–114

CHAPTER 52

Food Safety: Pesticides, Industrial Chemicals, Toxins, Antimicrobial Preservatives/Irradiation, and Indirect Food Additives

16. US Environmental Protection Agency. *Exposure and Human Health Reassessment of 2,3,7,8-Tetrachlorodibenzo-p-Dioxin (TCDD) and Related Compounds.* Washington, DC: US Environmental Protection Agency; 2000. Publication 600/P-00/001Be. Available at: http://cfpub.epa.gov/ncea/cfm/part1and2.cfm/ActType-default. Accessed April 17, 2003

17. US General Accounting Office. *Environmental Health Risks: Information on EPA's Draft Reassessment of Dioxins.* Washington, DC; US General Accounting Office; 2002. Publication GAO-02–515. Available at: http://www.gao.gov/main.htm. Accessed April 17, 2003

18. US Environmental Protection Agency. Health effects of PCBs. Available at: http://epa.gov/opptintr/pcb/effects.html. Accessed March 7, 2003

19. US Environmental Protection Agency. Mercury study report to congress. Available at: http://www.epa.gov/oar/mercury.html. Accessed April 17, 2003

20. Harada M. Congenital Minamata disease: intrauterine methylmercury poisoning. *Teratology.* 1978;18:285–288

21. Cox C, Clarkson TW, Marsh DO, Amin-Zaki L, Tikriti S, Myers GG. Dose-response analysis of infants prenatally exposed to methyl mercury: an application of a single compartment model to single-strand hair analysis. *Environ Res.* 1989;49:318–332

22. Grandjean P, Weihe P, White RF, et al. Cognitive deficit in 7-year-old children with prenatal exposure to methylmercury. *Neurotoxicol Teratol.* 1997;19:417–428

23. Rice DC, Gilbert SG. Effects of developmental exposure to methyl mercury on spatial and temporal visual function in monkeys. *Toxicol Appl Pharmacol.* 1990;102: 151–163

24. Michigan Department of Community Health 2002. Michigan Fish Advisory. Available at: http://www.michigan.gov/mdch/0,1607,7-132-2944-13110-,00.html. Accessed April 17, 2003

25. Center for Food Safety and Applied Nutrition. *Consumer Advisory for Pregnant Women and Women of Childbearing Age Who May Become Pregnant About the Risks of Mercury in Fish.* US Food and Drug Administration; March 2001. Available at: http://vm.cfsan.fda.gov/~dms/admehg.html. Accessed March, 2003

26. Aschner M. Manganese: brain transport and emerging research needs. *Environ Health Perspect.* 2000;108(suppl 3):429–432

27. Schettler T, Stein J, Reich F, Valenti M, Wallinga D. *In Harm's Way: Toxic Threats to Child Development.* Cambridge, MA: Greater Boston Physicians for Social Responsibility; 2000:59–68. Available at: http://psr.igc.org/ihw.htm. Accessed April 16, 2003

28. Center for Food Safety and Applied Nutrition. *Foodborne Pathogenic Microorganisms and Natural Toxins Handbook (Bad Bug Book).* US Food and Drug Administration. Available at: http://vm.cfsan.fda.gov/~mow/intro.html. Accessed April 16, 2003

29. Tan LJ. *Diagnosis and Management of Foodborne Illnesses: A Primer for Physicians.* Chicago, IL: American Medical Association; 2001

30. Center for Food Safety and Applied Nutrition. *Patulin in Apple Juice, Apple Juice Concentrates and Apple Juice Products.* Washington, DC: US Food and Drug Administration; 2001

31. Center for Food Safety and Applied Nutrition. *Background Paper in Support of Fumonisin Levels in Corn and Corn Products Intended for Human Consumption.* US Food and Drug Administration; November 9, 2001. Available at: http://vm.cfsan.fda.gov/~dms/fumonbg3.html. Accessed April 16, 2003

32. Council for Agricultural Science and Technology. *Naturally Occurring Antimicrobials in Food.* Ames, IA: Council for Agricultural Science and Technology; 1998. Task Force Report 132.

33. American Academy of Pediatrics Committee on Environmental Health. Technical report: irradiation of food. *Pediatrics.* 2000;106:1505–1510

34. International Atomic Energy Agency. *Facts About Food Irradiation.* Available at: http://www.iaea.org/icgfi/documents/publications.htm. Accessed March 13, 2003

35. World Health Organization. *Safety and Nutritional Adequacy of Irradiated Food.* Geneva, Switzerland: World Health Organization; 1994.

36. Urbain WM. Ionizing radiation. In: *Food Irradiation.* Orlando, FL: Academic Press Inc; 1986:1–22

37. US Department of Health and Human Services, Food and Drug Administration. Irradiation in the production, processing, and handling of food. *Fed Regist.* 1986;51:13376–13399

38. World Health Organization. *High-Dose Irradiation: Wholesomeness of Food Irradiated With Doses Above 10 kGy.* Geneva, Switzerland: World Health Organization; 1999. WHO Technical Report Series No. 890. Available at: http://www.who.int/fsf/Documents/newdoc.htm. Accessed April 17, 2003

39. Diehl JF. *Safety of Irradiated Food.* 2nd ed. New York, NY: Marcel Dekker; 1995

40. World Health Organization. *WHO Golden Rules for Safe Food Preparation.* Available at: http://www.who.int/fsf/goldenrules.htm. Accessed April 16, 2003

41. Murano EA, ed. *Food Irradiation: A Source Book.* Ames, IA: Iowa State University Press; 1995

42. American Academy of Pediatrics. *Pediatric Nutrition Handbook.* Kleinman RE, ed. 4th ed. Elk Grove Village, IL: American Academy of Pediatrics; 1998

43. US Food and Drug Administration, Center for Food Safety and Applied Nutrition. *The List of "Indirect" Additives Used in Food Contact Substances.* Available at: http://vm.cfsan.fda.gov/~dms/opa-indt.html. Accessed April 16, 2003

44. US Food and Drug Administration, Center for Food Safety and Applied Nutrition. *Toxicological Principles for the Safety of Food Ingredients.* Redbook 2000. October 2001. Available at: http://vm.cfsan.fda.gov/~redbook/red-toca.html. Accessed May 16, 2003

45. US Food and Drug Administration, Center for Food Safety and Applied Nutrition, Office of Premarket Approval. *Toxicological Testing of Food Additives.* 1983, Updated 1997. Available at: http://vm.cfsan.fda.gov/~dms/opa-tg1.html. Accessed May 16, 2003

46. US Food and Drug Administration, Center for Food Safety and Applied Nutrition, Office of Premarket Approval. *Guidance for Submitting Requests Under 21 CFR 170.39. Threshold of Regulation for Substances Used in Food-Contact Articles.* Available at: http://vm.csfan.fda.gov/~dms/opa-gg2.html. Accessed April 16, 2003

47. US Food and Drug Administration, Center for Food Safety and Applied Nutrition, Office of Premarket Approval. *Recommendations for Chemistry Data for Indirect Food Additives Petitions.* Available at: http://vm.cfsan.fda.gov/~dms/opa-cg5.html. Accessed May 16, 2003

48. Kaiser J. Endocrine disrupters. Panel cautiously confirms low-dose effects. *Science.* 2000;290:695–697

49. McNeal TP, Biles JE, Begley TH, Craun JC, Hopper ML, Sack CA. Determination of suspected endocrine disruptors in foods and food packaging. In: Keith LH, Jones-Lepp TL, Needham LL, eds. *Analysis of Environmental Endocrine Disruptors.* Washington, DC: American Chemical Society; 2000:33–52

50. MAFF UK. *Phthalates in Infant Formulae.* Number 83, March 1996. Available at: http://archive.food.gov.uk/maff/archive/food/infsheet/1996/no83/83phthal.htm. Accessed April 16, 2003

51. MAFF UK. *Phthalates in Infant Formulae—Follow-up Survey.* Number 168, December 1998. Available at: http://archive.food.gov.uk/maff/archive/food/infsheet/1998/no168/168phtha.htm. Accessed April 16, 2003

52. US Department of Health and Human Services. Memorandum. *Phthalates in Infant Formula—Assignment Summary.* December 19, 1996. Consumer Safety Officer, OFP/Domestic Programs Branch, HFS-636

53

New Food Ingredients

The nature of the food we eat evolves in response to new knowledge in health and nutrition, changing consumer demands, and changes designed to improve the production, shelf life, or sensory characteristics of foods. These changes in foods and food ingredients are developed through a variety of traditional methods (eg, plant and animal breeding, fermentation), addition of new ingredients designed for specific food functional or health benefits, and newer technologies (eg, biotechnology).

Biotechnology

New methods of bioengineering foods through genetic modification (GM) of plants and animals, including recombinant DNA (rDNA) and transgenic techniques, represent a continuum from the more traditional plant and animal breeding techniques.[1-4] Traditional breeding typically consists of hybridization between varieties of the same species and screening for progeny with desired characteristics. Such hybridization can only introduce traits found in close relatives. These techniques require extensive backcrossing with the parent line to eliminate mutations unlinked to that responsible for the desired phenotype and undesirable traits in extraneous genetic material introduced along with that encoding the desired trait. Biotechnology involves the isolation and subsequent introduction of discrete DNA segments containing the gene(s) of interest into recipient (host) plants or animals. The DNA segments can come from any organism (microbial, animal, or plant). These techniques are more precise (although not necessarily safer) than traditional cross-breeding approaches because they introduce only the gene or genes of interest with little or no extraneous DNA materials. Therefore, they increase the potential for better-characterized and more predictable foods. However, because of the wider variety of potential source organisms for the DNA segments, substances may be introduced into bioengineered foods that cannot be introduced by traditional breeding. Thus, there is a greater likelihood that some of the new substances will be significantly different from substances that have a history of safe use in food.

For purposes of this chapter, the terms "foods derived from biotech-nology," "genetically modified foods," or "bioengineered foods" will be used interchangeably to describe foods or food ingredients that are, or are derived from, plants and animals that have been modified (engineered) through the use of rDNA techniques.

Regulation

When consumed by humans, GM products are regulated as foods and food additives.[1-5] As such, they must meet the same types of safety and labeling regulations as foods and food ingredients produced under more traditional means. Use of biotechnology to transfer genes that encode pharmaceutical proteins, oral vaccines, and enzymes for human or animal use will require that these products meet regulatory requirements for biologics, drugs, or veterinary drugs, even when foods are used as the delivery vehicle (eg, bananas contain-ing vaccines). In some cases, residual substances from a GM drug- or vaccine-producing plant or animal may enter the food supply (eg, rbST [recombinant bovine somatotropin] milk as a consequence of its use as an animal drug). In these cases, regulatory evaluations must include considerations of human food exposures and safety. Plant products bioengineered to contain substances with pesticidal properties to improve agronomic properties must meet require-ments of both the Environmental Protection Agency (EPA) and the Food and Drug Administration (FDA).

Safety

All plant and animal breeding techniques have the potential for unintentional-ly introducing undesired new characteristics into foods.[1-4,6,7] This may occur either from bringing extraneous genetic material encoding trait(s) additional to the desired trait(s), or from introducing mutations (such as deletions, amplifi-cations, insertions, rearrangements, or DNA base-pair changes) into the native genetic material. Newly introduced DNA may physically insert into a transcrip-tionally active site on the chromosome and may, thereby, inactivate a host gene or alter control of its expression. The introduced gene product or a metabolic product affected by the genetic change may interact with other cellular process-es. Pleiotropic effects (multiple effects resulting from a single genetic change) may also occur. Altered expression of an enzyme at high levels may lead to secondary biochemical effects (eg, altered metabolic flux resulting in changing metabolic patterns). Biotechnology products have the additional potential to introduce substances into foods that cannot be introduced by traditional breeding. These techniques can, therefore, present more complex and novel safety issues than are seen with more conventional processes and often require nontraditional approaches to evaluating safety.

Safety concerns with GM foods can be categorized as relatively low or relatively high. A recent expert consultation of the Food and Agriculture Organization and the World Health Organization of the United Nations (FAO/WHO) concluded that the concept of "substantial equivalence" is a practical, science-based approach for evaluating the safety of many GM foods.[6,7] The goal of this approach is to ensure that the GM food, and any substances that have been introduced into the food as a result of GM, is "as safe as its traditional counterpart" when such a counterpart exists. This approach is deemed useful because of the practical difficulties in obtaining meaningful information from conventional toxicological studies on the safety of whole foods. For example, use of whole foods as a test substance in animal studies is difficult because the (a) bulkiness of the food dilutes the nutritional value of the diet causing adverse effects unrelated to the genetic modification, (b) satiety of the diet is adversely affected resulting in reduced food intake, and (c) bulk and satiety effects limit the dose response range to low multiples of the amounts that might be present in the human diet. However, the FAO/WHO expert panel also recognized that the "substantial equivalence" approach is not always sufficient and that animal testing is needed in cases where (a) the GM food is expected to make a significant dietary contribution, (b) there is an absence of history of consumption of the novel gene product, or (c) the genetic modification affects several metabolic pathways. In these cases, animal testing is recommended, starting with appropriate isolated substances and also including testing of the whole food in a form that reflects the food as it will be consumed by humans.

Safety concerns are least likely to be raised in GM foods if the proteins or other substances produced by the transferred genetic material do not differ significantly from other substances commonly found in food and are already present at generally comparable or greater levels in currently consumed foods.[1,2,6] An example would be insertion of the GmFad2-1 gene into the soybean genome to produce a high oleic acid soybean oil. Comparability to historic uses of foods will include such factors as the content of significant nutrients, naturally occurring toxicants, antinutrients, and prior safe use.

Transferred genetic material (ie, DNA) is generally not considered to raise safety concerns.[1,2,6] All food, rDNA-derived or otherwise, contains large amounts of DNA. Individuals consume approximately 0.1 to 1.0 g/d of DNA when eating conventional foods.[7] The added DNA from GM foods is estimated to contribute <1/250 000 of this ingested quantity of DNA. Normally, ingested DNA is rapidly digested in the gastrointestinal tract. Thus, evaluating the digestibility of the DNA in a GM food provides useful insight into the possibility of a gene transfer. In general, the FAO/WHO concluded that horizontal gene transfer from GM foods to gut microorganisms or human cells is a possibility. A few recent reports have shown antibiotic resistance genes transferring in human mouth and gut from animal microbial sources to human gut bacteria. This genetic material has not been shown to incorporate into human DNA. For gene transfer from a GM food to gut microflora or human cells to occur, all of the following events need to occur: (1) the relevant gene would need to be released, (2) the gene would need to survive plant and gastrointestinal tract nucleases, (3) the gene would have to compete for uptake with dietary DNA, (4) the recipient or mammalian cells would have to be competent for transformation, (5) the gene would have to survive their restrictive enzymes, and (6) the gene would have to be inserted into the host DNA by rare repair or recombination events.

Safety concerns are more likely to be raised if the modified food will contain substances that are significantly different from, or are present in food at a significantly higher level than, counterpart substances historically consumed in food.[1,2,6] Examples of these types of safety concerns include the potential for (a) introducing a food allergen that would not be expected to be in a particular food, (b) an expression of allergens at higher concentrations than they would otherwise be expressed, (c) compositional changes that would affect the nutritional quality of the food by altering nutrient levels, bioavailability, or stability of relied-upon nutrients, (d) increasing the level of naturally occurring toxicants, or (e) producing new metabolic pathways that would result in the synthesis of toxicants not normally found in a food.

A potential consequence of transferring genetic material from one source into another is the possibility of introducing a food allergen that would not be expected to be in a particular food.[1,2,4,6,7] This is because genes code for proteins, and virtually all allergens are proteins (although only a small subset of proteins are allergens). Thus, by increasing the range of potential proteins that can be introduced into food over that possible by traditional breeding, there is an increased potential for introducing an allergen into a GM food that could have an allergenic characteristic completely different from that of its conventional counterpart. Also, bioengineering can be used to express proteins at higher concentrations than they would otherwise be expressed, and these higher concentrations may increase the potential for such proteins to be allergenic. If the allergen was moved into a food product that never before produced that allergen, the susceptible consumer population would not know to avoid that food. For example, a gene from a Brazil nut plant was introduced into a soy plant to improve the protein content of soybeans for use in animal feed. The seed was never commercialized, however, because when the company tested the soybeans for allergenicity, they found that people allergic to Brazil nuts were also allergic to the GM soy.

Most common allergic reactions are mediated by allergen-specific IgE antibodies. The FAO/WHO recommends that the potential for allergenicity be evaluated if (a) the source of transferred material contains known allergens or an amino acid sequence homology similar to known allergens, (b) there is immunoreactivity to the IgE of blood serum of humans with known allergenicity to the source material, and (c) the substance is resistant to the effect of pH and digestion (unlike other dietary proteins, most allergens are resistant to gastric acidity and digestive proteases). Additionally, allergens that are labile to heat and processing should be allowed only if the GM food is always eaten in cooked or processed food.[7]

Genetic modifications have the potential to activate cryptic pathways synthesizing unknown or unexpected toxicants, or to increase expression from active pathways that ordinarily produce low or undetectable levels of toxicants.[1,2,6,7] Plants are known to naturally produce a number of toxicants and antinutritional factors (eg, protease inhibitors, hemolytic agents, and neurotoxins), which often serve the plant as natural defense compounds against pests or pathogens. Additionally, plants, like other organisms, have metabolic pathways that no longer function due to mutations that occurred during evolution. Such silent pathways may be activated by mutations, chromosomal rearrangements, or new regulatory regions introduced during breeding, and toxicants not associated with a plant species may be produced. Many of these toxicants are present in today's foods at levels that do not cause acute toxicity. Others require proper preparation to make them safe. To be considered safe and approved, new GM foods should not have significantly higher levels of toxicants than present in other edible varieties of the counterpart food.

The safety of antibiotic resistance selectable markers has been the focus of considerable discussion.[1,4,6–9] For research purposes, scientists enhance their ability to isolate plant cells that have taken up and stably incorporated the desired genes by physically linking the desired gene to a selectable marker gene, such as a gene that specifies the production of a substance that inactivates antibiotics. By linking the selectable marker gene to another gene that specifies a desired trait, scientists can identify and select plants that have taken up and express the desired genes. Selectable marker genes that produce enzymes that inactivate clinically useful antibiotics have the potential of reducing the therapeutic efficacy of the antibiotic when taken orally if the enzyme in the food inactivates the antibiotic. These genes may be expressed in the transgenic plant.

The kanamycin resistance gene is one of the most widely used selectable plant marker genes in GM foods. The kanamycin resistance gene specifies the information for the production of the enzyme, aminoglycoside 3^{1-} phosphotransferase II. The common name for this enzyme is kanamycin (or neomycin) phosphotransferase II (rNPT II). The kanamycins phosphotransferse II enzyme modifies aminoglycoside antibiotics, including kanamycin, neomycin, and geeticin (G418), chemically inactivating the antibiotic and rendering the cells that produce the kanamycin resistance gene produce refractory or resistant to the antibiotic. Plant cells that have received and stably express the kanamycin resistance gene survive and replicate on laboratory media in the presence of the antibiotic, kanamycin. Plant cells that did not take up and express the introduced kanamycin resistance gene will be killed by the antibiotic. Both the kanamycin resistance gene and its product, the kanamycin phosphotransferase II enzyme protein, are in foods derived from plants in which the maker gene has been used unless removed through special techniques.

The World Health Organization (1993)[9] and the FDA[8] reviewed safety issues associated with the use of selective antibiotic resistance genes in GM plants. They found no evidence that markers currently in use pose a health risk; but they recommended that genes that confer resistance to drugs with specific medical use or limited alternative therapies should not be used in widely disseminated rDNA biotechnology foods. They concluded that safety assessments for the presence of these genes in food products should include such factors as (1) an assessment of the potential toxicity of the protein, (2) an assessment of whether the protein has the potential to elicit allergenic reactions, and (3) an assessment of whether the presence in food of the enzyme or protein encoded by the antibiotic resistance marker gene would compromise the therapeutic efficiency of orally administered antibiotic. Safety evaluations should also consider whether the antibiotic is an important medication, frequently used, orally administered, unique, and has selective pressure for transformation to occur, as well as the background level of resistance to the antibiotic in bacterial populations and the availability of alternative effective therapies. If the information suggests that the presence of the marker gene or gene in the GM food could compromise the use of the relevant antibiotic(s), the marker gene or gene product should not be present in finished food. For example, certain antibiotics are the only drug available to treat certain clinical conditions (eg, vancomycin for treating certain staphylococcal infections). Marker genes that encode resistance to such antibiotics should not be used in GM foods. It should be noted also that antibiotic resistance is increasing rapidly and drugs that are currently not important to humans may become important. Thus, it may come to pass that all antibiotic resistance marker genes should not be incorporated into GM foods.

Because of the novel safety concerns raised by the use of the kanamycin resistance gene in such products as the FLAVR SAVR tomato (Calgene), the FDA reviewed evidence on the safety of this gene via the food additive petition process.[10] The evidence showed that, like other dietary proteins, the marker gene used to confer kanamycin resistance is rapidly degraded when subjected to conditions that simulate mammalian digestion. Based on this evidence, the FDA concluded that DNA for kanamycin resistance was not different from other rDNA in its digestibility. A food additive regulation authorized the use of rNPT II in canola, cotton, and tomatoes (see Table 53.1).

Purpose of Biotechnology Changes

To date, the use of bioengineering applications for food products primarily has been for agronomic purposes[3,11,12] (Table 53.1). However, increasingly, there is also interest in using biotechnology to improve benefits to consumers.

Agronomic uses of biotechnology include those uses that (a) increase crop productivity through increased resistance to herbicides, insects, or viruses, (b) increase shelf life through delayed fruit ripening, (c) affect fertility to control against cross-fertilization in field conditions or alter seed viability, (d) increase milk production in dairy cows, or (e) increase the bioavailability of phosphates in animal feeds[11,12] (see Table 53.1).

The use of recombinant bovine growth hormone or somatotropin to increase milk production in dairy animals was approved in 1993 for use as an animal drug.[13] The product contains a recombinant bGH (rbGH), which is essentially the same as bGH (pituitary derived). To grant approval of this product as an animal drug, the FDA determined, among other things, that food

Table 53.1.
Examples of Marketed Food Products Developed Through Biotechnology[3,11]

Food(s)	Intended Effects	Gene, Gene Product, or Gene Fragments	Source
Corn, Rice, Cotton, Canola, Flax, Soybean, Sugar Beet, Radicchio	Herbicide resistance to glufosinate	Phosphinothricin acetyltransferase (PAT)	*Streptomyces viridochromogenes or hygroscopicus*
Corn, Cotton, Sugar Beet, Canola, Soybean	Herbicide resistance to glyphosphate	5-Enolpyruvylshikimate-3-phosphate synthase (EPSPS); or glyphospate oxidoreductase (GOX)	*Agrobacterium* sp. Strain CP4; *Ochrobactrum anthropi; achromobacter* strain BAA
Canola, Cotton	Herbicide resistance to bromoxynil	Nitrilase	*Klepsilla ozaenae or pneumoniae* Subsp. *Ozaenae*
Flax, Cotton	Herbicide resistance to sulfonylurea	Acetolactate synthase (csr-1) (ALS)	*Arabidopsis; Nicotiana tabacum* cv. *Xanthi*
Corn, Tomato, Potato, Cotton	Insect resistance*	CryIF, CryIAb, CryIAc, CryIIIA, Cry9C proteins	*Bacillus thuringiensis*
Potato, Squash, Papaya	Virus resistance*	Plant virus coat proteins or mosaic viruses; potato leafroll virus replicase	Potato virus Y, potato leafroll virus, cucumber mosaic virus, zucchini yellow mosaic virus, watermelon mosaic virus 2, papaya ringspot virus
Cantaloupe, Tomato	Delayed fruit ripening	S-adenosylmethionine hydrolase	*Escherichia coli* bacteriophage T3
Tomato	Delayed fruit ripening	Gene fragment for amino cyclopropane carboxylic acid synthase (ACCS); polygalacturonase (PG) or the antisense PG gene	Tomato

Table 53.1.
Examples of Marketed Food Products Developed Through Biotechnology[3],[11] *(continued)*

Food(s)	Intended Effects	Gene, Gene Product, or Gene Fragments	Source
Tomato	Delayed fruit ripening	1-aminocyclopropane-1-carboxylic acid deaminase (ACCD)	*Pseudomonas chloraphis*
Tomato, Cotton, Canola	Antibiotic resistance marker that inactivates aminoglycosides (kanamycin, neomycin, geeticin)	Amino glycoside 3'-phosphotransferase II encoded *kanr* gene from the transposon Tn[5]	*Escherichia coli*
Corn, Canola, Radicchio, Canola	Male sterility; Fertility restorer	Barnase; Barstar	*Bacillus amyloliquefaciens*
Corn	Male sterility	DNA adenine methylase (DAM)	*Escherichia coli*
Canola	Degradation of phytate in animal feed	Phytase	*Aspergillus niger* van Tieghem
Dairy Products	Increase milk production in dairy animals		Recombinant bovine growth hormone (rbGH) or somatotropin (rbST)[†]
Soybean	To produce a high oleic acid soybean oil)	GmFad2-1 gene (to suppress endogenous GmFad2-1 gene which encodes delta-12 desaturase)	Soybean
Canola	To produce high laurate canola oil	12:0 acyl carrier protein thioesterase	*Umbellularia californica* (California Bay)

*Foods that contain an introduced pesticidal substance are regulated by both the Environmental Protection Agency (EPA) and the Food and Drug Administration (FDA).
†Regulated as an animal drug, taking into account safety for humans when dairy products from treated cows are consumed as foods.

products from cows treated with rbGH are safe for consumption by humans. This conclusion, however, is controversial. Subsequent to the FDA's approval, Canada's Health Department concluded that results of a 90-day oral rat toxicity study and the report of an antibody response to oral rbGH suggested possible adverse health effects of this product.[14] Therefore, Canada did not approve the use of rbGH or rbGST as an animal drug. After the Canadian decision, the FDA conducted a comprehensive audit of the human food safety used to support the 1993 rbGH approval, including the studies that Canada relied on in making its finding of safety concerns. Based on this audit, the FDA concluded that the Canadian reviewers did not interpret the study results correctly and that there are no new scientific concerns about the safety of milk from cows treated with rbGH. The FDA, therefore, reconfirmed its determination that safety had been established and that long-term studies were not necessary for assessing the safety of rbGH. The FDA's decision was based on evidence that showed that bGH is biologically inactive in humans even if ingested, rbGH is orally inactive, and bGH and rbGH are biologically indistinguishable.

Considerable controversy has also arisen over the use of the Cry9C gene to produce toxicity to certain insects (ie, Starlink Corn).[15] Prior to October 2001, plants containing the Cry9C proteins had been approved by EPA only for corn earmarked for animal feed and industrial uses. Approval had not been given for human consumption due to unresolved questions about the potential of Cry9C to cause allergic reactions. In approving this product for animal feed use, the EPA required Starlink's developer, Aventis, to ensure that the GM corn did not enter into the food supply. However, some of the GM corn became mingled with corn destined for human consumption (eg, taco shells). The presence of an unapproved pesticide in food means that the food is adulterated. Therefore, the manufacturer recalled contaminated products from the market. On October 16, 2001, the EPA, based on a review of scientific evidence demonstrating that *Bacillus thuringiensis* is not toxic to humans or other animals, approved corn genetically modified with *B thuringiensis* for 7 years for use in human food.

Although not yet approved for human use, scientists have created a genetically engineered variety of Atlantic salmon that grows to market weight in about 18 months, compared to the 24 to 30 months that it normally takes for fish to reach that size.[16,17] The idea for the fast-growing salmon was discovered by accident 20 years ago when a researcher in Canada accidentally froze a tank filled with flounder. When the tank was thawed out, the flounder were still alive. This species has a gene that produces a protein that works like antifreeze. Researchers isolated and copied the part of the flounder DNA that works like a genetic switch to turn on the production of the antifreeze protein. They then attached the flounder's gene to a previously isolated gene from Chinook salmon that produces a growth-stimulating hormone and inserted the new combination into fertilized salmon eggs. In the resulting salmon, the flounder's genetic switch produces a continuous supply of salmon growth hormone that accelerates the fish's development. The resulting fish do not become larger than conventional salmon; they simply grow faster. If approved, these products will be regulated similarly to rbST in that they will need to meet regulatory requirements for safety and efficacy as a veterinary drug and also establish safety for use of these salmon as human food.

Consumer Benefits

Bioengineering can also be used to develop foods that are designed to provide direct benefits to consumers (eg, improved quality or nutritional and health benefits of foods).[7,11,12] For example, rDNA techniques have been used to modify the nutrient composition of plants (eg, increase carotenoid content of rice), improve the healthfulness of foods (eg, decaffeinated coffee beans fresh off the tree), and increase characteristics desired by consumers (eg, fruit solids, fruit sweetness, prolonged shelf life). Transgenic animals may also be modified to produce GM foods. Examples include fish that produce more α-3 fatty acids, or trout with pink muscle tissue.

Two plants that serve as sources of food oils have been modified to change their fatty acid composition (see Table 53.1). Soybeans have been modified to produce soybean oil higher in oleic acid and lower in linoleic and linolenic acids, so that use of these oils in margarines and shortenings will not require hydrogenation and the resultant production of *trans* fatty acids. This will also reduce the potential for oxidation during shelf life. The canola (rapeseed) is genetically modified to increase the content of lauric and myristic fatty acids in their oils to make them functionally useful as a replacement for lauric oils such as palm kernel oil. These modified oil-producing plants were determined by the manufacturers to not be different from their traditional counterparts in anti-nutritional factors, allergen content, and other components with potential safety concerns (eg, isoflavones in soy). To avoid confusion with the traditional plants, these plants were given distinctive names—"high oleic acid soybean oil" and "laurate canola oil."

Macronutrient Substitutes

Macronutrient substitutes are added to foods in place of their usual macronutrients (eg, fat or sugars) to provide a potential health benefit.[18] The primary functions of these ingredients are to provide calorie, fat, or sugar reduction in familiar foods. Macronutrient substitutes can also add bulk to food, provide texture, and serve as carriers for the flavors in the product. The use of these substitutes to provide health benefits for children and adolescents has been inadequately studied. As such, they should not form a significant part of a child's diet.

Carbohydrate Replacements

Carbohydrate replacements include materials that reduce carbohydrate calories without loss of sweetness, reduce the cariogenic potential of a food, and add bulking or sensory properties to compensate for reductions in sugar content. These ingredients include a range of ingredients, such as artificial sweeteners, sugar alcohols, and complex carbohydrates, that serve as bulking agents.

Artificial Sweeteners

Artificial sweeteners are many times sweeter than sugar. Therefore, it takes less of them to create the same sweetness, resulting in negligible calories to achieve the same sweetening effect. To date, 4 sugar substitutes have been approved for use in a variety of foods—saccharin, aspartame, acesulfame K, and sucralose. Several other sweeteners are under FDA review—cyclamate, neotame, and alitame.[19]

Saccharin was discovered in 1879 and was used to help compensate for sugar rationing during both world wars. Saccharin is the chemical 1,2-benzisothiazolin-3-one–1,1– dioxide ($C_7H_5NO_3S$) and specified salts. It is 300 times sweeter than sugar. Because of animal studies suggesting saccharin caused bladder cancer in rats, the FDA proposed in 1977 to ban the use of saccharin as a food additive. Congress responded by passing the Saccharin Study and Labeling Act that placed a moratorium on any ban of the sweetener while additional safety studies were conducted. Also, the law originally required that any foods containing saccharin must carry a label that stated, "Use of this product may be hazardous to your health. This product contains saccharin which has been determined to cause cancer in laboratory animals." Congress has extended the moratorium against banning the use of saccharin several times, most recently renewing it until 2002. However, in 2001, Congress repealed the requirement for the warning label.

Aspartame is the chemical 1-methyl N-L-aspartyl-L-phenylalanine ($C_{14}H_{18}N_2O_5$). Aspartame is sold under trade names such as NutraSweet and Equal. Aspartame is 180 times sweeter than sugar. Because aspartame contains phenylalanine, its use is potentially harmful to phenylketonurics. Therefore, all products containing aspartame are required to bear a warning that the product contains phenylalanine.

Acesulfame potassium, also called Acesulfame K, is also known by its trade name Sunett. It is about 200 times sweeter than sugar. Acesulfame K is the potassium salt of 6-methyl-1,2,3-oxathiazine-4(3H)-one-2,2-dioxide.

Sucralose is the chemical 1,6-dichloro-1,6-D-fructofuranosyl-4-chloro-4-deoxy-D-galactopyranoside. Sucralose is 600 times sweeter than sugar. It is also known by its trade name, Splenda. Sucralose tastes and looks like sugar because it is made from table sugar. Because it cannot be digested, it adds no calories.

Sugar Alcohols

Sugar alcohols are used as anti- or reduced-cariogenic substitutes for sugars, as reduced calorie substitutes for starch or sugar, and as bulking agents when starch or sugar is removed from foods.[18] Sugar alcohols are naturally present in fruits and vegetables. For commercial food ingredient purposes, they are generally prepared by the catalytic hydrogenation of the parent sugars.

The digestion, absorption, and metabolism of the sugar alcohols differ among the alcohols and are generally less complete than that of the parent sugars. Bioavailability in the upper gastrointestinal tract varies significantly among the alcohols. The portion of the ingested sugar alcohols that reaches the colon undergoes anerobic fermentation by the colonic microflora to product methane, hydrogen, and short-chain fatty acids. Fermentation in the colon generates some usable energy but generally less than would be obtained from the parent sugar. The production of short-chain fatty acids and lactic acid also lowers the pH of colonic material and may change the species distribution of colonic microorganisms. The reduced- and anti-cariogenic properties of sugar alcohols, as compared with the caloric sweeteners, is related to their resistance to fermentation by the oral microflora and production of reduced quantities of plaque.

Mannitol. Approximately 25% of ingested D-mannitol is absorbed via passive diffusion.[18] Once absorbed, it is oxidized by mannitol dehydrogenase or L-iditol 2-dehydrogenase to fructose and undergoes normal fructose metabolism. The net energy value of mannitol may be as low as 1.5 kcal/g.

Sorbitol. Approximately 50% of ingested sorbitol is absorbed through passive diffusion in the small intestine and up to 85% of this is metabolized.[18] Sorbitol is absorbed more slowly than glucose. When consumed in large quantities, a laxative effect may be observed. Approximately 50% of ingested sorbitol reaches the colon where it is rapidly fermented to short-chain fatty acids, hydrogen, and methane. Estimates of the caloric value of sorbitol range from 2.0 to 3.9. kcal/g.

Xylitol. The absorption of xylitol occurs by simple diffusion and from 13% to 95%.[18] The unabsorbed xylitol is completely fermented in the colon. Most of the absorbed xylitol is metabolized in the liver. The metabolizable energy from xylitol is about 2.5 to 2.9 kcal/g.

Erythritol. Erythritol has a unique metabolic fate in animals, presumably because of its low molecular weight. The sugar alcohol is almost completely absorbed in the small intestine and quantitatively excreted unchanged in the urine.[18] The result is a bulking agent with no caloric value.

Isomalt. Isomalt is an equimolar mixture of α-D-glucopyranosyl-1-6-D-sorbitol (GPS) and α-D-glucopyranosyl-1,5-mannitol (GPM).[18] Although both components are slowly hydrolyzed by various glucan 1,4-α-glucosidases, including jejunal mucosal enzymes, most of the energy derived from GPS and GPM is a result of fermentation in the colon. The caloric value is approximately 3 kcal/g.

Lactitol. Lactitol is rapidly hydrolyzed to D-galactose and D-sorbitol by microbial enzymes; however, hydrolysis in the gastrointestinal tract is slow.[18] Lactitol undergoes little or no absorption in the stomach or small intestine. Lactitol in the colon is readily fermented. Lactitol is estimated to provide approximately 2 kcal/g.

Maltitol. In the stomach, maltitol is hydrolyzed to glucose and sorbitol, both of which are readily absorbed.[18] A substantial portion of maltitol reaches the large intestine and is fermented to short-chain fatty acids. The net energy value for maltitol is approximately 3 kcal/g.

Other Carbohydrate Bulking Agents

Carbohydrate-based bulking agents can be used to replace sugar, starch, or fat in foods. Low molecular weight materials (eg, polydextrose) are used as sucrose replacements in syrup confections and baked product applications.[18] Some complex mixtures of carbohydrate polymers can function as low-calorie bulking agents because of their ability to hold several times their weight and, thus, reduce the amount of carbohydrate or fat in a food (eg, gums). Some of these complex carbohydrate polymer mixtures also are measured analytically as dietary fibers (eg, cellulose, hemicelluloses, pectins, gums, mucilages, and lignins). The bulk provided by some of these polymers reduces transit time in the bowel. The complex carbohydrate bulking agents are poorly digested by normal gastrointestinal enzymes in the upper gastrointestinal tract, but many are fermented by the colonic microflora to shorter chain fatty acids.

Reduced Starch Hydrolysates are mixtures of monomeric, dimeric, and oligomeric polyols.[18] They are prepared by partial hydrolysis of starch followed by hydrogenation. On ingestion, they are hydrolyzed to glucose, sorbitol, and maltitol, with insignificant portions of the hydrolysis products reaching the colon. Their rate of absorption and metabolism is similar to maltitol but slower than sorbitol. Where the hydrogenated starch hydrolysates reach the colon, they are completely fermented to short-chain fatty acids. The net energy value of the hydrolysates is approximately 3 to 4 kcal/g.

Polydextrose is a low molecular weight, randomly bonded polymer of glucose, sorbitol, and citric or phosphoric acid.[18,20] Polydextrose is only partially metabolized by humans and is not fermented by the colonic microflora. The caloric availability of polydextrose in humans is 1 kcal/g. Laxation can occur when polydextrose is consumed at high levels; thus, food products delivering more than 15 g per serving must be labeled accordingly.

Pectins are complex galacturonoglycans composed primarily of polymers of D-galacturonic acid. Frequently, the polymers include arabinans, arabinogalactan, and galactans. Pectins are found primarily in the cell walls of plants. Pectins are slowly degraded and fermented by microflora in the large intestine and colon.

β-Glucans are complex carbohydrate materials composed of glucose polymers containing both $\beta(1\rightarrow3)$ and $\beta(1\rightarrow4)$ linkages.[18] Barley and oats are both excellent sources of β-glucans. Concentrated amounts of β-glucans in oats have been marketed commercially as Oatrim.[18,20] The mouthfeel of this ingredient mimics that of triglycerides, thus serving as a lower calorie alternative to fats.

Galactomannans are complex carbohydrate bulking agents composed of $\beta(1\rightarrow4)$-D-mannopyranosyl chains with $\beta(1\rightarrow6)$-D galactopyranosyl units attached at carbon 6 of the mannoses.[18] Major sources of galactomannan are guar gum and carob gum. These are frequently used in low-calorie foods to emulate the texture of the fat that has been removed.

Cellulose refers to a group of complex carbohydrates whose primary structure is a $\beta(1\rightarrow4)$ glucan.[18] It also includes a number of chemically modified celluloses (eg, carboxymethylcellulose, microcrystalline cellulose, and methyl-cellulose). The derivatized celluloses can be used in foods as functional bulking agents, binders, stabilizers in frozen food systems, and thickeners. Cellulose acts as a noncaloric insoluble bulking agent and fat mimetic in a variety of food applications.

Resistant starch is indigestible.[18] Its resistance occurs in several ways. The cell wall of the plant may make the starch inaccessible for digestive enzymes (eg, milled grains and seeds). Differences in the crystalline patterns of starch in the granule can affect its susceptibility to enzymatic digestion (eg, raw bananas and potato starch). Finally, cooking or processing resistant starch-containing foods may initially make the resistant starch digestible (eg, potatoes, cereals, legumes). However, upon cooling, the starch can recrystallize to an indigestible form. Resistant starch content is high in food products processed under relatively high moisture contents such as boiling, baking, or autoclaving. Significant amounts of resistant starch may escape digestion in the small intestine and pass into the colon where it is fermented. Resistant starch in the large intestine may share some of the health benefits attributed to dietary fiber.

Fat Replacers

Three types of substitutes have been developed to replace fat.[18,20] Fat mimetics are proteins or carbohydrates that imitate the organoleptic or physical properties of fat. Therefore, they provide 4 kcal/g rather than the 9 kcal/g provided by food fats. Fat substitutes are synthetic or enzymatically modified lipids that chemically resemble conventional fats. They can replace food fat on a gram for gram basis while providing no, or significantly fewer, calories than food fat. Structured triglycerides are similar to conventional fats in that they contain fatty acids attached to a glycerol backbone. However, they are designed to provide fewer calories than normal (<9 kcal/g) by substituting poorly absorbed fatty acids and short-chain fatty acids with lower caloric value than the usual fatty acids found in foods.[18,20]

Fat Mimetics

The typical constituents of fat mimetics are carbohydrates (eg, starch, cellulose, pectin, protein, hydrophilic colloids, dextrins, polydextrose) (see earlier discussions on carbohydrate ingredients) and proteins (eg, egg, milk, whey, soy, gelatin, and wheat gluten).[18,20] These materials are frequently microparticulated to emulate the particle size and mouthfeel of emulsified fats. Most of the fat mimetic materials are fully digestible, providing 4 kcal/g as compared to the

9 kcal/g for the food fats they replace. However, some mimetics are not digested (eg, cellulose, seaweed, some gums) so they contribute no calories. Many fat mimetics are highly hydrated; thus, part of the caloric advantage comes from the replacement of fat with water. One of the mimetics, Simplesse, is manufactured from whey protein concentrate by a patented microparticulation process. It retains any antigenic/allergenic properties of the parent protein.

Fat Substitutes

Fat substitutes are macromolecules that can replace food fat on a one-to-one basis.[18,20] Olestra is one example of a fat substitute. Olestra contains a mixture of octa-, hepta-, and hexa-esters of sucrose with fatty acids derived from edible fats and oils. It is formed by chemical transesterification or interesterification of sucrose with 6 to 8 conventional food fatty acids. Because humans lack enzymes to break the sucrose/fatty acid bonds, Olestra is not absorbed or metabolized. Therefore, Olestra provides no calories. However, because this is a non-absorbed lipid, products containing Olestra are required to add vitamins A, D, E, and K to compensate for any interference with the absorption of these fat-soluble vitamins. These added nutrients, since they are unlikely to be physiologically available, will not be considered in nutrient declarations in the food label Nutrition Facts box but will be listed in the ingredient list. Products are also required to carry a warning label for potential gastrointestinal effects.

Structured Lipids

Structured lipids are triglycerides that are designed to provide fewer than 9 kcal/g.[18,20] Examples of structured lipids include Caprenin (Procter and Gamble), Salatrim (Nabisco/Cultour), and medium-chain triglycerides.

Caprenin is a reduced-calorie fat. Its caloric reduction is achieved by esterifying 2 medium-chain fatty acids (caprylic and capric) and behenic acid to a glycerol backbone. Because behenic acid is only partially absorbed and caprylic and capric acids are more readily metabolized than other longer-chain fatty acids, caprenin provides only 5 kcal/g.

Salatrim represents a family of low-calorie fats composed of a mixture containing at least one short-chain fatty acid (eg, C2:0, C3:0, C4:0) and at least one long-chain fatty acid (predominately C18:0) attached to the glycerol backbone.[18,20] Because short-chain fatty acids have a lower caloric value than long-chain fatty acids, and because stearic acid is incompletely absorbed, the caloric value of Salatrim is about five ninths the value of conventional fats.

Medium-chain triglycerides predominately contain saturated fatty acids of chain length C8:0 (caprylic) and C11:0 (capric) with traces of C6:0 and

C12:0 fatty acids.[18,20] Medium-chain triglycerides are absorbed intact into the intestine as free fatty acids, without the need for enzymes or bile salts. They bind to serum albumin and are transported to the liver via the portal system. They are oxidized to ketone bodies in the liver. They are less likely to be stored in adipose tissue. They have been used clinically in enteral and parenteral diets for individuals with lipid absorption, digestion, or transport disorders. They provide about 8.3 kcal/g.

References

1. US Food and Drug Administration. Statement of policy: foods derived from new plant varieties. *Fed Regist.* 1992;57:22964–23001

2. US Food and Drug Administration. Premarket notice concerning bioengineeered foods; proposed rule. *Fed Regist.* 2001;66:4706–4738

3. Institute of Food Technologies. Introduction. In: *IFT Expert Report on Biotechnology and Foods.* Chicago, IL: Institute of Food Technologies; 2000

4. National Research Council, Board on Agriculture and Natural Resources, Committee on Genetically Modified Pest-Protected Plants. *Genetically Modified Pest-Protected Plants: Science and Regulation.* Washington, DC: National Academy Press; 2000

5. Formanek R Jr. Proposed rules issued for bioengineered foods. *FDA Consumer Magazine.* March-April 2001. Available at: http://www.fda.gov/fdac/features/2001/201_food.html. Accessed May 16, 2003

6. IFT expert report on biotechnology and foods. Human food safety evaluation of rDNA biotechnology-derived foods. *Food Technology.* 2000;54:53–61

7. Joint FAO/WHO Expert Consultation on Foods Derived from Biotechnology. *Safety Aspects of Genetically Modified Foods of Plant Origin.* Geneva, Switzerland: World Health Organization; 2000. Available at: http://www.who.int/fsf/GMfood/FAOWHO_Consultation_report_2000.html. Accessed April 17, 2003

8. US Food and Drug Administration. *Guidance for Industry: Use of Antibiotic Resistance Marker Genes in Transgenic Plants.* September 4, 1998. Available at: http://vm.cfsan.fda.gov/~dms/opa-armg.html. Accessed May 16, 2003

9. World Health Organization. *Health Aspects of Marker Genes in Genetically Modified Plants.* Report of WHO Workshop. Geneva, Switzerland: World Health Organization; 1993. Publication WHO/FNU/FOS/93.6

10. Aminoglycoside 3′-phosphotransferase II. 21 CFR §173.170

11. US Food and Drug Administration. *List of Completed Consultations on Bioengineered Foods.* October 2002. Available at: http://vm.cfsan.fda.gov/~lrd/biocon.html. Accessed April 16, 2003

12. Institute of Food Technologies. Benefits and concerns associated with recombinant DNA biotechnology-derived foods. In: *IFT Expert Report on Biotechnology and Foods.* Chicago, IL: Institute of Food Technologies; 2000

13. US Food and Drug Administration. *Report on the Food and Drug Administration's Review of the Safety of Recombinant Bovine Somatotropin.* Available at: http://www.fda.gov/ cvm/index/bst/rbrptfnl.htm. Accessed May 16, 2003

14. US Food and Drug Administration, Center for Veterinary Medicine. *CVM Update: Update on Human Food Safety of BST.* February 5, 1999. Available at: http://www.fda.gov/cvm/index/updates/bstsafup.html. Accessed May 16, 2003

15. US Environmental Protection Agency. *Biotechnology Corn Approved for Continued Use.* October 16, 2001. Available at: http://yosemite1.epa.gov/opa/admpress.nsf/b1ab9f485b098972852562e7004dc686/8db7a83e66e0f7d085256ae7005d6ec2?OpenDocument. Accessed May 16, 2003

16. US Food and Drug Administration. *Questions and Answers About Transgenic Fish.* Available at: http://www.fda.gov/cvm/index/consumer/transgen.htm. Accessed May 16, 2003

17. Lewis C. A new kind of fish story: the coming of biotech animals. *FDA Consumer Magazine.* January-February, 2001. Available at: http://www.fda.gov/fdac/features/2001/101_fish.html. Accessed May 16, 2003

18. Finley JW, Leveille GA. Macronutrient substitutes. In: Ziegler EE, Filer LJ Jr, eds. *Present Knowledge in Nutrition.* 7th ed. Washington, DC: International Life Sciences Institute; 1996:581–595

19. Henken J. Sugar substitutes: Americans opt for sweetness and lite. US Food and Drug Administration. *FDA Consumer Magazine.* November-December 1999

20. Akoh CC. Fat replacers: scientific status summary. *Food Technology.* 1998;52:47–53

Appendix A

Table A–1.
Representative Values for Constituents of Human Milk*

CONSTITUENT (Per Liter)*	EARLY MILK (<28 d postpartum)	MATURE MILK (≥28 d postpartum)
Energy (kcal)		650–700
Carbohydrate		
Lactose (g)	20–30	67
Glucose (g)	0.2–1.0	0.2–0.3
Oligosaccharides (g)	22–24	12–14
Total Nitrogen (g)	3.0	1.9
Nonprotein nitrogen (g)	0.5	0.45
Protein nitrogen (g)	2.5	1.45
Total Protein (g)	16	9–12.6
Total casein (g)		
β-casein (g)	3.8	5.7
κ-casein (g)	2.6	4.4
Whey proteins		6.7
α-Lactalbumin (g)	3.62	3.26
Lactoferrin (g)	3.53	1.94
Serum albumin (g)	0.39	0.41
SIgA (g)	2.0	1.0
IgM (g)	0.12	0.2
IgG (g)	0.34	0.05
Amino Acids (g)†		
Alanine	0.65–1.71	0.26–0.42
Arginine	1.16–1.42	0.25–0.40
Aspartic acid	1.18–3.52	0.54–0.92
Cystine	0.47–1.41	0.11–0.23

Table A–1.
Representative Values for Constituents of Human Milk*, *continued*

CONSTITUENT (Per Liter)*	EARLY MILK (<28 d postpartum)	MATURE MILK (≥28 d postpartum)
Glutamic acid+glutamine	2.03–4.75	1.26–1.97
Glycine	0.36–1.42	0.10–0.27
Histidine	0.41–0.67	0.15–0.25
Isoleucine	0.43–1.27	0.33–0.57
Leucine	1.48–2.80	0.82–0.94
Lysine	0.72–2.06	0.30–0.90
Methionine	0.16–0.45	0.09–0.19
Phenylalanine	0.50–1.52	0.26–0.36
Proline	0.93–2.51	0.57–1.05
Serine	1.27–2.59	0.42–0.62
Threonine	0.65–1.94	0.32–0.42
Tryptophan	0.25–0.42	0.09–0.17
Tyrosine	0.76–0.54	0.31–0.47
Valine	0.88–1.66	0.35–0.51
Total Lipids (%)	2	3.5
Triglyceride (% total lipids)	97–98	97–98
Cholesterol‡ (% total lipids)	0.7–1.3	0.4–0.5
Phospholipids (% total lipids)	1.1	0.6–0.8
Fatty Acids (weight %)	88	88
Total % saturated fatty acids	43–44	44–45
C12:0		5
C14:0		6
C16:0		20
C18:0		8
Total % monounsaturated fatty acids		40
C18: 1ω-9	32	31
Total % polyunsaturated acids (PUFA)	13	14–15

Table A–1.
Representative Values for Constituents of Human Milk*, *continued*

CONSTITUENT (Per Liter)*	EARLY MILK (<28 d postpartum)	MATURE MILK (≥28 d postpartum)
Total ω-3	1.5	1.5
C18: 3ω-3	0.7	0.9
C22: 5ω-3	0.2	0.1
C22: 6ω-3	0.5	0.2
Total ω-6	11.6	13.06
C18: 2ω-6	8.9	11.3
C20: 4ω-6	0.7	0.5
C22: 4ω-6	0.2	0.1
Water-Soluble Vitamins		
Ascorbic Acid (mg)		80–100
Thiamin (μg)	20	200
Riboflavin (μg)		400–600
Niacin (mg)	0.5	1.8–6.0
Vitamin B_6 (mg)		0.09–0.31
Folate (μg)		80–140
Vitamin B_{12} (μg)		0.5–1.0
Pantothenic Acid (mg)		2.0–2.5
Biotin (μg)		5–9
Fat-Soluble Vitamins		
Retinol (mg)	2	0.3–0.6
Carotenoids (mg)	2	0.2–0.6
Vitamin K (μg)	2–5	2–3
Vitamin D (μg)		0.33
Vitamin E (mg)	8–12	3–8
Major Minerals		
Calcium (mg)	250	200–250
Magnesium (mg)	30–35	30–35

Table A–1.
Representative Values for Constituents of Human Milk*, *continued*

CONSTITUENT (Per Liter)*	EARLY MILK (<28 d postpartum)	MATURE MILK (≥28 d postpartum)
Phosphorus (mg)	120–160	120–140
Sodium (mg)	300–400	120–250
Potassium (mg)	600–700	400–550
Chloride (mg)	600–800	400–450
Trace Minerals		
Iron (mg)	0.5–1.0	0.3–0.9
Zinc (mg)	8–12	1–3
Copper (mg)	0.5–0.8	0.2–0.4
Manganese (mg)	5–6	3
Selenium (mg)	40	7–33
Iodine (mg)		150
Fluoride (mg)		4–15

*All nutrient values except for amino acids are adapted from Picciano MF. Appendix: Representative values for constituents of human milk. *Pediatr Clin North Am.* 2001;48:263–272.

The values are expressed per liter of milk with the exception of lipids that are expressed as a percentage on the basis of milk volume or weight of total lipids. Values are expressed as mean values or ranges of means.

†Adapted from George DR, De Francesca BA. Human milk in comparison to cow milk. In: Lebenthal E, ed. *Textbook of Gastroenterology and Nutrition in Infancy and Childhood.* 2nd ed. New York, NY: Raven Press; 1989:242–243.

‡The cholesterol content of human milk ranges from 100 to 200 mg/L in most samples of human milk after day 21 of lactation.

Appendix B

Table B–1.
Cytotoxic Drugs That May Interfere With Cellular Metabolism of the Nursing Infant

Drug	Reason for Concern, Reported Sign or Symptom in Infant, or Effect on Lactation	Reference No.
Cyclophosphamide	Possible immune suppression; unknown effect on growth or association with carcinogenesis; neutropenia	26, 27
Cyclosporine	Possible immune suppression; unknown effect on growth or association with carcinogenesis	28, 29
Doxorubicin*	Possible immune suppression; unknown effect on growth or association with carcinogenesis	30
Methotrexate	Possible immune suppression; unknown effect on growth or association with carcinogenesis; neutropenia	31

* Drug is concentrated in human milk.

Table B–2.
Drugs of Abuse for Which Adverse Effects on the Infant During Breastfeeding Have Been Reported*

Drug	Reported Effect or Reasons for Concern	Reference No.
Amphetamine†	Irritability, poor sleeping pattern	32
Cocaine	Cocaine intoxication: irritability, vomiting, diarrhea, tremulousness, seizures	33
Heroin	Tremors, restlessness, vomiting, poor feeding	34
Marijuana	Only 1 report in literature; no effect mentioned; very long half-life for some components	35
Phencyclidine	Potent hallucinogen	36

*The Committee on Drugs strongly believes that nursing mothers should not ingest drugs of abuse, because they are hazardous to the nursing infant and to the health of the mother.
†Drug is concentrated in human milk.

Table B–3.
Radioactive Compounds That Require Temporary Cessation of Breastfeeding*

Compound	Recommended Time for Cessation of Breastfeeding	Reference No.
Copper 64 (^{64}Cu)	Radioactivity in milk present at 50 h	37
Gallium 67 (^{67}Ga)	Radioactivity in milk present for 2 wk	38
Indium 111 (^{111}In)	Very small amount present at 20 h	39
Iodine 123 (^{123}I)	Radioactivity in milk present up to 36 h	40, 41
Iodine 125 (^{125}I)	Radioactivity in milk present for 12 d	42
Iodine 131 (^{131}I)	Radioactivity in milk present 2–14 d, depending on study	43–46
Iodine[131]	If used for treatment of thyroid cancer, high radioactivity may prolong exposure to infant	47, 48
Radioactive sodium	Radioactivity in milk present 96 h	49
Technetium 99m (^{99m}Tc), ^{99m}Tc macroaggregates, ^{99m}Tc O$_4$	Radioactivity in milk present 15 h to 3 d	41, 50–55

*Consult nuclear medicine physician before performing diagnostic study so that radionuclide that has the shortest excretion time in breast milk can be used. Before study, the mother should pump her breast and store enough milk in the freezer for feeding the infant; after study, the mother should pump her breast to maintain milk production but discard all milk pumped for the required time that radioactivity is present in milk. Milk samples can be screened by radiology departments for radioactivity before resumption of nursing.

Table B–4.
Drugs for Which the Effect on Nursing Infants Is Unknown but May Be of Concern*

Drug	Reported or Possible Effect	Reference No.
Anti-anxiety		
Alprazolam	None	57
Diazepam	None	58–62
Lorazepam	None	63
Midazolam	–	64
Perphenazine	None	65
Prazepam†	None	66
Quazepam	None	67
Temazepam	–	68
Antidepressants		
Amitriptyline	None	69, 70
Amoxapine	None	71
Bupropion	None	72
Clomipramine	None	73
Desipramine	None	74, 75

Table B–4.
Drugs for Which the Effect on Nursing Infants Is Unknown but May Be of Concern*, *continued*

Drug	Reported or Possible Effect	Reference No.
Dothiepin	None	76, 77
Doxepin	None	78
Fluoxetine	Colic, irritability, feeding and sleep disorders, slow weight gain	79–87
Fluvoxamine	–	88
Imipramine	None	74
Nortriptyline	None	89, 90
Paroxetine	None	91
Sertraline†	None	92, 93
Trazodone	None	94
Antipsychotic		
Chlorpromazine	Galactorrhea in mother; drowsiness and lethargy in infant; decline in developmental scores	95–98
Chlorprothixene	None	99
Clozapine†	None	100
Haloperidol	Decline in developmental scores	101–104
Mesoridazine	None	105
Trifluoperazine	None	104
OTHERS		
Amiodarone	Possible hypothyroidism	106
Chloramphenicol	Possible idiosyncratic bone marrow suppression	107, 108
Clofazimine	Potential for transfer of high percentage of maternal dose; possible increase in skin pigmentation	109
Lamotrigine	Potential therapeutic serum concentrations in infant	110
Metoclopramide†	None described; dopaminergic blocking agent	111, 112
Metronidazole	In vitro mutagen; may discontinue breastfeeding for 12–24 h to allow excretion of dose when single-dose therapy given to mother	113, 114
Tinidazole	See metronidazole	115

*Psychotropic drugs, the compounds listed under anti-anxiety, antidepressant, and antipsychotic categories, are of special concern when given to nursing mothers for long periods. Although there are very few case reports of adverse effects in breastfeeding infants, these drugs do appear in human milk and, thus, could conceivably alter short-term and long-term central nervous system function.[56] See discussion in text of psychotropic drugs.
†Drug is concentrated in human milk relative to simultaneous maternal plasma concentrations.

Table B–5.
Drugs That Have Been Associated With Significant Effects on Some Nursing Infants and Should Be Given to Nursing Mothers With Caution*

Drug	Reported Effect	Reference No.
Acebutolol	Hypotension; bradycardia; tachypnea	116
5-Aminosalicylic acid	Diarrhea (1 case)	117–119
Atenolol	Cyanosis; bradycardia	120–124
Bromocriptine	Suppresses lactation; may be hazardous to the mother	125, 126
Aspirin (salicylates)	Metabolic acidosis (1 case)	127–129
Clemastine	Drowsiness, irritability, refusal to feed, high-pitched cry, neck stiffness (1 case)	130
Ergotamine	Vomiting, diarrhea, convulsions (doses used in migraine medications)	131
Lithium	One-third to one-half therapeutic blood concentration in infants	132–134
Phenindione	Anticoagulant: increased prothrombin and partial thromboplastin time in 1 infant; not used in United States	135
Phenobarbital	Sedation; infantile spasms after weaning from milk containing phenobarbital, methemoglobinemia (1 case)	136–140
Primidone	Sedation, feeding problems	136, 137
Sulfasalazine (salicylazosulfapyridine)	Bloody diarrhea (1 case)	141

* Blood concentration in the infant may be of clinical importance.

Table B–6.
Maternal Medication Usually Compatible With Breastfeeding*

Drug	Reported Sign or Symptom in Infant or Effect on Lactation	Reference No.
Acetaminophen	None	142–144
Acetazolamide	None	145
Acitretin	–	146
Acyclovir†	None	147, 148
Alcohol (ethanol)	With large amounts, drowsiness, diaphoresis, deep sleep, weakness, decrease in linear growth, abnormal weight gain; maternal ingestion of 1 g/kg daily decreases milk ejection reflex	4, 149–152

Table B–6.
Maternal Medication Usually Compatible With Breastfeeding*, *continued*

Drug	Reported Sign or Symptom in Infant or Effect on Lactation	Reference No.
Allopurinol	–	153
Amoxicillin	None	154
Antimony	–	155
Atropine	None	156
Azapropazone (apazone)	–	157
Aztreonam	None	158
B$_1$ (thiamin)	None	159
B$_6$ (pyridoxine)	None	160–162
B$_{12}$	None	163
Baclofen	None	164
Barbiturate	See Table B–5	
Bendroflumethia-zide	Suppresses lactation	165
Bishydroxycoum-arin (dicumarol)	None	166
Bromide	Rash, weakness, absence of cry with maternal intake of 5.4 g/d	167
Butorphanol	None	168
Caffeine	Irritability, poor sleeping pattern, excreted slowly; no effect with moderate intake of caffeinated beverages (2–3 cups per day)	169–174
Captopril	None	175
Carbamazepine	None	176, 177
Carbetocin	None	178
Carbimazole	Goiter	83, 179, 180
Cascara	None	181
Cefadroxil	None	154
Cefazolin	None	182
Cefotaxime	None	183
Cefoxitin	None	183
Cefprozil	–	184
Ceftazidime	None	185

Table B–6.
Maternal Medication Usually Compatible With Breastfeeding*, *continued*

Drug	Reported Sign or Symptom in Infant or Effect on Lactation	Reference No.
Ceftriaxone	None	186
Chloral hydrate	Sleepiness	187
Chloroform	None	188
Chloroquine	None	189–191
Chlorothiazide	None	192, 193
Chlorthalidone	Excreted slowly	194
Cimetidine†	None	195, 196
Ciprofloxacin	None	197, 198
Cisapride	None	199
Cisplatin	Not found in milk	30
Clindamycin	None	200
Clogestone	None	201
Codeine	None	144, 156, 202
Colchicine	–	203–205
Contraceptive pill with estrogen/ progesterone	Rare breast enlargement; decrease in milk production and protein content (not confirmed in several studies)	206–213
Cycloserine	None	214
D (vitamin)	None; follow up infant's serum calcium level if mother receives pharmacologic doses	215–217
Danthron	Increased bowel activity	218
Dapsone	None; sulfonamide detected in infant's urine	191, 219
Dexbromphenira- mine maleate with *d*-isoephedrine	Crying, poor sleeping patterns, irritability	220
Diatrizoate	None	221
Digoxin	None	222, 223
Diltiazem	None	224
Dipyrone	None	225
Disopyramide	None	226, 227
Domperidone	None	228
Dyphylline†	None	229
Enalapril	–	230

Table B–6.
Maternal Medication Usually Compatible With Breastfeeding*, *continued*

Drug	Reported Sign or Symptom in Infant or Effect on Lactation	Reference No.
Erythromycin†	None	231
Estradiol	Withdrawal, vaginal bleeding	232
Ethambutol	None	214
Ethanol (cf. Alcohol)	–	
Ethosuximide	None, drug appears in infant serum	176, 233
Fentanyl	–	234
Fexofenadine	None	235
Flecainide	–	236, 237
Fleroxacin	One 400-mg dose given to nursing mothers; infants not given breast milk for 48 h	238
Fluconazole	None	239
Flufenamic acid	None	240
Fluorescein	–	241
Folic acid	None	242
Gadopentetic (Gadolinium)	None	243
Gentamicin	None	244
Gold salts	None	245–249
Halothane	None	250
Hydralazine	None	251
Hydrochlorothiazide	–	192, 193
Hydroxychloroquine†	None	252, 253
Ibuprofen	None	254, 255
Indomethacin	Seizure (1 case)	256–258
Iodides	May affect thyroid activity; see iodine	259
Iodine	Goiter	259
Iodine (povidone-iodine, eg, in a vaginal douche)	Elevated iodine levels in breast milk, odor of iodine on infant's skin	259
Iohexol	None	97
Iopanoic acid	None	260

Table B–6.
Maternal Medication Usually Compatible With Breastfeeding*, *continued*

Drug	Reported Sign or Symptom in Infant or Effect on Lactation	Reference No.
Isoniazid	None; acetyl (hepatotoxic) metabolite secreted but no hepatotoxicity reported in infants	214, 261
Interferon-α	–	262
Ivermectin	None	263, 264
K_1 (vitamin)	None	265, 266
Kanamycin	None	214
Ketoconazole	None	267
Ketorolac	–	268
Labetalol	None	269, 270
Levonorgestrel	–	271–274
Levothyroxine	None	275
Lidocaine	None	276
Loperamide	–	277
Loratadine	None	278
Magnesium sulfate	None	279
Medroxyprogesterone	None	201, 280
Mefenamic acid	None	281
Meperidine	None	61, 282
Methadone	None	283–287
Methimazole (active metabolite of carbimazole)	None	288, 289
Methohexital	None	61
Methyldopa	None	290
Methyprylon	Drowsiness	291
Metoprolol†	None	120
Metrizamide	None	292
Metrizoate	None	97
Mexiletine	None	293, 294
Minoxidil	None	295
Morphine	None; infant may have measurable blood concentration	282, 296–298
Moxalactam	None	299

Table B–6.
Maternal Medication Usually Compatible With Breastfeeding*, *continued*

Drug	Reported Sign or Symptom in Infant or Effect on Lactation	Reference No.
Nadolol†	None	300
Nalidixic acid	Hemolysis in infant with glucose-6-phosphate dehydrogenase (G-6-PD) deficiency	301
Naproxen	–	302
Nefopam	None	303
Nifedipine	–	304
Nitrofurantoin	Hemolysis in infant with G-6-PD deficiency	305
Norethynodrel	None	306
Norsteroids	None	307
Noscapine	None	308
Ofloxacin	None	198
Oxprenolol	None	309, 310
Phenylbutazone	None	311
Phenytoin	Methemoglobinemia (1 case)	138, 176, 312
Piroxicam	None	313
Prednisolone	None	314, 315
Prednisone	None	316
Procainamide	None	317
Progesterone	None	318
Propoxyphene	None	319
Propranolol	None	320–322
Propylthiouracil	None	323
Pseudoephedrine†	None	324
Pyridostigmine	None	325
Pyrimethamine	None	326
Quinidine	None	191, 327
Quinine	None	296
Riboflavin	None	159
Rifampin	None	214
Scopolamine	–	156
Secobarbital	None	328
Senna	None	329

Table B–6.
Maternal Medication Usually Compatible With Breastfeeding*, *continued*

Drug	Reported Sign or Symptom in Infant or Effect on Lactation	Reference No.
Sotalol	–	237, 330
Spironolactone	None	331
Streptomycin	None	214
Sulbactam	None	332
Sulfapyridine	Caution in infant with jaundice or G-6-PD deficiency and ill, stressed, or premature infant; appears in infant's milk	333, 334
Sulfisoxazole	Caution in infant with jaundice or G-6-PD deficiency and ill, stressed, or premature infant; appears in infant's milk	335
Sumatriptan	None	336
Suprofen	None	337
Terbutaline	None	338
Terfenadine	None	235
Tetracycline	None; negligible absorption by infant	339, 340
Theophylline	Irritability	169, 341
Thiopental	None	139, 342
Thiouracil	None mentioned; drug not used in United States	343
Ticarcillin	None	344
Timolol	None	310
Tolbutamide	Possible jaundice	345
Tolmetin	None	346
Trimethoprim/ sulfamethoxazole	None	347, 348
Triprolidine	None	324
Valproic acid	None	176, 349, 350
Verapamil	None	351
Warfarin	None	352
Zolpidem	None	353

* Drugs listed have been reported in the literature as having the effects listed or no effect. The word "none" means that no observable change was seen in the nursing infant while the mother was ingesting the compound. Dashes indicate no mention of clinical effect on the infant. It is emphasized that many of the literature citations concern single case reports or small series of infants.
† Drug is concentrated in human milk.

Table B–7.
Food and Environmental Agents: Effects on Breastfeeding

Agent	Reported Sign or Symptom in Infant or Effect on Lactation	Reference No.
Aflatoxin	None	354–356
Aspartame	Caution if mother or infant has phenylketonuria	357
Bromide (photographic laboratory)	Potential absorption and bromide transfer into milk; see Table B–6	358
Cadmium	None reported	359
Chlordane	None reported	360
Chocolate (theobromine)	Irritability or increased bowel activity if excess amounts (≥16 oz/d) consumed by mother	169, 361
DDT, benzene hexachlorides, dieldrin, aldrin, hepatachlorepoxide	None	362–370
Fava beans	Hemolysis in patient with G-6-PD deficiency	371
Fluorides	None	372, 373
Hexachlorobenzene	Skin rash, diarrhea, vomiting, dark urine, neurotoxicity, death	374, 375
Hexachlorophene	None; possible contamination of milk from nipple washing	376
Lead	Possible neurotoxicity	377–380
Mercury, methylmercury	May affect neurodevelopment	381–383
Methylmethacrylate	None	384
Monosodium glutamate	None	385
Polychlorinated biphenyls and polybrominated biphenyls	Lack of endurance, hypotonia, sullen, expressionless facies	386–390
Silicone	Esophageal dysmotility	17–22
Tetrachloroethylene cleaning fluid (perchloroethylene)	Obstructive jaundice, dark urine	391
Vegetarian diet	Signs of B_{12} deficiency	392

References

1. American Academy of Pediatrics, Committee on Drugs. The transfer of drugs and other chemicals into human breast milk. *Pediatrics.* 1983;72:375–383
2. American Academy of Pediatrics, Committee on Drugs. Transfer of drugs and other·chemicals into human milk. *Pediatrics.* 1989;84:924–936

3. American Academy of Pediatrics, Committee on Drugs. Transfer of drugs and other chemicals into human milk. *Pediatrics*. 1994;93:137–150

4. Bisdom W. Alcohol and nicotine poisoning in nurslings. *JAMA*. 1937;109:178

5. Ferguson BB, Wilson DJ, Schaffner W. Determination of nicotine concentrations in human milk. *Am J Dis Child*. 1976;130:837–839

6. Luck W, Nau H. Nicotine and cotinine concentrations in the milk of smoking mothers: influence of cigarette consumption and diurnal variation. *Eur J Pediatr*. 1987;146:21–26

7. Luck W, Nau H. Nicotine and cotinine concentrations in serum and milk of nursing mothers. *Br J Clin Pharmacol*. 1984;18:9–15

8. Luck W, Nau H. Nicotine and cotinine concentrations in serum and urine of infants exposed via passive smoking or milk from smoking mothers. *J Pediatr*. 1985;107:816–820

9. Labrecque M, Marcoux S, Weber JP, Fabia J, Ferron L. Feeding and urine cotinine values in babies whose mothers smoke. *Pediatrics*. 1989;83:93–97

10. Schwartz-Bickenbach D, Schulte-Hobein B, Abt S, Plum C, Nau H. Smoking and passive smoking during pregnancy and early infancy: effects on birth weight, lactation period, and cotinine concentrations in mother's milk and infant's urine. *Toxicol Lett*. 1987;35:73–81

11. Schulte-Hobein B, Schwartz-Bickenbach D, Abt S, Plum C, Nau H. Cigarette smoke exposure and development of infants throughout the first year of life: influence of passive smoking and nursing on cotinine levels in breast milk and infant's urine. *Acta Paediatr*. 1992;81:550–557

12. Hopkinson JM, Schanler RJ, Fraley JK, Garza C. Milk production by mothers of premature infants: influence of cigarette smoking. *Pediatrics*. 1992;90:934–938

13. Little RE, Lambert MD III, Worthington-Roberts B, Ervin CH. Maternal smoking during lactation: relation to infant size at one year of age. *Am J Epidemiol*. 1994;140:544–554

14. Boshuizen HC, Verkerk PH, Reerink JD, Herngreen WP, Zaadstra BM, Verloove-Vanhorick SP. Maternal smoking during lactation: relation to growth during the first year of life in a Dutch birth cohort. *Am J Epidemiol*. 1998;147:117–126

15. Steldinger R, Luck W, Nau H. Half lives of nicotine in milk of smoking mothers: implications for nursing. *J Perinat Med*. 1988;16:261–262

16. Woodward A, Douglas RM, Graham NM, Miles H. Acute respiratory illness in Adelaide children: breast feeding modifies the effect of passive smoking. *J Epidemiol Community Health*. 1990;44:224–230

17. Levine JJ, Ilowite NT. Sclerodermalike esophageal disease in children breast-fed by mothers with silicone breast implants. *JAMA*. 1994;271:213–216

18. Levine JJ, Trachtman H, Gold DM, Pettei MJ. Esophageal dysmotility in children breast-fed by mothers with silicone breast implants: long-term follow-up and response to treatment. *Dig Dis Sci*. 1996;41:1600–1603

19. LeVier RR, Harrison MC, Cook RR, Lane TH. What is silicone? *Plast Reconstr Surg.* 1993;92:163–167
20. Berlin CM Jr. Silicone breast implants and breast-feeding. *Pediatrics.* 1994;94:547–549
21. Kjoller K, Mclaughlin JK, Friis S, et al. Health outcomes in offspring of mothers with breast implants. *Pediatrics.* 1998;102:1112–1115
22. Semple JL, Lugowski SJ, Baines CJ, Smith DC, McHugh A. Breast milk contamination and silicone implants: preliminary results using silicon as a proxy measurement for silicone. *Plast Reconstr Surg.* 1998;102:528–533
23. *Physicians' Desk Reference.* Montvale, NJ: Medical Economics Company; 2001
24. US Pharmacopeia. *USP DI 2001: Information for the Health Care Professional, Volume I.* Hutchinson TA, ed. Englewood, CO: Micromedex; 2001
25. US Pharmacopeia. *USP Dictionary of USAN and International Drug Names.* Rockville, MD: US Pharmacopeia; 2000
26. Wiernik PH, Duncan JH. Cyclophosphamide in human milk. *Lancet.* 1971;1:912
27. Amato D, Niblett JS. Neutropenia from cyclophosphamide in breast milk. *Med J Aust.* 1977;1:383–384
28. Flechner SM, Katz AR, Rogers AJ, Van Buren C, Kahan BD. The presence of cyclosporine in body tissue and fluids during pregnancy. *Am J Kidney Dis.* 1985;5:60–63
29. Nyberg G, Haljamae, Frisenette-Fich C, Wennergren M, Kjellmer I. Breast-feeding during treatment with cyclosporine. *Transplantation.* 1998;65:253–255
30. Egan PC, Costanza ME, Dodion P, Egorin MJ, Bachur NR. Doxorubicin and cisplatin excretion into human milk. *Cancer Treat Rep.* 1985;69:1387–1389
31. Johns DG, Rutherford LD, Leighton PC, Vogel CL. Secretion of methotrexate into human milk. *Am J Obstet Gynecol.* 1972;112:978–980
32. Steiner E, Villen T, Hallberg M, Rane A. Amphetamine secretion in breast milk. *Eur J Clin Pharmacol.* 1984;27:123–124
33. Chasnoff IJ, Lewis DE, Squires L. Cocaine intoxication in a breast-fed infant. *Pediatrics.* 1987;80:836–838
34. Cobrinik RW, Hood RT Jr, Chusid E. The effect of maternal narcotic addiction on the newborn infant: review of literature and report of 22 cases. *Pediatrics.* 1959;24:288–304
35. Perez-Reyes M, Wall ME. Presence of delta9-tetrahydrocannabinol in human milk. *N Engl J Med.* 1982;307:819–820
36. Kaufman KR, Petrucha RA, Pitts FN Jr, Weekes ME. PCP in amniotic fluid and breast milk: case report. *J Clin Psychiatry.* 1983;44:269–270
37. McArdle HJ, Danks DM. Secretion of copper 64 into breast milk following intravenous injection in a human subject. *J Trace Elem Exp Med.* 1991;4:81–84
38. Tobin RE, Schneider PB. Uptake of 67Ga in the lactating breast and its persistence in milk: case report. *J Nucl Med.* 1976;17:1055–1056
39. Butt D, Szaz KF. Indium-111 radioactivity in breast milk. *Br J Radiol.* 1986;59:80

40. Hedrick WR, Di Simone RN, Keen RL. Radiation dosimetry from breast milk excretion of radioiodine and pertechnetate. *J Nucl Med.* 1986;27:1569–1571
41. Rose MR, Prescott MC, Herman KJ. Excretion of iodine-123-hippuran, technetium-99 m-red blood cells, and technetium-99 m-macroaggregated albumin into breast milk. *J Nucl Med.* 1990;31:978–984
42. Palmer KE. Excretion of 125I in breast milk following administration of labelled fibrinogen. *Br J Radiol.* 1979;52:672–673
43. Honour AJ, Myant NB, Rowlands EN. Secretion of radioiodine in digestive juices and milk in man. *Clin Sci.* 1952;11:447–462
44. Karjalainen P, Penttila IM, Pystynen P. The amount and form of radioactivity in human milk after lung scanning, renography and placental localization by 131 I labelled tracers. *Acta Obstet Gynecol Scand.* 1971;50:357–361
45. Bland EP, Docker MF, Crawford JS, Farr RF. Radioactive iodine uptake by thyroid of breast-fed infants after maternal blood-volume measurements. *Lancet.* 1969;2:1039–1041
46. Nurnberger CE, Lipscomb A. Transmission of radioiodine (I^{131}) to infants through human maternal milk. *JAMA.* 1952;150:1398–1400
47. Robinson PS, Barker P, Campbell A, Henson P, Surveyor I, Young PR. Iodine-131 in breast milk following therapy for thyroid carcinoma. *J Nucl Med.* 1994;35:1797–1801
48. Rubow S, Klopper J, Wasserman H, Baard B, van Niekerk M. The excretion of radiopharmaceuticals in human breast milk: additional data and dosimetry. *Eur J Nucl Med.* 1994;21:144–153
49. Pommerenke WT, Hahn PF. Secretion of radio-active sodium in human milk. *Proc Soc Exp Biol Med.* 1943;52:223–224
50. O'Connell ME, Sutton H. Excretion of radioactivity in breast milk following 99Tcm-Sn polyphosphate. *Br J Radiol.* 1976;49:377–379
51. Berke RA, Hoops EC, Kereiakes JC, Saenger EL. Radiation dose to breast-feeding. *J Nucl Med.* 1973;14:51–52
52. Vagenakis AG, Abreau CM, Braverman LE. Duration of radioactivity in the milk of a nursing mother following 99 mTc administration. *J Nucl Med.* 1971;12:188
53. Wyburn JR. Human breast milk excretion of radionuclides following administration of radiopharmaceuticals. *J Nucl Med.* 1973;14:115–117
54. Pittard WB III, Merkatz R, Fletcher BD. Radioactive excretion in human milk following administration of technetium Tc 99 m macroaggregated albumin. *Pediatrics.* 1982;70:231–234
55. Maisels MJ, Gilcher RO. Excretion of technetium in human milk. *Pediatrics.* 1983;71:841–842
56. American Academy of Pediatrics, Committee on Drugs. Psychotropic drugs in pregnancy and lactation. *Pediatrics.* 1982;69:241–244
57. Oo CY, Kuhn RJ, Desai N, Wright CE, McNamara PJ. Pharmacokinetics in lactating women: prediction of alprazolam transfer into milk. *Br J Clin Pharmacol.* 1995;40:231–236

58. Patrick MJ, Tilstone WJH, Reavey P. Diazepam and breast-feeding. *Lancet.* 1972;1:542–543
59. Cole AP, Hailey DM. Diazepam and active metabolite in breast milk and their transfer to the neonate. *Arch Dis Child.* 1975;50:741–742
60. Dusci LJ, Good SM, Hall RW, Ilett KF. Excretion of diazepam and its metabolites in human milk during withdrawal from combination high dose diazepam and oxazepam. *Br J Clin Pharmacol.* 1990;29:123–126
61. Borgatta L, Jenny RW, Gruss L, Ong C, Barad D. Clinical significance of methohexital, meperidine, and diazepam in breast milk. *J Clin Pharmacol.* 1997;37:186–192
62. Dencker SJ, Johansson G, Milsom I. Quantification of naturally occurring benzodiazepine-like substances in human breast milk. *Psychopharmacology (Berl).* 1992;107:69–72
63. Summerfield RJ, Nielson MS. Excretion of lorazepam into breast milk. *Br J Anaesth.* 1985;57:1042–1043
64. Matheson I, Lunde PK, Bredesen JE. Midazolam and nitrazepam in the maternity ward: milk concentrations and clinical effects. *Br J Clin Pharmacol.* 1990;30:787–793
65. Olesen OV, Bartels U, Poulsen JH. Perphenazine in breast milk and serum. *Am J Psychiatry.* 1990;147:1378–1379
66. Brodie RR, Chasseaud LF, Taylor T. Concentrations of N-descyclopropylmethylprazepam in whole-blood, plasma, and milk after administration of prazepam to humans. *Biopharm Drug Dispos.* 1981;2:59–68
67. Hilbert JM, Gural RP, Symchowicz S, Zampaglione N. Excretion of quazepam into human breast milk. *J Clin Pharmacol.* 1984;24:457–462
68. Lebedevs TH, Wojnar-Horton RE, Yapp P, et al. Excretion of temazepam in breast milk. *Br J Clin Pharmacol.* 1992;33:204–206
69. Bader TF, Newman K. Amitriptyline in human breast milk and the nursing infant's serum. *Am J Psychiatry.* 1980;137:855–856
70. Erickson SH, Smith GH, Heidrich F. Tricyclics and breast feeding. *Am J Psychiatry.* 1979;136:1483–1484
71. Gelenberg AJ. Single case study. Amoxapine, a new antidepressant, appears in human milk. *J Nerv Ment Dis.* 1979;167:635–636
72. Briggs GG, Samson JH, Ambrose PJ, Schroeder DH. Excretion of bupropion in breast milk. *Ann Pharmacother.* 1993;27:431–433
73. Schimmell MS, Katz EZ, Shaag Y, Pastuszak A, Koren G. Toxic neonatal effects following maternal clomipramine therapy. *Clin Toxicol.* 1991;29:479–484
74. Sovner R, Orsulak PJ. Excretion of imipramine and desipramine in human breast milk. *Am J Psychiatry.* 1979;136:451–452
75. Stancer HC, Reed KL. Desipramine and 2-hydroxydesipramine in human breast milk and the nursery infant's serum. *Am J Psychiatry.* 1986;143:1597–1600
76. Rees JA, Glass RC, Sporne GA. Serum and breast-milk concentrations of dothiepin [letter]. *Practitioner.* 1976;217:686

77. Ilett KF, Lebedevs TH, Wojnar-Horton RE, et al. The excretion of dothiepin and its primary metabolites in breast milk. *Br J Clin Pharmacol.* 1992;33:635–639

78. Kemp J, Ilett KF, Booth J, Hackett LP. Excretion of doxepin and N-desmethyldoxepin in human milk. *Br J Clin Pharmacol.* 1985;20:497–499

79. Burch KJ, Wells BG. Fluoxetine/norfluoxetine concentrations in human milk. *Pediatrics.* 1992;89:676–677

80. Lester BM, Cucca J, Andreozzi L, Flanagan P, Oh W. Possible association between fluoxetine hydrochloride and colic in an infant. *J Am Acad Child Adolesc Psychiatry.* 1993;32:1253–1255

81. Burch KJ, Wells BG. Fluoxetine/norfluoxetine concentrations in human milk. *Pediatrics.* 1992;89:676–677

82. Taddio A, Ito S, Koren G. Excretion of fluoxetine and its metabolite, norfluoxetine, in human breast milk. *J Clin Pharmacol.* 1996;36:42–47

83. Brent NB, Wisner KL. Fluoxetine and carbamazepine concentrations in a nursing mother/infant pair. *Clin Pediatr (Phila).* 1998;37:41–44

84. Isenberg KE. Excretion of fluoxetine in human breast milk. *J Clin Psychiatry.* 1990;51:169

85. Nulman I, Koren G. The safety of fluoxetine during pregnancy and lactation. *Teratology.* 1996;53:304–308

86. Yoshida K, Smith B, Craggs M, Kumar RC. Fluoxetine in breast-milk and developmental outcome of breast-fed infants. *Br J Psychiatry.* 1998;172:175–178

87. Chambers CD, Anderson PO, Thomas RG, et al. Weight gain in infants breastfed by mothers who take fluoxetine. *Pediatrics.* 1999;104(5). Available at: http://www.pediatrics.org/cgi/content/full/104/5/e61. Accessed December 20, 2000

88. Wright S, Dawling S, Ashford JJ. Excretion of fluvoxamine in breast milk. *Br J Clin Pharmacol.* 1991;31:209

89. Wisner KL, Perel JM. Serum nortriptyline levels in nursing mothers and their infants. *Am J Psychiatry.* 1991;148:1234–1236

90. Wisner KL, Perel JM. Nortriptyline treatment of breast-feeding women. *Am J Psychiatry.* 1996;153:295

91. Stowe ZN, Cohen LS, Hostetter A, Ritchie JC, Owens MJ, Nemeroff CB. Paroxetine in human breast milk and nursing infants. *Am J Psychiatry.* 2000;157:185–189

92. Epperson CN, Anderson GM, McDougle CJ. Sertraline and breast-feeding. *N Engl J Med.* 1997;336:1189–1190

93. Stowe ZN, Owens MJ, Landry JC, et al. Sertraline and desmethylsertraline in human breast milk and nursing infants. *Am J Psychiatry.* 1997;154:1255–1260

94. Verbeeck RK, Ross SG, McKenna EA. Excretion of trazodone in breast milk. *Br J Clin Pharmacol.* 1986;22:367–370

95. Polishuk WZ, Kulcsar SA. Effects of chlorpromazine on pituitary function. *J Clin Endocrinol Metab.* 1956;16:292

96. Wiles DH, Orr MW, Kolakowska T. Chlorpromazine levels in plasma and milk of nursing mothers. *Br J Clin Pharmacol.* 1978;5:272–273

97. Nielsen ST, Matheson I, Rasmussen JN, Skinnemoen K, Andrew E, Hafsahl G. Excretion of iohexol and metrizoate in human breast milk. *Acta Radiol.* 1987;28:523–526

98. Ohkubo T, Shimoyama R, Sugawara K. Determination of chlorpromazine in human breast milk and serum by high-performance liquid chromatography. *J Chromatogr.* 1993;614:328–332

99. Matheson I, Evang A, Overo KF, Syversen G. Presence of chlorprothixene and its metabolites in breast milk. *Eur J Clin Pharmacol.* 1984;27:611–613

100. Barnas C, Bergant A, Hummer M, Saria A, Fleischhacker WW. Clozapine concentrations in maternal and fetal plasma, amniotic fluid, and breast milk. *Am J Psychiatry.* 1994;151:945

101. Stewart RB, Karas B, Springer PK. Haloperidol excretion in human milk. *Am J Psychiatry.* 1980;137:849–850

102. Whalley LJ, Blain PG, Prime JK. Haloperidol secreted in breast milk. *Br Med J (Clin Res Ed).* 1981;282:1746–1747

103. Ohkubo T, Shimoyama R, Sugawara K. Measurement of haloperidol in human breast milk by high-performance liquid chromatography. *J Pharm Sci.* 1992;81:947–949

104. Yoshida K, Smith B, Craggs M, Kumar RC. Neuroleptic drugs in breast milk: a study of pharmacokinetics and of possible adverse effects in breast-fed infants. *Psychol Med.* 1998;28:81–91

105. Ananth J. Side effects in the neonate from psychotropic agents excreted through breast-feeding. *Am J Psychiatry.* 1978;135:801–805

106. Plomp TA, Vulsma T, de Vijlder JJ. Use of amiodarone during pregnancy. *Eur J Obstet Gynecol Reprod Biol.* 1992;43:201–207

107. Havelka J, Hejzlar M, Popov V, Viktorinova D, Prochazka J. Excretion of chloramphenicol in human milk. *Chemotherapy.* 1968;13:204–211

108. Smadel JE, Woodward TE, Ley HL Jr, et al. Chloramphenicol Chloromycetin) in the treatment of tsutsugamushi disease (scrub typhus). *J Clin Invest.* 1949;28:1196

109. Venkatesan K, Mathur A, Girdhar A, Girdhar BK. Excretion of clofazimine in human milk in leprosy patients. *Lepr Rev.* 1997;68:242–246

110. Tomson T, Ohman I, Vitols S. Lamotrigine in pregnancy and lactation: a case report. *Epilepsia.* 1997;38:1039–1041

111. Gupta AP, Gupta PK. Metoclopramide as a lactogogue. *Clin Pediatr (Phila).* 1985;24:269–272

112. Kauppila A, Arvela P, Koivisto M, Kivinen S, Ylikorkala O, Pelkonen O. Metoclopramide and breast feeding: transfer into milk and the newborn. *Eur J Clin Pharmacol.* 1983;25:819–823

113. Erickson SH, Oppenheim GL, Smith GH. Metronidazole in breast milk. *Obstet Gynecol.* 1981;57:48–50

114. Heisterberg L, Branebjerg PE. Blood and milk concentrations of metronidazole in mothers and infants. *J Perinat Med.* 1983;11:114–120

115. Evaldson GR, Lindgren S, Nord CE, Rane AT. Tinidazole milk excretion and pharmacokinetics in lactating women. *Br J Clin Pharmacol*. 1985;19:503–507

116. Boutroy MJ, Bianchetti G, Dubruc C, Vert P, Morselli PL. To nurse when receiving acebutolol: is it dangerous for the neonate? *Eur J Clin Pharmacol*. 1986;30:737–739

117. Nelis GF. Diarrhoea due to 5-aminosalicylic acid in breast milk. *Lancet*. 1989;1:383

118. Jenss H, Weber P, Hartmann F. 5-Aminosalicylic acid its metabolite in breast milk during lactation [letter]. *Am J Gastroenterol*. 1990;85:331

119. Klotz U, Harings-Kaim A. Negligible excretion of 5-aminosalicylic acid in breast milk. *Lancet*. 1993;342:618–619

120. Liedholm H, Melander A, Bitzen PO, et al. Accumulation of atenolol and metoprolol in human breast milk. *Eur J Clin Pharmacol*. 1981;20:229–231

121. Schimmel MS, Eidelman AI, Wilschanski MA, Shaw D Jr, Ogilvie RJ, Koren G. Toxic effects of atenolol consumed during breast feeding. *J Pediatr*. 1989;114:476–478

122. Thorley KJ, McAinsh J. Levels of the beta-blockers atenolol and propanolol in the breast milk of women treated for hypertension in pregnancy. *Biopharm Drug Dispos*. 1983;4:299–301

123. Kulas J, Lunell NO, Rosing U, Steen B, Rane A. Atenolol and metoprolol. A comparison of their excretion into human breast milk. *Acta Obstet Gynecol Scand Suppl*. 1984;118:65–69

124. White WB, Andreoli JW, Wong SH, Cohn RD. Atenolol in human plasma and breast milk. *Obstet Gynecol*. 1984;63:42S–44S

125. Kulski JK, Hartmann PE, Martin JD, Smith M. Effects of bromocriptine mesylate on the composition of the mammary secretion in non-breast-feeding women. *Obstet Gynecol*. 1978;52:38–42

126. Katz M, Kroll D, Pak I, Osimoni A, Hirsch M. Puerperal hypertension, stroke, and seizures after suppression of lactation with bromocriptine. *Obstet Gynecol*. 1985;66:822–824

127. Clark JH, Wilson WG. A 16-day-old breast-fed infant with metabolic acidosis caused by salicylate. *Clin Pediatr (Phila)*. 1981;20:53–54

128. Levy G. Salicylate pharmacokinetics in the human neonate. In: Marselli PL, ed. *Basic and Therapeutic Aspects of Perinatal Pharmacology*. New York, NY: Raven Press; 1975:319

129. Jamali F, Keshavarz E. Salicylate excretion in breast milk. *Int J Pharm*. 1981;8:285–290

130. Kok TH, Taitz LS, Bennett MJ, Holt DW. Drowsiness due to clemastine transmitted in breast milk. *Lancet*. 1982;1:914–915

131. Fomina PI. Untersuchungen uber den Ubergang des aktiven agens des Mutterkorns in die milch stillender Mutter. *Arch Gynecol*. 1934;157:275

132. Schou M, Amdisen A. Lithium and pregnancy. 3. Lithium ingestion by children breast-fed by women on lithium treatment. *Br Med J*. 1973;2:138

133. Tunnessen WW Jr, Hertz CG. Toxic effects of lithium in newborn infants: a commentary. *J Pediatr*. 1972;81:804–807

134. Sykes PA, Quarrie J, Alexander FW. Lithium carbonate and breast-feeding. *Br Med J.* 1976;2:1299

135. Eckstein HB, Jack B. Breast-feeding and anticoagulant therapy. *Lancet.* 1970;1:672–673

136. Nau H, Rating D, Hauser I, Jager E, Koch S, Helge H. Placental transfer and pharmacokinetics of primidone and its metabolites phenobarbital, PEMA and hydroxyphenobarbital in neonates and infants of epileptic mothers. *Eur J Clin Pharmacol.* 1980;18:31–42

137. Kuhnz W, Koch S, Helge H, Nau H. Primidone and phenobarbital during lactation period in epileptic women: total and free drug serum levels in the nursed infants and their effects on neonatal behavior. *Dev Pharmacol Ther.* 1988;11:147–154

138. Finch E, Lorber J. Methaemoglobinaemia in newborn probably due to phenytoin excreted in human milk. *J Obstet Gynaecol Br Emp.* 1954;61:833–834

139. Tyson RM, Shrader EA, Perlman HH. Drugs transmitted through breast milk. II. Barbiturates. *J Pediatr.* 1938;13:86–90

140. Knott C, Reynolds F, Clayden G. Infantile spasms on weaning from breast milk containing anticonvulsants. *Lancet.* 1987;2:272–273

141. Branski D, Kerem E, Gross-Kieselstein E, Hurvitz H, Litt R, Abrahamov A. Bloody diarrhea-a possible complication of sulfasalazine transferred through human breast milk. *J Pediatr Gastroenterol Nutr.* 1986;5:316–317

142. Berlin CM Jr, Yaffe SJ, Ragni M. Disposition of acetaminophen in milk, saliva, and plasma of lactating women. *Pediatr Pharmacol (New York).* 1980;1:135–141

143. Bitzen PO, Gustafsson B, Jostell KG, Melander A, Wahlin-Boll E. Excretion of paracetamol in human breast milk. *Eur J Clin Pharmacol.* 1981;20:123–125

144. Findlay JW, DeAngelis RL, Kearney MF, Welch RM, Findlay JM. Analgesic drugs in breast milk and plasma. *Clin Pharmacol Ther.* 1981;29:625–633

145. Soderman P, Hartvig P, Fagerlund C. Acetazolamide excretion into human breast milk. *Br J Clin Pharmacol.* 1984;17:599–600

146. Rollman O, Pihl-Lundin I. Acitretin excretion into human breast milk. *Acta Derm Venereol.* 1990;70:487–490

147. Lau RJ, Emery MG, Galinsky RE. Unexpected accumulation of acyclovir in breast milk with estimation of infant exposure. *Obstet Gynecol.* 1987;69:468–471

148. Meyer LJ, de Miranda P, Sheth N, Spruance S. Acyclovir in human breast milk. *Am J Obstet Gynecol.* 1988;158:586–588

149. Binkiewicz A, Robinson MJ, Senior B. Pseudo-Cushing syndrome caused by alcohol in breast milk. *J Pediatr.* 1978;93:965–967

150. Cobo E. Effect of different doses of ethanol on the milk-ejecting reflex in lactating women. *Am J Obstet Gynecol.* 1973;115:817–821

151. Kesaniemi YA. Ethanol and acetaldehyde in the milk and peripheral blood of lactating women after ethanol administration. *J Obstet Gynaecol Br Commonw.* 1974;81:84–86

152. Little RE, Anderson KW, Ervin CH, Worthington-Roberts B, Clarren SK. Maternal alcohol use during breast-feeding and infant mental and motor development at one year. *N Engl J Med.* 1989;321:425–430

153. Kamilli I, Gresser U. Allopurinol and oxypurinol in human breast milk. *Clin Investig.* 1993;71:161–164

154. Kafetzis DA, Siafas CA, Georgakopoulos PA, Papadatos CJ. Passage of cephalosporins and amoxicillin into the breast milk. *Acta Paediatr Scand.* 1981;70:285–288

155. Berman JD, Melby PC, Neva FA. Concentration of Pentostam in human breast milk. *Trans R Soc Trop Med Hyg.* 1989;83:784–785

156. Sapeika N. Excretion of drugs in human milk: review. *J Obstet Gynaecol Br Emp.* 1947;54:426–431

157. Bald R, Bernbeck-Betthauser EM, Spahn H, Mutschler E. Excretion of azpropazone in human breast milk. *Eur J Clin Pharmacol.* 1990;39:271–273

158. Fleiss PM, Richwald GA, Gordon J, Stern M, Frantz M, Devlin RG. Aztreonam in human serum and breast milk. *Br J Clin Pharmacol.* 1985;19:509–511

159. Nail PA, Thomas MR, Eakin R. The effect of thiamin and riboflavin supplementation on the level of those vitamins in human breast milk and urine. *Am J Clin Nutr.* 1980;33:198–204

160. Roepke JL, Kirksey A. Vitamin B6 nutriture during pregnancy lactation. I. Vitamin B6 intake, levels of the vitamin in biological fluids, condition of the infant at birth. *Am J Clin Nutr.* 1979;32:2249–2256

161. West KD, Kirksey A. Influence of vitamin B6 intake on the content of the vitamin in human milk. *Am J Clin Nutr.* 1976;29:961–969

162. Greentree LB. Dangers of vitamin B6 in nursing mothers. *N Engl J Med.* 1979;300:141–142

163. Samson RR, McClelland DB. Vitamin B12 in human colostrum and milk. Quantitation of the vitamin and its binder and the uptake of bound vitamin B12 by intestinal bacteria. *Acta Paediatr Scand.* 1980;69:93–99

164. Eriksson G, Swahn CG. Concentrations of baclofen in serum and breast milk from a lactating woman. *Scand J Clin Lab Invest.* 1981;41:185–187

165. Healy M. Suppressing lactaton with oral diuretics. *Lancet.* 1961;1:1353

166. Brambel CE, Hunter RE. Effect of dicumarol on the nursing infant. *Am J Obstet Gynecol.* 1950;59:1153

167. Tyson RM, Shrader EA, Perlman HH. Drugs transmitted through breast milk. III. Bromides. *J Pediatr.* 1938;13:91–93

168. Pittman KA, Smyth RD, Losada M, Zighelboim I, Maduska AL, Sunshine A. Human perinatal distribution of butorphanol. *Am J Obstet Gynecol.* 1980;138:797–800

169. Berlin CM Jr. Excretion of the methylxanthines in human milk. *Semin Perinatol.* 1981;5:389–394

170. Tyrala EE, Dodson WE. Caffeine secretion into breast milk. *Arch Dis Child.* 1979;54:787–800

171. Hildebrandt R, Gundert-Remy U. Lack of pharmacological active saliva levels of caffeine in breast-fed infants. *Pediatr Pharmacol (New York)*. 1983;3:237–244

172. Berlin CM Jr, Denson HM, Daniel CH, Ward RM. Disposition of dietary caffeine in milk, saliva, and plasma of lactating women. *Pediatrics*. 1984;73:59–63

173. Ryu JE. Caffeine in human milk and in serum of breast-fed infants. *Dev Pharmacol Ther*. 1985;8:329–337

174. Ryu JE. Effect of maternal caffeine consumption on heart rate and sleep time of breast-fed infants. *Dev Pharmacol Ther*. 1985;8:355–363

175. Devlin RG, Fleiss PM. Captopril in human blood and breast milk. *J Clin Pharmacol*. 1981;21:110–113

176. Nau H, Kuhnz W, Egger JH, Rating D, Helge H. Anticonvulsants during pregnancy and lactation. Transplacental, maternal and neonatal pharmacokinetics. *Clin Pharmacokinet*. 1982;7:508–543

177. Pynnonen S, Kanto J, Sillanpaa M, Erkkola R. Carbamazepine: placental transport, tissue concentrations in foetus and newborn, and level in milk. *Acta Pharmacol Toxicol (Copenh)*. 1977;41:244–253

178. Silcox J, Schulz P, Horbay GL, Wassenaar W. Transfer of carbetocin into human breast milk. *Obstet Gynecol*. 1993;82:456–459

179. Cooper DS. Antithyroid drugs: to breast-feed or not to breast-feed. *Am J Obstet Gynecol*. 1987;157:234–235

180. Lamberg BA, Ikonen E, Osterlund K, et al. Antithyroid treatment of maternal hyperthyroidism during lactation. *Clin Endocrinol (Oxf)*. 1984;21:81–87

181. Tyson RM, Shrader EA, Perlman HH. Drugs transmitted through breast milk. I. Laxatives. *J Pediatr*. 1937;11:824–832

182. Yoshioka H, Cho K, Takimoto M, Maruyama S, Shimizu T. Transfer of cefazolin into human milk. *J Pediatr*. 1979;94:151–152

183. Dresse A, Lambotte R, Dubois M, Delapierre D, Kramp R. Transmammary passage of cefoxitin: additional results. *J Clin Pharmacol*. 1983;23:438–440

184. Shyu WC, Shah VR, Campbell DA, et al. Excretion of cefprozil into human breast milk. *Antimicrob Agents Chemother*. 1992;36:938–941

185. Blanco JD, Jorgensen JH, Castaneda YS, Crawford SA. Ceftazidime levels in human breast milk. *Antimicrob Agents Chemother*. 1983;23:479–480

186. Bourget P, Quinquis-Desmaris V, Fernandez H. Ceftriaxone distribution and protein binding between maternal blood and milk postpartum. *Ann Pharmacother*. 1993;27:294–297

187. Lacey JH. Dichloralphenazone and breast milk. *Br Med J*. 1971;4:684

188. Reed CB. A study of the conditions that require the removal of the child from the breast. *Surg Gynecol Obstet*. 1908;6:514

189. Soares R, Paulini E, Pereira JP. Da concentracao e eliminacao da cloroquina atraves da circulacao placentaria e do leite materno, de pacientes sob regime do sal loroquinado. *Rev Bras Malariol Doencas Trop*. 1957;9:19

190. Ogunbona FA, Onyeji CO, Bolaji OO, Torimiro SE. Excretion of chloroquine and desethylchloroquine in human milk. *Br J Clin Pharmacol.* 1987;23:473–476

191. Edstein MD, Veenendaal JR, Newman K, Hyslop R. Excretion of chloroquine, dapsone and pyrimethamine in human milk. *Br J Clin Pharmacol.* 1986;22:733–735

192. Werthmann MW Jr, Krees SV. Excretion of chlorothiazide in human breast milk. *J Pediatr.* 1972;81:781–783

193. Miller EM, Cohn RD, Burghart PH. Hydrochlorothiazide disposition in a mother and her breast-fed infant. *J Pediatr.* 1982;101:789–791

194. Mulley BA, Parr GD, Pau WK, Rye RM, Mould JJ, Siddle NC. Placental transfer of chlorthalidone and its elimination in maternal milk. *Eur J Clin Pharmacol.* 1978;13:129–131

195. Somogyi A, Gugler R. Cimetidine excretion into breast milk. *Br J Clin Pharmacol.* 1979;7:627–629

196. Oo CY, Kuhn RJ, Desai N, McNamara PJ. Active transport of cimetidine into human milk. *Clin Pharmacol Ther.* 1995;58:548–555

197. Gardner DK, Gabbe SG, Harter C. Simultaneous concentrations of ciprofloxacin in breast milk and in serum in mother and breast-fed infant. *Clin Pharm.* 1992;11:352–354

198. Giamarellou H, Kolokythas E, Petrikkos G, Gazis J, Aravantinos D, Sfikakis P. Pharmacokinetics of three newer quinolones in pregnant and lactating women. *Am J Med.* 1989;87(suppl):49S–51S

199. Hofmeyr GJ, Sonnendecker EW. Secretion of the gastrokinetic agent cisapride in human milk. *Eur J Clin Pharmacol.* 1986;30:735–736

200. Smith JA, Morgan JR, Rachlis AR, Papsin FR. Clindamycin in human breast milk [letter]. *Can Med Assoc J.* 1975;112:806

201. Zacharias S, Aguilera E, Assenzo JR, Zanartu J. Effects of hormonal and nonhormonal contraceptives on lactation and incidence of pregnancy. *Contraception.* 1986;33:203–213

202. Meny RG, Naumburg EG, Alger LS, Brill-Miller JL, Brown S. Codeine and the breastfed neonate. *J Hum Lact.* 1993;9:237–240

203. Milunsky JM. Breast-feeding during colchicine therapy for familial Mediterranean fever [letter]. *J Pediatr.* 1991;119:164

204. Ben-Chetrit E, Scherrmann J-M, Levy M. Colchicine in breast milk of patients with familial Mediterranean fever. *Arthritis Rheum.* 1996;39:1213–1217

205. Guillonneau M, Aigrain EJ, Galliot M, Binet MH, Darbois Y. Colchicine is excreted at high concentrations in human breast milk. *Eur J Obstet Gynecol Reprod Biol.* 1995;61:177–178

206. Nilsson S, Mellbin T, Hofvander Y, Sundelin C, Valentin J, Nygren KG. Long-term follow-up of children breast-fed by mothers using oral contraceptives. *Contraception.* 1986;34:443–457

207. Nilsson S, Nygren KG. Transfer of contraceptive steroids to human milk. *Res Reprod.* 1979;11:1–2

208. American Academy of Pediatrics, Committee on Drugs. Breast-feeding and contraception. *Pediatrics*. 1981;68:138–140
209. Barsivala VM, Virkar KD. The effect of oral contraceptives on concentration of various components of human milk. *Contraception*. 1973;7:307–312
210. Borglin NE, Sandholm LE. Effect of oral contraceptives on lactation. *Fertil Steril*. 1971;22:39–41
211. Curtis EM. Oral-contraceptive feminization of a normal male infant: report of a case. *Obstet Gynecol*. 1964;23:295–296
212. Kora SJ. Effect of oral contraceptives on lactation. *Fertil Steril*. 1969;20:419–423
213. Toaff R, Ashkenazi H, Schwartz A, Herzberg M. Effects of oestrogen and progestagen on the composition of human milk. *J Reprod Fertil*. 1969;19:475–482
214. Snider DE Jr, Powell KE. Should women taking antituberculosis drugs breast-feed? *Arch Intern Med*. 1984;144:589–590
215. Cancela L, Le Boulch N, Miravet L. Relationship between the vitamin D content of maternal milk and the vitamin D status of nursing women and breast-fed infants. *J Endocrinol*. 1986;110:43–50
216. Rothberg AD, Pettifor JM, Cohen DF, Sonnendecker EW, Ross FP. Maternal-infant vitamin D relationships during breast-feeding. *J Pediatr*. 1982;101:500–503
217. Greer FR, Hollis BW, Napoli JL. High concentrations of vitamin D2 in human milk associated with pharmacologic doses of vitamin D2. *J Pediatr*. 1984;105:61–64
218. Greenhalf JO, Leonard HS. Laxatives in the treatment of constipation in pregnant and breast-feeding mothers. *Practitioner*. 1973;210:259–263
219. Dreisbach JA. Sulphone levels in breast milk of mothers on sulphone therapy. *Lepr Rev*. 1952;23:101–106
220. Mortimer EA Jr. Drug toxicity from breast milk [letter]? *Pediatrics*. 1977;60:780–781
221. FitzJohn TP, Williams DG, Laker MF, Owen JP. Intravenous urography during lactation. *Br J Radiol*. 1982;55:603–605
222. Loughnan PM. Digoxin excretion in human breast milk. *J Pediatr*. 1978;92:1019–1020
223. Levy M, Granit L, Laufer N. Excretion of drugs in human milk. *N Engl J Med*. 1977;297:789
224. Okada M, Inoue H, Nakamura Y, Kishimoto M, Suzuki T. Excretion of diltiazem in human milk [letter]. *N Engl J Med*. 1985;312:992–993
225. Zylber-Katz E, Linder N, Granit L, Levy M. Excretion of dipyrone metabolites in human breast milk. *Eur J Clin Pharmacol*. 1986;30:359–361
226. MacKintosh D, Buchanan N. Excretion of disopyramide in human breast milk [letter]. *Br J Clin Pharmacol*. 1985;19:856–857
227. Hoppu K, Neuvonen PJ, Korte T. Disopyramide and breast feeding [letter]. *Br J Clin Pharmacol*. 1986;21:553
228. Hofmeyr GJ, van Idlekinge B. Domperidone and lactation [letter]. *Lancet*. 1983;1:647

229. Jorboe CH, Cook LN, Malesic I, Fleischaker J. Dyphylline elimination kinetics in lactating women: blood to milk transfer. *J Clin Pharmacol.* 1981;21:405–410

230. Redman CW, Kelly JG, Cooper WD. The excretion of enalapril and enalaprilat in human breast milk. *Eur J Clin Pharmacol.* 1990;38:99

231. Matsuda S. Transfer of antibiotics into maternal milk. *Biol Res Pregnancy Perinatol.* 1984;5:57–60

232. Nilsson S, Nygren KG, Johansson ED. Transfer of estradiol to human milk. *Am J Obstet Gynecol.* 1978;132:653–657

233. Koup JR, Rose JQ, Cohen ME. Ethosuximide pharmacokinetics in a pregnant patient and her newborn. *Epilepsia.* 1978;19:535–539

234. Steer PL, Biddle CJ, Marley WS, Lantz RK, Sulik PL. Concentration of fentanyl in colostrum after an analgesic dose. *Can J Anaesth.* 1992;39:231–235

235. Lucas BD Jr, Purdy CY, Scarim SK, Benjamin S, Abel SR, Hilleman DE. Terfenadine pharmacokinetics in breast milk in lactating women. *Clin Pharmacol Ther.* 1995;57:398–402

236. McQuinn RL, Pisani A, Wafa S, et al. Flecainide excretion in human breast milk. *Clin Pharmacol Ther.* 1990;48:262–267

237. Wagner X, Jouglard J, Moulin M, Miller AM, Petitjean J, Pisapia A. Coadministration of flecainide acetate and sotalol during pregnancy: lack of teratogenic effects, passage across the placenta, and excretion in human breast milk. *Am Heart J.* 1990;119:700–702

238. Dan M, Weidekamm E, Sagiv R, Portmann R, Zakut H. Penetration of fleroxacin into breast milk and pharmacokinetics in lactating women. *Antimicrob Agents Chemother.* 1993;37:293–296

239. Force RW. Fluconazole concentrations in breast milk. *Pediatr Infect Dis J.* 1995;14:235–236

240. Buchanan RA, Eaton CJ, Koeff ST, Kinkel AW. The breast milk excretion of flufenamic acid. *Curr Ther Res Clin Exp.* 1969;11:533–538

241. Mattern J, Mayer PR. Excretion of fluorescein into breast milk. *Am J Ophthalmol.* 1990;109:598–599

242. Retief FP, Heyns AD, Oosthuizen M, Oelofse R, van Reenen OR. Aspects of folate metabolism in lactating women studied after ingestion of 14C-methylfolate. *Am J Med Sci.* 1979;277:281–288

243. Rofsky NM, Weinreb JC, Litt AW. Quantitative analysis of gadopentetate dimeglumine excreted in breast milk. *J Magn Reson Imaging.* 1993;3:131–132

244. Celiloglu M, Celiker S, Guven H, Tuncok Y, Demir N, Erten O. Gentamicin excretion and uptake from breast milk by nursing infants. *Obstet Gynecol.* 1994;84:263–265

245. Bell RA, Dale IM. Gold secretion in maternal milk [letter]. *Arthritis Rheum.* 1976;19:1374

246. Blau SP. Letter: metabolism of gold during lactation. *Arthritis Rheum.* 1973;16:777–778

247. Gottlieb NL. Suggested errata. *Arthritis Rheum.* 1974;17:1057
248. Ostensen M, Skavdal K, Myklebust G, Tomassen Y, Aarbakke J. Excretion of gold into human breast milk. *Eur J Clin Pharmacol.* 1986;31:251–252
249. Bennett PN, Humphries SJ, Osborne JP, Clarke AK, Taylor A. Use of sodium aurothiomalate during lactation. *Br J Clin Pharmacol.* 1990;29:777–779
250. Cote CJ, Kenepp NB, Reed SB, Strobel GE. Trace concentrations of halothane in human breast milk. *Br J Anaesth.* 1976;48:541–543
251. Liedholm H, Wahlin-Boll E, Hanson A, Ingemarsson I, Melander A. Transplacental passage and breast milk concentrations of hydralazine. *Eur J Clin Pharmacol.* 1982;21:417–419
252. Ostensen M, Brown ND, Chiang PK, Aarbakke J. Hydroxychloroquine in human breast milk. *Eur J Clin Pharmacol.* 1985;28:357
253. Nation RL, Hackett LP, Dusci LJ, Ilett KF. Excretion of hydroxychloroquine in human milk. *Br J Clin Pharmacol.* 1984;17:368–369
254. Townsend RJ, Benedetti T, Erickson SH, Gillespie WR, Albert KS. A study to evaluate the passage of ibuprofen into breast-milk. *Drug Intell Clin Pharm.* 1982;16:482–483
255. Townsend RJ, Benedetti TJ, Erickson SH, et al. Excretion of ibuprofen into breast milk. *Am J Obstet Gynecol.* 1984;149:184–186
256. Eeg-Olofsson O, Malmros I, Elwin CE, Steen B. Convulsions in a breast-fed infant after maternal indomethacin [letter]. *Lancet.* 1978;2:215
257. Fairhead FW. Convulsions in a breast-fed infant after maternal indomethacin [letter]. *Lancet.* 1978;2:576
258. Lebedevs TH, Wojnar-Horton RE, Yapp P, et al. Excretion of indomethacin in breast milk. *Br J Clin Pharmacol.* 1991;32:751–754
259. Postellon DC, Aronow R. Iodine in mother's milk [letter]. *JAMA.* 1982;247:463
260. Holmdahl KH. Cholecystography during lactation. *Acta Radiol.* 1955;45:305–307
261. Berlin CM, Lee C. Isoniazid and acetylisoniazid disposition in human milk, saliva and plasma [abstr]. *Fed Proc.* 1979;38:426
262. Kumar AR, Hale TW, Mock RE. Transfer of interferon alfa into human breast milk. *J Hum Lact.* 2000;16:226–228
263. Ogbuokiri JE, Ozumba BC, Okonkwo PO. Ivermectin levels in human breast milk. *Eur J Clin Pharmacol.* 1993;45:389–390
264. Ogbuokiri JE, Ozumba BC, Okonkwo PO. Ivermectin levels in human breast milk. *Eur J Clin Pharmacol.* 1994;46:89–90
265. Dyggve HV, Dam H, Sondergaard E. Influence on the prothrombin time of breast-fed newborn babies of one single dose of vitamin K1 or synkavit given to the mother within 2 hours after birth. *Acta Obstet Gynecol Scand.* 1956;35:440–444
266. Von Kries R, Shearer M, McCarthy PT, Haug M, Harzer G, Goebel U. Vitamin K-1 content of maternal milk: Influence of the stage of lactation, lipid composition, and vitamin K-1 supplements given to the mother. *Pediatr Res.* 1987;22:513–517

267. Moretti ME, Ito S, Koren G. Disposition of maternal ketoconazole in breast milk. *Am J Obstet Gynecol.* 1995;173:1625–1626

268. Wischnik A, Manth SM, Lloyd J, Bullingham R, Thompson JS. The excretion of ketorolac tromethamine into breast milk after multiple oral dosing. *Eur J Clin Pharmacol.* 1989;36:521–524

269. Lunell HO, Kulas J, Rane A. Transfer of labetalol into amniotic fluid and breast milk in lactating women. *Eur J Clin Pharmacol.* 1985;28:597–599

270. Atkinson H, Begg EJ. Concentration of beta-blocking drugs in human milk [letter]. *J Pediatr.* 1990;116:156

271. Diaz S, Herreros C, Juez G, et al. Fertility regulation in nursing women: VII. Influence of Norplant levonorgestrel implants upon lactation and infant growth. *Contraception.* 1985;32:53–74

272. Shaaban MM, Odlind V, Salem HT, et al. Levonorgestrel concentrations in maternal and infant serum during use of subdermal levonorgestrel contraceptive implants, Norplant by nursing mothers. *Contraception.* 1986;33:357–363

273. Shikary ZK, Betrabet SS, Patel ZM, et al. ICMR task force study on hormonal contraception. Transfer of levonorgestrel (LNG) administered through different drug delivery systems from the maternal circulation into the newborn infant's circulation via breast milk. *Contraception.* 1987;35:477–486

274. McCann MF, Moggia AV, Higgins JE, Potts M, Becker C. The effects of a progestin-only oral contraceptive (levonorgestrel 0.03 mg) on breast-feeding. *Contraception.* 1989;40:635–648

275. Mizuta H, Amino N, Ichihara K, et al. Thyroid hormones in human milk and their influence on thyroid function of breast-fed babies. *Pediatr Res.* 1983;17:468–471

276. Zeisler JA, Gaarder TD, De Mesquita SA. Lidocaine excretion in breast milk. *Drug Intell Clin Pharm.* 1986;20:691–693

277. Nikodem VC, Hofmeyr GJ. Secretion of the antidiarrhoeal agent operamide oxide in breast milk. *Eur J Clin Pharmacol.* 1992;42:695–696

278. Hilbert J, Radwanski E, Affrime MB, Perentesis G, Symchowicz S, Zampaglione N. Excretion of loratadine in human breast milk. *J Clin Pharmacol.* 1988;28:234–239

279. Cruikshank DP, Varner MW, Pitkin RM. Breast milk magnesium and calcium concentrations following magnesium sulfate treatment. *Am J Obstet Gynecol.* 1982;143:685

280. Hannon PR, Duggan AK, Serwint JR, Vogelhut JW, Witter F, DeAngelis C. The influence of medroxyprogesterone on the duration of breast-feeding in mothers in an urban community. *Arch Pediatr Adolesc Med.* 1997;151:490–496

281. Buchanan RA, Eaton CJ, Koeff ST, Kinkel AW. The breast milk excretion of mefenamic acid. *Curr Ther Res Clin Exp.* 1968;10:592–597

282. Wittels B, Scott DT, Sinatra RS. Exogenous opioids in human breast milk and acute neonatal neurobehavior: a preliminary study. *Anesthesiology.* 1990;73:864–869

283. Blinick G, Inturrisi CE, Jerez E, Wallach RC. Methadone assays in pregnant women and progeny. *Am J Obstet Gynecol.* 1975;121:617–621

284. Blinick G, Wallach RC, Jerez E, Ackerman BD. Drug addiction in pregnancy and the neonate. *Am J Obstet Gynecol.* 1976;125:135–142

285. Wojnar-Horton RE, Kristensen JH, Yapp P, Ilett KF, Dusci LJ, Hackett LP. Methadone distribution and excretion into breast milk of clients in a methadone maintenance programme. *Br J Clin Pharmacol.* 1997;44:543–547

286. Geraghty B, Graham EA, Logan B, Weiss EL. Methadone levels in breast milk. *J Hum Lact.* 1997;13:227–230

287. McCarthy JJ, Posey BL. Methadone levels in human milk. *J Hum Lact.* 2000;16:115–120

288. Cooper DS, Bode HH, Nath B, Saxe V, Maloof F, Ridgway EC. Methimazole pharmacology in man: studies using or newly developed radioimmunoassay for methimazole. *J Clin Endocrinol Metab.* 1984;58:473–479

289. Azizi F. Effect of methimazole treatment of maternal thyrotoxicosis on thyroid function in breast-feeding infants. *J Pediatr.* 1996;128:855–858

290. White WB, Andreoli JW, Cohn RD. Alpha-methyldopa disposition in mothers with hypertension and in their breast-fed infants. *Clin Pharmacol Ther.* 1985;37:387–390

291. Shore MF. Drugs can be dangerous during pregnancy and lactations. *Can Pharm J.* 1970;103:358

292. Ilett KF, Hackett LP, Paterson JW, McCormick CC. Excretion of metrizamide in milk. *Br J Radiol.* 1981;54:537–538

293. Lownes HE, Ives TJ. Mexiletine use in pregnancy and lactation. *Am J Obstet Gynecol.* 1987;157:446–447

294. Lewis AM, Patel L, Johnston A, Turner P. Mexiletine in human blood and breast milk. *Postgrad Med J.* 1981;57:546–547

295. Valdivieso A, Valdes G, Spiro TE, Westerman RL. Minoxidil in breast milk [letter]. *Ann Intern Med.* 1985;102:135

296. Terwilliger WG, Hatcher RA. The elimination of morphine and quinine in human milk. *Surg Gynecol Obstet.* 1934;58:823–826

297. Robieux I, Koren G, Vandenbergh H, Schneiderman J. Morphine excretion in breast milk and resultant exposure of a nursing infant. *J Toxicol Clin Toxicol.* 1990;28:365–370

298. Oberlander TF, Robeson P, Ward V, et al. Prenatal and breast milk morphine exposure following maternal intrathecal morphine treatment. *J Hum Lact.* 2000;16:137–142

299. Miller RD, Keegan KA, Thrupp LD, Brann J. Human breast milk concentration of moxalactam. *Am J Obstet Gynecol.* 1984;148:348–349

300. Devlin RG, Duchin KL, Fleiss PM. Nadolol in human serum and breast milk. *Br J Clin Pharmacol.* 1981;12:393–396

301. Belton EM, Jones RV. Haemolytic anaemia due to nalidixic acid. *Lancet.* 1965;2:691

302. Jamali F, Stevens DR. Naproxen excretion in milk and its uptake by the infant. *Drug Intell Clin Pharm.* 1983;17:910–911

303. Liu DT, Savage JM, Donnell D. Nefopam excretion in human milk. *Br J Clin Pharmacol.* 1987;23:99–101

304. Ehrenkranz RA, Ackerman BA, Hulse JD. Nifedipine transfer into human milk. *J Pediatr.* 1989;114:478–480

305. Varsano I, Fischl J, Shochet SB. The excretion of orally ingested nitrofurantoin in human milk. *J Pediatr.* 1973;82:886–887

306. Laumas KR, Malkani PK, Bhatnagar S, Laumas V. Radioactivity in the breast milk of lactating women after oral administration of 3H-norethynodrel. *Am J Obstet Gynecol.* 1967;98:411–413

307. Pincus G, Bialy G, Layne DS, Paniagua M, Williams KI. Radioactivity in the milk of subjects receiving radioactive 19-norsteroids. *Nature.* 1966;212:924–925

308. Olsson B, Bolme P, Dahlstrom B, Marcus C. Excretion of noscapine in human breast milk. *Eur J Clin Pharmacol.* 1986;30:213–215

309. Sioufi A, Hillion D, Lumbroso P, et al. Oxprenolol placental transfer, plasma concentrations in newborns and passage into breast milk. *Br J Clin Pharmacol.* 1984;18:453–456

310. Fidler J, Smith V, De Swiet M. Excretion of oxprenolol and timolol in breast milk. *Br J Obstet Gynaecol.* 1983;90:961–965

311. Leuxner E, Pulver R. Verabreichung von irgapyrin bei schwangeren und wochnerinnen. *MMW Munch Med Wochenschr.* 1956;98:84–86

312. Mirkin B. Diphenylhydantoin: placental transport, fetal localization, neonatal metabolism, and possible teratogenic effects. *J Pediatr.* 1971;78:329–337

313. Ostensen M. Piroxicam in human breast milk. *Eur J Clin Pharmacol.* 1983;25:829–830

314. McKenzie SA, Selley JA, Agnew JE. Secretion of prednisolone into breast milk. *Arch Dis Child.* 1975;50:894–896

315. Greenberger PA, Odeh YK, Frederiksen MC, Atkinson AJ Jr. Pharmacokinetics of prednisolone transfer to breast milk. *Clin Pharmacol Ther.* 1993;53:324–328

316. Katz FH, Duncan BR. Entry of prednisone into human milk. *N Engl J Med.* 1975;293:1154

317. Pittard WB III, Glazier H. Procainamide excretion in human milk. *J Pediatr.* 1983;102:631–633

318. Diaz S, Jackanicz TM, Herreros C, et al. Fertility regulation in nursing women: VIII. Progesterone plasma levels and contraceptive efficacy of a progesterone-releasing vaginal ring. *Contraception.* 1985;32:603–622

319. Kunka RL, Venkataramanan R, Stern RM, Ladik CF. Excretion of propoxyphene and norpropoxyphene in breast milk. *Clin Pharmacol Ther.* 1984;35:675–680

320. Levitan AA, Manion JC. Propranolol therapy during pregnancy and lactation. *Am J Cardiol.* 1973;32:247

321. Karlberg B, Lundberg D, Aberg H. Letter: excretion of propranolol in human breast milk. *Acta Pharmacol Toxicol (Copenh)*. 1974;34:222–224

322. Bauer JH, Pape B, Zajicek J, Groshong T. Propranolol in human plasma and breast milk. *Am J Cardiol*. 1979;43:860–862

323. Kampmann JP, Johansen K, Hansen JM, Helweg J. Propylthiouracil in human milk: revision of a dogma. *Lancet*. 1980;1:736–737

324. Findlay JW, Butz RF, Sailstad JM, Warren JT, Welch RM. Pseudoephedrine and triprolidine in plasma and breast milk of nursing mothers. *Br J Clin Pharmacol*. 1984;18:901–906

325. Hardell LI, Lindstrom B, Lonnerholm G, Osterman PO. Pyridostigmine in human breast milk. *Br J Clin Pharmacol*. 1982;14:565–567

326. Clyde DF, Shute GT, Press J. Transfer of pyrimethamine in human milk. *J Trop Med Hyg*. 1956;59:277

327. Hill LM, Malkasian GD Jr. The use of quinidine sulfate throughout pregnancy. *Obstet Gynecol*. 1979;54:366–368

328. Horning MG, Stillwell WG, Nowlin J, Lertratanangkoon K, Stillwell RN, Hill RM. Identification and quantification of drugs and drug metabolites in human breast milk using gas chromatography mass spectrometry computer methods. *Mod Probl Paediatr*. 1975;15:73–79

329. Werthmann MW JR, Krees SV. Quantitative excretion of Senokot in human breast milk. *Med Ann Dist Columbia*. 1973;42:4–5

330. Hackett LP, Wojnar-Horton RE, Dusci LJ, Ilett KF, Roberts MJ. Excretion of sotalol in breast milk. *Br J Clin Pharmacol*. 1990;29:277–278

331. Phelps DL, Karim Z. Spironolactone: relationship between concentrations of dethioacetylated metabolite in human serum milk. *J Pharm Sci*. 1977;66:1203

332. Foulds G, Miller RD, Knirsch AK, Thrupp LD. Sulbactam kinetics and excretion into breast milk in postpartum women. *Clin Pharmacol Ther*. 1985;38:692–696

333. Jarnerot G, Into-Malmberg MB. Sulphasalazine treatment during breast feeding. *Scand J Gastroenterol*. 1979;14:869–871

334. Berlin CM Jr, Yaffe SJ. Disposition of salicylazosulfapyridine (Azulfidine) and metabolites in human breast milk. *Dev Pharmacol Ther*. 1980;1:31–39

335. Kauffman RE, O'Brien C, Gilford P. Sulfisoxazole secretion into human milk. *J Pediatr*. 1980;97:839–841

336. Wojnar-Horton RE, Hackett LP, Yapp P, Dusci LJ, Paech M, Ilett KF. Distribution and excretion of sumatriptan in human milk. *Br J Clin Pharmacol*. 1996;41:217–221

337. Chaiken P, Chasin M, Kennedy B, Silverman BK. Suprofen concentrations in human breast milk. *J Clin Pharmacol*. 1983;23:385–390

338. Lindberberg C, Boreus LO, de Chateau P, Lindstrom B, Lonnerholm G, Nyberg L. Transfer of terbutaline into breast milk. *Eur J Respir Dis Suppl*. 1984;134:87–91

339. Tetracycline in breast milk. *Br Med J*. 1969;4:791

340. Posner AC, Prigot A, Konicoff NG. Further observations on the use of tetracycline hydrochloride in prophylaxis and treatment of obstetric infections. In: Welch H, Marti-Ibanez F, eds. *Antibiotics Annual 1954–1955.* New York, NY: Medical Encyclopedia Inc; 1955:594

341. Yurchak AM, Jusko WJ. Theophylline secretion into breast milk. *Pediatrics.* 1976;57:518–520

342. Andersen LW, Qvist T, Hertz J, Mogensen F. Concentrations of thiopentone in mature breast milk and colostrum following an induction dose. *Acta Anaesthesiol Scand.* 1987;31:30–32

343. Williams RH, Kay GA, Jandorf BJ. Thiouracil: its absorption, distribution, and excretion. *J Clin Invest.* 1944;23:613–627

344. von Kobyletzki D, Dalhoff A, Lindemeyer H, Primavesi CA. Ticarcillin serum and tissue concentrations in gynecology and obstetrics. *Infection.* 1983;11:144–149

345. Moiel RH, Ryan JR. Tolbutamide orinase in human breast milk. *Clin Pediatr.* 1967;6:480

346. Sagranes R, Waller ES, Goehrs HR. Tolmetin in breast milk. *Drug Intell Clin Pharm.* 1985;19:55–56

347. Arnauld R. Etude du passage de la trimethoprime dans le lait maternel. *Ouest Med.* 1972;25:959

348. Miller RD, Salter AJ. The passage of trimethoprim/sulpha-methoxazole into breast milk and its significance. Proceedings of the 8th International Congress of Chemotherapy, Athens. *Hellenic Soc Chemother.* 1974;1:687

349. Alexander FW. Sodium valproate and pregnancy. *Arch Dis Child.* 1979;54:240

350. von Unruh GE, Froescher W, Hoffman F, Niesen M. Valproic acid in breast milk: how much is really there? *Ther Drug Monit.* 1984;6:272–276

351. Anderson P, Bondesson U, Mattiasson I, Johansson BW. Verapamil and norvera-pamil in plasma and breast milk during breast feeding. *Eur J Clin Pharmacol.* 1987;31:625–627

352. Orme ML, Lewis PJ, de Swiet M, et al. May mothers given warfarin breast-feed their infants? *Br Med J.* 1977;1:1564–1565

353. Pons G, Francoual C, Guillet P, et al. Zolpidem excretion in breast milk. *Eur J Clin Pharmacol.* 1989;37:245–248

354. Wild CP, Pionneau FA, Montesano R, Mutiro CF, Chetsanga CJ. Aflatoxin detected in human breast milk by immunoassay. *Int J Cancer.* 1987;40:328–333

355. Maxwell SM, Apeagyei F, de Vries HR, et al. Aflatoxins in breast milk, neonatal cord blood and sera of pregnant women. *J Toxicol Toxin Rev.* 1989;8:19–29

356. Zarba A, Wild CP, Hall AJ, et al. Aflatoxin M1 in human breast milk from The Gambia, west Africa, quantified by combined monoclonal antibody immunoaffinity chromatography HPLC. *Carcinogenesis.* 1992;13:891–894

357. Stegink LD, Filer LJ Jr, Baker GL. Plasma, erythrocyte human milk levels of free amino acids in lactating women administered aspartame or lactose. *J Nutr.* 1979;109:2173–2181

358. Mangurten HH, Kaye CI. Neonatal bromism secondary to maternal exposure in a photographic laboratory. *J Pediatr.* 1982;100:596–598

359. Radisch B, Luck W, Nau H. Cadmium concentrations in milk and blood of smoking mothers. *Toxicol Lett.* 1987;36:147–152

360. Miyazaki T, Akiyama K, Kaneko S, Horii S, Yamagishi T. Chlordane residues in human milk. *Bull Environ Contam Toxicol.* 1980;25:518–523

361. Resman BH, Blumenthal P, Jusko WJ. Breast milk distribution of theobromine from chocolate. *J Pediatr.* 1977;91:477–480

362. Wolff MS. Occupationally derived chemicals in breast milk. *Am J Ind Med.* 1983;4:259–281

363. Egan H, Goulding R, Roburn J, Tatton JO. Organo-chlorine pesticide residues in human fat and human milk. *Br Med J.* 1965;2:66–69

364. Quinby GE, Armstrong JF, Durham WF. DDT in human milk. *Nature.* 1965;207:726–728

365. Bakken AF, Seip M. Insecticides in human breast milk. *Acta Paediatr Scand.* 1976;65:535–539

366. Adamovic VM, Sokic B, Smiljanski MJ. Some observations concerning the ratio of the intake of organochlorine insecticides through food and amounts excreted in the milk of breast-feeding mothers. *Bull Environ Contam Toxicol.* 1978;20:280–285

367. Savage EP, Keefe TJ, Tessari JD, et al. National study of chlorinated hydrocarbon insecticide residues in human milk, USA. I. Geographic distribution of dieldrin, heptachlor, heptachlor epoxide, chlordane, oxychlordane, and mirex. *Am J Epidemiol.* 1981;113:413–422

368. Wilson DJ, Locker DJ, Ritzen CA, Watson JT, Schaffner W. DDT concentrations in human milk. *Am J Dis Child.* 1973;125:814–817

369. Bouwman H, Becker PJ, Cooppan RM, Reinecke AJ. Transfer of DDT used in malaria control to infants via breast milk. *Bull World Health Organ.* 1992;70:241–250

370. Stevens MF, Ebell GF, Psaila-Savona P. Organochlorine pesticides in Western Australian nursing mothers. *Med J Aust.* 1993;158:238–241

371. Emanuel B, Schoenfeld A. Favism in a nursing infant. *J Pediatr.* 1961;58:263–266

372. Simpson WJ, Tuba J. An investigation of fluoride concentration in the milk of nursing mothers. *J Oral Med.* 1968;23:104–106

373. Esala S, Vuori E, Helle A. Effect of maternal fluorine intake on breast milk fluorine content. *Br J Nutr.* 1982;48:201–204

374. Dreyfus-See G. Le passage dans le lait des aliments ou medicaments absorbes par denourrices. *Rev Med Interne.* 1934;51:198

375. Ando M, Hirano S, Itoh Y. Transfer of hexachlorobenzene (HCB) from mother to newborn baby through placenta and milk. *Arch Toxicol.* 1985;56:195–200

376. West RW, Wilson DJ, Schaffner W. Hexachlorophene concentrations in human milk. *Bull Environ Contam Toxicol.* 1975;13:167–169

377. Rabinowitz M, Leviton A, Needelman H. Lead in milk and infant blood: a dose-response model. *Arch Environ Health*. 1985;40:283–286

378. Sternowsky JH, Wessolowski R. Lead and cadmium in breast milk. Higher levels in urban vs rural mothers during the first 3 months of lactation. *Arch Toxicol*. 1985;57:41–45

379. Namihira D, Saldivar L, Pustilnik N, Carreon GJ, Salinas ME. Lead in human blood and milk from nursing women living near a smelter in Mexico City. *J Toxicol Environ Health*. 1993;38:225–232

380. Baum CR, Shannon MW. Lead in breast milk. *Pediatrics*. 1996;97:932

381. Koos BJ, Longo LD. Mercury toxicity in the pregnant woman, fetus, and newborn infant. A review. *Am J Obstet Gynecol*. 1976;126:390–409

382. Amin-Zaki L, Elhassani S, Majeed MA, Clarkson TW, Doherty RA, Greenwood MR. Studies of infants postnatally exposed to methylmercury. *J Pediatr*. 1974;85:81–84

383. Pitkin RM, Bahns JA, Filer LJ Jr, Reynolds WA. Mercury in human maternal and cord blood, placenta, and milk. *Proc Soc Exp Biol Med*. 1976;151:565–567

384. Hersh J, Bono JV, Padgett DE, Mancuso CA. Methyl methacrylate levels in the breast milk of a patient after total hip arthroplasty. *J Arthroplasty*. 1995;10:91–92

385. Stegink LD, Filer LJ Jr, Baker GL. Monosodium glutamate: effect on plasma and breast milk amino acid levels in lactating women. *Proc Soc Exp Biol Med*. 1972;140:836–841

386. Miller RW. Pollutants in breast milk: PCBs and cola-colored babies [editorial]. *J Pediatr*. 1977;90:510–511

387. Rogan WJ, Bagniewska A, Damstra T. Pollutants in breast milk. *N Engl J Med*. 1980;302:1450–1453

388. Wickizer TM, Brilliant LB, Copeland R, Tilden R. Polychlorinated biphenyl contamination of nursing mothers' milk in Michigan. *Am J Public Health*. 1981;71:132–137

389. Brilliant LB, Van Amburg G, Isbister J, Bloomer AW, Humphrey H, Price H. Breast-milk monitoring to measure Michigan's contamination with polybrominated biphenyls. *Lancet*. 1978;2:643–646

390. Wickizer TM, Brilliant LB. Testing for polychlorinated biphenyls in human milk. *Pediatrics*. 1981;68:411–415

391. Bagnell PC, Ellenberg HA. Obstructive jaundice due to a chlorinated hydrocarbon in breast milk. *Can Med Assoc J*. 1977;117:1047–1048

392. Higginbottom MC, Sweetman L, Nyhan WL. A syndrome of methylmalonic aciduria, homocystinuria, megaloblastic anemia neurologic abnormalities in a vitamin B12-deficient breast-fed infant of a strict vegetarian. *N Engl J Med*. 1978;299:317–323

Appendix C

The Standing Committee on the Scientific Evaluation of Dietary Reference Intakes of the Food and Nutrition Board, Institute of Medicine, National Academy of Sciences, has undertaken a comprehensive expansion of the periodic reports called Recommended Dietary Allowances (RDAs) into a set of 4 nutrient-based values known as Dietary Reference Intakes (DRIs). These reference values include the Estimated Average Requirement (EAR), RDA, Adequate Intake (AI), and the Tolerable Upper Intake Level (UL). If sufficient scientific evidence is not available to calcuate an RDA, a reference intake called an AI is provided instead. Recommended dietary allowances and AIs are levels of intake recommended for individuals. They should reduce the risk of developing a condition that is associated with the nutrient in question that has a negative functional outcome. The DRIs apply to the apparently healthy general population. They are based on nutrient balance studies, the nutrient intakes of breastfed infants and healthy adults, biochemical measurement of tissue saturation or molecular function, and extrapolation from animal models. Unfortunately, only limited data are available on vitamin requirements in infants and children because of ethical, cost, and time concerns. Meeting the recommended intakes for the nutrients would not necessarily provide enough for individuals who are already malnourished, nor would they be adequate for certain disease states marked by increased nutritional requirements.

Table C-1.
Dietary Reference Intakes: Recommended Intakes for Individuals, Food and Nutrition Board, The National Academies of Sciences

	Infants 0–6 mo	Infants 7–12 mo	Children 1–2 y	Children 3–8 y	Males 9–13 y	Males 14–18 y	Females 9–13 y	Females 14–18 y	Pregnancy 14–18	Lactation 14–18
Active PAL k EER (kcal/d)	Male 570 Female 520 (3 mo)	Male 743 Female 676 (9 mo)	Male 1046 Female 992 (24 mo)	Male 1742 Female 1642 (6y)	2279 (11 y)	3152 (16 y)	2071 (11 y)	2368 (16 y)	1st trimester 2368 2nd trimester 2708 3rd trimester 2820 (16 y)	1st 6 mo 2698 2nd 6 mo 2768
Carbohydrates l			130	130	130	130	130	130	175	210
Total Fiber	ND n	ND	19	25	31	48	26	26	28	29
AI (g/d) m Fat	31	30	ND	ND	ND	ND	ND	ND	ND	ND
n-6 Polyunsaturated Fatty Acids (g/d) (Linoleic Acid)	4.4	4.6	7	10	12	16	10	11	13	13
n-3 Polyunsaturated Fatty Acids (g/d) (α-Linoleic Acid)	0.5	0.5	0.7	0.9	1.2	1.6	1.0	1.1	1.4	1.3
Protein (g/kg/d)		1.5	1.10	0.95	0.95	0.85	0.95	.085		
Vitamin A (μg/d) a	400*	500*	300	400	600	900	600	700	750	1200
Vitamin C (mg/d)	40*	50*	15	25	45	75	45	65	80	115
Vitamin D (μg/d) b,c	5*	5*	5*	5*	5*	5*	5*	5*	5*	5*
Vitamin E (mg/d) d	4*	5*	6	7	11	15	11	15	15	19
Vitamin K (μg/d)	2.0*	2.5*	30*	55*	60*	75*	60*	75*	75*	75*

Table C-1.
Dietary Reference Intakes: Recommended Intakes for Individuals, Food and Nutrition Board, The National Academies of Sciences, *continued*

	Infants 0–6 mo	Infants 7–12 mo	Children 1–2 y	Children 3–8 y	Males 9–13 y	Males 14–18 y	Females 9–13 y	Females 14–18 y	Pregnancy 14–18	Lactation 14–18
Thiamin (mg/d)	0.2*	0.3*	0.5	0.6	0.9	1.2	0.9	1.0	1.4	1.4
Riboflavin (mg/d)	0.3*	0.4*	0.5	0.6	0.9	1.3	0.9	1.0	1.4	1.6
Niacin (mg/d)[e]	2*	4*	6	8	12	16	12	14	18	17
Vitamin B₆ (mg/d)	0.1*	0.3*	0.5	0.6	1.0	1.3	1.0	1.2	1.9	2.0
Folate (µg/d)[f]	65*	80*	150	200	300	400	300	400[g]	600[h]	500
Vitamin B₁₂ (mg/d)	0.4*	0.5*	0.9	1.2	1.8	2.4	1.8	2.4	2.6	2.8
Pantothenic Acid (mg/d)	1.7*	1.8*	2*	3*	4*	5*	4*	5*	6*	7*
Biotin (µg/d)	5*	6*	8*	12*	20*	25*	20*	25*	30*	35*
Choline[i] (mg/d)	125*	125*	200*	250*	375*	550*	375*	400*	450*	550*
Calcium (mg/d)	210*	270*	500*	800*	1300*	1300*	1300*	1300*	1300*	1300*
Chromium (µg/d)	0.2*	5.5*	11*	15*	25*	35*	21*	24*	29*	44
Copper (µg/d)	200*	220*	340	440	700	890	700	890	1000	1300
Fluoride (mg/d)	0.01*	0.5*	0.7*	1*	2*	3*	2*	2*	3*	3*

Table C–1.
Dietary Reference Intakes: Recommended Intakes for Individuals, Food and Nutrition Board, The National Academies of Sciences, *continued*

	Infants 0–6 mo	Infants 7–12 mo	Children 1–2 y	Children 3–8 y	Males 9–13 y	Males 14–18 y	Females 9–13 y	Females 14–18 y	Pregnancy 14–18	Lactation 14–18
Iodine (µg/d)	110*	130*	90	90	120	150	120	150	220	290
Iron (mg/d)	0.27*	11	7	10	8	11	8	15	27	10
Magnesium (mg/d)	30*	75*	80	130	240	410	240	360	400	360
Manganese (mg/d)	0.003*	0.6*	1.2*	1.5*	1.9*	2.2*	1.6*	1.6*	2.0*	2.6*
Molybdenum (µg/d)	2*	3*	17	22	34	43	34	43	50	50
Phosphorus (mg/d)	100*	275*	460	500	1250	1250	1250	1250	1250	1250
Selenium (µg/d)	15*	20*	20	30	40	55	40	55	60	70
Zinc (mg/d)	2*	3	3	5	8	11	8	9	13	14

NOTE: This table (taken from the DRI reports, see www.nap.edu presents Recommended Dietary Allowances (RDAs) in **bold type** and Adequate Intakes (AIs) are in ordinary type followed by an asterisk (*). RDAs and AIs may both be used as goals for individual intake. RDAs are set to meet the needs of almost all individuals in a group. For healthy breastfed infants, the AI is the mean intake. The AI for other life stage and gender groups is believed to cover needs of all individuals in the group, but lack of data or uncertainty in the data prevent being able to specify with confidence the percentage of individuals covered by this intake.

a As retinol activity equivalents (RAEs). 1 RAE = 1 µg retinol, 12 µg β-carotene, 24 µg α-carotene, or 24 µg β-cryptoxanthin in foods. To calculate RAEs from retinol equivalents (REs) of provitamin A carotenoids in foods, divide the REs by 2. For preformed vitamin A in foods or supplements and for provitamin A carotenoids in supplements, 1 RE = 1 RAE.

b Cholecalciferol. 1 µg cholecalciferol = 40 IU vitamin D.

c In the absence of adequate exposure to sunlight.

d As α-tocopherol. α-Tocopherol includes RRR-α-tocopherol, the only form of α-tocopherol that occurs naturally in foods, and the 2R-stereoisomeric forms of α-tocopherol (RRR-, RSR-, RRS-, and RSS-α-tocopherol) that occur in fortified foods and supplements. It does not include the 2S-stereoisomeric forms of α-tocopherol (SRR-, SSR-, SRS-, and SSS-α-tocopherol), also found in fortified foods and supplements.

e As niacin equivalents (NE). 1 mg of niacin = 60 mg of tryptophan; 0–6 months-preformed niacin (not NE).

f As dietary folate equivalents (DFE). 1 DFE=1 µg food folate=0.6 µg of folic acid from fortified food or as a supplement consumed with food=0.5 µg of a supplement taken on an empty stomach.

g In view of evidence linking folate intake with neural tube defects in the fetus, it is recommended that all women capable of becoming pregnant consume 400 μg from supplements or fortified foods in addition to intake of food folate from the diet.

h It is assumed that women will continue consuming 400 μg from supplements or fortified food until their pregnancy is confirmed and they enter prenatal care, which ordinarily occurs after the end of the preconceptional period—the critical time for formation of the neural tube.

i Although AIs have been set for choline, there are few data to assess whether a dietary supply of choline is needed at all stages of the life cycle, and it may be that the choline requirement can be met by endogenous synthesis at some of these stages.

j For healthy moderately active American and Canadians.

k PAL = physical activity letter, EER = estimated energy requirement, TEE = total energy expenditure. The intake that meets the average energy expenditure of individuals at the reference height, weight, and age.

l RDA = Recommended Dietary Allowance. The intake that meets the nutrient need of almost all (97–98 percent) of individuals in a group.

m AI = Adequate Intake. The observed average or experimentally determined intake by a defined population or subgroup that appears to sustain a defined nutritional status, such as growth rate, normal circulating nutrient values, or other functional indicators of health. The AI is used if sufficient scientific evidence is not available to derive an EAR. For healthy infants receiving human milk, the AI is the mean intake. The AI is not equivalent to an RDA. Based on 14g/1000 kcal of required energy.

n ND = not determined. The observed average or experimentally determined intake by a defined population or subgroup that appears to sustain a defined nutritional status, such as growth rate, normal circulating nutrient values, or other functional indicators of health. The AI is used if sufficient scientific evidence is not available to derive an Estimated Average Requirement (EAR). For healthy infants receiving human milk, the AI is the mean intake. The AI is not equivalent to an RDA.

No determined biological function in humans has been identified for the nutrients: Silicon and Vanadium.

Table C–2.
Dietary Reference Intakes (DRIs): Tolerable Upper Intake Levels (UL[a]), Food and Nutrition Board, The National Academies of Sciences

	Infants 0–6 mo	Infants 7–12 mo	Children 1–3 y	Children 4–8 y	Males/Females 9–13 y	Males/Females 14–18 y	Pregnancy ≤18	Lactation ≤18
Vitamin A (μg/d)[b]	600	600	600	900	1700	2800	2800	2800
Vitamin C (mg/d)	ND[f]	ND	400	650	1200	1800	1800	1800
Vitamin D (μg/d)	25	25	50	50	50	50	50	50
Vitamin E (mg/d)[c,d]	ND	ND	200	300	600	800	800	800
Vitamin K (μg/d)	ND	ND	ND	ND	ND	ND	ND	ND
Thiamin (mg/d)	ND	ND	ND	ND	ND	ND	ND	ND
Riboflavin (mg/d)	ND	ND	ND	ND	ND	ND	ND	ND
Niacin (mg/d)[d]	ND	ND	10	15	20	30	30	30
Vitamin B6 (mg/d)	ND	ND	30	40	60	80	80	80
Folate (μg/d)[d]	ND	ND	300	400	600	800	800	800
Vitamin B12 (mg/d)	ND	ND	ND	ND	ND	ND	ND	ND

Table C–2.
Dietary Reference Intakes (DRIs): Tolerable Upper Intake Levels (UL[a]), Food and Nutrition Board, The National Academies of Sciences, *continued*

	Infants 0–6 mo	Infants 7–12 mo	Children 1–3 y	Children 4–8 y	Males/Females 9–13 y	Males/Females 14–18 y	Pregnancy ≤18	Lactation ≤18
Pantothenic Acid (mg/d)	ND	ND	ND	ND	ND	ND	ND	ND
Biotin (μg/d)	ND	ND	ND	ND	ND	ND	ND	ND
Choline (mg/d)	ND	ND	1.0	1.0	2.0	3.0	3.0	3.0
Carotenoids[e]	ND	ND	ND	ND	ND	ND	ND	ND
Arsenic[b]	ND	ND	ND	ND	ND	ND	ND	ND
Boron (mg/d)	ND	ND	3	6	11	17	17	17
Calcium (mg/d)	ND	ND	2.5	2.5	2.5	2.5	2.5	2.5
Chromium (μg/d)	ND	ND	ND	ND	ND	ND	ND	ND
Copper (μg/d)	ND	ND	1000	3000	5000	8000	8000	8000
Fluoride (mg/d)	.07	.09	1.3	2.2	10	10	10	10
Iodine (μg/d)	ND	ND	200	300	600	900	900	900
Iron (mg/d)	40	40	40	40	40	45	45	45

Table C–2.
Dietary Reference Intakes (DRIs): Tolerable Upper Intake Levels (UL[a]), Food and Nutrition Board, The National Academies of Sciences, *continued*

	Infants 0–6 mo	Infants 7–12 mo	Children 1–3 y	Children 4–8 y	Males/Females 9–13 y	Males/Females 14–18 y	Pregnancy ≤18	Lactation ≤18
Magnesium (mg/d)[c]	ND	ND	65	110	350	350	350	350
Manganese (mg/d)	ND	ND	2	3	6	9	9	9
Molybdenum (μg/d)	ND	ND	300	600	1100	1700	1700	1700
Nickel (mg/d)	ND	ND	0.2	0.3	0.6	1.0	1.0	1.0
Phosphorus (mg/d)	ND	ND	3	3	4	4	3.5	4
Selenium (μg/d)	45	60	90	150	280	400	400	400
Silicon[d]	ND	ND	ND	ND	ND	ND	ND	ND
Vanadium (mg/d)[e]	ND	ND	ND	ND	ND	ND	ND	ND
Zinc (mg/d)	4	5	7	12	23	34	34	34

[a] UL = The maximum level of daily nutrient intake that is likely to pose no risk of adverse effects. Unless other wise specified, the UL represents total intake from food, water, and supplements. Due to lack of suitable data, ULs could not be established for vitamin K, thiamin, riboflavin, vitamin B_{12}, pantothenic acid, biotin, or carotenoids. In the absences of ULs, extra caution may be warranted in consuming levels above recommended intakes.

[b] As preformed vitamin A only.

[c] As α-tocopherol; applies to any form of supplemental α-tocopherol.

[d] The ULs for vitamin E, niacin, and folate apply to synthetic forms obtained from supplements, fortified foods, or a combination of the two.

[e] β–Carotene supplements are advised only to serve as a provitamin A source for individuals at risk of vitamin A deficiency.

[f] ND = Not determinable due to lack of data of adverse effects in this age group and concern with regard to lack of ability to handle excess amounts.

Table C–3.
Nutrition During Pregnancy[1]

Dietary Reference Intakes (DRIs) During Pregnancy[1]						
	Females			**Pregnancy**		
Life Stage Group	14–18 y	19–30 y	31–50 y	≤18 y	19–30 y	31–50 y
Calcium (mg/d)	1300*	1000*	1000*	1300*	1000*	1000*
Phosphorus (mg/d)	1250	700	700	1,250	700	700
Magnesium (mg/d)	360	310	320	400	350	360
Vitamin A (μg/d)	700	700	700	750	770	770
Vitamin D (μg/d)[a,b]	5*	5*	5*	5*	5*	5*
Fluoride (mg/d)	3*	3*	3*	3*	3*	3*
Thiamin (mg/d)	1.0	1.1	1.1	1.4	1.4	1.4
Riboflavin (mg/d)	1.0	1.1	1.1	1.4	1.4	1.4
Niacin (mg/d)[c]	14	14	14	18	18	18
Vitamin B_6 (mg/d)	1.2	1.3	1.3	1.9	1.9	1.9
Folate (μg/d)[d]	400[g]	400[g]	400[g]	600[h]	600[h]	600[h]
Vitamin B_{12} (μg/d)	2.4	2.4	2.4	2.6	2.6	2.6
Pantothenic Acid (mg/d)	5*	5*	5*	6*	6*	6*
Biotin (μg/d)	25*	30*	30*	30*	30*	30*
Choline[e] (mg/d)	400*	425*	425*	450*	450*	450*
Vitamin C (mg/d)	65	75	75	80	85	85
Vitamin E[f] (mg/d)	15	15	15	15	15	15
Iron (mg/d)	15	18	18	27	27	27
Zinc (mg/d)	9	8	8	13	11	11
Copper (μg/d)	890	900	900	1000	1000	1000
Selenium (μg/d)	55	55	55	60	60	60
Iodine (μg/d)	150	150	150	220	220	220

Institute of Medicine.[35,37,49,54]

* Adequate Intakes (AI).

[a] As cholecalciferol. 1 μg cholecalciferol = 40 IU vitamin D.

[b] In the absence of adequate exposure to sunlight.

[c] As niacin equivalents (NE). 1 mg of niacin = 60 mg of tryptophan.

[d] As dietary folate equivalents (DFE). 1 DFE = 1 μg food folate = 0.6 μg of folic acid from fortified food or as a supplement consumed with food = 0.5 μg of a supplement taken on an empty stomach.

[e] Although AIs have been set for choline, there are few data to assess whether a dietary supply of choline is needed at all stages of the life cycle, and it may be that the choline requirement can be met by endogenous synthesis at some of these stages.

[f] As α-tocopherol. α-Tocopherol includes *RRR*-α-tocopherol, the only form of α-tocopherol that occurs naturally in foods, and the 2*R*-stereoisomeric forms of α-tocopherol (*SRR*-, *SSR*-, *SRS*, and *SSS*-α-tocopherol), also found in fortified foods and supplements.

g In view of evidence linking folate intake with neural tube defects in the fetus, it is recommended that all women capable of becoming pregnant consume 400 μg from supplements or fortified foods in addition to intake of food folate from a varied diet.

h It is assumed that women will continue consuming 400 μg from supplements or fortified food until their pregnancy is confirmed and they enter prenatal care, which ordinarily occurs after the end of the periconceptional period—the critical time for formation of the neural tube.

1a 35.   Institute of Medicine. Vitamin A. In: *Dietary Intakes for Vitamin A, Vitamin K, Arsenic, Boron, Chromium, Copper, Iodine, Iron, Manganese, Molybdenum, Nickel, Silicon, Vanadium, and Zinc.* National Academy Press; 2001:65–126

1b 37.   Institute of Medicine FNB. Dietary Reference Intakes for Calcium, Phosphorus, Magnesium, Vitamin D, and Fluoride. Washington, DC: Institute of Medicine; 1997

1c 49.   Institute of Medicine FNB. Dietary Reference Intakes for Thiamin, Riboflavin, Niacin, Vitamin B$_6$, Folate, Vitamin B$_{12}$, Pantothenic Acid, Biotin, and Choline. Washington, DC: Institute of Medicine; 1998

1d 54.   Institute of Medicine FNB. Dietary Reference Intakes for Vitamin C, Vitamin E, Selenium, and Carotenoids. Washington, DC: Institute of Medicine; 2000

Appendix D

Table D–1.
Recommended Nutrient Levels of Infant Formulas (per 100 kcal)
(From the American Academy of Pediatrics Committee on Nutrition 1982 Task Force and 1987 FDA Recommendations)

Nutrient	Range	
	Lowest Adequate	Not to Exceed*
Protein, g	1.8†	4.5†
Fat, g	3.3 (30% of cal)	6 (54% of cal)
Including essential fatty acid (linoleate), mg	300 (2.7% of cal)	
Vitamins		
A, IU	250 (75 μg)‡	750 (225 μg)‡
D, IU	40 (1 μg)§	100 (2.5 μg)§
K, μg‖	4	...
E, IU	0.7 (0.5 mg)¶ at least 0.71 U (0.5 mg)/g linoleic acid	... ...
C (ascorbic acid), mg	8	...
B₁ (thiamine), μg	40	...
B₂ (riboflavin), μg	60	...
B₆ (pyridoxine), μg	35 (15 μg/g of protein)	...
B₁₂, μg	0.15	...
Niacin, μg	250 (or 0.8 mg niacin equivalents)	...
Folic acid, μg	4	
Pantothenic acid, μg	300	...
Biotin, μg	1.5#	
Choline, mg	7#	
Inositol, mg	4#	

Table D–1.
Recommended Nutrient Levels of Infant Formulas (per 100 kcal)
(From the American Academy of Pediatrics Committee on Nutrition 1982 Task Force and 1987
FDA Recommendations), *continued*

Nutrient	Range	
	Lowest Adequate	Not to Exceed*
Minerals**		
Calcium, mg	60††	...
Phosphorus, mg	30††	...
Magnesium, mg	6	...
Iron, mg	0.15	3.0‡‡
Iodine, μg	5	25
Zinc, mg	0.5	...
Copper, μg	60	...
Manganese, μg	5	...
Sodium, mg	20 (5.8 mEq)	60 (17.5 mEq)
Potassium, mg	80 (13.7 mEq)	200 (34.3 mEq)
Chloride, mg	55 (10.4 mEq)	150 (28.3 mEq)
Selenium, μg§§	3	...

* Where no upper limit is given, toxic effects are not well defined. The Task Force is concerned that massive excesses may have adverse consequences.
† At least nutritionally equivalent to casein quality recommended as outlined in Statement: Commentary on breastfeeding and infant formulas, including proposed standards for formulas. *Pediatrics.* 1976;57:278–285.
‡ Retinol equivalents.
§ Cholecalciferol.
‖ Any vitamin K added shall be in the form of phylloquinone.
¶ d-α-tocopherol equivalents.
# Average present in milk-based formulas; should be included in this amount in other formulas.
** Formula should be made with water low in fluoride and, in any case, should contain less than 45 μg/100 kcal. For explanation, see Committee on Nutrition Statement: Fluoride supplementation. Pediatrics. 1986;77:758–761.
†† Calcium-phosphorus ratio should be no less than 1.1 or more than 2.
‡‡ Prudence indicates that there should be an upper limit on iron. If formula is labeled infant formula with iron, it must contain not less than 1 mg/100 kcal.
§§ Selenium is not included in the 1987 recommendations. The safe range is very narrow.

Table D–2.
Recommendations of the Expert Panel for Nutrient Levels in Infant Formulas

Nutrients (Units)[1]		LSRO (1998)	FDA (1985)
Energy (kcal/dl)	minimum	63	*
	maximum	71	*
Total Fat (g) [% energy]	minimum	4.4 [40]	3.3 [30]
	maximum	6.4 [57.2]	6.0 [54]
Essential fats (all *cis*-; as % of total fatty acids): Linoleic acid; LA α-Linoleic acid; ALA Ratio LA:ALA	minimum	8 1.75 16:1	2.7 * *
Linoleic acid; LA α-Linoleic acid; ALA Ratio LA: ALA	maximum	35 4.0 6:1	* * *
Protein (g)	minimum	1.7[2]	1.8
	maximum	3.4[3]	4.5
Carnitine (mg)	mininum	1.2	*
	maximum	2.0	*
Taurine (mg)**	minimum	0	*
	maximum	12	*
Nucleotides (mg)**	minimum	0	*
	maximum	16	*
Choline (mg)	minimum	7	7.0
	maximum	30	*
Inositol (mg)	minimum	4	4.0
	maximum	40	*
Total Carbohydrate (g)	minimum	9	*
	maximum	13	*

Table D–2.
Recommendations of the Expert Panel for Nutrient Levels in Infant Formulas, *continued*

Nutrients (Units)[1]		LSRO (1998)	FDA (1985)
MINERALS			
Calcium (mg)	minimum	50[4]	80[4]
	maximum	140	*
Phosphorus (mg)	minimum	20[4,5]	30[4]
	maximum	70[5]	*
Magnesium (mg)	minimum	4	6.0
	maximum	17	*
Iron (mg)	minimum	0.2	0.15
	maximum	1.65	3.0
Zinc (mg)	mininum	0.4	0.5
	maximum	1.0	*
Manganese (μg)	minimum	1.0	5.0
	maximum	100	*
Copper (μg)	minimum	60	60
	maximum	160	*
Iodine (μg)	minimum	8	5.0[6]
	maximum	35	*
Sodium (mg)	minimum	25	20
	maximum	50	60
Potassium (mg)	minimum	60	80
	maximum	160	200
Chloride (mg)	minimum	50	55
	maximum	160	150
Selenium (μg)	minimum	1.5	
	maximum	5.0	
Fluoride (μg)**	minimum	0	
	maximum	60	
VITAMINS			
Vit. A (IU)	minimum	200	250
	maximum	500	750
Vit. D (IU)	minimum	40	40
	maximum	100	100

Table D-2.
Recommendations of the Expert Panel for Nutrient Levels in Infant Formulas, *continued*

Nutrients (Units)[1]		LSRO (1998)	FDA (1985)
Vit. E (mg α-TE/g PUFA)[7]	minimum	0.5	0.7[8]
	maximum	5	*
Vit. K$_1$ (μg)	minimum	1.0	4.0
	maximum	25	*
Vit. B$_1$: Thiamin (μg)	minimum	30	40
	maximum	200	*
Vit. B$_2$: Riboflavin (μg)	minimum	80	60
	maximum	300	*
Vit. B$_3$: Niacin (μg)	mininum	550	250
	maximum	2000	*
Vit B$_6$: Pyridoxine (μg)	minimum	30	35[9]
	maximum	130	*
Vit. B$_{12}$: Cobalamin (μg)	minimum	0.08	0.15
	maximum	0.7	*
Folic acid (μg)	minimum	11	4.0
	maximum	40	*
Pantothenic acid (μg)	minimum	300	300
	maximum	1200	*
Biotin (μg)	minimum	1.0	1.5
	maximum	15	*
Vit. C: Ascorbic acid (mg)	minimum	6	8.0
	maximum	15	*

* No values specified.
** The inclusion of these substances in this table does not constitute an endorsement of their use in formulas intended for term infants, rather it is a recognition of apparent safety at levels defined by the maximum.
[1] Units expressed per 100 kcal of formula unless otherwise noted.
[2] Refers to true protein (α-amino nitrogen x 6.25)
[3] Refers to crude protein (total nitrogen x 6.25)
[4] Calcium to phosphorus ratio must be no less than 1.1 nor more than 2.0.
[5] Indicates available (nonphytate) phosphorus.
[6] Previous specifications recommended soy-based formulas contain 10–20 μg/100 kcal.
[7] To contain no less than 0.5 mg α-TE/100 kcal.
[8] Specifications indicated that vitamin E also be expressed as 0.7 IU per g of linoleic acid.
[9] Vitamin B$_6$ also expressed as 15 μg per g of protein formula.

Appendix E

Table E–1.
Human Milk, Cow Milk, and Goat Milk

	g/100 mL			mg/100 mL Source				Source		Osmolality (m Osm/kg of H₂0) and General Comments
	Pro	Fat	CHO	Na / K	Ca / P	Fe	CHO	Fat		
Human Milk (Mature) (20 kcal/30 mL)	0.9	3.9	6.7	12–25 / 40–55	20–25 / 12–14	<0.1	Lactose Glucose Oligosaccarhides	Human Milk Fat		(260–300) Whey:casein ratio is 60:40.
Evaporated Whole Milk (43 kcal/30 mL)	7.0	8.0	10.7	113 / 322	278 / 216	0.2	Lactose	Butterfat		Milk is diluted and dextrose added to make a 20 calorie per oz formula.
Skim Milk (11 kcal/30 mL)	3.5	0.2	5.0	53 / 171	128 / 104	Trace	Lactose	Trace Butterfat		(279) Deficient in essential fatty acids. Not recommended for children <2 y.
2% Milk (15 kcal/30 mL)	3.4	2.0	5.0	51 / 159	125 / 98	Trace	Lactose	Butterfat		(279) Used to moderately reduce calories and fat. Not recommended for infants <2 y.
Whole Milk (19 kcal/30 mL)	3.3	3.4	4.8	50 / 156	123 / 96	Trace	Lactose	Butterfat		(279) Whey:casein ratio is 18:82. Not recommended for infants <1 y.
Goat Milk (21 kcal/30 mL)	3.7	4.3	4.6	51 / 210	138 / 114	Trace	Lactose	Butterfat		(267) Fat more readily digested than fat in cow milk. Used rarely for intolerance to cow milk. Not appropriate for use in infancy, as it is inadequate in folate and other essential nutrients.

Table E–2.
Cow Milk-Based Infant Formulas (per Liter)

per liter unless otherwise stated	Enfamil®/ Enfamil® with Iron (Mead Johnson®, Evansville IN)*	Enfamil®/ AR Liquid Only (Mead Johnson®, Evansville, IN)	Enfamil® Lacto-Free®* (Mead Johnson®, Evansville, IN)	Enfamil® Lipil (Mead Johnson®, Evansville, IN)*	NAN®* (Nestle, Glendale, CA)	Store Brand Milk-based Formula† (Wyeth Nutritionals)	Good Start Supreme®* (Nestle, Glendale, CA)	Good Start® Essentials (Nestle, Glendale, CA)	Good Start® Supreme with DHA & ARA (Nestle, Glendale, CA)
Energy, kcal	680	680	680	680	676	672	676	676	676
Protein, g	14.5	16.9	14.3	14.5	15	15	15	15	15
Casein, % of total protein	40	82	82	40	40	40	0	40	
Whey, % of total protein	60	18	18	60	60	60	100‡	60	100
Fat, g	36	35	36	36	35	36	35	35	35
Polyunsaturated, %	19	19	19	20	22	17.7	22	22	24
Monounsaturated, %	38	38	38	37	33	37.3	33	33	32
Saturated, %	43	43	43	43	45	45	45	45	44
Oils	Palm olein, high-oleic sunflower, coconut, and soy	Palm olein, high-oleic sunflower, coconut, and soy	Palm olein, soy, coconut, and high-oleic sunflower	Palm olein, high-oleic sunflower, soy, and coconut DHA, ARA	Palm olein, soy, coconut, high-oleic sunflower, and safflower	Palm, high-oleic, coconut and soybean, safflower, or sunflower	Palm olein, soy, coconut, and high-oleic safflower	Palm olein, soy, coconut, high-oleic safflower	Palm olein, soy, coconut, high-oleic safflower, DHA, ARA
Carbohydrate, g	73	74	73	73	76	72	76	76	76
	Lactose	Lactose, rice, starch, and maltodextrin	Corn syrup solids	Lactose	Lactose, corn syrup	Lactose	Lactose, corn maltodextrins		
Osmolality mOsm/kg	300	240	200	300	299	290	260		

Table E–2.
Cow Milk-Based Infant Formulas (per Liter), *continued*

per liter unless otherwise stated	Enfamil®/ Enfamil® with Iron (Mead Johnson®, Evansville IN)*	Enfamil®/ AR Liquid Only (Mead Johnson®, Evansville, IN)	Enfamil® Lacto-Free®* (Mead Johnson®, Evansville, IN)	Enfamil® Lipil (Mead Johnson®, Evansville, IN)*	NAN®* (Nestle, Glendale, CA)	Store Brand Milk-based Formula† (Wyeth Nutritionals)	Good Start Supreme®* (Nestle, Glendale,CA)	Good Start® Essentials (Nestle, Glendale,CA)	Good Start® Supreme with DHA & ARA (Nestle, Glendale,CA)
Minerals									
Calcium, mg	530	530	550	530	510	420	435	503	435
Phosphorus, mg	360	360	370	360	286	280	245	286	245
Magnesium, mg	54	54	54	54	48	45	48	48	48
Iron, mg	4.7/12.2§	12.2	12.2	12.2	10.2	12	10.2	10.2	10.2
Zinc, mg	6.8	6.8	6.8	6.8	5.4	5	5.4	5.4	5.4
Manganese, μg	101	101	101	100	48	100	48	48	48
Copper, μg	510	510	510	510	544	470	544	544	544
Iodine, μg	68	68	101	68	82	60	82	68	82
Sodium, mEq	8	11.7	8.7	8	7.10	6.4	7.10	6.78	7.10
Potassium, mEq	18.7	18.7	18.9	18.7	17.44	14.4	17.44	17.08	17.44
Chloride, mEq	12.1	14.4	12.7	12.1	12.48	10.7	12.48	11.33	12.48
Vitamins									
A, IU	2000	2000	2000	2000	2027	2000	2039	2040	2039
D, IU	410	410	410	410	405	400	408	408	408
E, IU	13.5	13.5	13.5	13.5	13.6	10	13.6	13.6	13.6
K, μg	54	54	54	54	54	55	54	54	54
Thiamine (B$_1$), μg	540	540	540	540	405	670	408	408	408

Table E–2.
Cow Milk-Based Infant Formulas (per Liter), *continued*

per liter unless otherwise stated	Enfamil®/Enfamil® with Iron (Mead Johnson®, Evansville IN)*	Enfamil® AR Liquid Only (Mead Johnson®, Evansville, IN)	Enfamil® Lacto-Free®* (Mead Johnson®, Evansville, IN)	Enfamil® Lipil (Mead Johnson®, Evansville, IN)*	NAN®* (Nestle, Glendale, CA)	Store Brand Milk-based Formula† (Wyeth Nutritionals)	Good Start Supreme®* (Nestle, Glendale, CA)	Good Start® Essentials (Nestle, Glendale, CA)	Good Start® Supreme with DHA & ARA (Nestle, Glendale, CA)
Riboflavin (B_2), μg	950	950	950	950	952	1000	952	952	952
Pyridoxine, μg	410	410	410	410	510	420	510	442	510
B_{12}, μg	2.0	2.0	2.0	2.0	1.7	1.0	1.7	1.5	1.7
Niacin, mg	6.8	6.8	6.8	6.8	5.1	5.0	5.1	5.1	5.1
Folic acid, μg	108	108	108	108	102	50	102	102	102
Pantothenic acid, mg	3.4	3.4	3.4	3.4	3.06	2.1	3.06	3.06	3.06
Biotin, μg	20	20	20	20	14.9	15	15	15	15
C (ascorbic acid), mg	81	81	81	81	61	55	61	61	61
Choline, mg	81	81	81	81	82	100	82	82	82
Inositol, mg	41	41	41	41	122	27	122	68	122
Linoleic acid, mg								6120	6118
Linolenic acid, mg								938	637
Selenium, μg								7	8
Nucleotides (added)								34	34

*Liquid and powder.
†With nucleotides.
‡Partially hydrolyzed.
§High iron.

Table E–2.
(continued)

per liter unless otherwise stated	Similac® Low Iron/with Iron* (Ross, Columbus, OH)	Similac® Lactose Free* (Ross, Columbus, OH)	Similac® PM 60/40 Powder Only (Ross, Columbus, OH) Prepared to 20 kcal/oz	Similac® with Iron 24 Liquid Only (Ross, Columbus OH)	Similac® Advance*
Energy, kcal	676	676	676	806	676
Protein, g	14	14	15	21.9	14
Casein, % of total protein	52	18	40	18	52
Whey, % of total protein	48	82	60	82	48
Fat, g	36.5	36.5	37.8	42.5	36.5
Polyunsaturated, %	24	37	39	37	
Monounsaturated %	39	17	18	17	
Saturated, %	37	46	43	46	
Oils	High-oleic safflower, coconut, and soy	Soy and coconut	Corn, coconut, and soy	Soy and coconut oils	High-oleic safflower, soy, coconut, <2% M. alpina and C. cohnii oils (0.15% DHA, 0.4% ARA)
Carbohydrate, g	73	72.3	68.9	85	73
	Lactose	Corn syrup solids and sucrose	Lactose	Lactose	Lactose
Osmolality mOsm/kg	300	200	300	380	300
Minerals					
Calcium, mg	527	568	378	726	527
Phosphorus, mg	284	378	189	565	284

Table E–2.
(continued)

per liter unless otherwise stated	Similac® Low Iron/with Iron* (Ross, Columbus, OH)	Similac® Lactose Free* (Ross, Columbus, OH)	Similac® PM 60/40 Powder Only (Ross, Columbus, OH) Prepared to 20 kcal/oz	Similac® with Iron 24 Liquid Only (Ross, Columbus OH)	Similac® Advance*
Magnesium, mg	41	41	40.5	56.5	40.5
Iron, mg	4.7/12.2§	12.2	4.7	14.5	12.2
Zinc, mg	5.1	5.1	5.07	6.05	5.1
Manganese, μg	34	34	34	40	34
Copper, μg	608	608	608	726	608
Iodine, μg	41	61	41	73	41
Sodium, mEq	7.1	8.8	7.1	11.9	6.8
Potassium, mEq	18.1	18.5	14.9	27.2	18.2
Chloride, mEq	12.4	12.4	11.2	18.4	12.2
Vitamins					
A, IU	2027	2027	2027	2419	2027
D, IU	405	405	405	484	405
E, IU	10.1	20.3	16.9	24.2	10.1
K, μg	54	54	54	65	54
Thiamine (B_1), μg	676	676	676	806	676
Riboflavin (B_2), μg	1014	1014	1014	1210	676
Pyridoxine, μg	405	405	405	484	405
B_{12}, μg	1.7	1.7	1.69	1.69	1.7

Table E–2.
(continued)

per liter unless otherwise stated	Similac® Low Iron/with Iron* (Ross, Columbus, OH)	Similac® Lactose Free* (Ross, Columbus, OH)	Similac® PM 60/40 Powder Only (Ross, Columbus, OH) Prepared to 20 kcal/oz	Similac® with Iron 24 Liquid Only (Ross, Columbus OH)	Similac® Advance*
Niacin, mg	7.1	7.1	7.1	8.5	7.1
Folic acid, μg	101	101	101	101	101
Pantothenic acid, mg	3.04	3.04	3	3.6	3.04
Biotin, μg	29.7	29.7	30.4	30.4	29.7
C (ascorbic acid), mg	61	61	61	61	61
Choline, mg	108	108	81	129	108
Inositol, mg	32	29	162.2	37.9	32

Table E–3.
Follow-up Formulas for Infant Feeding (per Liter)

	Similac® 2* (Ross, Columbus, OH)	Good Start® 2 Essentials (Nestle, Glendale, CA)†	Good Start® 2 Essentials Soy (Nestle, Glendale, CA)	Enfamil® Next-Step (Mead Johnson, Evansville, IN)	Store Brand Formula for Older Infants (Wyeth Nutritionals)†	Enfamil® Next-Step® Soy Powder (Mead Johnson)	Isomil® 2 (Ross Columbus, OH)
Energy, kcal	676	676	676	680	680	680	676
Protein, g	14*	17.5	21	17.6	18	22‡	16‡
Casein, % of total calories	52	82	0	82	50	...	NA
Whey, %	48	18	0	18	50	...	NA
Fat, g	37	28	29	34	6	30	37
Polyunsaturated, %	24	22	22	19	14.5	19	24
Monounsaturated %	39	33	33	38	41.3	38	39
Saturated, %	37	45	45	40	44.2	40	37
Predominant oil	High-oleic safflower and coconut and soy oils	Palm, olein, soy, coconut, and high-oleic safflower	Palm olein, soy, coconut, and high-oleic safflower	Palm olein, soy, coconut, and high-oleic sunflower	Oleo, coconut, high-oleic, and soy oils	Palm olein, soy, coconut, and high-oleic sunflower	High-oleic safflower, coconut, and soy oils
Carbohydrate, g	72§	89§	80	75§	69§	80‖	70‖
Osmolality mOsm/kg	300	200		270	280	260	200
Minerals							
Calcium, mg	797	810	902	810	816	780	912
Phosphorus, mg	432	540	602	570	571	610	608
Magnesium, mg	40.5	54	67	54	67	54	50.7
Iron, mg	12.2	12.5	12.1	12.2	12	12.2	12.2

Table E–3.
Follow-up Formulas for Infant Feeding (per Liter), *continued*

	Similac® 2* (Ross, Columbus, OH)	Good Start® 2 Essentials (Nestle, Glendale, CA)†	Good Start® 2 Essentials Soy (Nestle, Glendale, CA)	Enfamil® Next-Step (Mead Johnson, Evansville, IN)	Store Brand Formula for Older Infants (Wyeth Nutritionals)†	Enfamil® Next-Step® Soy Powder (Mead Johnson)	Isomil® 2 (Ross Columbus, OH)
Zinc, mg	5.1	5.4	6	6.1	6.0	8.1	5.1
Manganese, µg	34	48	247	47	40	169	169
Copper, µg	608	571	802	610	580	510	507
Iodine, µg	41	67	100	54	69	101	101
Sodium, mEq	7.1	11.48	11.04	12.2	9.6	13	12.9
Potassium, mEq	18.1	23.36	20.26	23	21.5	26	18.7
Chloride, mEq	12.4	17.15	14.92	16.3	15.7	19.2	11.8
Vitamins							
A, IU	2027	1692	2006	2000	2500	2000	2027
D, IU	405	405	402	410	440	417	405
E, IU	20.3	13.5	19.5	13.5	13.6	13.5	10.1
K, µg	54	54	53	54	67	54	74
Thiamine (B₁), µg	676	540	535	680	1000	540	405
Riboflavin (B₂), µg	1014	945	628	1010	1500	610	608
Pyridoxine, µg	405	436	468	410	600	610	405
B₁₂, µg	1.7	1.7	2.1	1.7	2	2	3.04
Niacin, mg	7.1	6.07	8.69	7.1	6.9	6.8	9.1
Folic acid, µg	101	104	107	101	10.2	108	101
Pantothenic acid, mg	3	3.24	3.14	3	3	3.4	5.1

Table E-3.
Follow-up Formulas for Infant Feeding (per Liter), *continued*

	Similac® 2* (Ross, Columbus, OH)	Good Start® 2 Essentials (Nestle, Glendale, CA)†	Good Start® 2 Essentials Soy (Nestle, Glendale, CA)	Enfamil® Next-Step (Mead Johnson, Evansville, IN)	Store Brand Formula for Older Infants (Wyeth Nutritionals)†	Enfamil® Next-Step® Soy Powder (Mead Johnson)	Isomil® 2 (Ross Columbus, OH)
Biotin, μg	29.7	14.5	52	30	20	20	30.4
C (ascorbic acid), mg	61	61	100	61	90	81	61
Choline, mg	108	81	81	108	100	81	54
Inositol, mg	31.8	125	81	32	27	115	33.8
Linoleic acid, mg		680	5750				
Linolenic acid, mg		60	780				
Selenium μg		13.6	13				

*Cow milk and soy isolate.
§For infants 4–12 months and older.
‡Soy protein isolate.
″Lactose and corn syrup.
‖Corn syrup solids and sucrose.

Table E–4.
Increasing the Caloric Density of Human Milk and Infant Formula

Human Milk		
kcal/oz	Milk Volume	Powdered Standard Infant Formula
24	4 oz	1¹/₄ tsp
30	4 oz	1 T
Infant Formula (Powdered)		
kcal/oz	Amount Powder	Volume Water
24	1¹/₄ c	29 oz (32/3 c)
30	1¹/₂ c	29 oz (32/3 c)
Infant Formula (Liquid Concentrate)		
kcal/oz	Volume Concentrate	Volume Water
24	13 oz (1 can)	8 oz (1 c)
28	13 oz (1 can)	5.5 oz (1 c)
30	13 oz (1 can)	4 oz (¹/₂ c)
Other Additives		
Medium-chain triglyceride oil contains 7.7 kcal/mL; 1 tsp contains 39 kcal. Vegetable oil contains 40 kcal/tsp. Polycose liquid contains 60 kcal/oz; Polycose powder contains 8 kcal/tsp.		

Appendix F

Table F-1.
Soy-Based Formulas (per Liter)

	Good Start® Essentials Soy (Nestle, Glendale, CA)	Prosobee® (Mead Johnson, Evansville, IN)	Isomil® (Ross, Columbus, OH)	Isomil® DF (Ross, Columbus, OH)	Store Brand Soy Infant Formula (Wyeth Nutritionals)
Energy, kcal	676	680	676	676	672
Protein, g	19	16.9	16.55	17.97	18
Source	100% soy protein isolate	Soy protein isolate	Soy protein isolate and L-Methionine	Soy protein isolate and L-Methionine	Soy protein isolate and L-Methionine
Fat, g	34	36	36.89	36.89	36
Polyunsaturated, %	22	19			17.7
Monounsaturated %	33	38			37.3
Saturated, %	45	40			45.0
Predominant oil	Palm olein, soy, coconut, and high-oleic safflower	Palm olein, soy, coconut, and high-oleic sunflower oils	High-oleic saf-flower, coconut, and soy oils	Soy and coconut oils	Palm, high-oleic, coconut, and soybean oils
Carbohydrate, g	74	72	69.6	69.6	69
	Corn maltodextrin and sucrose	Corn syrup solids	Corn syrup solids and sucrose	Corn syrup and sucrose	Corn syrup solids and sucrose
Osmolality mOsm/kg	200	200	200	240	220
Minerals					
Calcium, mg	704	710	709	709	600
Phosphorus, mg	423	560	507	507	420
Magnesium, mg	74	74	50.7	50.7	67
Iron, mg	12.1	12.2	12.2	12.2	12

Table F–1.
Soy-Based Formulas (per Liter), *continued*

	Good Start Essentials Soy® (Nestle, Glendale, CA)	Prosobee® (Mead Johnson, Evansville, IN)	Isomil® (Ross, Columbus, OH)	Isomil® DF (Ross, Columbus, OH)	Store Brand Soy Infant Formula (Wyeth Nutritionals)
Zinc, mg	6	8.1	5.07	5.07	5
Manganese, μg	228	169	169	203	200
Copper, μg	805	510	507	507	470
Iodine, μg	101	101	101	101	60
Sodium, mEq	10.22	10.4	12.9	12.9	8.7
Potassium, mEq	19.95	21	18.7	18.7	17.9
Chloride, mEq	13.45	15.2	11.8	11.8	10.7
Vitamins					
A, IU	2012	2000	2027	2027	2000
D, IU	402	410	405	405	400
E, IU	20.1	13.5	10.1	20.3	10
K, μg	54	54	74	74	55
Thiamine (B_1), μg	402	540	405	405	670
Riboflavin (B_2), μg	631	610	608	608	1000
Pyridoxine, μg	402	410	405	405	420
B_{12}, μg	2.1	2	3.04	3.04	2
Niacin, mg	8.72	6.8	9.1	9.1	5

Table F–1.
Soy-Based Formulas (per Liter), *continued*

	Good Start Essentials Soy® (Nestle, Glendale, CA)	Prosobee® (Mead Johnson, Evansville, IN)	Isomil® (Ross, Columbus, OH)	Isomil® DF (Ross, Columbus, OH)	Store Brand Soy Infant Formula (Wyeth Nutritionals)
Folic acid, μg	107	108	101	101	50
Pantothenic acid, mg	3.15	3.4	5.1	5.1	3.0
Biotin, μg	52	20	30.4	30.4	35
C (ascorbic acid), mg	107	81	61	61	55
Choline, mg	80	81	54	54	85
Inositol, mg	121	41	33.8	33.8	27
Linoleic acid, mg	6171				
Linolenic acid, mg	891				
Selenium, μg	20.1				

Appendix G

Table G–1.
Amino Acid/Protein Hydrolysate-Based Formulas for Infants—Nutrition Information Comparison Chart (per Liter)

	Neocate (SHS North America, Rockville, MD)	Alimentum® (Ross, Columbus, OH)	Enfamil® Nutramigen® (Mead Johnson, Evansville, IN)	Enfamil® Pregestimil® (Mead Johnson, Evansville, IN)
Form	Powder Unflavored	Liquid* Unflavored	Powder† Unflavored	Powder† Unflavored
Energy, kcal	670	676	680	680
Protein, equivalent g	20.95	18.6	19.3	19.3
Protein source	Free amino acids	Hydrolyzed casein	Hydrolyzed casein	Hydrolyzed casein
Carbohydrate, g	79	68.9	75	69
Fat, g	30.4	37.4	34	38
Linoleic acid, mg	4500	12 838	5800	8000
Energy Distribution				
Carbohydrate	47%	41%	44%	41%
Protein	12%	11%	11%	11%
Fat	41%	48%	45%	48%
LCT	95%	67%	100%	45%
MCT	5%	33%	0%	55%
% Total energy from essential fatty acids	7.7	17.1	8.5	11.7
Osmolality mOsm/kg	375	370	260	340
Minerals				
Calcium, mg	826	709	640	780
Phosphorus, mg	619	507	430	510
Magnesium, mg	82	50.7	74	74
Iron, mg	12.5	12.2	12.2	12.2
Zinc, mg	11.22	5.07	6.8	6.8
Manganese, μg	60	54	169	169

Table G–1.
Amino Acid/Protein Hydrolysate-Based Formulas for Infants—Nutrition Information
Comparison Chart (per Liter), *continued*

	Neocate (SHS North America, Rockville, MD)	Alimentum® (Ross, Columbus, OH)	Enfamil® Nutramigen® (Mead Johnson, Evansville, IN)	Enfamil® Pregestimil® (Mead Johnson, Evansville, IN)
Copper, μg	822	507	510	510
Iodine, μg	104	101	101	101
Sodium, mEq	11	12.9	13.9	13.9
Potassium, mEq	26	20.6	18.9	18.9
Chloride, mEq	15	15.2	16.3	16.3
Vitamins				
A, IU	2720	2027	2000	2600
D, IU	578	304	340	340
E, IU	7.6	20.3	13.5	27
K, μg	58	101	54	81
Thiamine (B$_1$), μg	616	405	540	540
Riboflavin (B$_2$), μg	916	608	610	610
Pyridoxine, μg	822	405	410	410
B$_{12}$, μg	1.15	3.04	2	2
Niacin, mg	10.3	9.1	6.8	6.8
Folic acid, μg	68.94	101	108	108
Pantothenic acid, mg	4.2	5.1	3.4	3.4
Biotin, μg	20.95	30.4	20	20
C (ascorbic acid), mg	62.58	61	81	81
Choline, mg	88.54	54	81	81
Inositol, mg	155	33.8	115	115

* Also available in powder form.
† Also available in liquid form.

Appendix H

Table H–1.
Formulas for Low-Birth-Weight and Prematurely Born Infants (per Liter)

	Similac® Special Care® 24* Liquid (Ross Laboratories, Columbus, Ohio)	Enfamil® Premature Lipil® 24*†‡ Liquid (Mead Johnson, Evansville, Indiana)	Neosure® Advance®†‡ 22 cal Liquid (Ross Laboratories Columbus, Ohio)	Enfacare®† 22 cal Liquid (Mead Johnson, Evansville, Indiana)
Energy, kcal	806	810	746	740
Protein, g	22*§	24*§	19.4§	21§
Fat, g	43.8‖	41¶	41	39
Polyunsaturated, g	8.3	10.3	–	–
Monounsaturated,g	3.5	4.5	–	–
Saturated, g	32	26.2	–	–
Linoleic acid, g	5.7	8.5	5.6	7.1
Carbohydrate, g	86.1#	90**	76.9	79
Minerals				
Calcium, mg	1460	1340	784	890
Phosphorus, mg	730	670	463	490
Magnesium, mg	100	55	67.2	59
Iron, mg	3.0	2	13.4	13.3
Zinc, mg	12.2	12.2	9.0	9.0
Manganese, μg	100	51	75	111
Copper, μg	2030	1010	896	890
Iodine, μg	50	200	112	111
Sodium, mEq	15	13.9	10.7	11.3
Potassium, mEq	27	21	27.1	20.2
Chloride, mEq	19	19.4	15.8	16.5

Table H–1.
Formulas for Low-Birth-Weight and Prematurely Born Infants (per Liter), *continued*

	Similac® Special Care® 24*	Enfamil® Premature Lipil® 24*†‡	Neosure® Advance®†‡ 22 cal	Enfacare®† 22 cal
	Liquid (Ross Laboratories, Columbus, Ohio)	Liquid (Mead Johnson, Evansville, Indiana)	Liquid (Ross Laboratories Columbus, Ohio)	Liquid (Mead Johnson, Evansville, Indiana)
Vitamins				
A, USP Units	10 081	10 100	3433	3330
D, USP Units	1210	2200	522	590
E, USP Units	32.3	51	27	30
K, μg	97	65	82	59
Thiamine (B$_1$), μg	2016	1620	1642	1480
Riboflavin (B$_2$), μg	5000	2400	1119	1480
Pyridoxine, μg	2016	1220	746	740
B$_{12}$, μg	4.4	2	3.0	2.2
Niacin, mg	40.3	32	14.5	14.8
Folic acid, μg	298	280	187	192
Pantothenic acid, mg	15.3	9.7	6.0	6.3
Biotin, μg	298	32	67	44
C (ascorbic acid), mg	298	162	112	118
Choline, mg	81	97	119	111
Inositol, mg	48.4	138	45	220

*24 cal/oz; 81 cal/dL.
†With nucleotides.
‡With DHA and ARA.
§Nonfat milk, whey protein concentrate.
||MCT oil, 50%; soy oil, 30%; coconut oil, 20%.
¶MCT oil, 40%; soy oil, 40%; coconut oil, 20%.
#Glucose polymers, 60%; lactose, 40%.
**Lactose, 50%; glucose polymers, 50%.

Table H–2.
Human Milk Fortifiers for Premature Infants Fed Human Milk—Nutrients Provided When Added to 100 mL of Human Milk

Nutrient	Enfamil Human Milk Fortifier (4 pkt) Mead Johnson, Evansville, IN	Similac Human Milk Fortifier (4 pkt) Ross Laboratories Columbus, OH	Similac Natural Care Fortifier (Liquid, 100 mL)* Ross Laboratories, Columbus, OH
Energy, kcal	14	14	80
Protein, g	1.1	1.0	2.2
Fat, g	0.65	0.36	4.4
Linoleic acid, mg	90	0	565
α-Linolenic acid, mg	11	0	
Carbohydrate, g	1.1	1.8	8.5
Vitamin A, IU	950	620	1,008
Vitamin D, IU	150	120	121
Vitamin E, IU	4.6	3.2	3.2
Vitamin K, μg	4.4	8.3	9.7
Vitamin C (ascorbate), mg	12	25	30
Thiamin, μg	150	233	202
Riboflavin, μg	220	417	500
Pyridoxine, μg	115	211	202
Niacin, mg	3	3.57	4
Pantothenate, mg	0.73	1.5	1.5
Biotin, μg	2.7	26	30
Folate, μg	25	23	30
Vitamin B_{12}, μg	0.18	0.64	0.44
Calcium, mg	90	117	169
Phosphorus, mg	45	67	94
Magnesium, mg	1	7	9.7
Iron, mg	1.44	0.35	.32
Zinc, mg	0.72	1	1.2
Manganese, μg	10	7.2	9.7
Copper, μg	44	170	202
Sodium, mEq	0.48	0.65	1.5
Potassium, mEq	0.51	1.6	2.7
Chloride, mEq	0.25	1.1	1.8

*Similac Natural Care is to be diluted 1:1 with human milk.

Appendix I

Table I–1.
Drugs Whose Absorption Is Increased by Food

Atovaquone (administer with a high-fat meal)
Cefpodoxime
Cefuroxime
Erythromycin
Griseofulvin (administer with a high-fat meal)
Hydralazine
Morphine sulfate
Nitrofurantoin
Tiagabine (absorption is prolonged in the presence of food)
Theophylline sustained release (increased rate of absorption with high-fat meal)

Table I–2.
Drugs Whose Absorption May Be Delayed by Food

(Drugs in this category should either be administered on an empty stomach, or taken consistently with regard to food.)
Acetaminophen
Amitriptyline
Ampicillin
Aspirin
Azithromycin
Cefaclor
Ceftibuten
Cephalexin
Cimetidine
Ciprofloxacin
Clindamycin
Digoxin

Table I–2.
Drugs Whose Absorption May Be Delayed by Food, *continued*

Diltiazem
Furosemide
Glipizide
Metronidazole
Penicillin
Sulfisoxazole
Trazodone
Valproic acid
Zafirlukast
Zalcitabine
Zidovudine

Table I–3.
Drugs That Should Be Administered on an Empty Stomach

Ampicillin
Amprenavir (avoid antacids and high-fat meals)
Azithromycin
Captopril
Ceftibuten
Cloxacillin
Dicloxacillin
Didanosine
Indinavir (high-fat, calories, and proteins significantly decrease absorption)
Iron (avoid milk and antacids)
Isoniazid
Ketoconazole
Loracarbef
Mycophenolate
Rifampin
Tacrolimus (separate antacids by at least 2 hours)
Tetracycline
Zafirlukast
Zalcitabine

Table I–4.
Miscellaneous Food-Nutrient Effects

Drug or Class	Nutrient	Comment
Albuterol	Glucose	May cause hyperglycemia
Amiloride	Potassium	May cause hyperkalemia
Amphotericin	Magnesium, potassium, sodium	Causes electrolyte wasting
Aspirin	Folate	May cause folate deficiency
	Iron	May cause iron deficiency anemia
Captopril	Potassium	May cause small increases in serum potassium
Ciprofloxacin	Enteral feeds	Enteral feeds may interfere with absorption
	Caffeine	May exaggerate effects of caffeine
Cisplatin	Magnesium	Causes magnesium depletion
Cholestyramine	Fat-soluble vitamins	May result in deficiency
Corticosteroids	Glucose	May cause hyperglycemia
Digoxin	Calcium	May cause arrhythmias due to inotropic effect
	Antacids, fiber	May decrease digoxin effects
Ethambutol	Aluminum salts	May decrease absorption of ethambutol
Furosemide	Calcium, magnesium, potassium, sodium	May cause electrolyte depletion
Gabapentin	Glucose	May cause fluctuations in glucose and weight gain
Glipizide, Glyburide	Alcohol	Disulfuram-like reaction with alcohol
Insulin	Concentrated sugar	Can increase insulin requirement
Isoniazid	Pyridoxine	Isoniazid is a B_6 antagonist
Isotretinoin	Vitamin A	May result in increased toxicity
Lithium	Sodium	Maintain constant sodium intake
	Caffeine	Caffeine may decrease lithium effects to avoid toxicity
Monoamine oxidase inhibitors	Tyramine	Dietary tyramine can cause hypertensive crisis
Methotrexate	Folic acid	Folic acid may decrease effects
Metronidazole	Alcohol	Causes disulfuram-like reaction
Mineral oil	Fat-soluble vitamins	May decrease absorption of fat-soluble vitamins
Nonsteroidal anti-inflammatory drugs	Potassium	May cause hyperkalemia in patients with renal impairment or on supplements, or potassium-sparing diuretics

Table I–4.
Miscellaneous Food-Nutrient Effects, *continued*

Drug or Class	Nutrient	Comment
Omeprazole, Lansoprozole	Acid	Acid-labile drug, administer with beads intact
Pancreatic enzymes	Calcium carbonate	May increase drug effect
	Magnesium hydroxide	
Phenobarbital	Protein	Be consistent with protein intake
	Vitamin C	Displaces drug from binding sites
	Vitamin D	Deficiency may result from malabsorption
Phenytoin	Enteral feeds	May interfere with phenytoin absorption
	Folate	High-dose folic acid may reverse drug effects
	Calcium	Phenytoin decreases absorption
	Vitamin D	May interfere with phenytoin metabolism
	Vitamin C	Displaces drug from binding sites
	Glucose	May cause hypoglycemia
Primidone	Folic acid	Megaloblastic anemia due to folate deficiency may occur
Propranolol	Vitamin C	May result in increased propranolol effects
Spironolactone	Potassium	May cause hyperkalemia, avoid supplements
Sulfasalazine	Folic acid	May inhibit absorption of folate
Terbutaline	Glucose, potassium	May cause hyperglycemia, hypokalemia
Theophylline	Caffeine	May cause increased theophylline toxicity
Thiazide diuretics	Magnesium, sodium, potassium	May cause electrolyte depletion
Trimethoprim	Folate	May cause folate depletion
Valproic acid	Carbonated beverages	Avoid carbonated beverages with syrup
	Carnitine	May cause carnitine deficiency with hyperammonemia
Warfarin	Vitamin K	May inhibit response to warfarin
	Vitamin E	May increase effects of warfarin
Zidovudine	Folic acid	May cause megaloblastic anemia
Zinc	Calcium, zinc, phytate	avoid foods high in these nutrients

Table I–5.
Drug-Grapefruit Juice Interactions

Drug	Effect of Grapefruit Juice on Drug Conc.	Clinical Significance	Onset	Documentation
Amlodipine	Increases	Minor	Delayed	Poor
Atorvastatin	Increases	Moderate	Rapid	Fair
Bexarotene	Increases	Moderate	Delayed	Poor
Busprione	Increases	Moderate	Rapid	Fair
Carbamazepine	Increases	Moderate	Rapid	Fair
Cisapride	Increases	Major	Rapid	Fair
Clomipramine	Increases	Moderate	Delayed	Fair
Cyclosprine	Increases	Moderate	Delayed	Good
Diazepam	Increases	Moderate	Rapid	Poor
Felodipine	Increases	Moderate	Rapid	Good
Indinavir	Decreases	No dose changes needed per manufacturer	NA	NA
Itraconazole	Decreases	Moderate	Rapid	Fair
Lovastatin	Increases	Moderate	Rapid	Fair
Methylprednisolone	Increases	Unknown	Unknown	Fair
Midazolam	Increases	Moderate	Rapid	Fair
Nifedipine	Increases	Moderate	Rapid	Good
Nimodipine	Increases	Moderate	Rapid	Poor
Nisoldipine	Increases	Moderate	Rapid	Fair
Omeprazole	Decreases	Minor	Rapid	Poor
Pimozide	Increases	Major	Rapid	Poor
Pravastatin	Increases	None	Unknown	Poor
Quinidine	Unknown	Moderate	Rapid	Fair
Saquinavir	Increases drug level	Minor	Rapid	Poor
Sertraline	Increases	Moderate	Delayed	Poor
Simvastatin	Increases	Moderate	Rapid	Fair
Sirolimus	Increases	Moderate	Delayed	Fair
Tacrolimus	Increases	Moderate	Delayed	Poor
Triazolam	Increases	Minor	Rapid	Fair

Bibliography

Harriet Lane Handbook

Kane G, Lipsky J. Drug-Grapefruit Juice Interactions. *Mayo Clinic Proceedings.* 2000;75:933–942

Kirk J. Significant Drug-Nutrient Interactions. *Am Fam Physician.* 1995;51:1175–1182

Maka D, Murphy L. Drug-Nutrient Interactions: A Review. *Advanced Practice in Acute & Critical Care.* 2000;11:580–588

Lacy C, et al. *Drug Information Handbook.* 7th Edition. Hudson, OH: Lexi-Comp Inc. MicroMedex on-line drug information; 1999–2000

Appendix J

Appendix J-1

SET I   **Birth to 36 months: Boys**
Length-for-age and Weight-for-age percentiles
Birth to 36 months: Boys
Head circumference-for-age and Weight-for-length percentiles
Birth to 36 months: Girls
Length-for-age and Weight-for-age percentiles
Birth to 36 months: Girls
Head circumference-for-age and Weight-for-length percentiles
2 to 20 years: Boys
Stature-for-age and Weight-for-age percentiles
2 to 20 years: Boys
Body mass index-for-age percentiles
2 to 20 years: Girls
Stature-for-age and Weight-for-age percentiles
2 to 20 years: Girls
Body mass index-for-age percentiles
Weight-for-stature percentiles: Boys
Weight-for-stature percentiles: Girls

SET II   **Birth to 36 months: Boys**
Length-for-age and Weight-for-age percentiles
Birth to 36 months: Boys
Head circumference-for-age and Weight-for-length percentiles
Birth to 36 months: Girls
Length-for-age and Weight-for-age percentiles
Birth to 36 months: Girls
Head circumference-for-age and Weight-for-length percentiles
2 to 20 years: Boys
Stature-for-age and Weight-for-age percentiles
2 to 20 years: Boys
Body mass index-for-age percentiles
2 to 20 years: Girls
Stature-for-age and Weight-for-age percentiles
2 to 20 years: Girls
Body mass index-for-age percentiles

Appendix J-2

Down Syndrome Girls Physical Growth: 1 to 36 months
Down Syndrome Boys Physical Growth: 1 to 36 months
Girls with Down Syndrome Physical Growth: 2 to 18 years
Boys with Down Syndrome Physical Growth: 2 to 18 years

Appendix J-1, SET I

Birth to 36 months: Boys
Length-for-age and Weight-for-age percentiles

NAME _____

RECORD # _____

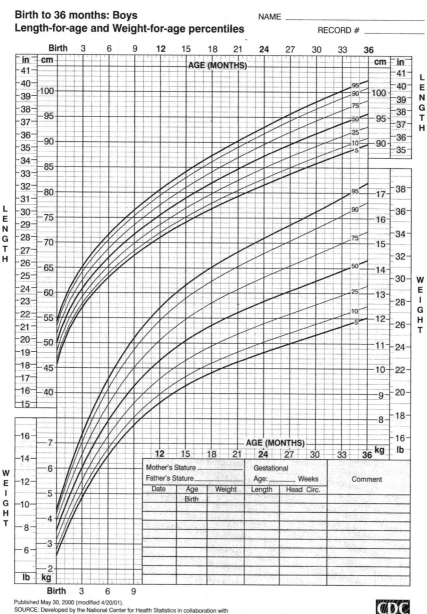

Published May 30, 2000 (modified 4/20/01).
SOURCE: Developed by the National Center for Health Statistics in collaboration with
the National Center for Chronic Disease Prevention and Health Promotion (2000).
http://www.cdc.gov/growthcharts

CDC
SAFER · HEALTHIER · PEOPLE™

Birth to 36 months: Boys
Head circumference-for-age and
Weight-for-length percentiles

NAME _____

RECORD # _____

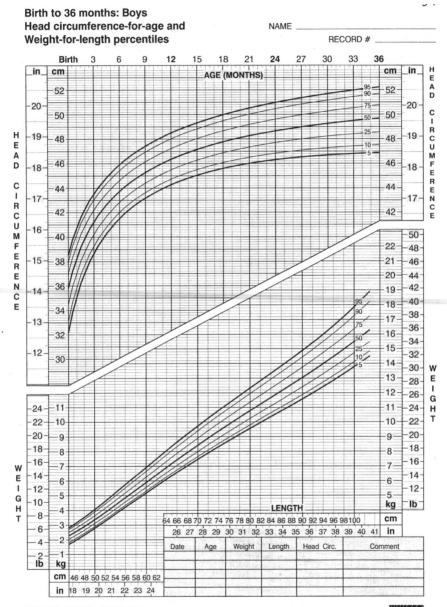

Published May 30, 2000 (modified 10/16/00).
SOURCE: Developed by the National Center for Health Statistics in collaboration with
the National Center for Chronic Disease Prevention and Health Promotion (2000).
http://www.cdc.gov/growthcharts

CDC
SAFER · HEALTHIER · PEOPLE™

Birth to 36 months: Girls
Length-for-age and Weight-for-age percentiles

NAME _____

RECORD # _____

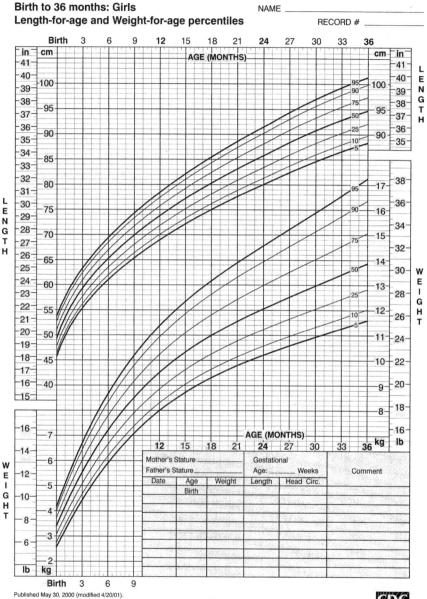

Published May 30, 2000 (modified 4/20/01).
SOURCE: Developed by the National Center for Health Statistics in collaboration with
the National Center for Chronic Disease Prevention and Health Promotion (2000).
http://www.cdc.gov/growthcharts

SAFER · HEALTHIER · PEOPLE™

Birth to 36 months: Girls
Head circumference-for-age and
Weight-for-length percentiles

NAME _____

RECORD # _____

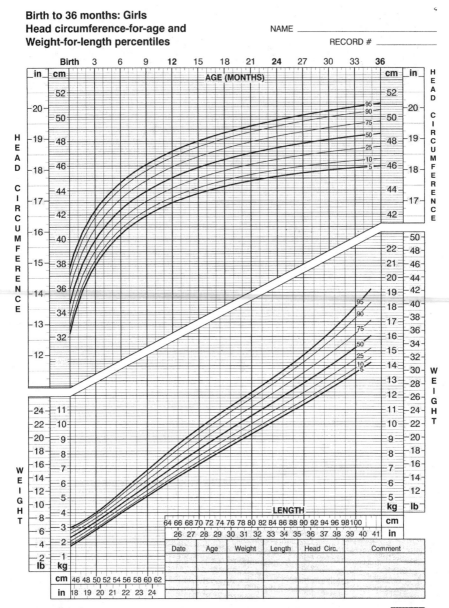

Published May 30, 2000 (modified 10/16/00).
SOURCE: Developed by the National Center for Health Statistics in collaboration with
the National Center for Chronic Disease Prevention and Health Promotion (2000).
http://www.cdc.gov/growthcharts

CDC
SAFER·HEALTHIER·PEOPLE™

2 to 20 years: Boys
Stature-for-age and Weight-for-age percentiles

NAME _____

RECORD # _____

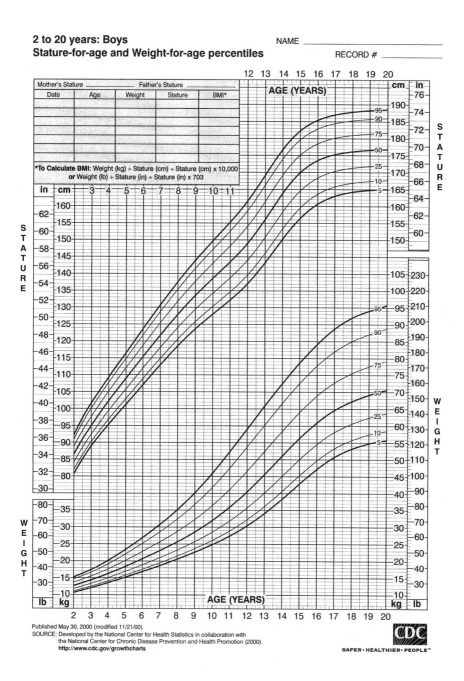

Published May 30, 2000 (modified 11/21/00).
SOURCE: Developed by the National Center for Health Statistics in collaboration with
the National Center for Chronic Disease Prevention and Health Promotion (2000).
http://www.cdc.gov/growthcharts

SAFER · HEALTHIER · PEOPLE™

2 to 20 years: Boys
Body mass index-for-age percentiles

NAME _____

RECORD # _____

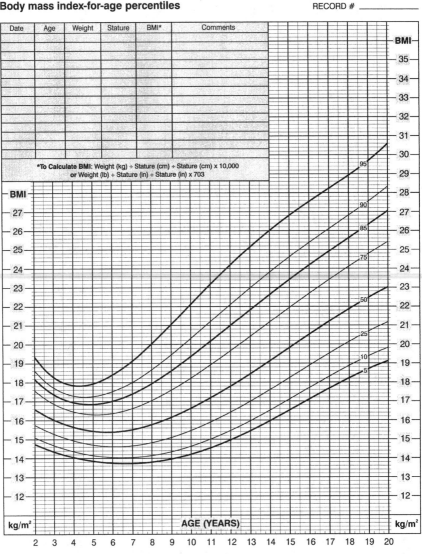

*To Calculate BMI: Weight (kg) ÷ Stature (cm) ÷ Stature (cm) x 10,000
or Weight (lb) ÷ Stature (in) ÷ Stature (in) x 703

SOURCE: Developed by the National Center for Health Statistics in collaboration with
the National Center for Chronic Disease Prevention and Health Promotion (2000).
http://www.cdc.gov/growthcharts

2 to 20 years: Girls
Stature-for-age and Weight-for-age percentiles

NAME _____

RECORD # _____

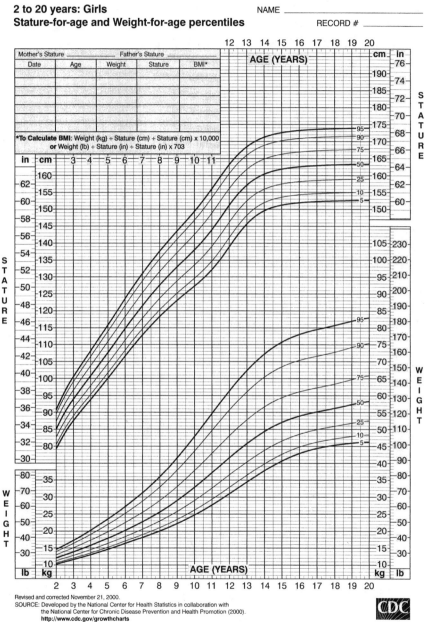

Revised and corrected November 21, 2000.
SOURCE: Developed by the National Center for Health Statistics in collaboration with
the National Center for Chronic Disease Prevention and Health Promotion (2000).
http://www.cdc.gov/growthcharts

2 to 20 years: Girls
Body mass index-for-age percentiles

NAME _____

RECORD # _____

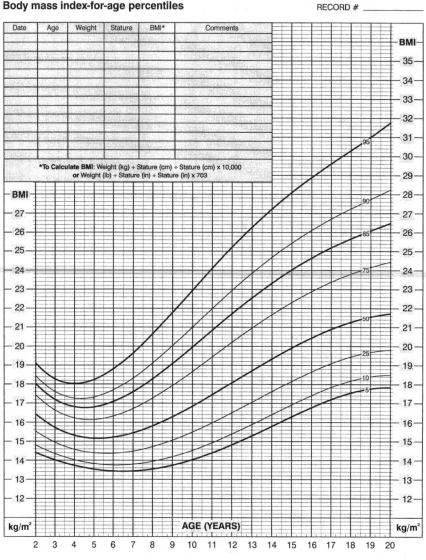

*To Calculate BMI: Weight (kg) ÷ Stature (cm) ÷ Stature (cm) x 10,000
or Weight (lb) ÷ Stature (in) ÷ Stature (in) x 703

SOURCE: Developed by the National Center for Health Statistics in collaboration with
the National Center for Chronic Disease Prevention and Health Promotion (2000).
http://www.cdc.gov/growthcharts

Weight-for-stature percentiles: Boys

NAME _____

RECORD # _____

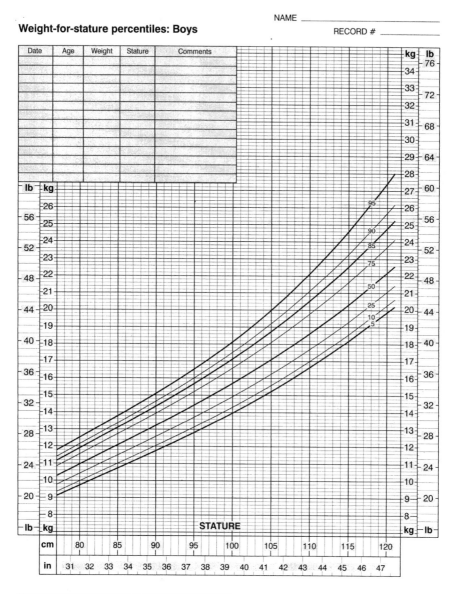

SOURCE: Developed by the National Center for Health Statistics in collaboration with
the National Center for Chronic Disease Prevention and Health Promotion (2000).
http://www.cdc.gov/growthcharts

NAME _____

Weight-for-stature percentiles: Girls

RECORD # _____

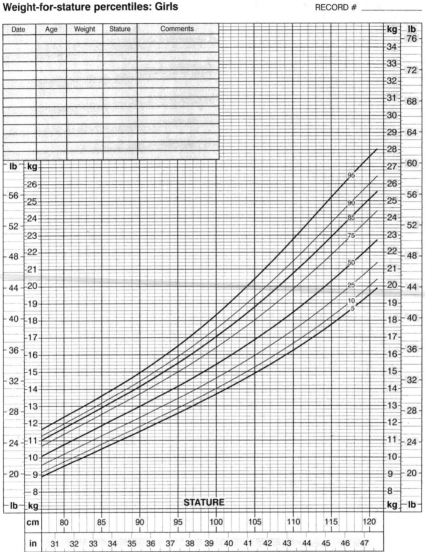

Date	Age	Weight	Stature	Comments

STATURE

cm 80 85 90 95 100 105 110 115 120

in 31 32 33 34 35 36 37 38 39 40 41 42 43 44 45 46 47

SOURCE: Developed by the National Center for Health Statistics in collaboration with
the National Center for Chronic Disease Prevention and Health Promotion (2000).
http://www.cdc.gov/growthcharts

Appendix J-1, SET II

Birth to 36 months: Boys
Length-for-age and Weight-for-age percentiles

NAME _____

RECORD # _____

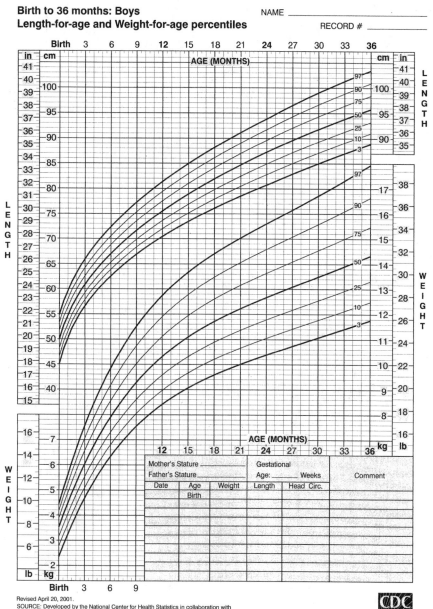

Revised April 20, 2001.
SOURCE: Developed by the National Center for Health Statistics in collaboration with
the National Center for Chronic Disease Prevention and Health Promotion (2000).
http://www.cdc.gov/growthcharts

Birth to 36 months: Boys
Head circumference-for-age and
Weight-for-length percentiles

NAME _____

RECORD # _____

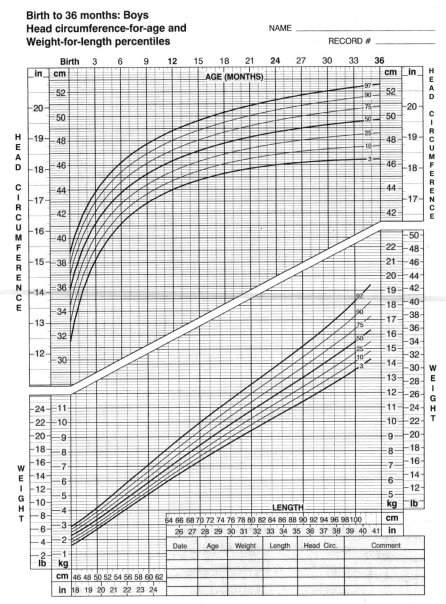

SOURCE: Developed by the National Center for Health Statistics in collaboration with
the National Center for Chronic Disease Prevention and Health Promotion (2000).
http://www.cdc.gov/growthcharts

Birth to 36 months: Girls
Length-for-age and Weight-for-age percentiles

NAME _____

RECORD # _____

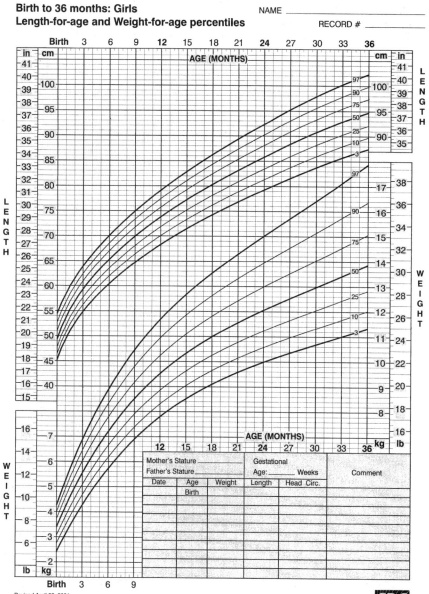

AGE (MONTHS)

Mother's Stature _____
Father's Stature _____

Gestational
Age: _____ Weeks

Comment

Date	Age	Weight	Length	Head Circ.	
Birth					

Revised April 20, 2001.
SOURCE: Developed by the National Center for Health Statistics in collaboration with
the National Center for Chronic Disease Prevention and Health Promotion (2000).
http://www.cdc.gov/growthcharts

CDC

Birth to 36 months: Girls
Head circumference-for-age and
Weight-for-length percentiles

NAME _____

RECORD # _____

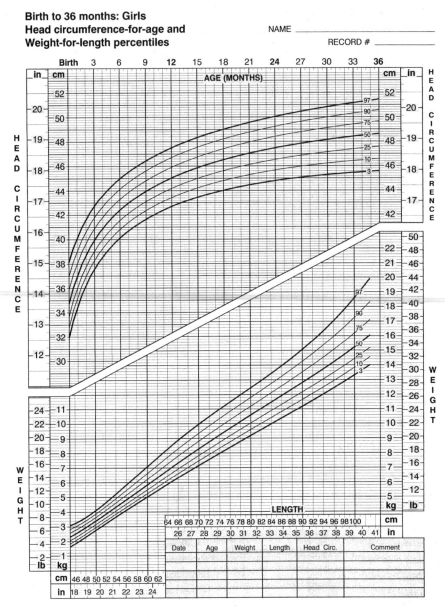

SOURCE: Developed by the National Center for Health Statistics in collaboration with
the National Center for Chronic Disease Prevention and Health Promotion (2000).
http://www.cdc.gov/growthcharts

2 to 20 years: Boys
Stature-for-age and Weight-for-age percentiles

NAME _____

RECORD # _____

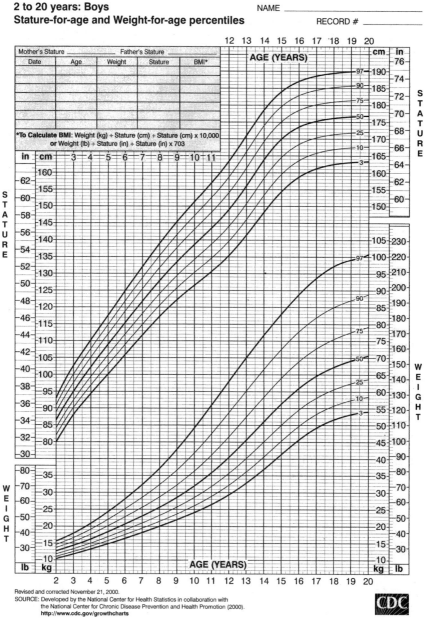

Revised and corrected November 21, 2000.
SOURCE: Developed by the National Center for Health Statistics in collaboration with
the National Center for Chronic Disease Prevention and Health Promotion (2000).
http://www.cdc.gov/growthcharts

2 to 20 years: Boys
Body mass index-for-age percentiles

NAME _____

RECORD # _____

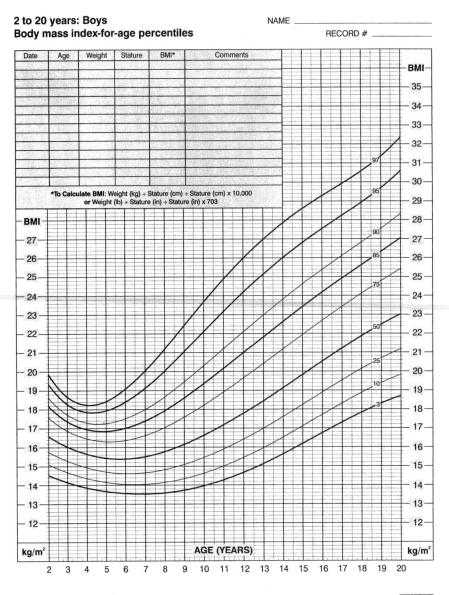

*To Calculate BMI: Weight (kg) ÷ Stature (cm) ÷ Stature (cm) x 10,000
or Weight (lb) ÷ Stature (in) ÷ Stature (in) x 703

AGE (YEARS)

kg/m²

SOURCE: Developed by the National Center for Health Statistics in collaboration with
the National Center for Chronic Disease Prevention and Health Promotion (2000).
http://www.cdc.gov/growthcharts

2 to 20 years: Girls
Stature-for-age and Weight-for-age percentiles

NAME _____

RECORD # _____

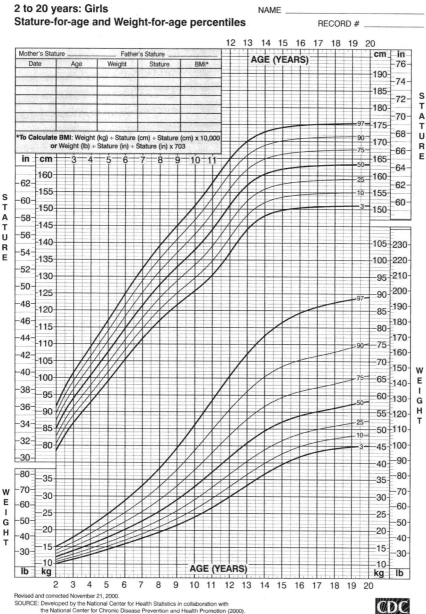

*To Calculate BMI: Weight (kg) ÷ Stature (cm) ÷ Stature (cm) x 10,000
or Weight (lb) ÷ Stature (in) ÷ Stature (in) x 703

Revised and corrected November 21, 2000.
SOURCE: Developed by the National Center for Health Statistics in collaboration with
the National Center for Chronic Disease Prevention and Health Promotion (2000).
http://www.cdc.gov/growthcharts

CDC

2 to 20 years: Girls
Body mass index-for-age percentiles

NAME _____

RECORD # _____

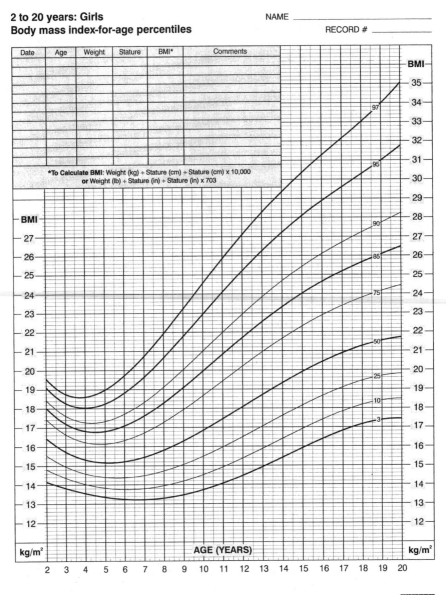

SOURCE: Developed by the National Center for Health Statistics in collaboration with
the National Center for Chronic Disease Prevention and Health Promotion (2000).
http://www.cdc.gov/growthcharts

Appendix J-2

**DOWN SYNDROME GIRLS
PHYSICAL GROWTH:
1 TO 36 MONTHS** NAME _____ RECORD # _____

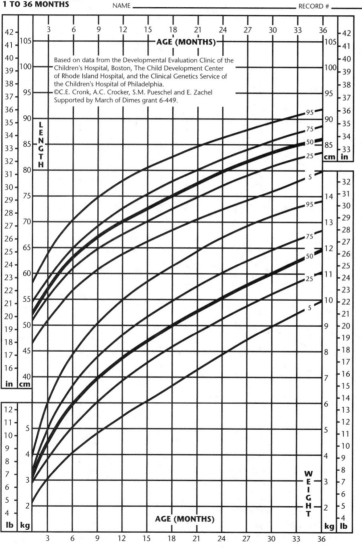

Based on data from the Developmental Evaluation Clinic of the
Children's Hospital, Boston, The Child Development Center
of Rhode Island Hospital, and the Clinical Genetics Service of
the Children's Hospital of Philadelphia.
©C.E. Cronk, A.C. Crocker, S.M. Pueschel and E. Zachel
Supported by March of Dimes grant 6-449.

Down syndrome, length and weight for girls, 1 to 36 months. From
Cronk C, Crocker AC, Siegfried M, et al. Growth charts for children with
Down syndrome: 1 month to 18 years of age. *Pediatrics.* 1988;81:102–110.

**DOWN SYNDROME BOYS
PHYSICAL GROWTH:
1 TO 36 MONTHS**   NAME _____   RECORD # _____

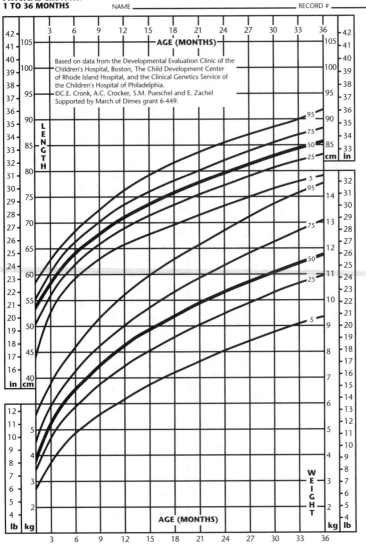

Down syndrome, length and weight for boys, 1 to 36 months. From
Cronk C, Crocker AC, Siegfried M, et al. Growth charts for children with
Down syndrome: 1 month to 18 years of age. *Pediatrics.* 1988;81:102–110.

GIRLS WITH DOWN SYNDROME
PHYSICAL GROWTH:
2 TO 18 YEARS   NAME _____ RECORD # _____

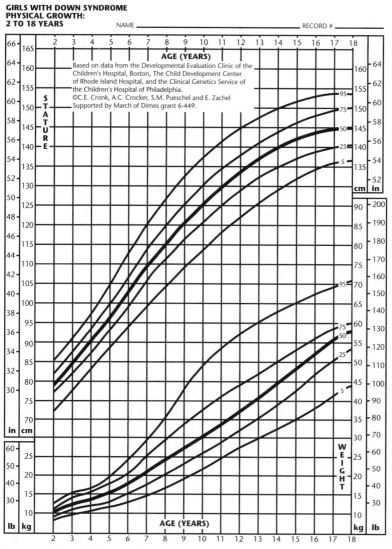

Down syndrome, height and weight for girls, 2 to 18 years. From
Cronk C, Crocker AC, Siegfried M, et al. Growth charts for children with
Down syndrome: 1 month to 18 years of age. *Pediatrics.* 1988;81:102–110.

BOYS WITH DOWN SYNDROME
PHYSICAL GROWTH:
2 TO 18 YEARS

NAME _____ RECORD # _____

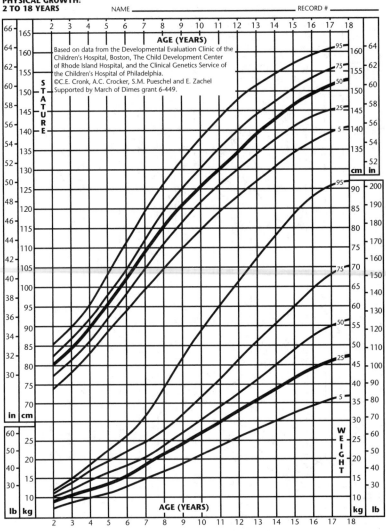

Based on data from the Developmental Evaluation Clinic of the Children's Hospital, Boston, The Child Development Center of Rhode Island Hospital, and the Clinical Genetics Service of the Children's Hospital of Philadelphia.
©C.E. Cronk, A.C. Crocker, S.M. Pueschel and E. Zachel
Supported by March of Dimes grant 6-449.

Down syndrome, height and weight for boys, 2 to 18 years. From Cronk C, Crocker AC, Siegfried M, et al. Growth charts for children with Down syndrome: 1 month to 18 years of age. *Pediatrics.* 1988;81:102–110.

Appendix K

Appendix K-1
  A. Low Birth Weight Growth Charts
  B. Very Low Birth Weight Growth Charts

Appendix K-2
  A. Intrauterine Growth Charts
     Canadian male singletons, crude curves
  B. Intrauterine Growth Charts
     Canadian female singletons, crude curves
  C. Intrauterine Growth Charts
     Canadian male singletons, corrected and smooth curves
  D. Intrauterine Growth Charts
     Canadian female singletons, corrected and smooth curves

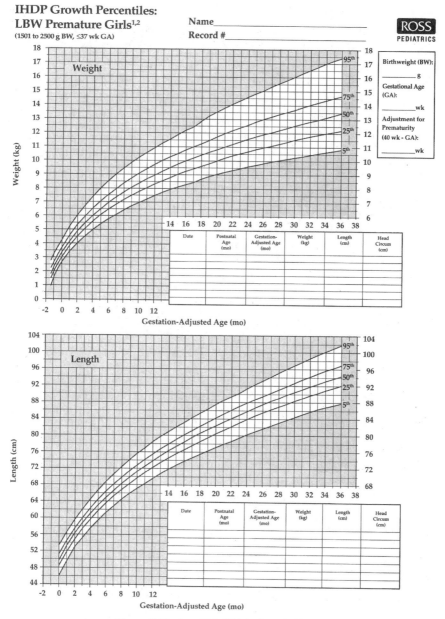

Figure K-1A. Low Birth Weight Growth Charts.

IHDP Growth Percentiles: LBW Premature Girls[1,2]

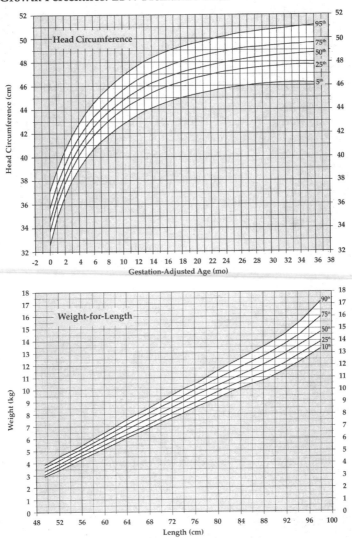

References
1. Guo SS, Roche AF, Chumlea WC, et al: Growth in weight, recumbent length, and head circumference for preterm low-birthweight infants during the first three years of life using gestation-adjusted ages. *Early Hum Dev* 1997;47:305-325.
2. Guo SS, Wholihan K, Roche AF, et al: Weight-for-length reference data for preterm, low-birth-weight infants. *Arch Pediatr Adolesc Med* 1996;150:964-970. Copyright: 1996, American Medical Association.

Acknowledgment
IHDP studies were supported by grants from the Robert Wood Johnson Foundation, Pew Charitable Trusts, and the Bureau of Maternal and Child Health, US Department of Health and Human Services. The IHDP growth percentile graphs were prepared by S.S. Guo and A.F. Roche, Wright State University, Yellow Springs, Ohio. IHDP, its sponsors and the investigators do not endorse specific products.

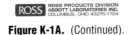

ROSS PRODUCTS DIVISION
ABBOTT LABORATORIES INC.
COLUMBUS, OHIO 43215-1724

Provided as a service of
Similac NeoSure™
Infant Formula With Iron

Figure K-1A. (Continued).

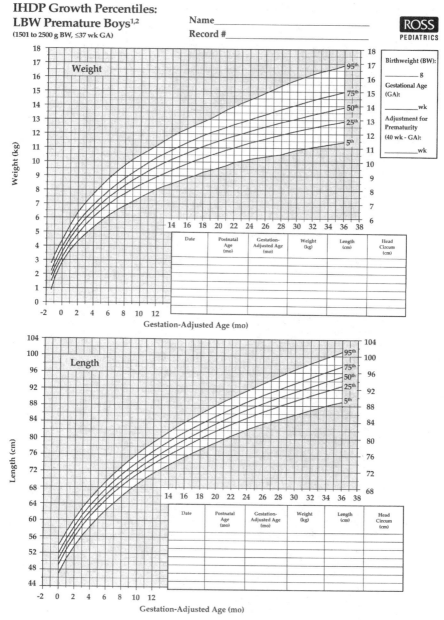

IHDP Growth Percentiles: LBW Premature Boys[1,2]
(1501 to 2500 g BW, ≤37 wk GA)

Figure K-1A. (Continued).

IHDP Growth Percentiles: LBW Premature Boys[1,2]

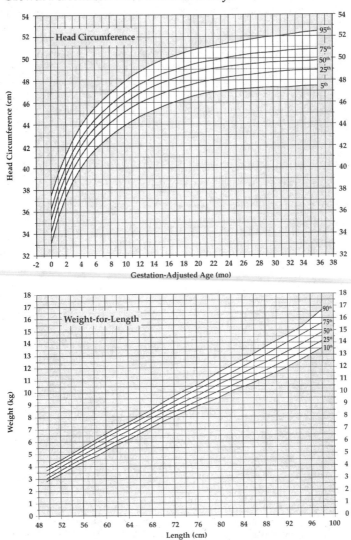

References

1. Guo SS, Roche AF, Chumlea WC, et al: Growth in weight, recumbent length, and head circumference for preterm low-birthweight infants during the first three years of life using gestation-adjusted ages. *Early Hum Dev* 1997;47:305-325.

2. Guo SS, Wholihan K, Roche AF, et al: Weight-for-length reference data for preterm, low-birth-weight infants. *Arch Pediatr Adolesc Med* 1996;150:964-970. Copyright: 1996, American Medical Association.

Acknowledgment

IHDP studies were supported by grants from the Robert Wood Johnson Foundation, Pew Charitable Trusts, and the Bureau of Maternal and Child Health, US Department of Health and Human Services. The IHDP growth percentile graphs were prepared by S.S. Guo and A.F. Roche, Wright State University, Yellow Springs, Ohio. IHDP, its sponsors and the investigators do not endorse specific products.

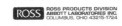

ROSS PRODUCTS DIVISION
ABBOTT LABORATORIES INC.
COLUMBUS, OHIO 43215-1724

Provided as a service of
Similac NeoSure™
Infant Formula With Iron

Figure K-1A. (Continued).

IHDP Growth Percentiles: VLBW Premature Girls[1,2]

(≤1500 g BW, ≤37 wk GA)

Name____________________

Record #____________________

ROSS PEDIATRICS

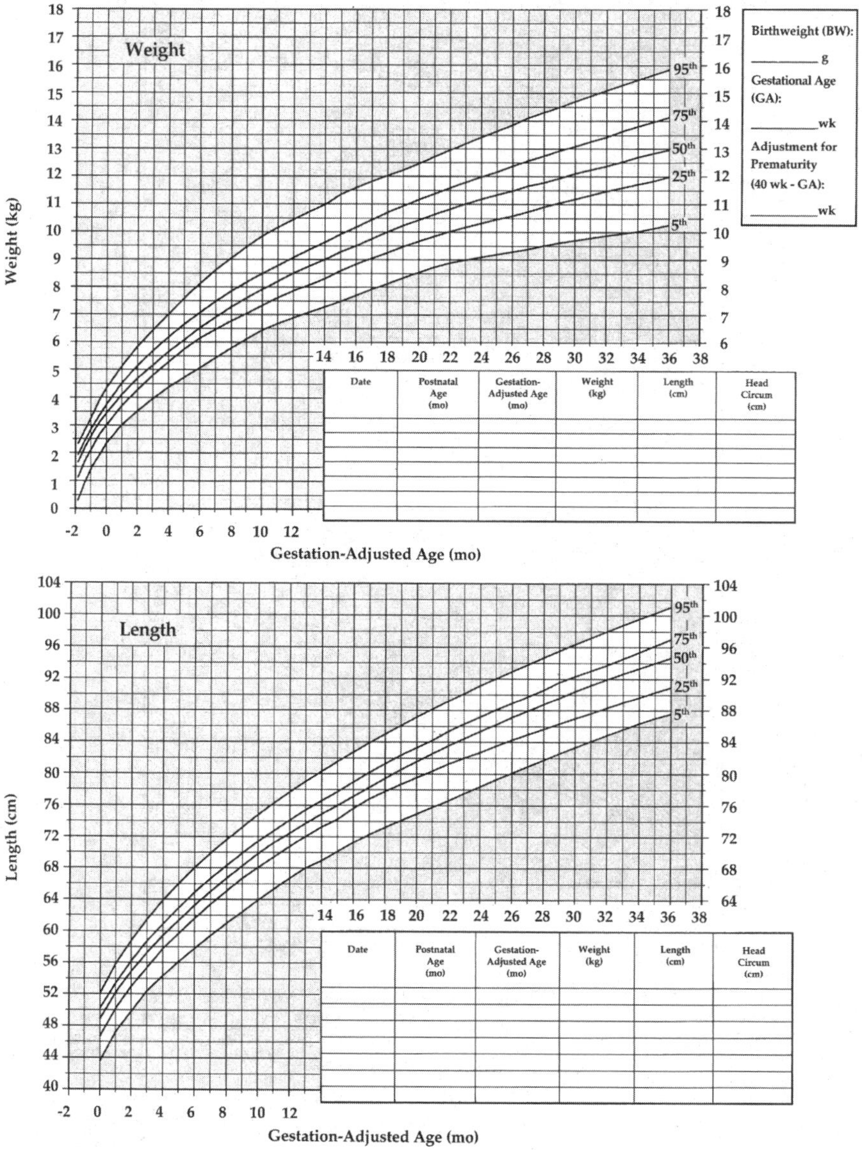
Weight
Weight (kg)
95th
75th
50th
25th
5th
Birthweight (BW): _____ g
Gestational Age (GA): _____ wk
Adjustment for Prematurity (40 wk - GA): _____ wk
Date
Postnatal Age (mo)
Gestation-Adjusted Age (mo)
Weight (kg)
Length (cm)
Head Circum (cm)
Gestation-Adjusted Age (mo)
Length
Length (cm)
Gestation-Adjusted Age (mo)

Figure K-1B. Very Low Brith Weight Growth Charts.

IHDP Growth Percentiles: VLBW Premature Girls[1,2]

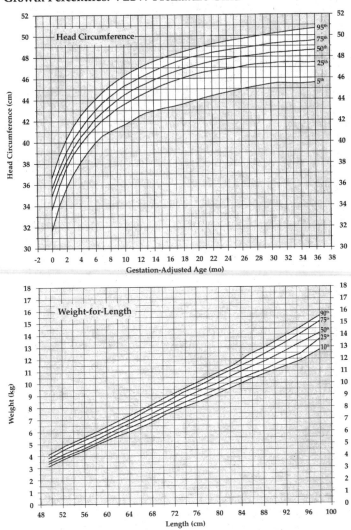

References

1. Guo SS, Roche AF, Chumlea WC, et al: Growth in weight, recumbent length, and head circumference for preterm low-birthweight infants during the first three years of life using gestation-adjusted ages. *Early Hum Dev* 1997;47:305-325.

2. Guo SS, Wholihan K, Roche AF, et al: Weight-for-length reference data for preterm, low-birth-weight infants. *Arch Pediatr Adolesc Med* 1996;150:964-970. Copyright: 1996, American Medical Association.

Acknowledgment

IHDP studies were supported by grants from the Robert Wood Johnson Foundation, Pew Charitable Trusts, and the Bureau of Maternal and Child Health, US Department of Health and Human Services. The IHDP growth percentile graphs were prepared by S.S. Guo and A.F. Roche, Wright State University, Yellow Springs, Ohio. IHDP, its sponsors and the investigators do not endorse specific products.

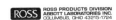 ROSS PRODUCTS DIVISION
ABBOTT LABORATORIES INC.
COLUMBUS, OHIO 43215-1724

Provided as a service of
Similac NeoSure™
Infant Formula With Iron

Figure K-1B. (Continued).

IHDP Growth Percentiles:
VLBW Premature Boys[1,2]
(≤1500 g BW, ≤37 wk GA)

Name_____

Record #_____

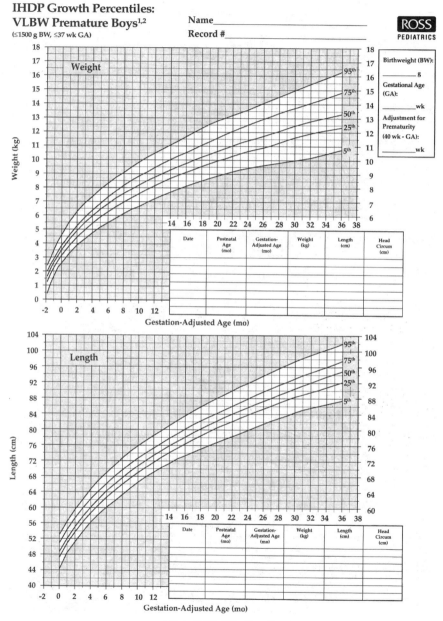

Birthweight (BW):

_____ g

Gestational Age (GA):

_____ wk

Adjustment for Prematurity (40 wk - GA):

_____ wk

Date	Postnatal Age (mo)	Gestation-Adjusted Age (mo)	Weight (kg)	Length (cm)	Head Circum (cm)

Figure K-1B. (Continued).

IHDP Growth Percentiles: VLBW Premature Boys[1,2]

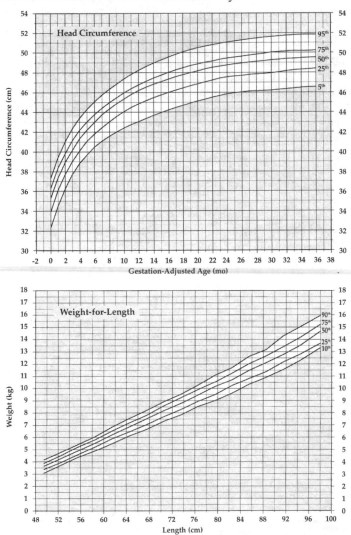

References

1. Guo SS, Roche AF, Chumlea WC, et al: Growth in weight, recumbent length, and head circumference for preterm low-birthweight infants during the first three years of life using gestation-adjusted ages. *Early Hum Dev* 1997;47:305-325.

2. Guo SS, Wholihan K, Roche AF, et al: Weight-for-length reference data for preterm, low-birth-weight infants. *Arch Pediatr Adolesc Med* 1996;150:964-970. Copyright: 1996, American Medical Association.

Acknowledgment

IHDP studies were supported by grants from the Robert Wood Johnson Foundation, Pew Charitable Trusts, and the Bureau of Maternal and Child Health, US Department of Health and Human Services. The IHDP growth percentile graphs were prepared by S.S. Guo and A.F. Roche, Wright State University, Yellow Springs, Ohio. IHDP, its sponsors and the investigators do not endorse specific products.

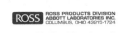

ROSS PRODUCTS DIVISION
ABBOTT LABORATORIES INC.
COLUMBUS, OHIO 43215-1724

Provided as a service of
Similac NeoSure™
Infant Formula With Iron

Figure K-1B. (Continued).

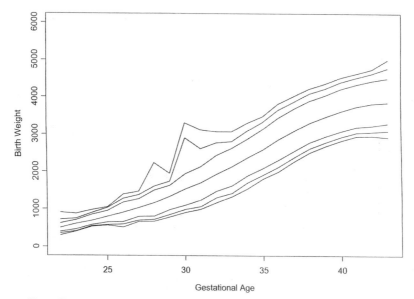

Figure K-2A. Intrauterine Growth Charts. Canadian male singletons, crude curves.

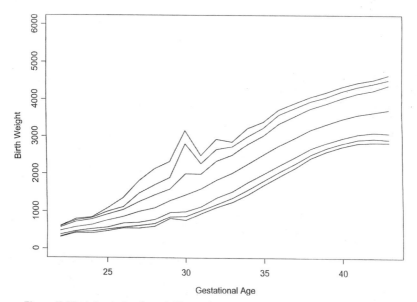

Figure K-2B. Intrauterine Growth Charts. Canadian female singletons, crude curves.

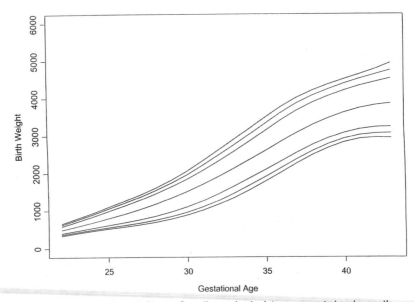

Figure K-2C. Intrauterine Growth Charts. Canadian male singletons, corrected and smooth curves.

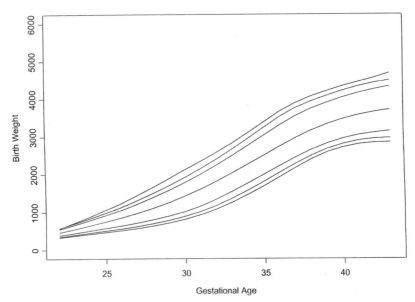

Figure K-2D. Intrauterine Growth Charts. Canadian female singletons, corrected and smooth curves.

Appendix L

Table L–1.
Arm Measurements

Mid-Upper-Arm-Circumference (MUAC) for Length or Height Reference Data									
Length/Height* (cm)	Boys			Combined Sexes			Girls			Length/Height* (cm)
	Median	−2 SD	−3 SD	Median	−2 SD	−3 SD	Median	−2 SD	−3 SD	
65.0	14.6	12.7	11.7	14.0	12.4	11.5	14.0	12.1	11.2	65.0
65.5	14.7	12.7	11.8	14.4	12.5	11.5	14.1	12.2	11.2	65.5
68.0	14.7	12.8	11.8	14.5	12.5	11.6	14.2	12.3	11.3	66.0
68.5	14.8	12.8	11.8	14.5	12.6	11.6	14.3	12.3	11.3	66.5
67.0	14.8	12.9	11.9	14.6	12.6	11.6	14.4	12.4	11.4	67.0
67.5	14.9	12.8	11.9	14.7	12.7	11.7	14.4	12.4	11.4	67.5
68.0	15.0	12.0	11.0	14.7	12.7	11.7	14.5	12.5	11.5	68.0
68.5	15.0	13.0	12.0	14.8	12.8	11.7	14.6	12.6	11.5	68.8
60.0	10.1	13.0	12.0	14.8	12.8	11.8	14.7	12.8	11.6	69.0
69.5	15.1	13.0	12.0	14.9	12.8	11.8	14.7	12.7	11.6	69.5
70.0	15.1	13.1	12.0	15.0	12.9	11.8	14.8	12.7	11.7	70.0
70.5	15.2	13.1	12.0	15.0	12.9	11.9	14.8	12.8	11.7	70.5
71.0	15.2	13.1	12.1	15.1	13.0	11.9	14.9	12.8	11.7	71.0
71.5	15.3	13.1	12.1	15.1	13.0	11.8	15.0	12.8	11.8	71.5
72.0	15.3	13.2	12.1	15.2	13.0	12.0	15.0	12.9	11.8	72.0
72.5	15.3	13.2	12.1	15.2	13.1	12.0	15.1	12.9	11.8	72.5
73.0	15.4	13.2	12.1	15.2	13.1	12.0	15.1	13.0	11.9	73.0
73.5	15.4	13.2	12.2	15.3	13.1	12.0	15.2	13.0	11.9	73.5
74.0	15.4	13.3	12.2	15.3	13.1	12.1	15.2	13.0	11.9	74.0
74.5	15.5	13.3	12.2	15.4	13.2	12.1	15.2	13.1	12.0	74.5
75.0	15.5	13.3	12.2	15.4	13.2	12.1	15.3	13.1	12.0	75.0
75.5	15.5	13.3	12.2	15.4	13.2	12.1	15.3	13.1	12.0	75.5
76.0	15.6	13.4	12.2	15.5	13.3	12.2	15.4	13.2	12.1	76.0

Table L–1.
Arm Measurements, *continued*

	Mid-Upper-Arm-Circumference (MUAC) for Length or Height Reference Data									
Length/ Height* (cm)	Boys			Combined Sexes			Girls			Length/ Height* (cm)
	Median	−2 SD	−3 SD	Median	−2 SD	−3 SD	Median	−2 SD	−3 SD	
76.5	15.6	13.4	12.3	15.5	13.3	12.2	15.4	13.2	12.1	76.5
77.0	15.6	13.4	12.3	15.5	13.3	12.2	15.4	13.2	12.1	77.0
77.5	15.6	13.4	12.3	15.6	13.3	12.2	15.5	13.3	12.1	77.5
78.0	15.7	13.4	12.3	15.6	13.4	12.2	15.5	13.3	12.2	78.0
78.5	15.7	13.4	12.3	15.6	13.4	12.3	15.6	13.3	12.2	78.5
79.0	15.7	13.5	12.3	15.6	13.4	12.3	15.6	13.3	12.2	79.0
79.5	15.7	13.5	12.4	15.7	13.4	12.3	15.6	13.4	12.2	79.5
80.0	15.8	13.5	12.4	15.7	13.4	12.3	15.6	13.4	12.3	80.0
80.5	15.8	13.5	12.4	15.7	13.5	12.3	15.7	13.4	12.3	80.5
81.0	15.8	13.6	12.4	15.8	13.5	12.4	15.7	13.5	12.3	81.0
81.5	15.8	13.6	12.4	15.8	13.5	12.4	15.7	13.5	12.3	81.5
82.0	15.9	13.6	12.4	15.8	13.5	12.4	15.8	13.5	12.3	82.0
82.5	15.9	13.6	12.5	15.8	13.6	12.4	15.8	13.5	12.4	82.5
83.0	15.9	13.6	12.5	15.9	13.6	12.4	15.8	13.5	12.4	83.0
83.5	15.9	13.6	12.5	15.9	13.6	12.5	15.8	13.6	12.4	83.5
84.0	15.9	13.7	12.5	15.9	13.6	12.5	15.9	13.6	12.4	84.0
84.5	16.0	13.7	12.5	15.9	13.6	12.5	15.9	13.6	12.5	84.5
85.0	16.0	13.7	12.5	15.9	13.6	12.5	15.9	13.6	12.5	85.0
85.5	16.0	13.7	12.6	16.0	13.7	12.5	15.9	13.6	12.5	85.5
86.0	16.0	13.7	12.6	16.0	13.7	12.5	15.9	13.7	12.5	86.0
86.5	16.0	13.7	12.6	16.0	13.7	12.6	16.0	13.7	12.5	86.5
87.0	16.1	13.8	12.6	16.0	13.7	12.6	16.0	13.7	12.6	87.0
87.5	16.1	13.8	12.6	16.0	13.7	12.6	16.0	13.7	12.6	87.5
88.0	16.1	13.8	12.6	16.1	13.8	12.6	16.0	13.7	12.6	88.0
88.5	16.1	13.8	12.7	16.1	13.8	12.6	16.1	13.8	12.6	88.5
89.0	16.1	13.8	12.7	16.1	13.8	12.7	16.1	13.8	12.6	89.0
89.5	16.2	13.9	12.7	16.1	13.8	12.7	16.1	13.8	12.7	89.5
90.0	16.2	13.9	12.7	16.2	13.9	12.7	16.1	13.8	12.7	90.0
90.5	16.2	13.9	12.8	16.2	13.9	12.7	16.2	13.8	12.7	90.5
91.0	16.2	13.9	12.8	16.2	13.9	12.7	16.2	13.9	12.7	91.0

Table L–1.
Arm Measurements, *continued*

Mid-Upper-Arm-Circumference (MUAC) for Length or Height Reference Data									
Length/ Height* (cm)	Boys			Combined Sexes			Girls			Length/ Height* (cm)
	Median	−2 SD	−3 SD	Median	−2 SD	−3 SD	Median	−2 SD	−3 SD	
91.5	16.3	14.0	12.8	16.2	13.9	12.8	16.2	13.9	12.7	91.5
92.0	16.3	14.0	12.8	16.3	13.9	12.8	16.2	13.9	12.8	92.0
92.5	16.3	14.0	12.9	16.3	14.0	12.8	16.2	13.9	12.8	92.5
93.0	16.3	14.0	12.9	16.3	14.0	12.8	16.3	14.0	12.8	93.0
93.5	16.4	14.1	12.9	16.3	14.0	12.9	16.3	14.0	12.8	93.5
94.0	16.4	14.1	12.9	16.4	14.0	12.9	16.3	14.0	12.8	94.0
94.5	16.4	14.1	13.0	16.4	14.1	12.9	16.3	14.0	12.9	94.5
95.0	16.4	14.1	13.0	16.4	14.1	12.9	16.4	14.1	12.9	95.0
95.5	16.5	14.2	13.0	16.4	14.1	13.0	16.4	14.1	12.9	95.5
96.0	16.5	14.2	13.0	16.5	14.1	13.0	16.4	14.1	12.9	96.0
96.5	16.5	14.2	13.1	16.5	14.2	13.0	16.4	14.1	13.0	96.5
97.0	16.5	14.2	13.1	16.5	14.2	13.0	16.5	14.1	13.0	97.0
97.5	16.6	14.3	13.1	16.5	14.2	13.1	16.5	14.2	13.0	97.5
98.0	16.6	14.3	13.1	16.6	14.2	13.1	16.5	14.2	13.0	98.0
98.5	16.6	14.3	13.2	16.6	14.3	13.1	16.5	14.2	13.1	98.5
99.0	16.7	14.3	13.2	16.6	14.3	13.1	16.6	14.3	13.1	99.0
99.5	16.7	14.4	13.	16.6	14.3	13.2	16.6	14.3	13.1	99.5
100.0	16.7	14.4	13.2	16.7	14.4	13.2	16.6	14.3	13.1	100.0
100.5	16.8	14.4	13.3	16.7	14.4	13.2	16.7	14.3	13.2	100.5
101.0	16.8	14.5	13.3	16.7	14.4	13.2	16.7	14.4	13.2	101.0
101.5	16.8	14.5	13.3	16.8	14.4	13.3	16.7	14.4	13.2	101.5
102.0	16.9	14.5	13.4	16.8	14.5	13.3	16.7	14.4	13.2	102.0
102.5	16.9	14.6	13.4	16.8	14.5	13.3	16.8	14.4	13.3	102.5
103.0	16.9	14.6	13.4	16.9	14.5	13.4	16.8	14.5	13.3	103.0
103.5	16.9	14.6	13.4	16.9	14.6	13.4	16.8	14.5	13.3	103.5
104.0	17.0	14.6	13.5	16.9	14.6	13.4	16.9	14.5	13.4	104.0
104.5	17.0	14.7	13.5	17.0	14.6	13.4	16.9	14.6	13.4	104.5
105.0	17.0	14.7	13.5	17.0	14.6	13.5	16.9	14.6	13.4	105.0
105.5	17.1	14.7	13.6	17.0	14.7	13.5	17.0	14.6	13.4	105.5
106.0	17.1	14.8	13.6	17.1	14.7	13.5	17.0	14.6	13.5	106.0

Table L–1.
Arm Measurements, *continued*

Mid-Upper-Arm-Circumference (MUAC) for Length or Height Reference Data									
Length/ Height* (cm)	Boys			Combined Sexes			Girls			Length/ Height* (cm)
	Median	–2 SD	–3 SD	Median	–2 SD	–3 SD	Median	–2 SD	–3 SD	
106.5	17.1	14.8	13.6	17.1	14.7	13.6	17.0	14.7	13.5	106.5
107.0	17.2	14.8	13.6	17.1	14.8	13.6	17.1	14.7	13.6	107.0
107.5	17.2	14.8	13.7	17.2	14.8	13.6	17.1	14.7	13.6	107.5
108.0	17.3	14.9	13.7	17.2	14.8	13.6	17.1	14.8	13.6	108.0
108.5	17.3	14.9	13.7	17.2	14.9	13.7	17.2	14.8	13.6	108.5
109.0	17.3	14.9	13.7	17.3	14.9	13.7	17.2	14.8	13.6	109.0
109.5	17.4	15.0	13.8	17.3	14.9	13.7	17.2	14.9	13.7	109.5
110.0	17.4	15.0	13.8	17.4	15.0	13.8	17.3	14.9	13.7	110.0
110.5	17.4	15.0	13.8	17.4	15.0	13.8	17.3	14.9	13.7	110.5
111.0	17.5	15.1	13.9	17.4	15.0	13.8	17.4	15.0	13.8	111.0
111.5	17.5	15.1	13.9	17.5	15.0	13.8	17.4	14.0	13.8	111.5
112.0	17.5	15.1	13.9	17.5	15.1	13.9	17.5	15.0	13.8	112.0
112.5	17.6	15.1	13.9	17.6	15.1	13.9	17.5	15.1	13.9	112.5
113.0	17.6	15.2	14.0	17.6	15.1	13.9	17.6	15.1	13.9	113.0
113.5	17.7	15.2	14.0	17.6	15.2	14.0	17.6	15.2	13.9	113.5
114.0	17.7	15.2	14.0	17.7	15.2	14.0	17.7	15.2	14.0	114.0
114.5	17.7	15.3	14.0	17.7	15.2	14.0	17.7	15.2	14.0	114.5
115.0	17.8	15.3	14.0	17.8	15.3	14.0	17.8	15.3	14.0	115.0
115.5	17.8	15.3	14.1	17.8	15.3	14.1	17.8	15.3	14.1	115.5
116.0	17.9	15.4	14.1	17.9	15.3	14.1	17.9	15.3	14.1	116.0
116.5	17.9	15.4	14.1	17.9	15.4	14.1	17.9	15.4	14.1	116.5
117.0	18.0	15.4	14.1	18.0	15.4	14.1	18.0	15.4	14.1	117.0
117.5	18.0	15.4	14.2	18.0	15.4	14.2	18.0	15.5	14.2	117.5
118.0	18.0	15.5	14.2	18.1	15.5	14.2	18.1	15.5	14.2	118.0
118.5	18.1	15.5	14.2	18.1	15.5	14.2	18.1	15.5	14.2	118.5
119.0	18.1	15.5	14.2	18.2	15.6	14.3	18.2	15.6	14.3	119.0
119.5	18.2	15.6	14.2	18.2	15.6	14.3	18.2	15.6	14.3	119.5
120.0	18.2	15.6	14.3	18.3	15.6	14.3	18.3	15.7	14.3	120.0
120.5	18.3	15.6	14.3	18.3	15.7	14.3	18.4	15.7	14.4	120.5
121.0	18.3	15.6	14.3	18.4	15.7	14.4	18.4	15.7	14.4	121.0

Table L–1.
Arm Measurements, *continued*

Mid-Upper-Arm-Circumference (MUAC) for Length or Height Reference Data									
Length/ Height* (cm)	Boys			Combined Sexes			Girls			Length/ Height* (cm)
	Median	–2 SD	–3 SD	Median	–2 SD	–3 SD	Median	–2 SD	–3 SD	
121.5	18.4	15.7	14.0	18.4	15.7	14.4	18.5	15.8	14.4	121.5
122.0	18.4	15.7	14.3	18.5	15.8	14.4	18.5	15.8	14.5	122.0
122.5	18.5	15.7	14.4	18.6	15.8	14.4	18.6	15.9	14.5	122.5
123.0	18.5	15.8	14.4	18.6	15.8	14.5	18.7	15.9	14.5	123.0
123.5	18.6	15.8	14.4	18.6	15.9	14.5	18.7	16.0	14.6	123.5
124.0	18.6	15.8	14.4	18.7	15.9	14.5	18.8	16.0	14.6	124.0
124.5	18.7	15.8	14.4	18.8	15.9	14.5	18.9	16.1	14.6	124.5
125.0	18.7	15.9	14.5	18.8	16.0	14.6	18.9	16.1	14.7	125.0
125.5	18.8	15.9	14.5	18.9	16.0	14.6	19.0	16.1	14.7	125.5
126.0	18.8	15.9	14.5	19.0	16.1	14.6	19.1	16.2	14.7	126.0
126.5	18.9	16.0	14.5	19.0	16.1	14.6	19.2	16.2	14.8	126.5
127.0	18.9	16.0	14.5	19.1	16.1	14.7	19.2	16.3	14.8	127.0
127.5	19.0	16.0	14.5	19.2	16.2	14.7	19.3	16.3	14.8	127.5
128.0	19.1	16.1	14.6	19.2	16.2	14.7	19.4	16.4	14.9	128.0
128.5	19.1	16.1	14.6	19.3	16.3	14.7	19.5	16.4	14.9	128.5
129.0	19.3	16.1	14.6	19.4	16.3	14.8	19.5	16.5	14.9	129.0
129.5	19.3	16.2	14.6	19.4	16.3	14.8	19.6	16.5	15.0	129.5
130.0	19.3	16.2	14.6	19.5	16.4	14.8	19.7	16.6	15.0	130.0
130.5	19.4	16.2	14.6	19.6	16.4	14.9	19.8	16.6	15.1	130.5
131.0	19.5	16.3	14.7	19.7	16.5	14.9	19.9	16.7	15.1	131.0
131.5	19.6	16.3	14.7	19.8	16.5	14.9	20.0	16.7	15.1	131.5
132.0	19.6	16.3	14.7	19.8	16.6	14.9	20.1	16.8	15.2	132.0
132.5	19.7	16.4	14.7	19.9	16.6	15.0	20.2	16.8	15.2	132.5
133.0	19.8	16.4	14.7	20.0	16.7	15.0	20.2	16.9	15.2	133.0
133.5	19.8	16.5	14.8	20.1	16.7	15.0	20.3	17.0	15.3	133.5
134.0	19.9	16.5	14.8	20.2	16.8	15.0	20.4	17.0	15.3	134.0
134.5	20.0	16.5	14.8	20.3	16.8	15.1	20.5	17.1	15.3	134.5
135.0	20.1	16.6	14.8	20.4	16.9	15.1	20.5	17.1	15.4	135.0
135.5	20.2	16.6	14.9	20.5	16.9	15.1	20.7	17.2	15.4	135.5
136.0	20.3	16.7	14.9	20.6	17.0	15.2	20.8	17.2	15.5	136.0

Table L–1.
Arm Measurements, *continued*

	Mid-Upper-Arm-Circumference (MUAC) for Length or Height Reference Data									
Length/ Height* (cm)	Boys			Combined Sexes			Girls			Length/ Height* (cm)
	Median	−2 SD	−3 SD	Median	−2 SD	−3 SD	Median	−2 SD	−3 SD	
136.5	20.4	16.7	14.9	20.7	17.0	15.2	20.9	17.3	15.5	136.5
137.0	20.5	16.8	14.9	20.8	17.1	15.2	21.1	17.4	15.5	137.0
137.5	20.5	16.8	15.0	20.9	17.1	15.3	21.2	17.4	15.6	137.5
138.0	20.7	16.9	15.0	21.0	17.2	15.3	21.3	17.5	15.6	138.0
138.5	20.8	16.9	15.0	21.1	17.3	15.3	21.4	17.6	15.7	138.5
139.0	20.9	17.0	15.0	21.2	17.3	15.4	21.5	17.6	15.7	139.0
139.5	21.0	17.0	15.1	21.3	17.4	15.4	21.6	17.7	15.7	139.5
140.0	21.1	17.1	15.1	21.4	17.4	15.4	21.7	17.8	15.8	140.0
140.5	21.2	17.2	15.2	21.5	17.5	15.5	21.8	17.9	15.8	140.5
141.0	21.3	17.2	15.2	21.7	17.6	15.5	22.0	17.9	15.9	141.0
141.5	21.5	17.3	15.2	21.8	17.6	15.6	22.1	18.0	15.9	141.5
142.0	21.6	17.4	15.3	21.9	17.7	15.6	22.2	18.0	15.9	142.0
142.5	21.7	17.5	15.3	22.0	17.8	15.7	22.4	18.1	16.0	142.5
143.0	21.9	17.5	15.4	22.2	17.9	15.7	22.5	18.2	16.0	143.0
143.5	22.0	17.6	15.4	22.3	17.9	15.8	22.7	18.3	16.1	143.5
144.0	22.1	17.7	15.5	22.5	18.0	15.8	22.8	18.4	16.1	144.0
144.5	22.3	17.8	15.5	22.6	18.1	15.9	22.9	18.4	16.2	144.5
145.0	22.4	17.9	15.6	22.6	18.2	15.9	23.1	18.5	16.2	145.0

Length below 85 cm, height = 85 cm. Reprinted with permission from: Mei et al. The development of a MUAC-for-height reference, including a comparison to other nutritional status screening indicators. *WHO Bull.* 1997;75:333–341.

Table L–2.
Arm Measurements

MUAC-for-Age Reference Data for Boys Aged 6–59 Months*							
Age, mo	−4 SD	−3 SD	−2 SD	−1 SD	Mean	+1 SD	+2 SD	+3 SD
6	10.3	11.5	12.6	13.8	14.9	16.1	17.3	18.4
7	10.4	11.6	12.7	13.9	15.1	16.3	17.5	18.6
8	10.5	11.7	12.8	14.0	15.2	16.4	17.6	18.8
9	10.5	11.7	12.9	14.2	15.4	16.6	17.8	19.0
10	10.6	11.8	13.0	14.2	15.5	16.7	17.9	19.1
11	10.6	11.9	13.1	14.3	15.6	16.8	18.0	19.3
12	10.7	11.9	13.2	14.4	15.7	16.9	18.1	19.4
13	10.7	12.0	13.2	14.5	15.7	17.0	18.2	19.5
14	10.8	12.0	13.3	14.5	15.8	17.1	18.3	19.6
15	10.8	12.1	13.3	14.6	15.9	17.1	18.4	19.7
16	10.8	12.1	13.4	14.6	15.9	17.2	18.5	19.8
17	10.8	12.1	13.4	14.7	16.0	17.3	18.6	19.8
18	10.8	12.1	13.4	14.7	16.0	17.3	18.6	19.9
19	10.9	12.2	13.5	14.8	16.1	17.4	18.7	20.0
20	10.9	12.2	13.5	14.8	16.1	17.4	18.7	20.0
21	10.9	12.2	13.5	14.8	16.1	17.5	18.8	20.1
22	10.9	12.2	13.5	14.8	16.2	17.5	18.8	20.1
23	10.9	12.2	13.5	14.8	16.2	17.6	18.9	20.2
24	10.9	12.3	13.6	14.8	16.2	17.6	18.9	20.2
25	10.9	12.3	13.6	14.9	16.3	17.6	18.9	20.3
26	10.9	12.3	13.6	14.9	16.3	17.6	19.0	20.3
27	10.9	12.3	13.6	15.0	16.3	17.7	19.0	20.4
28	10.9	12.3	13.6	15.0	16.3	17.7	19.1	20.4
29	10.9	12.3	13.7	15.0	16.4	17.7	19.1	20.4
30	10.9	12.3	13.7	15.0	16.4	17.8	19.1	20.5
31	11.0	12.3	13.7	15.1	16.4	17.8	19.2	20.5
32	11.0	12.3	13.7	15.1	16.5	17.8	19.2	20.6
33	11.0	12.4	13.7	15.1	16.5	17.9	19.2	20.6
34	11.0	12.4	13.8	15.1	16.5	17.9	19.3	20.6
35	11.0	12.4	13.8	15.2	16.5	17.9	19.3	20.7
36	11.0	12.4	13.8	15.2	16.6	18.0	19.3	20.7
37	11.0	12.4	13.8	15.2	16.6	18.0	19.4	20.8

Table L–2.
Arm Measurements, *continued*

MUAC-for-Age Reference Data for Boys Aged 6–59 Months*							
Age, mo	–4 SD	–3 SD	–2 SD	–1 SD	Mean	+1 SD	+2 SD	+3 SD
38	11.0	12.4	13.8	15.2	16.6	18.0	19.4	20.8
39	11.1	12.5	13.9	15.3	16.7	18.1	19.5	20.9
40	11.1	12.5	13.9	15.3	16.7	18.1	19.5	20.9
41	11.1	12.5	13.9	15.3	16.7	18.1	19.6	21.0
42	11.1	12.5	13.9	15.4	16.8	18.2	19.6	21.0
43	11.1	12.5	14.0	15.4	16.8	18.2	19.7	21.1
44	11.1	12.5	14.0	15.4	16.8	18.3	19.7	21.1
45	11.1	12.6	14.0	15.4	16.9	18.3	19.8	21.2
46	11.1	12.6	14.0	15.5	16.9	18.4	19.8	21.3
47	11.1	12.6	14.0	15.5	17.0	18.4	19.9	21.3
48	11.1	12.6	14.1	15.5	17.0	18.4	19.9	21.4
49	11.1	12.6	14.1	15.6	17.0	18.5	20.0	21.4
50	11.1	12.6	14.1	15.6	17.1	18.5	20.0	21.5
51	11.1	12.6	14.1	15.6	17.1	18.6	20.1	21.6
52	11.1	12.6	14.1	15.6	17.1	18.6	20.1	21.6
53	11.1	12.6	14.1	15.7	17.2	18.7	20.2	21.7
54	11.1	12.6	14.2	15.7	17.2	18.7	20.2	21.8
55	11.1	12.6	14.2	15.7	17.2	18.8	20.3	21.8
56	11.1	12.6	14.2	15.7	17.3	18.8	20.4	21.9
57	11.1	12.6	14.2	15.8	17.3	18.9	20.4	22.0
58	11.1	12.6	14.2	15.9	17.3	18.9	20.5	22.1
59	11.1	12.6	14.2	15.9	17.4	19.0	20.6	22.2

* Reprinted with permission from: de Onis, et al. The development of MUAC-for-age reference data recommended by a WHO expert committee. *WHO Bull.* 1997;75:11–18.

Table L–3.
Arm Measurements

MUAC-for-Age Reference Data for Girls Aged 6–59 Months*							
Age, mo	−4 SD	−3 SD	−2 SD	−1 SD	Mean	+1 SD	+2 SD	+3 SD
6	9.2	10.4	11.5	12.7	13.9	15.0	16.2	17.4
7	9.4	10.6	11.8	13.0	14.1	15.3	16.5	17.7
8	9.6	10.8	12.0	13.2	14.4	15.6	16.8	18.0
9	9.8	11.0	12.2	13.4	14.6	15.8	17.0	18.2
10	9.9	11.1	12.3	13.6	14.8	16.0	17.2	18.4
11	10.0	11.3	12.5	13.7	15.0	16.2	17.4	18.6
12	10.1	11.4	12.6	13.9	15.1	16.4	17.6	18.8
13	10.2	11.5	12.7	14.0	15.2	16.5	17.7	19.0
14	10.3	11.6	12.8	14.1	15.4	16.6	17.9	19.2
15	10.4	11.7	12.9	14.2	15.5	16.7	18.0	19.3
16	10.4	11.7	13.0	14.3	15.6	16.8	18.1	19.4
17	10.5	11.8	13.1	14.4	15.7	16.9	18.2	19.5
18	10.5	11.8	13.1	14.4	15.7	17.0	18.3	19.6
19	10.6	11.9	13.2	14.5	15.8	17.1	18.4	19.7
20	10.6	11.9	13.2	14.5	15.8	17.2	18.5	19.8
21	10.6	11.9	13.3	14.6	15.9	17.2	18.5	19.8
22	10.7	12.0	13.3	14.6	15.9	17.3	18.6	19.9
23	10.7	12.0	13.3	14.7	16.0	17.3	18.6	20.0
24	10.7	12.0	13.4	14.7	16.0	17.4	18.7	20.0
25	10.7	12.0	13.4	14.7	16.1	17.4	18.7	20.1
26	10.7	12.1	13.4	14.7	16.1	17.4	18.8	20.1
27	10.7	12.1	13.4	14.8	16.1	17.5	18.8	20.2
28	10.7	12.1	13.4	14.8	16.1	17.5	18.8	20.2
29	10.7	12.1	13.5	14.8	16.2	17.5	18.9	20.3
30	10.8	12.1	13.5	14.8	16.2	17.6	18.9	20.3
31	10.8	12.1	13.5	14.9	16.2	17.6	19.0	20.3
32	10.8	12.1	13.5	14.9	16.3	17.6	19.0	20.4
33	10.8	12.2	13.5	14.9	16.3	17.7	19.0	20.4
34	10.8	12.2	13.6	14.9	16.3	17.7	19.1	20.5
35	10.8	12.2	13.6	15.0	16.3	17.7	19.1	20.5
36	10.8	12.2	13.6	15.0	16.4	17.8	19.2	20.6
37	10.8	12.2	13.6	15.0	16.4	17.8	19.2	20.6

Table L–3.
Arm Measurements, *continued*

MUAC-for-Age Reference Data for Girls Aged 6–59 Months*							
Age, mo	−4 SD	−3 SD	−2 SD	−1 SD	Mean	+1 SD	+2 SD	+3 SD
38	10.9	12.2	13.6	15.0	16.4	17.8	19.2	20.6
39	10.9	12.3	13.7	15.1	16.5	17.9	19.3	20.7
40	10.9	12.3	13.7	15.1	16.6	17.9	19.3	20.7
41	10.9	12.3	13.7	15.1	16.6	18.0	19.4	20.8
42	10.9	12.3	13.8	15.2	16.6	18.0	19.4	20.8
43	10.9	12.4	13.8	15.2	16.6	18.1	19.5	20.9
44	10.9	12.4	13.8	15.2	16.7	18.1	19.5	21.0
45	11.0	12.4	13.8	15.3	16.7	18.1	19.6	21.0
46	11.0	12.4	13.9	15.3	16.7	18.2	19.6	21.1
47	11.0	12.4	13.9	15.3	16.8	18.2	19.7	21.2
48	11.0	12.4	13.9	15.4	16.8	18.3	19.8	21.2
49	11.0	12.5	13.9	15.4	16.9	18.3	19.8	21.3
50	11.0	12.5	14.0	15.4	16.9	18.4	19.9	21.4
51	11.0	12.5	14.0	15.5	17.0	18.4	19.9	21.4
52	11.0	12.5	14.0	15.5	17.0	18.5	20.0	21.5
53	11.0	12.5	14.0	15.5	17.0	18.6	20.1	21.6
54	11.0	12.5	14.0	15.6	17.1	18.6	20.1	21.7
55	11.0	12.5	14.1	15.6	17.1	18.7	20.2	21.7
56	11.0	12.5	14.1	15.6	17.2	18.7	20.3	21.8
57	11.0	12.5	14.1	15.7	17.2	18.8	20.3	21.9
58	11.0	12.5	14.1	15.7	17.3	18.8	20.4	22.0
59	11.0	12.5	14.1	15.7	17.3	18.9	20.5	22.1

* Reprinted with permission from: de Onis, et al. The development of MUAC-for-age reference data recommended by a WHO expert committee. *WHO Bull.* 1997;75:11–18.

Appendix M

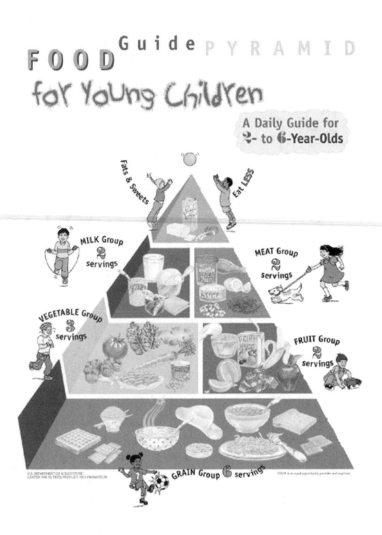

Figure M–1. Food Guide Pyramid for Young Children: A Daily Guide for 2- to 6-Year-Olds
U.S. Department of Agriculture
Center for Nutrition Policy and Promotion

Table M–1.
US Department of Agriculture Center for Nutrition Policy and Promotion

What counts as one serving?	
Grain Group	**Vegetable Group**
1 slice of bread	1/2 c chopped raw of cooked vegetables
1/2 c cooked rice or pasta	1 c raw leafy vegetables
1/2 c cooked cereal	
1 oz ready-to-eat cereal	
Fruit Group	**Milk Group**
1 piece of fruit or melon wedge	1 c milk or yogurt
3/4 c juice	2 oz of cheese
1/2 c canned fruit	
1/4 c dried fruit	
Meat Group	**Fats and Sweets**
2 to 3 oz cooked lean meat, poultry, or fish	Limit calories from these
1/2 c cooked dried beans or 1 egg counts as 1 oz lean meat	
2 tbsp of peanut butter counts as 1 oz of meat	

Four- to 6-year-olds can eat these serving sizes. Offer 2- to 3-year-olds less, except for milk. Two- to 6-year-old children need a total of 2 servings from the milk group each day.

Appendix N

Table N–1.
Iron Content of Selected Foods*

Food	Serving	Iron (mg)
Baked Goods		
Bagel, plain, toasted	1 each	2.83
Bread, mixed grain	1 piece	.90
Bread, white, soft	1 piece	1.08
Bread, whole wheat	1 piece	1.30
English muffins, plain, toasted	1 each	1.53
Chips and Snacks		
Corn chips	1 oz	.37
Chex mix	1 oz (2/3 c)	6.92
Fruit Leather (Fruit Roll-Up)	1 each	.549
Trail mix, regular	1 oz	.86
Dairy and Dairy Products		
Cream cheese, low fat	1T	.252
Creamer (non-dairy), Mocha Mix		.06
Eggs		
Boiled, large, chopped	1 lg	.59
Fruits and Fruit Juices		
Apricots, dried, halves	10 each	1.65
Avocado, California	1 med	2.04
Fig, dried	10 each	4.17
Peach, dried, halves	10 each	5.28
Pineapple, canned in juice	1 c, packed	.70
Prunes, dried	10 each	2.08
Prune juice, canned	8 fl oz	3.02
Raisins	2/3 c	2.08
Tomato juice	6 oz	1.06

Table N–1.
Iron Content of Selected Foods*, *continued*

Food	Serving	Iron (mg)
Grains and Grain Products		
Amaranth, grain	1 c	14.8
Cereal, Cold		
40% Bran flakes, Post	1 oz (2/3 c)	8.10
100% Bran	1/2 c	3.44
All-Bran, Kellogg's	1/2 c	4.50
Cheerios, General Mills	1 c	8.10
Grape Nuts, Post	2 oz (1/2 c)	8.10
Total, General Mills	3/4 c	18.0
Shredded Wheat, Nabisco	1 c	1.44
Wheaties, General Mills	1 c	8.10
Cereals, Hot		
Corn grits, white, enriched, ckd	1 c	1.55
Cream of Wheat, instant, cooked	3/4 c	9.05
Spaghetti, enriched	1c	1.96
Wheat germ, toasted	1/4 c	10.3
Meats (Edible Portion Only)		
Beef	1 oz	.770
Chicken breast, skinless, roasted	1 each	.89
Clams, steamed/boiled, (or can) sm	9 (3 oz)	23.78
Oysters, eastern, canned	3 oz	5.70
Nuts and Seeds		
Almonds, whole, dried	1 oz (24 each)	1.02
Cashew, dry roasted	1 oz	1.70
Mixed nuts, dry roasted w/peanuts	1 c	5.08
Pistachio, dried	1 c	8.69
Sesame seeds, whole, roasted, toasted	1 T	1.31
Sesame butter/tahini, from roasted & toasted kernels	1 T	1.34
Sunflower seeds, dried	1 oz	1.40
Vegetables and Legumes		
Beet greens, boiled	1 c	2.74
Broccoli, boiled	1/2 c	.66

Table N–1.
Iron Content of Selected Foods*, *continued*

Food	Serving	Iron (mg)
Chard, Swiss – chopped & boiled	1/2 c	1.99
Collard, frozen, boiled	1/2 c	.95
Garbanzo/chickpea, canned	1 c	3.24
Great northern beans, canned	1 c	4.11
Green beans, frozen, boiled	1/2 c	.60
Kidney beans, canned	1 c	3.15
Mushrooms, raw, pieces	1/2 c	.43
Mustard greens, frozen, boiled	1/2 c	.84
Pinto beans, cooked	1 c	4.46
Potatoes, baked (microwaved) w/skin	1 each	2.50
Soybean tofu, raw, firm	1/2 c	13.19
Vegetarian Foods		
Dinner Cuts, Loma Linda Foods	2 slices	2
Linketts, Loma Linda Foods	1 link	2
Nuteena, Loma Linda Foods	3/8" slice	2
Tender Bits, Loma Linda Foods	6 pieces	4
Vegeburger, Loma Linda Foods	1/4 c	2
Breakfast Patties, Morningstar Farms	1 pattie	10
Grillers, Morningstar Farms	1 pattie	6
Breakfast Sandwich-Bagel/Scramblers/ Pattie/cheese Morningstar Farms	1 sandwich	45
Bolono, Worthington Foods	3 slices	10
Frichik, Worthington Foods	2 pieces	6
Prime Stakes, Worthington Foods	1 piece	2
Prosage Links, Worthington Foods	2 links	8
Miscellaneous (Spices, etc)		
Basil, dried	1 tsp	.42
Caraway seed	1 tsp	.32
Oregano, ground	1 tsp	.88
Parsley, fresh, chopped	1/2 c	1.86
Thyme, ground	1 tsp	1.24
Yeast, Brewer's	1T	1.38

*Adapted from Hodgkin G, Maloney S, eds. *Loma Linda University Diet Manual: Handbook Supporting Vegetarian Nutrition.* Loma Linda, CA: Loma Linda University Press; 2003.

References

1. Yip R, Dallman PR. Iron, In: Ziegler EE, Filer LJ Jr, eds. *Present Knowledge in Nutrition.* 7th ed. Washington, DC: ILSI Press; 1996
2. Kasdan TS. Nutritional care in anemia. In: Mahan LK, Escott-Stump S. *Krause's Food, Nutrition, & Diet Therapy.* 9th ed. Philadelphia, PA: W.B. Saunders Co; 1996
3. Salonen JY, Nyyssonen K, Korpela H, et al. High stored iron levels are associated with excess risk of myocardial infarction in Eastern Finish men. Circulation. 1992; 86:803–811
4. Herbert V. Everyone should be tested for iron disorders. *J Am Diet Assoc.* 1992;92:1502–1509
5. Pennington JAT. *Bowes and Church's Food Values of Portions Commonly Used.* 17th ed. Philadelphia, PA: J.B. Lippincott; 1998

Table N–2.
Calcium Content of Foods, mg per Serving*

100±	150±	200±	250±
15 Brazil nuts	1 c ice cream	1 c beet greens	1 c almonds
6 medium stalks broccoli	1 c oysters	1 oz cheddar or Muenster cheese	1 oz Swiss or Parmesan cheese
2 c instant farina	1 c cooked rhubarb	3 oz sardines with bones	1 c cooked dandelion greens
1 c cooked kale	1 c cooked spinach		1 c milk
1 tbsp blackstrap molasses	1 oz feta or mozzarella cheese		1/2 c cooked ricotta cheese
3 tbsp light (reg) molasses	1/2 c cooked chopped collards		
1 c cooked navy beans	3 oz canned salmon with bones		
3.5 oz soybean curd (tofu)			
3.5 oz sunflower seeds			
5 tbsp maple syrup			
1 c cottage cheese, regular or low fat			

*Plus-minus signs indicate approximately.

Table N-3.
Zinc Content of Common Household Portions of Selected Foods*

Food	Portion	Zinc, mg	Protein, g
Fish (flounder, tuna, salmon)	3 oz	0.58	22.89
Oysters	3 oz	77.51	6.00
Crab	3 oz	6.48	16.46
Poultry			
Dark meat	3 oz	2.20	22.08
Light meat	3 oz	0.87	25.34
Beef	3 oz	4.60	26.82
Pork	3 oz	4.40	26.72
Bologna	3 oz	1.70	13.02
Liver (chicken, beef, pork)	3 oz	4.90	23.48
Whole egg	1 large	0.70	6.07
Dried beans and lentils	1/2 c	0.95	7.70
Milk	1 c	0.93	8.03
Cheese (cheddar)	1 oz	0.88	7.05
Bread			
White	1 slice	0.15	2.97
Wheat	1 slice	0.47	2.69
Rice			
White	1/2 c	0.35	2.00
Brown	1/2 c	0.60	1.80
Cornmeal (cooked)	1/2 c	0.15	1.50
Oatmeal (cooked)	1/2 c	0.58	3.00
Bran flakes (40%)	1 oz	1.16	3.20
Corn flakes	1 oz	0.03	0.95

*From United States Department of Agriculture. *Agricultural Handbooks;* 1976–1988.

Table N–4.
Saturated and Polyunsaturated Fat and Cholesterol Content of Common Foods*

Foods	Quantity	Saturated Fat, g	Polyunsaturated Fat, g	Cholesterol, mg	kcal
Almonds (roasted, salted, shelled)	12	2	2	0	100
Bacon (cured, cooked)	2 slices	4	1	30	90
Beef, lean	3 oz	4	0	80	170
Bread	1 slice	0	0	0	70
Butter	1 tbsp	6	1	35	125
Cheese					
Cheddar	1 oz	5	0	30	100
Cottage, creamed	1/2 c	2	0	20	55
Cream or spread	1 oz	5	0	30	100
Chicken (with skin)	3 oz	2	1	75	140
Coconut (dried, sweetened)	2 tbsp	5	0	0	100
Corn oil	1 tbsp	2	7	0	125
Cottonseed oil	1 tbsp	3	6	0	125
Egg					
Whole	1 medium	2	0	215	81
White	1 medium	0	0	5	16
Yolk	1 medium	2	0	215	65
Fish (fillet or flounder, sole)	3 1/2 oz	0	0	60	90
Hamburger (80% lean)	3 oz	10	0	80	250
Ice cream (10% fat)	1/2 c	5	0	30	100
Lamb (lean leg)	3 oz	4	0	80	170
Lard and other animal fats	1 tbsp	6	1	12	125
Liver (beef)	3 oz	5	1	400	170
Margarine					
Regular (hydrogenated)	1 tbsp	3	2	...	100
Liquid oil	1 tbsp	4	2	...	100
Milk					
Whole	1 c	5	0.2	30	160

Table N–4.
Saturated and Polyunsaturated Fat and Cholesterol Content of Common Foods*, *continued*

Foods	Quantity	Saturated Fat, g	Polyunsaturated Fat, g	Cholesterol, mg	kcal
2%	1 c	2	0.2	20	115
Skimmed	1 c	0	0	5	90
Olive oil	1 tbsp	1	1	0	125
Oysters (Eastern)	3 1/2 oz	1	1	60	110
Peanut oil	1 tbsp	2	3	0	125
Pork (lean)	3 oz	5	0	80	180
Safflower oil	1 tbsp	1	9	0	125
Salmon, king (canned)	3 1/2 oz	4	4	40	200
Shrimp (canned in wet pack)	3 1/2 oz	0	0	150	90
Soybean oil	1 tbsp	2	7	0	125
Sweetbreads (calf)	3 oz	5	1	400	170
Tuna fish, canned in vegetable oil	3 1/2 oz	0	0	60	90
Turkey (light meat)	3 oz	<1	1	65	140

*A low-cholesterol, low-fat diet should limit cholesterol intake to 300 mg/d, have less than 35% of calories as fat, and have polyunsaturated fats at least equal to saturated fats. Monounsaturated fat, hence total fat, is not included except under kcal.

Table N–5.
Sodium Content of Foods, mg per Serving

500	250	200	100	50
1/8 tsp salt	2 oz canned sardines or salmon	1 slice regular bread	1/2 c of the following unsalted vegetables: beet greens, frozen mixed peas and car-rots, Swiss chard	1/2 c of the following fresh, frozen, or canned vegetables, canned without salt:
3/4 tsp monosodium glutamate	1/2 c regularly seasoned spinach, beets, celery, kale, or white turnips	2 thin slices bacon, crisp and drained	1 oz frozen fish fillets	1 artichoke (edible base and leaves),
1/2 bouillon cube	1 oz salami	1/2 c canned carrots or seasoned vegetables not listed elsewhere	3/4 c milk (6 oz)	beets, carrots, celery, dandelion greens, kale,
1/2 c tomato juice	1 hard roll	1/2 c frozen peas or lima beans	1/2 c pasta cooked in salted water	mustard greens, peas (blackeyed), spinach, succo-
1 average serving 1/2 c, eg, of cooked rice, spaghetti, noodles, hominy, seasoned with salt	1/2 c rice or grits cooked in salted water	1 oz natural cheddar cheese	1 oz tuna, drained (not rinsed)	tash, turnip greens, turnip (white)
1/2 c drained sauerkraut	3 oz shrimp (fresh) cooked in salted water	1 tbsp catsup		
1 average frankfurter (1 1/2 oz)		5 saltine crackers		
1 oz turkey luncheon meat				

Appendix O

Table O–1.
Selected Enteral Products for Special Indications*

Product	Energy, kcal/L	Protein Source, g/L	Carbohydrate Source, g/L	Fat Source, g/L	Fiber g/L	Purpose
Advera†	1280	Soy protein hydrolysate, Na caseinate / 60	Maltodextrin, sucrose, soy fiber / 215.8	Canola, medium chain triglycerides (MCT) and sardine oils / 22.8	8.9	High-calorie, high-protein complete formula, designed for people with HIV or AIDS
Additions‡	526/ 100 g	Na caseinate, whey protein isolate / 31.6/ 100 g	Corn syrup solids / 47.4/ 100 g	Canola oil, soy lecithin / 26.3/ 100 g		Neutral-flavored powdered blend of protein, carbohydrate, and fat used to supplement regular food
Alitraq†	1000	Soy hydrolysate, amino acids, whey protein concentrate, lactalbumin hydrolysate / 52.5	Maltodextrin, sucrose, fructose / 165	Safflower and MCT (53%) oils / 15.5		Elemental formula with added glutamine, designed for patients with impaired GI function
Amin-aid§	1956	Essential amino acids + histidine / 19.4	Maltodextrin, sucrose / 366	Partially hydrogenated soybean oil, lecithin / 46.2		Essential amino acid and calorie supplement for patients with renal failure—contains no vitamins or minerals

Table 0–1.
Selected Enteral Products for Special Indications*, *continued*

Product	Energy, kcal/L	Protein Source, g/L	Carbohydrate Source, g/L	Fat Source, g/L	Fiber g/L	Purpose
Boost‖ (with fiber)	1010	Milk-protein concentrate 43	Corn syrup solids, sucrose (soy fiber, acacia, microcrystalline cellulose) 173 (178)	Canola, high-oleic sunflower, and corn oils 18	(11.1)	Nutritionally complete liquid food, lactose-free
Boost High Protein‖	1010	Milk-protein concentrate, Na and Ca caseinate 61	Corn syrup solids, sucrose 139	Canola, high-oleic sunflower, and corn oils 23		High-protein, nutritionally complete oral supplement
Boost Plus‖	1520	Na and Ca caseinate 59	Corn syrup solids, sucrose 200	Canola, high-oleic sunflower, and corn oils 58		High-calorie, nutritionally complete oral supplement
Casec‖	380/ 100 g	Ca caseinate 90/ 100 g		Soy lecithin 2/ 100 g		Concentrated, intact, powdered protein supplement
Choice dm beverage‖	930	Ca and Na caseinate, milk-protein concentrate 39	Maltodextrin, sucrose, soy fiber, acacia, microcrystalline cellulose 93	Canola, high-oleic sunflower, and corn oils 43	11	Fiber-containing oral supplement, designed for people with diabetes
Choice dm TF‖	1060	Milk protein concentrate, casein 45	Maltodextrin, microcrystalline cellulose, soy fiber, acacia 119	Canola, high-oleic sunflower, corn, and MCT (10%) oils 51	14.4	Nutritionally complete tube feeding with fiber for patients with abnormal glucose tolerance

Table O-1.
Selected Enteral Products for Special Indications*, *continued*

Product	Energy, kcal/L	Protein Source, g/L	Carbohydrate Source, g/L	Fat Source, g/L	Fiber g/L	Purpose
Citrotein¶	730	Pasteurized egg white solids	41	Sucrose, maltodextrins	120	Mono and diglycerides, soybean oil	1.6		Clear, fruit-flavored liquid nutrition, low in fat, lactose and gluten free
Compleat¶	1070	Beef, Ca caseinate	43	Hyrolyzed cornstarch, fruits, vegetables	140	Canola oil, beef	37	4.3	Blenderized tube feed formulated from traditional foods
Compleat Pediatric¶	1000	Beef, Na and Ca caseinate	38	Hydrolyzed cornstarch, fruites, vegetables, apple juice	130	High-oleic sunflower, soybean, MCT (18%) oils	39	4.4	Intact protein, formulated from traditional foods including meats, vegetables, and fruit
Comply‖	1500	Na and Ca caseinate	60	Maltodextrin	180	Canola, high-oleic sunflower, MCT (20%), and corn oils	61		Nutritionally complete, high-calorie formula for tube feeding
Criticare HN‖	1060	Casein hydrolysate, amino acids	38	Maltodextrin, modified cornstarch	220	Safflower oil, emulsifiers	5.3		Ready to use elemental formula—50% small peptides, 50% amino acids
Crucial‡	1500	Hydrolyzed casein, L-arginine	94	Maltodextrin	135	MCT oil (50%), deodorized fish oil, soy oil, soy lecithin	68		High-calorie and protein peptide-based formula designed for critically ill patients
Deliver 2.0‖	2000	Na and Ca caseinate	75	Corn syrup	200	Soy and MCT (30%) oils	101		High-calorie and high-nitrogen complete liquid diet

Table 0–1.
Selected Enteral Products for Special Indications*, _continued_

Product	Energy, kcal/L	Protein Source, g/L	Carbohydrate Source, g/L	Fat Source, g/L	Fiber g/L	Purpose
DiabetiSource¶	1000	Ca caseinate, beef	Maltodextrin, fructose, vegetables, fruits	High-oleic sunflower, canola, and beef oils	49	4.3	Traditional food ingredients, designed for abnormal glucose tolerance
Elecare†	1000	Free L-amino acids	Corn syrup solids	High-oleic safflower, MCT (33%), and soy oils	48		Complete amino-acid based diet for children >1 year of age with intact protein intolerance
EO28 Extra (flavored)#	886 (854)	Free amino acids	Dried glucose syrup (Sugar, sodium saccharin, dried glucose syrup)	MCT (35%), canola, hybrid safflower oils	118 (110)	35	Nutritionally complete elemental diet for adults and children >5 years of age with GI impairment
Duocal#	490/ 100 g		Hydrolyzed cornstarch	Corn, coconut, MCT (35%) oils	73	22	Powdered carbohydrate and fat supplement
Enlive†	1250	Whey protein isolate	Maltodextrin, sucrose		267	0	High-calorie fat-free clear liquid oral supplement
Ensure Fiber with FOS†	1060	Na and Ca caseinate, soy protein isolate	Maltodextrin, sucrose, soy fiber, oat fiber, fructo-oligosaccharides	High-oleic safflower, canola, and corn oils	177	26	11.8	Complete or supplemental nutrition with fiber and FOS
Ensure†	1060	Ca caseinate, soy protein isolate, whey protein concentrate	Corn syrup, sucrose, maltodextrin	Corn, high-oleic safflower, and canola oils	167	25	Nutritionally complete oral supplement

Table 0–1.
Selected Enteral Products for Special Indications*, continued

Product	Energy, kcal/L	Protein Source, g/L	Carbohydrate Source, g/L	Fat Source, g/L	Fiber g/L	Purpose
Ensure High Calcium	950	Ca and Na caseinates, soy protein isolate	51	Sucrose, maltodextrin	131	High-oleic safflower, canola, and soy oils	25		Supplemental high protein oral nutrition with 1,688 mg Ca/L
Ensure High Protein	950	Ca and Na caseinates, soy protein isolate	51	Sucrose, maltodextrin	131	High-oleic safflower, canola, and soy oils	25		High-protein complete oral nutritional supplement
Ensure Light	850	Ca caseinate	42	Sucrose, maltodextrin	141	High-oleic safflower and canola oils	13		Lower calorie, lower fat nutritionally complete oral supplement
Ensure Plus†	1500	Na and Ca caseinate, soy protein isolate	55	Corn syrup, maltodextrin, sucrose	211	High-oleic safflower, canola, and corn oils	48		High-calorie, complete oral supplement
Ensure Plus HN-flavored (unflavored RTH) †	1500	Na and Ca caseinate, soy protein isolate	62 (63)	Maltodextrin, sucrose (maltodextrin)	200 (204)	Corn oil (high-oleic safflower, canola, and MCT [20%] oils	50 (49)		High-calorie, high-nitrogen nutritionally complete liquid for oral supplementation or tube feeding
f.a.a	1000	Free amino acids	50	Maltodextrin, cornstarch	176	Soybean and MCT (25%) oils	11.2		Low-fat elemental diet with 20% of calories from free amino acids
FiberSource Standard¶	1200	Soy concentrate, soy isolate	43	Corn syrup, hydrolyzed cornstarch	170	Canola and MCT (20%) oils	39	10	Higher calories, contains soluble and insoluble fiber
FiberSource HN¶	1200	Soy isolate, soy concentrate	53	Corn syrup, hydrolyzed cornstarch	160	Canola and MCT (20%) oils	39	10	Higher calories and protein, contains soluble and insoluble fiber

Table 0–1.
Selected Enteral Products for Special Indications* , continued

Product	Energy, kcal/L	Protein Source, g/L	Carbohydrate Source, g/L	Fat Source, g/L	Fiber g/L	Purpose
Glucerna†	1000	Na and Ca caseinate	41.8	Maltodextrin, fructose, soy flour	95.6	High-oleic safflower and canola oils, soy lecithin	54.4	14.1	Supplemental or complete tube feeding or oral nutrition for patients with abnormal glucose tolerance
Glytrol‡	1000	Ca and K caseinate	45	Maltodextrin, cornstarch, fructose, gum arabic, pectin, soy polysaccharides	100	Canola, high-oleic safflower and MCT (20%) oils, soy lecithin	47.5	15	Fiber containing, fat and CHO designed for better glucose control
HepaticAid§	1176	L-amino acids	44	Maltodextrin, sucrose	169	Partially hydrogenated soybean oil, lecithin, mono and diglycerides	36		High-branched chain amino acid and calorie supplement for patients with chronic liver disease—contains no vitamins or minerals
Immun-Aid§	1000	Lactalbumin, supplemental amino acids	80	Maltodextrin	120	MCT (50%) and canola oils	22		High-nitrogen, nutritionally complete feeding for immuno-compromised patients
Impact (with fiber)¶	1000	Na and Ca caseinate, L-arginine	56	Hydrolyzed cornstarch	130 (140)	Palm kernel and sunflower oil, menhaden oil	28	(10)	High protein designed for critically ill patients

Table O–1.
Selected Enteral Products for Special Indications*, *continued*

Product	Energy, kcal/L	Protein Source, g/L	Carbohydrate Source, g/L		Fat Source, g/L		Fiber g/L	Purpose
Impact Glutamine¶	1300	Wheat protein hydrolysate, free amino acids, sodium caseinate	78	Maltodextrin	150	Palm kernal, menhaden, and sunflower oils	43		High-glutamine (15 g/L), immune-enhancing enteral formula for critically ill patients
Intensical‖‖	1300	Casein hydrolysate, L-arginine	81	Maltodextrin, modified cornstarch	150	Canola, MCT (25%), high oleic sunflower, corn, refined menhaden oils	42		Complete elemental nutrition for highly metabolically stressed patients
Impact 1.5¶	1500	Na and Ca caseinate, L-arginine	84	Hydrolyzed cornstarch	140	Palm kernal and sunflower oil, menhaden and MCT (55%) oil	69		High-calorie and protein designed for critically ill patients
Isocal‖‖	1060	Ca and Na caseinate, soy protein isolate	34	Maltodextrin	135	Soy and MCT (20%) oils	44		Nutritionally complete, isotonic, tube feeding formula
Isocal HN‖‖	1060	Na and Ca caseinate, soy protein isolate	44	Maltodextrin	124	Soy and MCT (40%) oils	45		Moderately high-nitrogen, isotonic, nutritionally complete tube feeding
Isocal HN Plus‖	1200	Milk protein concentrate, casein	54	Maltodextrin	156	Canola, MCT (30%), high-oleic sunflower and corn oils	40		Moderately high-nitrogen 1.2 calorie/mL nutritionally complete tube feeding

Table 0–1.
Selected Enteral Products for Special Indications*, continued

Product	Energy, kcal/L	Protein Source, g/L	Carbohydrate Source, g/L	Fat Source, g/L	Fiber g/L	Purpose
Isosource Standard¶	1200	Soy isolate 43	Corn syrup, hydrolyzed cornstarch 170	Canola and MCT (20%) oils 39		High-calorie soy protein formula
Isosource 1.5 Cal¶	1500	Na and Ca caseinate 68	Hydrolyzed cornstarch, sugar 170	Canola, MCT (30%), and soybean oils 65	8	High calorie, high nitrogen, contains soluble and insoluble soy fiber
Isosource HN¶	1200	Soy isolate 53	Corn syrup, hydrolyzed cornstarch 160	Canola and MCT (20%) oils 39		High-nitrogen, high-calorie soy protein formula
Isosource VHN¶	1000	Na and Ca caseinate 62	Hydrolyzed cornstarch 130	Canola and MCT (50%) oils 29	10	High nitrogen, isotonic, contains soluble and insoluble fiber
Jevity†	1060	Na and Ca caseinate 44.3	Maltodextrin, soy fiber, corn syrup 155	High oleic safflower, canola, and MCT (20%) oils 34.7	14.4	Isotonic, fiber-containing nutritionally complete tube feeding formula
Jevity Plus†	1200	Na and Ca caseinate 56	Corn syrup, maltodextrin, fructo-oligosaccharides, fiber blend 173	High oleic safflower, canola, and MCT (19%) oils 39.3	12	Higher calorie, high-protein fiber-containing tube feeding
Kindercal (with fiber)‖	1060	milk-protein concentrate 30	Maltodextrin, sugar 135	Canola, high-oleic sunflower, corn, and MCT (20%) oils 44	(6.3)	Nutritionally complete, lactose free oral beverage for children 1–10 years

Table O–1.
Selected Enteral Products for Special Indications*, *continued*

Product	Energy, kcal/L	Protein Source, g/L	Carbohydrate Source, g/L	Fat Source, g/L	Fiber g/L	Purpose
Kindercal TF (with fiber)ǁ	1060	Milk protein concentrate	30	Sugar, maltodextrin	135	Canola, high-oleic sunflower, MCT (20%), and corn oils	44	(6.3)	Nutritionally complete, isotonic, lactose-free tube feeding for children 1–10 years of age
Lipisorb Liquidǁ	1350	Na and Ca caseinate	57	Maltodextrin, sucrose	161	MCT (85%) and soy oils	57		Nutritionally complete MCT formulation for patients with fat malabsorption
MCT oilǁ	115 kcal/ tbsp 8.3 kcal/g	...	0	...	0	Fractionated coconut oil	934		Fat supplement or substitute for patients with long-chain fatty acid malabsorption—directly absorbed into portal vein
Magnacal Renalǁ	2000	Na and Ca caseinate	75	Maltodextrins, sucrose	200	Canola, high oleic sunflower, MCT (20%) and corn oils	101		Very high-calorie complete oral- or tube-feeding formula designed for patients on hemodialysis
Meritene¶ (mixed with whole milk)	1080	Nonfat and whole milk	69	Lactose, corn syrup solids, sucrose	120	Milk fat	34		High-protein oral supplement, concentrated with vitamins and minerals, low in fat and cholesterol, high calcium, gluten free, mix with whole or skim milk

Table 0–1.
Selected Enteral Products for Special Indications*, continued

Product	Energy, kcal/L	Protein Source, g/L	Carbohydrate Source, g/L	Fat Source, g/L	Fiber g/L	Purpose
Microlipid‖	4500	…	0	Safflower oil	506		50% fat emulsion for special dietary use in oral or tube-feeding formulas
Moducal‖	375 kcal/ 100 g	…	Maltodextrin	95 g/ 100 g			Powdered, low osmolality calorie supplement consisting of glucose polymers
Modulen IBD‡	1000	Acid casein	Sugar	108	Milk fat, MCT (25%) and corn oils	46	Oral intact protein formula designed for people with Crohn's disease
Neocate Jr.#	1000	Free amino acids	Corn syrup solids	104	MCT (35%), canola, hybrid safflower oils	50	Nutritionally complete elemental formula for children >1 year with severe GI impairment; more vitamins and minerals than Neocate 1+
Neocate 1+#	1000	Free amino acids	Corn syrup solids	146	MCT (35%), canola, hybrid safflower oils	35	Elemental diet suitable for children >1 year with protein hypersensitivity or allergy
Nepro†	2000	Ca, Mg, and Na caseinate, milk protein isolate	Corn syrup, sucrose, fructo-oligosac-charides	222.3	High-oleic safflower and canola oils	95.6	Very high-calorie complete oral or tube feeding designed for dialysis patients

Table O–1.
Selected Enteral Products for Special Indications*, continued

Product	Energy, kcal/L	Protein Source, g/L		Carbohydrate Source, g/L	Fat Source, g/L		Fiber g/L	Purpose
NovaSource Pulmonary¶	1500	Na and Ca caseinates	75	Corn syrup, sugar	150	Canola and MCT (20%) oils	68	8	High-calorie and nitrogen formula, designed for pulmonary patients
NovaSource Renal¶	2000	Na and Ca caseinate, L-arginine	74	Corn syrup, fructose	200	High oleic sunflower, corn, and MCT (14%) oils	100		Very high-calorie, vitamin and mineral profile specifically formulated for dialysis patients, TetraBrik® Pak
NovaSource 2.0¶	2000	Ca and Na caseinate	90	Corn syrup solids, sucrose, maltodextrin	220	Canola and MCT (20%) oils	87.5		Very high calorie, high nitrogen, reduced level of sodium, TetraBrik® Pak
NuBasics‡	1000	Ca caseinate	35	Corn syrup solids, sucrose	132.4	Canola and corn oils, soy lecithin	36.8		Oral supplement, lactose free, gluten-free
NuBasics Plus‡	1500	Ca caseinate	52.4	Corn syrup solids, sucrose	176.4	Canola and corn oils, soy lecithin	64.8		High-calorie, lactose-free oral supplement
NuBasics 2.0‡	2000	Ca and K caseinate	80	Corn syrup solids, maltodextrin, sucrose	196	MCT oil (75%), canola, soy lecithin, corn oils	106		Very high calorie, 75% of fat from MCT
NuBasics VHP‡	1000	Ca and K caseinate	62.4	Corn syrup solids, sucrose	112.8	Canola and corn oils, soy lecithin	33.2		High-protein, lactose-free oral supplement

Table 0–1.
Selected Enteral Products for Special Indications*, _continued_

Product	Energy, kcal/L	Protein Source, g/L	Carbohydrate Source, g/L	Fat Source, g/L	Fiber g/L	Purpose
Nutren 1.0 (fiber)‡	1000	Ca and K caseinate	40	Maltodextrin, corn syrup solids (soy polysaccharides)	127	Canola, MCT (25%), corn oils, soy lecithin	38	(14)	Complete liquid nutrition, fiber for management of diarrhea or constipation
Nutren 1.5‡	1500	Ca and K caseinate	60	Maltodextrin	169.2	MCT (50%), canola, corn oils, soy lecithin	67.6		High calorie for fluid restriction, 50% MCT oil
Nutren 2.0‡	2000	Ca and K caseinate	80	Corn syrup solids, maltodextrin, sucrose	196	MCT (75%), canola, soy lecithin, corn oils	106		Very high calorie, severe fluid restriction, 75% MCT oil
Nutren Jr (fiber)‡	1000	Casein, whey	30	Maltodextrin, sucrose (soy polysaccharides)	127.5	MCT (25%), canola, and soybean oils, soy lecithin	42	(6)	Balanced formula designed to meet needs of children ages 1–10 years
NutriFocus	1500	Na caseinate, milk protein isolate, soy protein isolate, arginine	62	Corn syrup, sucrose, fiber blend, fructo-oligosaccharides	215	Canola, corn, and high-oleic safflower oils	49	10.5	High-calorie, high-protein oral supplement used for wound healing

Table O–1.
Selected Enteral Products for Special Indications*, *continued*

Product	Energy, kcal/L	Protein Source, g/L	Carbohydrate Source, g/L	Fat Source, g/L		Fiber g/L	Purpose
NutriHep‡	1500	L-amino acids, whey protein (50% BCAA)	Maltodextrin, modified corn starch	290	MCT (66%), canola, soy lecithin, and corn oils	21.2		High branched-chain amino acids, low aromatic and ammonogenic amino acids
NutriRenal‡	2000	Ca and K caseinate	Corn syrup solids, maltodextrin, sucrose	205	MCT (50%), canola, corn oils	104		High-calorie, high-biological protein, designed for the patient on dialysis
NutriVent‡	1500	Ca and K caseinate	Maltodextrin	100	Canola, MCT (40%), corn oils, soy lecithin	94		High fat content, deigned to reduce CO_2 production
Optimental†	1000	Soy protein hydrolysate, partially hydrolyzed Na caseinate, free arginine	Maltodextrin, sucrose, fructooligosaccharides	139	Sardine oil/MCT structured lipid, canola, and soybean oils	28		Complete elemental oral or tube-feeding formula designed for patients with malabsorptive conditions
Osmolite†	1060	Na and Ca caseinates, soy protein isolate	Maltodextrin	151	High-oleic safflower, canola, and MCT (20%) oils	35		Isotonic, low residue complete nutrition for oral or tube-feeding use

Table O–1.
Selected Enteral Products for Special Indications*, *continued*

Product	Energy, kcal/L	Protein Source, g/L		Carbohydrate Source, g/L		Fat Source, g/L		Fiber g/L	Purpose
Osmolite HN†	1060	Na and Ca caseinates, soy protein isolate	44	Maltodextrin	144	High-oleic safflower, canola, and MCT (20%) oils	35		Isotonic, nutritionally complete, high-nitrogen, mild-flavored liquid for oral or tube feeding
Osmolite HN Plus†	1200	Na and Ca caseinates	56	Maltodextrin	158	High-oleic safflower, canola, MCT (19%) oils	39		High-calorie, high-nitrogen complete oral or tube feeding
Oxepa	1500	Na and Ca caseinates	63	Sucrose, maltodextrin	106	Canola, MCT (25%), borage and refined deodorized sardine oils	94		High-calorie complete tube-feeding formula for patients with lung injury
Pediasure and Pediasure Enteral (with fiber)†	1000	Na caseinate, whey protein concentrate	30	Maltodextrin, sucrose	110 (114)	High-oleic safflower, soy, and MCT (20%) oils	50	(5)	Complete oral or tube feeding designed for patients ages 1–10 years
Pediatric EO28#	1000	Free amino acids	25	Maltodextrin, sucrose	146	MCT (33%), canola, high-oleic safflower oils	35		Ready-to-feed, flavored elemental liquid for children >1 year old with severe GI impairment
Pepdite One+ (banana-flavored)#	1000	Soy and pork hydrolysates, free amino acids	31	Corn syrup solids (sucrose, aspartme)	106	MCT (35%), canola, safflower oils	50		Semi-elemental formula for children >1 year old with severe GI impairment

Table O–1.
Selected Enteral Products for Special Indications*, *continued*

Product	Energy, kcal/L	Protein Source, g/L	Carbohydrate Source, g/L	Fat Source, g/L	Fiber g/L	Purpose
Peptamen (oral)‡	1000	Enzymatically hydrolyzed whey	40	Maltodextrin, cornstarch (sucrose)	127	MCT (70%), soybean, soy lecithin	39		Peptide-based, isotonic, designed for general malabsorption
Peptamen 1.5 (oral)‡	1500	Enzymatically hydrolyzed whey	60	Maltodextrin, cornstarch (sucrose)	191	MCT (70%), soybean, soy lecithin	58.5		High-calorie, peptide-based, high %-age MCT oil designed for malabsorption
Peptamen VHP (oral)‡	1000	Enzymatically hydrolyzed whey	62.5	Maltodextrin, cornstarch (sucrose)	104.5	MCT (70%), soybean, soy lecithin	39.2		High-protein, peptide-based, high %-age MCT oil designed for general malabsorption
Peptamen, Jr. (oral)‡	1000	Enzymatically hydrolyzed whey	30	Maltodextrin, cornstarch (sucrose)	137.6	MCT (60%), soybean, and canola oils, soy lecithin	38.5		Designed for children aged 1–10 years, peptide-based, 60% of fat from MCT oil
Perative†	1300	Partially hydrolyzed Na caseinate, lactalbumin hydrolysate, l-arginine	66.6	Maltodextrin	177.2	Canola, MCT (40%), and corn oils	37.4		Higher calorie, 40% of fat from MCT oil, designed for metabolically stressed patients
PFD 2‖	400/ 100 g powder	26 mg taurine/100 g powder	0	Corn syrup solids, sugar, modified cornstarch	88/ 100 g	Soy oil	4.8/ 100 g		Protein-free powdered supplement providing calories, vitamins, and minerals

1046

Table 0-1.
Selected Enteral Products for Special Indications*, _continued_

Product	Energy, kcal/L	Protein Source, g/L	Carbohydrate Source, g/L	Fat Source, g/L	Fiber g/L	Purpose
Polycose†	380/100 g powder, 2000/L liquid	0	Glucose polymers from corn-starch, 94/100 g, 500/L	...	0		CHO calorie supplement, available in powder or liquid
Portagen (20 kcal/oz Dilution)||	67.6/100 mL	Sodium caseinate 2.3 g/100 mL	Corn syrup solids, sucrose 7.7 g/100 mL	MCT (86%) and corn oils 3.2 g/100 mL		Nutritionally complete for infants and children <2 years With inefficient conventional fat digestion or malabsorption, 3.6% kcal for linoleic acid
ProBalance†	1200	Ca and K caseinate 54	Maltodextrin, corn syrup solids, polysaccharides, gum arabic 156	Canola, MCT (20%), and corn oils, soy lecithin 40.8	10	Higher calorie, fiber containing for the mature adult
Product 3232A||	500/100 g powder	Casein hydrolysate 22 g/100 g	Modified tapioca starch 33 g/100 g	MCT (85%) and corn oils 33 g/100 g		Protein hydrolysate formula free of mono- and disaccharides for use with added carbohydrate
Product 80056||	500/100 g powder	Taurine added 0	Corn syrup solids, modified tapioca starch 72/100 g	corn oil 23/100 g		Protein-free formula base for use with added protein, sodium, potassium, and chloride

Table O–1.
Selected Enteral Products for Special Indications*, *continued*

Product	Energy, kcal/L	Protein Source, g/L	Carbohydrate Source, g/L	Fat Source, g/L	Fiber g/L	Purpose
ProMod†	4.2/g	Whey protein concentrate with lecithin	75/ 100 g	<10/ 100 g	<9/ 100 g	Powdered protein supplement
Promote† (with fiber)	1000	Sodium and calcium caseinate, soy protein isolate	62.5	Maltodextrin, sucrose (oat and soy fiber)	130 (138)	High-oleic safflower, canola, MCT (19%) oil, soy lecithin	26 (28)	(14.4)	High-protein complete oral or tube feeding
Protain XL‖	1000	Na and Ca caseinate	57	Maltodextrin, soy fiber	145	Canola, high oleic sunflower, MCT (20%) and corn oils	30	9.1	Nutritionally complete high protein, fiber containing, designed to aid with wound healing
Pulmocare†	1500	Na and Ca caseinates	62.6	Sucrose, maltodextrin	106	Canola, MCT (20%), high oleic safflower and corn oils	93.3		High-fat, low-carbohydrate complete oral or tube feeding designed for pulmonary patients
Reabilan‡	1000	Enzymatically hydrolyzed casein and whey	31.5	Corn syrup solids, corn starch	131.5	MCT (50%), soybean and canola oils, soy lecithin, glyceryl monostearate	40.5		Peptide based, low nitrogen, 50% of oil from MCT

Table 0–1.
Selected Enteral Products for Special Indications*, _continued_

Product	Energy, kcal/L	Protein Source, g/L		Carbohydrate Source, g/L		Fat Source, g/L		Fiber g/L	Purpose
Reabilan HN‡	1333	Enzymatically hydrolyzed casein and whey	57.9	Corn syrup solids, corn starch	158	MCT (50%), soybean and canola oils, soy lecithin, glyceryl monostearate	54		Higher calorie, peptide-based, 50% og oil from MCT, designed for GI impairment
Renalcal Diet‡	2000	Essential and select non-essential amino acids, whey protein	34.4	Maltodextrin, modified corn starch	290.4	MCT (70%), canola, and corn oils, soy lecithin	82.4		Very high calorie, low protein designed to maintain positive nitrogen balance, added histidine for renal failure, negligible electrolytes
Replete (with fiber)‡	1000	Ca and K caseinate	62.4	Maltodextrin, corn syrup solids (soy polysaccharides)	113.2	Canola and MCT (25%) oils, soy lecithin	34	(14)	High-protein, elevated vitamin and mineral profile designed for wound healing
Resource Diabetic¶	1060	Na and Ca caseinate, soy protein isolates	63	Hydrolyzed corn starch	100	High oleic sunflower and soybean oils	47	13	Fiber containing, designed for diabetics, TetraBrik® Pak
ReSource Fruit Beverage¶	1060	Whey protein isolate	38	Sugar, corn syrup			0		Fat-free clear liquid nutritional supplement

Table O–1.
Selected Enteral Products for Special Indications*, *continued*

Product	Energy, kcal/L	Protein Source, g/L	Carbohydrate Source, g/L		Fat Source, g/L		Fiber g/L	Purpose
ReSource Just for Kids (with fiber)¶	1000	Na and Ca caseinate, whey protein concentrate	30	Hydrolyzed corn starch, sucrose, fructose (chocolate only) 230	High oleic sunflower, soybean and MCT (20%) oils	50	(6)	Complete formula designed for children aged 1–10 years, available with fiber, TetraBrik® Pak
ReSource Plus¶	1520	Na and Ca caseinates, soy protein isolate	55	Corn syrup solids, sugar 110	High oleic sunflower and corn oils	46		High calorie, lactose and gluten free, TetraBrik® Pak
ReSource Standard¶	1060	Na and Ca caseinates, soy protein isolates	38	Corn syrup, sugar 220	High oleic sunflower and corn oils	25		Nutritionally balanced, lactose and gluten free, TetraBrik® Pak
ReSource 2.0¶	2000	Ca and Na caseinates	89	Corn syrup, sucrose, maltodextrin 170	canola and MCT (20%) oils	89		Very high calorie, designed for medication pass supplement programs, pouch pak
Respalor‖	1500	Na and Ca caseinate	75	maltodextrin, sugar 215	Canola, high oleic sunflower, corn and MCT (30%) oils	68		High calorie, designed for patients with limited respiratory function, COPD
SandoSource Peptide¶	1000	Casein hydrolysate, free amino acids, Na caseinate	50	Hydrolyzed corn starch 146	MCT (54%) and soybean oils, hydroxylated lecithin	17		High-protein, semi-elemental, low-fat formula

Note: The carbohydrate column shows two values per row (g/L). Reading by horizontal alignment: ReSource Just for Kids 230/110, ReSource Plus 110/220, ReSource Standard 220/170, ReSource 2.0 170/215, Respalor 215/146, SandoSource Peptide 146/160.

Table 0–1.
Selected Enteral Products for Special Indications*, *continued*

Product	Energy, kcal/L	Protein Source, g/L	Carbohydrate Source, g/L	Fat Source, g/L	Fiber g/L	Purpose
Subdue‖	1000	Hydrolyzed whey protein concentrate or casein hydrolysate	50	Maltodextrin, modified corn starch, sugar 130	MCT (52%), canola, high oleic sunflower, and corn oils 34		Ready-to-use liquid peptide-based formula designed for malabsorption problems
Subdue Plus‖	1500	Hydrolyzed whey protein concentrate	76	Maltodextrin, modified corn starch 186	MCT (47%), canola, high oleic sunflower, and corn oils 51		High-calorie, peptide-based liquid designed for impaired GI function
Suplena†	2000	Na and Ca caseinates	30	Maltodextrin, sucrose	High-oleic safflower and soy oils 95.6		Very high-calorie, low-protein complete formula for renal failure
Tolerex¶	1000	Free amino acids	21	Maltodextrin, modified corn starch 255.2	Safflower oils 1.5		Nutritionally complete, truly elemental diet, low fat
Traumacal‖	1500	Na and Ca caseinate	82	Corn syrup, sucrose 230	Soy and MCT (30%) oils 68		High calorie, high nitrogen for metabolically stressed patients
TwoCal HN†	2000	Na and Ca caseinates	84	Maltodextrin, sucrose, fructo-oligosaccharides 142	High oleic safflower, MCT (19%) and canola oils 91		Complete very high-calorie feeding with fructo-oligosaccharides

Table O–1.
Selected Enteral Products for Special Indications*, continued

Product	Energy, kcal/L	Protein Source, g/L	Carbohydrate Source, g/L	Fat Source, g/L	Fiber g/L	Purpose
Ultracal‖	1060	Milk protein concentrate, casein	Maltodextrin, microcrystalline cellulose, soy fiber, acacia	219	Canola, MCT (40%), high oleic sunflower, and corn oils	39	14.4	Nutritionally complete tube feeding formula with dietary fiber
Ultracal HN Plus‖	1200	Milk protein concentrate, casein	Maltodextrin, microcrystalline cellulose, soy fiber, acacia	142	Canola, MCT (30%), high oleic sunflower, and corn oils	40	10.5	Moderately high-nitrogen, nutritionally complete tube-feeding formula with dietary fiber
Vital High Nitrogen†	1000	Partially hydrolyzed whey, meat, soy, free essential amino acids	Maltodextrin, sucrose	156	Safflower and MCT (45%) oils	10.8		Nutritionally complete, peptide-based formula for patients with impaired GI function
Vivonex T.E.N.¶	1000	Free amino acids	Maltodextrin, modified corn starch	185	Safflower oil	2.8		Free amino acids plus additional glutamine, deigned for GI impairment
Vivonex Plus¶	1000	Free amino acids	Maltodextrin, modified corn starch	210	Soybean oil	6.7		High-nitrogen, very low-fat elemental diet; additional glutamine arginine and BCAA
Vivonex Pediatric¶	800	Free amino acids	Maltodextrin, modified corn starch	190	MCT (68%) and soybean oils	24		Nutritionally complete, elemental formula for children, can be flavored with Vivonex Flavor Packets

Table 0–1.
Selected Enteral Products for Special Indications* , *continued*

Product	Energy, kcal/L	Protein Source, g/L		Carbohydrate Source, g/L		Fat Source, g/L		Fiber g/L	Purpose
Vivonex RTF¶	1000	Free amino acids	50	Maltodextrin, modified corn starch	130	Soybean and MCT (40%) oils	12		Ready-to-use high-nitrogen, low-fat elemental diet for use in stressed, catabolic patients
					175				

*Composition of products as of December 2002.
†Ross Products Division, Abbott Laboratories, Columbus, OH.
‡Nestle Clinical Nutrition, Deerfield, IL.
§B. Braun, Irvine, CA.
‖Mead Johnson Nutritionals, Evansville, IN.
¶Novartis Nutrition Corp., Minneapolis, MN.
#Scientific Hospital Supplies North America, Gaithersburg, MD.

Table O–2.
Enteral Products Grouped by Usage Indication

Standard adult oral	Boost, Ensure High Calcium, Ensure, Ensure Light, NuBasics, ReSource Standard
Standard adult tube feeding	FiberSource Standard, Isocal, Isosource Standard, Jevity, Nutren 1.0, Osmolite, Ultracal
High-protein oral	Boost High Protein, Ensure High Protein, Ensure Plus HN, Meritene, NuBasics VHP
High-protein tube feeding	FiberSource HN, Isocal HN, Isosource HN, Jevity Plus, Osmolite HN, Osmolite HN Plus, ProBalance, Promote, Ultracal HN Plus
1.5 cal/mL	Boost Plus, Comply, Ensure Plus, NuBasics Plus, Nutren 1.5, ReSource Plus
2.0 cal/mL	Deliver 2.0, NovaSource 2.0, NuBasics 2.0, Nutren 2.0, ReSource 2.0, TwoCal HN
Standard pediatric (>1 year of age)	Kindercal, Kindercal TF, Nutren Jr., Pediasure, ReSource Just For Kids
Blenderized	Compleat, Compleat Pediatric
Clear fortified liquid	Citrotein, Enlive, ReSource Fruit Beverage
Peptide-based adult	Alitraq, Criticare HN, Peptamen, Peptamen 1.5, Peptamen VHP, Perative, SandoSource Peptide, Vital High Nitrogen
Peptide-based pediatric	Pepdite One+, Peptamen Jr.
Free amino acid adult	EO28 Extra, Tolerex, Vivonex T.E.N., Vivonex Plus, Vivonex RTF
Free amino acid pediatric (>1 year of age)	Elecare, Neocate Junior, Neocate One+, Pediatric EO28, Vivonex Pediatric
Immune enhancing	Immun-Aid, Impact, Impact 1.5, Impact Glutamine
Wound healing	Crucial, Intensical, Isosource VHN, NutriFocus, Protain XL, Reabilan, Reabilan HN, Replete, Traumacal
Diabetes	Choice dm beverage, Choice dm TF, DiabetiSource, Glucerna, Glytrol, ReSource Diabetic
Kidney disease	Amin-Aid, Magnacal Renal, Nepro, NovaSource Renal, NutriRenal, Renalcal Diet, Suplena
Liver disease	Hepatic-Aid, NutriHep
Pulmonary disease	Isosource 1.5, NovaSource Pulmonary, NutriVent, Oxepa, Pulmocare, Respalor
HIV/AIDS	Advera
Inflammatory bowel disease	Modulen, Optimental, Subdue, Subdue Plus
Fat malabsorption	Lipisorb, Portagen
Carbohydrate modulars	Moducal, Polycose
Protein modulars	Casec, ProMod
Calorie enhancers	Additions, Duocal, PFD2, Product 3232A, Product 80056
Fat modulars	MCT oil, Microlipid

Table O–3.
Energy and Protein Content of Selected Energy-Dense Foods*

Energy, kcal	Protein, g	
Instant breakfast powder (1 packet)	130	7
Mixed with 1 c whole milk	280	15
Powdered milk (1 tbsp)	33	3
Evaporated milk (1 tbsp)	25	1
Cheese (1 oz)	100	7
Peanut butter (1 tbsp)	95	4
Butter or margarine† (1 tsp)	45	0

*See also Appendix P.
†Not the "spreads," which have a lot of air and water added and therefore are lower in kcal.

Table O-4.
Source for Medical Food Modules for Treatment of Inborn Errors of Metabolism

	AppliedNutrition	Cambrooke Foods	Dietary Specialties
	273 Franklin Ave Randolph, NJ 07869 Tel: 800/605–0410 Fax: 201/262–6707 Web site: www.medicalfood.com	2 Central St Framingham, MA 01701 Tel: 508/276–1800 Fax: 630/839–7413 E-mail: info@cambrookefoods.com Web site: www.cambrookefoods.com	1248 Sussex Turnpike, Unit C–1 Randolph, NJ 07869 Tel: 888/640–2800 Fax: 973/895–3742 Web site: www.dietspec.com
Medical Protein Modules	beverage powder bars		
Low-Protein Substitute Modules	confectionary	bagels, breads, snacks, sweets, pasta, mixes, cheese	mixes, cookies, pasta, bread, snacks, sauces, spreads, dessert mixes
	Ener-G-Foods	Glutino	Kingsmill Foods
	PO Box 84487 Seattle, WA 98124–5787 Tel: 800/331–5222 206/767–6660 Fax: 206/764–3398 E-mail: samiii@ener-g.com Web site: www.ener-g.com	1118 Berlier St Laval, Quebec Canada H71 3R9 Tel: 800/363–3438 Fax: 450/629–7689 E-mail: info@glutino.com Web site: www.glutino.com	1399 Kennedy Rd, #17 Scarborough, ON Canada M1P 1L6 Tel: 416/755–1124 Fax: 416/755–4486 E-mail: kingsmill@kingsmillfoods.com Web site: www.kingsmillfoods.com
Medical Protein Modules			
Low-Protein Substitute Modules	pasta, cheese, milk substitutes, mixes, cookies, crackers, soup mix, egg replacer	pastas, cookies, crackers	mixes, cookies, egg replacer, jellies

Table 0–4.
Source for Medical Food Modules for Treatment of Inborn Errors of Metabolism, *continued*

	Liv-N-Well Distributors	Mead Johnson	Med-Diet
	#1–7900 River Rd Richmond, British Columbia Canada V6X 1X7 Tel: 604/270-8474 877/270-8479 (orders only) Fax: 604/270-8477 E-mail: zeno@direct.ca Web site: www.liv-n-well.com	2400 West Lloyd Expressway Evansville, IN 47721–0001 Tel: 812/429-6399 Fax: 812/429-7189 Web site: www.meadjohnson.com	3600 Holly Ln, Suite 80 Plymouth, MN 55447 Tel: 800/633-3438 Fax: 763/550-2022 E-mail: meddiet@med-diet.com Web site: www.med-diet.com
Medical Protein Modules		beverage powders	
Low-Protein Substitute Modules	pastas, cookies, crackers, mixes		pastas, cookies, crackers, sauce mixes, baking mix, soup mix

	Ross Products Division/Abbott Laboratories	SHS North America	Specialty Food Shop
	585 Cleveland Columbus, OH 43215–1724 Tel: 800/551-5838 Web site: www.ross.com/productHandbook/metabolic.asp	PO Box 117 Gaithersburg, MD 20877–0117 Tel: 301/315-5500 800/365-7354 Fax: 301/315-5519 Web site: www.shsna/com	555 University Ave Toronto, Ontario Canada, M5G 1X8 Tel: 800/737-7976 Fax: 416/977-8394 E-mail: sfs@sickkids.on.ca Web site: www.sickkids.on.ca/sfs_site/
Medical Protein Modules	beverage powders beverage solutions	beverage powders, bars, capsules	
Low-Protein Substitute Modules		pastas, baking mix, confectionaries, cookies, crackers, cereal, milk substitute	pastas, mixes, crackers, soups, sauces, cookies

Appendix P

Table P-1.
Sports/Nutrition Bars

Product (gram weight)	Calories	Protein	Fat (saturated fat)	Fiber	Sodium	Calcium (%DV)	Iron (%DV)	Folic Acid (%DV)	Vitamin C (%DV)
Atkins' Advantage (60 g)	250	18 g	13 g (8 g)	1 g	197 mg	69%	0	60%	60%
Balance (50 g)	200	15 g	6 g (3.5 g)	2 g	190 mg	8%	20%	20%	100%
Balance Gold (50 g)	210	15 g	7 g (4 g)	<1 g	90 mg	10%	20%	20%	100%
Balance Outdoor (50 g)	200	15 g	6 g (1.5 g)	3 g	140 mg	8%	15%	0	0
Clif (68 g)	250	10 g	4 g (1.5 g)	5 g	170 mg	25%	30%	20%	100%
Clif's Luna Bar (48 g)	180	10 g	4 g (3 g)	2 g	50 mg	35%	35%	100%	100%
GeniSoy (61.5 g)	230	14 g	5 g (3 g)	1 g	150 mg	25%	25%	25%	25%
IronMan Hi Energy Bar (56.8 g)	230	16 g	8 g (1.5 g)	1 g	220 mg	20%	50%	50%	50%
IronMan Nutrition Bar (56.8 g)	230	17 g	7 g (3 g)	0	230 mg	25%	50%	50%	50%
Kashi GoLean (78 g)	280	13 g	5 g (4 g)	6 g	85 mg	10%	8%	0	0
MetRx (30 g)	110	6 g	1.5 g (0.5 g)	0	35 mg	10%	2%	100%	100%
PowerBar (65 g)	230	10 g	2.5 g (0.5 g)	3 g	90 mg	30%	35%	100%	100%
PowerBar Essentials (53 g)	180	10 g	4 g (2 g)	3 g	100 mg	50%	25%	50%	100%
PowerBar Harvest (65 g)	240	7 g	4 g (0.5 g)	4 g	80 mg	15%	15%	50%	100%
PowerBar Protein Plus (78 g)	290	24 g	5 g (3 g)	1 g	140 mg	40%	35%	100%	100%
Think! (57 g)	223	10 g	9 g (2 g)	1 g	174 mg	20%	10%	0%	5%
TigerSport (65 g)	230	10 g	2 g (0.5 g)	3 g	90 mg	30%	35%	100%	100%
Tigers Milk (35 g)	140	4 g	3 g (1.5 g)	2 g	35 mg	50%	30%	100%	25%
Worldwide Sport Nutrition Bar (78 g)	290	34 g	5 g (3 g)	<1 g	35 mg	50%	50%	50%	50%
Zone Perfect (50 g)	210	14 g	7 g (4 g)	1 g	320 mg	6%	0	40%	200%

Appendix Q

Table Q–1.
Common Fast-Food Meals Chosen by Young Children
Meal 1

Meal components	Calories	Protein (g)	Fat (g)	% calories from fat	Sodium (mg)	Calcium (mg)
Cheeseburger	~300	15	13	39%	820	20
Small French fries	~210	3	10	43%	135	10
Soda (12 oz)	~150	—	—	—	35	—
TOTAL MEAL	~660	18	23	32%	990	30

Meal 2

Meal components	Calories	Protein (g)	Fat (g)	% calories from fat	Sodium (mg)	Calcium (mg)
Chicken nuggets	~290	19	~16	~50%	520	13
Small French Fries	~210	3	10	43%	135	10
Soda (12 oz)	~150	—	—	—	35	—
TOTAL MEAL	~650	22	26	36%	690	23

Better Option for Fast-Food Meal for Young Children
Meal 3

Meal components	Calories	Protein (g)	Fat (g)	% calories from fat	Sodium (mg)	Calcium (mg)
1 pizza slice (thin crust medium cheese pizza)	~200	11	8	38%	435	145
Garden salad	35	—	—	—	—	4
Lite vinaigrette dressing (1 oz)	~30	~1	~1	—	150	6
Diet soda (12 oz)	—	—	—	—	35	—
TOTAL MEAL	265	12	9	31%	620	155

Table Q–2.
Common Fast-Food Meals Chosen by Adolescents
Meal 1

Meal components	Calories	Protein (g)	Fat (g)	% calories from fat	Sodium (mg)	Calcium (mg)
Whopper with cheese	730	33	46	57%	1190	250
Medium French fries	370	5	20	49%	238	—
Soda (16 oz)	~200	—	—	—	47	—
TOTAL MEAL	1300	38	66	46%	1475	250

Meal 2

Meal components	Calories	Protein (g)	Fat (g)	% calories from fat	Sodium (mg)	Calcium (mg)
Grilled chicken sandwich with mayonnaise	440	27	20	41%	1040	6
Medium French fries	370	5	20	49%	~240	—
Soda (16 oz)	~200	—	—	—	47	—
TOTAL MEAL	1010	32	40	36%	1327	6

<u>Better Option for Fast-Food Meal Adolescents</u>

Meal 3

Meal components	Calories	Protein (g)	Fat (g)	% calories from fat	Sodium (mg)	Calcium (mg)
2 pizza slice (thin crust medium cheese pizza)	~400	22	16	38%	870	290
Garden salad	35	—	—	—	—	4
Fat-free vinaigrette dressing (59 mL)	50	—	—	—	330	—
Diet soda (16 oz)	—	—	—	—	47	—
TOTAL MEAL	485	22	16	~30%	1247	294

Appendix R

Nomogram for estimation of children's body surface area from height and body mass*

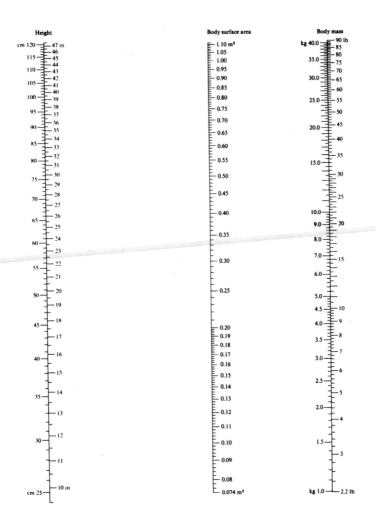

*From the formula of Du Bois and Du Bois. *Arch Intern Med.* 1916;17:863. $S = M^{0.425} \times H^{0.725} \times 71.84$; $\log S = \log M \times 0.425 + \log H \times 0.725 = 1.8564$ [S: body surface area (in cm^2); M: body (mass in kg); H: height (in cm)].

Figure R–1. Body surface area of children. (From Lentner C, ed. *Geigy Scientific Tables.* 8th ed. vol. 5. Basel, Switzerland: Ciba-Geigy; 1990:105–106.)

Nomogram for estimation of children's body surface area from height and body mass*

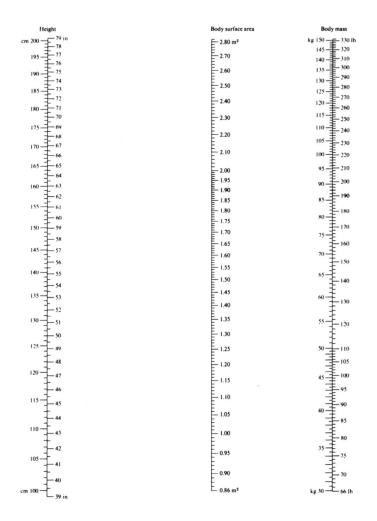

*From the formula of Du Bois and Du Bois. *Arch Intern Med.* 1916;17:863. $S = M^{0.425} \times H^{0.725} \times 71.84$; log S = log $M \times 0.425 + \log H \times 0.725 = 1.8564$ [S: body surface area (in cm^2); M: body (mass in kg); H: height (in cm)]

Figure R–2. Body surface area of children. (From Lentner C, ed. *Geigy Scientific Tables.* 8th ed. vol. 5. Basel, Switzerland: Ciba-Geigy; 1990:105–106.)

Appendix S

Table S–1.
Conversions From Conventional Units to Système International (SI) Units*

Component	System	Reference Range, Conventional Units	Conventional Units	Conversion Factor (Multiply by)	Reference Range, SI Units	SI Units
Acetaminophen (therapeutic)	Serum, plasma	10–30	μg/mL	6.62	70–200	μmol/L
Acetoacetic acid	Serum, plasma	<1	mg/dL	0.098	<0.1	mmol/L
Acetone	Serum, plasma	<2.0	mg/dL	0.172	<0.34	mmol/L
Acetylcholinesterase	Red blood cells	30–40	U/g of hemoglobin	0.0645	2.13–2.63	MU/mol of hemoglobin
Acid phosphatase (prostatic)	Serum	0.0–0.6	U/L	1.0	0.0–0.6	U/L
Activated partial thrombo-plastin time (APTT)	Whole blood	25–40	s	1.0	25–40	s
Adenosine deaminase	Serum	11.5–25.0	U/L	1.0	11.5–25.0	U/L
Adrenocorticotropic hormone (ACTH) (see Corticotropin)	Plasma					
Alanine	Serum	1.87–5.89	mg/dL	112.2	210–661	μmol/L
Alanine amino-transferase (ALT, previously SGPT)	Serum	10–40	U/L	1.0	10–40	U/L
Albumin	Serum	3.5–5.0	g/dL	10	35–50	g/L
Alcohol (see Ethanol, Isopropanol, Methanol)						

Table S–1.
Conversions From Conventional Units to Système International (SI) Units*, _continued_

Component	System	Reference Range, Conventional Units	Conventional Units	Conversion Factor (Multiply by)	Reference Range, SI Units	SI Units
Alcohol dehydrogenase	Serum	<2.8	U/L	1.0	<2.8	U/L
Aldolase	Serum	1.0–7.5	U/L	1.0	1.0–7.5	U/L
Aldosterone	Serum, plasma	7–30	ng/dL	0.0277	0.19–0.83	nmol/L
	Urine	3–20	μg/24 h	2.77	8–55	nmol/d
Alkaline phosphatase	Serum	50–120	U/L	1.0	50–120	U/L
Alprazolam (therapeutic)	Serum, plasma	10–50	ng/mL	3.24	32–162	nmol/L
Aluminum	Serum	0–6	ng/mL	0.0371	0.00–0.22	nmol/L
Amikacin (therapeutic) (peak)	Serum, plasma	20–30	μg/mL	1.71	34–52	μmol/L
Aminobutyric acid (α-aminobutyric acid)	Plasma	0.08–0.36	mg/dL	97	8–35	μmol/L
Amiodarone (therapeutic)	Serum, plasma	0.5–2.5	μg/mL	1.55	0.8–3.9	μmol/L
Aminolevulinic acid (δ-aminolevulinic acid)	Urine	1.0–7.0	mg/24 h	7.626	8–53	μmol/L
Amitriptyline (therapeutic)	Serum, plasma	80–250	ng/mL	3.61	289–903	nmol/L
Ammonia (as NH_3)	Plasma	15–45	μg/dL	0.714	11–32	μmol/L
Amobarbital (therapeutic)	Serum	1–5	μg/mL	4.42	4–22	μmol/L
Amoxapine (therapeutic)	Plasma	200–600	ng/mL	1.0	200–600	μg/L

Table S–1.
Conversions From Conventional Units to Système International (SI) Units*, _continued_

Component	System	Reference Range, Conventional Units	Conventional Units	Conversion Factor (Multiply by)	Reference Range, SI Units	SI Units
Amylase	Serum	25–85	U/L	1.0	25–85	U/L
Androstenedione						
Adult male	Serum	75–205	ng/dL	0.0349	2.6–7.2	nmol/L
Adult female	Serum	85–275	ng/dL	0.0349	3.0–9.6	nmol/L
Angiotensin I	Plasma	<25	pg/mL	1.0	<25	ng/L
Angiotensin II	Plasma	10–60	pg/mL	1.0	10–60	ng/L
Angiotensin-converting enzyme (ACE)	Serum	8–52	U/L	1.0	8–52	U/L
Anion gap Na+–(C1−=HCO$_3$−)	Serum, plasma	8–16	mEq/L	1.0	8–16	nmol/L
Antidiuretic hormone (ADH, vasopressin) (varies with osmolality) 285–290 mOsm/kg	Plasma	1–5	pg/mL	0.926	0.9–4.6	pmol/L
Antithrombin III	Plasma	21–30	mg/dL	10	210–300	mg/L
α1-Antitrypsin	Serum	126–226	mg/dL	0.01	1.26–2.26	g/L
Apolipoprotein A						
Male	Serum	80–151	mg/dL	0.01	0.8–1.5	g/L
Female	Serum	80–170	mg/dL	0.01	0.8–1.7	g/L
Apolipoprotein B						
Adult male	Serum, plasma	50–123	mg/dL	0.01	0.5–1.2	g/L
Adult female	Serum, plasma	25–120	mg/dL	0.01	0.25–1.20	g/L
Arginine	Plasma	0.37–2.40	mg/dL	57.4	21–138	μmol/L

Table S–1.
Conversions From Conventional Units to Système International (SI) Units*, *continued*

Component	System	Reference Range, Conventional Units	Conventional Units	Conversion Factor (Multiply by)	Reference Range, SI Units	SI Units
Arsenic (As)	Whole blood	<23	μg/L	0.0133	<0.31	μmol/L
Acute poisoning	Whole blood	600–9300	μg/L	0.0133	7.98–123.7	μmol/L
Ascorbate, ascorbic acid (see Vitamin C)						
Asparagine	Plasma	0.40–0.91	mg/dL	75.7	30–69	μmol/L
Aspartate amino transferase (AST, previously SGOT)	Serum	20–48	U/L	1.0	20–48	U/L
Aspartic acid	Plasma	<0.3	mg/dL	75.1	<25	μmol/L
Atrial natriuretic hormone	Plasma	20–77	pg/mL	1.0	20–77	ng/L
Bands (see White blood cell count)						
Barbiturates (see Pentobarbital, Phenobarbital, Thiopental)						
Basophils (see White blood cell count)						
Benzodiazepines (see Alprazolam, Chlordiazepoxide, Diazepam, Lorazepam)						

Table S–1.
Conversions From Conventional Units to Système International (SI) Units*, continued

Component	System	Reference Range, Conventional Units	Conventional Units	Conversion Factor (Multiply by)	Reference Range, SI Units	SI Units
Bicarbonate	Plasma	21–28	mEq/L	1.0	21–28	mmol/L
Bile acids (total)	Serum	0.3–2.3	µg/mL	2.448	0.73–5.63	µmol/L
Bilirubin						
Total	Serum	0.3–1.2	mg/dL	17.1	5–21	µmol/L
Direct (conjugated)	Serum	<0.2	mg/dL	17.1	<3.4	µmol/L
Biotin	Whole blood, serum	200–500	pg/mL	0.0041	0.82–2.05	nmol/L
Bismuth	Whole blood	1–12	µg/L	4.785	4.8–57.4	nmol/L
Blood gases						
Pco_2	Arterial blood	35–45	mm Hg	1.0	35–45	mm Hg
pH	Arterial blood	7.35–7.45	...	1.0	7.35–7.45	...
Po_2	Arterial blood	80–100	mm Hg	1.0	80–100	mm Hg
Bromide	Serum	<5	mg/dL	0.125	<0.63	mmol/L
C1 esterase inhibitor	Serum	12–30	mg/dL	0.01	0.12–0.30	g/L
C3 complement	Serum	1200–1500	µg/mL	0.001	1.2–1.5	g/L
C4 complement	Serum	350–600	µg/mL	0.001	0.35–0.60	g/L
Cadmium (nonsmoker)	Whole blood	0.3–1.2	µg/L	8.897	2.7–10.7	nmol/L
Calcitonin	Serum, plasma	<19	pg/mL	1.0	<19	ng/L
Calcium						
Ionized	Serum	4.60–5.08	mg/dL	0.25	1.15–1.27	mmol/L
	Serum	2.30–2.54	mEq/L	0.50	1.15–1.27	mmol/L

Table S–1.
Conversions From Conventional Units to Système International (SI) Units*, *continued*

Component	System	Reference Range, Conventional Units	Conventional Units	Conversion Factor (Multiply by)	Reference Range, SI Units	SI Units
Calcium, continued						
Total	Serum	8.2–10.2	mg/dL	0.25	2.05–2.55	mmol/L
Normal diet	Urine	<250	mg/24 h	0.025	<6.2	mmol/d
Carbamazepine (therapeutic)	Serum, plasma	8–12	µg/mL	4.23	34–51	µmol/L
Carbon dioxide	Serum, plasma, venous blood	22–28	mEq/L	1.0	22–28	mmol/L
Carboxyhemoglobin (carbon monoxide) (as proportion of hemoglobin saturation)						
Nonsmoker	Whole blood	<2.0	%	0.01	<0.02	Proportion of 1.0
Toxic	Whole blood	>20	%	0.01	>0.2	Proportion of 1.0
Carcinoembryonic antigen (CEA)	Serum	<3.0	ng/mL	1.0	<3.0	µg/L
β-Carotene	Serum	10–85	µg/dL	0.0186	0.2–1.6	µmol/L
Ceruloplasmin	Serum	20–40	mg/dL	10	200–400	mg/L
Chloramphenicol (therapeutic)	Serum	10–25	µg/mL	3.1	31–77	µmol/L
Chlordiazepoxide (therapeutic)	Serum, plasma	0.7–1.0	µg/mL	3.34	2.3–3.3	µmol/L
Chloride	Serum, plasma	96–106	mEq/L	1.0	96–106	mmol/L
	CSF	118–132	mEq/L	1.0	118–132	mmol/L

Table S–1.
Conversions From Conventional Units to Système International (SI) Units*, _continued_

Component	System	Reference Range, Conventional Units	Conventional Units	Conversion Factor (Multiply by)	Reference Range, SI Units	SI Units
Chlorpromazine (therapeutic)	Plasma	50–300	ng/mL	3.14	157–942	nmol/L
Chlorpropamide (therapeutic)	Plasma	75–250	mg/L	3.61	270–900	μmol/L
Cholecalciferol (see Vitamin D)						
Cholesterol (total)						
Desirable	Serum	<200	mg/dL	0.02586	<5.17	mmol/L
Borderline high	Serum	200–239	mg/dL	0.02586	5.17–6.18	mmol/L
High	Serum	≥240	mg/dL	0.02586	≥6.21	mmol/L
Cholesterol, high-density lipoproteins (HDL) (see High-density lipoprotein cholesterol)						
Cholesterol, low-density lipoproteins (LDL) (see Low-density lipoprotein cholesterol)						
Cholesterol esters (as plasma fraction of total cholesterol)	Plasma	60–75	%	0.01	0.60–0.75	Proportion of 1.0
Chromium	Whole blood	0.7–28.0	μg/L	19.2	13.4–538.6	nmol/L

Table S–1.
Conversions From Conventional Units to Système International (SI) Units*, continued

Component	System	Reference Range, Conventional Units	Conventional Units	Conversion Factor (Multiply by)	Reference Range, SI Units	SI Units
Citrate	Serum	1.2–3.0	mg/dL	52.05	60–160	μmol/L
Citrulline	Plasma	0.2–1.0	mg/dL	57.1	12–55	μmol/L
Clonazepam (therapeutic)	Serum	10–50	ng/mL	3.17	32–158	nmol/L
Coagulation factor I (fibrinogen)	Plasma	0.15–0.35	g/dL	29.41	4.4–10.3	μmol/L
	Plasma	150–350	mg/dL	0.01	1.5–3.5	g/L
Coagulation factor II (prothrombin)	Plasma	70–130	%	0.01	0.70–1.30	Proportion of 1.0
Coagulation factor V	Plasma	70–130	%	0.01	0.70–1.30	Proportion of 1.0
Coagulation factor VII	Plasma	60–140	%	0.01	0.60–1.40	Proportion of 1.0
Coagulation factor VIII	Plasma	50–200	%	0.01	0.50–2.00	Proportion of 1.0
Coagulation factor IX	Plasma	70–130	%	0.01	0.70–1.30	Proportion of 1.0
Coagulation factor X	Plasma	70–130	%	0.01	0.70–1.30	Proportion of 1.0
Coagulation factor XI	Plasma	70–130	%	0.01	0.70–1.30	Proportion of 1.0
Coagulation factor XII	Plasma	70–130	%	0.01	0.70–1.30	Proportion of 1.0
Cobalt	Serum	4.0–10.0	μg/L	16.97	67.9–169.7	nmol/L
Cocaine (toxic)	Serum	>1000	ng/mL	3.3	>3300	nmol/L
Codeine (therapeutic)	Serum	10–100	ng/mL	3.34	33–334	nmol/L
Copper	Serum	70–140	μg/dL	0.1574	11.0–22.0	μmol/L
Coproporphyrin	Urine	<200	μg/24 h	1.527	<300	nmol/d
Corticotropin	Plasma	<120	pg/mL	0.22	<26	pmol/L
Cortisol	Plasma	5–25	μg/dL	27.59	140–690	nmol/L
	Urine	30–100	μg/24 h	2.759	80–280	nmol/d

Table S–1.
Conversions From Conventional Units to Système International (SI) Units*, *continued*

Component	System	Reference Range, Conventional Units	Conventional Units	Conversion Factor (Multiply by)	Reference Range, SI Units	SI Units
Cotinine (smoker)	Plasma	16–145	ng/mL	5.68	91–823	nmol/L
C peptide	Serum	0.5–2.5	ng/mL	0.333	0.17–0.83	nmol/L
Creatine	Serum	0.1–0.4	mg/dL	76.25	8–31	μmol/L
Creatine Kinase (CK)	Serum	50–200	U/L	1.0	50–200	U/L
Creatine kinase-MB fraction (isoenzymes; proportion of total CK)	Serum Serum	<6 <10	% U/L	0.01 1.0	<0.06 <10	Proportion of 1.0 U/L
Creatine	Serum, plasma	0.6–1.2	mg/dL	88.4	53–106	μmol/L
	Urine	1–2	g/24 h	8.8	8.8–17.7	mmol/d
Creatinine clearance	Serum, urine	75–125	mL/min	0.01667	1.24–2.08	mL/s
Cyanide (toxic)	Whole blood	>1.0	μg/mL	38.4	>38.4	μmol/L
Cyanocobalamin (see Vitamin B_{12})						
Cyclic adenosine monophosphate (cAMP)	Plasma	4.6–8.6	ng/mL	3.04	14–26	nmol/L
Cystine	Plasma	0.40–1.40	mg/dL	83.3	33–117	μmol/L
Dehydroepiandrosterone (DHEA) (unconjugated, adult male)	Plasma, serum	180–1250	ng/dL	3.47	6.2–43.3	nmol/L

Table S–1.
Conversions From Conventional Units to Système International (SI) Units*, *continued*

Component	System	Reference Range, Conventional Units	Conventional Units	Conversion Factor (Multiply by)	Reference Range, SI Units	SI Units
Dehydroepiandro-sterone sulfate (DHEA-S) (adult male)	Plasma, serum	50–450	μg/dL	0.027	1.6–12.2	μmol/L
Desipramine (therapeutic)	Plasma, serum	50–200	ng/mL	3.75	170–700	nmol/L
Diazepam (therapeutic)	Plasma, serum	100–1000	ng/mL	0.00351	0.35–3.51	μmol/L
Digoxin (therapeutic)	Plasma	0.5–2.0	ng/mL	1.281	0.6–2.6	nmol/L
Disopyramide (therapeutic)	Plasma, serum	2.8–7.0	mg/L	2.95	8–21	μmol/L
Doxepin (therapeutic)	Plasma, serum	150–250	ng/mL	3.58	540–890	nmol/L
Electrophoresis (protein) Proportion of total protein						
Albumin	Serum	52–65	%	0.01	0.52–0.65	Proportion of 1.0
α₁-Globulin	Serum	2.5–5.0	%	0.01	0.025–0.05	Proportion of 1.0
α₂-Globulin	Serum	7.0–13.0	%	0.01	0.07–0.13	Proportion of 1.0
β-Globulin	Serum	8.0–14.0	%	0.01	0.08–0.14	Proportion of 1.0
γ-Globulin	Serum	12.0–22.0	%	0.01	0.12–0.22	Proportion of 1.0
Concentration						
Albumin	Serum	3.2–5.6	g/dL	10.0	32–56	g/L
α₁-Globulin	Serum	0.1–0.4	g/dL	10.0	1–10	g/L

Table S-1.
Conversions From Conventional Units to Système International (SI) Units*, *continued*

Component	System	Reference Range, Conventional Units	Conventional Units	Conversion Factor (Multiply by)	Reference Range, SI Units	SI Units
Electrophoresis, Concentration, *continued*						
α_2-Globulin	Serum	0.4–1.2	g/dL	10.0	4–12	g/L
β-Globulin	Serum	0.5–1.1	g/dL	10.0	5–11	g/L
γ-Globulin	Serum	0.5–1.6	g/dL	10.0	5–16	g/L
Eosinophils (see White blood cell count)						
Epinephrine	Plasma	<60	pg/mL	5.46	<330	pmol/L
	Urine	<20	μg/24 h	5.46	<109	nmol/d
Erythrocyte count (see Red blood cell count)						
Erythrocyte sedimentation rate	Whole blood	0–20	mm/h	1.0	0–20	mm/h
Erythropoietin	Serum	5–36	mU/mL	1.0	5–36	IU/L
Estradiol (E_2, unconjugated) (varies with age and menstrual cycle)	Serum	30–400	pg/mL	3.67	110–1470	pmol/L
Estriol (E_3, unconjugated) (varies with length of gestation)	Serum	5–40	ng/mL	3.47	17.4–138.8	nmol/L
Estrogens (total)	Serum	60–400	pg/mL	1.0	60–400	ng/L

Table S–1.
Conversions From Conventional Units to Système International (SI) Units*, *continued*

Component	System	Reference Range, Conventional Units	Conventional Units	Conversion Factor (Multiply by)	Reference Range, SI Units	SI Units
Estrone (E₁) (varies with day of menstrual cycle)	Plasma, serum	1.5–25.0	ng/dL	37	55–925	pmol/L
Ethanol (ethyl alcohol)	Serum, whole blood	<100	mg/dL	0.2171	<21.7	mmol/L
Ethchlorvynol (toxic)	Plasma, serum	>20	μg/mL	6.92	>138	μmol/L
Ethylene glycol (toxic)	Plasma, serum	>30	mg/dL	0.1611	>5	mmol/L
Fatty acids (nonesterified)	Plasma	300–480	μEq/L	1.00	300–480	μmol/L
Fecal fat (as stearic acid)	Stool	2.0–6.0	g/d	1.0	2–6	g/d
Ferritin	Plasma	15–200	ng/mL	1.0	15–200	μg/L
α₁-Fetoprotein	Serum	<10	ng/mL	1.0	<10	μg/L
Fibrinogen (see Coagulation factor I)	Plasma	0.15–0.35	g/dL	29.41	4.4–10.3	μmol/L
Fibrin breakdown products (fibrin split products)	Serum	<10	μg/mL	1.0	<10	mg/L
Fluoride	Whole blood	<0.05	mg/dL	0.5263	<0.027	mmol/L
Folate (folic acid)	Red blood cells	166–640	ng/mL	2.266	376–1450	nmol/L
	Serum	5–25	ng/mL	2.266	11–57	nmol/L

Table S–1.
Conversions From Conventional Units to Système International (SI) Units*, continued

Component	System	Reference Range, Conventional Units	Conventional Units	Conversion Factor (Multiply by)	Reference Range, SI Units	SI Units
Follicle-stimulating hormone (FSH) (follitropin)	Serum	1–100	mIU/mL	1.0	1–100	IU/L
	Urine	5–30	IU/24 h	1.0	5–30	IU/d
Fructosamine	Serum	1.5–2.7	mmol/L	1.0	1.5–2.7	mmol/L
Fructose	Serum	1–6	mg/dL	55.5	55.5–333	μmol/L
Galactose	Plasma, serum	<20	mg/dL	0.0555	<1.10	mmol/L
Gastrin (fasting)	Serum	<100	pg/mL	0.477	47.7	pmol/L
Gentamicin (therapeutic)	Serum	6–10	μg/mL	2.1	12–21	μmol/L
Glucagon	Plasma	20–100	pg/mL	1.0	20–100	ng/L
Glucose	Serum, plasma	70–110	mg/dL	0.05551	3.9–6.1	mmol/L
	CSF	50–80	mg/dL	0.05551	2.8–4.4	mmol/L
Glucose 6 phosphate dehydrogenase	Red blood cells	10–14	U/g of hemoglobin	0.0645	0.65–0.90	MU/mol of hemoglobin
Glutamic acid	Plasma	0.2–2.8	mg/dL	67.97	15–190	μmol/L
Glutamine	Plasma	6.1–10.2	mg/dL	68.42	420–700	μmol/L
γ-Glutamyltransferase (GGT; γ-glutamyl transpeptidase)	Serum	0–30	U/L	1.0	0–30	U/L
Glutethimide (therapeutic)	Plasma, serum	<6	μg/mL	4.60	<28	μmol/L
Glycerol (free)	Serum	<1.5	mg/dL	0.1086	<0.16	mmol/L
Glycine	Plasma	0.9–4.2	mg/dL	133.3	120–560	μmol/L

Table S–1.
Conversions From Conventional Units to Système International (SI) Units*, *continued*

Component	System	Reference Range, Conventional Units	Conventional Units	Conversion Factor (Multiply by)	Reference Range, SI Units	SI Units
Glycosylated hemoglobin (glycated hemoglobin; hemoglobin A_1, A_{1c})	Whole blood	4–7	% of total hemoglobin	0.01	0.04–0.07	Proportion of total hemoglobin
Gold (therapeutic)	Serum	100–200	µg/dL	0.05077	5.1–10.2	µmol/L
Growth hormone (GH, somatotropin)	Plasma, serum	<20	ng/mL	44	<880	pmol/L
Haloperidol (therapeutic)	Serum, plasma	5–20	ng/mL	2.6	13–52	nmol/L
Haptoglobin	Serum	40–180	mg/dL	0.01	0.4–1.8	g/L
Hematocrit						
Adult male	Whole blood	41–50	%	0.01	0.41–0.50	Proportion of 1.0
Adult female	Whole blood	35–45	%	01	0.35–0.45	Proportion of 1.0
Hemoglobin						
Mass concentration						
Adult male	Whole blood	14.0–17.5	g/dL	10.0	140–175	g/L
Adult female	Whole blood	12.0–15.0	g/dL	10.0	120–150	g/L
Substance concentration (Hb [Fe])						
Adult male	Whole blood	13.6–17.2	g/dL	0.6206	8.44–10.65	mmol/L
Adult female	Whole blood	12.0–15.0	g/dL	0.6206	7.45–9.30	mmol/L

Table S-1.
Conversions From Conventional Units to Système International (SI) Units*, *continued*

Component	System	Reference Range, Conventional Units	Conventional Units	Conversion Factor (Multiply by)	Reference Range, SI Units	SI Units
Hemoglobin, continued						
Mean corpuscular hemoglobin (MCH)						
Mass concentration	Red blood cells	27–33	pg	1.0	27–33	pg
Substance concentration (Hb [Fe])	Red blood cells	27–33	pg	0.06206	1.70–2.05	fmol
Mean corpuscular hemoglobin concentration (MCHC)						
Mass concentration	Red blood cells	33–37	g/dL	10	330–370	g/L
Hemoglobin A$_{1c}$ (see Glycosylated hemoglobin)						
Hemoglobin A$_2$	Whole blood	2.0–3.0	%	0.01	0.02–0.03	Proportion of 1.0
High-density lipoprotein cholesterol (HDL-C)						
Male	Plasma	35–65	mg/dL	0.02586	0.91–1.68	mmol/L
Female	Plasma	35–80	mg/dL	0.02586	0.91–2.07	mmol/L
Histidine	Plasma	0.5–1.7	mg/dL	64.5	32–110	μmol/L
Homocysteine (total)	Plasma, serum	5–15	μmol/L	1.0	5–15	μmol/L
Homovanillic acid	Urine	<8	mg/24 h	5.489	<45	μmol/d

Table S–1.
Conversions From Conventional Units to Système International (SI) Units*, *continued*

Component	System	Reference Range, Conventional Units	Conventional Units	Conversion Factor (Multiply by)	Reference Range, SI Units	SI Units
Human chorionic gonadotropin (HCG) (adult female, not pregnant)	Serum	<3	mIU/mL	1.0	<3	IU/L
Hydroxybutyric acid (as β-hydroxybutyric acid)	Serum	0.21–2.81	mg/dL	96.05	20–270	μmol/L
5-Hydroxyindoleacetic acid (5-HIAA)	Urine	<25	mg/24 h	5.23	<131	μmol/d
17 α-Hydroxy-progesterone (adult female)	Serum	20–300	ng/dL	0.03	0.6–9.0	nmol/L
Hydroxyproline	Plasma	<0.55	mg/dL	76.3	<42	μmol/L
Imipramine (therapeutic)	Plasma	150–250	ng/mL	3.57	536–893	nmol/L
Immunoglobin A (IgA)	Serum	113–563	mg/dL	0.01	1.1–5.6	g/L
Immunoglobin D (IgD)	Serum	0.5–3.0	mg/dL	10	5–30	mg/L
Immunoglobin E (IgE)	Serum	0.01–0.04	mg/dL	10	0.1–0.4	mg/L
Immunoglobin G (IgG)	Serum	800–1800	mg/dL	0.01	8.0–18.0	g/L
Immunoglobin M (IgM)	Serum	54–222	mg/dL	0.01	0.5–2.2	g/L
Insulin	Plasma	11–240	μU/mL	7.175	79–1722	pmol/L
Insulin C peptide (see C peptide)						

Table S–1.
Conversions From Conventional Units to Système International (SI) Units*, *continued*

Component	System	Reference Range, Conventional Units	Conventional Units	Conversion Factor (Multiply by)	Reference Range, SI Units	SI Units
Insulinlike growth factor	Plasma	130–450	ng/mL	1.0	130–450	ng/mL
Ionized calcium (see Calcium)						
Iron (total)	Serum	60–150	μg/dL	0.179	10.7–26.9	μmol/L
Iron binding capacity	Serum	250–400	μg/dL	0.179	44.8–71.6	μmol/L
Isoleucine	Plasma	0.5–1.3	mg/dL	76.24	40–100	μmol/L
Isoniazid (therapeutic)	Plasma	1–7	μg/mL	7.29	7–51	μmol/L
Isopropanol (toxic)	Plasma, serum	>400	mg/L	0.0166	>6.64	mmol/L
Lactate (lactic acid)	Arterial blood	3–7	mg/dL	0.1110	0.3–0.8	mmol/L
	Venous blood	4.5–19.8	mg/dL	0.1110	0.5–2.2	mmol/L
Lactate dehydrogenase (LDH)	Serum	50–200	U/L	1.0	50–200	U/L
Lactate dehydrogenase isoenzymes						
LD$_1$	Serum	17–27	%	0.01	0.17–0.27	Proportion of 1.0
LD$_2$	Serum	27–37	%	0.01	0.27–0.37	Proportion of 1.0
LD$_3$	Serum	18–25	%	0.01	0.18–0.25	Proportion of 1.0
LD$_4$	Serum	3–8	%	0.01	0.03–0.08	Proportion of 1.0
LD$_5$	Serum	0–5	%	0.01	0.00–0.05	Proportion of 1.0
Lead	Whole blood	<25	μg/dL	0.0483	<1.21	μmol/L
Leucine	Plasma	1.0–2.3	mg/dL	76.3	75–175	μmol/L

Table S–1.
Conversions From Conventional Units to Système International (SI) Units*, *continued*

Component	System	Reference Range, Conventional Units	Conventional Units	Conversion Factor (Multiply by)	Reference Range, SI Units	SI Units
Leukocyte count (see White blood cell count)						
Lidocaine (therapeutic)	Serum, plasma	1.5–6.0	µg/mL	4.27	6.4–25.6	µmol/L
Lipase	Serum	14–280	mIU/mL	1.0	14–280	U/L
Lipoprotein(a) [Lp(a)]	Serum, plasma	10–30	mg/dL	0.01	0.1–0.3	g/L
Lithium (therapeutic)	Serum	0.6–1.2	mEq/L	1.0	0.6–1.2	mmol/L
Lorazepam (therapeutic)	Serum, plasma	50–240	ng/mL	3.11	156–746	nmol/L
Low-density lipoprotein cholesterol (LDL-C)	Plasma	60–130	mg/dL	0.025–86	1.55–3.37	mmol/L
Luteinizing hormone (LH)	Serum	6–30	mIU/mL	1.0	6–30	IU/L
Lymphocytes (see White blood cell count)						
Lysine	Plasma	1.2–3.5	mg/dL	68.5	80–240	µmol/L
Lysozyme (muramidase)	Serum	4–13	mg/L	1.0	4–13	mg/L
Magnesium	Serum	1.5–2.5	mg/dL	0.4114	0.60–0.95	mmol/L
	Serum	1.3–2.1	mEq/L	0.50	0.65–1.05	mmol/L
Manganese	Whole blood	10–12	µg/L	18.2	182–218	nmol/L
Maprotiline (therapeutic)	Plasma	200–600	ng/mL	1.0	200–600	µg/L
Mean corpuscular hemoglobin (see Hemoglobin)						

Table S–1.
Conversions From Conventional Units to Système International (SI) Units*, *continued*

Component	System	Reference Range, Conventional Units	Conventional Units	Conversion Factor (Multiply by)	Reference Range, SI Units	SI Units
Mean corpuscular hemoglobin concentration (see Hemoglobin)						
Meperidine (therapeutic)	Serum, plasma	0.4–0.7	μg/mL	4.04	1.6–2.8	μmol/L
Meprobamate (therapeutic)	Serum	6–12	μg/mL	4.58	28–55	μmol/L
Mercury	Whole blood	0.6–59.0	μg/L	4.99	3.0–294.4	nmol/L
Metanephrines (total)	Urine	<1.0	mg/24 h	5.07	<5	μmol/d
Methadone (therapeutic)	Serum, plasma	100–400	ng/mL	0.00323	0.32–1.29	μmol/L
Methanol	Whole blood, serum	<1.5	mg/L	0.0312	<0.05	mmol/L
Methaqualone (therapeutic)	Serum, plasma	2–3	μg/mL	4.00	8–12	μmol/L
Methemoglobin	Whole blood	<0.24	g/dL	155	<37.2	μmol/L
	Whole blood	<1.0	% of total hemoglobin	0.01	<0.01	Proportion of total hemoglobin
Methionine	Plasma	0.1–0.6	mg/dL	67.1	6–40	μmol/L
Methsuximide (therapeutic)	Serum	10–40	μg/mL	5.29	53–212	μmol/L
Methyldopa (therapeutic)	Serum, plasma	1–5	μg/mL	4.73	5–24	μmol/L

Table S–1.
Conversions From Conventional Units to Système International (SI) Units*, *continued*

Component	System	Reference Range, Conventional Units	Conventional Units	Conversion Factor (Multiply by)	Reference Range, SI Units	SI Units
Metoprolol (therapeutic)	Serum, plasma	75–200	ng/mL	3.74	281–748	nmol/L
β₂-Microglobulin	Serum	<2	μg/mL	85	<170	nmol/L
Morphine	Serum, plasma	10–80	ng/mL	3.50	35–280	nmol/L
Muramidase (see Lysozyme)						
Myoglobin	Serum	5–70	μg/L	1.0	5–70	μg/L
Niacin (nicotinic acid)	Urine	2.4–6.4	mg/24 h	7.30	17.5–46.7	μmol/d
Nickel	Whole blood	1.0–28.0	μg/L	17	17–476	nmol/L
Nicotine (smoker)	Plasma	0.01–0.05	mg/L	6.16	0.062–0.308	μmol/L
Nitrogen (nonprotein)	Serum	20–35	mg/dL	0.714	14.3–25.0	mmol/L
Norepinephrine	Plasma	110–410	pg/mL	5.91	650–2423	nmol/L
	Urine	15–80	μg/24 h	5.91	89–473	nmol/d
Nortriptyline (therapeutic)	Serum, plasma	50–150	ng/mL	3.80	190–570	nmol/L
Ornithine	Plasma	0.4–1.4	mg/dL	75.8	30–106	μmol/L
Osmolality	Serum	275–295	mOsm/kg H₂O	1.0	275–295	mmol/kg H₂O
	Urine	250–900	mOsm/kg H₂O	1.0	250–900	mmol/kg H₂O
Osteocalcin	Serum	3.0–13.0	ng/mL	1.0	3.0–13.0	μg/L
Oxalate	Serum	1.0–2.4	mg/L	11.4	11–27	μmol/L
Oxazepam (therapeutic)	Serum, plasma	0.2–1.4	μg/mL	3.49	0.7–4.9	μmol/L
Oxygen, partial pressure (Po₂)	Arterial blood	80–100	mm Hg	1.0	80–100	mm Hg

Table S–1.
Conversions From Conventional Units to Système International (SI) Units*, continued

Component	System	Reference Range, Conventional Units	Conventional Units	Conversion Factor (Multiply by)	Reference Range, SI Units	SI Units
Pantothenic acid (see Vitamin B$_3$)						
Parathyroid hormone						
Intact	Serum	10–50	pg/mL	0.1053	1.1–5.3	pmol/L
N-terminal specific	Serum	8–24	pg/mL	0.1053	0.8–2.5	pmol/L
C-terminal (mid-molecule)	Serum	0–340	pg/mL	0.1053	0–35.8	pmol/L
Pentobarbital (therapeutic)	Serum, plasma	1–5	μg/mL	4.42	4.0–22	μmol/L
Pepsinogen I pH (see Blood gases)	Serum	28–100	ng/mL	1.0	28–100	μg/L
Phenobarbital (therapeutic)	Serum, plasma	15–40	μg/mL	4.31	65–172	μmol/L
Phenylalanine	Plasma	0.6–1.5	mg/dL	60.5	35–90	μmol/L
Phenytoin (therapeutic)	Serum, plasma	10–20	μg/mL	3.96	40–79	μmol/L
Phosphorus (inorganic)	Serum	2.3–4.7	mg/dL	0.3229	0.74–1.52	mmol/L
	Urine	0.9–1.3	g/24 h	32.29	29–42	mmol/L
Phospholipid phosphorus (total)	Serum	8.0–11.0	mg/dL	0.3229	2.58–3.55	mmol/L
Placental lactogen (5- to 38-wk gestation)	Serum	0.5–11	μg/mL	46.30	23–509	nmol/L
Plasminogen	Plasma	20	mg/dL	10	200	mg/L
	Plasma	80–120	%	0.01	0.80–1.20	Proportion of 1.0

Table S-1.
Conversions From Conventional Units to Système International (SI) Units*, *continued*

Component	System	Reference Range, Conventional Units	Conventional Units	Conversion Factor (Multiply by)	Reference Range, SI Units	SI Units
Plasminogen activator inhibitor	Plasma	<15	IU/mL	1.0	15	IU/L
Platelet count (thrombocytes)	Whole blood	150–450	x10³/μL	10⁶	150–450	x10⁹/L
Porphobilinogen deaminase	Red blood cells	>7.0	nmol/s/L	1.0	>7.0	nmol · s⁻¹ · L⁻
Porphyrins (total)	Urine	<320	nmol/L	1.0	<320	nmol/L
Potassium	Plasma	3.5–5.0	mEq/L	1.0	3.5–5.0	mmol/L
Pregnanediol	Urine	<2.6	mg/24 h	3.12	<8	μmol/d
Pregnanetriol	Urine	<2.5	mg/24 h	2.97	<7.5	μmol/d
Primidone (therapeutic)	Plasma	5–12	μg/mL	4.58	23–55	μmol/L
Procainamide (therapeutic)	Serum, plasma	4–10	μg/mL	4.23	17–42	μmol/L
Progesterone (first trimester)	Serum	>1000	ng/dL	0.0318	>32	nmol/L
Prolactin (nonlactating subject)	Serum	1–25	ng/mL	1.0	1–25	μg/L
Proline	Plasma	1.2–3.9	mg/dL	86.9	104–340	μmol/L
Propoxyphene (therapeutic)	Serum	0.1–0.4	μg/mL	2.946	0.3–1.2	μmol/L
Propanolol (therapeutic)	Serum	50–100	ng/mL	3.86	190–390	nmol/L
Prostate-specific antigen	Serum	<4.0	ng/mL	1.0	<4.0	ng/mL

Table S-1.
Conversions From Conventional Units to Système International (SI) Units*, *continued*

Component	System	Reference Range, Conventional Units	Conventional Units	Conversion Factor (Multiply by)	Reference Range, SI Units	SI Units
Prostatic acid phosphatase (see Acid phosphatase)						
Protein (total)	Serum	6.0–8.0	g/dL	10.0	60–80	g/L
Prothrombin time (PT)	Plasma	10–13	s	1.0	10–13	s
Protoporphyrin	Red blood cells	15–50	mg/dL	0.0177	0.27–0.89	μmol/L
Pyridoxine (see Vitamin B_6)						
Pyruvate (as pyruvic acid)	Whole blood	0.3–0.9	mg/dL	113.6	34–102	μmol/L
Quinidine (therapeutic)	Serum	2.0–5.0	μg/mL	3.08	6.2–15.4	μmol/L
Red blood cell count						
Female	Whole blood	3.9–5.5	$\times10^6/\mu$L	$\times10^6$	3.9–5.5	$\times10^{12}$/L
Male	Whole blood	4.6–6.0	$\times10^6/\mu$L	$\times10^6$	4.6–6.0	$\times10^{12}$/L
Red cell folate (see Folate)						
Renin	Plasma	1.0–6.0	ng/mL/h	.077	0.77–4.6	nmol • L^{-1} • h^{-1}
Reticulocyte count	Whole blood	25–75	$\times10^3/\mu$L	10^6	25–75	$\times10^9$/L
	Whole blood	0.5–1.5	% of red blood cells	0.01	0.005–0.015	Proportion of red blood cells
Retinol (see Vitamin A)						
Riboflavin (see Vitamin B_2)						
Salicylates (therapeutic)	Serum, plasma	15–30	mg/dL	0.07240	1.08–2.17	mmol/L

Table S–1.
Conversions From Conventional Units to Système International (SI) Units*, _continued_

Component	System	Reference Range, Conventional Units	Conventional Units	Conversion Factor (Multiply by)	Reference Range, SI Units	SI Units
Sedimentation rate (see Erythrocyte sedimentation rate)						
Selenium	Whole blood	58–234	μg/L	0.0127	0.74–2.97	μmol/L
Serine	Plasma	0.7–2.0	mg/dL	95.2	65–193	μmol/L
Serotonin (5-hydroxytryptamine)	Whole blood	50–200	ng/mL	0.00568	0.28–1.14	μmol/L
Sex hormone binding globulin	Serum	0.5–1.5	μg/dL	34.7	17.4–52.1	nmol/L
Sodium	Plasma	136–142	mEq/L	1.0	136–142	mmol/L
Somatostatin	Plasma	<25	pg/mL	1.0	<25	ng/L
Somatomedin C (see Insulinlike growth factor)						
Strychnine (toxic)	Whole blood	>0.5	mg/L	2.99	>1.5	μmol/L
Substance P	Plasma	<240	pg/mL	1.0	<240	ng/L
Sulfmethemoglobin	Whole blood	<1.0	% of total	0.01	<0.010	Proportion of total hemoglobin
Taurine	Plasma	0.3–2.1	mg/dL	80	24–168	μmol/L
Testosterone	Plasma, serum	300–1200	ng/dL	0.0347	10.4–41.6	nmol/L
Theophylline (therapeutic)	Plasma, serum	10–20	μg/mL	5.55	56–111	μmol/L

1093

Table S–1.
Conversions From Conventional Units to Système International (SI) Units*, *continued*

Component	System	Reference Range, Conventional Units	Conventional Units	Conversion Factor (Multiply by)	Reference Range, SI Units	SI Units
Thiamin(e) (see Vitamin B$_1$)						
Thiocyanate (nonsmoker)	Plasma, serum	1–4	mg/L	17.2	17–69	μmol/L
Thiopental (therapeutic)	Plasma, serum	1–5	μg/mL	4.13	4–21	μmol/L
Thioridazine (therapeutic)	Plasma, serum	1.0–1.5	μg/mL	2.70	2.7–4.1	μmol/L
Threonine	Plasma	0.9–2.5	mg/dL	84	75–210	μmol/L
Thrombocytes (see Platelet count)						
Thyroglobulin	Serum	3–42	ng/mL	1.0	3–42	μg/L
Thyrotropin (thyroid-stimulating hormone, TSH)	Serum	0.5–5.0	μIU/mL	1.0	0.5–5.0	μIU/L
Thyroxine						
Free (FT$_4$)	Serum	0.9–2.3	ng/dL	12.87	12–30	pmol/L
Total (T$_4$)	Serum	5.5–12.5	μg/dL	12.87	71–160	nmol/L
Thyroxine-binding globulin (TBG)	Serum	10–26	μg/dL	10	100–260	μg/L
Tissue plasminogen activator	Plasma	<0.04	IU/mL	1000	<40	IU/L
Tobramycin (therapeutic)	Plasma, serum	5–10	μg/mL	2.14	10–21	μmol/L
Tocainide (therapeutic)	Plasma, serum	4–10	μg/mL	5.20	21–52	μmol/L

Table S–1.
Conversions From Conventional Units to Système International (SI) Units*, continued

Component	System	Reference Range, Conventional Units	Conventional Units	Conversion Factor (Multiply by)	Reference Range, SI Units	SI Units
α-Tocopherol (see Vitamin E)						
Tolbutamide (therapeutic)	Plasma	80–240	μg/mL	3.70	296–888	μmol/L
Transferrin (siderophilin)	Serum	200–380	mg/dL	0.01	2.0–3.8	g/L
Triglycerides (as triolein)	Plasma, serum	10–190	mg/dL	0.01129	0.11–2.15	mmol/L
Triiodothyronine						
Free (FT₃)	Serum	260–480	pg/dL	0.0154	4.0–7.4	pmol/L
Resin uptake	Serum	25–35	%	0.01	0.25–0.35	Proportion of 1.0
Total (T₃)	Serum	70–200	ng/dL	0.0154	1.08–3.14	nmol/L
Troponin I (cardiac)	Serum	<0.6	mg/mL	1.0	<0.6	μg/L
Troponin T (cardiac)	Serum	<0.2	μg/L	1.0	<0.2	μg/L
Tryptophan	Plasma	0.5–1.5	mg/dL	48.97	25–73	μmol/L
Tyrosine	Plasma	0.4–1.6	mg/dL	55.19	20–90	μmol/L
Urea nitrogen	Serum	8–23	mg/dL	0.357	2.9–8.2	μmol/L
Uric acid	Serum	4.0–8.5	mg/dL	0.0595	0.24–0.51	μmol/L
Urobilinogen	Urine	0.05–2.5	mg/24 h	1.693	0.1–4.2	μmol/d
Valine	Plasma	1.7–3.7	mg/dL	85.5	145–315	μmol/L
Valproic acid (therapeutic)	Plasma, serum	50–100	μg/mL	6.93	346–693	μmol/L
Vancomycin (therapeutic)	Plasma, serum	20–40	μg/mL	0.690	14–28	μmol/L

Table S–1.
Conversions From Conventional Units to Système International (SI) Units*, _continued_

Component	System	Reference Range, Conventional Units	Conventional Units	Conversion Factor (Multiply by)	Reference Range, SI Units	SI Units
Vanillylmandelic acid (VMA)	Urine	2.1–7.6	mg/24 h	5.046	11–38	μmol/d
Vasoactive intestinal polypeptide	Plasma	<50	pg/mL	1.0	<50	ng/L
Verapamil (therapeutic)	Plasma, serum	100–500	ng/mL	2.2	220–1100	nmol/L
Vitamin A	Serum	30–80	μg/dL	0.0349	1.05–2.80	μmol/L
Vitamin B$_1$	Whole blood	2.5–7.5	μg/dL	29.6	74–222	nmol/L
Vitamin B$_2$	Plasma, serum	4–24	μg/dL	26.6	106–638	nmol/L
Vitamin B$_3$	Whole blood	0.2–1.8	μg/mL	4.56	0.9–8.2	μmol/L
Vitamin B$_6$	Plasma	5–30	ng/mL	4.046	20–121	nmol/L
Vitamin B$_{12}$	Serum	160–950	pg/mL	0.7378	118–701	pmol/L
Vitamin C	Plasma, serum	0.4–1.5	mg/dL	56.78	23–85	μmol/L
Vitamin D						
1,25-Dihydroxy vitamin D	Plasma, serum	16–65	pg/mL	2.6	42–169	pmol/L
25-Hydroxy vitamin D	Plasma, serum	14–60	ng/mL	2.496	35–150	nmol/L
Vitamin E	Plasma, serum	0.5–1.8	mg/dL	23.22	12–42	μmol/L
Vitamin K	Plasma, serum	0.13–1.19	ng/mL	2.22	0.29–2.64	nmol/L
Warfarin (therapeutic)	Plasma, serum	1.0–10	μg/mL	3.24	3.2–32.4	μmol/L

Table S–1.
Conversions From Conventional Units to Système International (SI) Units*, continued

Component	System	Reference Range, Conventional Units	Conventional Units	Conversion Factor (Multiply by)	Reference Range, SI Units	SI Units
White blood cell count	Whole blood	4.5–11.0	x10³/μL	10^6	4.5–11.0	x10⁹/L
Differential count						
Neutrophils	Whole blood	1800–7800	/μL	10^6	1.8–7.8	x10⁹/L
Bands	Whole blood	0–700	/μL	10^6	0.00–0.70	x10⁹/L
Lymphocytes	Whole blood	1000–4800	/μL	10^6	1.0–4.8	x10⁹/L
Monocytes	Whole blood	0–800	/μL	10^6	208>0.80	x10⁹/L
Eosinophils	Whole blood	0–450	/μL	10^6	0.00–0.45	x10⁹/L
Basophils	Whole blood	0–200	/μL	10^6	0.00–0.20	x10⁹/L
Differential count (number fraction)						
Neutrophils	Whole blood	56	%	0.01	0.56	Proportion of 1.00
Bands	Whole blood	3	%	0.01	0.03	Proportion of 1.00
Lymphocytes	Whole blood	34	%	0.01	0.34	Proportion of 1.00
Monocytes	Whole blood	4	%	0.01	0.04	Proportion of 1.00
Eosinophils	Whole blood	2.7	%	0.01	0.027	Proportion of 1.000
Basophils	Whole blood	0.3	%	0.01	0.003	Proportion of 1.000
Xylose absorption test (25-g dose)	Whole blood	25–40	mg/dL	0.066–61	1.67–2.66	mmol/L
Zidovudine (therapeutic)	Plasma, serum	0.15–0.27	μg/mL	3.7	0.56–1.01	μmol/L
Zinc	Serum	50–150	μg/dL	0.153	7.7–23.0	μmol/L

Table S–1.
Conversions From Conventional Units to Système International (SI) Units*, *continued*

* Reprinted with permission from the *American Medical Association Manual of Style: A Guide for Authors and Editors*. 9th ed. Chicago, IL: AMA; 1998:486–503. Copyright 1998, American Medical Association. The information in this table is from the following sources: (1) Tietz NW, ed. *Clinical Guide to Laboratory Tests*. 3rd ed. Philadelphia, Pa: WB Saunders Co; 1995; (2) Jacobs DS, Demott WR, Grady HJ, Horvat RT, Huestis DW, Kasten BL, eds. *Laboratory Test Handbook*. 4th ed. Hudson, Ohio: Lexi-Comp Inc; 1996; (3) Henry JB, ed. *Clinical Diagnosis and Management by Laboratory Methods*. 19th ed. Philadelphia, Pa: WB Saunders Co; 1996; (4) Laposata M. *SI Unit Conversion Guide*. Boston, Mass: NEJM Books; 1992. The reference values are provided for illustration only and are not intended to be comprehensive or definitive. Each laboratory determines its won values, and reference ranges are highly method dependent. Reference values given are for adults, unless otherwise specified. For some entries for which specific molecular masses are not known (eg, proteins), reference values in SI are given as mass amounts per liter.

Appendix T

Table T–1.
Exchange Lists for Diabetic Diets*

Groups/Lists	Carbohydrate, g	Protein, g	Fat, g	Calories
Carbohydrate Group				
Starch	15	3	1 or less	80
Fruit	15	...	...	60
Milk				
Skim	12	8	0–3	90
Low-fat	12	8	5	120
Whole	12	8	8	150
Other carbohydrates	15	varies	varies	varies
Vegetables	5	2	...	25
Meat and Meat Substitute Group				
Very lean	...	7	0–1	35
Lean	...	7	3	55
Medium-fat	...	7	5	75
High-fat	...	7	8	100
Fat Group	...	...	**5**	**45**

*From the American Diabetes Association, Inc, Framingham, MA, and the American Dietetic Association, Chicago, IL. *Exchange Lists for Meal Planning*; 1995

Table T–2.
Food Exchange Lists

<table>
<tr><th>Starch List</th></tr>
<tr><td>

Cereals, grains, pasta, breads, crackers, snacks, starchy vegetables, and cooked beans, peas, and lentils are starches. In general, one starch is:

- 1/2 cup of cooked cereal, grain, or starchy vegetable. 1/3 cup of cooked rice or pasta
- 1 oz of a bread product, such as 1 slice of bread
- 3/4 to 1 oz of most snack foods (Some snack foods may also have added fat.)

</td></tr>
</table>

Table T–2.
Food Exchange Lists, *continued*

Nutrition Tips

1. Most starch choices are good sources of B vitamins.
2. Foods made from whole grains are good sources of fiber
   - A serving from the bread list, on average, has 1 gram of fiber
   - A serving from the cereals and grains list or the crackers and snacks list, on average, has 2 grams of fiber
   - A serving from the starchy vegetables list, on average, has 3 grams of fiber.
3. Beans, peas, and lentils are good sources of protein and fiber
   - A serving from this food group, on average, has 6 grams of fiber.

Selection Tips

1. Choose starches made with little fat as often as you can.
2. Starchy vegetables prepared with fat count as one starch and one fat.
3. For many starchy foods (eg, bagels, muffins, dinner rolls, buns), a general rule of thumb is 1 oz equals 1 carbohydrate serving. However, bagels or muffins range widely in size. Check the size you eat. Also, use the Nutrition Facts on food labels when available.
4. Beans, peas, and lentils are also found on the meat and meat substitutes list.
5. A waffle or pancake is about the size of a compact disc (CD) and about 1/4 inch thick.
6. Because starches often swell in cooking, a small amount of uncooked starch will become a much larger amount of cooked food.
7. Most of the serving sizes are measured or weighed after cooking.
8. For specific information, check Nutrition Facts on the food label.

Starch List
One starch exchange equals: 15 grams of carbohydrate, 3 grams of protein, 0–1 grams of fat and 80 calories.

Bread	
Bagel, 4 oz 1/4 (1 oz)	1/4 (1 oz)
Bread, reduced-calorie	2 slices (1 1/2 oz)
Bread, white, whole-wheat, pumpernickel, rye	1 slice (1 oz)
Bread sticks, crisp, 4 inch × 1/2 inch	4 (2/3 oz)
English muffin	1/2
Hot dog bun or hamburger bun	1/2 (1 oz)
Naan, 8 × 2 inch	1/4
Pancake, 4 inch across, 1/4 inch thick	1
Pita, 6 inch across	1/2
Roll, plain, small	1 (1 oz)
Raisin bread, unfrosted	1 slice (1 oz)
Tortilla, corn, 6 inch across	1
Tortilla, flour, 6 inch across	1

Table T–2.
Food Exchange Lists, *continued*

Bread, *continued*	
Tortilla, flour, 10 inch across	1/3
Waffle, 4 inch square or across, reduced-fat	1
Cereals and Grains	
Bran cereals	1/2 cup
Bulgur	1/2 cup
Cereals, cooked	1/2 cup
Cereals, unsweetened, ready-to-eat	3/4 cup
Cornmeal (dry)	3 Tbsp
Couscous	1/3 cup
Flour (dry)	3 Tbsp
Granola, low-fat	1/4 cup
Grape-Nuts®	1/4 cup
Grits	1/2 cup
Kasha	1/2 cup
Millet	1/3 cup
Musesli	1/4 cup
Oats	1/2 cup
Pasta	1/3 cup
Puffed cereal	1 1/2 cups
Rice, white or brown	1/3 cup
Shredded Wheat®	1/2 cup
Sugar-frosted cereal	1/2 cup
Wheat germ	3 Tbsp
Starchy Vegetables	
Baked beans	1/3 cup
Corn	1/2 cup
Corn on cob, large	1/2 cob (5 oz)
Mixed vegetables with corn, peas, or pasta	1 cup
Peas, green	1/2 cup
Plantain	1/2 cup
Potato, boiled	1/2 cup or 1/2 medium (3 oz)
Potato, baked with skin	1/4 large (3 oz)

Table T–2.
Food Exchange Lists, *continued*

Starchy Vegetables, *continued*	
Potato, mashed	1/2 cup
Squash, winter (acorn, butternut, pumpkin)	1 cup
Yam, sweet potato, plain	1/2 cup
Crackers and Snacks	
Animal crackers	8
Graham cracker, 2 1/2 inch square	3
Matzoh	3/4 oz
Melba toast	4 slices
Oyster crackers	24
Popcorn (popped, no fat added, or low-fat microwave)	3 cups
Pretzels	3/4 oz
Rice cakes, 4 inch across	2
Saltine-type crackers	6
Snack chips, fat-free or baked (tortilla, potato)	15–20 (3/4 oz)
Whole-wheat crackers, no fat added	2–5 (3/4 oz)
Beans, Peas, and Lentils (count as 1 starch exchange, plus 1 very lean meat exchange)	
Beans and peas (garbanzo, pinto, kidney, white, split, black-eyed)	1/2 cup
Lima beans	2/3 cup
Lentils	1/2 cup
Miso~	3 Tbsp
~ = 400 mg or more sodium per exchange.	
Common Measurements	
3 tsp = 1 Tbsp	4 oz = 1/2 cup
4 Tbsp = 1/4 cup	8 oz = 1 cup
5 1/3 Tbsp = 1/3 cup	1 cup = 1/2 pint
Starchy Foods Prepared with Fat (count as 1 starch exchange, plus 1 fat exchange)	
Biscuit, 2 1/2 inch across	1
Chow mein noodles	1/2 cup
Corn bread, 2 inch cube	1 (2 oz)
Crackers, round butter type	6

Table T–2.
Food Exchange Lists, *continued*

Starchy Foods Prepared with Fat, *continued*	
Croutons	1 cup
French-fried potatoes (oven-baked) (see also the fast foods list)	3 oz
Granola	1/4 cup
Hummus	1/3 cup
Muffin	1 small (1 1/2 oz)
Popcorn, microwaved	3 cups
Sandwich crackers, cheese or peanut butter filling	3
Snack chips (potato, tortilla)	9–13 (3/4 oz)
Stuffing, bread (prepared)	1/3 cup
Taco shell, 6 in. across	2
Waffle, 4 inch square or across	1
Whole-wheat crackers, fat added	4–6 (1 oz)

Fruit List

Fresh, frozen, canned, and dried fruits and fruit juices are on this list. In general, one fruit exchange is:
- 1 small fresh fruit (4 oz)
- 1/2 cup of canned or fresh fruit or unsweetened fruit juice
- 1/4 cup of dried fruit

Nutrition Tips

1. Fresh, frozen, and dried fruits have about 2 grams of fiber per choice. Fruit juices contain very little fiber.
2. Citrus fruits, berries, and melons are good sources of vitamin C.

Selection Tips

1. Count 1/2 cup cranberries or rhubarb sweetened with sugar substitutes as free foods.
2. Read the Nutrition Facts on the food label. If one serving has more than 15 grams of carbohydrate, you will need to adjust the size of the serving you eat or drink.
3. Portion sizes for canned fruits are for the fruit and a small amount of juice.
4. Whole fruit is more filling than fruit juice and may be a better choice.
5. Food labels for fruits may contain the words "no sugar added" or "unsweetened." This means that no sucrose (table sugar) has been added.
6. Generally, fruit canned in extra light syrup has the same amount of carbohydrate per serving as the "no sugar added" or the juice pack. All canned fruits on the fruit list are based on one of these three types of pack.

Table T–2.
Food Exchange Lists, *continued*

Fruit	
Apple, unpeeled, small	1 (4 oz)
Applesauce, unsweetened	1/2 cup
Apples, dried	4 rings
Apricots, fresh	4 whole (5 1/2 oz)
Apricots, dried	8 halves
Apricots, canned	1/2 cup
Banana, small	1 (4 oz)
Blackberries	3/4 cup
Blueberries	3/4 cup
Cantaloupe, small	1/3 melon (11 oz) or 1 cup cubes
Cherries, sweet, fresh	12 (3 oz)
Cherries, sweet, canned	1/2 cup
Dates	3
Figs, fresh	1 1/2 large or 2 medium (3 1/2 oz)
Figs, dried	1 1/2
Fruit cocktail	1/2 cup
Grapefruit, large	1/2 (11 oz)
Grapefruit sections, canned	3/4 cup
Grapes, small	17 (3 oz)
Honeydew melon	1 slice (10 oz) or 1 cup cubes
Kiwi	1 (3 1/2 oz)
Mandarin oranges, canned	3/4 cup
Mango, small	1/2 fruit (5 1/2 oz) or 1/2 cup
Nectarine, small	1 (5 oz)
Orange, small	1 (6 1/2 oz)
Papaya	1/2 fruit (8 oz) or 1 cup cubes
Peach, medium, fresh	1 (4 oz)
Peaches, canned	1/2 cup
Pear, large, fresh	1/2 (4 oz)

Table T–2.
Food Exchange Lists, *continued*

Fruit, continued	
Pears, canned	1/2 cup
Pineapple, fresh	3/4 cup
Pineapple, canned	1/2 cup
Plums, small	2 (5 oz)
Plums, canned	1/2 cup
Plums, dried (prunes)	3
Raisins	2 Tbsp
Raspberries	1 cup
Strawberries	1 1/4 cup whole berries
Tangerines, small	2 (8 oz)
Watermelon	1 slice (13 1/2 oz) or 1 1/4 cup cubes
Fruit Juice, Unsweetened	
Apple juice/cider	1/2 cup
Cranberry juice cocktail	1/3 cup
Cranberry juice cocktail, reduced-calorie	1 cup
Fruit juice blends, 100% juice	1/3 cup
Grape juice	1/3 cup
Grapefruit juice	1/2 cup
Orange juice	1/2 cup
Pineapple juice	1/2 cup
Prune juice	1/3 cup

MILK LIST

Different types of milk and milk products are on this list. Cheeses are on the meat and meat sub-stitutes list and cream and other dairy fats are on the fat list. Based on the amount of fat they contain, milks are divided into fat-free/low-fat milk, reduced-fat milk, and whole milk. One choice of these includes:

	Carbohydrate (grams)	Protein (grams)	Fat (grams)	Calories
Fat-free/low-fat (1/2% or 1%)	12	8	0–3	90
Reduced-fat (2%)	12	8	5	120
Whole	12	8	8	150

Table T–2.
Food Exchange Lists, *continued*

Nutrition Tips

1. Milk and yogurt are good sources of calcium and protein. Check the Nutrition Facts on the food label.
2. The higher the fat content of milk and yogurt, the greater the amount of saturated fat and cholesterol. Choose lower-fat varieties.
3. For those who are lactose intolerant, look for lactose-reduced or lactose-free varieties of milk. Check the food label for total amount of carbohydrate per serving.

Selection Tips

1. 1 cup equals 8 fluid oz or 1/2 pint.
2. Look for chocolate milk, rice milk, frozen yogurt, and ice cream on the sweets, desserts, and other carbohydrates list.
3. Nondairy creamers are on the free foods list.

Fat-Free and Low-Fat Milk (0–3 grams fat per serving)	
Fat-free milk	1 cup
1/2% milk	1 cup
1% milk	1 cup
Buttermilk, low-fat or fat-free	1 cup
Evaporated fat-free milk	1/2 cup
Fat-free dry milk	1/3 cup dry
Soy milk, low-fat or fat-free	1 cup
Yogurt, fat-free, flavored, sweetened with nonnutritive sweetener and fructose	2/3 cup (6 oz)
Yogurt, plain fat-free	2/3 cup (6 oz)
Reduced-Fat (5 grams fat per serving)	
2% milk	1 cup
Soy milk	1 cup
Sweet acidophilus milk	1 cup
Yogurt, plain low-fat	3/4 cup
Whole Milk (8 grams fat per serving)	
Whole milk	1 cup
Evaporated whole milk	1/2 cup
Goat's milk	1 cup
Kefir	1 cup
Yogurt, plain (made from whole milk)	3/4 cup

Table T–2.
Food Exchange Lists, *continued*

Sweets, Desserts, and Other Carbohydrates List

You can substitute food choices from this list for a starch, fruit, or milk choice on your meal plan. Some choices will also count as one or more fat choices.

Nutrition Tips

1. These foods can be substituted for other carbohydrate-containing foods in your meal plan, even though they contain added sugars or fat. However, they do not contain as many important vitamins and minerals as the choices on the starch, fruit, or milk list.
2. When choosing these foods, include foods from the other lists to eat balanced meals.

Selection Tips

1. Because many of these foods are concentrated sources of carbohydrate and fat, saturated fat, and *trans* fat, the portion sizes are often very small.
2. Look for the words "hydrogenated" or "partially hydrogenated" on the ingredient label. The lower down on the list these words appear, the fewer *trans* fats there are.
3. Be sure to check the Nutrition Facts on the food label. It will be your most accurate source of information.
4. Many fat-free or reduced-fat products made with fat replacers contain carbohydrate. When eaten in large amounts, they may need to be counted. Talk with your dietitian to determine how to count these in your meal plan.
5. Look for fat-free salad dressings in smaller amounts on the free foods list.

Food Serving	Size	Exchanges per Serving
Angel food cake, unfrosted	1/12th cake (about 2 oz)	2 carbohydrates
Brownie, small unfrosted	2 inch square (about 1 oz)	1 carbohydrate, 1 fat
Cake, unfrosted	2 inch square (about 1 oz)	1 carbohydrate, 1 fat
Cake, frosted	2 inch square (about 2 oz)	2 carbohydrates, 1 fat
Cookie or sandwich cookie with crème filling	2 small (about 2/3 oz)	1 carbohydrate, 1 fat
Cookies, sugar-free	3 small or 1 large (3/4–1 oz)	1 carbohydrate, 1–2 fats
Cranberry sauce, jellied	1/4 cup	1 1/2 carbohydrates
Cupcake, frosted	1 small (about 2 oz)	2 carbohydrates, 1 fat
Doughnut, plain cake	1 medium (1 1/2 oz)	1 1/2 carbohydrates, 2 fats
Doughnut, glazed	3 3/4 inch across (2 oz)	2 carbohydrates, 2 fats
Energy, sport, or breakfast bar	1 bar (1 1/3 oz)	1 1/2 carbohydrates, 0–1 fat
Energy, sport, or breakfast bar	1 bar (2 oz)	2 carbohydrates, 1 fat
Fruit cobbler	1/2 cup (3 1/2 oz)	3 carbohydrates, 1 fat
Fruit juice bars, frozen, 100% juice	1 bar (3 oz)	1 carbohydrate
Fruit snacks, chewy (pureed fruit concentrate)	1 roll (3/4 oz)	1 carbohydrate

Table T–2.
Food Exchange Lists, *continued*

Food	Serving Size	Exchanges per Serving
Fruit spreads, 100% fruit	1 1/2 Tbsp	1 carbohydrate
Gelatin, regular	1/2 cup	1 carbohydrate
Gingersnaps	3	1 carbohydrate
Granola or snack bar, regular or low-fat	1 bar (1 oz)	1 1/2 carbohydrates
Honey	1 Tbsp	1 carbohydrate
Ice cream	1/2 cup	1 carbohydrate, 2 fats
Ice cream, light.	1/2 cup	1 carbohydrate, 1 fat
Ice cream, low-fat	1/2 cup	1 1/2 carbohydrates
Ice cream, fat-free, no sugar added	1/2 cup	1 carbohydrate
Jam or jelly, regular	1 Tbsp	1 carbohydrate
Milk, chocolate, whole	1 cup	2 carbohydrates, 1 fat
Pie, fruit, 2 crusts	1/6 of 8-inch commercially prepared pie	3 carbohydrates, 2 fats
Pie, pumpkin or custard	1/8 of 8-inch commercially prepared pie	2 carbohydrates, 2 fats
Pudding, regular (made with reduced-fat milk)	1/2 cup	2 carbohydrates
Pudding, sugar-free or sugar-free and fat-free (made with fat-free milk)	1/2 cup	1 carbohydrate
Reduced-calorie meal replacement (shake)	1 can (10–11 oz)	1 1/2 carbohydrates, 0–1 fat
Rice milk, low-fat or fat-free, plain	1 cup	1 carbohydrate
Rice milk, low-fat, flavored	1 cup	1 1/2 carbohydrates
Salad dressing, fat-free~	1/4 cup	1 carbohydrate
Sherbet, sorbet	1/2 cup	2 carbohydrates
Spagetti sauce or pasta sauce, canned~	1/2 cup	1 carbohydrate, 1 fat
Sports drinks	8 oz (1 cup)	1 carbohydrate
Sugar	1 Tbsp	1 carbohydrate
Sweet roll or Danish	1 (2 1/2 oz)	2 1/2 carbohydrates, 2 fats
Syrup, light	2 Tbsp	1 carbohydrate
Syrup, regular	1 Tbsp	1 carbohydrate
Syrup, regular	1/4 cup	4 carbohydrates
Vanilla wafers	5	1 carbohydrate, 0–1 fat
Yogurt, frozen, fat-free	1/3 cup	1 carbohydrate
Yogurt, low-fat with fruit	1 cup	3 carbohydrates, 0–1 fat

~ = 400 mg or more of sodium per exchange.

Table T–2.
Food Exchange Lists, *continued*

Nonstarchy Vegetable List

Vegetables that contain small amounts of carbohydrate and calories are on this list. Vegetables contain important nutrients. Try to eat at least 2 or 3 vegetable choices each day. In general, one vegetable exchange is:

1/2 cup of cooked vegetables or vegetable juice

1 cup of raw vegetables

If you eat 3 cups or more of raw vegetables or 1 1/2 cups of cooked vegetables at one meal, count them as 1 carbohydrate choice.

Nutrition Tips

1. Fresh and frozen vegetables have less added salt than canned vegetables. Drain and rinse canned vegetables if you want to remove some salt.
2. Choose more dark green and dark yellow vegetables, such as spinach, broccoli, romaine, carrots, chilies, and peppers.
3. Broccoli, Brussels sprouts, cauliflower, greens, peppers, spinach, and tomatoes are good sources of vitamin C.
4. Vegetables contain 1 to 4 grams of fiber per serving.

Selection Tips

1. A 1-cup portion of broccoli is a portion about the size of a light bulb.
2. Tomato sauce is different from spaghetti sauce, which is on the sweets, desserts, and other carbohydrates list.
3. Canned vegetables and juices are available without added salt.
4. Starchy vegetables such as corn, peas, winter squash, and potatoes that contain larger amounts of calories and carbohydrates are on the starch list.

Nonstarchy Vegetable List

One vegetable exchange (1/2 cup cooked or 1 cup raw) equals: 5 grams of carbohydrate, 2 grams of protein, 0 grams of fat, and 25 calories.

Artichoke
Artichoke hearts
Asparagus
Beans (green, wax, Italian)
Bean sprouts
Beets
Broccoli
Brussels sprouts
Cabbage
Carrots
Cauliflower
Celery
Cucumber

Table T–2.
Food Exchange Lists, *continued*

Eggplant
Green onions or scallions
Greens (collard, kale, mustard, turnip)
Kohlrabi
Leeks
Mixed vegetables (without corn, peas, or pasta)
Mushrooms
Okra
Onions
Pea pods
Peppers (all varieties)
Radishes
Salad greens (endive, escarole, lettuce, romaine, spinach)
Sauerkraut~
Spinach
Summer squash
Tomato
Tomatoes, canned
Tomato sauce~
Tomato/vegetable juice~
Turnips
Water chestnuts
Watercress
Zucchini
~ = 400 mg or more sodium per exchange.
Meat and Meat Substitutes List

Meat and meat substitutes that contain both protein and fat are on this list. In general, one meat exchange is:

- 1 oz of meat, fish, poultry, or cheese
- 1/2 cup of beans, peas, or lentils

Based on the amount of fat they contain, meats are divided into very lean, lean, medium-fat, and high-fat lists. This is done so you can see which ones contain the least amount of fat. One ounce (one exchange) of each of these includes:

Table T–2.
Food Exchange Lists, *continued*

	Carbohydrate (grams)	Protein (grams)	Fat (grams)	Calories
Very lean	0	7	0–1	35
Lean	0	7	3	55
Medium-fat	0	7	5	75
High-fat	0	7	8	100

Nutrition Tips

1. Choose very lean and lean meat choices whenever possible. Items from the high-fat group are high in saturated fat, cholesterol, and calories and can raise blood cholesterol levels.
2. Beans, peas, and lentils are good sources of fiber, about 3 grams per serving.
3. Some processed meats, seafood, and soy products may contain carbohydrate when consumed in large amounts. Check the Nutrition Facts on the label to see if the amount is close to 15 grams. If so, count it as a carbohydrate choice as well as a meat choice.

Selection Tips

1. Weigh meat after cooking and removing bones and fat. Four ounces of raw meat is equal to 3 oz of cooked meat. Some examples of meat portions are:
- 1 oz cheese = 1 meat choice and is about the size of a 1-inch cube or 4 cubes the size of dice
- 2 oz meat = 2 meat choices, such as:
  1 small chicken leg or thigh
  1/2 cup cottage cheese or tuna
- 3 oz meat = 3 meat choices and is about the size of a deck of cards, such as:
  1 medium pork chop
  1 small hamburger
  1/2 of a whole chicken breast
  1 unbreaded fish fillet
2. Limit your choices from the high-fat group to three times per week or less.
3. Most grocery stores stock Select and Choice grades of meat. The Select grades of meat are the leanest. The Choice grades contain a moderate amount of fat, and Prime cuts of meat have the highest amount of fat.
4. "Hamburger" may contain added seasoning and fat, but ground beef does not.
5. Read labels to find products that are low in fat and cholesterol (5 grams of fat or less per serving).
6. Dried beans, peas, and lentils are also found on the starch list.
7. Peanut butter, in smaller amounts, is also found on the fat list.
8. Bacon, in smaller amounts, is also found on the fat list.
9. Don't be fooled by ground beef packages that say X% lean (eg, 90% lean). This is the percentage of fat by weight, NOT the percentage of calories from fat. A 3.5-oz patty of this raw ground beef has about half of its calories from fat.
10. Meatless burgers are in the combination foods list (3 oz of soy based burger = 1/2 carbohydrate + 2 very lean meats; 3 oz of vegetable and starch-based burger = 1 carbohydrate + 1 lean meat).

Table T–2.
Food Exchange Lists, *continued*

Very Lean Meat and Substitutes List	
• One very lean meat exchange is equal to anyone of the following items:	
Poultry: Chicken or turkey (white meat, no skin), Cornish hen (no skin)	14
Fish: Fresh or frozen cod, flounder, haddock, halibut, trout, lox (smoked salmon)~; tuna fresh or canned in water	1 oz
Shellfish: Clams, crab, lobster, scallops, shrimp, imitation shellfish	1 oz
Game: Duck or pheasant (no skin), venison, buffalo, ostrich	1 oz
Cheese with 1 gram of fat or less per ounce: Fat-free or low-fat cottage cheese	1/4 cup
Fat-free cheese	1 oz
Other: Processed sandwich meats with 1 gram of fat or less per ounce, such as deli thin, shaved meats, chipped beef~, turkey ham	1 oz
Egg whites	2
Egg substitutes, plain	1/4 cup
Hot dogs with 1 gram of fat or less per ounce~	1 oz
Kidney (high in cholesterol)	1 oz
Sausage with 1 gram of fat or less per ounce	1 oz
Count the following items as one very lean meat and one starch exchange.	
Beans, peas, lentils (cooked)	1/2 cup
~ = 400 mg or more sodium per exchange.	
Meal Planning Tips	
1. Bake, roast, broil, grill, poach, steam, or boil meat and fish rather than frying.	
2. Place meat on a rack so the fat will drain off during cooking.	
3. Use a nonstick spray and a nonstick pan to brown or fry foods.	
4. Trim off visible fat or skin before or after cooking.	
5. If you add flour, bread crumbs, coating mixes, fat, or marinades when cooking, ask your dietitian how to count it in your meal plan.	
• One lean meat exchange is equal to anyone of the following items:	
Beef: USDA Select or Choice grades of lean beef trimmed of fat, such as round, sirloin, and flank steak; tenderloin; roast (rib, chuck, rump); steak (T-bone, porterhouse, cubed); ground round	1 oz
Pork: Lean pork, such as fresh ham; canned, cured, or boiled ham; Canadian bacon ~; tenderloin, center loin chop	1 oz
Lamb: Roast, chop, or leg	1 oz
Veal: Lean chop, roast	1 oz

Table T–2.
Food Exchange Lists, *continued*

Poultry: Chicken, turkey (dark meat, no skin), chicken (white meat, with skin), domestic duck or goose (well-drained off fat, no skin)	1 oz
Fish:	
Herring (uncreamed or smoked)	1 oz
Oysters	6 medium
Salmon (fresh or canned), catfish	1 oz
Sardines (canned)	2 medium
Tuna (canned in oil, drained)	1 oz
Game: Goose (no skin), rabbit	1 oz
Cheese: 4.5%-fat cottage cheese	1/4 cup
Grated Parmesan	2 Tbsp
Cheeses with 3 grams of fat or less per ounce	1 oz
Other:	
Hot dogs with 3 grams of fat or less per ounce~	1 1/2 oz
Processed sandwich meat with 3 grams of fat or less per ounce, such as turkey pastrami or kielbasa	1 oz
Liver, heart (high in cholesterol)	1 oz
Medium-Fat Meat and Substitutes List	
• One medium-fat meat exchange is equal to anyone of the following items:	
Beef: Most beef products fall into this category (ground beef, meatloaf, corned beef, short ribs, Prime grades of meat trimmed of fat, such as prime rib)	1 oz
Pork: Top loin, chop, Boston butt, cutlet	1 oz
Lamb: Rib roast, ground	1 oz
Veal: Cutlet (ground or cubed, unbreaded)	1 oz
Poultry: Chicken (dark meat, with skin), ground turkey or ground chicken, fried chicken (with skin)	1 oz
Fish: Any fried fish product	1 oz
Cheese with 5 grams or less fat per ounce: Feta	1 oz
Mozzarella	1 oz
Ricotta	1/4 cup (2 oz)
Other: Egg (high in cholesterol, limit to 3 per week)	1
Sausage with 5 grams of fat or less per ounce	1 oz
Tempeh	1/4 cup
Tofu	4 oz or 1/2 cup

Table T–2.
Food Exchange Lists, *continued*

High-Fat Meat and Substitutes List	
Remember these items are high in saturated fat, cholesterol, and calories and may raise blood cholesterol levels if eaten on a regular basis.	
• One high-fat meat exchange is equal to anyone of the following items:	
Pork: Spareribs, ground pork, pork sausage	1 oz
Cheese: All regular cheeses, such as American~, cheddar, Monterey Jack, Swiss	1 oz
Other: Processed sandwich meats with 8 grams of fat or less per ounce, such as bologna, pimento loaf, salami	1 oz
Sausage, such as bratwurst, Italian, knockwurst, Polish, smoked	1 oz
Hot dog (turkey or chicken)~	1 (10/lb)
Bacon	3 slices (20 slices/lb)
Peanut butter (contains unsaturated fat)	1 Tbsp
• Count the following items as 1 high-fat meat plus 1 fat exchange:	
Hot dog (beef, pork, or combination)~	1 (10/lb)
~ = 400 mg or more sodium per exchange.	

Fat List

Fats are divided into three groups, based on the main type of fat they contain: monounsaturated, polyunsaturated, and saturated. Monounsaturated and polyunsaturated fats in the foods we eat are linked with good health benefits. Saturated fats and fats called *trans* fatty acids (or *trans* unsaturated fatty acids) are linked with heart disease. In general, one fat exchange is:

- 1 teaspoon of regular margarine or vegetable oil
- 1 tablespoon of regular salad dressing

Nutrition Tips

1. All fats are high in calories. Limit serving sizes for good nutrition and health.
2. Nuts and seeds contain small amounts of fiber, protein, and magnesium.
3. If blood pressure is a concern, choose fats in the unsalted form to help lower sodium intake, such as unsalted peanuts.

Selection Tips

1. Check the Nutrition Facts on food labels for serving sizes. One fat exchange is based on a serving size containing 5 grams of fat.
2. The Nutrition Facts on food labels usually list total fat grams and saturated fat grams per serving. When most of the calories come from saturated fat, the food fits into the saturated fats list.
3. Occasionally the Nutrition Facts on food labels will list monounsaturated and/or polyunsaturated fats in addition to total and saturated fats. If more than half the total fat is monounsaturated, the food fits into the monounsaturated fats list; if more than half is polyunsaturated, the food fits into the polyunsaturated fats list.

Table T–2.
Food Exchange Lists, *continued*

4. When selecting fats to use with your meal plan, consider replacing saturated fats with monounsaturated fats.
5. When selecting regular margarine, choose those with liquid vegetable oil as the first ingredient. Soft margarines are not as saturated as stick margarines and are healthier choices.
6. Avoid foods on the fat list (such as margarines) listing hydrogenated or partially hydrogenated fat as the first ingredient because these foods will contain higher amounts of *trans* fatty acids.
7. When selecting reduced-fat or lower-fat margarines, look for liquid vegetable oil as the second ingredient. Water is usually the first ingredient.
8. When used in smaller amounts, bacon and peanut butter are counted as fat choices. When used in larger amounts, they are counted as high-fat meat choices.
9. Fat-free salad dressings are on the sweets, desserts, and other carbohydrates list and the free foods list.
10. See the free foods list for nondairy coffee creamers, whipped topping, and fat-free products, such as margarines, salad dressings, mayonnaise, sour cream, cream cheese, and nonstick cooking spray.

Monounsaturated Fats List	
Avocado, medium	2 Tbsp (1 oz)
Oil (canola, olive, peanut)	1 tsp
Olives: ripe (black)	10 large
green, stuffed~	
Nuts: almonds, cashews	6 nuts
mixed (50% peanuts)	6 nuts
peanuts	10 nuts
pecans	4 halves
Peanut butter, smooth or crunchy	1/2 Tbsp
Sesame seeds	2 tsp
Tahini or sesame paste	2 tsp
Polyunsaturated Fats List	
Margarine: stick, tub or squeeze	1 tsp
Lower-fat spread (30% to 50% vegetable oil)	1 Tbsp
Mayonnaise: regular	1 tsp
Reduced-fat	1 Tbsp
Nuts: walnuts, English	4 halves
Oil (corn, safflower, soybean)	1 tsp
Salad dressing: regular~	1 Tbsp
Reduced-fat	2 Tbsp

Table T–2.
Food Exchange Lists, *continued*

Polyunsaturated Fats List, continued	
Miracle Whip Salad Dressing®:	
Regular	2 tsp
Reduced-fat	1 Tbsp
Seeds: pumpkin, sunflower	1 Tbsp
~ = 400 mg or more sodium per exchange	
Saturated Fats List	
Bacon, cooked	1 slice (20 slices/lb)
Bacon, grease	1 tsp
Butter: stick	1 tsp
whipped	2 tsp
reduced-fat	1 Tbsp
Chitterlings, Boiled	2 Tbsp (1/2 oz)
Coconut, sweetened, shredded	2 Tbsp
Coconut milk	1 Tbsp
Cream, half and half	2 Tbsp
Cream cheese:	
regular	1 Tbsp (1/2 oz)
reduced-fat	1 1/2 Tbsp (3/4 oz)
Fatback or salt pork,~see below*	
Shortening or lard	1 tsp
Sour cream: regular	2 Tbsp
reduced-fat	3 Tbsp
*Use a piece 1 inch × 1 inch × 1/4 inch if you plan to eat the fatback cooked with vegetables. Use a piece 2 inch × 1 inch × 1/2 inch when eating only the vegetables with the fatback removed.	
Free Foods List	
A free food is any food or drink that contains less than 20 calories or less than or equal to 5 grams of carbohydrate per serving. Foods with a serving size listed should be limited to 3 servings per day. Be sure to spread them out throughout the day. If you eat all 3 servings at one time, it could raise your blood glucose level. Foods listed without a serving size can be eaten whenever you like.	
Fat-Free or Reduced-Fat Foods	
Cream cheese, fat-free	1 Tbsp (1/2 oz)
Creamers, nondairy, liquid	1 Tbsp
Creamers, nondairy, powdered	2 tsp

Table T–2.
Food Exchange Lists, *continued*

Fat-Free or Reduced- Fat Foods, continued	
Mayonnaise, fat-free	1 Tbsp
Mayonnaise, reduced-fat	1 tsp
Margarine spread, fat-free	4 Tbsp
Margarine spread, reduced-fat	1 tsp
Miracle Whip@, fat-free	1 Tbsp
Miracle Whip@, reduced-fat	1 tsp
Nonstick cooking spray	
Salad dressing, fat -free or low-fat	1 Tbsp
Salad dressing, fat-free, Italian	2 Tbsp
Sour cream, fat-free, reduced-fat	1 Tbsp
Whipped topping, regular	1 Tbsp
Whipped topping, light or fat-free	2 Tbsp
Sugar-Free Foods	
Candy, hard, sugarfree	1 candy
Gelatin dessert, sugar-free	
Gelatin, unflavored	
Gum-sugar-free	
Jam or jelly, light	2 tsp
Sugar substitutes*	
Syrup, sugar-free	2 Tbsp
*Sugar substitutes, alternatives, or replacements that are approved by the Food and Drug Administration (FDA) are safe to use. Common brand names include:	
Equal@ (aspartame)	
Splenda@ (sucralose)	
Sprinkle Sweet@ (saccharin)	
Sweet One@ (acesulfame K)	
Sweet-10@ (saccharin)	
Sugar Twin@ (saccharin)	
Sweet 'N Low@ (saccharin)	
Drinks	
Bouillon, broth, consomme~	
Bouillon or broth, low-sodium	
Carbonated or mineral water	

Table T–2.
Food Exchange Lists, *continued*

Drinks, continued	
Club soda	
Cocoa powder	
Unsweetened	1 Tbsp
Coffee	
Diet soft drinks, sugar-free	
Drink mixes, sugar-free	
Tea	
Tonic water, sugar-free	
Condiments	
Catsup	1 Tbsp
Horseradish	
Lemon juice	
Lime juice	
Mustard	
Pickle relish	1 Tbsp
Pickles, dill~	1 1/2 medium
Pickles, sweet (bread and butter)	2 slices
Pickles, sweet (gherkin)	3/4 oz
Salsa	1/4 cup
Soy sauce, regular or light~	1 Tbsp
Taco sauce	1 Tbsp
Vinegar	
Yogurt	2 Tbsp
Seasonings	
Flavoring extracts	
Garlic	
Herbs, fresh or dried	

Table T–2.
Food Exchange Lists, *continued*

Seasonings, continued
Pimento
Spices
Tabasco® or hot pepper sauce
Wine, used in cooking
Worcestershire sauce
Be careful with seasonings that contain sodium or are salts, such as garlic or celery salt, and lemon pepper.
~ = 400 mg or more of sodium per exchange.

Combination Foods List

Many of the foods we eat are mixed together in various combinations. These combination foods do not fit into anyone exchange list. Often it is hard to tell what is in a casserole dish or prepared food item. This is a list of exchanges for some typical combination foods. This list will help you fit these foods into your meal plan. Ask your dietitian for information about any other combination foods you would like to eat.

Food	Serving Size	Exchanges per Serving
Entrees		
Tuna noodle casserole, lasagna, spaghetti with meatballs, chili with beans, macaroni and cheese~	1 cup (8 oz)	2 carbohydrates, 2 medium-fat meats
Chow mein (without noodles or rice)~	2 cups (16 oz)	1 carbohydrate, 2 lean meats
Tuna or chicken salad	1/2 cup (3 1/2 oz)	1/2 carbohydrate, 2 lean meats, 1 fat
Frozen entrees and meals		
Dinner-type meal	Generally 14–17 oz	3 carbohydrates, 3 medium-fat meats, 3 fats
Meatless burger, Soy based	3 oz	1/2 carbohydrate, 2 lean meats
Meatless burger, Vegetable and starch based	3 oz	1 carbohydrate, 1 lean meat
Pizza, cheese, Thin crust~	1/4 of 12 inch (6 oz)	2 carbohydrates, 2 medium-fat meats, 1 fat

Table T–2.
Food Exchange Lists, *continued*

Food	Serving Size	Exchanges per Serving
Pizza, meat topping, Thin crust~	1 (7 oz)	2 1/2 carbohydrates, 1 medium-fat meat, 3 fats
Entree or meal with less than 340 calories~	About 8–11 oz	2–3 carbohydrates, 1–2 lean meats
Soups		
Bean~	1 cup	1 carbohydrate, 1 very lean meat
Cream (made with water)!	1 cup (8 oz)	1 carbohydrate, 1 fat
Instant~	6 oz prepared	1 carbohydrate
Instant with beans/Lentils~	8 oz prepared	2 1/2 carbohydrates, 1 very lean meat
Split pea (made with water)~	1/2 cup (4 oz)	1 carbohydrate
Tomatoe (made with water)~	1 cup (8 oz)	1 carbohydrate
Vegetable beef, Chicken noodle, or other broth-type	1 cup (8 oz)	1 carbohydrate

~ = 400 mg or more sodium per exchange.

Fast Foods* List

Food	Serving Size	Exchange per Serving
Burrito with beef~	1 (5–7 oz)	3 carbohydrates, 1 medium-fat meat, 1 fat
Chicken nuggets~	6	1 carbohydrate, 2 medium-fat meats, 1 fat
Chicken breast and wing, breaded and fried~	1	1 carbohydrate, 4 medium-fat meats, 2 fats
Chicken sandwich, grilled~	1	2 carbohydrates, 3 very lean meats
Chicken wings, hot~	6 (5 oz)	1 carbohydrate, 3 medium fat meats, 4 fats
Fish sandwich/tartar sauce~	1	3 carbohydrates, 1 medium-fat meat, 3 fats

Table T–2.
Food Exchange Lists, *continued*

Food	Serving Size	Exchanges per Serving
French fries~	1 medium serving (5 oz)	4 carbohydrates, 4 fats
Hamburger, regular	1	2 carbohydrates, 2 medium-fat meats
Hamburger, large~	1	2 carbohydrates, 3 medium-fat meats 1 fat
Hot dog with bun~	1	1 carbohydrate, 1 high-fat meat, 1 fat
Individual pan pizza~	1	5 carbohydrates, 3 medium-fat meats, 3 fats
Pizza, cheese, thin crust~	1/4 12 inch (about 6 oz)	2 1/2 carbohydrates, 2 medium-fat meats
Pizza, meat, thin crust~	1/4 12 inch (about 6 oz)	2 1/2 carbohydrates 2 medium-fat meats, 1 fat
Soft-serve cone	1 small (5 oz)	2 1/2 carbohydrates, 1 fat
Submarine sandwich~	1 sub (6 inch)	3 carbohydrates, 1 vegetable, 2 medium-fat meats, 1 fat
Submarine sandwich~ (less than 6 grams fat)	1 sub (6 inch)	2 1/2 carbohydrates, 2 lean meats
Taco, hard or soft shell~	1 (3–3 1/2 oz)	1 carbohydrate, 1 medium-fat meat, 1 fat

~ = 400 mg or more of sodium per exchange.
*Ask at your fast-food restaurant for nutrition information about your favorite fast foods or check Web sites.

Appendix U

Table U–1.
Beverages and Alcoholic Drinks
Calories and Selected Electrolytes (per fluid ounce)*

Beverage	Energy, kcal	Sodium, mg	Potassium, mg	Phosphorous, mg
Regular Soft Drinks				
Cola or pepper	12–14	0–2.3	0–1.5	3.3–6.2
Decaffeinated cola or pepper	12–15	0–2.3	0–1.5	3.3–6.2
Lemon-lime (clear)	12.3	3.4	0.3	0.0
Orange	14.9	3.7	0.6	0.3
Other citrus	10–16	0.8–4.1	0–10.0	0–0.1
Root beer	12.6	4.0	0.3	0.0
Ginger ale	10.4	2.1	0.3	0.0
Tonic water	10.4	1.2	0.0	0.0
Other	12–18	0–3.5	0–2.0	0–7.8
Diet Soft Drinks				
Diet cola or pepper	<1	0–5.2	0–5.0	2.1–4.7
Decaffeinated diet cola or pepper	<1	0–6.0	0–10.0	2.1–4.7
Diet lemon-lime	<1	0–7.9	0–6.9	0-trace
Diet root beer	<2	3.3–8.5	0–3.0	0–1.6
Other diet	<6	0–8.0	0.3–10.1	0-trace
Club soda, seltzer, and sparkling water	0	0–8.1	0–0.5	0–0.1
Apricot nectar, canned	17.6	0.9	35.8	2.8
Apple juice, unsweetened	14.6	0.9	36.9	2.2
Cranberry juice cocktail, bottled	18.0	0.6	5.7	0.6
Grape juice, canned, unsweetened	19.3	0.9	41.7	3.5

Table U–1.
Beverages and Alcoholic Drinks
Calories and Selected Electrolytes (per fluid ounce)*, *continued*

Beverage	Energy, kcal	Sodium, mg	Potassium, mg	Phosphorous, mg
Grapefruit juice, canned, unsweetened	11.7	0.3	47.3	3.4
Orange juice, raw	14.0	0.3	62.0	5.3
Pear nectar, canned	18.7	1.2	4.1	0.9
Peach nectar, canned	16.8	2.2	12.4	1.9
Pineapple juice, canned, unsweetened	17.5	0.3	41.9	2.5
Tomato juice, canned, without salt added	5.2	3.0	66.9	5.8
Alcohol				
Beer	12.2	1.49	7.4	3.6
Gin, rum, vodka, whiskey (80 proof)	64.2	0.3	0.6	1.1
Dessert wine	37.2–45.1	2.7	27.1	2.7
Table wine	20.7	2.4	26.3	4.1

* Based on data from US Department of Agriculture, Agricultural Research Service. 2001. USDA Nutrient Database for Standard Reference, Release 14. Nutrient Data Laboratory Home Page, http://www.nal.usda.gov/fnic/foodcomp. Other data obtained from *About Soft Drinks*. National Soft Drink Association. 25 January 2002. http://www.nsda.org/softdrinks/ingredients.html.

Appendix V

Table V–1.
Sources of Dietary Fiber

Food	Fiber (g/100 g)	Fiber (g/serving)	Food	Fiber (g/100 g)	Fiber (g/serving)
Fruits			Prunes	11.9	11.9/11 dried prunes
Apple (without skin)	2.1	2.9/1 medium-sized apple	Raisins	8.7	2.2/packet
Apple (with skin)	2.5	3.5/1 medium-sized apple	Raspberries	5.1	6.3/1 c
Apricot (fresh)	1.7	1.8/3 apricots	Strawberries	2.0	3.0/1 c
Apricot (dried)	8.1	10.5/1 c	Watermelon	0.3	1.3/4 × 8-in wedges
Banana	2.1	2.5/1 banana	**Juices**		
Blueberries	2.7	3.9/1 c	Apple	0.3	0.74/1 c
Cantaloupe	1.0	2.7/half edible portion	Grapefruit	0.4	1.0/1 c
Cherries, sweet	1.2	1.2/15 cherries	Grape	0.5	1.3/1 c
Dates	7.6	13.5/1 c (chopped)	Orange	0.4	1.0/1 c
Grapefruit	1.3	1.6/half edible portion	Papaya	0.6	1.5/1 c
Grapes	1.3	2.6/10 grapes	**Vegetables Cooked**		
Oranges	2.0	2.6/1 orange	Asparagus, cut	1.5	1.5/7 spears
Peach (with skin)	2.1	2.1/1 peach	Beans, string green	2.6	3.4/1 c
Peach (without skin)	1.4	1.4/1 peach	Broccoli	2.8	5.0/1 stalk
Pear (with skin)	2.8	4.6/1 pear	Brussel sprouts	3.0	4.6/7–8 sprouts
Pear (without skin	2.3	3.8/1 pear	Cabbage, red	2.0	2.9/1 c (cooked)
Pineapple	1.4	2.2/1 c (diced)	Cabbage, white	2.0	2.9/1 c (cooked)
Plums, damsons	1.7	1.7/3 plums	Carrots	3.0	4.6/ 1 c

Table V–1.
Sources of Dietary Fiber, *continued*

Food	Fiber (g/100 g)	Fiber (g/serving)	Food	Fiber (g/100 g)[a]	Fiber (g/serving)
Cauliflower	1.7	2.1/1 c	Onions, sliced	1.3	1.3/1 c
Corn, canned	2.8	4.5/1 c	Peppers, green, sliced	1.3	1.0/1 pod
Kale leaves	2.6	2.9/1 c (cooked)	Tomato	1.5	1.8/1 tomato
Parsnip	3.5	5.4/ 1 c (cooked)	Spinach	4.0	8.0/1 c (chopped)
Peas	4.5	7.2/1 c (cooked)	**Legumes**		
Potato (without skin)	1.0	1.4/1 boiled	Baked beans, Tomato sauce	7.3	18.6/1 c
Potato (with skin)	1.7	2.3/1 boiled	Dried peas, Cooked	4.7	4.7/half c (cooked)
Spinach	2.3	4.1/1 c (raw)	Kidney beans, Cooked	7.9	7.4/half c (cooked)
Squash, summer	1.6	3.4/1 c (cooked, diced)	Lima beans, Cooked/canned	5.4	2.6/half c (cooked)
Sweet potatoes	2.4	2.7/1 baked (5×2 inches)	Lentils, cooked	3.7	1.9/half c (cooked)
Turnip	2.2	3.4/1 c (cooked, diced)	Navy beans, cooked	6.3	3.1/half c (cooked)
Zucchini	2.0	4.2/1 c (cooked, diced)	**Breads, Pastas, and Flours**		
Uncooked Vegetables			Bagels	1.1	1.1/half bagel
Bean sprout soy	2.6	2.6/1 c	Bran muffins	6.3	6.3/muffin
Celery, diced	1.5	3.7/1 large stalk	Cracked wheat	4.1	4.1/slice
Cucumber with skin	0.8	0.2/6–8 slices	Crisp bread, rye	14.9	
Lettuce, sliced	1.5	20/1 wedge iceberg	Crisp bread, wheat	12.9	
Mushrooms, sliced	2.5	0.8/half c (sliced)	French bread	2.0	0.67/slice

Table V–1.
Sources of Dietary Fiber, *continued*

Food	Fiber (g/100 g)	Fiber (g/serving)	Food	Fiber (g/100 g)	Fiber (g/serving)
Italian bread	1.0	0.33/slice	**Flours and Grains**		
Mixed grains	3.7		Bran, corn	62.2	18.7/oz
Oatmeal	2.2	5.3/1 c	Bran, oat	27.8	8.3/oz
Pita bread (5in.)	0.9		Bran, wheat	41.2	12.4/oz
Pumpernickel bread	3.2	1.0/slice	Rolled oats	5.7	13.7/1 c (cooked)
Raisin bread	2.2	0.55/slice	Rye flour (72%)	4.5	5.2/1 c
White bread	2.2	0.55/slice	Rye flour (100%)	12.8	15.4/1 c
Whole-wheat bread	5.7	1.66/slice	Wheat flour		
Pasta and Rice Cooked			Whole meal	8.9	10.6/1 c (100%)
Macaroni	0.8	1.0/1 c (cooked)	Brown (85%) White (72%)	7.3 2.9	8.8 1 c 2.9/1 c
Rice, brown	1.2	2.4/1 c (cooked)	**Nuts**		
Rice, polished	0.3	0.6/1 c	Almonds	7.2	3.6/half c
Spaghetti (regular)	0.8	1.0/1 c (cooked)	Peanuts	8.1	(slivered) 11.7/1 c
Spaghetti (whole wheat)	2.8	3.0/1 c (cooked)	Filberts	6.0	2.8/half c

Appendix W

Table W–1.
Recommended Dietary Fluoride Supplement* Schedule

Age	Fluoride concentration in community drinking water†		
	<0.3 ppm	0.3–0.6 ppm	>6 ppm
0–6 months	None	None	None
6 months–3 years	0.25 mg/d	None	None
3–6 years	0.50 mg/d	0.25 mg/d	None
6–16 years	1.0 mg/d	0.50 mg/d	None

*Sodium fluoride (2.2 mg sodium fluoride contains 1 mg fluoride ion).
†1.0 parts per million (ppm) = 1 mg/L

Sources:

Meskin LH, ed. Caries diagnosis and risk assessment: a review of preventive strategies and management. *J Am Dent Assoc.* 1995;126(suppl):1S–24S

American Academy of Pediatric Dentistry. Special issue: reference manual 1994–95. *Pediatr Dent.* 1995;16(special issue):1–96

American Academy of Pediatrics Committee on Nutrition. Fluoride supplementation for children: interim policy recommendations. *Pediatrics.* 1995;95:777

Appendix X

Table X–1.
Carbohydrate Content of Juices

Fruit or Juice	Fructose	Glucose	Sucrose	Sorbitol
Prune	14.0	23.0	0.6	12.7
Pear	6.6	1.7	1.7	2.1
Sweet cherry	7.0	7.8	0.2	1.4
Peach	1.1	1.0	6.0	0.9
Apple	6.0	2.3	2.5	0.5
Grape	6.5	6.7	0.6	trace
Strawberry	2.2	2.3	0.9	0.0
Raspberry	2.0	1.9	1.9	0.0
Blackberry	3.4	3.2	0.2	0.0
Pineapple	1.4	2.3	7.9	0.0
Orange	2.4	2.4	4.7	0.0

AAP News. February 1991;7:2.

Appendix Y

Table Y–1.
Ketogenic Diet: Sample Menus

Ketogenic meals are made up of 4 major components:
Fat—butter, margarine, mayonnaise, oil (unsaturated fats are recommended)
Protein—eggs, fish, cheese, beef, chicken, bacon, sausage…
Carbohydrate—fruits or vegetables
Cream—heavy whipping cream with 36% to 40% fat
1100 kcals 4:1 ratio
3 meals 1 snack
Bacon Fruit
16 g Bacon, Oscar Mayer
11 g Cantaloupe
16 g Fat A or 21 g Fat B
30 g Heavy Cream
Cheeseburger Vegetable
12 g Beef, Regular Ground
10 g Cheese, Kraft Deli Deluxe
10 g Tomato, Raw
10 g Pickle, Dill
16 g Fat A or 21 g Fat B
30 g Heavy Cream
Egg Salad Vegetable
20 g Hard-Cooked Egg Yolk
17 g Hard-Cooked Egg White
10 g Tomato, Raw
10 g Romaine Lettuce Raw
20 g Hellman's Mayonnaise
30 g Heavy Cream

Table Y–1.
Ketogenic Diet: Sample Menus, *continued*

Internet Resources:
www.stanford.edu/group/ketodiet/
www.hopkinsmedicine.org/ketodiet.html
www.efa.org/answerplace/epusa/ketogenic.html
www.php.com/dosig/ketogenic
www.charliefoundation.org/

Appendix Z

Table Z-1.
Brand-Specific Composition of Common Pediatric Parenteral Amino Acid Solutions

Product (Manufacturer)	Solutions Designed for Infants		Standard Solutions Suitable for Ages 1 Year and Above				
	Aminosyn PF (Abbott)	TrophAmine (B. Braun/McGaw)	Aminosyn (Abbott)	Aminosyn II (Abbott)	FreAmine III (B. Braun/McGaw)	Novamine (Baxter)	Travasol (Baxter)
Nitrogen mg per 100 mL of 1% solution	152	155	157	153	153	158	165
Amino acids (essentialy, mg per 100 mL of 1% solution							
Isoleucine	76	82	72	66	69	50	60
Leucine	120	140	94	100	91	69	73
Lysine	68	82	72	105	73	79	58
Methionine	18	34	40	17	53	50	40
Phenylalanine	43	48	44	30	56	69	56
Threonine	51	42	52	40	40	50	42
Tryptophan	18	20	16	20	15	17	18
Valine	67	78	80	50	66	64	58
Amino acids (nonessential) mg per 100 mL of 1% solution							
Alanine	70	54	128	99	71	145	207
Arginine	123	120	98	102	95	98	115
Histidine	31	48	30	30	28	60	48

Table Z-1.
Brand-Specific Composition of Common Pediatric Parenteral Amino Acid Solutions, *continued*

Product (Manufacturer)	Solutions Designed for Infants		Standard Solutions Suitable for Ages 1 Year and Above				
	Aminosyn PF (Abbott)	TrophAmine (B. Braun/McGaw)	Aminosyn (Abbott)	Aminosyn II (Abbott)	FreAmine III (B. Braun/McGaw)	Novamine (Baxter)	Travasol (Baxter)
Proline	81	68	86	72	112	60	68
Serine	50	38	42	53	59	39	50
Taurine	7	2.5	–	–	–	–	–
Tyrosine	4	4.4	4.4	27	–	2.6	4
Glycine	39	36	128	50	140	69	103
Glutamic Acid	62	50	–	74	–	50	–
Aspartic Acid	53	32	–	70	–	29	–
Cysteine	–	< 1.6	–	–	< 2.4	–	–
N-ac-L-tyrosine	–	24	–	–	–	–	–

Table Z–2.
Currently Available Intravenous Fat Emulsions (in the United States)

PRODUCT AND DISTRIBUTOR	OIL (%)		FATTY ACID CONTENT (%)				
	SAFFLOWER	SOYBEAN	LINOLEIC	OLEIC	PALMITIC	LINOLENIC	STEARIC
Intralipid* 10% (Clintec)		10	50	26	10	9	3.5
Intralipid* 20% (Clintec)		20	50	26	10	9	3.5
Intralipid* 30% (Clintec)		30	50	26	10	9	3.5
Liposyn II† 10% (Abbott)	5	5	65.8	17.7	8.8	4.2	3.4
Liposyn II† 20% (Abbott)	10	10	65.8	17.7	8.8	4.2	3.4
Liposyn III† 10% (Abbott)		10	54.5	22.4	10.5	8.3	4.2
Liposyn III† 20% (Abbott)		20	54.5	22.4	10.5	8.3	4.2

PRODUCT AND DISTRIBUTOR	EGG YOLK PHOSPHOLIPIDS (%)	GLYCERINE (%)	KCAL/ ML	OSMOLARITY (mOsm/L)	PHOSPHOLIPID/ TRIGLYCERIDE (PL/TG) RATIO
Intralipid* 10% (Clintec)	1.2	2.25	1.1	260	0.12
Intralipid* 20% (Clintec)	1.2	2.25	2	260	0.06
Intralipid* 30% (Clintec)	1.2	1.7	3	200	0.04
Liposyn II† 10% (Abbott)	1.2	2.5	1.1	276	0.12
Liposyn II† 20% (Abbott)	1.2	2.5	2	258	0.06
Liposyn III† 10% (Abbott)	1.2	2.5	1.1	284	0.12
Liposyn III† 20% (Abbott)	1.2	2.5	2	292	0.06

*Store at 25°C (77°F) or below; do not freeze.
†Store at 30°C (86°F) or below; do not freeze.

Subject Index